Stedman's

SURGERY

WORDS

INCLUDES
ANATOMY,
ANESTHESIA, &
PAIN MANAGEMENT
Fourth Edition

Stedman's

SURGERY

WORDS

INCLUDES
ANATOMY,
ANESTHESIA, &
PAIN MANAGEMENT
Fourth Edition

Wolters Kluwer | Lippincott Williams & Wilkins
Health
Philadelphia • Baltimore • New York • London
Buenos Aires • Hong Kong • Sydney • Tokyo

Publisher: Julie K. Stegman
Editorial Manager: Eric Branger
Associate Managing Editor: Erin M. Cosyn
Manufacturing Coordinator: Margie Orzech-Zeranko
Typesetter: Aptara, Inc.
Printer & Binder: Data Reproductions Corporation

Copyright © 2009 Lippincott Williams & Wilkins
351 West Camden Street
Baltimore, Maryland 21201-2436

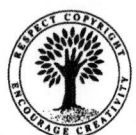

Fourth Edition, 2009

Library of Congress Cataloging-in-Publication Data

Stedman's surgery words : includes anatomy, anesthesia & pain management. – 4th ed.
    p. ; cm. – (Stedman's word book series)
  Includes bibliographical references.
  ISBN 978-0-7817-9008-6
  1. Surgery–Terminology.   I. Stedman, Thomas Lathrop, 1853–1938.   II. Title: Surgery
words.   III. Series: Stedman's word books.
  [DNLM: 1. Surgery–Terminology–English. WO 15 S8124 2009]
  RD16.S74 2009
  617.001′4–dc22   2008008838

09 10 11 12
1 2 3 4 5 6 7 8 9 10

Contents

Acknowledgments

An important part of our editorial process is the involvement of medical transcriptionists—as advisors, reviewers, and/or editors.

We extend special thanks to Ellen Atwood and Patricia Lee White, CMT, for editing the manuscript, helping resolve many difficult questions, and contributing material for the appendix sections. We are grateful to our MT Editorial Advisory Board members, including Sandy Kovacs, CMT, AHDI-F; Terry B. Lary, CMT; Helen Littrell, IMT; and Wendy Ryan, RHIT, who were instrumental in the development of this reference. They recommended sources and shared their valuable judgment, insight, and perspective.

We also extend thanks to Janet West for working on the appendices. Additional thanks to Helen Littrell, IMT for performing the final prepublication review. Other important contributors to this edition include Cheryl Ackerman; Kimberly Adams, CMT; Susan Bartolucci, CMT, FAAMT; Jeanne Bock, CSR, MT; Shemah Fletcher; Rhonda S. Hase; Diane S. Heath, CMT; Robin Koza; Wendy Ryan, RHIT; and Jenifer F. Walker, MA.

And, as always, Kathy Cadle played an integral role in the process by reviewing the content files for format and updating the database.

As with all our *Stedman's* word references, this resource incorporates the suggestions and expertise of our many contacts in the medical transcriptionist community. Thanks to all of our advisory board participants, reviewers, and editors; AAMT meeting attendees; and others who have written to us with requests and comments—keep talking, and we'll keep listening.

Editor's Preface

New transcriptionists may wonder why "ops" are deemed so difficult; I certainly thought I knew enough to type them, back in the greenhorn days. Then I rather quickly realized that the savvy transcriptionist needs to be well-versed in the deepest knowledge, those things that experienced people "just know," things that may not even be written down, or are only contained in one venerable resource no longer in print. An obstetrician would not perform a heart transplantation and an eye surgeon does not venture deep into the brain. But, an MT who is skilled in surgical reports must understand terms common to lancing a boil, then switch to those of complex maxillofacial reconstruction with the click of a mouse.

Surgery is dynamic: the biggest, most dramatic, most all-encompassing portion of medical transcription. Ophthalmologic, plastic, and neurosurgery are the oldest known procedures, having been practiced by so-labeled "primitive" peoples for eons, although it is unknown if a report was dictated. With such a long history, the types, improvements, variations, and minutiae of surgery and its adjuncts are endless. Eponyms are now strung like pearls in front of a procedure's description as newer techniques augment the traditional. Necessary knowledge includes grounding in all the aspects of medicine, such as disease and condition names; drugs and therapies before, during, and after surgery; and laboratory and diagnostic tests. In some specialties, drugs and diagnostics are an integral part of the operative procedure. Technology is producing not only new equipment and techniques, but also novel, living materials that replace diseased and malfunctioning organs and structures. This topic is so huge we need 3, even 4, separate books to adequately cover the myriad basics: *Stedman's Medical and Surgical Equipment Words, Fifth Edition*; *Stedman's Anatomy & Physiology Words, Second Edition*; *Stedman's Medical Eponyms, Second Edition;* and this work, *Stedman's Surgery Words, Includes Anatomy, Anesthesia, & Pain Management, Fourth Edition.*

Surgery dictators add special flavor to their reports, with wide extremes ranging from precisely enunciated technical language all the way to reports composed entirely of abbreviations and acronyms. Some doctors give us written templates that they follow punctiliously. Another variety is a sort of verbal template, almost a chant, nearly unintelligible to the user. Hardest of all for the MT may be those surgeons who, despite style rules we all want to adhere to, insist on certain terms being typed in a way at wide variance with those rules.

Anesthesiologists are key. Originally requiring the administration of a few drugs and gases, anesthesia has become a complex multidrug, multi-faceted, highly individualized specialty. Depth and type of anesthesia are tailored to individual patient needs and type of operation, with various innovations in sedation and induced coma assisting in trauma and severe medical illness recovery. When the acute pain of surgery or trauma does not gradually resolve and fade away, anesthesiologists develop treatment protocols for chronic pain states, widening their field of contact from surgeons to physiatry, respiratory therapy to psychiatry.

Many other specialist physicians, nurses, technicians, and allied health personnel are involved in patient preparation for and recovery from surgery. Currently, dictated reports are not required from each professional involved in patient care before, during, or after surgery. That may well come someday as the demand for accurate, careful documentation continues to evolve, and surgery expands to involve even more subspecialties.

Thus, mastery of the art of surgical transcription includes not only a massively broad knowledge base, but also the ability to efficiently search qualified reference materials, such as *Stedman's Word Books*. Calling on accumulated understanding and inner sense to quickly recognize and transcribe a new, obscure, or unintelligible term is a skill built over time and with exposure. Knowing which reference to consult, which category of term, which variation on a theme to look for aids in speedily completing an accurate report.

This fourth edition of *Stedman's Surgery Words, Includes Anatomy, Anesthesia, & Pain Management* with its companion volume, *Stedman's Medical & Surgical Equipment Words, Fifth Edition* will quickly become the premier reference for medical transcriptionists. You will find the arcane, unusual, and most importantly, practical information logically ordered in a standardized, easy-to-use format.

Special thanks to Patricia White, who suddenly, valiantly leapt into the midst of this book's needs shortly after completing a challenging project. Janet West provided valuable insight and new material for the appendices, and earns my appreciation and admiration. Thanks especially to Erin Cosyn for her innovations in dealing with some new technical surprises, and to the online editor Kathy Cadle who turns the squiggles into crisp typescript. The entire team at Stedman's, many whose names never appear in print, are held in high esteem for their commitment to providing dependable, quality reference products for medical transcriptionists and others who rely on *Stedman's Word Books*. Most importantly, thanks to the many medical transcriptionists who make their needs known, and in particular to those who serve on the editorial advisory board. With your input, we are able provide resources suitable to your locale along with the national and international.

Ellen Atwood
March 20, 2008

Publisher's Preface

Stedman's Surgery Words, Includes Anatomy, Anesthesia, & Pain Management, Fourth Edition, offers an authoritative assurance of quality and exactness to the wordsmiths of the healthcare professions—medical transcriptionists, medical editors and copyeditors, health information management personnel, court reporters, and the many other users and producers of medical documentation.

We have received many requests for updates to *Stedman's Surgery Words*. As a result, we have published this new edition that includes surgical, anatomical, anesthesia, and pain management terminology. As with the previous edition, we have opted to omit equipment terminology. You will find *Stedman's Medical & Surgical Equipment Words, Fifth Edition* to be an excellent companion source for verifying equipment terminology.

In *Stedman's Surgery Words, Includes Anatomy, Anesthesia, & Pain Management, Fourth Edition* users will find thousands of words as they relate to the specialties of surgery, gross anatomy, anesthesia, and pain management. Users will also find terms for protocols, diagnostic and therapeutic procedures, new techniques, lab tests, clinical research terms, as well as abbreviations with their expansions. The appendix sections provide anatomical illustrations with useful captions and labels, sample reports, common terms by procedure, a pain glossary, pain management techniques, an explanation of dermatomes, American Academy of Pain Management (AAPM)-accredited pain programs, drugs commonly used in pain practice, drugs used for anesthesia, drugs by indication, anesthesia methods, common suture techniques and materials, common surgical intubation techniques, and common surgical fluids.

This compilation of more than 100,000 entries, fully cross-indexed for quick access, was built from a base vocabulary of approximately 66,000 medical words, phrases, abbreviations, and acronyms. The extensive A-Z list was developed from the database of *Stedman's Medical Dictionary, 28th Edition,* and supplemented by terminology found in current medical literature (see References on page xix).

We at Lippincott Williams & Wilkins strive to provide you with the most up-to-date and accurate word references available. Your use of this word book will prompt new editions, which we will publish as often as updates and revisions justify. We welcome your suggestions for improvements, changes, corrections, and additions—whatever will make this *Stedman's* product more useful to you. Please visit us online at www.stedmans.com to submit your suggestions and recommendations.

Explanatory Notes

Medical transcription is an art as well as a science. Both approaches are needed to correctly interpret the dictation of a physician, whose language is a product of education, training, and experience. This variety in medical language means that there are several acceptable ways to express certain terms, including jargon. *Stedman's Surgery Words, Includes Anatomy, Anesthesia, & Pain Management, Fourth Edition* provides variant spellings and phrasings for many terms. These elements, in addition to complete cross-indexing, make *Stedman's Surgery Words, Includes Anatomy, Anesthesia, & Pain Management, Fourth Edition* a valuable resource for determining the validity of terms as they are encountered.

Alphabetical Organization

Alphabetization of main entries is letter by letter as spelled, ignoring punctuation, spaces, prefixed numbers, or other characters. For example:

chlormerodrin accumulation test
2-chloroprocaine
Cho anterior cruciate ligament reconstruction

Terms beginning or ending with Greek letters show the Greek letters spelled out and listed alphabetically. For example:

beta
    b. adrenoreceptor
    b. hemolytic streptococci infection

In subentry alphabetization, the abbreviated singular form or the spelled-out plural form of the noun main entry word is ignored.

Format and Style

All main entries are in **boldface** to expedite locating a sought-after term, to enhance distinction between main entries and subentries, and to relieve the textual density of the pages.

Irregular plurals and variant spellings are shown on the same line as the singular or preferred form of the word. For example:

---

acetabulum, pl. **acetabula**
discectomy, diskectomy

Hyphenation

As a rule of style, multiple eponyms (e.g., Mears-Rubash approach) are hyphenated. Also, hyphens have been added between a manufacturer and one or more eponyms (e.g., Vital-Metzenbaum dissecting scissors). Please note that in many cases, hyphenation is a question of style, not of accuracy, and thus is a matter of choice.

Possessives

Possessive forms have been dropped in this reference for the sake of consistency and conformance with the guidelines of the American Association for Medical Transcription (AAMT) and other groups. Please note, however, that in many cases, retaining the possessive, like hyphenating, is a question of style, not of accuracy, and thus is a matter of choice. To form the possessive of a word, simply add the apostrophe or apostrophe "s" to the end of the word.

Cross-indexing

The word list is in an index-like main entry-subentry format that contains two combined alphabetical listings:

(1) A *noun* main entry-subentry organization, which is typical of the A-Z section of medical dictionaries like *Stedman's*:

mallet
   m. finger deformity
   m. fracture
   m. toe deformity

reconstruction
   mandibular r.
   r. method
   microsurgical r.

(2) An *adjective* main entry-subentry organization, which lists words and phrases as you hear them. The main entries are the adjectives or modifiers in a multiword term. The subentries are the nouns around which the terms are constructed and to which the adjectives or modifiers pertain:

mucinous
   m. adenocarcinoma
   m. ascites
   m. cystic neoplasm (MCN)

regional
   r. anesthetic technique
   r. block
   r. flap

This format provides the user with more than one way to locate and identify a multiword term. For example:

end
   e. expiratory

expiratory
   end e.

algorithm
   registration a.

registration
   r. algorithm

It also allows the user to see together all terms that contain a particular descriptor, as well as all types, kinds, or variations of a noun entity. For example:

hand
   h. massage
   radial club h.
   h. ratio

knee
   k. anatomy
   k. arthroplasty
   descending artery of k.

Wherever possible, abbreviations are separately defined and cross-referenced. For example:

ICU
   intensive care unit
intensive
   i. care unit (ICU)
unit
   intensive care u. (ICU)

References

In addition to the manufacturers' literature we gather at various medical meetings, scientific reports from hospitals, and the lists of our MT Editorial Advisory Board members (from their daily transcription work), we used the following sources for new terms in *Stedman's Surgery Words, Includes Anatomy, Anesthesia, & Pain Management, Fourth Edition.*

Books

Abram SE, Haddox JD. *The Pain Clinic Manual, 2nd Edition*. Philadelphia: Lippincott Williams & Wilkins, 2000.

Ballantyne GH, Marescaux J, Giulianotti PC, eds. *Primer of Robotic & Telerobotic Surgery*. Philadelphia: Lippincott Williams & Wilkins, 2004.

Ballantyne JC, ed. *The Massachusetts General Handbook of Pain Management, 3rd Edition*. Philadelphia: Lippincott Williams & Wilkins, 2005.

Barash PG, Cullen BF, Stoelting RK. *Handbook of Clinical Anesthesia, 5th Edition*. Philadelphia: Lippincott Williams & Wilkins, 2005.

Cheng DCH, David TE, eds. *Perioperative Care in Cardiac Anesthesia and Surgery*. Baltimore: Lippincott Williams & Wilkins, 2005.

Chung KW. *Gross Anatomy, 5th Edition*. Philadelphia: Lippincott Williams & Wilkins, 2005.

Corman ML. *Colon and Rectal Surgery, 5th Edition*. Philadelphia: Lippincott Williams & Wilkins, 2005.

Drake E. *Sloane's Medical Word Book, 4th Edition*. Philadelphia: Saunders, 2001.

Fischer JE, Bland KI, Callery MP, Clagett GP, Jones DB, eds. *Mastery of Surgery, 5th Edition*. Philadelphia: Lippincott Williams & Wilkins, 2006.

General Surgery/GI Words and Phrases. Modesto, CA: Health Professions Institute, 2001.

Greenfield LJ, Mulholland MW, Oldham KT, Zelenock GB, Lilemoe KD. *Surgery: Scientific Principles and Practice, 3rd Edition*. Philadelphia: Lippincott Williams & Wilkins, 2001.

Hiatt JL, Gartner LP. *Textbook of Head and Neck Anatomy, 3rd Edition*. Philadelphia: Lippincott Williams & Wilkins, 2000.

Hollinshead WH. *Anatomy for Surgeons, The Head and Neck, 3rd Edition*. Philadelphia: Lippincott Williams & Wilkins, 1982.

Inabnet WB, DeMaria EJ, Ikramuddin S, eds. *Laparoscopic Bariatric Surgery*. Philadelphia: Lippincott Williams & Wilkins, 2005.

Jaffe RA, Samuels SI, eds. *Anesthesiologist's Manual of Surgical Procedures, 3rd Edition*. Philadelphia: Lippincott Williams & Wilkins, 2004.

Kalimi R, Faber LP, eds. *Clinical Scenarios in Thoracic Surgery*. Philadelphia: Lippincott Williams & Wilkins, 2004.

Lance LL. *Quick Look Drug Book 2002*. Baltimore: Lippincott Williams & Wilkins, 2002.

Lawrence PF, Bell RF, Dayton MT, Ahmed MI, eds. *Essentials of General Surgery, 4th Edition*. Philadelphia: Lippincott Williams & Wilkins, 2005.

Loeser JD, Butler SH, Chapman CR, Turk DC. *Bonica's Management of Pain, 3rd Edition*. Philadelphia: Lippincott Williams & Wilkins, 2000.

McCaffery M, Pasero C. *Pain Clinic Manual, 2nd Edition*. Philadelphia: Saunders, 1999.

Mulholland, MW, Doherty GA, eds. *Complications in Surgery, 5th Edition*. Philadelphia: Lippincott Williams & Wilkins, 2005.

Nirula, R. *High-Yield Surgery, 2nd Edition*. Baltimore: Lippincott Williams & Wilkins, 2005.

Olson T. *A.D.A.M. Student Atlas of Anatomy*. Philadelphia: Lippincott Williams & Wilkins, 1996.

Pain Management Made Incredibly Easy! Philadelphia: Lippincott Williams & Wilkins, 2003.

Schwartz SI, Shires GT, Spencer FC, Galloway AC. *Principles of Surgery, 7th Edition*. Columbus: McGraw-Hill, 1998.

Shapiro FE. *Manual of Office-Based Anesthesia Procedures*. Baltimore: Lippincott Williams & Wilkins, 2007.

Slinger PD, ed. *Progress in Thoracic Anesthesia*. Philadelphia: Lippincott Williams & Wilkins, 2004.

Stedman's Medical Dictionary, 28th Edition. Baltimore: Lippincott Williams & Wilkins, 2000.

Taylor J. *Comprehensive Sports Injury Management: From Examination of Injury to Return to Sport*. Austin: Pro-Ed, 2003.

Tessier C. *The AAMT Book of Style*. Modesto, CA: AAMT, 1995.

Tessier C. *The Surgical Word Book, 2nd Edition*. Philadelphia: Saunders, 1991.

Upchurch Jr, GR, Henke PK, eds. *Clinical Scenarios in Vascular Surgery*. Philadelphia: Lippincott Williams & Wilkins, 2005.

Valentine JR, Wind GG. *Anatomic Exposures in Vascular Surgery, 2nd Edition*. Philadelphia: Lippincott Williams & Wilkins, 2003.

Vera Pyle's Current Medical Terminology, 10th Edition. Modesto, CA: Health Professions Institute, 2005.

Washington Manual of Surgery, 4th Edition. Baltimore: Lippincott Williams & Wilkins, 2005.

Whyte-Ferguson L, Gerwin R, eds. *Clinical Mastery in the Treatment of Myofascial Pain*. Philadelphia: Lippincott Williams & Wilkins, 2005.

CD

Lippincott's Interactive Anesthesia Library v3.0. Philadelphia: Lippincott Williams & Wilkins, 2001.

Image Sources

Abraham SE and Haddox JD. *The Pain Clinic Manual, 2nd Edition*. Philadelphia: Lippincott Williams & Wilkins, 2000.

Agur AMR, Lee MJ. *Grant's Atlas of Anatomy, 10th Edition*. Baltimore: Lippincott Williams & Wilkins, 1999.

Caldwell S, Pikesville, MD. From *Stedman's Medical Dictionary, 27th Edition*. Baltimore: Lippincott Williams & Wilkins, 2000.

Cousins MJ, Bridenbaug PO eds. *Neural Blockade in Clinical Anesthesia and Management of Pain*. Philadelphia: Lippincott-Raven Publishers, 1997.

Georgiade NG, Riefkohl R, Levine LS, Georgiade, GS. *Plastic, Maxillofacial and Reconstructive Surgery, 3rd Edition*. Baltimore: Williams & Wilkins, 1996.

LifeART Emergency 4, CD-ROM. Baltimore: Lippincott Williams & Wilkins.

LifeART Nursing 1-2, CD-ROM. Baltimore: Lippincott Williams & Wilkins.

LifeART Pediatrics 1, CD-ROM. Baltimore: Lippincott Williams & Wilkins.

LifeART Super Anatomy Collections 3-8, CD-ROM. Baltimore: Lippincott Williams & Wilkins.

MediClip Clinical Cardiopulmonary, CD-ROM. Baltimore: Lippincott Williams & Wilkins.

MediClip Human Anatomy 1-3, CD-ROM. Baltimore: Lippincott, Williams & Wilkins.

Mikki Senkarik, San Antonio, TX. From Pillitteri A, PhD, RN, PNP. *Maternal & Child Health Nursing: Care of the Childbearing & Childrearing Family, 3rd Edition*. Philadelphia: Lippincott Williams & Wilkins, 1998.

Mikki Senkarik, San Antonio, TX. From *Stedman's Medical Dictionary, 27th Edition*. Baltimore: Lippincott Williams & Wilkins, 2000.

Neil O. Hardy of Westport, CT and Susan Caldwell of Pikesville, MD. From *Stedman's Medical Dictionary, 27th edition*. Baltimore: Lippincott Williams & Wilkins, 2000.

Smeltzer SC & Bare BG. *Brunner & Suddarth's Textbook of Medical Surgical-Nursing, 8th Edition*. Philadelphia: JB Lippincott Company, 1996.

Ward L of Salt Lake City, UT. From Fuller J, RN, PhD & Schaller-Ayers J, RN, MNSc, PhD. *A Nursing Approach, 2nd Edition*. Philadelphia: J.B. Lippincott Company, 1994.

Willis MC. *Medical Terminology: The Language of Health Care*. Baltimore: Williams Wilkins, 1996.

Journals

Anesthesia & Analgesia. Baltimore: Lippincott Williams & Wilkins, 2005–2007.

Anesthesiology. Baltimore: Lippincott Williams & Wilkins, 2001–2007.

Annals of Surgery. Baltimore: Lippincott Williams & Wilkins, 1999–2007.

Clinical Journal of Pain. Baltimore: Lippincott Williams & Wilkins, 1999–2007.

Colon and Rectal Surgery. Baltimore: Lippincott Williams & Wilkins, 2004–2005.

Computer Aided Surgery. New York: John Wiley & Sons, Inc., 1997–2000.

Journal of the American College of Surgeons. New York: Elsevier Science, 1997–2007.

Laparoscopic Update. Baltimore: Lippincott Williams & Wilkins, 1998–2001.

Latest Word. Philadelphia: Saunders, 1999–2001.

Surgical Laparoscopy Endoscopy & Percutaneous Techniques. Baltimore: Lippincott Williams & Wilkins, 1999–2007.

Topics in Pain Management. Baltimore: Lippincott Williams & Wilkins, 2001–2007.

Websites

http://www.aapainmanage.org./search/FacilSearch.php

http://carecure.rutgers.edu/spinewire/Articles/SpinalLevels.html

http://my.webmd.com/index

http://surgery.medscape.com/Home/Topics/surgery/surgery.html

http://www.aapainmange.org

http://www.anesthesiology.org

http://www.asahq.org

http://www.aspmn.org

http://www.centerwatch.com

http://www.facs.org

http://www.gasnet.com

http://www.hpisum.com

http://www.laparoscopy.com

http://www.lapsurgery.com

http://www.mtdaily.com
http://www.mtdesk.com
http://www.mtmonthly.com
http://www.nccn.org/patients/patient_gls/_english/_pain/3_treatment.asp
http://www.nci.nih.gov/cancertopics/treatment/types-of-treatment
http://www.pain.com
http://www.sciwire.com
http://www.sls.org
http://www.theasgs.org
http://www.ussurg.com
http://www.webmd.com

a.
   arteria
   artery
A
   acromion
   ampere
   anesthesia
aa.
   arteriae
AA
   anterior apical
     AA segment
AAA
   abdominal aortic aneurysm
     AAA stent-graft
AAC
   acute acalculous cholecystitis
AACLR
   arthroscopic anterior cruciate ligament
     reconstruction
AAD
   acute aortic dissection
   atlantoaxial dislocation
AADSN
   acquired immunodeficiency
     virus-associated distal sensory
     neuropathy
AAI
   A-line ARX index
   A-line autoregressive index
   atlantoaxial instability
AAL
   anterior axillary line
AANA
   American Association of Nurse
     Anesthetists
$(A-a)O_2$
   alveolar-arterial oxygen gradient
AAR
   automated anesthesia record
AARF
   atlantoaxial rotatory fixation
Aaron sign
AAS
   atlantoaxial subluxation
AAST
   American Association for the Surgery
     of Trauma
ab
   a. externo filtering operation
   a. externo incision
   a. interno incision
AB
   anterior basal
     AB segment

Ab
   abortion
   antibody
ABA
   American Board of Anesthesiology
Abbe
   A. flap
   A. intestinal anastomosis
   A. lip-switch flap
   A. vaginal construction
Abbe-Estlander
   A.-E. flap
   A.-E. vascularized lip flap
Abbe-McIndoe
   A.-M. total endoscopic vaginal
     reconstruction procedure
   A.-M. vaginal reconstruction
**Abbe-McIndoe-Williams vaginoplasty
procedure**
**Abbe-Wharton-McIndoe vaginal
reconstruction procedure**
Abbott
   A. esophagogastroscopy
   A. esophagogastrostomy
   A. knee approach
   A. Pain Manager II
   A. scoliosis treatment method
**Abbott-Carpenter posterior knee
approach**
Abbott-Gill
   A.-G. epiphysial plate exposure
   A.-G. osteotomy
Abbott-Lucas shoulder operation
abbreviated
   a. injury scale (AIS)
   A. Injury Score (AIS)
ABC
   airway, breathing, circulation
   aspiration biopsy cytology
ABD
   abduction
   autologous blood donation
abdomen
   accordion a.
   acute surgical a.
   aperture of a.
   boatlike a.
   boat-shaped a.
   carinate a.
   concave a.
   diffusely tender a.
   distended a.
   doughy a.
   exquisitely tender a.
   fascia of a.

abdomen (*continued*)
    flabby a.
    flat a.
    hostile a.
    hyperdistended a.
    hyperresonant a.
    navicular a.
    nondistended a.
    obliterated a.
    pendulous a.
    postlymphangiography a.
    postsurgical a.
    protuberant a.
    prune-belly a.
    resonant a.
    scaphoid a.
    soft a.
    splinting of a.
    stiff a.
    surgical a.
    tympanitic a.

abdominal
    a. abscess
    a. adhesiolysis
    a. adipose tissue
    a. agitation
    a. air collection
    a. angina
    a. angiography
    a. aorta
    a. aortic aneurysm (AAA)
    a. aortic artery
    a. aortic plexus
    a. aortic sympathic plexus
    a. aponeurosis
    a. approach
    a. apron
    a. binder
    a. brace position
    a. canal
    a. carcinoma
    a. cardiac reflex
    a. cavity
    a. circulation
    a. colectomy
    a. colic
    a. compartment syndrome (ACS)
    a. complication
    a. content
    a. cramp
    a. cutaneous nerve entrapment
      syndrome
    a. decompression
    a. distention
    a. domain
    a. drainage
    a. evisceration
    a. examination

a. exploration
a. external oblique muscle
a. fasciocutaneous flap
a. fat
a. fat pad
a. film
a. fissure
a. fluid collection
a. fluid wave
a. girth
a. guarding
a. gunshot wound
a. gutter
a. hemorrhage
a. hydatid disease
a. hysterectomy
a. hysteropexy
a. hysterotomy
a. imaging
a. impalement
a. incisional hernia
a. incision dehiscence
a. intercostal hernia
a. internal oblique muscle
a. iron deposition
a. irradiation
a. kidney
a. lavage
a. lipectomy
a. lymph node biopsy
a. malignancy
a. midline incisional hernioplasty
a. migraine
a. muscle deficiency syndrome
a. myomectomy
a. nephrectomy
a. ostium
a. panniculus
a. paracentesis
a. peritoneum
a. pool
a. pregnancy
a. pressure
a. pressure technique
a. procedure
a. proctocolectomy
a. pull-through
a. pulse
a. rectopexy
a. reflux
a. region
a. respiration
a. respiratory motion
a. rigidity
a. ring
a. sac
a. sacrocolpopexy
a. sacropexy

a. salpingo-oophorectomy
a. salpingotomy
a. section
a. sonography
a. space
a. splenectomy
a. stoma
a. stool
a. structure
a. tap
a. tenderness
A. Trauma Index (ATI)
a. tumor
a. vascular accident
a. view
a. viscera
a. viscus
a. volume
a. wall anomaly
a. wall closure
a. wall fistula
a. wall hernia
a. wall incision
a. wall lifting
a. wall mass
a. wall mobility
a. wall rhabdomyosarcoma
a. wall venous pattern
a. wound closure
a. x-ray (AXR)
a. zone
abdominalis
abdominal-perineal resection
(APR)
abdominal-sacral colpoperineopexy
abdominis
abdominocentesis
abdominocystic
abdominogenital
abdominohysterectomy
abdominohysterotomy
abdominoinguinal incision
abdominojugular reflux
abdominopelvic
a. abscess
a. cavity
a. irradiation
a. mass
a. splanchnic nerve
a. viscus
abdominoperineal
a. excision
a. proctectomy
a. resection (APR)
abdominoplasty
abdominosacral resection
abdominoscopy
abdominoscrotal

abdominothoracic
a. arch
a. incision
abdominovaginal hysterectomy
abdominovesical
abducens nerve (*var. of* abducent nerve)
abducent nerve [CN VI], abducens
nerve
abduction (ABD)
a. deformity
a. external rotation test
a. osteotomy
a. traction technique
abduction-external
a.-e. rotation (AER)
a.-e. rotation fracture
abductor
a. digiti minimi opponensplasty
a. digiti quinti opponensplasty
a. hallucis muscle
a. longus muscle
a. magnus muscle
a. osteotomy
a. pollicis brevis muscle
a. pollicis longus muscle
a. pollicis longus tendon
abductorplasty
Camitz palmaris longus a.
flexor pollicis longus a.
Smith flexor pollicis longus a.
abductory wedge osteotomy
Aberdeen knot
Abernethy
A. external iliac artery ligation
A. fascia
A. sarcoma
aberrancy
acceleration-dependent a.
aberrant
a. bile duct
a. bronchial origin
a. ductule
a. ganglion
a. goiter
a. lymphatic drainage
a. node
a. obturator artery
a. obturator vein
a. pancreas
a. regeneration
a. third nerve degeneration
a. tissue
a. umbilical
a. umbilical stoma
a. vessel
aberration
angle of a.
chromatic lens a.

aberration (*continued*)
- color a.
- coma a.
- curvature a.
- dioptric a.
- distantial a.
- distortion a.
- hemodynamic a.
- intraventricular a.
- lateral a.
- lens a.
- longitudinal a.
- meridional a.
- monochromatic a.
- newtonian a.
- oblique a.
- optic a.
- regeneration a.
- sexual a.
- spherical lens a.
- ventricular a.

ABG
- arterial blood gas

ability
- tumor-targeting a.

Abiomed BVS 500 VAD

ablate

ablatio
- a. placentae
- a. retinae

ablation
- accessory conduction a. (ACA)
- adrenal a.
- androgen a.
- atrioventricular junctional a.
- carbon dioxide laser plaque a.
- catheter a.
- catheter-based a.
- celiac alcohol a.
- cold forceps a.
- cold snare a.
- contact laser a.
- continuous wave laser a.
- coronary rotational a.
- cryogenic a.
- cryosurgical a.
- direct current shock a.
- electrical catheter a.
- endometrial a.
- endoscopic mucosal a.
- ethanol a.
- excimer laser a.
- fast-pathway radiofrequency a.
- His bundle a.
- homogeneous a.
- Kent bundle a.
- laparoscopic uterine nerve a. (LUNA)
- laparoscopic uterosacral nerve a. (LUNA)
- Livewire TC cardiac a.
- marrow a.
- mucosal a.
- Nd:YAG laser a.
- needle a.
- neoadjuvant total androgen a.
- nerve rootlet a.
- organ a.
- ovarian a.
- panretinal a.
- parathyroid tumor a.
- percutaneous ethanol a.
- percutaneous radical cryosurgical a.
- percutaneous radiofrequency catheter a.
- percutaneous tumor a.
- peripheral panretinal a.
- photothermal laser a.
- pituitary a.
- plasma-mediated a.
- pulsed laser a.
- radiofrequency a. (RFA)
- radiofrequency catheter a. (RFCA)
- radiofrequency thermal a. (RFTA)
- radiofrequency tissue a. (RFTA)
- radioiodine a.
- rectoscopic endometrial a.
- renal cyst a.
- rollerball endometrial a. (REA)
- rotational a.
- slow-pathway radiofrequency a.
- stereotactic surgical a.
- surgical estrogen a.
- temperature-controlled radiofrequency tissue a. (TCRFTA)
- a. therapy
- thermal a.
- thyroid nodule a.
- tissue a.
- toric a.
- transcatheter a.
- transurethral needle a. (TUNA)
- tumor a.
- valve a.
- visual laser a.

ablative
- a. cardiac surgery
- a. laser angioplasty
- a. laser therapy
- a. procedure
- a. technique

ABMT, ABMTx
- autologous bone marrow transplant

ABMTR
- Autologous Bone and Marrow Transplant Registry

abnormal
    a. bleeding
    a. clotting
    a. cytology
    a. fetal urogenital tract
    a. mammogram
    a. parathyroid gland
    a. preoperative localization
     signal
abnormality
    anatomic a.
    bleeding a.
    calyceal a.
    clotting a.
    cytologic a.
    dislocation contour a.
    diverticulation a.
    DNA ploidy a.
    electrical activation a.
    electrolyte a.
    extremity a.
    genetic a.
    ictal a.
    limb reduction a.
    mammographic a.
    migration a.
    mucosal a.
    nondermatomal sensory a.
     (NDSA)
    nonpalpable mammographic a.
    oral cavity a.
    persistent breast a.
    pulmonary vascular a.
    regional wall motion a. (RWMA)
    renal a.
    reproductive tract a.
    rostrocaudal extent signal a.
    segmental wall motion a.
     (SWMA)
    sensory a.
    skeletal a.
    soft tissue a.
    structural a.
    suspicious a.
    tissue texture a. (TTA)
    urinary tract a.
    vascular a.
    ventilation/perfusion a.
    ventricular depolarization a.
abnormally
    a. feeding blood vessel
    a. hyperplastic gland
ABO barrier
aborad, aboral
aboral (*var. of* aborad)
abortion (Ab)
    menstrual extraction a.
abortive infection
above-elbow amputation (AEA)

above-knee
    a.-k. amputation (AKA)
    a.-k. amputation conversion
ABPC
    argon beam plasma coagulation
ABPI
    ankle-brachial pressure index
ABPM
    ambulatory blood pressure monitoring
    American Board of Pain Medicine
ABPS
    Attitudes to Back Pain Scale
abraded wound
Abraham iridotomy
Abraham-Pankovich tendo calcaneus
   repair
Abrami disease
abrasion
    a. arthroplasty
    bobby-pin a.
    a. chondroplasty
    corneal a.
    perioperative corneal a.
    traumatic corneal a.
abrasive
    a. brush biopsy
    a. point
Abrikosov tumor
abrupt hemodynamic collapse
abruptio placentae (AP)
Abruzzini incision
ABS
    American Board of Surgery
abscess
    abdominal a.
    abdominopelvic a.
    actinomycotic brain a.
    acute a.
    amebic hepatic a.
    anal a.
    anastomotic a.
    anorectal a.
    aponeurotic a.
    appendiceal a.
    arthrifluent a.
    axillary a.
    Bezold a.
    bicameral a.
    blind a.
    bone a.
    bowel a.
    brain a.
    breast a.
    Brodie metaphysial a.
    buccal space a.
    button a.
    caseous a.
    cerebral a.
    chronic subareolar a.

abscess (*continued*)
    cold a.
    collar-button a.
    colonic a.
    corneal a.
    crypt a.
    cuff a.
    deep interloop a.
    diffuse a.
    Douglas a.
    draining a.
    dry a.
    echinococcal liver a.
    encapsulated brain a.
    enteroperitoneal a.
    epidural a.
    extradural a.
    fecal a.
    fluctuant a.
    a. formation
    frontal a.
    gallbladder wall a.
    gas a.
    gas-forming liver a.
    gravitation a.
    growth plate a.
    hepatic a.
    Highmore a.
    horseshoe a.
    hot a.
    hypostatic a.
    infraorbital space a.
    intermesenteric a.
    intersphincteric a.
    intraabdominal a.
    intradural a.
    intrahepatic a.
    intramural a.
    intramuscular a.
    intraosseous a.
    intraperitoneal a.
    ischiorectal a.
    kidney a.
    lacunar a.
    liver a.
    local a.
    localized a.
    lumbar epidural a.
    mesentery a.
    metaphysial a.
    metastatic a.
    midpalmar a.
    migrating a.
    miliary a.
    missile track a.
    multiple diffuse intrahepatic a.'s
    necrotic a.
    pancreatic a.
    parahepatic a.

    paranephric a.
    parapharyngeal space a.
    pelvic a.
    perforating a.
    perianal a.
    perianal fistula a.
    periappendiceal a.
    peridiverticular a.
    periesophageal a.
    perihepatic a.
    perineal a.
    perinephric a.
    perirectal a.
    peritoneal cavity a.
    periumbilical a.
    periureteral a.
    periurethral a.
    phlegmonous a.
    pilonidal a.
    point of a.
    postoperative a.
    premasseteric space a.
    prevertebral space a.
    pterygomandibular space a.
    pyogenic a.
    pyogenic hepatic a.
    residual a.
    retrocecal a.
    retroperitoneal a.
    retroperitoneal iliopsoas a.
    retrorectal a.
    ring a.
    a. ring
    satellite a.
    soft tissue a.
    space of Retzius a.
    spinal epidural a. (SEA)
    splenic a.
    stercoral a.
    sterile a.
    stitch a.
    subdiaphragmatic a.
    subdural a.
    subgaleal a.
    subhepatic a.
    sublingual space a.
    submandibular space a.
    submasseteric space a.
    submental space a.
    subperiosteal a.
    subphrenic a.
    supralevator perirectal a.
    tuberculous a.
    tuboovarian a.
    wandering a.
    wound a.

abscise

abscission
    corneal a.

absence
    microscopic a.
absent
    a. bowel sounds
    a. bow tie sign
    a. gag reflex
    a. peristalsis
    a. respiration
Absidia **infection**
absolute (A)
    a. construction
    a. curative resection
    a. humidity
    a. noncurative resection
absorbable surgical suture
absorbent
    a. point
    a. vessel
absorptiometry
absorption
    external a.
    nutrient a.
    reservoir mucosal a.
    systemic a.
absorptive cell
abut
abutment
    implant a.
    screw-type a.
    subperiosteal implant a.
ABx
    antibiotic
AC
    acromioclavicular
ACA
    anterior cerebral artery
    anterior choroidal artery
    anterior communicating artery
ACAD
    atherosclerotic carotid artery
    disease
acalculous cholecystitis
acantha
acanthion
acanthocytosis
acanthoid
acantholysis
ACBE
    air-contrast barium enema
accelerans
accelerated
    a. arteriolar gas embolization
    a. atherosclerosis
    a. respiration
    a. transplant rejection
acceleration
    angular a.
    growth a.
    a. injury

    tibial a.
    a. time
acceleration/deceleration injury
acceleration-dependent aberrancy
accelerator
    a. fiber
    linear a. (LINAC)
    a. nerve
accelerometer
    TOF-Watch SX a.
acceleromyographic train-of-four ratio
acceleromyography
accentuation
access
    cavity a.
    a. cavity
    central venous a.
    cutdown a.
    a. emergency
    exit a.
    extrahepatic a.
    a. flap
    minimally invasive surgical a.
    a. needle
    percutaneous a.
    peritoneal a.
    a. preparation
    root canal a.
    side-entry a.
    surgical a.
    transcervical tubal a.
    transcutaneous a.
    transjugular liver a.
    vascular a.
    venous a.
    ventricular a.
accessible lesion
accessory
    a. adrenal
    a. areolar gland of Montgomery
    a. breast
    a. cephalic vein
    a. conduction ablation (ACA)
    a. duct stenting
    a. muscle activity
    a. nerve
    a. nerve root
    a. nerve trunk
    a. nipple
    a. obturator artery
    a. palatine canal
    a. pancreas
    a. pancreatic duct
    a. papillotomy
    a. parotid gland
    a. plantar ligament
    a. process
    a. root canal
    a. spleen

accessory (*continued*)
    a. suprarenal gland
    a. thyroid gland
    a. tubercle
    a. venous sinus of Verga
    a. volar ligament
accident
    abdominal vascular a.
    cerebrovascular a. (CVA)
    intraoperative vascular a.
    vascular a.
accidental
    a. decannulation
    a. esophageal intubation
    a. hemorrhage
    a. hypothermia
    a. pulp exposure
accommodation
    a. curve
    a. disorder
    a. reflex
accordion
    a. abdomen
    a. graft
    a. sign
accretion line
accumulation
    collagen a.
    third space fluid a.
accuracy
    diagnostic a.
    subvoxel a.
ACDF
    anterior cervical discectomy and
    fusion
ACE
    antegrade continence enema
Ace-Colles frame technique
acellular
    a. mass
    a. pannus tissue
acentric relation
acestoma
acetabular
    a. artery
    a. augmentation graft
    a. branch
    a. cavity
    a. cup arthroplasty
    a. cup extractor
    a. extensile approach
    a. lip
    a. notch
    a. protrusio deformity
    a. reinforcement ring
    a. retractor
    a. rim fracture
acetabuli
    protrusio a.

acetabuloplasty
    Pemberton a.
    shelf a.
acetohydroxamic acid irrigation
acetowhite
    a. lesion
    a. test
acetylcholine receptor
acetylsalicylic
    a. acid (ASA)
    a. acid-induced gastric ulceration
achalasia
    a. balloon dilation
    esophageal a.
    idiopathic a.
    a. of cardia
Aches and Pains Scale
Achilles
    A. bursa
    A. tendon
    A. tendon rupture
Achillis
    Banks open slide lengthening of
    tendo A.
    bursa A.
    Gaines and Ford technique for
    determining adequate lengthening
    of tendo A.
    Garbarino and Clancy geometrical
    method for calculating lengthening
    of tendo A.
    Pierrot and Murphy transplantation
    of insertion of tendo A.
    tendo A.
    White slide lengthening of tendo
    A.
achondrogenesis
achondroplasia
    homozygous a.
achondroplastic dwarfism
achondroplasty
achromic patch
acid
    acetylsalicylic a. (ASA)
    amino a.
    aromatic amino a.'s
    a. aspiration
    deoxyribonucleic a. (DNA)
    a. etch bonding technique
    gastric chloric a.
    a. gland
    a. hemolysis
    hepatobiliary iminodiacetic a.
    (HIDA)
    long-chain fatty a.'s
    medium-chain fatty a.'s
    mefenamic a.
    a. peptic disease
    phenylethylbarbituric a.

polyglycolic a. (PGA)
a. reflux
retinoic a.
stomach a.
acid-base
a.-b. balance
a.-b. disturbance
a.-b. equilibrium
a.-b. homeostasis
a.-b. status
a.-b. value
acid-etched restoration
acidification treatment
acidosis
concomitant a.
hepatocellular a.
hyperchloremic metabolic a.
lactic a.
local a.
metabolic a.
renal tubular a.
Acier stainless steel suture
acinar tissue
acini (*pl. of* acinus)
acinic
a. cell carcinoma
a. cell tumor grading
acinose (*var. of* acinous)
acinous, acinose
a. cell carcinoma
a. gland
acinus, *pl.* **acini**
lobular a.
Ackerman-Proffitt classification of malocclusion
ACL
anterior cruciate ligament
ACL reconstruction
ACL repair
ACLS
advanced cardiac life support
ACM
Arnold-Chiari malformation
acneform, acneiform
a. lesion
a. rash
acneiform (*var. of* acneform)
ACoA
anterior communicating artery
AComA
anterior communicating artery
acorn treatment
Acosta endometriosis classification
acoustic
a. canal
a. foramen
a. method
a. monitor
a. nerve

a. neuroma
A. Neuroma Registry
a. pharyngometry
a. pressure
a. quantification
a. reflection measurement
a. reflectometry
a. rhinometry
a. shadowing
a. stimulation study
a. stimulation test
AC-PC
anterior commissure-posterior commissure
AC-PC line
ACPS
acrocephalopolysyndactyly
acquired
a. centric relation
a. cornification disorder
a. deformity
a. diverticulum
a. eccentric jaw relation
a. eventration
a. hernia
a. immunodeficiency virus-associated distal sensory neuropathy (AADSN)
a. neurologic dysfunction
a. postintubation stenosis
a. thoracic chondrodystrophy syndrome
acquisition
image a.
multiple gated a. (MUGA)
acral lentiginous melanoma (ALM)
Acrel ganglion
acrobrachycephaly
acrocephalia (*var. of* acrocephaly)
acrocephalic
acrocephalopolysyndactyly (ACPS)
acrocephalosyndactyly (type I-IV)
acrocephalous
acrocephaly, acrocephalia
acrocyanosis
acrodermatitis continua
acrodysplasia
acrofacial syndrome
acromegalia (*var. of* acromegaly)
acromegaly, acromegalia
acromial
a. arterial network
a. artery
a. articular facies
a. articular surface
a. branch
a. bursa
a. extremity
a. process

acromioclavicular (AC)
a. articulation
a. disc
a. injury classification
a. joint dislocation
a. joint repair
a. ligament
a. pin fixation
a. space
acromiocoracoid
acromiohumeral
acromion (A)
acromionectomy
Armstrong a.
acromioplasty
anterior a.
McLaughlin a.
McShane-Leinberry-Fenlin a.
Neer a.
acromioscapular
acromiothoracic
a. approach
a. artery
acroosteolysis
ACS
abdominal compartment syndrome
acute coronary syndrome
American College of Surgeons
ACT
activated clotting time
activated coagulation time
anticoagulant therapy
ACTH
adrenocorticotropic hormone
Acticoat
Actinomyces luteus
actinomycetoma
actinomycoma
actinomycotic brain abscess
actinomyoma
action
anesthesia a.
ball valve a.
a. line
nonstereospecific a.
a. of anesthetic
peripheral antinociceptive a.
stereospecific a.
Actiq
activated
a. clotting time (ACT)
a. coagulation time (ACT)
a. protein C resistance
activating solution
activation
baroreflex a.
cortical a.
egg a.
hemostatic a.

hypothalamic a.
a. map-guided surgical resection
a. moment
neuronal nicotinic receptor a.
neutrophil a.
presynaptic and postsynaptic
nicotinic a.
very late a.
activation-sequence mapping
activator modification
active
a. appliance therapy
a. assistive motion therapy
a. chronic inflammation
a. core cooling
a. hemorrhage
a. reciprocation
a. source of bleeding
a. specific immunotherapy
a. systemic bacterial infection
actively bleeding varix
activity
accessory muscle a.
antithrombotic a.
atrial a.
a. avoidance
channel a.
duodenal migrating a.
ectopic a.
efferent nerve a.
inspiratory intercostal a.
jejunal fasting motor a.
mitotic a.
motor a.
opioid antinociceptive a.
a. pattern analysis
postprandial motor a.
pulseless electrical a. (PEA)
serotonergic a.
sympathetic nerve a. (SNA)
actuation
direct mechanical ventricular a.
Acufex bioabsorbable Suretac suture
acuminata (*pl. of* acuminatum)
acuminatum, *pl.* **acuminata**
condyloma a.
acuology
acupoint
extra 1 a.
Zusanli a.
acupressure
Korean hand a.
acupuncture
a. anesthesia
auricular a.
French energetic a.
Japanese a.
neuroanatomic a.
regular body a.

A

acusection
acustimulation antiemetic prophylaxis
acute
- a. abscess
- a. acalculous cholecystitis (AAC)
- a. allergic extrinsic alveolitis
- a. allograft rejection
- a. and chronic inflammation
- a. and postherpetic neuralgia
- a. aortic dissection (AAD)
- a. blood transfusion
- a. calculous cholecystitis
- a. cardiac event
- a. cellular rejection
- a. circulatory failure
- a. colonic pseudoobstruction
- a. compression triad
- a. coronary syndrome (ACS)
- a. digestive bleeding
- a. disconnection syndrome
- a. embolic arterial occlusion
- a. fracture
- a. gastric mucosal lesion
- a. graft-versus-host disease
- a. headache
- a. hemolytic transfusion reaction
- a. hemorrhagic inflammation
- a. hemorrhagic ulceration
- a. hepatic coma
- a. hepatic rupture
- a. herpetic neuralgia
- a. inflammatory exudate
- a. inflammatory membrane
- a. intermittent porphyria
- a. intestinal obstruction
- a. ischemic stroke
- a. isovolemic hemodilution
- a. limb ischemia
- A. Low Back Pain Screening Questionnaire (ALBPSQ)
- a. lung injury
- a. lung rejection
- a. mesenteric venous thrombosis
- a. nephrotoxicity
- a. normovolemic hemodilution (ANH)
- a. normovolemic hemodilution transfusion
- a. opioid tolerance
- a. pain
- a. pain service
- a. pancreatitis
- A. Physiology and Chronic Health Evaluation II (APACHE II)
- a. physiology prognostic scoring index
- a. presentation
- a. pulmonary edema, hypotension, shock resuscitation algorithm
- a. pyogenic membrane
- a. quadriplegic myopathy
- a. radiation pneumonitis
- a. recurrent headache
- a. recurrent rhabdomyolysis
- a. rejection
- a. rejection of liver transplant
- a. respiratory distress syndrome (ARDS)
- a. respiratory failure
- a. severe isovolemic anemia
- a. subdural hematoma
- a. suppurative thyroiditis
- a. surgical abdomen
- a. symptom
- a. toxicity
- a. traumatic lesion
- a. tubular necrosis
- a. tumor lysis syndrome (ATLS)
- a. vascular rejection
- a. wound
- a. wound granulation tissue

Acutrol suture
acystia
AD
　　anterior displacement
adactylia (*var. of* adactyly)
adactylous
adactyly, adactylia
ADAM
　　Aneurysm Detection and Management
adamantine membrane
adamantinoblastoma
adamantinocarcinoma
adamantinoma
adamantinum
Adam iridectomy
Adamkiewicz
　　artery of A.
Adams
　　A. hallux valgus interphalangeus correction procedure
　　A. hip operation
　　A. position
Adam's apple
adaptable
adaptation
　　arterial a.
　　a. disease
　　a. syndrome of Selye
adaptational approach
adaptive
　　a. correction
　　a. relaxation
adaxial
ADD
　　adduction
addiction
　　a. acknowledgment scale

addiction (*continued*)
    opioid therapy a.
    a. potential scale
    A. Severity Index
Addison point
additional canal
additive interaction
additivity
adduction (ADD)
    a. deformity
    a. osteotomy
    a. traction technique
adduction-internal
    a.-i. rotation
    a.-i. rotation deformity
adductor
    a. canal
    a. hiatus
    a. longus muscle rupture
    a. magnus
    a. magnus tendon
    a. pollicis
    a. tenotomy
adductovarus deformity
adenectomy
adenoacanthoma
adenoameloblastoma
adenocarcinoma
    alveolar a.
    ampullary a.
    anaplastic a.
    anular a.
    appendiceal a.
    bile duct a.
    bronchial a.
    bronchiolar a.
    bronchioloalveolar a.
    bronchogenic a.
    cervical a.
    colonic a.
    colorectal a.
    cystic a.
    duct cell a.
    duodenal a.
    endometrial a.
    esophageal a.
    gastric a.
    infiltrating duct a.
    invasive a.
    kidney a.
    medullary a.
    mesonephric a.
    metastatic a.
    mucinous a.
    ovarian clear cell a.
    pancreatic a.
    peritoneal a.
    primary a.
    prostatic a.

    renal a.
    sebaceous a.
    secretory a.
    serous a.
    signet-ring a.
    spontaneous a.
    stomach a.
    sweat gland a.
    undifferentiated a.
    uterine a.
    vaginal a.
    vulvar adenoid cystic a.
adenochondroma
adenocystic carcinoma
adenocystoma
adenodiastasis
adenoepithelioma
adenofibroma
adenofibromyoma
adenohypophyseal (*var. of*
  adenohypophysial)
adenohypophysial, adenohypophyseal
adenohypophysis
adenoid
    a. cystic carcinoma
    a. pad
    a. squamous cell carcinoma
    a. tumor
adenoidal pad
adenoidal-pharyngeal-conjunctival virus
adenoidectomy
    lateral a.
    tonsillectomy and a. (T&A)
adenoleiomyofibroma
adenolipoma
adenolymphocele
adenolymphoma
adenolysis
adenoma (A), *pl.* **adenomas,**
  adenomata
    adnexal a.
    adrenal a.
    bile duct a.
    bronchial a.
    colonic a.
    colorectal a.
    double a.'s
    ductal a.
    duodenal a.
    ectopic parathyroid a.
    fibroid a.
    glucocorticoid-producing
     adrenal a.
    hepatic a.
    hyperfunctioning a.
    a. hyperplastic polyp ratio
    kidney a.
    malignant a.
    monoclonal a.

a. of breast
papillary a.
parathyroid a.
pituitary a.
pleomorphic a.
prostatic a.
renal a.
a. sebaceum
sessile a.
single a.
small intestine a.
sporadic pituitary a.
sweat gland a.
thyroid a.
a. to nonadenoma ratio
toxic a.
tracheal a.
tubulovillous a.
upper a.
well-localized a.
adenomas (*pl. of* adenoma)
adenomata (*pl. of* adenoma)
adenomatosis
endocrine a.
adenomatous
a. hyperplasia
a. polyp
a. polyposis coli (APC)
adenomectomy
adenomyosarcoma
adenopathy
axillary a.
bulky a.
cervical a.
metastatic a.
retroperitoneal a.
adenosarcoma
adenose
adenosine
a. diphosphate
a. monophosphate
(AMP)
adenosine-regulating agent
adenosis
sclerosing a.
adenosquamous carcinoma
adenotomy
adenotonsillectomy
adenoviral
a. infection
a. transfer
adenovirus infection
adequate hydration
adherence obstruction
adherent
a. clot catheter
a. leukoma
a. zone
adhesed

adhesiectomy
adhesiolysis
abdominal a.
adhesion
anomalous mesenteric a.
attic a.
banjo-string a.
a. barrier
cell-cell a.
cell-extracellular matrix a.
dense a.
fibrinous a.
fibrous a.
filmy a.
a. formation
hard a.
intraabdominal a.
intraperitoneal a.
laparoscopic lysis of a.'s
a. lysis
lysis of a.'s
matted a.
membranous a.
a. molecule
peritoneal a.
piano-wire a.
primary a.
secondary a.
serologic a.
tenacious a.
adhesiotomy
adhesive
a. arachnoiditis
a. band
a. bandage
a. bonding
a. capsulitis
a. disease
a. ileus
a. inflammation
a. otitis media
a. peritonitis
a. resin-bonded bridge
a. resin-bonded cast restoration
a. small bowel obstruction
a. syndrome
tissue a.
adipectomy
adipocele
adipodermal graft
adipolysis
adipose
a. body
a. capsule
a. connective tissue
a. fold
a. graft
a. infiltration
a. tissue extract

aditus
    laryngeal a.
adjunct
    perioperative a.
    surgical a.
    a. therapy
adjunctive
    a. balloon angioplasty
    a. chemotherapy
    a. screw fixation
    a. sedation
    a. suppressive medical therapy
adjustable
    a. gastric banding
    a. pressure limiting (APL)
    a. ring gastroplasty
    a. suture strabismus surgery
adjuvant
    anesthesia a.
    a. chemoradiation therapy
    a. chemotherapy
    a. diagnostic modality
    a. drug therapy
    a. irradiation
    a. nephrectomy
    a. radiotherapy
    a. regimen
    a. therapy
Adkins
    A. spinal fusion
    A. technique spinal arthrodesis
Adler operation
admaxillary gland
admedial, admedian
admedian (*var. of* admedial)
admin
    administration
administered
    spinally a.
administration (admin)
    altering route of a.
    buccal drug a.
    concomitant a.
    drug a.
    epidural a.
    Food and Drug A. (FDA)
    interpleural a.
    intraocular a.
    intraoperative clonidine a.
    intraperitoneal drug a.
    intraspinal a.
    intrathecal a.
    intravenous a.
    oral a.
    oxygen a.
    parenteral a.
    postischemic a.
    preischemic a.
    route of a.

    sequential a.
    transdermal a.
    transmucosal a.
    transnasal a.
    vasodilator a.
admit
    same-day a.
admixture
    a. lesion
    venous a.
adnexa, *pl. of* **adnexum**
adnexal
    a. adenoma
    a. carcinoma
    a. infection
    a. mass
    a. metastasis
adnexectomy
adnexopexy
adnexum, *pl.* **adnexa**
    ocular adnexa
ADPKD
    autosomal dominant polycystic kidney disease
adrenal
    a. ablation
    accessory a.
    a. adenoma
    a. androgen
    a. body
    a. branch
    a. capsule
    a. carcinoma
    a. cortex
    a. cystic mass
    a. feminization syndrome
    a. gland
    a. gland biopsy
    a. gland tumor
    a. hemorrhage
    a. incidentaloma
    a. insufficiency
    Marchand a.
    a. medulla graft
    a. medulla transplant
    a. metastasis
    a. pathology
    a. pheochromocytoma
    a. primary aldosteronism
    a. vein
    a. vein sampling
adrenalectomy
    bilateral total a.
    complete a.
    endoscopic a.
    ipsilateral a.
    laparoscopic a.
    laparoscopic anterior a.
    laparoscopic posterior a.

laparoscopic transperitoneal a.
open a. (OA)
open anterior a.
open thoracoabdominal a.
transperitoneal laparoscopic a.
unilateral a.
adrenergic
alpha a.
alpha-1 a.
alpha-2 a.
adrenic
adrenoceptor blocker
adrenocortical
a. carcinoma
a. extract
adrenocorticotropic hormone (ACTH)
adrenoprival
adrenoreceptor
alpha a.
beta a.
Adson
A. anterior transperitoneal approach
A. test
A. thoracic outlet maneuver
Adson-Coffey scalenotomy
adsorption theory of narcosis
adsternal
adterminal
adult
a. cardiovascular surgery
a. familial hyaline membrane
  disease
a. intussusception
a. patient
a. polycystic liver disease
a. population
a. recipient
a. scoliosis surgery
a. wandering spleen
adulthood astrocytoma
adult-to-adult
a.-t.-a. live donor liver transplantation
a.-t.-a. living related donor living
  transplant
advance
a. directive
a. to regular diet
advanced (adv, ADV)
a. cardiac life support (ACLS)
a. cardiac mapping
a. disease
a. hyperspectral analysis
a. local invasion
a. retroperitoneal rhabdomyosarcoma
a. therapeutic endoscopy
a. trauma life support (ATLS)
a. tumor perforation
advancement
Baker patellar a.

a. flap
a. flap graft
Johnson pronator a.
Le Fort III facial a.
mandibular osteotomy a.
mucosal a.
a. of rectal flap
a. procedure
transanal pouch a.
V-Y a.
advancer
rotator cuff a.
Advantiv Safety I.V.
catheter
adventitia
adverse
a. effect
a. event
a. outcome
a. prognostic sign
A–E
oxygen cylinder A–E.
AEA
above-elbow amputation
Aeby
A. muscle
A. plane
AED
automatic external defibrillator
AEP
auditory evoked potential
AEP monitor
AER
abduction-external rotation
aerobe
gram-negative a.
aerobic
a. exercise
a. flora
a. gram-negative organism
a. infection
a. metabolism
a. respiration
aerobilia
aerocele
aerocystoscopy
aerodigestive tract
aerodynamic size
aerosol
inhalation a.
respirable a.
a. therapy
aerosolized
a. medication
a. pollutant exposure
Aesculap AG
AESOP
Automated Endoscopic System for
Optimal Positioning

AESOP (*continued*)
    AESOP robotic voice-activated camera controller
AESOP-assisted laparoscopic surgery
aesthetic (*var. of* esthetic)
    a. procedure
    a. reconstruction
    a. rhinoplasty
    a. surgery
aesthetics (*var. of* esthetics)
A-exotropia
AFBG
    aortofemoral bypass graft
AFF
    atrial fibrillation-flutter
affect
    congruent a.
affective
    a. component
    a. disorder
afferens
afferent
    a. blockade
    a. clot
    a. glomerular arteriole
    a. jejunal limb
    a. jejunostomy
    a. limb
    a. limb syndrome
    a. loop syndrome (ALS)
    a. lymphatic vessel
    pancreatojejunostomy a.
    PJA a.
    a. projection
    a. spinal
    a. spinal signaling
    a. vagal
    a. vasodilation
AFH
    anterior facial height
AFib
    atrial fibrillation
afibrinogenemia
afterload
    decreased a.
    a. reduction
afterloading technique
afterpain
AFX
    air-fluid exchange
A/G
    antigen
AG
    Aesculap AG
Ag
    antigen
    silver
aganglionic rectum

aganglionosis
    total colonic a.
age (A)
    fertilization a.
    age, metastases, extent, size (AMES)
Agee force-couple splint reduction
agenesis
    gallbladder a.
    tracheal a.
agenetic fracture
agent
    adenosine-regulating a.
    alpha-adrenergic a.
    alpha-sympatholytic a.
    anesthetic induction a.
    antiadhesion a.
    antibacterial a.
    antifibrinolytic a.
    antifungal a.
    antimicrobial a.
    antimotility a.
    antineoplastic a.
    beta-sympathomimetic a.
    cavity lining a.
    chemoprevention a.
    chemopreventive a.
    endogenous algogenic a.
    gastric protection a.
    hemostatic a.
    inhalation a.
    inhaled a.
    membrane stabilizing a.
    neuroleptic a.
    neurolytic a.
    neuromuscular blocking a. (NMBA)
    oral antimotility a.
    prothrombogenic a.
    selective relaxant binding a.
    sympatholytic a.
    sympathomimetic a.
    thrombolytic a.
    topical antibacterial a.
    topical hemostatic a.
    triggering a.
    vasodilator a.
    ventilation a.
    volatile anesthetic a.
age-related macular degeneration (ARMD)
agglutinant
agglutinate
aggregate gland
aggregation
    platelet a.
aggressive
    a. lesion
    a. renal angiomyolipoma
    a. surgical approach

aging degenerative change
agitation
    abdominal a.
    emergence a.
Agliette supracondylar osteotomy
aglossia-adactylia syndrome
aglossostomia
agminate gland
agnathia
agnathous
Agnew
    A. canthoplasty
    A. lacrimal sac operation
Agnew-Verhoeff incision
AgNOR
    argyrophilic nucleolar organizer region
agonadal
agonal
    a. clot
    a. respiration
agonist
    alpha-1 adrenergic a.
    alpha-2 adrenergic a.
    alpha adrenergic receptor a.
    alpha-2 adrenoreceptor a.
    beta adrenergic a.
    beta receptor a.
    muscarinic a.
    opioid a.
    sigma receptor a.
    synthetic opioid receptor a.
    vanilloid a.
agoraphobia
Agrikola operation
ahaustral
Ahern knot
AHI
    Arthritis Helplessness Index
AICA
    anterior inferior cerebellar artery
aid
    on-site first a.
AIH
    artificial insemination homologous
    artificial insemination husband
AIIS
    anterior inferior iliac spine
AIOD
    aortoiliac occlusive disease
air
    bowel loop a.
    a. collection
    colonic a.
    a. critical care transport
    a. cyst
    a. detector clamp
    a. embolism
    a. embolus
    a. enema

a. entrainment
a. entry
a. exchange
expired a.
extrapleural a.
free a.
a. injection
inspired a.
a. insufflation
intramural colonic a.
intramyocardial a.
intraperitoneal a.
a. leak
minimal a.
oxygen in a.
a. plethysmography
a. sac
a. sinus
a. space
a. space disease
a. test
a. vesicle
air-bone-tissue boundary
airborne infection
airbrasive technique
air-contrast barium enema (ACBE)
Aird pancreas exploration maneuver
air-filled loop
air-fluid
    a.-f. exchange (AFX)
    a.-f. line
air-gap technique
airplane position
Airtraq laryngoscope
airway
    airway, breathing, circulation (ABC)
    a. caliber
    Combitube esophagotracheal a.
    a. compromise
    a. elastance
    esophageal obturator a. (EOA)
    esophagotracheal a.
    failed a.
    a. fire
    a. gas monitoring
    intubating laryngeal mask a. (ILMA,
        I-LMA)
    large mask a.
    laryngeal mask a. (LMA)
    loss of a.
    a. management
    nasal a.
    nasopharyngeal a. (NPA)
    a. obstruction
    a. occlusion technique
    oral pharyngeal a. (OPA)
    oropharyngeal a. (OPA)
    a. pathology
    a. pattern

airway (*continued*)
    pediatric a.
    perilaryngeal a. (PLA)
    pharyngeal a.
    a. pressure (AWP)
    a. pressure release ventilation
      (APRV)
    a. protection
    a. reactivity
    a. reflex
    a. responsiveness
    a. score
    a. shape
    a. shunt
    a. smooth muscle
    a. stenosis
    a. suction
    supraglottic a. (SGA)
    surgical a.
    a. tone
AIS
    abbreviated injury scale
    Abbreviated Injury Score
Aitken epiphysial fracture
 classification
AJCC
    American Joint Committee on Cancer
    AJCC TNM tumor classification
Ajmalin liver injury
AKA
    above-knee amputation
Åkerlund deformity
Akin
    A. bunionectomy
    A. procedure
    A. proximal phalangeal osteotomy
Akiyama procedure
Al
    aluminum
ala, *pl.* **alae**
    sacral a.
Alabama Breast Cancer Project
alae (*pl. of* ala)
alanine aminotransferase (ALT)
Alanson amputation
alar
    a. base reduction
    a. cartilage
    a. fascia
    a. fold
    a. groove
    a. incision
    a. lamina
    a. ligament
    a. reconstruction
    a. spine
    a. wedge excision
alarm
alba, *pl.* **albae**

albae (*pl. of* alba)
Albarran
    A. gland
    A. y Dominguez tubule
Albee spinal fusion
albendazole therapy
Albert
    A. suture
    A. suture technique
Albert-Lembert
    A.-L. gastroplasty
    A.-L. suture
Albinus muscle
ALBPSQ
    Acute Low Back Pain Screening
    Questionnaire
Albrecht bone
Albright-Chase arthroplasty
Albright synovectomy
albugineotomy
albumin
    radiolabeled serum a.
Albumisol
Alcian blue stain
Alcock canal
alcohol
    a. dependence scale
    a. fixation
    a. used disorders identification test
alcohol-fixed gastric biopsy
alcoholic
    a. cirrhosis
    a. coma
    a. liver
    a. liver disease (ALD)
Alcon suture
ALD
    alcoholic liver disease
Alden loop gastric bypass
Alder-Reilly anomaly
aldosterone-producing carcinoma
aldosteronism
    adrenal primary a.
aldosteronoma
    unilateral a.
Aldrete score
Aldridge-Studdefort urethral suspension
Aldridge urethral sling procedure
alendronate
alertness/sedation score
Alexander
    A. incision
    A. musculoskeletal relaxation
    technique
    A. perineal prostatectomy
    A. suprapubic prostatectomy
Alexander-Adams
    A.-A. hysteropexy
    A.-A. uterine suspension

Alfenta
alfentanil
Alfieri stitch
algesimeter
Al-Ghorab
    A.-G. modification
    A.-G. procedure
alginate
algiomotor
algodystrophy
algology
algorithm
    acute pulmonary edema,
      hypotension, shock resuscitation a.
    difficult airway a.
    narrow-complex supraventricular
      tachycardia resuscitation a.
    nonrigid registration a.
    PALS pulseless arrest a.
    registration a.
    ventricular fibrillation/pulseless
      ventricular tachycardia
      resuscitation a.
algoscopy
alien hand sign
aligner
    incision a.
alignment
    extramedullary a.
    normal anatomic a.
alimentarium
    systema a.
alimentary
    a. apparatus
    a. canal
    a. limb
    a. tract
    a. tract duplication
alimentation
    central venous a.
    enteral a.
    forced a.
    intravenous a.
    parenteral a.
    peripheral intravenous a.
    rectal a.
    total parenteral a. (TPA)
alinasal
A-line
    A-l. AEP index
    A-l. ARX index (AAI)
    A-l. auditory evoked potential
      index
    A-l. autoregressive index (AAI)
aliquorrhea
    spontaneous a.
aliquot
alkaline
    a. phosphatase-antiphosphatase

    a. reflux
    a. reflux gastritis (ARG)
Alken renal stone approach
alkylation resistance
allantoic
    a. circulation
    a. sac
Allen
    A. blood supply to hand test
    A. choledochojejunostomy
    A. correction
    A. lung volume reduction
    A. scalenous anterior syndrome
      maneuver
allergen exposure
allergic
    a. bronchopulmonary aspergillosis
    a. fungal sinusitis
    a. inflammation
    a. manifestation
    a. shock
allergy
    latex a.
Allgöwer-Donati suture
Allgöwer stitch
alligator skin
all-inside repair
Allis
    A. hip dislocation maneuver
    A. sign
Allis-Abramson breast biopsy
Allison
    A. antireflux procedure
    A. antireflux technique
    A. gastroesophageal reflux repair
    A. GE reflux correction
    A. hiatal hernia repair
Allman acromioclavicular injury
  classification
allocation
    dynamic storage a.
    fresh tissue a.
    a. of treatment
    static storage a.
    storage a.
allodynia
    brush-induced a.
    cold a.
    compression-evoked a.
    mechanical a.
    thermal a.
allodynic pain
allogeneic (*var. of* allogenic)
allogenic, allogeneic
    a. blood
    a. blood component
    a. blood transfusion
    a. bone
    a. bone graft

allogenic (*continued*)
    a. bone marrow
    a. fetal graft
    a. transplant
allogenous bone graft
allograft
    a. corneal rejection
    cryopreserved heart-valve a.
    a. extraction
    femoral cortical ring a.
    functioning a.
    hepatic a.
    intestinal a.
    liver a.
    a. monitoring
    organ a.
    osteoarticular a.
    osteochondral a.
    pancreaticoduodenal a.
    renal a.
    strut a.
    a. transplant
    a. vasculopathy
allografting
    nerve a.
    peripheral nerve a.
allokeratoplasty
allongement
allopathic keratoplasty
alloplastic chin augmentation
alloplasty
all-or-nothing phenomenon
allotransplantation, homotransplantation, homotransplant
    inlet a.
    liver a.
alloy restoration
Allport operation
ALM
    acral lentiginous melanoma
ALND
    axillary lymph node dissection
alone
    pancreas transplant a. (PTA)
    pancreatic transplantation a. (PTA)
Alonso-Lej choledochal cyst classification
alopecia
    pressure a.
    traction a.
ALP
    argon laser photocoagulation
alpha
    a. adrenergic
    a. adrenergic receptor agonist
    a. adrenoreceptor
alpha-1
    a.-1 adrenergic
    a.-1 adrenergic agonist
    a.-1 adrenergic antagonist

alpha-2
    a.-2 adrenergic
    a.-2 adrenergic agonist
    a.-2 adrenergic receptor
    a.-2 adrenergic receptor antagonist
    a.-2 adrenoreceptor agonist
alpha-adrenergic
    a.-a. agent
    a.-a. antagonist
    a.-a. receptor
alpha-loop maneuver
alpha-stat blood gas management
alpha-sympatholytic agent
Alport syndrome
already-threaded suture
ALS
    afferent loop syndrome
ALT
    alanine aminotransferase
    argon laser trabeculopexy
    argon laser trabeculoplasty
    serum ALT
Altemeier
    A. perineal rectal pullthrough procedure
    A. repair of rectal prolapse
alteration
    dentin crystal a.
alterative inflammation
altercursive intubation
altered gene product
altering route of administration
alternate-day therapy
alternating suture technique
alternation
alternative
    cost-effective a.
    a. introduction site
    a. medicine
    a. surgical approach
    therapeutic a.
    a. therapy
    a. treatment
altitude simulation study
ALTK
    automated lamellar therapeutic keratoplasty
ALTP
    argon laser trabeculoplasty
altruistic donor
aluminum (Al)
    a. cranioplasty
    implant alloy a.
    a. toxicity
Alvarado iliac fossa pain score
alveodental suppuration
alveolar
    a. adenocarcinoma
    a. artery

a. body
a. canal
a. carbon dioxide pressure
a. cavity
a. cell carcinoma
a. concentration
a. dead space
a. dead-space fraction
a. diffusion measurement
a. echinococcosis
a. ectasia
a. end-capillary difference
a. fistula
a. fluid transport
a. gas equation
a. hemorrhage
a. hyperventilation
a. hypoventilation
a. index
a. nerve
a. partial pressure
a. plateau
a. plate fenestration
a. point
a. point-meatus plane
a. point-nasal point line
a. point-nasion line
a. process
a. process fracture
a. recruitment
a. rhabdomyosarcoma
a. sac
a. socket wall fracture
a. tumor
a. ventilation
a. ventilation per minute
a. yoke
alveolar-arterial (A-a)
    a.-a. oxygen gradient $((A-a)O_2)$
    a.-a. pressure difference $(p(A-a)O_2)$
alveolarization
alveolectomy
    partial a.
alveoli (*pl. of* alveolus)
alveolitis
    acute allergic extrinsic a.
    chronic extrinsic a.
    extrinsic allergic a.
alveolobasilar line
alveolocapillary
    a. membrane
    a. partial pressure gradient
alveolodental membrane
alveololabial groove
alveolomerotomy
alveolonasal line
alveoloplasty
    interradicular a.
    intraseptal a.

alveolotomy
alveolus, *pl.* **alveoli**
alveoplasty
alvine calculus
alvinolith
Alvis cataract operation
AM
    anterior midpapillary
        AM segment
amalgam
    a. condensation
    a. restoration
Amato body
amaurosis
    intoxication a.
    pressure a.
Amberg lateral sinus line
ambient
    a. cisterna
    a. oxygen concentration
    a. temperature
ambiguous external genitalia
amblyopia
    deprivation a.
    eclipse a.
    a. ex anopsia
    exertional a.
ambulant (*var. of* ambulatory)
ambulation
    independent a.
ambulatory, ambulant
    a. anesthesia
    a. blood pressure monitoring (ABPM)
    a. gynecologic laparoscopy
    a. hemorrhoidectomy
    a. patient
    a. pneumoperitoneum
    a. setup
    a. surgery
    a. surgery center
AMC
    arthrogryposis multiplex congenita
AMD
    arthroscopic microdiscectomy
amebiasis
amebic
    a. colitis
    a. cyst
    a. hepatic abscess
    a. infection
    a. perforation
    a. peritonitis
ameboma, amoeboma
ameliorating myocardial stunning liposomal coenzyme
amelioration

ameloblastic
a. carcinoma
a. fibroma
ameloblastoma
America
Infectious Disease Society of A.
(IDSA)
American
A. Association for Surgery of
Trauma Organ Injury Scale
classification
A. Association for the Surgery of
Trauma (AAST)
A. Association of Nurse
Anesthetists (AANA)
A. Board of Anesthesiology
(ABA)
A. Board of Pain Medicine
(ABPM)
A. Board of Surgery (ABS)
A. College of Surgeons (ACS)
A. Draeger Vapor
A. Heart Association classification
A. Joint Committee on Cancer
(AJCC)
A. laryngectomy technique
A. Pain Society (APS)
A. Pediatric Surgical Association
(APSA)
A. Rheumatism Association index
A. silk suture
A. Society for Aesthetic Plastic
Surgery (ASAPS)
A. Society for Bariatric Surgery
(ASBS)
A. Society for Colon and Rectal
Surgeons (ASCRS)
A. Society for Gastrointestinal
Endoscopy (ASGE)
A. Society of Anesthesiologists
(ASA)
A. Society of Anesthesiologists
classification
A. Society of Anesthesiologists
Physical Status Classification
(ASAPSC)
A. Society of Anesthesiologists
status
A. Society of Anesthesiology score
A. Society of Colon and Rectal
Surgeons
A. Society of Regional Anesthesia
and Pain Medicine (ASRA)
A. Society of Transplant Surgeons
(ASTS)
A. Surgical Association (ASA)
A. Thoracic Society (ATS)
A. Urological Association symptom
index

Ames
A. criteria
A. mutagenic chemical test
AMES
age, metastases, extent, size
ametropia
position a.
amidation
amide
a. analogue
a. local anesthetic
amino acid
aminoglycoside
a. toxicity
a. tubular necrosis
aminotransferase
alanine a. (ALT)
amitriptyline
AML
angiomyolipoma
Ammon
A. canthoplasty
A. cheek flap blepharoplasty
A. dacryocystostomy
AMN
angiomyoneuroma
amnesia
patch a.
amnestic effect
amniocele
amnioinfusion
amnioma
amnion
a. ring
a. rupture
amnionic (*var. of* amniotic)
amnioscopy
amniotic, amnionic
a. band amputation
a. cavity
a. fluid embolism
a. fold
a. hernia
a. infection syndrome
a. membrane
a. sac
amniotomy
amobarbital
A-mode
amplitude modulation
amoeboma (*var. of* ameboma)
amotivation
depression-related a.
AMP
adenosine monophosphate
assisted medical procreation
ampere (A)
amphibolic, amphibolous
a. fistula

amphibolous (*var. of* amphibolic)
amphipathic molecules
amphoric respiration
Amplatz coronary catheterization technique
amplitude
    a. modulation (A-mode)
    a. of fusion
    plethysmographic pulse wave a.
amplitude-summation interferential current
ampulla, *pl.* **ampullae**
    a. ductus deferentis
    duodenal a.
    hepatopancreatic a.
    a. of Vater
    rectal a.
    Thoma a.
ampullae (*pl. of* ampulla)
ampullaris
ampullary
    a. adenocarcinoma
    a. aneurysm
    a. cancer
    a. carcinoma
    a. granulation tissue
    a. lesion
    a. sulcus
    a. tumor
ampullectomy
ampulloma
amputation
    above-elbow a. (AEA)
    above-knee a. (AKA)
    Alanson a.
    amniotic band a.
    Béclard a.
    below-elbow a. (BEA)
    below-knee a. (BKA)
    Berger interscapular a.
    Bier a.
    bilateral a.
    birth a.
    bloodless a.
    border ray a.
    Boyd ankle a.
    Bunge a.
    Burgess below-knee a.
    Callander a.
    central ray a.
    cervical a.
    chop a.
    Chopart a.
    circular open a.
    closed flap a.
    congenital above-elbow a.
    congenital below-elbow a.
    consecutive a.
    disarticular a.

dry a.
extremity a.
Farabeuf a.
fingertip a.
fishmouth a.
forearm a.
forequarter a.
Gordon-Taylor hindquarter a.
Gritti-Stokes a.
guillotine a.
hand a.
hindfoot a.
hindquarter a.
immediate a.
incomplete a.
index ray a.
interilioabdominal a.
interinnominoabdominal a.
intermediate a.
interpelviabdominal a.
interphalangeal a.
interscapular a.
intrapyretic a.
intrauterine a.
Jaboulay a.
Kendrick method below-knee a.
King-Steelquist hindquarter a.
Lisfranc a.
major a.
Manchester prolapsed uterus
    cervical a.
minor a.
multiple ray a.
neuropathic pain from a.
open a.
pathologic a.
penile a.
Pirogoff a.
primary a.
pulp a.
quadruple a.
ray a.
rectangular a.
root a.
secondary a.
shoulder a.
Sorondo-Ferré hindquarter a.
spontaneous a.
1-stage a.
2-stage Syme a.
supracondylar a.
Syme ankle disarticulation a.
tarsal a.
tarsometatarsal a.
tendinomyoplastic a.
tertiary a.
through-knee a.
transcarpal a.
transiliac a.

amputation (*continued*)
    transmetatarsal a.
    transpelvic a.
    traumatic a.
    Tripier foot a.
    Wagner modification of Syme a.
    Wagner 2-stage Syme a.
    Wilms a.
amputee
    unilateral a.
Amreich vaginal extirpation
Amsler operation
Amspacher-Messenbaugh
    A.-M. closing wedge osteotomy
    A.-M. cubitus varus correction
     technique
Amstutz-Wilson osteotomy
Amussat
    A. incision
    A. transverse abdominal incision
     operation
    A. valve
    A. valvula
amygdaline
amygdalohippocampectomy
amygdalotomy
amyloid
    a. angiopathy
    a. kidney
    a. oral cavity disease
anabolic
    a. hormone
    a. hormone supplementation
    a. response
anabolism
    muscle a.
anaclitic therapy
anacrotic notch
anadidymus
anaerobe
anaerobic, anaerobiotic
    a. glycosis
    a. ocular infection
    a. respiration
anaerobiotic (*var. of* anaerobic)
anaeroplasty
anagenesis
Anagnostakis entropion operation
anal
    a. abscess
    a. anastomosis
    a. canal
    a. canal artery
    a. canal rhythmic contraction
    a. canal staining
    a. cancer
    a. cleft
    a. column
    a. condyloma

    a. continence
    a. crypt
    a. dilation
    a. electrical stimulation
    a. endoscopy
    a. fascia
    a. fissure
    a. fistula
    a. fistulotomy
    a. foreign body
    a. high pressure zone
    a. HPZ
    a. incontinence
    a. manometry
    a. orifice
    a. pecten
    a. pouch
    a. region
    a. resting pressure
    a. seton
    a. sinus
    a. sphincter injury
    a. sphincter reconstruction
    a. sphincter repair
    a. sphincter squeeze pressure
    a. squamous intraepithelial lesion
     (ASIL)
    a. stretch
    a. tag
    a. transition zone (ATZ)
    a. triangle
    a. ulceration
    a. verge
analgesia
    ceiling a.
    conduction a.
    dermatomal level of a.
    dual-action a.
    epidural a.
    fixed-dose patient-controlled a.
     (FDPCA)
    inhalation a.
    interpleural a.
    intrathecal opioid labor a.
    multimodal a.
    neuraxial a.
    opioid a.
    parenteral a.
    parturient-controlled epidural a.
    patient-controlled a. (PCA)
    patient-controlled epidural a. (PCEA)
    patient-controlled epidural with
     intravenous a.
    patient-controlled intranasal a.
     (PCINA)
    patient-controlled regional a. (PCRA)
    perineal a.
    perioperative a.
    a. permeation

pinprick a.
postoperative a.
preemptive a.
preoperative a.
rescue a.
site-specific a.
spinal a.
stimulation-induced a. (SIA)
stress-induced a.
supplementary a.
thoracic epidural a.
tracheal topical a.
analgesia-induced PGID
analgesic, analgetic
a. abuse headache
a. effect
a. index
a. infusion
intranasal a.
intrathecal a.
intravenous a.
narcotic a.
nonopioid a.
NSAID a.
opioid a.
oral a.
parenteral a.
pediatric a.
postoperative a.
selective spinal a.
spinal a.
transdermal a.
analgetic (*var. of* analgesic)
analog (*var. of* analogue)
analogous
analogue, analog
amide a.
capsaicin a.
nonamide a.
somatostatin a.
analyses (*pl. of* analysis)
analysis, *pl.* **analyses**
activity pattern a.
advanced hyperspectral a.
antinociception a.
bioimpedance a.
blood gas a.
body composition a.
combined a.
deformity a.
displacement a.
failure a.
fixed-dose a.
frozen section a.
histopathologic a.
hyperspectral a.
image a.
immunohistochemical a.
isobologram a.

isobolographic a.
mutation a.
neutron activation a.
peak pressure a.
pressure-volume a.
pulse contour a.
retrospective a.
saturation a.
sound a.
total space a.
visual a.
volumetric a.
analytic, analytical
Late Effects of Normal
Tissue — Subjective, Objective,
Management, A. (LENT-SOMA)
a. method
a. reconstruction
analytical (*var. of* analytic)
analyzer, analyzor
oxygen a.
patient state a.
platelet function a.
analyzor (*var. of* analyzer)
anaphylactoid reaction
anaphylactoid-type reaction
anaphylaxis
eosinophilic chemotactic factor of a.
anaplastic
a. adenocarcinoma
a. astrocytoma
a. carcinoma
a. ependymoma
anapophysis
anastole
anastomose
anastomosed graft
anastomoses (*pl. of* anastomosis)
anastomosis, *pl.* **anastomoses**
Abbe intestinal a.
anal a.
antecolic a.
antiperistaltic a.
aortic a.
arterial a.
arteriolovenular a.
arteriovenous a. (AVA)
Baffe a.
Béclard a.
beveled a.
bidirectional superior cavopulmonary
a.
biliary-enteric a.
biliary-intestinal a.
biliodigestive a.
Billroth I, II gastrointestinal a.
bladder neck-to-urethra a.
bowel a.
Brackin ureterointestinal a.

anastomosis (*continued*)
    Braun a.
    carotid-basilar a.
    carotid-vertebral a.
    cavopulmonary a.
    cecorectal a.
    cervical a.
    cervical esophagogastric a.
    choledochocholedochostomy
      side-to-side a.
    circular a.
    Clado a.
    cobra-head a.
    Coffey ureterointestinal a.
    coloanal a.
    colocolic a.
    colocolonic a.
    coloendoanal a.
    colonic pouch anal a.
    colorectal a.
    conjoined a.
    cornual a.
    Couvelaire ileourethral a.
    cross-facial nerve graft a.
    crucial a.
    cruciate a.
    crunch-stick a.
    crushing a.
    curved end-to-end a.
    D-D a.
    delayed direct coloanal a.
    delta-shaped a.
    diamond a.
    dismembered a.
    distal a.
    duct-to-duct a.
    duct-to-mucosa a.
    elliptical a.
    endoanal a.
    end-to-back bowel a.
    end-to-end a. (EEA)
    end-to-end ileoanal a.
    end-to-end splenoadrenal a.
    end-to-side a. (ESA)
    end-weave a.
    esophageal-jejunal a.
    esophagocolic a.
    esophagogastric a.
    extended end-to-end a.
    extraabdominal a.
    extracorporeal a.
    extrapleural a.
    extravesical a.
    fishmouth a.
    flexor tendon a.
    Fontan atriopulmonary a.
    Furniss a.
    Galen a.
    gastroduodenal a.

gastrointestinal a. (GIA)
gastrojejunal a.
genicular a.
Glenn a.
graft a.
Haight a.
handmade a.
handsewn a.
hand-sutured ileoanal a.
heel-toe a.
hepatojejunal a.
Hofmeister a.
Hofmeister-Pólya a.
Horsley a.
Hoyer a.
H-shaped ileal pouch-anal a.
hypoglossal facial nerve a.
Hyrtl a.
ileal pouch-anal a. (IPAA)
ileal pouch-distal rectal a.
ileal-sigmoid a.
ileoanal a. (IAA)
ileorectal a. (IRA)
ileosigmoid a. (ISA)
ileotransverse colon a.
ileovesical a.
intercoronary a.
intermesenteric arterial a.
intestinal a.
intracorporeal a.
intragastric a.
intrathoracic a.
intrathoracic esophagogastric a.
intravesical a.
invaginating a.
isoperistaltic a.
jejunoduodenal a.
jejunoileal a.
jejunojejunal a.
J-pouch ileoanal a.
J-shaped ileal pouch-anal a.
Kocher a.
Kugel a.
Lane ileorectal a.
laparoscopic bilioenteric a.
2-layer a.
LeDuc a.
leptomeningeal a.
Lich-Gregoir a.
longitudinal side-to-side a.
lymphaticovenous a.
Martin-Gruber a.
Maunsell-Weir coloanal a.
mechanical a.
mesocaval a.
microneurovascular a.
microsurgical tubocornual a.
microvascular surgical a.
mucosa-to-mucosa a.

Nakayama a.
nerve a.
nondismembered a.
omega jejunoduodenal a.
onlay patch a.
pancreatic a.
pancreaticojejunal a.
pancreatogastric a.
pancreatogastrointestinal a.
pancreatogastrostomy a. (PGA)
pancreatojejunostomy a. (PJA)
Parks ileoanal a.
percutaneous portocaval a.
Politano-Leadbetter a.
Pólya a.
portacaval a.
portal-systemic a.
portoportal a.
portopulmonary venous a.
portosystemic a.
Potts a.
Potts-Smith a.
precapillary a.
primary end-to-end a.
primary thyrotracheal a.
pyeloileocutaneous a.
rectosigmoid a.
Riche-Cannieu a.
right-angled end-to-side a.
Riolan a.
Roux-en-Y hepaticojejunal a.
Schmidel a.
Schoemaker a.
side-to-side a.
spinal accessory nerve-facial
  nerve a.
splenoadrenal a.
splenorenal venous a.
S-shaped ileal pouch-anal a.
STA-MCA a.
stapled coloanal a.
stapled ileal pouch-anal a.
stapled ileoanal a.
stapled vascular a.
stenotic esophagogastric a.
subcutaneous a.
Sucquet a.
Sucquet-Hoyer a.
supraoptic a.
suture a.
sutureless bowel a.
Swenson rectosigmoidectomy with
  coloanal a.
temporal-cerebral arterial a.
tension-free a.
terminoterminal a.
transanal mucosectomy with
  handsewn a.
transureteroureteral a.

triple a.
ureterocolonic a.
ureteroileal a.
ureterosigmoid a.
ureterotubal a.
ureteroureteral a.
urethrovesical a.
valved conduit a.
vascular a.
venous a.
venous-to-venous a. (VVA)
vesicourethral a.
von Haberer-Finney a.
Waterston extrapericardial a.
wide elliptical a.
wide-open a.
W-shaped ileal pouch-anal a.
Z-shaped a.

anastomotic
a. abscess
a. aneurysm
a. area
a. branch
a. breakdown
a. complication
a. complication rate
a. dehiscence
a. disruption
a. edge
a. failure
a. fiber
a. fistula
a. flow
a. healing
a. hemorrhage
a. leak
a. leakage
a. operation
a. stoma
a. stricture
a. stricture formation
a. stricture rate
a. stump
a. stump leak
a. suture line
a. ulceration
a. vein

anatomic, anatomical
a. abnormality
a. barrier
a. dead space
a. diagnosis
a. equator
a. event
a. fracture
a. fracture reduction principle
a. imaging
a. imaging information
a. insertion

anatomic (*continued*)
    a. integrity
    a. localization
    a. pathology
    a. plane
    a. porous replacement (APR)
    a. porous replacement fixation
    a. radical retropubic prostatectomy
    a. repair
    a. resection
    a. situation
    a. snuffbox
    a. sphincter
    a. structure
    a. tooth
    a. tubercle
anatomical (*var. of* anatomic)
    a. root
anatomicosurgical
anatomist
anatomy
    anomalous a.
    biliary a.
    Billroth II a.
    cervicothoracic pedicle a.
    congenitally altered a.
    coronary vessel a.
    dental a.
    designed after natural a. (DANA)
    fetal intracranial a.
    gingival a.
    immune system a.
    intracranial a.
    intrahepatic a.
    knee a.
    Lowsley lobar a.
    native coronary a.
    neurovascular a.
    normal planar MR a.
    pathological a.
    pedicle a.
    peritoneal a.
    plantar compartmental a.
    retropubic a.
    surgical a.
    topographic a.
    vascular a.
    zonal a.
anatrophic
    a. nephrolithotomy
    a. nephroscopy
    a. nephrotomy
Ancap braided silk suture
anchor
    a. mastopexy
    a. molar
    suture a.
anchorage
    extramaxillary a.

    extraoral a.
    gastrophrenic a.
anchoring point
anchovy tendon interposition
   procedure
ancillary circuit
ancipital, ancipitate, ancipitous
ancipitate (*var. of* ancipital)
ancipitous (*var. of* ancipital)
anconal, anconeal
anconeal
anconeus
    a. arthroplasty
    a. muscle
    a. muscle flap
AND
    axillary node dissection
Andersch
    A. ganglion
    A. nerve
Anderson
    A. abnormal mixed head position
      correction procedure
    A. ankle fusion
    A. modification of Berndt-Harty
      osteochondral talar lesion
      classification
Anderson-D'Alonzo odontoid fracture
   classification
Anderson-Fowler
    A.-F. calcaneal displacement
      osteotomy
    A.-F. laparoscopic colon resection
      procedure
Anderson-Hutchins unstable tibial shaft
   fracture
Anderson-Hynes pyeloplasty
Andrews
    A. iliotibial band reconstruction
    A. strangulated hernia repair
      technique
Andrews-type nonorthodontic normal
   crown angulation
androblastoma
androgen
    a. ablation
    adrenal a.
    excess a.
    a. receptor blockade
androgenic obesity
androgenization
android pelvis
Andy Gump deformity
anecdotal procedure
anechoic tissue
Anel
    A. aneurysm operation
    A. arterial ligation method
    A. lacrimal fistula operation

anemia

    acute severe isovolemic a.
    cold autoimmune hemolytic a.
    Fanconi a.
    hereditary hemolytic a.
    macrocytic a.
    megaloblastic a.
    microcytic hypochromic a.
    a. of hemodialysis
    warm autoimmune hemolytic a.

anergia

anergy nutritional assessment

anesthesia (A)

    a. action
    acupuncture a.
    a. adjuvant
    ambulatory a.
    ankle block a.
    axillary block a.
    balanced a.
    barbiturate burst-suppression a.
    basal a.
    Bier block a.
    BIS-guided general a.
    block a.
    bolus intravenous a.
    brachial a.
    a. breathing circuit
    bypass a.
    cardiac a.
    cardiovascular a.
    caudal a.
    centroneuroaxis a.
    cervical a.
    circle absorption a.
    closed circuit a.
    cocaine a.
    coinduction of a.
    combined epidural and general a.
    combined spinal-epidural a. (CSEA)
    come-and-go a.
    compression a.
    computer-assisted a.
    conduction a.
    continuous epidural a.
    continuous lumbar peridural a.
    continuous spinal a.
    controlled hypotensive a.
    corneal a.
    Crile-Matas regional a.
    crossed a.
    deep volatile a.
    dental a.
    depth of a.
    diagnostic a.
    differential spinal a.
    digital block a.
    direct vein a.
    dissociated a.

    dissociative a.
    a. dolorosa
    ear a.
    electric a.
    endotracheal a.
    epidural a. (EA)
    examination under a. (EUA)
    extradural a.
    failed a.
    fast-track a.
    fast-track cardiac a.
    field block a.
    fitness for general a.
    fractional epidural a.
    fractional spinal a.
    general a.
    general endotracheal a.
    geriatric a.
    girdle a.
    glove a.
    graded spinal a.
    gustatory a.
    gynecologic a.
    high spinal a.
    hydrate microcrystal theory of a.
    hyperbaric spinal a.
    hypnosis a.
    hypobaric spinal a.
    hypotensive a.
    hypothermic a.
    hysteric a.
    induction of a.
    infiltration a.
    infraorbital a.
    inhalant a.
    inhalational a.
    inhalation mask a.
    insufflation a.
    intercostal a.
    interpleural a.
    intracavitary a.
    intraligamentary a.
    intramedullary a.
    intranasal a.
    intraoral a.
    intraorbital a.
    intraosseous a.
    intraperitoneal a.
    intrapulpal a.
    intraspinal a.
    intrathecal a.
    intratracheal a.
    intravenous block a.
    intravenous regional a. (IVRA)
    intravenous sedation a.
    isobaric spinal a.
    laryngeal a.
    laryngotracheal a. (LTA)
    ligamental a.

anesthesia (*continued*)
  local a.
  low central venous pressure a.
  low spinal a.
  low thoracic level epidural a.
  lumbar epidural a. (LEA)
  1-lung a.
  MAC a.
  management of a.
  maternal a.
  modified van Lint a.
  monitored anesthesia care a.
  muscular a.
  neonatal a.
  nerve block a.
  nerve compression a.
  neuraxial a.
  neuroleptanalgesia a.
  neurosurgical a.
  newborn a.
  nonrebreathing a.
  nose a.
  O'Brien a.
  obstetric a.
  ocular microtremor during general a.
  olfactory a.
  open drop a.
  ophthalmic a.
  ophthalmologic a.
  opioid a.
  orbital a.
  oropharyngeal a.
  orthopedic a.
  outpatient a.
  painful a.
  paracervical block a.
  paravertebral a.
  parenteral a.
  patient-controlled a. (PCA)
  pediatric radiotherapy a.
  peribulbar a.
  peridural a.
  perineal a.
  perineural a.
  periodontal ligament a.
  peripheral nerve block a.
  pharyngeal a.
  Ponka technique for local a.
  postcesarean a.
  postoperative a.
  preemptive a.
  preperitoneal a.
  presacral a.
  pressure a.
  pudendal a.
  rapid-sequence induction of a.
  rebreathing a.
  a. record
  rectal a.

  refrigeration a.
  regional a.
  retrobulbar a.
  risk management of a.
  sacral a.
  saddle block a.
  segmental epidural a.
  segmental peridural spinal a.
  selective a.
  semiclosed a.
  semiopen a.
  single-breath induction of a.
  single-shot spinal a.
  spinal a. (SA)
  splanchnic a.
  stellate ganglion block a.
  stocking a.
  stocking-glove a.
  subarachnoid a.
  supraclavicular brachial block a.
  surgical a.
  tactile a.
  therapeutic a.
  thermal a.
  thermic a.
  thoracic a.
  thoracic epidural a. (TEA)
  throat a.
  a. time
  to-and-fro a.
  toe-block a.
  topical oropharyngeal a. (TOPA)
  total intravenous a. (TIVA)
  total spinal a.
  transdermal a.
  traumatic a.
  ultrasound-guided regional a.
  unilateral a.
  unmonitored local a.
  urologic a.
  van Lint a.
  variable-dose patient-controlled a.
    (VDPCA)
  visceral a.
  volatile a.
anesthesia-induced PGID
anesthesiologist
  American Society of A.'s (ASA)
anesthesiology
  American Board of A. (ABA)
  critical care a.
  a. critical care medicine
anesthetic
  action of a.
  amide local a.
  a. and fluid management
  a. approach
  a. binding site
  a. block

a. blockade
cardiac a.
a. circuit
a. consideration
a. cutoff
a. degradation
a. depth
a. emergence
epidural a.
ester local a.
eutectic mixture of local a.'(EMLA)
flammable a.
a. gas
gas a.
a. gas exposure
a. gas mixture
general a.
halogenated volatile a.
a. hepatitis
a. hepatotoxicity
hyperbaric local a.
a. immediate recovery
a. index
a. induction
a. induction agent
inhaled a.
injection of local a.
instillation of a.
intradermal a.
intramuscular a.
intraperitoneal a.
intrathecal a.
intravenous a.
local a.
low-dose a.
a. management
a. monitoring
multiple-mechanism inhaled a.
multiple-site inhaled a.
opioid a.
oral a.
pediatric a.
polymer a.
a. potency
potent inhaled a.
a. preconditioning
preoperative a.
primary a.
a. reaction
a. record
rectal a.
regional a.
ring block digital a.
a. risk
secondary a.
a. shock
single-mechanism inhaled a.
single-site inhaled a.
a. solubility

spinal a.
a. system
a. technique
a. time
a. tolerance
topical a.
total intravenous a. (TIVA)
trace a.
a. vapor
volatile a.
walking epidural a.
anesthetic/hypnotic
anesthetic-induced postconditioning
anesthetist
American Association of Nurse A.'s (AANA)
certified registered nurse a. (CRNA)
nurse a.
anesthetization
anesthetize
aneuploid cell line
aneurysm
abdominal aortic a. (AAA)
ampullary a.
anastomotic a.
anterior circulation a.
aortic a.
aortoiliac a.
arterial a.
arteriosclerotic a.
arteriovenous a.
atherosclerotic a.
axial a.
axillary artery a.
basilar artery a.
basilar bifurcation a.
basilar tip a.
Bérard a.
berry a.
bifurcation a.
celiac artery a.
circulation a.
clavicular fracture a.
a. clip ligation
coiled intracranial a.
complex intracranial a.
compound a.
congenital cerebral a.
consecutive a.
cylindroid a.
dental mycotic abdominal a.
descending aortic a.
A. Detection and Management (ADAM)
diffuse a.
dissecting a.
ectatic a.
endogenous a.
endovascular a.

aneurysm (*continued*)
    exogenous a.
    false a.
    femoral artery a.
    fusiform a.
    hernial a.
    iliac artery a.
    inflammatory abdominal aortic a.
    infraclinoid a.
    infrarenal aortic a.
    intracranial a.
    isolated iliac artery a.
    juxtarenal a.
    a. management
    miliary a.
    mitral valve a.
    mycotic a.
    mycotic abdominal a.
    pararenal aortic a.
    peripheral a.
    phantom a.
    posterior circulation a.
    Pott a.
    a. repair
    ruptured abdominal aortic a.
    saccular a.
    serpentine a.
    splanchnic artery a.
    splenic artery a. (SAA)
    staged repair of extensive aortic a.
    subclavian artery a.
    supraclinoid a.
    thoracic a.
    thoracoabdominal a.
    thoracoabdominal aortic a.
    a. tissue
    traction a.
    traumatic false a.
    true a.
    tubular a.
    varicose a.
aneurysmal, aneurysmatic
    a. dilatation
    a. dilation
    a. disease
    a. hematoma
    a. hemorrhage
    a. rupture
    a. sac
    a. tissue
    a. varix
aneurysmatic (*var. of* aneurysmal)
aneurysmectomy
    aortic a.
    conventional aortic a.
    elective a.
    laparoscopic-assisted a.
    Matas a.
aneurysmoplasty

aneurysmorrhaphy
aneurysmotomy
angel's kiss malformation
Angelucci cataract operation
angel-wing deformity
angiectasia, angiectasis
angiectasis (*var. of* angiectasia)
angiectatic
angiectopia
angiitis, angitis
    hypersensitivity a.
    necrotizing a.
angina
    abdominal a.
    intestinal a.
    unstable a. (UA, USA)
angio
    angiogram
    angiographic
    angiography
angioblastic lymphadenopathy
angioblastoma
angiocatheter with looped polypropylene suture
angiocentric
    a. immunoproliferative lesion
    a. lymphoproliferative lesion
angiodysplastic lesion
angioembolization
angioendothelioma
angiofibrolipoma
angiofibroma
    facial a.
    juvenile a.
angiogenesis
    therapeutic a.
    tumor a.
angiogram (angio)
    mesenteric a.
    multigated a. (MUGA)
angiographic (angio)
    a. demonstration
    a. embolization
    a. evaluation
    a. intervention
    a. result
    a. road-mapping technique
    a. study
angiographically occult intracranial vascular malformation (AOIVM)
angiography (ang, ANG, angio)
    abdominal a.
    arterial a.
    computed tomographic hepatic a.
    fluorescein a.
    magnetic resonance a. (MRA)
    mesenteric a.
    on-table a.
    selective a.

A

angioimmunoblastic lymphadenopathy
angioinvasive lesion
angiokeratoma
angioleiomyoma
angiolipofibroma
angiolipoma
angiolith
angiolithic
angiolysis
angioma, *pl.* angiomata, angiomas
    arterial a.
    bleeding a.
    capillary a.
    cavernous a.
    cerebral a.
    cherry a.
    conjunctival a.
    gastric a.
    orbital a.
    pulmonary a.
    a. serpiginosum
    spider a.
    spinal a.
    strawberry a.
    superficial a.
    telangiectatic a.
    tufted a.
    venous a.
angiomas (*pl. of* angioma)
angiomata (*pl. of* angioma)
angiomatosis
    skeletal-extraskeletal a.
angiomatous neoplastic tissue
Angiomax
angiomyofibroma
angiomyolipoma (AML)
    aggressive renal a.
    asymptomatic a.
    hemorrhagic a.
    malignant a.
    renal a.
    uncomplicated a.
    visceral a.
angiomyoma
angiomyoneuroma (AMN)
angiomyxoma
angioneurectomy
angioneuromyoma
angioneurotomy
angio-osteohypertrophy syndrome
angiopathy
    amyloid a.
    radiation a.
angioplany
angioplasty
    ablative laser a.
    adjunctive balloon a.
    aortoiliac a.
    balloon catheter a.

    balloon coarctation a.
    balloon coronary a.
    balloon dilation a.
    balloon laser a.
    bootstrap 2-vessel a.
    brachiocephalic vessel a.
    carotid a.
    complementary balloon a.
    coronary artery a.
    coronary balloon a.
    culprit lesion a.
    excimer laser coronary a. (ELCA)
    facilitated a.
    high-risk a.
    holmium: yttrium-aluminum-garnet
      laser a.
    Ho:YAG laser a.
    iliac artery a.
    infrapopliteal transluminal a.
    Kinsey rotation atherectomy
      extrusion a.
    kissing balloon a.
    laser-assisted balloon a. (LABA)
    Linton patch a.
    low-speed rotational a.
    Osypka rotational a.
    patch-graft a.
    percutaneous a.
    percutaneous balloon a.
    percutaneous low-stress a.
    percutaneous transluminal a. (PTA)
    percutaneous transluminal coronary
      a. (PTCA)
    percutaneous transluminal renal a.
    peripheral balloon a.
    peripheral laser a.
    postcoronary a.
    renal a.
    rescue a.
    rotational a.
    salvage balloon a.
    subclavian vein patch a.
    thermal/perfusion balloon a.
    tibial a.
    tibioperoneal trunk a.
    tibioperoneal vessel a.
    transluminal coronary a.
    vein patch a.
    vibrational a.
angioplasty-related vessel occlusion
angioproliferative lesion
angioreticuloma
angiorrhaphy
angiorrhexis
angiosarcoma
angioscopy
    fluorescein fundus a.
    percutaneous transluminal a.
angioscotoma

angiostomy
angiotelectasia (*var. of* angiotelectasis)
angiotelectasis, angiotelectasia
angiotensin
    a. II-induced vascular contraction
    a. II receptor antagonist
angiotensinogen
angiotomy
angitis (*var. of* angiitis)
angle
    anomaly a.
    anorectal a.
    anterior angulation a.
    axial line a.
    biorbital a.
    a. bisection technique
    Böhler calcaneal a.
    Broca basilar a.
    Broca facial a.
    buccoocclusal line a.
    calcaneal inclination a.
    calcaneal-second metatarsal angle
      inclination a.
    cardiohepatic a.
    cavity line a.
    costal a.
    Daubenton a.
    declination a.
    deformity a.
    distobuccal line a.
    distobuccoocclusal point a.
    distolabial line a.
    distolabioincisal point a.
    distolingual line a.
    distolinguoincisal point a.
    distoocclusal point a.
    duodenojejunal a.
    elevation a.
    epigastric a.
    facial a.
    filtration a.
    Frankfort mandibular incisor a.
      (FMIA)
    Frankfort mandibular plane a.
    hepatic-renal a.
    hepatorenal a.
    hypsiloid a.
    incisal mandibular plane a.
    infrasternal a.
    iridocorneal a.
    Jacquart facial a.
    labioincisal line a.
    line a.
    linguoincisal line a.
    linguoocclusal line a.
    Louis a.
    Ludwig a.
    lumbosacral a.
    magnetization precession a.

    A. malocclusion classification
    mandibular incisor a.
    mandibular plane a.
    mesiobuccal line a.
    mesiobuccoocclusal point a.
    mesiolabial line a.
    mesiolabioincisal point a.
    mesiolingual line a.
    mesiolinguoincisal point a.
    mesiolinguo-occlusal point line a.
    mesioocclusal line a.
    metafacial a.
    nail-to-nail bed a.
    occipital a.
    occlusal plane a.
    a. of aberration
    a. of femoral torsion
    a. of His
    a. of orientation
    a. of reflection
    ophryospinal a.
    parietal a.
    pelvivertebral a.
    Pirogoff a.
    point a.
    pubic a.
    Quatrefages a.
    Serres a.
    sharp a.
    sphenoidal a.
    splenorenal a.
    sternal a.
    sternoclavicular a.
    a. stitch
    subpubic a.
    substernal a.
    superior a.
    a. suture technique
    talocalcaneal a.
    tip a.
    Topinard facial a.
    tracheal bifurcation a.
    venous a.
    xiphicostal a.
    Y a.
angled blade plate fixation
Anglo-Saxon nomenclature
angular
    a. acceleration
    a. artery
    a. deformity
    a. incision
    a. line
    a. notch
    a. osteotomy
    a. phenolization
    a. position
    a. spine
    a. vein

angularis
    incisura a.
angulated
    a. fracture
    a. lesion
angulation
    Andrews-type nonorthodontic normal
      crown a.
    anterior a.
    apex dorsal a.
    bracket slot a.
    built-in a.
    caudal a.
    coronal a.
    crown a.
    a. deformity
    a. fracture
    horizontal a.
    kyphotic a.
    limb length a.
    lower incisor a.
    a. motion
    a. osteotomy
    palmar a.
    plantar a.
    radius of a.
    RAO a.
    rectoanal a.
    right anterior oblique a.
    screw a.
    upper incisor a.
    valgus a.
    vertical a.
    volar a.
anguli (*pl. of* angulus)
angulus, *pl.* **anguli**
ANH
    acute normovolemic hemodilution
anhepatic
    a. phase
    a. stage of liver transplant
anhydration
anhydrous facial foundation
ani (*pl. of* anus)
animation
    suspended a.
anisocoria
    postoperative a.
anisotropic
    a. rotation
    a. tissue
ankle
    a. block
    a. blockade
    a. block anesthesia
    a. brachial blood pressure ratio
    a. dislocation
    dorsiflexion of a.
    a. fusion

    lateral joint of a.
    a. mortise diastasis
    a. mortise fracture
    a. region
ankle-brachial
    a.-b. pressure index (ABPI)
    a.-b. pressure measurement
ankyloglossia superior syndrome
ankylosing spondylitis
ankylosis
    extraarticular a.
    extracapsular a.
Ann
    A. Arbor
    A. Arbor classification of Hodgkin
      disease staging
    A. Arbor Hodgkin disease
      classification
    A. Arbor Hodgkin lymphoma (stage
      I, IE, II, IIE, IIIE, IIIS, IIISE,
      IV)
annexectomy
annexopexy
annular (*var. of* anular)
annuloplasty (*var. of* anuloplasty)
annulorrhaphy
annulotomy
annulus (*var. of* anulus)
ano
    fistula in a. (FIA)
anociassociation
anococcygeal
    a. body
    a. ligament
anocutaneous
    a. line
    a. stimulation
anoderm
anoderm-preserving hemorrhoidectomy
anodyne
anogenital raphe
anomalad
    Pierre Robin a.
anomalous
    a. anatomy
    a. fixation
    a. innominate artery compression
      syndrome
    a. insertion
    a. junction of pancreatobiliary duct
    a. mesenteric adhesion
    a. position
    a. rectification
    a. vertebral artery
anomaly
    abdominal wall a.
    Alder-Reilly a.
    a. angle
    anorectal a.

anomaly (*continued*)
    arterial a.
    atrioventricular connection a.
    atrioventricular junction a.
    Axenfeld a.
    branchial a.
    cardiac a.
    cervical a.
    chest a.
    Chiari a.
    coexisting anomalies
    coloboma a.
    congenital conotruncal a.
    conjoined nerve-root a.
    conotruncal a.
    coronary artery a.
    craniofacial a.
    Cruveilhier-Baumgarten a.
    dental a.
    dentofacial a.
    diaphragmatic a.
    double-inlet ventricle a.
    Duane a.
    duplication a.
    dysgnathic a.
    Ebstein a.
    Ebstein cardiac a.
    Ebstein congenital a.
    eugnathic a.
    facet a.
    fetal cardiac a.
    fetal chest a.
    fetal gastrointestinal a.
    fetal vascular a.
    fixation a.
    Freund a.
    gastrointestinal a.
    genetic a.
    genitourinary a.
    gestant a.
    hand a.
    heart a.
    intracranial dural vascular a.
    jugular bulb a.
    kidney a.
    Kimerle a.
    Klippel-Feil a.
    lacrimal angle duct a.
    laryngeal a.
    limb reduction a.
    maxillofacial a.
    megadolichovertebrobasilar a.
    Michel a.
    Möbius a.
    Mondini a.
    morning glory optic disc a.
    motor a.
    müllerian duct a.
    nevoid a.

numerary renal a.
occipitoatlantoaxial a.
oculocephalic vascular a.
a. of Zahn
oral a.
orthopedic a.
osseous a.
Peters a.
Poland a.
postsurgical motor a.
presacral a.
pulmonary valve a.
pulmonary venous connection a.
pulmonary venous return a.
renal a.
reticulate pigmented a.
root a.
segmentation a.
Shone a.
Sprengel a.
structural a.
Taussig-Bing a.
tracheobronchial a.
Uhl a.
umbilical cord a.
Undritz a.
urinary tract a.
urogenital a.
uterine a.
VACTERL a.
vaginal a.
vascular a.
ventricular inflow a.
viscerobronchial cardiovascular a.
vitelline duct a.

anoplasty
    cutback a.
    a. flap
    House advancement a.
    House flap a.
    Martin a.
    a. treatment
    Y-V a.

anopsia
    amblyopia ex a.

anorchia (*var. of* anorchism)
anorchism, anorchia
anorectal
    a. abscess
    a. angle
    a. anomaly
    a. carcinoma
    a. disorder
    a. fistula
    a. flexure
    a. foreign body
    a. function test
    a. impalement
    a. junction

a. line
a. malformation
a. manometry
a. melanoma
a. mucosal prolapse
a. myectomy
a. outlet obstruction
a. pain
a. ring
a. sepsis
a. septum
a. space
a. sphincter
a. surgery
a. variceal bleeding
anorectoplasty
Laird-McMahon a.
posterior sagittal a. (PSARP)
anorectovaginoplasty
anorectum
anorexia
anorexigenic effect
anoscopy
anosigmoidoscopy
anosmia
anosmic
anospinal
anotia
anovesical
anovulation
persistent a.
anoxemia
anoxia
anoxic a.
diffusion a.
histotoxic a.
stagnant a.
anoxic
a. anoxia
a. preconditioning phenomenon
ANP
atrial natriuretic peptide
ANS
autonomic nervous system
ansa, *pl.* **ansae**
a. cervicalis
a. cervicalis nerve
a. cervicalis root
Haller a.
a. subclavia
Vieussens a.
ansae (*pl. of* ansa)
anserina
cutis a.
anserine bursa
anserinus
Anson-McVay
A.-M. hernia repair
A.-M. inguinal hernia operation

ansotomy
ant.
anterior
antagonist (antag)
alpha-adrenergic a.
alpha-1 adrenergic a.
alpha-2 adrenergic receptor a.
angiotensin II receptor a.
antimuscarinic a.
beta-receptor a.
nonselective opioid receptor a.
opiate receptor a.
opioid a.
receptor a.
antagonistic
a. drug interaction
a. muscle
antagonize
antalgesia
antalgic
a. gait
a. medication
antebrachial
a. fascia
a. flexor retinaculum
a. reflex
a. region
antecolic
a. anastomosis
a. approach
a. duodenoileostomy
a. long-loop isoperistaltic
gastrojejunostomy
a. position
a. Roux limb
antecubital
a. approach
a. arteriovenous fistula
a. space
antegrade
a. approach
a. catheterization
a. continence enema (ACE)
a. continence enema procedure
a. direction
a. double balloon-double wire
technique
a. method
a. nailing
a. passage
a. puncture
a. tracheal gas insufflation
a. transcystic sphincterotomy
**antegrade/retrograde cardioplegia
technique**
antemortem clot
antenatal dislocation
antenna procedure
antepartum hemorrhage

anteposition
anteprostate
anterior (ant.)
- a. abdominal injury
- a. abdominal wall
- a. acromioplasty
- a. acromioplasty approach
- a. and posterior (A&P)
- a. and posterior repair
- a. angulation
- a. angulation angle
- a. antebrachial region
- a. aortic wall
- a. apical
- a. apical segment
- a. aspiration
- a. auricular artery
- a. auricular groove
- a. auricular muscle
- a. auricular nerve
- a. axillary approach
- a. axillary fold
- a. axillary line (AAL)
- a. basal (AB)
- a. basal branch
- a. basal segment
- a. brachial region
- a. calcaneal osteotomy
- a. capsulolabral reconstruction
- a. capsulotomy
- a. carotid artery
- a. cavernous sinus syndrome
- a. cecal artery
- a. cerebral artery (ACA)
- a. cervical approach
- a. cervical discectomy and fusion (ACDF)
- a. cervical intertransverse muscle
- a. cervical spine surgery
- a. cervical surgery vocal cord damage
- a. cervicothoracic junction surgery
- a. chest wall syndrome
- a. choroidal artery
- a. ciliary artery
- a. circulation aneurysm
- a. circumflex humeral artery
- a. clear space
- a. clinoid process
- a. column
- a. column fracture
- a. column osteosynthesis
- a. commissure-posterior commissure (AC-PC)
- a. commissure-posterior commissure line
- a. communicating artery (AComA)
- a. complete dislocation
- a. condylar canal
- a. condyloid foramen
- a. cord
- a. cord compression
- a. cornea
- a. corneal curvature
- a. corpectomy
- a. correction
- a. cortex
- a. costotransverse ligament
- a. cranial base
- a. cranial fossa
- a. cruciate ligament (ACL)
- a. cruciate ligament reconstruction
- a. cutaneous branch
- a. cutaneous nerve
- a. cyst
- a. descending artery
- a. discectomy
- a. displacement
- a. epineurotomy
- a. esophagus
- a. ethmoidal nerve
- a. ethmoidectomy
- a. extensile approach
- a. extradural clinoidectomy
- a. extraperitoneal approach
- a. extremity
- a. facial height (AFH)
- a. focal point
- a. fontanelle
- a. fundoplasty
- a. gastropexy
- a. gastrotomy
- a. great vessel
- a. ground bundle
- a. helical rim free flap
- a. hip dislocation
- a. humeral circumflex artery
- a. incision
- a. inferior cerebellar artery (AICA)
- a. inferior iliac spine (AIIS)
- a. inferior pancreaticoduodenal artery
- a. inferior segment
- a. inguinal herniorrhaphy
- a. innominate osteotomy
- a. innominate rotation
- a. intercostal artery
- a. intermuscular septum
- a. internal fixation
- a. internal stabilization
- a. intraoccipital joint
- a. knee region
- a. labial artery
- a. labial commissure
- a. labial nerve
- a. labrum periosteum shoulder arthroscopic lesion
- a. limiting ring

a. lingual gland
a. lip
a. lower cervical spine surgery
a. lumbar vertebral interbody fusion
a. mediastinal artery
a. mediastinal fat
a. mediastinal mass
a. mediastinum
a. meningeal artery
a. metallic fixation
a. midpapillary (AM)
a. midpapillary level
a. midpapillary segment
a. nasal meatus
a. nephrectomy
a. oblique position
a. oblique projection
a. parietal artery
a. partial laryngectomy
a. pelvic exenteration
a. plate fixation
a. Pólya gastrectomy procedure
a. primary division
processus clinoideus a.
a. puncture
a. quadriceps musculocutaneous flap technique
a. radicular artery
a. rectopexy
a. rectus fascia
a. rectus muscle
a. rectus sheath
a. rectus sheath wall
a. resection
a. retraction
a. retroperitoneal decompression
a. retroperitoneal flank approach
a. rhizotomy
a. root
a. sandwich patch technique
a. scalene compression syndrome
a. scalene muscle
a. sclerotomy
a. screw fixation
a. scrotal nerve
a. semicircular canal
a. seromyotomy
a. serratus muscle
a. sheath
a. short-segment stabilization
a. shoulder dislocation
a. spinal artery (ASA)
a. spinal artery syndrome
a. spinal fixation
a. spinal fusion (ASF)
a. stabilization procedure
a. sternoclavicular ligament
a. sternomastoid approach
a. superior alveolar artery

a. superior iliac spine (ASIS)
a. superior pancreatiocoduodenal artery
a. superior segment
a. supraclavicular nerve
a. surgical exposure
a. synechia formation
a. talofibular ligament rupture
a. temporal artery
a. thoracic wall
a. thoracotomy
a. tibial bursa
a. tibialis tendon
a. tibial muscle
a. tibial recurrent artery
a. tibiotalar ligament
a. transabdominal approach
a. transhepatic approach
a. translation
a. transoral approach
a. transperitoneal approach
a. transthoracic approach
a. tubercle
a. ulnar recurrent artery
a. urethra
a. uveitis
a. vaginal fornix
a. vaginal trunk
a. vertical canal
a. view
a. vitrectomy
a. wound
anterior-inferior dislocation
anterior-posterior (AP)
a.-p. compression
a.-p. fusion with SSI
anterocrural celiac plexus block
anterograde
a. direction
a. transseptal technique
anterolateral (AL)
a. approach
a. compression fracture
a. cordotomy
a. dislocation
a. fontanelle
a. neck
a. prefrontal cortex
a. thalamostriate artery
a. thoracotomy
a. thoracotomy incision
a. tractotomy
anterolisthesis
anteromedial
a. arm
a. bundle
a. incision
a. retropharyngeal approach
a. thalamostriate artery

anteroposterior (AP)
    a. chest x-ray
    a. compression
    a. correction
    a. nail
    a. projection
    a. translation
anterosuperior external ilium
  movement
antevesical hernia
anthelix (*var. of* antihelix)
anthracosis
anthropoid pelvis
anthropometric evaluation
anthropometry
antiadhesion agent
antianalgesia
antiangiogenic effect
antiantibody formation
antiarrhythmic therapy
antibacterial agent
antibasement membrane
antibiotic (ABx)
    a. bead pouch
    broad-spectrum a.
    perioperative a.
    postoperative a.
    prophylactic a.
    prophylactic intravenous a.
    a. prophylaxis
    systemic a.
    a. therapy
    topical a.
antibiotic-impregnated catheter
antibody (Ab)
    a. formation
    fungal a.
    HCV a.
    heparin-associated antiplatelet a.'s
    unfractionated heparin a.
antibody-coated suture
anticalculous
anticholinergic medication
anticipated blood loss
anticipatory coarticulation
anticoagulant
    a. effect
    lupus a.
    a. monitoring
    oral a.
    a. therapy (ACT)
anticoagulation
    a. monitoring
    a. monitoring requirement
    oral a.
    prophylactic a.
    a. protocol
    systemic a.
    a. therapy

anticonvulsant
anticus
antidepressant
    atypical a.
antidote
antidromic stimulation
antiembolic position
antiemetic
    prophylactic a.
    a. prophylaxis
    rescue a.
    a. therapy
antiepileptic
    a. drug
    a. medication
antifibrinolytic
    a. agent
    a. drug
antifungal
    a. agent
    a. esophageal infection
    a. prophylaxis
    a. regimen
    a. therapy
    a. treatment
antifungal-resistant opportunistic infection
antigen (Ag)
    cancer a. 19-9 (CA19-9)
    carcinoembryonic a. (CEA)
    CTL-inducing peptide a.
    human leukocyte a. (HLA)
    Lewis Y a.
    proliferating cell nuclear a.
      (PCNA)
    serum carcinoembryonic a.
    tumor a.
antigen-extracted allogeneic bone
antigenic modulation
antiglaucoma surgery
antiglomerular
    a. basement membrane
    a. basement membrane antibody
    disease
antigravity muscles
antihelix, anthelix
antihemophilic
antihemorrhagic
antihistamine
antihormonal therapy
antiincontinence procedure
antiinflammatory medication
antilymphocyte globulin
antilymphoid therapy
antimesenteric
    a. enterotomy
    a. fat pad
    a. incision
    a. side
antimetabolite

antimicrobial
    a. agent
    a. therapy
antimotility agent
antimuscarinic antagonist
antimycotic
antineoplastic agent
antinephritic
antineural autoantibody testing
antiniad
antinial
antinion
antinociception
    a. analysis
    intrathecal a.
antinociceptive
antioxidant
    a. defense
    a. reserve capacity
antiperistaltic
    a. anastomosis
    a. loop
    a. operation
antiphospholipid antibody syndrome
antiplatelet
    a. protocol
    a. regimen
antipsychotic
antipyogenic
antireflux
    a. flap-valve mechanism
    a. operation
    a. procedure
    a. surgery
    a. therapy
    a. ureteral implantation technique
antirefluxing colonic conduit
antiretroviral
    a. drug
    a. toxic neuropathy (ATN)
antisaccade
antisense
antisialagogue
antispasmodic therapy
antitension line (ATL)
antithrombin III plasma level
antithromboembolic prophylaxis
antithrombogenic material
antithrombotic
    a. activity
    a. therapy
antitorque suture
antitragicus muscle
antitragus
anti-Trendelenburg position
antitubular basement membrane
antiviral
    a. prophylaxis
    a. therapy

antral
    a. biopsy
    a. edema
    a. exclusion
    a. irrigation
    a. lavage
    a. membrane
    a. sphincter
    a. stenting
    a. tumor
    a. web
antrectomy
    Roux-en-Y biliary bypass
      with a.
antroduodenectomy
antropyloric canal
antroscopy
antrostomy
    inferior meatal a.
    intraoral a.
    nasal a.
antrotomy
antrum
    a. cardiacum
    gastric a.
    mastoid a.
    maxillary a.
    a. of Highmore
    pyloric a.
    Willis a.
Antyllus arterial ligation method
anular, annular
    a. adenocarcinoma
    a. cartilage
    a. constricting lesion
    a. corneal graft operation
    a. pancreas
    a. sphincter
anuli (*pl. of* anulus)
anuloplasty, annuloplasty
    a. band insertion
    Carpentier a.
    DeVega tricuspid valve a.
    Gerbode a.
    isolated a.
    mitral band a.
    prosthetic ring a.
    reduction a.
    tricuspid valve a.
    Wooler-type a.
anulus, annulus, *pl.* **anuli**
    Haller a.
    mitral valve a.
    tricuspid valve a.
anum
    per a.
anuria
anuric

anus, *pl.* **ani**
 artificial a.
 ectopic a.
 imperforate a. (IA)
 vaginal ectopic a.
anusitis
anxiety
 dental a.
 a. disorder
anxiolytic
Anzemet
AO
 Arbeitsgemeinschaft für
 Osteosynthesefragen
  AO classification
  AO dynamic compression plate
   construct
  AO external fixation
  AO procedure
  AO rigid fixation
  AO spinal internal fixation
  AO technique
AOD
 arterial occlusive disease
AOIVM
 angiographically occult intracranial
 vascular malformation
aorta (Ao), *pl.* **aortae**
 abdominal a.
 appendicular a.
 arcuate a.
 coarctation of a.
 deep articular a.
 dissection of a.
 infrarenal a.
 infrarenal abdominal a.
 proximal a.
 pseudocoarctation of a.
 recoarctation of a.
 supraceliac a.
 thoracic a.
aortae (*pl. of* aorta)
aortectomy
aortic
 a. anastomosis
 a. aneurysm
 a. aneurysmal disease
 a. aneurysmectomy
 a. aneurysm tissue
 a. arch
 a. arch disease
 a. atheromatous
  disease
 a. bifurcation
 a. blood pressure
 a. body
 a. body tumor
 a. clamping
 a. conduit

a. cross-clamping
a. cuff
a. dicrotic notch pressure
a. dissection
a. endograft
a. foramen
a. graft placement
a. hiatus
a. hypoplasia
a. insufficiency
a. intramural hematoma
a. knob
a. laceration
a. neck
a. nipple
a. node metastasis
a. occlusion
a. occlusive disease
a. patch
a. perfusion
a. pressure gradient
a. pullback pressure
a. reconstructive surgery
a. regurgitation murmur
a. ring
a. root reconstruction
a. root replacement (ARR)
a. root velocity waveform
a. rupture
a. sac
a. stenosis
a. stump blow-out
a. transection
a. valve area
a. valve atresia
a. valve disease
a. valve gradient
a. valve insufficiency
a. valve leaflet
a. valve repair
a. valve replacement (AVR)
a. valve resistance
a. valve restenosis
a. valve velocity profile
a. valvoplasty
a. valvotomy
a. wall
a. wall deterioration
aorticopulmonary (*var. of*
 aortopulmonary)
aorticorenal ganglion
aortic-pulmonic window
aortoannular ectasia
aortobifemoral bypass
aortocaval fistula
aortocoronary
aortoduodenal fistula
aortoenteric fistula
aortoesophageal fistula

aortofemoral
> a. bypass
> a. bypass graft (AFBG)

aortogastric fistula

aortograft duodenal fistula

aortogram
> flush a.

aortoiliac
> a. aneurysm
> a. angioplasty
> a. bypass
> a. endarterectomy
> a. occlusive disease
> (AIOD)

aortoplasty
> patch a.

aortopulmonary, aorticopulmonary
> a. fenestration
> a. window (APW)

aortorenal
> a. bypass
> a. reconstruction
> a. reimplantation

aortorrhaphy

aortosigmoid fistula

aortotomy

A&P
> anterior and posterior
> A&P projection
> A&P repair

AP
> airway pressure
> anterior-posterior
> anteroposterior

APACHE
> Acute Physiology and Chronic Health
> Evaluation
> APACHE II
> APACHE III
> APACHE IV

apatite calculus

APC
> adenomatous polyposis coli

APD
> automated percutaneous discectomy

apellous

aperistalsis

aperta
> spina bifida a.

Apert syndrome

aperture
> inferior pelvic a.
> inferior thoracic a.
> laryngeal a.
> lateral cerebral a.
> a. of abdomen
> superior pelvic a.
> superior thoracic a.
> upper thorax a.

apex, *pl.* **apices**
> corneal a.
> a. dorsal angulation
> a. fracture
> lateral a.

Apgar score

aphakia
> extracapsular a.

aphakic correction

apheresis, pheresis
> continuous endotoxin a.

aphthous
> a. ulcer
> a. ulceration

aphthous-type lesion

apical
> anterior a. (AA)
> a. ballooning syndrome
> a. canal
> a. fenestration
> a. gland
> a. infection
> inferior a. (IA)
> lateral a. (LA)
> a. left ventricular puncture
> a. lordotic projection
> a. lordotic view
> a. polar nephrectomy
> a. ramification
> a. segment
> septal a. (SA)
> a. space
> a. suture
> a. transverse

apically repositioned flap in mucogingival surgery

apiceotomy (*var. of* apicotomy)

apices (*pl. of* apex)

apicoectomy

apicolysis
> extrapleural a.
> Semb a.

apicoposterior segment

apicoposterius

apicostomy

apicotomy, apiceotomy

APL
> adjustable pressure limiting
> APL valve

Apley
> A. compression test
> A. sign
> A. torn meniscus
> maneuver

apnea
> induced a.
> obstructive a.
> postextubation a.
> posthyperventilation a.

apnea (*continued*)
    postoperative a.
    succinylcholine-related a.
apnea-induced hemoglobin
  desaturation
apneic
    a. arrest
    a. oxygenation
    a. threshold
apneusis, apneustic breathing
apneustic
    a. breathing
    a. respiration
    a. ventilation
apocrine
    a. carcinoma
    a. gland
    a. metaplasia
apolipoprotein lipase
APOLT
    auxiliary partial orthotopic liver
    transplant
      APOLT technique
aponeurectomy
aponeurorrhaphy
aponeuroses (*pl. of* aponeurosis)
aponeurosis, *pl.* **aponeuroses**
    abdominal a.
    Denonvilliers a.
    epicranial a.
    external oblique a.
    internal oblique a.
    Petit a.
    temporal a.
    thoracolumbar a.
    transversus abdominis a.
    triangular a.
    Vulpius and Strofel inverted V slide
      lengthening of distal
      gastrocnemius/soleus a.
aponeurotic
    a. abscess
    a. closure
    a. defect
    a. flap
    a. layer
aponeurotica
aponeurotomy
apophysary (*var. of* apophysial)
apophyseal (*var. of* apophysial)
apophysial, apophyseal, apophysary
    a. fracture
    a. point
apophysis
    iliac a.
    ring a.
    slipped vertebral a.
    temporal a.
    vertebral ring a.

apophysitis
    calcaneal a.
apoplectic coma
apoplexy
apoptosis
    hepatic a.
    morphine-induced lymphocyte a.
    pulmonary a.
    resuscitation-induced pulmonary a.
    selective lectin-triggered a.
apoptotic
    a. endothelial cell death
    a. mechanism
apostaxis
apotreptic therapy
apparatus, *pl.* **apparatus**
    alimentary a.
    digestive a.
    genitourinary a.
    hyoid a.
    a. hyoideus
    lacrimal a.
    a. lacrimalis
    temperature exchange a.
    Tillaux a.
    urinary a.
    urogenital a.
apparent short leg syndrome
(ASLS)
appearance
    batwing a.
    beads-on-a-string a.
    beefy a.
    cobblestone a.
    coiled spring a.
    collar-bone a.
    corkscrew a.
    dewy a.
    gland a.
    granular a.
    ground-glass a.
    hobnailed a.
    honeycombed a.
    lead-pipe a.
    macroscopic a.
    mammographic a.
    meaty a.
    moth-eaten a.
    mottled a.
    nutmeg a.
    onion peel a.
    sausage-shaped a.
    signet-ring a.
    speckled a.
    spoke-wheel a.
    steamy a.
    string-of-beads a.
    tigroid a.
    whorled a.

A

appendage
    epiploic a.
    omental a.
    testicular a.
    vermiform a.
    vesicular a.
appendectomy (appy), appendicectomy
    auricular a.
    colonoscopic a.
    emergency a.
    emergent a.
    incidental a.
    a. incision
    interval a.
    inversion a.
    inversion-ligation a.
    laparoscopic a. (lap appy)
    laser-assisted a.
    McBurney a.
    needlescopic a.
    negative a.
    open a.
    percutaneous a.
    Weir a.
appendical (*var. of* appendiceal)
appendiceal, appendical
    a. abscess
    a. adenocarcinoma
    a. cancer
    a. colic
    a. CT
    a. fecalith
    a. gangrene
    a. intussusception
    a. mass
    a. mucocele
    a. opening
    a. orifice
    a. perforation
    a. vascular arcade
appendicectomy (*var. of* appendectomy)
appendices (*pl. of* appendix)
appendicitis
    chronic a.
    epiploic a.
    gangrenous a.
    ruptured a.
appendicocele
appendicocystostomy
    continent cutaneous a.
    dismembered reimplanted a.
    nonplicated a.
    orthotopic a.
    plicated a.
    reversed reimplanted a.
appendicoenterostomy
appendicolithiasis, appendolithiasis
appendicolysis

appendicostomy
appendicovesicostomy
    Mitrofanoff a.
appendicular
    a. aorta
    a. artery
    a. colic
    a. mucosal intussusception
    a. muscle
    a. skeleton
    a. vein
appendix, *pl.* **appendices**
    cecal a.
    ensiform a.
    epiploic a.
    a. mucocele
    pelvic a.
    perforated a.
    smoldering a.
    vermiform a.
    a. vermiformis
appendolithiasis (*var. of* appendicolithiasis)
apperceptive mass
applanation
    a. pressure
    tension by a.
    a. tonometry
apple
    Adam's a.
apple-core lesion
apple-peel deformity
appliance modification
application
    arch bar a.
    cast a.
    clip a.
    cold a.
    force a.
    frame a.
    heat a.
    ice a.
    interpleural a.
    laparoscopic clip a.
    paraffin film a.
    paraspinal rod a.
    pilot a.
    topical iodine a.
    traction a.
    transverse fixator a.
Appolito
    A. intestinal operation
    A. suture
    A. suture technique
apponensplasty
appose
apposition
    stent a.
    a. suture technique

approach

Abbott-Carpenter posterior knee a.
Abbott knee a.
abdominal a.
acetabular extensile a.
acromiothoracic a.
adaptational a.
Adson anterior transperitoneal a.
aggressive surgical a.
Alken renal stone a.
alternative surgical a.
anesthetic a.
antecolic a.
antecubital a.
antegrade a.
anterior acromioplasty a.
anterior axillary a.
anterior cervical a.
anterior extensile a.
anterior extraperitoneal a.
anterior retroperitoneal flank a.
anterior sternomastoid a.
anterior transabdominal a.
anterior transhepatic a.
anterior transoral a.
anterior transperitoneal a.
anterior transthoracic a.
anterolateral a.
anteromedial retropharyngeal a.
axillary a.
Bailey-Badgley anterior cervical a.
Banks-Laufman a.
basal subfrontal a.
Bennett posterior shoulder a.
Berger-Bookwalter posterior a.
Berke lateral orbital wall a.
bilateral ilioinguinal a.
bilateral sacroiliac a.
Bosworth posterior femur a.
Boyd elbow a.
Boyd-Sisk shoulder a.
brachial artery a.
Brackett-Osgood posterior hip a.
Brodsky-Tullos-Gartsman posterior
  shoulder joint a.
Broomhead medial ankle a.
Brown knee a.
Brown lateral knee a.
Bruser knee a.
Bruser lateral knee a.
Bryan-Morrey elbow a.
Bryan-Morrey extensive posterior a.
buccopharyngeal a.
buttonhole a.
Caldwell-Luc sinus a.
Callahan enterolateral hip a.
Campbell posterior shoulder a.
Campbell posterolateral a.
Carnesale acetabular extensile a.

Carnesale hip a.
case-by-case a.
Cave hip a.
Cave knee a.
central a.
cerebellopontine angle a.
cervical a.
cervicothoracic a.
Clairmont a.
closed a.
Cloward cervical disc a.
cochleovestibular a.
Codman saber-cut shoulder a.
Colonna-Ralston ankle a.
Colonna-Ralston medial a.
combined anterior and posterior a.
combined laparoscopic and
  thoracoscopic a.
combined low cervical and
  transthoracic a.
combined neurosurgical-external
  sinus a.
combined
  presigmoid-transtransversarium
  intradural a.
combined transsylvian and middle
  fossa a.
consortial a.
Coonse-Adams knee a.
costotransversectomy a.
Cubbins shoulder a.
curved a.
deltoid-splitting shoulder a.
deltopectoral a.
Dickinson a.
disease-based a.
distal interphalangeal joint a.
dorsal finger a.
dorsal midline a.
dorsalward a.
dorsolateral a.
dorsomedial a.
dorsoplantar a.
dorsoradial a.
dorsorostral a.
dorsoulnar a.
double-doughnut a.
double-seton modified surgical a.
Duran aortic vegetation a.
DuVries plantar fasciotomy a.
elbow a.
Endius posterior keyhole pedicle
  screw a.
endoscopic a.
endovascular a.
ethmoidal a.
extended iliofemoral a.
extended subfrontal a.
extensive a.

extensive posterior a.
extrabursal a.
extracapsular a.
extracavitary a.
extralaryngeal a.
extraperitoneal a.
extrapharyngeal a.
extrapleural a.
extravesical Lich a.
extreme lateral transcondylar a.
Fahey hip arthrotomy a.
far lateral inferior suboccipital a.
fascial sling a.
femoral artery a.
Fernandez extensile anterior a.
flank a.
foraminal a.
fornix a.
Fowler-Philip retrocalcaneal
  exostosis a.
frontal cortical a.
frontotemporal a.
gasless laparoscopic a.
Gatellier-Chastang ankle a.
Gatellier-Chastang posterolateral a.
Gibson posterior hip a.
Gordon a.
Guleke-Stookey lumbar fusion a.
Hardinge lateral hip a.
Harmon cervical a.
Harmon modified posterolateral a.
Harmon shoulder a.
Harris anterolateral ankle a.
Harris lateral trigeminal
  neurolytic a.
Hay lateral hip a.
Henderson posterolateral tibia a.
Henderson posteromedial knee a.
Henry anterior strap a.
Henry anterolateral a.
Henry extensile a.
Henry posterior interosseous
  nerve a.
Henry radial a.
high cervical anterior
  retropharyngeal a.
Hoffmann a.
Hoppenfeld-Deboer orthopaedic a.
Howorth a.
humeral a.
idiographic a.
Iliff blepharoptosis a.
iliofemoral a.
ilioinguinal acetabular a.
inferior extradural a.
inferior-lateral endonasal
  transsphenoidal a.
inferior transvermian a.
infralabyrinthine a.

inframammary a.
infratemporal fossa a.
infratentorial supracerebellar a.
inguinal a.
interfascial a.
interforniceal a.
interhemispheric a.
interscalene a.
intracapsular a.
intradural a.
intranasal a.
intrapleural a.
intratentorial supracerebellar a.
inverted-U a.
Ivor Lewis esophagogastrectomy a.
Japanese a.
Kave knee a.
keyhole a.
Kikuchi-MacNob-Moreau anterior
  cervical disectomy a.
Kocher curved L a.
Kocher-Gibson posterolateral a.
Kocher-Langenbeck posterior
  proximal femur and acetabulum a.
Kocher lateral J a.
Koenig-Schaefer medial a.
Kraske parasacral a.
Kugel hernia repair a.
labioglossomandibular a.
labiomandibular a.
laparoscopic common bile duct
  exploration transcystic a.
lateral deltoid splitting a.
lateral extracavitary a.
lateral Gatellier-Chastang ankle a.
lateral J a.
lateral Kocher a.
Leslie-Ryan anterior axillary a.
lesser sac a.
Letournel-Judet acetabular a.
limbal a.
lingual a.
Lortat-Jacob pediatric GERD a.
low cervical a.
Ludloff medial open reduction
  hip a.
lumbar a.
lumbar transforaminal a.
Mayo a.
McConnell extensile knee a.
McConnell median and ulnar
  nerve a.
McFarland-Osborne lateral hip a.
McLaughlin a.
McWhorter posterior shoulder a.
medial extradural a.
medial parapatellar capsular a.
midlateral a.
midline a.

approach (*continued*)
    midline medial a.
    midline spinal a.
    minianterior thoracotomy a.
    minimally invasive a.
    Minkoff-Jaffe-Menendez posterior knee a.
    Mize-Bucholz-Grogen posterolateral femur a.
    modified surgical a.
    Molesworth-Campbell elbow a.
    Moore posterior hip a.
    multidisciplinary a.
    multiple-stage a.
    neurosurgical a.
    nonoperative a.
    occipitocervical a.
    Ollier arthrodesis a.
    Ollier lateral hip a.
    open laparoscopic a.
    open lung a.
    operative a.
    orbitozygomatic temporopolar a.
    oropharyngeal a.
    Osborne posterior hip a.
    osteoplastic flap a.
    otomicrosurgical transtemporal a.
    palatal a.
    palmar a.
    paramedian a.
    pararectus a.
    parasacral a.
    paraspinal a.
    parietooccipital a.
    patella turndown a.
    percutaneous endoscopic a.
    percutaneous transhepatic a.
    peroral a.
    Perry extensile anterior distal humerus a.
    petrosal a.
    Pfannenstiel transverse a.
    Phemister medial epiphysiodesis a.
    piggyback a.
    plantar a.
    Pogrund lateral meniscectomy a.
    portal vein a.
    posterior costotransversectomy a.
    posterior extraperitoneal a.
    posterior inverted-U a.
    posterior laparoscopic a.
    posterior lumbar a.
    posterior midline a.
    posterior occipitocervical a.
    posterior radial a.
    posterior shoulder a.
    posterior transolecranon a.
    posterolateral a.
    posteromedial a.

    preperitoneal a.
    presigmoid-transtransversarium intradural a.
    proprioceptive neuromuscular facilitation a.
    proximal interphalangeal joint a.
    pterional a.
    pulp a.
    Putti posterior knee a.
    rapid-volume a.
    Redman a.
    Reinert acetabular extensile a.
    retrocolic a.
    retrocrural a.
    retrograde endoscopic a.
    retrograde femoral a.
    retrolabyrinthine presigmoid a.
    retroperitoneal a. (RPA)
    retropharyngeal a.
    retrosigmoid a.
    retrosternal a.
    rhinoseptal a.
    Risdon submandibular a.
    Roberts a.
    robotic a.
    Roos transaxillary 1st rib resection a.
    Rowe posterior shoulder a.
    Royle posterior hemivertebra a.
    saber-cut a.
    sacral-foraminal a.
    sacroiliac a.
    sacroperineal a.
    screw-plate a.
    semilateral a.
    sensorimotor stimulation a.
    skin-sparing mastectomy a.
    skull base a.
    Smith-Petersen anterior hip a.
    Smith-Petersen-Cave-Van Gorder anterolateral hip a.
    Smith-Robinson cervical disc a.
    somatic gene-transfer a.
    Somerville anterior hip a.
    Southwick-Robinson anterior cervical a.
    Spetzler anterior transoral a.
    split-heel a.
    split-patellar a.
    stabilization a.
    staged a.
    standard open a.
    sternum-splitting a.
    subchoroidal a.
    subclavicular a.
    subfrontal a.
    subfrontal-transbasal a.
    sublabial midline rhinoseptal a.
    suboccipital-subtemporal a.

suboccipital-transmeatal a.
subtemporal-intradural a.
superior-intradural a.
supine-oblique a.
supracerebellar a.
supraclavicular a.
supraduodenal a.
supraorbital-pterional a.
supratentorial a.
surgical a.
suspended-pedicle a.
Swedish a.
sylvian a.
takedown abdominal a.
Taylor combined spinal-epidural
  anesthesia a.
therapeutic a.
Thompson anterolateral hip a.
Thompson anteromedial
  shoulder a.
Thompson posterior radial a.
thoracic a.
thoracoabdominal extrapleural a.
thoracoabdominal intrapleural a.
thoracolumbar retroperitoneal a.
thoracolumbar transdiaphragmatic a.
thoracoscopic a.
thoracotomy a.
thumb metacarpophalangeal joint a.
tongue-splitting transmandibular a.
totally extraperitoneal a.
transabdominal a.
transacromial a.
transanal a.
transantral a.
transantral ethmoidal a.
transaxillary a.
transbrachioradialis a.
transcallosal transventricular a.
transcanine a.
transcavernous transpetrous apex a.
transcerebellar hemispheric a.
transcervical a.
transclavicular a.
transcoccygeal a.
transcochlear a.
transcortical transventricular a.
transcranial frontal-temporal-orbital a.
transcranial-supraorbital a.
transcubital a.
transcystic a.
transdiaphragmatic a.
transduodenal a.
transfibular a.
transfrontal a.
transgluteal a.
transhepatic a.
transhiatal esophagectomy a.
translabyrinthine and suboccipital a.

transmandibular-glossopharyngeal a.
transmastoid a.
transmeatal a.
transmural a.
transolecranon a.
transoral a.
transpalatal a.
transpapillary a.
transpedicular a.
transperitoneal a.
transpleural a.
transradial a.
transrectal a.
transseptal a.
transsinus a.
transsphenoidal a.
transsphincteric a.
transsternal a.
transsylvian a.
transtentorial a.
transthoracic a.
transtorcular a.
transtrochanteric a.
transvaginal a.
transvenous a.
transventricular a.
transverse a.
transxiphoid a.
trapdoor a.
triradiate acetabular extensile a.
triradiate transtrochanteric a.
unilateral sacroiliac a.
vaginal wall a.
VATS a.
Virginia Mason pancreatic
  cancer a.
volar finger a.
volar midline a.
volar radial a.
volar ulnar a.
volarward a.
Wadsworth elbow a.
Wadsworth posterolateral a.
Wagoner posterior spinal a.
Watson-Jones anterolateral total
  hip a.
Wiltberger anterior cervical a.
Wiltse-Spencer paraspinal a.
Yee posterior shoulder a.
York-Mason rectourinary fistula a.
Zazapen-Gamidov anteromedial lesser
  trochanter a.
zig-zag a.
Z-plasty a.

approx
approximate
approximate (approx)
  a. entropy
  a. lethal concentration

approximation
- Friedewald a.
- skin a.
- successive a.
- a. suture technique
- tissue a.
- vocal fold a.
- wound a.

appy
- appendectomy

APR
- abdominal-perineal resection
- abdominoperineal resection
- anatomic porous replacement
- APR cement fixation

aprepitant

aproctia

apron
- abdominal a.
- fatty a.
- a. flap
- a. flap incision
- a. skin incision

aprotinin

APRV
- airway pressure release ventilation

APS
- American Pain Society

APSA
- American Pediatric Surgical Association

APW
- aortopulmonary window

aquapuncture

aquatic
- a. stabilization program
- a. therapy

Aquavan injection

aqueduct
- Cotunnius a.
- sylvian a.
- a. veil

aqueductal intubation

aqueductus

aqueous
- a. extract
- a. exudation
- a. humor
- a. solution
- a. vein

Ar
- argon

arachnoid
- a. cyst
- a. granulation
- a. hemorrhage
- a. mater encephali
- a. membrane
- a. retrocerebellar pouch

- a. space
- a. villus

arachnoidea mater encephali

arachnoiditis
- adhesive a.
- chemical a.

ARAMIS
- Arthritis, Rheumatism, and Aging Medical Information System

Arantius
- A. body
- canal of A.
- A. duct
- A. ligament
- plate of A.

Arbeitsgemeinschaft
- A. für Osteosynthesefragen (AO)
- A. für Osteosynthesefragen classification

Arbor
- Ann A.

arborization
- a. block
- pattern a.
- pulmonary a.

Arbuthnot Lane disease

arc
- bregmatolambdoid a.
- flexion-extension a.
- mobile a.
- nasobregmatic a.
- nasooccipital a.
- reflex a.
- Riolan a.

arcade
- appendiceal vascular a.
- gastroepiploic a.
- intestinal arterial a.
- omental a.
- pancreaticoduodenal arterial a.
- Riolan a.

arch
- abdominothoracic a.
- aortic a.
- arterial a.
- axillary a.
- a. bar
- a. bar application
- crural a.
- deep crural a.
- deep palmar a.
- double aortic a.
- expansion of the a.
- extramedullary alignment a.
- femoral a.
- a. fracture
- hemal a.
- iliopectineal a.
- interrupted aortic a.

jugular venous a.
Langer a.
a. maneuver
neural a.
palatoglossal a.
posterior a.
prepancreatic a.
pubic a.
Simon expansion a.
superciliary a.
superficial palmar a.
supraorbital a.
tendinous a.
transverse aponeurotic a.
Treitz a.
vertebral a.
wire a.
zygomatic a.

arch-and-slouch position
archenteronoma
archicerebellum
architectural pattern
architecture
lesion a.
tissue a.
arch-loop-whorl
arciform vein of kidney
arctation
arcuata
arcuate
a. aorta
a. artery
a. eminence
a. incision
a. line
a. nerve fiber bundle
a. pubic ligament
a. suture technique
a. transverse keratotomy
a. vein
a. zone
arcuation
arcuatum
arcuatus
arcus
corneal a.
ARDS
acute respiratory distress syndrome
area
anastomotic a.
aortic valve a.
articulation a.
bare a.
body surface a. (BSA)
cortical a.
cribriform a.
cross-sectional a.
crural a.
denture foundation a.

end-diastolic cross-sectional a.
end-systolic a.
end-systolic cross-sectional a.
fusion a.
gastric a.
graft a.
jejunal puncture a.
Kiesselbach a.
Killian-Jamieson a.
Laimer a.
laser controlled a.
left ventricular end-diastolic a.
(LVEDa)
left ventricular end-systolic a.
(LVESa)
Little a.
a. medullovasculosa
mitral valve a.
Panum fusion a.
paraglottic a.
periaqueductal gray a.
pericolostomy a.
pressure a.
pressure-sensitive a.
proliferation a.
pulmonary valve a.
right crural a.
skip a.
Stroud pectinated a.
tissue-bearing a.
total body surface a. (TBSA)
total graft a.
tricuspid valve a.
a. under curve (AUC)
valve orifice a.
visual association a.
voluntary a.
area-length method
areflexia
detrusor a.
areola, *pl.* **areolae**
areolae (*pl. of* areola)
areolar
a. complex
a. connective tissue
a. gland
a. incision
a. mastopexy
areola-sparing mastectomy
ARG
alkaline reflux gastritis
argatroban
arginine-vasopressin
argon (Ar)
a. beam coagulation
a. beam plasma coagulation (ABPC)
a. gas cryoablation
a. laser endophotocoagulation
a. laser iridectomy

argon (*continued*)
    a. laser photocoagulation (ALP)
    a. laser therapy
    a. laser trabeculopexy (ALT)
    a. laser trabeculoplasty (ALT, ALTP)
Argyll-Robertson
    A.-R. glaucomatous eye trepanning
    A.-R. suture technique
argyrophilic
    a. nucleolar organizer region (AgNOR)
    a. nucleolar organizer region staining
Aria coronary bypass
Aries-Pitanguy
    A.-P. breast reduction
    A.-P. mammaplasty
Arion operation
Arlt
    A. epicanthus repair
    A. eyelid repair
    A. line
    A. operation
    A. suture technique
Arlt-Jaesche
    A.-J. excision
    A.-J. eyelash transplant
arm
    anteromedial a.
    batwing a.
    brawny a.
    dissected tissue a.
    endosteal implant a.
    a. flap
    a. position
    posterior a.
armamentarium
    endodontic a.
ARMD
    age-related macular degeneration
arm-extension position
Armistead
    A. distraction osteogenesis technique
    A. ulnar lengthening operation
Armstrong acromionectomy
Arneth polymorphonuclear neutrophil classification
Arnold
    A. body
    A. bundle
    A. canal
    A. ganglion
    A. nerve
    A. tract
Arnold-Chiari
    A.-C. deformity
    A.-C. malformation (ACM)
    A.-C. syndrome

aromatic amino acids (AAA)
Aronson-Prager supracondylar humerus fracture pinning technique
around-the-clock (ATC)
    a.-t.-c. dosing
    a.-t.-c. oral maintenance bronchodilator therapy
ARR
    aortic root replacement
arrangement
    hepatocyte a.
    lesion a.
array
    cytometric bead a.
    epidural electrode a.
    subdural electrode a.
arrector, *pl.* **arrectores**
    a. pili muscle
arrectores (*pl. of* arrector)
arrest
    apneic a.
    cardiac a.
    circulatory a.
    deep hypothermia and circulatory a. (DHCA)
    deep hypothermic circulatory a. (DHCA)
    hypothermic circulatory a.
    hypothermic hypokalemic cardioplegic a. (HHCA)
    imminent cardiac a.
    profoundly hypothermic circulatory a. (PHCA)
    secondary a.
    traumatic cardiac a.
    vagal a.
arrested-heart
    a.-h. revascularization
    a.-h. revascularization technique
arrhenoblastoma
Arrhigi
    point of A.
arrhythmia
    atrial a.
    exercise-induced a.
    supraventricular a.
arrhythmogenic
Arrowhead operation
Arroyo
    A. cataract extraction
    A. dacryostomy
    A. encircling suture
    A. keratoplasty
    A. knee arthrodesis
    A. tenotomy
Arruga
    A. cataract extraction
    A. dacryostomy
    A. encircling suture

A. keratoplasty
A. retinal reattachment operation
A. tenotomy
Arruga-Berens ophthalmologic operation
arsenal
therapeutic a.
ART
assisted reproductive technique
artefact (*var. of* artifact)
arteria (a.), *pl.* **arteriae (aa.)**
a. calcarina
a. cystica
a. deferentialis
a. tuberis cinerei
a. zygomatico-orbitalis
arteriae (aa.) (*pl. of* arteria)
arterial (a.)
a. adaptation
a. anastomosis
a. aneurysm
a. angiography
a. angioma
a. anomaly
a. arch
a. bleeding
a. bleeding site
a. blood
a. blood collection
a. blood gas (ABG)
a. blood pressure
a. blood pressure monitor
a. branch
a. cannulation
a. cannulation anesthetic technique
a. carbon dioxide
a. carbon dioxide pressure
a. catheterization
a. cerebral circle
a. chemoembolization
a. circulation
a. compression syndrome
a. decortication
a. dicrotic notch pressure
a. disorder
a. embolectomy
a. embolization
a. entry site
a. flap
a. groove
a. hemorrhage
a. hypertension
a. inflow
a. injury
a. insufficiency ulcer
a. lactate level
a. limb salvage procedure
a. mean line
a. occlusion

a. occlusive disease (AOD)
a. oxygen desaturation
a. oxygen saturation (SaO_2)
a. oxyhemoglobin saturation
a. partial pressure
a. partial pressure of CO_2 ($PaCO_2$)
a. reconstructive procedure
a. reconstructive surgery
a. revascularization
a. ring
a. silk suture
a. steal syndrome
a. stenosis
a. supply
a. switch operation (ASO)
a. switch procedure
a. system
a. thrombosis
a. transfusion
umbilical a. (UA)
a. vein
a. wall dissection
a. web
a. wedge
arterial-arterial fistula
arterial-enteric fistula
arterialization
arterialized flap
arterial-portal fistula
arterial-selective intravenous vasodilator
arteriectomy
arteriobiliary fistula
arteriocapillary
arteriococcygeal gland
arteriogram
arteriographic presence
arteriography
visceral biplanar a.
arteriola (*var. of* arteriole), *pl.* **arteriolae**
arteriolae (*pl. of* arteriola)
arteriolar attenuation
arteriole, arteriola
afferent glomerular a.
capillary a.
copper-wire a.
efferent glomerular a.
silver-wire a.
arteriolith
arteriolovenular anastomosis
arterionephrosclerosis
arterioplasty
arterioportal fistula
arterioportobiliary fistula
arteriorrhaphy
arteriorrhexis
arteriosa
arteriosclerosis obliterans (ASO)

arteriosclerotic
    a. aneurysm
    a. gangrene
    a. kidney
arteriosinusoidal penile fistula
arteriostenosis
arteriosum
arteriosus
    ductus a.
    patent ductus a. (PDA)
arteriotomy
    brachial a.
    end-to-side a.
arteriovenosa
arteriovenous (AV)
    a. anastomosis (AVA)
    a. aneurysm
    a. dialysis
    a. fistula (AVF)
    a. hemofiltration
    a. malformation (AVM)
    a. subclavian fistula
arteritis
    giant cell a.
    inflammatory a.
    lymphocytic a.
    Takayasu a.
    temporal a.
artery (a.), arteria
    abdominal aortic a.
    aberrant obturator a.
    accessory obturator a.
    acetabular a.
    acromial a.
    acromiothoracic a.
    alveolar a.
    anal canal a.
    angular a.
    anomalous vertebral a.
    anterior auricular a.
    anterior carotid a.
    anterior cecal a.
    anterior cerebral a. (ACA)
    anterior choroidal a.
    anterior ciliary a.
    anterior circumflex humeral a.
    anterior communicating a. (ACoA, AComA)
    anterior descending a. (ADA)
    anterior humeral circumflex a.
    anterior inferior cerebellar a. (AICA)
    anterior inferior pancreaticoduodenal a.
    anterior intercostal a.
    anterior labial a.
    anterior mediastinal a.
    anterior meningeal a.
    anterior parietal a.
    anterior radicular a.
    anterior spinal a. (ASA)
    anterior superior alveolar a.
    anterior superior pancreatiocoduodenal a.
    anterior temporal a.
    anterior tibial recurrent a.
    anterior ulnar recurrent a.
    anterolateral thalamostriate a.
    anteromedial thalamostriate a.
    appendicular a.
    arcuate a.
    ascending cervical a.
    ascending pharyngeal a.
    atherosclerotic carotid a.
    axillary a.
    basilar a.
    blood supply a.
    brachial a.
    brachiocephalic trunk a.
    bronchial a.
    buccal a.
    buccinator a.
    calcaneal a.
    calcareous a.
    calcarine a.
    callosomarginal a.
    caroticotympanic a.
    carpal a.
    caudal pancreatic a.
    cecal a.
    celiac a.
    celiacomesenteric a.
    central retinal a.
    central sulcal a.
    cerebellar a.
    cerebral a.
    cervicovaginal a.
    choroidal a.
    ciliary a.
    cilioretinal a.
    circumflex femoral a.
    circumflex humeral a.
    circumflex iliac a.
    circumflex scapular a.
    coarctation of pulmonary a.
    colic a.
    collateral digital a.
    common femoral a. (CFA)
    common femoral artery-superficial femoral a. (CFA-SFA)
    common hepatic a.
    common iliac a.
    common interosseous a.
    common palmar digital a.
    common peroneal a.
    common plantar digital a.
    communicating a.
    companion a.

copper-wire a.
cortical a.
costocervical a.
cricothyroid a.
cystic a.
deep auricular a.
deep brachial a.
deep cervical a.
deep circumflex inguinal a.
deep epigastric a.
deep femoral a.
deep profunda brachial a.
deep temporal a.
deferential a.
descending genicular a.
descending palatine a.
descending scapular a.
digital collateral a.
diploic a.
D-loop transposition of great a.'s
dolichoectatic a.
dorsal digital a. (DDA)
dorsal interosseous a.
dorsal pancreatic a.
dorsal scapular a.
dorsal thoracic a.
a. ectasia
ectatic carotid a.
endometrial spiral a.
epigastric a.
esophageal a.
ethmoidal a.
external acoustic meatus a.
external carotid a. (ECA)
external carotid artery-posterior
  cerebral a. (ECA-PCA)
external iliac a. (EIA)
external mammary a.
external maxillary a.
external pudendal a.
external spermatic a.
extradural vertebral a.
facial a.
femoral a.
first metacarpal a.
frontal a.
gastric a.
gastroduodenal a. (GDA)
gastroepiploic a. (GEA)
gastroomental a.
genicular a.
gingival a.
gonadal a.
great anastomotic a.
greater palatine a.
great pancreatic a.
great radicular a.
great superior pancreatic a.
helicine a.

hepatic a.
Huebner recurrent a.
humeral a.
hyaloid a.
hypogastric a.
hypoglossal a.
hypophysial a.
ileal a.
ileocolic a.
iliac a.
iliofemoral flap a.
iliolumbar a.
inferior alveolar a.
inferior carotid a.
inferior cerebral a.
inferior epigastric a. (IEA)
inferior gluteal a.
inferior hemorrhoidal a.
inferior hypophysial a.
inferior internal parietal a.
inferior labial a.
inferior laryngeal a.
inferior lateral genicular a.
inferior medial genicular a.
inferior mesenteric a.
inferior pancreatic a.
inferior pancreaticoduodenal a.
inferior phrenic a.
inferior rectal a.
inferior suprarenal a.
inferior thoracic a.
inferior thyroid a.
inferior ulnar collateral a.
inferior vesical a.
infragenicular popliteal a. (IGPA)
infraorbital a.
infrascapular a.
innominate a.
insular a.
intercostal a.
interlobular a.
intermediate temporal a.
internal auditory a.
internal carotid a. (ICA)
internal iliac a.
internal mammary a. (IMA)
internal maxillary a.
internal pudendal a.
internal rectal a.
internal spermatic a.
internal thoracic a.
intestinal a.
intramural a.
a. island flap
jejunal a.
labyrinthine a.
lacrimal a.
left carotid a. (LCA)
left colic a.

artery (*continued*)
    left coronary a. (LCA)
    left gastric a.
    left gastroomental a.
    left internal thoracic a.
    left pulmonary a.
    left vertebral a.
    lenticulostriate a.
    lesser palatine a.
    lienal a.
    a. ligation
    lingual a.
    long thoracic a.
    lower thyroid a.
    lowest lumbar a.
    lowest thyroid a.
    lumbar a.
    major a.
    marginal a.
    masseteric a.
    maxillary a.
    mediastinal a.
    medium-sized a.
    medullary spinal a.
    mental a.
    mesenteric a.
    metacarpal a.
    metatarsal a.
    Michal II direct anastomosis of
        inferior epigastric artery to dorsal
        penile a.
    middle cerebral a. (MCA)
    middle colonic a.
    muscular a.
    musculophrenic a.
    mylohyoid a.
    Neubauer a.
    nutrient a.
    obturator a.
    occipital a.
    a. occlusion
    a. of Adamkiewicz
    a. of pancreatic tail
    a. of tuber cinereum
    a. of Willis
    ophthalmic a.
    orbitofrontal a.
    ovarian a.
    palmar interosseous a.
    palpebral a.
    pancreatic a.
    pancreaticoduodenal a.
    parathyroid a.
    parietal a.
    parietooccipital a.
    pericallosal a.
    pericardiacophrenic a.
    perineal a.
    peroneal a.

    persistent sciatic a. (PSA)
    petrosal a.
    pontine a.
    popliteal a.
    postcentral sulcal a.
    posterior alveolar a.
    posterior auricular a.
    posterior cecal a.
    posterior cerebral a. (PCA)
    posterior choroidal a.
    posterior circumflex humeral a.
    posterior communicating a. (PCoA)
    posterior humeral circumflex a.
    posterior inferior cerebellar a.
        (PICA)
    posterior inferior
        pancreaticoduodenal a.
    posterior intercostal a.
    posterior interosseous a.
    posterior labial a.
    posterior mediastinal a.
    posterior meningeal a.
    posterior pancreaticoduodenal a.
    posterior parietal a.
    posterior radicular a.
    posterior spinal a. (PSA)
    posterior superior alveolar a.
    posterior superior
        pancreaticoduodenal a.
    posterior temporal a.
    posterior tibial recurrent a.
    posterior ulnar recurrent a.
    posterolateral central a.
    posteromedial central a.
    precentral sulcal a.
    precuneal a.
    prerolandic a.
    princeps cervicis a.
    princeps pollicis a.
    profunda brachii a.
    profunda cervicalis a.
    proper hepatic a.
    proper palmar digital a.
    proper plantar digital a.
    pterygoid a.
    pubic a.
    pulmonary a.
    pyloric a.
    radial a.
    radial collateral a.
    radial index a.
    radial recurrent a.
    radicular a.
    a. reconstruction
    recurrent interosseous a.
    recurrent radial a.
    recurrent ulnar a.
    renal a.
    retroduodenal a.

retroesophageal a.
retrograde vascularization of superior
  mesenteric a.
right carotid a. (RCA)
right colic a.
right coronary a. (RCA)
right femoral a. (RFA)
right internal thoracic a. (RITA)
right middle suprarenal a.
right obturator a.
right replaced hepatic a.
right subclavian a.
right testicular a.
right vertebral a.
rolandic a.
scrotal a.
second lumbar a.
sheathed a.
short central a.
short gastric a.
sigmoid a.
sphenopalatine a.
spinal a.
splenic a.
a. stenosis
sternal a.
sternocleidomastoid a.
sternomastoid a.
striate a.
stylomastoid a.
subclavian a.
subcostal a.
sublingual a.
submental a.
subscapular circumflex a.
subscapular a.
sulcal a.
superficial brachial a.
superficial cervical a.
superficial circumflex iliac a.
superficial epigastric a.
superficial external pudendal a.
superficial femoral a. (SFA)
superficial palmar a.
superficial perineal a.
superficial temporal a. (STA)
superficial temporal artery to middle
  cerebral a. (STA-MCA)
superficial temporalis a.
superficial volar a.
superior alveolar a.
superior cerebellar a.
superior epigastric a.
superior gluteal a.
superior hemorrhoidal a.
superior hypophysial a.
superior intercostal a.
superior internal parietal a.
superior labial a.

superior lateral genicular a.
superior medial genicular a.
superior mesenteric a. (SMA)
superior pancreaticoduodenal a.
superior phrenic a.
superior rectal a.
superior suprarenal a.
superior thoracic a.
superior thyroid a.
superior ulnar collateral a.
superior vesical a.
supraduodenal a.
supragenicular popliteal a. (SGPA)
supraorbital a.
suprascapular a.
supratrochlear a.
supreme intercostal a.
sural a.
temporal a.
testicular a.
thoracoabdominal a.
thoracoacromial a.
thoracodorsal a.
thymic a.
thyrocervical a.
tibial a.
tortuous intercostal a.
transposition of the great arteries
  (TGA)
transverse cervical a.
transverse facial a.
transverse pancreatic a.
transverse scapular a.
ulnar a.
umbilical a. (UA)
urethral a.
uterine a. (UA)
vaginal a.
vertebral a.
visceral a.
volar interosseous a.
Wilkie a.
zygomaticofacial a.
zygomaticoorbital a.

arthralgia
asymmetric a.
recurrent a.
arthrifluent abscess
arthritides (*pl. of* arthritis)
arthritis, *pl.* **arthritides**
gonococcal a.
A. Helplessness Index (AHI)
hemophilic a.
juvenile rheumatoid a. (JRA)
Lyme a.
pisotriquetral a.
psoriatic a.
pyogenic a.
reactive a.

arthritis (*continued*)
    Arthritis, Rheumatism, and Aging
      Medical Information System
      (ARAMIS)
    rheumatoid a. (RA)
    scaphotrapezial trapezoid a.
    septic a.
    tuberculous a.
arthrocele
arthrodesis
    Adkins technique spinal a.
    Arroyo knee a.
    atlantoaxial a.
    Batchelor-Brown extraarticular
      subtalar a.
    beak modification with triple a.
    Brockman-Nissen wrist a.
    Charnley compression a.
    compression a.
    Enneking resection a.
    excisional a.
    extension injury posterior
      atlantoaxial a.
    extraarticular a.
    Gallie ankle a.
    tarsometatarsal truncated-
      wedge a.
    tibiocalcaneal a.
    tibiotalocalcaneal a.
    triple a.
    truncated tarsometatarsal wedge a.
    truncated-wedge a.
arthrodial
    a. articulation
    a. cartilage
    a. joint
arthroereisis (*var. of* arthrorisis)
**arthrographic capsular distention and
rupture technique**
**arthrogryposis multiplex congenita
(AMC)**
arthrologia (*var. of* arthrology)
arthrology, arthrologia
arthropathy
    cuff tear a.
    hemophilic a.
    hydroxyapatite a.
    osteopulmonary a.
    rotator cuff a.
arthrophyte
arthroplasty
    abrasion a.
    acetabular cup a.
    Albright-Chase a.
    anconeus a.
    Ashworth hand a.
    Ashworth implant a.
    Aufranc cup a.
    Austin-Moore a.

autogenous interpositional
    shoulder a.
Bechtol a.
bipolar hip a.
Bryan a.
Campbell interpositional a.
Campbell resection a.
capitellocondylar total elbow a.
capsular interposition a.
carpometacarpal a.
Carroll a.
cemented total hip a.
cementless total hip a.
Charnley total hip a.
Clayton forefoot a.
Colonna trochanteric a.
condylar implant a.
constrained ankle a.
constrained shoulder a.
convex condylar implant a.
Coonrad-Morrey total elbow a.
Coonrad total elbow a.
Cracchiolo forefoot a.
Crawford-Adams cup a.
Cubbins a.
cuff tear a.
débridement a.
Dewar-Barrington a.
distraction a.
duToit-Roux a.
Eaton implant a.
Eaton volar plate a.
Eden-Hybbinette a.
elbow a.
Ewald capitellocondylar total
    elbow a.
Ewald-Walker kinematic knee a.
excision a.
fascial a.
finger joint a.
forefoot a.
Gristina-Webb total shoulder a.
Gunston a.
Harmon suppurative hip a.
Harrington total hip a.
Head hip a.
Helal flap a.
hemiresection interposition a.
hip a.
Hungerford-Krackow-Kenna
    knee a.
ICLH double-cup a.
Imperial College of London
    double-cup a.
implant a.
Inglis triaxial total elbow a.
Insall-Burstein-Freeman knee a.
interpositional elbow a.
interpositional shoulder a.

intracapsular temporomandibular joint a.
Jones resection a.
Keller resection a.
knee a.
Kocher-McFarland hip a.
Larmon forefoot a.
Magnuson-Stack shoulder a.
Mann-DuVries a.
Matchett-Brown hip a.
Mayo modified total elbow a.
Mayo resection a.
metacarpophalangeal joint a.
Meuli a.
Millender a.
Miller-Galante knee a.
modified mold and surface replacement a.
mold acetabular a.
monospherical total shoulder a.
Morrey-Bryan total elbow a.
Mould a.
Mueller hip a.
Mumford-Gurd a.
NEB hip a.
Neer unconstrained shoulder a.
New England Baptist hip a.
Niebauer trapeziometacarpal a.
noncemented total hip a.
Post total shoulder a.
prosthetic a.
proximal femoral resection-interposition a.
Putti-Platt a.
resection a.
revision hip a.
Rizzoli a.
rotator cuff tear a.
Schlein elbow a.
semiconstrained total elbow a.
shoulder a.
Silastic lunate a.
silicone implant a.
silicone rubber a.
silicone wrist a.
Smith-Petersen cup a.
Speed a.
Stanmore shoulder a.
Steffee thumb a.
Suave-Kapandji a.
surface replacement hip a.
Swanson convex condylar a.
Swanson radial head implant a.
Swanson silicone wrist a.
tendon interposition a.
total ankle a. (TAA)
total articular replacement a. (TARA)
total articular resurfacing a. (TARA)

total elbow a. (TEA)
total hip a. (THA)
total knee a. (TKA)
total patellofemoral joint a.
total shoulder a. (TSA)
total wrist a. (TWA)
trapeziometacarpal silicone a.
triaxial total elbow a.
Tupper a.
ulnar hemiresection interposition a.
unconstrained shoulder a.
unicompartmental knee a. (UKA)
Vaino metacarpophalangeal joint a.
volar plate a.
Volz a.
Wilson-McKeever a.

arthrorisis, arthroereisis

arthroscopic
a. abrasion chondroplasty
a. anterior cruciate ligament reconstruction (AACLR)
a. augmentation
a. entry portal
a. examination
a. laser surgery
a. meniscectomy
a. microdiscectomy (AMD)
a. stitch
a. synovectomy

arthroscopy (scope)
a. and débridement
diagnostic and operative a.
laser a.
midcarpal a.
needle a.
operative a.
radiocarpal a.
Ringer a.
total knee a. (TKA)

arthrosia
exanthesis a.

arthrotomy
diagnostic arthroscopy, operative arthroscopy, possible operative a.
Magnuson-Stack shoulder a.
operative a.
parapatellar a.

articular
a. bone loss
a. branch
a. capsule
a. cartilage
a. cartilage lesion
a. cavity
a. crescent
a. crest
a. facet
a. fragment
a. manifestation

articular (*continued*)
    a. mass separation fracture
    a. pillar fracture
    a. process
    a. recurrent nerve
    a. surface
    a. vascular circle
    a. vascular network
articulate
articulated
articulation
    acromioclavicular a.
    a. area
    arthrodial a.
    atlantoaxial a.
    atlantooccipital a.
    balanced a.
    bicondylar a.
    calcaneocuboid a.
    carpometacarpal a.
    Chopart a.
    condylar a.
    coracoclavicular a.
    costochondral a.
    coxofemoral a.
    cricothyroid a.
    a. curve
    dental a.
    deviant a.
    a. disorder
    glenohumeral a.
    humeral a.
    humeroradial a.
    humeroulnar a.
    incudomalleolar a.
    a. index
    infantile a.
    intercarpal a.
    interchondral a.
    intermetacarpal a.
    interphalangeal a.
    Lisfranc a.
    mandibular a.
    metacarpophalangeal a.
    metatarsocuneiform a.
    metatarsophalangeal a.
    a. of pisiform bone
    patellofemoral a.
    peg-and-socket a.
    place of a.
    proximal radioulnar a.
    radiocapitellar a.
    radiocarpal a.
    radioulnar a.
    sacroiliac a.
    scapuloclavicular a.
    secondary a.
    spheroid a.
    sternocostal a.

    subtalar a.
    superior tibial a.
    talocalcaneal a.
    talocalcaneonavicular a.
    tarsometatarsal a.
    temporomandibular joint a.
    a. test
    tibiofemoral a.
    tibiofibular a.
    triquetropisiform a.
    trochoid a.
    Vermont spinal fixator a.
articulationes carpometacarpeae
articulatory procedure
artifact, artefact
    pacemaker a.
artificial
    a. anus
    a. classification cavity
    a. disc
    a. endocrine pancreas
    a. erection test
    a. fat pad
    a. fistulation
    a. insemination homologous (AIH)
    a. insemination husband (AIH)
    a. intravaginal insemination
    a. kidney
    a. method
    a. nose
    a. respiration
    a. sphincter
    a. ventilation
    a. vertebral body
Arvidsson dimension-length method
ARX
    autoregressive
    ARX index
arycorniculata
    synchondrosis a.
aryepiglottic
    a. fold
    a. muscle
arytenoepiglottidean fold
arytenoid
    a. cartilage
    a. gland
    a. muscle
    paired a.
arytenoidal
arytenoidectomy
arytenoidopexy
    King a.
aryvocalis
    musculus a.
ASA
    acetylsalicylic acid
    American Society of Anesthesiologists
    American Surgical Association

anterior spinal artery
    ASA classification I-IV
    ASA physical status
ASA-induced gastric ulceration
ASAPS
    American Society for Aesthetic Plastic
    Surgery
ASAPSC
    American Society of Anesthesiologists
    Physical Status Classification
ASBS
    American Society for Bariatric Surgery
ascendens
    cervicalis a.
ascending
    a. anterior branch
    a. aortic pressure
    a. cervical artery
    a. colon
    a. lumbar vein
    a. mesocolon
    a. nociceptive pathway
    a. pathway
    a. pathway of pain projection
    a. pharyngeal artery
    a. pharyngeal plexus
    a. posterior branch
    a. technique
Ascher
    A. glass-rod phenomenon
    A. syndrome
Aschoff body
ascites
    bile a.
    blood-tinged a.
    chyliform a.
    chylous a.
    cloudy a.
    exudative a.
    fatty a.
    a. formation
    gelatinous a.
    hemorrhagic a.
    intractable a.
    marked a.
    massive a.
    milky a.
    mucinous a.
    mucoid a.
    myxedema a.
    pancreatic a.
    progressive a.
    pseudochylous a.
    recurrent a.
    refractory a. (RA)
    straw-colored a.
    transudative a.
    tumor a.
ascitic fluid

ascitogenous
ASCRS
    American Society for Colon and
    Rectal Surgeons
ASCUS
    atypical squamous cells of
    undetermined significance
ASD
    atrial septal defect
Aselli
    A. gland
    A. pancreas
asepsis
aseptic
    a. peritonitis
    a. surgery
    a. technique
asepticism
ASF
    anterior spinal fusion
ASGE
    American Society for Gastrointestinal
    Endoscopy
ASHD
    atherosclerotic heart disease
Ashford retracted nipple operation
Ashhurst-Bromer ankle fracture
   classification
ash-leaf
    a.-l. patch
    a.-l. spot
Ashman beat
Ashworth
    A. hand arthroplasty
    A. implant arthroplasty
ASIF
    Association for the Study of Internal
    Fixation
    ASIF screw fixation technique
ASIL
    anal squamous intraepithelial lesion
ASIS
    anterior superior iliac spine
Ask-Upmark kidney
ASLS
    apparent short leg syndrome
Asnis cannulated screw fixation
   technique
ASO
    arterial switch operation
    arteriosclerosis obliterans
aspect
    buccal a.
    dorsal a.
    inferomedial a.
    laminar cortex posterior a.
    medial a.
    medicolegal a.
    paraspinous a.

aspect (*continued*)
    physiologic a.
    plantar a.
    posterior a.
    posterolateral a.
    puriform a.
    spinous a.
    volar a.
aspergilloma formation
aspergillosis
    allergic bronchopulmonary a.
Aspergillus **infection**
aspermatogenic
aspermia
asphyxia
asphyxial
asphyxiant
asphyxiate
asphyxiating thoracic dysplasia
asphyxiation
    intrapartum a.
aspirate
    endotracheal a.
    percutaneous a.
    transtracheal a.
aspirated foreign body
aspiration
    acid a.
    anterior a.
    a. biopsy cytology
    bone marrow a.
    breast cyst a.
    cataract a.
    Cavitron ultrasound a.
    cervical a.
    cold knife cone a.
    corporeal a.
    CT-directed needle a.
    CT-guided fine-needle a.
    CT scan-guided needle a.
    cyst a.
    diagnostic a.
    endoscopic transesophageal
      fine-needle a.
    epididymal sperm a.
    EUS-guided fine-needle a.
    fine-needle a. (FNA)
    fluid a.
    foreign body a.
    full-thickness rectal a.
    gastric fluid a.
    guided fine-needle a.
    hematoma a.
    Hürthle fine-needle a.
    iliac crest bone a.
    image-guided pancreatic core a.
    irrigation and a. (I&A)
    joint a.
    lateral a.

    meconium a.
    medial a.
    menstrual a.
    Michele vertebral a.
    microscopic epididymal sperm a.
    microsurgical epididymal sperm a.
      (MESA)
    mineral oil a.
    mucosal needle a.
    myringotomy with a.
    needle a.
    a. needle biopsy
    negative a.
    a. of cortex
    percutaneous balloon a.
    percutaneous CT-guided a.
    percutaneous epididymal sperm a.
      (PESA)
    percutaneous fine-needle a.
      (PFNA)
    peritoneal a.
    pleural fluid a.
    a. pneumonia
    a. pneumonitis
    a. portal
    preoperative percutaneous a.
    a. prophylaxis
    pulmonary a.
    real-time endoscopic
      ultrasound-guided fine-needle a.
    recurrent a.
    seminal vesicle a.
    silent a.
    sonography-guided a.
    sperm a.
    stereotactic a.
    suction a.
    suprapubic needle a.
    tracheal a.
    transbronchial needle a. (TBNA)
    transthoracic needle a. (TTNA)
    transtracheal a. (TTA)
    ultrasonic a.
    ultrasound-guided fine-needle a.
    uterine a.
    vacuum a.
    vertebral a.
    vitreous a.
aspirator
    handgun a.
asplenia
asplenic state
ASRA
    American Society of Regional
    Anesthesia and Pain Medicine
assay
    cell-based a.
    chemotaxis a.
    coagulation factor a.

intraoperative intact parathyroid hormone a.
intraoperative iPTH a.
intraoperative parathyroid hormone a.
a. normalization
platelet function a.
radioligand binding a.
rapid intraoperative parathormone a.
rapid intraoperative parathormone immunoradiometric a.

assessment
anergy nutritional a.
awake neurological a.
computer-assisted a.
cytological a.
echocardiographic a.
electronic momentary a.
endoscopic color Doppler a.
extrapyramidal function a.
functional capacities a.
global pain a. (GPA)
histologic a.
intraoperative a.
jugular bulb catheter placement a.
Migraine Disability A. (MIDAS)
noninvasive a.
nutritional a.
pain a.
peritoneal cytological a.
sequential organ failure a. (SOFA)
weight estimation and a.

Assézat triangle
assimilation
a. pelvis
a. sacrum

assist
Certified Surgical Technologist, First A. (CSTFA)
hand a.
Registered Nurse, First A. (RNFA)
Suture A.

assistance
laparoscopic a.

assist-control mode ventilation
assisted
a. circulation
a. expiration
hand a.
a. medical procreation (AMP)
a. reproduction technology
a. reproductive technique (ART)
a. respiration
a. ventilation

associated
a. injury
a. myofascial trigger point

association
American Pediatric Surgical A. (APSA)

American Surgical A. (ASA)
a. cortex
a. fiber
A. for the Study of Internal Fixation (ASIF)
law of a.
a. mechanism
megacystis-megaureter a.
Minimally Invasive Robotics A. (MIRA)
noncausal a.
a. time
a. tract
VATER a.

asterion
asternal
asteroid body
asthenia
asthma
exercise-induced a. (EIA)
extrinsic a.

asthmatic
steroid-dependent a.

asthmoid respiration
astigmatic keratotomy
astigmatism
corneal a.
a. correction

Astler-Coller
A.-C. (A, B1, B2, C1, C2) colorectal carcinoma classification
A.-C. modification
A.-C. modification of Dukes classification

astragalar
astragalocalcanean
astragaloscaphoid
astragalotibial
Astrand
A. 30-beat stopwatch method
A. 6-minute submaximal cycle ergometer test

astriction
astringent
astroblastoma
astrocyte
fibrillary a.

astrocytoma
adulthood a.
anaplastic a.
giant cell a.
high-grade a.
subependymal giant cell a.

ASTS
American Society of Transplant Surgeons

Astwood-Coller staging

asymmetric, asymmetrical
- a. arthralgia
- a. gradient coil
- a. hyperplasia
- a. parathyroid enlargement
- a. surgery
- a. unit membrane

asymmetrical (*var. of* asymmetric)

asymmetry
- chiral a.

asymptomatic
- a. angiomyolipoma
- a. cholecystitis
- a. disease
- a. infection
- a. mass
- a. neoplasm
- a. patient

asynchronism

asynclitic position

ataractic

Atasoy
- A. palmar flap
- A. triangular advancement flap
- A. volar V-Y flap
- A. V-Y technique

Atasoy-Kleinert hand advancement flap

Atasoy-type flap

atavistic epiphysis

ataxia, ataxy
- respiratory a.
- transient a.

ataxy (*var. of* ataxia)

ATC
- around-the-clock
- ATC dosing

atelectasis

atherectomy
- Auth a.
- coronary angioplasty versus excisional a.
- coronary rotational a.
- directional coronary a.
- excisional a.
- high-speed rotational a. (HSRA)
- a. index
- Kinsey a.
- percutaneous coronary rotational a. (PCRA)
- rotational coronary a.
- Simpson a.
- transluminal extraction a.

atheroembolism
- peripheral a.

atheroma embolism

atheromatous
- a. plaque
- a. vessel

atherosclerosis
- accelerated a.
- carotid a.

atherosclerotic
- a. aneurysm
- a. carotid artery
- a. carotid artery disease (ACAD)
- a. carotid artery lesion
- a. heart disease (ASHD)
- a. plaque
- a. renal artery stenosis

athletic pubalgia

ATI
- Abdominal Trauma Index

Atkin epiphysial fracture

Atkinson
- A. cataract extraction technique
- A. lid block

atlantad

atlantal, atloid
- a. fracture

atlantica

atlantis

atlantoaxial, atloaxoid
- a. arthrodesis
- a. articulation
- a. dislocation (AAD)
- a. fracture-dislocation
- a. fusion
- a. instability (AAI)
- a. joint
- a. lesion
- a. rotatory fixation (AARF)
- a. stabilization
- a. subluxation (AAS)

atlantoepistrophic

atlantooccipital, atlooccipital
- a. articulation
- a. extension
- a. fusion
- a. joint
- a. joint dislocation
- a. ligament
- a. membrane
- a. stabilization
- a. transection

atlantoodontoid

atlas

atlas-axis combination fracture

atloaxoid

atloid (*var. of* atlantal)

atlooccipital (*var. of* atlantooccipital)

ATLS
- acute tumor lysis syndrome
- advanced trauma life support

atm
- atmosphere

atmosphere (atm)
    a.'s of pressure
    oxygen-enriched a.
ATN
    acute tubular necrosis
    antiretroviral toxic neuropathy
atomic mass
atomizer
atonia (*var. of* atony)
atonic bladder
atony, atonia
    gastric a.
atopic line
atrabiliaris
    glandula a.
atrabiliary capsule
Atraloc suture
atraumatic
    a. coronary artery bypass
    a. suture technique
atresia
    aortic valve a.
    biliary a.
    distal a.
    duodenal a.
    esophageal a.
    extrahepatic biliary a.
    intestinal a.
    perinatal biliary a.
    pulmonary a.
    urethral a.
atretocystia
atretogastria
atria (*pl. of* atrium)
atrial
    a. activation mapping
    a. activity
    a. arrhythmia
    a. baffle operation
    a. balloon septostomy
    a. defibrillation threshold
    a. dissociation
    a. dysrhythmia
    a. ectopic tachycardia
    a. electrogram
    a. extrastimulus method
    a. fibrillation (Afib)
    a. fibrillation-flutter (AFF)
    a. filling pressure
    a. natriuretic peptide
    (ANP)
    a. pacing transesophageal
    a. ring
    a. septal defect (ASD)
    a. septal resection
    a. septectomy
    a. stasis index
atrial-well technique
atriocaval shunt

atriocommissuropexy
atriodextrofascicular tract
atriofascicular tract
atrionodal bypass tract
atriopulmonary connection
atriotomy
    pursestring a.
atrioventricular (AV)
    a. bundle
    a. canal
    a. canal defect
    a. conduction tissue
    a. connection anomaly
    a. dissociation
    a. junctional ablation
    a. junction anomaly
    a. malformation
    a. nodal function
    a. node
    a. reentry tachycardia
    a. ring
    a. septal defect (AVSD)
    a. sulcus
    a. valve insufficiency
atrium, *pl.* **atria**
atrophia (*var. of* atrophy)
atrophic
    a. excavation
    a. fenestration
    a. fracture
    a. inflammation
    a. kidney
    a. skin
atrophy, atrophia
    brown a.
    cortical a.
    crypt a.
    endometrial a.
    exhaustion a.
    gastric a.
    graft a.
    healed yellow a.
    intestinal villous a.
    mammary a.
    mucosal a.
    multiple system a.
    muscular a.
    optic nerve a.
    peroneal muscle a.
    pressure a.
    scapular peroneal a.
    skeletal muscle a.
    traction a.
    villous a.
    vocal cord a.
    yellow a.
atropine
ATS
    American Thoracic Society

attached
    a. cranial section
    a. craniotomy
    a. gingiva extension
attack
    recurrent a.
    transient ischemic a. (TIA)
attenuating tissue
attenuation
    arteriolar a.
    beam a.
    broadband a.
    a. correction
    digital beam a.
    heterogeneous a.
    high a.
    interaural a.
    a. level
    a. of tendon
    signal a.
    ultrasonic a.
attic adhesion
Attitudes to Back Pain Scale (ABPS)
attorney
    power of a. (POA)
atypia
    nuclear a.
atypical
    a. antidepressant
    a. dislocation
    a. hyperplasia
    a. junction
    a. mycobacterial infection
    a. regeneration
    a. squamous cells of undetermined significance (ASCUS)
ATZ
    anal transition zone
Au
    gold
AUC
    area under curve
    postprandial AUC
Auchincloss modified radical mastectomy
audioanalgesia
auditory
    a. canal
    a. closure
    a. evoked potential (AEP)
    a. method
    a. tract
    a. tube
    a. tube nerve
auditus
Auerbach
    A. ganglion
    A. plexus
Aufranc cup arthroplasty
Aufrecht sign

augmentation
    alloplastic chin a.
    arthroscopic a.
    bladder a.
    bone marrow a.
    breast a.
    chin a.
    connective tissue a.
    a. cystoplasty
    demucosalized a.
    donor-specific bone marrow a.
    endoscopic breast a.
    extraarticular a.
    gastroileac a.
    a. genioplasty
    gingival a.
    a. graft
    hamstring ligament a.
    ileocecocystoplasty bladder a.
    iliotibial band graft a.
    Leach-Schepsis-Paul a.
    Mainz pouch a.
    a. mammaplasty
    a. plaque
    reverse a.
    simultaneous areolar mastopexy and breast a. (SAMBA)
    slotted acetabular a.
    submucosal urethral a.
    synthetic a.
    a. therapy
    thiol a.
    transumbilical breast a. (TUBA)
    ureteral bladder a.
augmented pain perception
augmentor nerve
aural fistula
Aureomycin suture
auricle
auricular
    a. acupuncture
    a. appendectomy
    a. canaliculus
    a. cartilage
    a. fissure
    a. ganglion
    a. index
    a. ligament
    a. muscle
    a. nerve
    a. notch
    a. point
    a. surface
    a. triangle
    a. tubercle
    a. vein
auriculocranial
auriculoinfraorbital plane
auriculomastoid

auriculotemporal nerve
auriculoventricular groove
auscultation
Austin
    A. bunionectomy
    A. Flint murmur
    A. Flint respiration
    A. osteotomy
Austin-Moore arthroplasty
Auth atherectomy
autoamputation
autoaugmentation
    bladder a.
autocastration
autocatheterism (*var. of*
  autocatheterization)
autocatheterization, autocatheterism
autocystoplasty
autocytolysis
autodilation
    Frank nonsurgical perineal a.
autodrainage
autogeneic graft
autogenic training
autogenous
    a. bone graft
    a. fascial heterograft
    a. interpositional shoulder
      arthroplasty
    a. keratoplasty
    a. strip
    a. tooth transplant
    a. vein
autograft
    cultured epithelial a.
    a. fusion
    a. harvesting
    parathyroid a.
    pulmonary a.
    Russell fibular head a.
autografting
autoimmune
    a. cirrhosis
    a. connective tissue disorder
    a. demyelination
    a. hepatitis
    a. neuropathy
autoimmunization
    surgical a.
autoinflation
autoinfusion
autokeratoplasty
autolesion
autologous
    a. blood
    a. blood clot pulmonary
      embolism
    a. blood donation (ABD)
    a. blood stem cell transplant

    a. blood unit
    A. Bone and Marrow Transplant
      Registry (ABMTR)
    a. bone marrow transplant (ABMT,
      ABMTx)
    a. clot
    a. internal jugular vein
    a. lymph node transplant
    a. melanoma system
    a. osteochondral allograft
      transplant
    a. osteochondral mosaicplasty
    a. ovarian transplant
    a. pericardial patch
    a. priming
    a. RBC unit
autolytic débridement
automated
    a. anesthesia record (AAR)
    a. boundary protection
    A. Endoscopic System for Optimal
      Positioning (AESOP)
    a. lamellar therapeutic keratoplasty
      (ALTK)
    a. large-core breast biopsy
    a. oscillometry
    a. percutaneous discectomy
      (APD)
automatic
    a. ectopic tachycardia
    a. external defibrillator (AED)
    a. muscle relaxation control
autonephrectomy
    silent a.
autonomic
    a. blockade
    a. dysreflexia
    a. dysregulation
    a. ganglion block
    a. modulation
    a. nerve
    a. nerve block
    a. nerve preservation
    a. nervous system (ANS)
    a. neurogenic bladder
    a. symptom
autonomicorum
    ganglia plexuum a.
autonomous function
autoplasty
autopod (*var. of* autopodium)
autopodium, autopod
autopsy
    laparoscopic a.
autoregressive (ARX)
autoregulation
    cerebral a.
autoreinfection
autorrhaphy

autoscopy
autosomal
    a. dominant polycystic kidney disease (ADPKD)
    a. recessive
Auto Suture
autosuture technique
autotransfusion
    massive a.
autotransplant
autotransplantation
    colostomy pyloric a.
    pancreatic a.
    posttraumatic a.
    pyloric a.
    renal a.
autotrophic fixation
autovaccination
Auvray incision
auxiliary
    a. canal
    a. partial orthotopic liver transplant (APOLT)
    a. transplant
AV
    arteriovenous
    atrioventricular
    AV bundle
    AV dissociation
    AV fistula
    AV malformation
    AV nodal modification
    AV node
AVA
    arteriovenous anastomosis
avascular
    a. fragment
    a. necrosis (AVN)
avascularization
average
    a. extubation time
    a. flow rate
    a. mean pressure
    moving time a.
AVF
    arteriovenous fistula
Avila technique
avium-intracellulare
    Mycobacterium a.-i. (MAI)
AVM
    arteriovenous malformation
AVN
    avascular necrosis
avoidance
    activity a.
    fear a.
    fear-related activity a.
    a. maneuver

AVR
    aortic valve replacement
AVSD
    atrioventricular septal defect
avulse
avulsed
    a. fragment
    a. wound
avulsion
    brachial plexus a.
    a. stress fracture
    a. technique
    a. trauma
awake
    a. craniotomy
    a. fiberoptic intubation
    a. intraoperative electrocorticography
    a. intubation
    a. laryngoscopy
    a. neurological assessment
    a. tracheotomy
awaken
    failure to a.
awakening
    planned a.
awareness
    body a.
    intraoperative a.
AWP
    airway pressure
AXB
    axillary block
AXBF
    axillobifemoral
Axenfeld
    A. anomaly
    A. suture technique
Axer
    A. lateral opening wedge osteotomy
    A. varus derotational osteotomy
Axer-Clark muscle-tendon transfer for elbow paralysis procedure
axes (*pl. of* axis)
axial
    a. aneurysm
    a. calcaneal projection
    a. compression
    a. compression injury
    a. compression principle
    a. compression test
    a. fixation
    a. flag flap
    a. hiatal hernia
    a. illumination
    a. inclination
    a. lesion
    a. line angle
    a. loading fracture

a. melanoma
a. muscle
a. pattern scalp flap
a. plane
a. point
a. rotation
a. rotation joint
a. section
a. sesamoid projection
a. skeleton
a. spin-echo image
a. surface cavity
axifugal
axilla, *pl.* **axillae**
  hot a.
  a. temperature
axillae (*pl. of* axilla)
axillary
a. abscess
a. adenopathy
a. approach
a. arch
a. artery
a. artery aneurysm
a. bed
a. block (AXB)
a. block anesthesia
a. block anesthetic technique
a. endoscopic reduction
a. envelope
a. fascia
a. fat pad
a. flap
a. fold
a. fossa
a. hematoma
a. hyperhidrosis
a. incision
a. insertion
a. line
a. lymphadenectomy
a. lymphadenopathy
a. lymph node dissection (ALND)
a. nerve
a. node dissection (AND)
a. node dissection mastectomy
a. node metastasis
a. node negative
a. perivascular technique
a. plexus
a. region
a. relapse
a. sheath
a. skin lesion
a. space
a. sweat gland
a. tail

a. tail of Spence
a. thoracotomy
a. triangle
a. vascular injury
a. vein
axilloaxillary bypass
axillobifemoral (AXBF)
a. bypass
a. bypass graft
axillofemoral
a. bypass
a. tunnel
axillounifemoral (AXUF)
a. bypass
axiobuccolingual plane
axiolabiolingual plane
axiomesiodistal plane
axis, *pl.* **axes**
basibregmatic a.
basicranial a.
basifacial a.
celiac a.
cephalocaudal a.
conjugate a.
craniofacial a.
facial a.
a. fixation
flexion-extension a.
a. fracture
hypothalamic-hypophysial-ovarian-
  endometrial a.
long a.
mesentericoportal a.
a. of rotation
pelvic a.
thoracic a.
thyroid a.
axis-atlas combination fracture
axofugal
axon
corticospinal a.
axonal
a. demyelination
a. injury
a. regeneration
axotomy
AXR
abdominal x-ray
AXUF
axillounifemoral
Aylett total colectomy
Ayre spatula-Zelsmyr cytobrush cervical specimen collection technique
azathioprine
azeotrope
azeotropic solution
azoospermia
obstructive a.

azotemia
    transient a.
azure lunula
azygoesophageal
    a. line
    a. recess

azygos
    a. artery of vagina
    a. continuation of IVC
    a. fissure
    a. vein
azygous

B
 B fibers
 B point
 B ring
Ba
 barium
 basion
Babcock
 B. rectal pullthrough
 B. suture technique
Babinski sign
BAC
 blood alcohol concentration
Bachmann
 B. bundle
 internodal tract of B.
back
 b. gunshot wound
 b. pain
 b. projection
back-and-forth suture technique
backbone
backcut incision
backfire fracture
backflow
 b. bleeding
 pyelovenous b.
background illumination
back-knee deformity
back-propagation neural network program
back-up position
backup self-inflating bag
backward
 b. coarticulation
 b. position
 backward, upward, rightward pressure (BURP)
backwash ileitis
Bacon-Babcock abdominal-anal incision
bacteremia, bacteriemia
 perioperative b.
bacteremic donor
bacteria (*pl. of* bacterium)
bacterial (bact)
 b. complication
 b. contamination
 b. endotoxin
 b. flora
 b. infection
 b. mucosal infiltration
 b. overgrowth
 b. pneumonia
 b. synergistic gangrene
 b. translocation

bactericidal concentration
bacteriemia (*var. of* bacteremia)
bacteriologic data
bacteriolysis
bacteriopexy
bacteriospermia
bacteriostasis
bacteriostatic barrier
bacterium, *pl.* **bacteria**
 probiotic bacteria
bacteriuria
Badal
 B. cicatricial entropion operation
 B. conical cornea operation
Badenoch urethroplasty
Badgley
 B. anterior cervical discectomy and fusion technique
 B. combination cervical discectomy and fusion procedure
 B. iliac wing resection
Bado Monteggia fracture classification
BaE
 barium enema
Baehr-Lohlein lesion
Baer cataract operation
Baffe anastomosis
baffle fenestration
bag
 backup self-inflating b.
 Bogota b.
 collapsible venous reservoir b.
 EndoCatch b.
 b. extraction
bag-and-mask ventilation
bagged mask ventilation
bag-of-bones technique
bag-valve-mask (BVM)
Bailey-Badgley
 B.-B. anterior cervical approach
 B.-B. cervical spine fusion
 B.-B. cervical spine interbody fusion technique
Bailey-Dubow
 B.-D. internal fixation technique
 B.-D. osteotomy
bailout valvoplasty
Bailyn classification
Bain
 B. circle
 B. circuit
Baker
 B. cyst
 B. patellar advancement
 B. pyridine extraction

Baker (*continued*)
    B. technique
    B. tongue in groove slide
      lengthening of distal aponeurosis
      of gastrocnemius
    B. translocation operation
    B. tube
Baker-Hill
    B.-H. osteotomy
    B.-H. posterior tibial tendon
      translocation operation
BAL
    bronchoalveolar lavage
Balacescu closing wedge osteotomy
Balacescu-Golden hallux valgus
  osteotomy technique
balance
    acid-base b.
    caloric b.
    extravascular fluid b.
    heat b.
    thermal b.
balanced
    b. anesthesia
    b. anesthetic technique
    b. articulation
    b. salt solution volume diuresis
balanic
balanitis
balanocele
balanoplasty
balanoposthitis
balanus
Balbiani body
Baldy uteropexy operation
Baldy-Webster
    B.-W. operation
    B.-W. uterine displacement repair
      procedure
    B.-W. uterine suspension
Balfour gastroenterostomy
Balkan nephrectomy
ball
    B. anal sensory nerve division
    ping-pong b.
    b. valve action
    b. wedge
ball-and-socket
    b.-a.-s. epiphysis
    b.-a.-s. joint
    b.-a.-s. trochanteric osteotomy
Ballard examination
8-ball hemorrhage
Ball-Hoffman operation
ballistics
balloon
    b. aortic valvoplasty
    b. aortic valvotomy
    b. atrial septostomy

    b. bronchoplasty
    b. catheter angioplasty
    b. catheter technique
    b. coarctation angioplasty
    b. compression
    b. coronary angioplasty
    b. counterpulsation
    b. dilation
    b. dilation angioplasty
    b. dilation valvoplasty
    b. dissection
    b. embolectomy
    b. epiphysis
    b. esophagoplasty
    b. expulsion test
    b. fenestration procedure
    b. inflation
    b. laser angioplasty
    b. mitral commissurotomy
    b. mitral valvoplasty
    b. mitral valvotomy
    b. occlusive intravascular lysis
      enhanced recanalization
    b. photodynamic therapy
    b. pulmonary valvoplasty
    b. pulmonary valvotomy
    b. rupture
    b. septectomy
    b. tamponade technique
    b. tricuspid valvotomy
    b. tube tamponade
    b. tuboplasty
    B. Valvuloplasty Registry
balloon-catheter and basket-retrieval
  technique
balloon-cell formation
balloon-occluded retrograde transvenous
  obliteration
ball-valve obstruction
BALT
    bronchial-associated lymphoid tissue
bamboo spine
banana
    b. fracture
    b. sign
band
    adhesive b.
    ciliary body b.
    Clado b.
    b. erosion
    fracture b.
    gastric b.
    iliotibial b. (ITB)
    b. keratopathy
    Ladd b.
    Lane b.
    laparoscopic adjustable gastric b.
      (LAGB)
    b. ligation

B

Maissiat b.
Marlex b.
Meckel b.
moderator b.
pecten b.
peritoneal b.
b. placement
b. sigmoidopexy
Simonart b.
b. slippage
Z b.
zonular b.
bandage
adhesive b.
compression b.
Esmarch b.
b. method
Band-Aid operation
band-assist device
bandeau defect
banded gastroplasty
Bandi knee procedure
banding
adjustable gastric b.
Kuzmak gastric b.
laparoscopic adjustable silicone gastric b.
laparoscopic gastric b.
open adjustable silicone gastric b.
bandy leg
Baner flap
Banff renal allograft rejection classification
Bangerter
B. method of pleoptics
B. pterygium operation
banjo-string adhesion
bank
blood b.
cryopreserved tissue b.
National Trauma Data B. (NTDB)
Banks open slide lengthening of tendo Achillis
shoulder dislocation bone b.
staple capsulorraphy bone b.
tissue b.
Traumatic Coma Data B.
Bankart
B. anterior capsolabral reconstruction
B. dislocated shoulder capsular repair
B. fracture
B. shoulder dislocation
B. shoulder lesion
B. shoulder procedure
B. shoulder repair
Bankart-Putti-Platt shoulder operation
banking

Banks-Laufman
B.-L. approach
B.-L. incision
B.-L. surgical exposure of extremities techniques
Bannayan-Riley-Ruvalcaba syndrome
Baptist
New England B. (NEB)
bar
arch b.
b. bolt fixation
Mercier b.
Passavant b.
b. resection
b. section
Baralyme
barber
b. chair position
b. pole stripe transfer
barbiturate
b. burst-suppression anesthesia
b. coma
barbiturate-related hyperalgesia
barbotage
Barcat distal hypospadias repair technique
Bard
B. endoscopic suturing
B. modified Kugel patch
bare
b. area
b. area diaphragm
b. scleral technique
bariatric
b. operation
b. patient
b. surgery
barium (Ba)
b. contrast x-ray
b. enema (BaE)
b. enema examination
b. enema finding
b. esophagram
b. peritonitis
b. swallow (BaS)
b. swallow study
Barkan
B. double cyclodialysis
B. goniotomy operation
B. membrane
B. trabeculotomy technique
Barkan-Cordes linear cataract operation
Barlow developmental hip dysplasia maneuver
Barnard heart transplant
baroceptor (*var. of* baroreceptor)
barogenic esophageal perforation
barometric pressure

baroreceptor, baroceptor
  b. nerve
  b. test
baroreflex
  b. activation
  b. response
  b. responsiveness
barostat method
barotrauma
Barr
  B. body
  B. open reduction and internal fixation
  B. tendon transfer operation
  B. tibial fracture fixation
barrage cryopexy
Barraquer
  B. enzymatic zonulolysis
  B. keratomileusis
  B. silk suture
  B. suture technique
  B. zonula ciliaris dissolution method
  B. zonulolysis
Barratt Impulsivity Scale
barrel
  b. staving
  wire-reinforced airway b.
barrel-shaped lesion
Barrett
  B. epithelium
  B. esophagus
  B. metaplasia
Barrie-Jones canaliculodacryorhinostomy
barrier
  ABO b.
  adhesion b.
  anatomic b.
  bacteriostatic b.
  blood-air b.
  blood-brain b. (BBB)
  blood-cerebral b.
  blood-cerebrospinal fluid b.
  blood-liquor b.
  blood-ocular b.
  blood-optic nerve b.
  blood-retinal b.
  blood-thymus b.
  blood-urine b.
  cerebrospinal fluid-brain b.
  elastic b.
  endothelial b.
  epithelial b.
  gastric mucosal b.
  integumentary b.
  Ioban protective skin b.
  b. layer
  b. method
  motion b.

  mucosal b.
  ocular b.
  pathologic b.
  physical b.
  physiologic b.
  placental b.
  posterior capsular zonular b.
  b. protection
  Seprafilm adhesion b.
  side-bending b.
  skin b.
  sterile field b.
  b. technique
  b. zone
Barriers Pain Questionnaire
Barrios lumbar discectomy
Barron
  B. hemorrhoidal banding technique
  B. ligation
Barsky
  B. bilateral cleft lips repair technique
  B. cleft closure
  B. cleft hand repair procedure
  B. macrodactyly reduction
Barth hernia
Bartholin
  B. cystectomy
  B. duct
  B. gland
Bartlett
  B. nail fold
  B. nail fold excision
Barton fracture
Barton-Smith fracture
BaS
  barium swallow
basad
basal
  b. anal canal pressure
  b. anal sphincter pressure
  b. anesthesia
  anterior b. (AB)
  b. body temperature
  b. cell carcinoma
  b. cell hyperplasia
  b. cell membrane
  b. cistern
  b. ganglia hematoma
  b. ganglion
  b. ganglionic lesion
  inferior b. (IB)
  b. iridectomy
  b. lamina
  lateral b. (LB)
  b. line
  b. neck fracture
  septal b. (SB)

B

b. skull fracture
b. sphincter
b. subfrontal approach
b. tentorial branch
b. vein
b. vein of Rosenthal
basaloid
bascule
cecal b.
base
anterior cranial b.
cavity preparation b.
cement b.
cranial b.
b. deficit
extension b.
fixation b.
b. line
b. medication
National Cancer Data B. (NCDB)
b. of bladder
b. plane
b. projection
saddle connector b.
tissue-supported b.
tissue-tissue-supported b.
b. wedge osteotomy
baseball
b. finger fracture
b. stitch
b. suture
b. suture technique
baseline capacity evaluation
basement
b. membrane
b. membrane zone
base-of-neck osteotomy
base-ring tilt
bas-fond
basialis
basialveolar
basibregmatic axis
basic
b. life support (BLS)
b. technique
basicranial axis
basifacial axis
basihyal, basihyoid
basihyoid (*var. of* basihyal)
basilar, basilaris
b. artery
b. artery aneurysm
b. artery migraine
b. bifurcation
b. bifurcation aneurysm
b. bone
b. cartilage
b. femoral neck fracture

b. fibrocartilage
b. index
b. invagination
b. lamina
b. membrane
b. osteotomy
b. process
b. skull fracture
b. suture
b. suture technique
b. tip aneurysm
b. venous plexus
b. venous sinus
b. vertebra
basilaris (*var. of* basilar)
basilar-type migraine
basilateral
basilic vein
basiliximab
basin
lymph node b.
nonclassic nodal b.
portal lymph node b.
regional lymph node b.
retropancreatic lymph node b.
basinasal line
basioccipital bone
basiocciput
basioglossus
basion (Ba)
basipetal
basipharyngeal canal
basis
basisphenoid bone
basitemporal
basivertebral vein
basket
b. extraction technique
b. fragmentation technique
b. impaction
stone b.
basketing technique
basket-weave vacuolation
basolateral membrane
basosquamous cell carcinoma
Bass method
Basset radical vulvectomy
Bassini
B. herniorrhaphy method
B. herniorrhaphy technique
B. inguinal hernia procedure
B. inguinal hernia repair
B. inguinal herniorrhaphy
B. operation
Bassini-Stetten hernia repair
bastard suture technique
basting suture
Batchelor-Brown extraarticular subtalar arthrodesis

Batch-Spittler-McFaddin
   B.-S.-M. knee disarticulation
   B.-S.-M. through-knee amputation
   technique
bat ear surgery
Bateman
   B. hemiarthroplasty
   B. modification
   B. modification of Mayer trapezius
   muscle
bath
   contrast b.
   sitz b.
bathing trunk nevus
Batista experimental open heart
   procedure
batrachian position
Batson plexus
Battle
   B. appendix operation
   B. incision
   B. sign
battledore incision
Battle-Jalaguier-Kammerer incision
batwing
   b. appearance
   b. arm
   b. deformity
Baudelocque extrauterine pregnancy
   removal
Bauer-Jackson traumatic chondral lesion
   classification
Bauer-Tondra-Trusler
   B.-T.-T. operation
   B.-T.-T. syndactyly skin release
   technique
Bauhin
   B. gland
   valve of B.
Baumann and Koch intramuscular
   lengthening of gastrocnemius and/or
   soleus
Baume dental classification
Baumgard-Schwartz tennis elbow
   technique
Baxter
   B. VAMP
   B. venous/arterial management
   protection
Baxter-D'Astous proximal femoral
   resection-interposition arthroplasty
   procedure
Bayne-Klug centralization
Baynton leg ulcer operation
bayonet
   b. canal
   b. dislocation
   b. fracture position
bayonet-curved canal

bayonet-type incision
BBB
   blood-brain barrier
   bundle branch block
BCDDP
   Breast Cancer Detection Demonstration
   Project
BCS
   breast-conserving surgery
BEA
   below-elbow amputation
beach chair position
bead
   b. bed
   b. chain study
   b. pouch
   b. technique filling
beads-on-a-string appearance
beak
   b. fracture
   b. modification
   b. modification with triple
   arthrodesis
   b. nail
beam
   b. attenuation
   fluoroscopy b.
Beard-Cutler eyelid reconstruction
Beard tarsectomy
beat
   Ashman b.
beating-heart bypass surgery
Beatson ovariotomy
beat-to-beat variation of fetal heart rate
Beau line
Bechterew (*var. of* Bekhterev)
Bechtol arthroplasty
Beck
   B. Depression Inventory, version II
   B. gastric opening method
   B. gastrostomy
   B. I cardiopericardiopexy
   B. II aorta to coronary sinus shunt
   B. triad
Beck-Carrel-Jianu gastrostomy
Beckenbaugh
   B. biaxial wrist implant technique
   B. correction
Becker
   B. muscular dystrophy
   B. otoplasty technique
Becker-type tardive muscular dystrophy
Beckwith-Wiedemann syndrome
Béclard
   B. amputation
   B. anastomosis
   B. hernia
   B. suture technique
   B. triangle

Becton
    B. fracture fixation technique
    B. open reduction
bed
    axillary b.
    bead b.
    bone graft b.
    fracture b.
    gastric b.
    graft b.
    hot axillary b.
    liver b.
    mud b.
    nail b.
    parotid b.
    tumor b.
    ulcer b.
    vascular b.
bedroom fracture
bedside laparoscopy
beefy appearance
Beer
    B. artificial pupil
    B. iridectomy
Begg light wire differential force orthodontic technique
behavior
    drug-seeking b.
    pain b.
behavioral
    b. inhibition system
    b. pain scale
    b. technique
    b. treatment
Behçet
    B. disease
    B. skin puncture test
    B. syndrome
behind-sternum column esophagoplasty
Bekhterev, Bechterew
    line of B.
bell
    B. muscle
    B. palsy
    B. respiratory nerve
    B. suture
bell-clapper deformity
Bell-Dally cervical dislocation
Bellemore-Barrett closing wedge osteotomy
bellied
2-bellied muscle
bellows classification
Bell-Tawse
    B.-T. open reduction technique
    B.-T. radial head procedure
belly
    b. bath therapy
    b. button augmentation mammaplasty

    occipital b.
    posterior b.
Belmont buddy fluid warmer
below-elbow amputation (BEA)
below-knee amputation (BKA)
Belsey
    B. esophagoplasty
    B. fundoplication method
    B. fundoplication procedure
    B. fundoplication technique
    B. IV fundoplasty
    B. Mark IV antireflux operation
    B. Mark IV cardioplasty
    B. Mark IV fundoplication
    B. Mark IV gastropexy
    B. Mark IV repair
    B. partial fundoplication
    B. 2/3 wrap fundoplication
belt
    b. loop gastropexy
    b. muscle
    b. radical prostatectomy technique
Belt-Fuqua hypospadias repair
Bence Jones body
bench
    b. examination
    b. surgery
    b. surgical technique
Benchekroun stoma
Benedict
    B. blind perforating gastroscope
    B. orbit operation
Benedict-Talbot body surface area method
Benelli lollipop mastopexy
Bengston method
benign
    b. bone lesion
    b. bone tumor
    b. duodenocolic fistula
    b. dysphagia
    b. esophageal disorder
    b. fasciculation
    b. germ cell tumor
    b. giant cell synovioma
    b. inflammatory disease
    b. liver cyst
    b. lymphoepithelial lesion
    b. lymphoproliferative lesion
    b. mass
    b. mesothelioma
    b. nature
    b. pain
    b. papillomavirus infection
    b. paroxysmal positional vertigo
    b. pneumatic colonoscopy complication
    b. process
    b. prostatic hyperplasia (BPH)

benign *(continued)*
    b. prostatic hypertrophy (BPH)
    b. reading
    b. stricture
    b. subcutaneous cyst
    b. vascular hamartoma
    b. vascular lesion
benign-acting renal cell carcinoma
Bennett
    B. classification
    B. comminuted fracture
    B. dislocation
    B. fracture-dislocation
    B. lesion
    B. nail biopsy
    B. posterior shoulder approach
Bentall
    B. aortic graft procedure
    B. composite graft technique
    B. inclusion technique
bent inner tube sign
bent-nail syndrome
benzodiazepine-induced hypoventilation
Bérard aneurysm
Berci-Shore choledochoscopy
Berens
    B. graft
    B. pterygium transplant operation
    B. sclerectomy
Berens-Smith
    B.-S. cataract operation
    B.-S. cul-de-sac restoration
Berger
    B. disease
    B. interscapular amputation
    B. interscapulothoracic amputation
      operation
    B. space
Berger-Bookwalter posterior approach
Bergey bacteria classification
Bergmann incision
Bergmann-Israel incision
Berke
    B. lateral orbital wall approach
    B. operation
Berke-Krönlein orbitotomy
Berke-Motais upper eyelid ptosis
  correction
Berman-Gartland
    B.-G. adduction of forepart of foot
      procedure
    B.-G. metatarsal osteotomy
Bernard
    B. canal
    B. duct
    B. lip reconstruction
    B. lip reconstruction procedure
    B. puncture
Bernard-Burlow cheiloplasty

Bernard-Soulier syndrome
Berndt-Harty osteochondral talar lesion
  classification
Bernese periacetabular osteotomy
Bernoulli effect
Bernstein GERD test
berry
    b. aneurysm
    B. ligament
Bertel position
Bertin column
Bertrandi suture technique
beta (β)
    b. adrenergic agonist
    b. adrenoreceptor
    b. hemolytic streptococcus infection
    b. oxidation pathway
    b. receptor agonist
beta-adrenergic
    b.-a. blockade
    b.-a. receptor
beta-2 adrenergic receptor
beta-blocker medication
beta-receptor antagonist
beta-sympathomimetic agent
betaxolol
betel carcinoma
Bethke
    B. iridectomy
    B. sacrococcygeal chordoma repair
Betoptic
Bevan
    B. abdominal incision
    B. orchiopexy
beveled anastomosis
bevel preparation
Beverly-Douglas lip-tongue adhesion
  technique
bezoar
    medication b.
Bezold abscess
Bezold-Jarisch reflex
BH Moore procedure
BH:VH
    body hematocrit to venous hematocrit
    ratio
Bi
    bismuth
biarticular
biasterionic
biaxial joint
BIB
    biliointestinal bypass
bicameral abscess
bicanalicular sphincter
bicarb
    carbon dioxide
    bicarbonate
bicarbonate (bicarb)

biceps
    b. interval lesion
    b. tendon
Bichat
    B. canal
    B. fat pad
    B. fossa
    B. membrane
bicipital
    b. groove
    b. rib
    b. ridge
bicipitoradial bursa
bicipitoradialis
    bursa b.
Bickel-Moe osteoid osteoma procedure
bicondylar
    b. articulation
    b. joint
    b. T-shaped fracture
    b. Y-shaped fracture
bicoronal
    b. incision
    b. scalp flap
bicortical screw fixation
bicycle spoke fracture
bidirectional
    b. Glenn shunt
    b. ligation
    b. superior cavopulmonary anastomosis
    b. tracheal gas insufflation (Bi-TGI)
Biebl loop
Bielschowsky
    B. ocular deviation method
    B. operation
    B. 3-step head-tilt test
    B. vertical strabismus maneuver
Bielschowsky-Parks head-tilt 3-step test
Bier
    B. amputation
    B. block
    B. block anesthesia
    B. reactive hyperemia method
Biesiadecki fossa
bifid
    b. penis
    b. rib
    b. thumb
    b. thumb deformity
bifida
    spina b.
bifocal fixation
bifoveal fixation
bifrontal
    b. craniotomy
    b. incision
bifurcated vascular graft

bifurcation
    b. aneurysm
    aortic b.
    basilar b.
    carotid artery b.
    coronary b.
    b. graft
    b. involvement
    b. lesion
    b. of root
    b. osteotomy
    portal b.
Bigelow
    B. litholapaxy
    B. posterior hip dislocation maneuver
    B. septum
bikini skin incision
bilabe
bilaminar membrane
bilateral
    b. adrenal hemorrhage
    b. amputation
    b. anterior thoracotomy
    b. bundle branch block
    b. headache
    b. ilioinguinal approach
    b. inguinal hernia
    b. inguinal hernia repair
    b. inguinal hernia repair method
    b. inguinal hernia repair procedure
    b. inguinal hernia repair technique
    b. interfacetal dislocation
    b. lithotomies
    b. lymphadenectomy
    b. myocutaneous graft
    b. neck dissection
    b. neck exploration
    b. nephroureterectomies
    b. resection
    b. sacroiliac approach
    b. salpingo-oophorectomy (BSO)
    b. sequential lung transplant
    b. subcostal incisions
    b. subcutaneous mastectomy
    b. temporary tarsorrhaphy
    b. torsion
    b. total adrenalectomy
    b. transabdominal incisions
    b. ureterostomy takedown
    b. vagotomies
    b. ventral rhizotomy
    b. V-Y Kutler flap
bilayered cellular matrix
bilayer patch hernia repair
bile
    b. acid circulation
    b. ascites
    b. duct

bile (*continued*)
    b. duct adenocarcinoma
    b. duct adenoma
    b. duct calculus
    b. duct cannulation
    b. duct carcinoma
    b. duct catheterization
    b. duct colic
    b. duct cystadenocarcinoma
    b. duct dilation
    b. duct epithelium
    b. duct exploration
    b. duct injury
    b. duct ligation
    b. duct lumen
    b. duct manipulation
    b. duct parasite
    b. duct pressure
    b. duct stricture
    b. duct wall
    b. encrustation
    b. fluid examination
    b. leak
    b. leakage
    b. papilla
    b. plug syndrome
    b. sample
    b. tract
    b. tract drainage
bile-stained cyst content
bilevel positive airway pressure (BiPAP)
bilharzial carcinoma
Bilhaut-Cloquet polydactyly procedure
biliaris
biliary
    b. anatomic variation
    b. anatomy
    b. atresia
    b. calculus
    b. canaliculus
    b. cannulation
    b. carcinoma
    b. cirrhosis
    b. colic
    b. conduit
    b. cystadenoma
    b. dilation
    b. drainage
    b. duct
    b. ductule
    b. dyskinesia
    b. endoprosthesis insertion
    b. endoscopy
    b. enteric bypass
    b. epithelium
    b. fistula
    b. injury
    b. leakage

    b. lithiasis
    b. lithotripsy
    b. pancreatitis
    b. pleuritis
    b. problem
    b. reconstruction
    b. saturation index
    b. secretion
    b. sludge
    b. sphincterotomy
    b. sphincterotomy and stent placement
    b. stenting
    b. stent patency
    b. stricture
    b. sump syndrome
    b. system
    b. tract
    b. tract cancer
    b. tract disease
    b. tract infection
    b. tract obstruction
    b. tract pressure
    b. tract stone
    b. tract torsion
    b. tract tumor
    b. tree
biliary-bronchial fistula
biliary-cutaneous fistula
biliary-duodenal
    b.-d. fistula
    b.-d. pressure gradient
biliary-enteric
    b.-e. anastomosis
    b.-e. anastomosis operation
    b.-e. fistula
biliary-intestinal anastomosis
biliocystic fistula
biliodigestive
    b. anastomosis
    b. origin
bilioenteric continuity
biliointestinal bypass (BIB)
biliopancreatic
    b. bypass
    b. diversion
    b. diversion with duodenal switch
    b. limb
biliopleural fistula
bilious
    b. colic
    b. empyema
    b. vomit
    b. vomiting
bilirubin
    b. concentration
    b. level
    serum b.
billowing mitral valve syndrome

Billroth
- B. I gastroduodenostomy
- B. I gastroduodenostomy method
- B. I partial gastrectomy
- B. II anatomy
- B. II gastrojejunostomy
- B. II pancreatoduodenectomy
- B. I, II gastrectomy
- B. I, II gastric procedure
- B. I, II gastroenterostomy
- B. I, II gastrointestinal anastomosis
- B. I, II gastrointestinal reconstruction
- B. I, II operation
- B. I, II technique
- splenic cord of B.

bilobar
- b. disease
- b. liver metastasis
- b. resection

bilobate, bilobed
bilobectomy
bilobed (*var. of* bilobate)
- b. polypoid lesion
- b. skin flap
- b. transposition flap

bilobular
bilocular, biloculate
- b. femoral hernia
- b. joint
- b. stomach

biloculate (*var. of* bilocular)
biloma
bimalleolar ankle fracture
bimanual
- b. palpation
- b. pelvic examination

bimastoid line
bimodal method
bimucosa
binaural
- b. fusion
- b. integration

binder
- abdominal b.
- chest b.

binding motif
Binet system of leukemia classification
Bing-Siebenmann malformation
Bing-Taussig heart procedure
binocular
- b. fixation
- b. fusion
- b. indirect ophthalmoscopy
- b. microscopy

bioabsorbable
- b. Dexon suture
- b. hernia plug
- b. membrane

bioartificial
- b. liver device
- b. liver support system

bioavailability
- nitric oxide b.

biobehavioral response
biochemical
- b. evidence
- b. mediator
- b. metastasis
- b. modulation
- b. stimulation

biocoherence
biocompatibility
- implant b.

biodegradable polymer scaffold
bioelectrical impedance spectroscopy (BIS)
bioelectric treatment
Bio-FASTak suture
biofeedback
- EMG b.
- thermal b.

biofilm production
bioimpedance
- b. analysis
- thoracic b.

biologic, biological
- b. effect
- b. fixation
- b. liver support
- b. marker

biological (*var. of* biologic)
biology
- cellular b.
- molecular b.

biomagnetic therapy
biomechanical preparation
bioprogressive technique
bioprosthesis
biopsy (Bx)
- abdominal lymph node b.
- abrasive brush b.
- adrenal gland b.
- alcohol-fixed gastric b.
- Allis-Abramson breast b.
- antral b.
- aspiration needle b.
- automated large-core breast b.
- Bennett nail b.
- bite b.
- blind percutaneous liver b.
- bone marrow aspiration and b.
- brain b.
- breast b.
- bronchial brush b.
- bronchoscopic needle b.
- brush b.
- *Campylobacter-like* organism b.

biopsy (*continued*)
catheter-guided b.
b. cavity
cervical cone b.
channel and core b.
chorionic villus b.
CLO b.
coin b.
cold cone b.
cold cup b.
colonoscopic b.
colorectal b.
computed tomography-guided b.
cone b.
core needle b.
corporal b.
cortical b.
Crosby-Kugler capsule for b.
CT-guided liver b.
CT-guided needle aspiration b.
cutting needle b.
cytobrush b.
cytologic b.
diagnostic b.
diathermic loop b.
digitally guided b.
direct-vision liver b.
Dunn b.
elliptical b.
embryo b.
endometrial b.
endomyocardial b.
endoscopic small-bowel b.
endoscopic sphenoidal b.
ERCP-guided b.
esophageal b.
excision b.
excisional b.
fetal liver b.
fetal skin b.
fine-needle aspiration b.
FNA b.
forage core b.
Fosnaugh nail b.
guided transcutaneous b.
guillotine needle b.
hilar b.
hot b.
ileal b.
iliac crest b.
image-guided breast b. (IGBB)
image-guided fine-needle
    aspiration b.
image-guided stereotactic brain b.
incisional b.
internal mammary node b.
intestinal b.
intramedullary tumor b.
intraoperative b.

jejunal b.
jumbo b.
Kevorkian punch b.
Keyes punch b.
kidney b.
kidney graft b.
laparoscopic liver b.
large-core needle aspiration b.
large-particle b.
lift-and-cut b.
liver b.
lumbar spine b.
lung b.
lymph node b.
mammary node b.
mediastinal lymph node b.
Menghini technique for percutaneous
    liver b.
minimally invasive b.
mirror-image breast b.
mucosal b.
multiple core b.
muscle b.
nasopharyngeal b.
native renal b.
needle core b.
needle-localized excisional b.
needle-localized open b. (NLOB)
negative breast b.
nerve b.
node b.
onion bulb changes on b.
open brain b.
open liver b.
open lung b.
open surgical b.
optic b.
out-of-phase endometrial b.
outpatient b.
pancreatic b.
paracollicular b.
parathyroid b.
pelvic aspiration b.
percutaneous excisional breast b.
percutaneous fine-needle aspiration b.
percutaneous fine-needle
    pancreatic b.
percutaneous native renal b.
percutaneous needle liver b.
percutaneous pancreas b.
pericardial b.
peritoneal b.
peroral intestinal b.
PET-guided b.
pinch b.
Pipelle b.
pleural b.
4-point b.
point-in-space stereotactic b.

positron emission tomography-guided b.
pouch b.
preoperative b.
punch b.
random bladder b.
rectal suction b.
renal b.
b. sample
saucerized b.
scalene fat pad b.
scalene lymph node b.
scalene node b.
scan-directed b.
Scher nail b.
secondary diagnostic b.
sentinel lymph node b. (SLNB)
sentinel node b. (SNB)
serial percutaneous liver b.
shave b.
single b.
b. site
skeletal b.
skin b.
skinny-needle b.
SLN b.
snap-frozen b.
snare excision b.
snare loop b.
sonoguided b.
b. specimen
spinal infection b.
sponge b.
stereotactic aspiration b.
stereotactic brain b.
stereotactic core breast b.
stereotactic-guided b.
stereotactic needle core b. (SNCB)
stereotactic percutaneous needle b.
strip b.
suction b.
supraclavicular lymph node b.
sural nerve b.
surface b.
surgical excision b.
synovial b.
systematic sextant b.
tangential b.
targeted brain b.
b. technique
temporal artery b. (TAB)
testicular b.
thin-needle b.
thoracic spine b.
thyroid needle b.
tissue b.
total b.
transbronchial lung b.
transcutaneous b.

transfemoral liver b.
transgastric fine-needle aspiration b.
transitional zone b.
transjugular hepatic b.
transjugular liver b.
transnasal b.
transpapillary b.
transrectal ultrasound-guided sextant b. (TRUS)
transthoracic needle aspiration b.
transthoracic percutaneous fine-needle aspiration b.
transvenous liver b.
trephine needle b.
trophectoderm b.
Tru-Cut needle b.
ultrasonography-guided fine-needle aspiration b.
ultrasound-guided anterior subcostal liver b.
ultrasound-guided automated large-core breast b.
ultrasound-guided core breast b.
ultrasound-guided core needle b. (US-CNB)
ultrasound-guided echo b.
ultrasound-guided fine-needle aspiration b. (US-FNAB)
ultrasound-guided needle b.
ultrasound-guided stereotactic b.
vacuum-assisted core b.
vaginal cone b.
Valls-Ottolenghi-Schajowicz bone neoplasm needle b.
ventricular endomyocardial b.
vertical lip b.
video-assisted excisional b.
Vim-Silverman technique for liver b.
b. volume
vulvar b.
Watson capsule b.
wedge hepatic b.
wedge liver b.
wire-guided breast b.
wound b.
Zaias nail b.
biopsy-proven metastasis
biorbital angle
BioSorb suture
biospectroscopy
biosurfactant
Biosyn synthetic monofilament suture
Biot
    B. breathing
    B. respiration
    B. ventilation
biotransformation
biotrauma

B

BiPAP
bilevel positive airway pressure
biparietal
b. diameter (BPD)
b. suture
b. suture technique
bipartition
facial b.
bipedicle dorsal flap
bipennate muscle
bipennatus
biperforate
biphase pin fixation
biphasic stridor
biplanar fluoroscopy
biplane
b. cineangiography
b. fluoroscopy
b. scan
b. trochanteric osteotomy
bipolar
b. ablation device
b. affective disorder
b. cauterization
b. coagulation
b. disorder
b. electrocautery
b. electrocoagulation
b. hip arthroplasty
BI-RADS
Breast Imaging Reporting and Data
System
BI-RADS abnormal mammogram
management classification
BI-RADS score
biramous
Bircher stomach reduction
Bircher-Weber traditional orthopaedic technique
Birch-Hirschfeld entropion operation
bird-beak deformity
bird's nest lesion
Birkett hernia
birth
b. amputation
b. canal
b. canal laceration
b. fracture
birthing position
Birt-Hoss-Dube syndrome
bis
BIS
bioelectrical impedance spectroscopy
bisacromial
bisaxillary
Bischof myelotomy
bisecting
b. angle cone position
b. angle technique

bisecting-the-angle technique
bisection
bisector line
bisegmentectomy
bisensory method
bisexual
BIS-guided general anesthesia
Bishop classification
Bishop-Koop ileostomy
bismuth (Bi)
B. benign bile duct stricture classification
B. bile duct stricture (type I-V) classification
B. classification I-IV of Klatskin tumor
b. line
B. type IV stricture
Bismuth-Corlette staging system
Bismuth-Strasberg biliary injury (type A-E) classification
bispectral
b. index (BIS)
b. index monitoring
bissac
hernia en b.
bisubcostal incision
bite
b. biopsy
b. plane
b. plane therapy
b. sign
bitemporal
16-bite nylon suture
biterminal
bitewing technique
Bi-TGI
bidirectional tracheal gas insufflation
biting pressure
bitrochanteric
biVAD
biventricular assist device
bivalent reversible direct thrombin inhibitor
bivalirudin
biventral
biventricular assist device (biVAD)
bizygomatic
Björk method of Fontan tricuspid atresia repair procedure
Björk-Shiley graft
BKA
below-knee amputation
black
b. blood clot
b. box warning
b. braided nylon suture
b. braided silk suture
B. carious lesion classification

B

b. epidermoidoma
b. line
b. patch syndrome
B. repair
b. silk bridle suture
b. silk sling suture
B. technique
Black-Broström staple technique
Blackburn technique
bladder
  atonic b.
  b. augmentation
  b. autoaugmentation
  autonomic neurogenic b.
  base of b.
  b. calculus
  b. carcinoma
  b. carcinoma classification
  b. catheterization
  b. chimney procedure
  b. distention
  b. diverticulectomy
  b. drainage
  b. dysfunction
  b. fistula
  b. flap
  b. flap hematoma
  b. hemorrhage
  b. hernia
  hyperreflexic b.
  hypertonic b.
  ileal b.
  b. laceration
  b. leak
  b. neck elevation test
  b. neck preserving technique
  b. neck suspension
  b. neck-to-urethra anastomosis
  neurogenic b.
  neuropathic b.
  orthotopic b.
  b. outlet reconstruction
  b. perforation
  poorly compliant b.
  b. pressure
  pseudoneurogenic b.
  reflex neurogenic b.
  b. replacement urinary pouch
  b. stone
  b. temperature
  trabeculated b.
  uninhibited neurogenic b.
  unstable b.
  urinary b.
  valve b.
bladder-drained pancreas transplant
blade
  b. atrial septostomy
  b. bone

inferior turbinate b.
b. plate fixation
shoulder b.
Blair
  B. cleft lip operation
  B. epicanthus repair
  B. fusion
  B. hypospadias technique
  B. incision
Blair-Brown
  B.-B. procedure
  B.-B. skin graft
Blair-Byars hypospadias technique
Blaivas classification of urinary
  incontinence
Blake drain
Blalock-Hanlon
  B.-H. atrial septectomy
  B.-H. operation
  B.-H. transposition of great vessels
  repair procedure
Blalock-Taussig
  B.-T. operation
  B.-T. shunt
  B.-T. shunt ligation
  B.-T. subclavian to pulmonary artery
  shunt procedure
blanchable red lesion
blanched cutaneous
  elevation
Blandin gland
Blandin-Nuhn gland
Bland onlay flap
blanket
  cooling b.
  Snuggle Warm b.
  b. suture
  b. suture technique
Blaschko line
Blasius
  B. duct
  B. lid flap
  operation
Blaskovics
  B. canthoplasty
  B. dacryostomy
  B. eyelid flap
  B. lid operation
  B. tarsectomy
blast
  b. gut injury
  b. lung injury
blastic
  b. lesion
  b. metastasis
blastocele, blastocoele
blastocoele (*var. of* blastocele)
blastocystic cavity
blastocytoma

blastolysis
blastoma
    pulmonary b.
blastotomy
Blatt
    B. capsulodesis
    B. capsulodesis procedure
**Blatt-Ashworth trapezium excision
  procedure**
bleb
    endothelial b.
    b. resection
**Bleck midcalf lengthening by recession
  technique**
bleed
bleeding
    abnormal b.
    b. abnormality
    active source of b.
    acute digestive b.
    b. angioma
    anorectal variceal b.
    arterial b.
    backflow b.
    celiac trunk b.
    chronic digestive b.
    colorectal b.
    concomitant b.
    b. controlled with direct pressure
    b. controlled with electrocautery
    digestive b.
    distal b.
    b. duodenal ulcer
    b. episode
    esophageal variceal b.
    esophagogastric variceal b.
    excessive b.
    external b.
    gastric variceal b.
    gastrointestinal b.
    implantation b.
    intraabdominal b.
    intracranial b.
    intraoperative b.
    intraparenchymal b.
    intrathoracic b.
    b. lesion
    massive lower gastrointestinal b.
    nonvariceal gastrointestinal b.
    occult b.
    painless rectal b.
    pinpoint gastric mucosal defect b.
    placentation b.
    b. point
    portal hypertensive b.
    postcoital b.
    postgastrectomy b.
    postmenopausal b.
    postoperative b.

postpolypectomy b.
retroperitoneal b.
b. risk
b. site
b. site ligation
b. site localization
staple-line b.
b. time
b. time coagulation panel
b. track
trocar wound b.
b. tumor
upper gastrointestinal b.
variceal b.
b. vessel
blenorrhagic inflammation
blepharal
blepharectomy
blepharochalasis repair
blepharon
blepharoplasty
    Ammon cheek flap b.
    Bossalino b.
    Budinger b.
    Davis-Geck b.
    Dupuy-Dutemps lower lid b.
    Fricke reconstructive b.
    reoperative b.
    von Ammon cheek flap b.
blepharoptosis repair
blepharorrhaphy
    Elschnig b.
blepharospasm, blepharospasmus
blepharospasmus (*var. of* blepharospasm)
blepharosphincterectomy
blepharotomy
blind
    b. abscess
    b. clamping
    b. dilation
    b. dissection
    b. end
    b. fistula
    b. foramen
    b. gut
    b. insertion
    b. lithotripsy
    b. loop of bowel
    b. loop syndrome (BLS)
    b. nasal intubation anesthetic
      technique
    b. nasotracheal intubation
    b. nasotracheal intubation anesthetic
      technique
    b. osteotomy
    b. percutaneous liver biopsy
    b. pouch syndrome
    b. rectal pouch
    b. upper esophageal pouch

blind-spot projection technique
blister
> fracture b.
> pressure b.
> subcorneal b.

bloc
> en b.

Bloch-Paul-Mikulicz extraperitoneal colon resection
block
> b. anesthesia
> anesthetic b.
> ankle b.
> anterocrural celiac plexus b.
> arborization b.
> Atkinson lid b.
> autonomic ganglion b.
> autonomic nerve b.
> axillary b. (AXB)
> Bier b.
> bilateral bundle branch b.
> brachial plexus b. (BPB)
> bundle branch b. (BBB)
> caudal b.
> celiac plexus b.
> central b.
> cervical medial branch b.
> cervical plexus b.
> ciliovitrectomy b.
> complete left bundle branch b.
> complete right bundle branch b.
> confirmatory bupivacaine b.
> continuous peripheral nerve b.
> continuous popliteal sciatic nerve b.
> controlled diagnostic b.
> coracoid infraclavicular brachial plexus b.
> deep peroneal nerve b.
> depolarization b.
> depolarizing b.
> diagnostic b.
> differential nerve b.
> differential spinal b.
> digital b.
> direct obturator nerve b.
> endplate-muscular b.
> epidural b.
> exit b.
> extradural b.
> fascia iliaca b.
> femoral nerve b. (FNB)
> field b.
> ganglion impar b.
> gasserian ganglion b.
> genitofemoral nerve b.
> glossopharyngeal nerve b.
> GON b.
> greater occipital nerve b.
> Hara infiltration b.

> b. height
> hepatic outflow b.
> His bundle heart b.
> iliohypogastric nerve b.
> ilioinguinal-iliohypogastric nerve b. (IINB)
> ilioinguinal nerve b.
> 3-in-1 b.
> incomplete right bundle branch b.
> indirect obturator nerve b.
> infiltration b.
> infraclavicular brachial plexus b.
> infraorbital nerve b.
> inguinal field b.
> inguinal perivascular b.
> b. injection
> intercostal fossa b.
> intercostal nerve b.
> interpleural b.
> interscalene brachial plexus b. (IBPB)
> intrapleural b.
> intravenous b.
> intravenous regional sympathetic b. (IRSB)
> Labat sciatic nerve b.
> laparoscopic celiac plexus pain b.
> left bundle branch b.
> lower extremity nerve b.
> lumbar plexus b.
> lumbar sympathetic b. (LSB)
> lytic nerve b.
> mandibular nerve b.
> maxillary nerve b.
> mental nerve b.
> modified coracoid approach infraclavicular brachial plexus b.
> motor point b.
> multiple-needle medial branch b.
> nerve b.
> neuraxial neurolytic b.
> neurolytic celiac plexus b. (NCPB)
> neuromuscular b.
> nondepolarizing b.
> obturator nerve b.
> occipital nerve b.
> b. osteotomy
> paracervical b. (PCB)
> parasternal b.
> paravertebral lumbar sympathetic b.
> penile b.
> percutaneous neurolytic intercostal b.
> peribulbar b.
> peripheral nerve b.
> phase I, II b.
> phrenic nerve b.
> 2-point nerve b.
> posterior tibial nerve b.
> preganglionic sympathetic b.

B

block (*continued*)
    prognostic b.
    psoas sheath b.
    ramus communicans b.
    regional b.
    retrobulbar nerve b.
    retrocrural celiac plexus b.
    right bundle branch b.
    ring b.
    saddle b.
    saphenous nerve b.
    scalp nerve b.
    sciatic-femoral nerve b.
    sciatic nerve b.
    selective obturator nerve b.
    sensory b.
    single injection ultrasound-assisted
      femoral nerve b.
    single-needle medial branch b.
    single-shot caudal b.
    single-shot conduction b.
    single-shot subarachnoid b.
    sinuatrial exit b.
    sinus exit b.
    skull b.
    spinal b.
    b. spread
    Steinberg infiltration b.
    stellate ganglion b. (SGB)
    subarachnoid b. (SAB)
    subclavian perivascular b.
    subdural b.
    sub-Tenon b.
    superficial peroneal branch b.
    superior hypogastric b.
    supine sciatic b.
    supraclavicular brachial b.
    suprascapular nerve b. (SSNB)
    sural nerve b.
    sympathetic nerve b.
    therapeutic nerve b.
    tibial augmentation b.
    tracheal b.
    transarterial axillary b.
    transsacrococcygeal ganglion impar
      b.
    transversus abdominis plane b.
    trigeminal nerve b.
    ultrasound-guided lumbar facet nerve
      b.
    upper extremity nerve b.
    uterosacral b.
    van Lint lid b.
    wrist b.
    yoke b.
blockade
    afferent b.
    androgen receptor b.
    anesthetic b.

    ankle b.
    autonomic b.
    beta-adrenergic b.
    central neuraxial b.
    cholinergic b.
    continuous sympathetic spinal b.
    depolarizing b.
    epidural neural b.
    fascia iliaca compartment b.
    flickering b.
    ganglionic b.
    gasserian ganglion b.
    interscalene b.
    intervertebral disc b.
    intravenous regional b.
    local anesthetic sympathetic b.
    lytic b.
    myoneural b.
    neuraxial b.
    neurogenic b.
    neurolytic b.
    neuromuscular b. (NMB)
    nondepolarizing b.
    occipital nerve b.
    onset of b.
    paravertebral somatic nerve b.
    penile b.
    preganglionic cardiac sympathetic b.
    pulmonary sympathetic b.
    regional b.
    residual neuromuscular b.
    segmental neural b.
    selective b.
    sensory b.
    sphenopalantine ganglion b.
    stellate ganglion b.
    sympathetic b.
    sympathetic ganglion b.
    temporary nerve b.
    transient motor b.
blockage
    complete b.
    ganglion b.
    prolonged neural b.
    shunt b.
blocker
    adrenoceptor b.
    endobronchial b.
    ganglion b.
    H2 b.
    sodium channel b.
    torque control endobronchial b.
    wire-guided endobronchial b.
blocking
    b. procedure
    tissue b.
    vecuronium neuromuscular b.
Block-Potts bowel clamp
Blom-Singer tracheoesophageal fistula

blood

    b. alcohol concentration (BAC)
    allogenic b.
    arterial b.
    autologous b.
    b. bank
    b. calculus
    b. cell count
    cerebral b.
    circulating b.
    b. clot
    b. coagulation
    b. coagulation disorder
    b. donation
    b. flow
    b. flow rate
    b. gas
    b. gas analysis
    b. gas exchange
    human placental umbilical cord b.
    intraoperatively donated autologous b.
    intravenous b.
    b. lactate
    b. loss
    b. marker
    maternal venous b.
    MV b.
    occult b.
    b. oxygenation level-dependent
    b. oxygenation level-dependent contrast
    oxygen concentration in pulmonary capillary b.
    oxygen saturation of hemoglobin of arterial b.
    b. patch
    b. patch injection
    b. perfusion
    preoperatively donated autologous b.
    b. pressure (BP)
    b. pressure monitoring
    b. pressure support
    b. product
    b. product transfusion
    pulmonary capillary b.
    b. substitute
    b. substitute resuscitation
    b. supply
    b. supply artery
    b. transfusion volume
    b. tumor
    UA b.
    umbilical artery b.
    umbilical vein b.
    b. urea nitrogen (BUN)
    UV b.
    b. vessel
    b. vessel formation
    b. vessel invasion
    b. vessel tumor

blood-air barrier

blood-borne

    b.-b. infection
    b.-b. metastasis

blood-brain

    b.-b. barrier (BBB)
    b.-b. equilibration time

blood-cerebral barrier

blood-cerebrospinal fluid barrier (BCB)

blood-gas partition coefficient

Bloodgood syndrome

bloodless

    b. amputation
    b. decerebration
    b. field
    b. operation
    b. phlebotomy
    b. zone of necrosis

bloodletting

    general b.
    local b.

blood-liquor barrier

blood-ocular barrier

blood-optic nerve barrier

blood-retinal barrier

bloodstream infection

blood-thymus barrier

blood-tinged

    b.-t. ascites
    b.-t. CSF

blood-urine barrier

bloody peritoneal fluid

Bloom-Raney

    B.-R. modification
    B.-R. modification of Smith-Robinson anterior discectomy and interbody fusion technique

blot hemorrhage

Blount

    B. displacement osteotomy
    B. technique for osteoclasis

blowhole

    b. decompressing colostomy
    b. ileostomy

blow-in fracture

blow-out

    aortic stump b.-o.
    b.-o. fracture

BLS

    basic life support
    blind loop syndrome

blue

    b. dome breast cyst
    b. dot sign
    b. line
    b. rubber bleb nevus syndrome
    b. staining

B

blue (*continued*)
    b. toe syndrome
    b. twisted cotton suture
    b. urticaria
blue-black monofilament suture
blue-gray lesion
Blumberg sign
Blumenbach clivus
Blumensaat line
Blumenthal lesion
Blumer shelf
Blumgart T-staging system
Blundell Jones technique
blunderbuss apical canal
blunt
    b. abdominal trauma
    b. and sharp dissection
    b. carotid injury
    b. dissection
    b. eversion carotid endarterectomy
    b. hepatic trauma
    b. liver injury
    b. torso injury
blur point
blush
    tumor b.
BM
  bowel movement
BMI
  body mass index
B-mode
  brightness modulation
    B-mode imaging
BMP
  bone morphogenetic protein
BMT
  bone marrow transplantation
BNP
  brain natriuretic peptide
BO
  bronchiolitis obliterans
Bo
  Bolton craniometric point
board
    Pediatric Surgery B.
    Vascular Surgery B.
board-certified surgeon
boardlike rigidity
Boari
    B. bladder flap
    B. bladder flap procedure
    B. ureteral flap repair
Boari-Ockerblad ureteral flap
Boas
    B. point
    B. sign
boatlike abdomen
boat nail
boat-shaped abdomen

Bobath therapeutic exercise method
bobby-pin abrasion
Bochdalek
    B. gap
    B. hernia
    B. ring
    B. valve
Bock
    B. ganglion
    B. nerve
Boden-Gibb tumor staging
body
    adipose b.
    adrenal b.
    alveolar b.
    Amato b.
    anal foreign b.
    anococcygeal b.
    anorectal foreign b.
    aortic b.
    Arantius b.
    Arnold b.
    artificial vertebral b.
    Aschoff b.
    aspirated foreign b.
    asteroid b.
    b. awareness
    Balbiani b.
    Barr b.
    Bence Jones b.
    Bracht-Wachter b.
    brassy b.
    cancer b.
    carotid b.
    cartilaginous loose b.
    b. cast syndrome
    caudate b.
    cavernous b.
    b. cavity
    b. cell mass
    central fibrous b.
    chromaffin b.
    chromatinic b.
    ciliary b.
    coccidian b.
    coccygeal b.
    colloid b.
    colonic foreign b.
    b. composition analysis
    compressed b.
    compressible cavernous b.
    corneal foreign b.
    Creola b.
    crescent b.
    cystoid b.
    cytoid b.
    dense b.
    duodenal foreign b.
    Dutcher b.

B

Ehrlich inner b.
Elschnig b.
esophageal foreign b.
esophageal Lewy b.
external geniculate b.
b. fat
fat b.
fibrous loose b.
b. fluid
foreign b.
Gamna-Gandy b.
gastric foreign b.
gelatin compression b.
geniculate b.
glomus b.
Goldmann-Larson foreign b.
Gordon elementary b.
b. habitus
Hamazaki-Wesenberg b.
Harting b.
Hassall b.
Heinz b.
Heinz-Ehrlich b.
b. hematocrit to venous hematocrit
  ratio (BH:VH)
hematoxylin b.
Henle b.
Hensen b.
Highmore b.
Hirano b.
Howell-Jolly b.
hyaline bodies
hyaloid b.
b. image
inclusion b.
infrapatellar fat b.
ingested foreign b.
intraarticular loose b.
intraluminal foreign b.
intraocular foreign b. (IOFB)
intraorbital foreign b.
intrauterine foreign b.
intravascular foreign b.
Jaworski b.
juxtaglomerular b.
juxtarestiform b.
Kelvin b.
Lallemand b.
Lallemand-Trousseau b.
Landolt b.
b. language
lateral geniculate b.
Lewy b.
Lieutaud b.
loose intraarticular b.
lower gastrointestinal tract foreign b.
Luys b.
malpighian b.
mamillary b.

Maragiliano b.
b. mass-dependent dose
b. mass index (BMI)
Maxwell b.
May-Hegglin b.
melon seed b.
metallic foreign b.
Michal I direct anastomosis of
  inferior epigastric artery to
  cavernous b.
mineral oil foreign b.
Mott b.
Müller duct b.
multilamellar b.
Neill-Mooser b.
newtonian b.
nigroid b.
b. of gallbladder
olivary b.
osteocartilaginous loose b.
osteochondral loose b.
owl's eye inclusion b.
pampiniform b.
pancreatic b.
Pappenheimer b.
paranephric b.
paraterminal b.
pectinate b.
pedunculated loose b.
perineal b.
pineal b.
pituitary b.
b. position
Prowazek-Greeff b.
psammoma b.
pubic b.
pyknotic b.
radiopaque foreign b.
rectal foreign b.
refractile b.
Reilly b.
removal of foreign b.
residual b.
restiform b.
retained foreign b.
rice b.
b. righting reflex
rigid b.
Rosenmüller b.
Ross b.
round b.
Rucker b.
sand b.
Sandström b.
Savage perineal b.
b. scanning
Schaumann b.
b. schema
Schiller-Duvall b.

body (*continued*)
    Seidelin b.
    selenoid b.
    b. side integration
    spongy b.
    S-shaped b.
    b. stalk
    striate b.
    suprarenal b.
    b. surface area (BSA)
    b. surface burned (BSB)
    b. surface laplacian mapping
    Symington anococcygeal b.
    b. temperature
    thoracic vertebral b.
    thrombogenic foreign b.
    thyroid b.
    tracheobronchial foreign b.
    trapezoid b.
    b. tumor
    upper gastrointestinal tract foreign b.
    vagal b.
    vaginal foreign b.
    vermiform b.
    vertebral b.
    vitreous foreign b.
    wall of b.
    b. weight
    Winkler b.
    wolffian b.
    X b.
    Y b.
    yellow b.
3-body wear
Boehler
    B. calcaneal view
    B. lumbosacral view
Boerema
    B. anterior gastropexy
    B. hernia repair
Boerhaave
    B. gland
    B. syndrome
Bogorad syndrome
Bogota bag
Bogros space
BOH
    bundle of His
Böhler calcaneal angle
Bohlman
    B. anterior cervical vertebrectomy
    B. triple-wire cervical fusion
      technique
Böhm spine and limb bony metastasis resection
Bohr
    B. effect
    B. equation
    B. isopleth method

Boitzy open reduction
bolster
    b. suture
    b. suture technique
bolstering partial posterior fundoplication
bolt
    b. fixation
    Richmond b.
Bolton craniometric point (Bo)
Bolton-nasion line
bolus
    fluid b.
    b. injection
    b. intravenous anesthesia
    b. intravenous anesthetic technique
    b. thermodilution (BTD)
Bonaccolto-Flieringa vitreous operation
bonded cast restoration
Bondek absorbable suture
bonding
    adhesive b.
bone
    b. abscess
    Albrecht b.
    allogenic b.
    antigen-extracted allogeneic b.
    articulation of pisiform b.
    b. autogenous graft
    basilar b.
    basioccipital b.
    basisphenoid b.
    blade b.
    b. block procedure
    breast b.
    Breschet b.
    b. bruise sign
    bundle b.
    calcaneal b.
    calf b.
    capitate b.
    central b.
    cheek b.
    b. chip
    b. chip graft
    collar b.
    compact b.
    3-cornered b.
    cornua of hyoid b.
    cortical b.
    coxal b.
    cranial b.
    cuboid b.
    cuneiform b.
    b. cyst excision
    b. cyst fracture probability
    b. destruction
    b. disease
    b. dissection
    b. distraction

dorsal talonavicular b.
ear b.
ectopic b.
enchondroma of b.
endochondral b.
epactal b.
epipteric b.
episternal b.
ethmoid b.
exoccipital b.
b. exposure
facial b.
first cuneiform b.
flank b.
b. flap
b. flap osteitis
Flower b.
b. formation
b. fragment
frontal b.
Goethe b.
b. graft bed
b. graft collapse
b. graft decompression
b. graft extrusion
b. graft incorporation
b. graft placement
b. graft repair
b. graft substitute
b. graft substitute graft
greater multangular b.
hamate b.
heel b.
hip b.
hollow b.
hooked b.
b. hunger
hyoid b.
iliac b.
incarial b.
b. ingrowth fixation
innominate b.
intermediate cuneiform b.
interparietal b.
irregular b.
ischial b.
jaw b.
jugal b.
Krause b.
lacrimal b.
lamellar b.
b. lavage
lentiform b.
lingual b.
long b.
b. loss
lower jaw b.
lunate b.
lyophilization of b.

b. marrow aspiration
b. marrow aspiration and biopsy
b. marrow augmentation
b. marrow dysfunction
b. marrow examination
b. marrow failure
b. marrow graft
b. marrow infiltration
b. marrow lesion
b. marrow pressure
b. marrow puncture
b. marrow transplantation (BMT)
b. mass
b. matrix
mesethmoid b.
metacarpal b.
b. metastasis
metatarsal b.
b. morphogenetic protein (BMP)
multangular b.
navicular b.
occipital b.
osteonal lamellar b.
osteoporotic b.
b. pain
palatine b.
parietal b.
b. peg graft
periotic b.
petrosal b.
pipe b.
Pirie b.
pisiform b.
pneumatic b.
postsphenoid b.
preinterparietal b.
presphenoid b.
pubic b.
pyramidal b.
b. regeneration
b. resection
Riolan b.
sacred b.
b. scan
scaphoid b.
second cuneiform b.
semilunar b.
sesamoid b.
shank b.
shin b.
short b.
sieve b.
sphenoid b.
sphenoidal turbinated b.
suprainterparietal b.
suprasternal b.
sutural b.
tail b.
talonavicular b.

B

bone (*continued*)
 b. tamp
 b. technique
 temporal b.
 thigh b.
 tongue b.
 triangular b.
 triquetral b.
 b. tumor
 turbinated b.
 tympanic b.
 tympanohyal b.
 unciform b.
 upper jaw b.
 Vesalius b.
 b. wax suture
 wedge b.
 b. wedge
 wormian b.
 yoke b.
 zygomatic b.
bone-cement interface
bone-holding clamp
bone-implant interface
bone-ligament dissection
bone-patellar tendon-bone preparation
bone-retinaculum-bone autograft graft
bone-screw interface strength
bone-tendon-bone graft
bone-to-bone graft
Bonferroni correction
Bonfiglio
 B. bone graft
 B. modification
 B. modification of Phemister bone
  graft of femoral neck technique
Bonfiglio-Bardenstein bone grafting of femoral head and neck technique
Bonnaire femoral neck screw fixation method
Bonner position
Bonnet
 B. capsule
 B. enucleation operation
Bonney
 B. abdominal hysterectomy
 B. urinary incontinence test
Bonola diaphyseal resection technique
bony
 b. bridge resection
 b. deformity
 b. demineralization
 b. dissection
 b. element destruction
 b. excrescence
 b. exposure
 b. fragment
 b. labyrinth
 b. landmark

 b. lesion
 b. mass
 b. metastasis
 b. necrosis
 b. necrosis and destruction
 b. procedure
 b. projection
 b. semicircular canal
 b. structure
Bonzel artificial pupil operation
book thoracotomy
Bookwalter retractor
boomerang-shaped lesion
boost technique
boot
 Unna b.
bootstrap
 b. dilation
 b. 2-vessel angioplasty
 b. 2-vessel technique
boot-top fracture
Boplant graft
Bora
 B. centralization
 B. operation
 B. technique
border
 frontal b.
 interosseous b.
 b. involvement
 mesenteric b.
 nasal b.
 occipital b.
 parietal b.
 b. ray amputation
 squamous b.
 b. tissue
 b. tissue movement
 b. tissue of Jacoby
 vermilion b.
borderline personality disorder
Borggreve
 B. limb rotation
 B. rotation-plasty
Borggreve-Hall tibial rotation plasty technique
Borg treadmill exertion scale
Borrmann
 B. gastric cancer (type I–IV)
  classification
 B. type I–IV gastric cancer
 B. type I–IV gastric carcinoma
BOS
 bronchiolitis obliterans syndrome
Bose
 B. hip resurfacing operation
 B. hip resurfacing procedure
 B. nail fold excision
Bosniak renal cystic disease classification

B

boss
    carpal b.
Bossalino blepharoplasty
bosselation
Bosworth
    B. femoroischial transplant
    B. fracture
    B. posterior femur approach
    B. spinal fusion
    B. tendo calcaneus repair
both-bone fracture
both-column fracture
Botox
Botox
    botulinum toxin
Böttcher
    B. canal
    B. space
botulinum
    b. toxin
    b. toxin A (BTA)
Bouchut respiration
bougienage technique
bounce point
boundary
    air-bone-tissue b.
    inferior b.
    nuclear-annular b.
    superior b.
boutonnière
    b. deformity
    b. hand dislocation
    b. incision
Bovero muscle
Bovie
    B. cauterization
    B. coagulation
bovinum
    cor b.
bowel
    b. abscess
    b. anastomosis
    blind loop of b.
    b. bypass
    b. bypass syndrome
    b. cleansing
    compliant b.
    b. continuity
    denuded b.
    dilated loop of b.
    b. dilation
    edematous b.
    b. fistula
    b. function
    ganglionated b.
    b. habits
    incarcerated intussuscepted b.
    b. injury
    b. lavage

    b. length
    b. loop
    b. loop air
    b. movement (BM)
    Noble surgical plication of b.
    obstructed b.
    b. obstruction
    b. perforation
    b. plication
    b. preparation
    prepared large b.
    b. refashioning procedure
    b. resection
    b. rest
    short b.
    b. sounds
    b. stoma
    supple b.
    b. transplant
    b. wall
    b. wall hematoma
    weakened b.
Bowen cavity primer
Bowers genital reassignment technique
bowing
    b. deformity
    b. fracture
bowleg deformity
Bowles breast conserving technique
Bowman
    B. gland
    B. membrane
    B. operation
    B. ptosis correction
    B. pupil excision
    B. space
    B. transconjunctival resection of the
      levator
bow-tie
    b.-t. knot
    b.-t. sign
    b.-t. stitch
boxer's fracture
box stitch
Boyce
    longitudinal nephrotomy of B.
    B. position
Boyce-Vest bladder exstrophy procedure
Boyd
    B. ankle amputation
    B. classification
    B. elbow approach
    B. hip disarticulation
    B. operation
    B. point
Boyd-Anderson
    B.-A. biceps tendon repair
    B.-A. distal biceps tendon repair
      technique

Boyd-Bosworth tennis elbow procedure
Boyden sphincter
Boyd-Griffin trochanteric fracture classification
Boyd-McLeod
    B.-M. tennis elbow procedure
    B.-M. tennis elbow technique
Boyd-Sisk
    B.-S. posterior capsulorrhaphy
    B.-S. shoulder approach
Boyer bursa
Boyes brachioradialis transfer technique
Boytchev shoulder procedure
Bozeman
    B. hysterocystocleisis
    B. position
    B. suture technique
BP
    blood pressure
BPB
    brachial plexus block
BPD
    biparietal diameter
    bronchopulmonary dysplasia
BPEC
    bipolar electrocoagulation
BPF
    bronchopleural fistula
    bronchopulmonary fistula
BPH
    benign prostatic hyperplasia
    benign prostatic hypertrophy
BPI
    Brief Pain Inventory
BPTT
    brachial plexus tension test
Braasch bulb technique
brachia (*pl. of* brachium)
brachial
    b. anesthesia
    b. arteriotomy
    b. artery
    b. artery approach
    b. fascia
    b. gland
    b. muscle
    b. plexopathy
    b. plexus
    b. plexus avulsion
    b. plexus block (BPB)
    b. plexus block anesthetic technique
    b. plexus infiltration
    b. plexus nerve
    b. plexus repair
    b. plexus tension test (BPTT)
    b. plexus traction injury
    b. region
brachialis

brachioaxillary
    b. bridge
    b. bridge graft fistula
brachiocephalic
    b. trunk
    b. trunk artery
    b. vein
    b. vessel angioplasty
brachiocephalicus
brachioplasty
brachioradialis flap
brachioradial muscle
brachiosubclavian
    b. bridge
    b. bridge graft
    b. bridge graft fistula (BSGF)
brachium, *pl.* **brachia**
Bracht-Wachter
    B.-W. body
    B.-W. lesion
brachybasocamptodactyly
brachybasophalangia
brachycheilia, brachychilia
brachychilia (*var. of* brachycheilia)
brachydactylia (*var. of* brachydactyly)
brachydactyly, brachydactylia
brachyfacial
brachygnathia
brachymorphic
brachypellic pelvis
brachyprosopic
brachyrhinia
brachyrhynchus
brachystaphyline
brachysyndactyly
brachytherapy
    endobronchial b.
    interstitial b.
bracing
    external b.
    fracture b.
bracket
    b. modification
    b. slot angulation
    b. wire localization
Brackett-Osgood posterior hip approach
Brackett-Osgood-Putti-Abbott posterior knee technique
Brackett osteotomy
Brackin
    B. incision
    B. technique
    B. ureterointestinal anastomosis
Bradford fusion
bradycinesia (*var. of* bradykinesia)
Brady-Jewett proximal radial resection technique
bradykinesia, bradycinesia
bradypnea

Bragg peak proton-beam therapy
braided
> b. Ethibond suture
> b. Mersilene suture
> b. Nurolon suture
> b. nylon suture
> b. polyamide suture
> b. polyester suture
> b. polyglactin suture
> b. silk suture
> b. suture
> b. Vicryl suture
> b. wire suture

braidlike lesion
Brailey supraorbital nerve stretching
brain
> b. abscess
> b. arteriovenous malformation
> b. biopsy
> b. concussion
> b. congestion
> b. contusion
> b. death
> b. edema
> b. herniation
> b. infection
> b. injury
> b. laceration
> B. LMA-insertion technique
> b. mass
> b. metastasis
> b. natriuretic peptide (BNP)
> b. neoplasm
> b. puncture
> b. region
> respirator b.
> b. revascularization
> b. stimulation
> b. temperature
> b. tissue oxygenation
> b. transplant
> b. tumor
> b. tumor headache
> B. Tumor Registry

brain-dead patient
brain-derived neurotrophic factor
brainstem, brain stem
> b. compression
> b. evoked response (BSER)
> b. hemorrhage
> b. hypoperfusion
> b. lesion

braking radiation
Bralon braided nylon suture
branch
> acetabular b.
> acromial b.
> adrenal b.
> anastomotic b.
> anterior basal b.
> anterior cutaneous b.
> arterial b.
> articular b.
> ascending anterior b.
> ascending posterior b.
> basal tentorial b.
> buccal b.
> capsular b.
> carotid sinus b.
> caudate b.
> celiac b.
> cervical b.
> clavicular b.
> communicating b.
> deep palmar b.
> deep plantar b.
> deltoid b.
> descending anterior b.
> descending posterior b.
> digastric b.
> dorsal b.
> epiploic b.
> esophageal b.
> external b.
> faucial b.
> frontal b.
> ganglionic b.
> gastric b.
> genital b.
> glandular b.
> gonadal b.
> hepatic b.
> iliac b.
> inferior temporal b.
> inguinal b.
> internal b.
> joint b.
> lateral calcaneal b.
> lateral nasal b.
> b. lesion
> lingual b.
> lingular b.
> lumbar b.
> major sinistral b.
> mammary b.
> marginal mandibular b.
> marginal tentorial b.
> mastoid b.
> medial cutaneous b.
> medial mammary b.
> mediastinal b.
> meningeal b.
> mental b.
> occipital b.
> omental b.
> orbital b.
> ovarian b.
> b. pad

B

branch (*continued*)
 palmar b.
 palpebral b.
 pancreatic b.
 parietal b.
 parotid b.
 pectoral b.
 perforating b.
 pericardial b.
 petrosal b.
 pharyngeal b.
 phrenicoabdominal b.
 posterior basal b.
 pterygoid b.
 pubic b.
 recurrent meningeal b.
 renal b.
 right b.
 saphenous b.
 sectorial b.
 sinuatrial nodal b.
 splenic b.
 sternal b.
 stylohyoid b.
 subscapular b.
 superficial b.
 superior cervical cardiac b.
 superior labial b.
 superior laryngeal nerve external b.
 suprahyoid b.
 sympathetic b.
 temporal b.
 thoracic cardiac b.
 thymic b.
 tonsillar b.
 tracheal b.
 tubal b.
 ulnar b.
 ureteral b.
 ureteric b.
 zygomatic b.
 zygomaticofacial b.
 zygomaticotemporal b.
branched
 b. calculus
 b. vascular graft
branchial
 b. anomaly
 b. cartilage
 b. cleft cyst
 b. cyst
 b. fistula
 b. sinus
branching
 b. canal
 b. morphogenesis
 b. tubule formation
branchiogenous cyst
branchiomeric muscles

Brand tendon transfer technique
Brantigan lung volume reduction
 procedure
Brantigan-Voshell posterior cruciate
 ligament procedure
Brasdor aneurysm ligation method
brassy body
Braun
 B. anastomosis
 B. gastric procedure
 B. shoulder tenotomy
Braune
 B. canal
 B. muscle
Braun-Jaboulay gastroenterostomy
Braun-Wangensteen graft
brawny
 b. arm
 b. induration
breach
 serosal b.
breakdown
 anastomotic b.
 epithelial b.
 muscle b.
 sepsis-induced muscle b.
break point
breakthrough pain (BTP)
breast
 b. abscess
 accessory b.
 adenoma of b.
 b. approach thyroidectomy
 b. augmentation
 b. biopsy
 b. biopsy tissue
 b. bone
 b. calcification
 b. cancer
 B. Cancer Detection Demonstration
  Project (BCDDP)
 b. cancer-related mutation
 b. cancer risk
 b. cancer risk prediction
 b. cancer-specific survival
 b. carcinoma
 comedocarcinoma of b.
 b. conservation therapy
  (BCT)
 b. contour
 b. cyst
 b. cyst aspiration
 b. discharge
 b. fibroma
 b. flap
 B. Imaging Reporting and Data
  System (BIRADS)
 b. implant
 b. incision

b. irradiation
b. lymphatic mapping
male b.
b. metastasis
b. mucocele
b. parenchyma
b. preservation
b. reconstruction
b. reduction
b. reduction technique
b. resection
b. size
b. skin envelope
b. stimulation contraction test
(BSCT)
supernumerary b.
breast-conserving
b.-c. method
b.-c. procedure
b.-c. surgery (BCS)
b.-c. technique
b.-c. therapy (BCT)
breast-lift mastopexy
breast-milk jaundice
breast-preservation therapy
breast-sparing mastectomy
breath
b. excretion test
machine-triggered b.
patient-triggered b.
b. stacking
breathing
apneustic b.
Biot b.
b. circuit
continuous positive pressure b.
(CPPB)
intermittent positive pressure b.
(IPPB)
b. lung
b. method
negative inspiratory b.
pattern of b.
positive-negative pressure b. (PNPB)
rescue b.
spontaneous b.
ventilator b.
work of b. (WOB)
breathing-focused relaxation
breech
b. extraction
b. head
bregma (Br)
bregma-mentum projection
bregmatic fontanelle
bregmatolambdoid arc
bregmatomastoid
b. suture
b. suture technique

Brenner
B. gastrojejunostomy technique
B. lung volume reduction
brephoplastic graft
Breschet
B. bone
B. canal
B. hiatus
Brescia-Cimino
B.-C. AV fistula
B.-C. graft
Breslow
B. melanoma thickness classification
B. thickness
Brett-Campbell tibial osteotomy
Breuer-Hering inflation reflex
Breuerton view
Brevibloc
brevis
extensor carpi radialis b. (ECRB)
extensor digitorum b. (EDB)
extensor pollicis b. (EPB)
Bricker
B. conduit
B. ileal conduit operation
B. ileoureterostomy procedure
B. ureteroileostomy
Brickner position
bridge
adhesive resin-bonded b.
brachioaxillary b.
brachiosubclavian b.
colostomy b.
conjugation b.
extension b.
fascial b.
Gaskell b.
b. graft
loop ostomy b.
membrane b.
mucosal b.
mylohyoid b.
B. operation
b. organ transplant
b. pedicle flap
b. pedicle flap operation
b. plate fixation
retention suture b.
suture b.
bridgelike
b. lesion
b. septum
bridging syndesmophyte
bridle
B. foot drop procedure
b. suture
b. suture technique
Brief Pain Inventory (BPI)
Briggs strabismus operation

Bright disease
brightness modulation (B-mode)
brim
    pelvic b.
    b. sign
Brinell hardness indenter point
Brisbane pediatric liver transplantation
  method
brisement therapy
Bristow-Helfet glenohumeral joint
  procedure
Bristow-May glenohumeral joint
  procedure
Bristow operation
brittle
    b. nail
    b. nail syndrome
broad
    b. fascia
    b. ligament hernia
    b. uterine ligament
broadband attenuation
Broadbent registration point
Broadbent-Woolf 4-limb Z-plasty
broadest muscle
broad-spectrum antibiotic (BSA)
Broca
    B. basilar angle
    B. facial angle
    B. pouch
    B. visual plane
Brock
    B. closed transventricular valvotomy
    B. incision
    B. infundibulectomy
    B. pulmonary valvotomy and
      infundibular resection procedure
Brockenbrough
    B. transseptal commissurotomy
    B. transseptal left heart
      catheterization technique
Brockhurst scleral buckle technique
Brockman incision
Brockman-Nissen wrist arthrodesis
Brödel bloodless line
Broders
    B. index
    B. index of malignant tumor
      classification
Brodie
    B. bursa
    B. metaphysial abscess
Brodie-Trendelenburg tourniquet test
Brodsky-Tullos-Gartsman posterior
  shoulder joint approach
Broesike fossa
Bromage motor block scale
bromide
    rocuronium b.

bromination
Bromley foreign body operation
Brom supravalvular aortic stenosis
  repair
    bromide
bronchi (pl. of bronchus)
bronchia (pl. of bronchium)
bronchial
    b. adenocarcinoma
    b. adenoma
    b. artery
    b. brush biopsy
    b. brushing
    b. carcinoma
    b. circulation
    b. fracture
    b. gland
    b. inflammation
    b. inhalation challenge test
    b. mucus transport
    b. respiration
    b. sleeve procedure
    b. sleeve resection
    b. tract
    b. tree
    b. vein
bronchial-associated lymphoid tissue
  (BALT)
bronchiogenic
bronchiolar adenocarcinoma
bronchiole
    respiratory b.
    terminal b.
bronchiolitis
    b. obliterans (BO)
    b. obliterans syndrome (BOS)
    obliterative b.
bronchioloalveolar
    b. adenocarcinoma
    b. carcinoma
bronchiolopulmonary
bronchiolus
bronchiomediastinalis
    truncus (lymphaticus) b.
bronchitis
bronchium, pl. bronchia
bronchoalveolar
    b. carcinoma
    b. lavage (BAL)
    b. lavage culture
bronchobiliary fistula
bronchocavernous respiration
bronchoconstriction
bronchodilatation (var. of bronchodilation)
bronchodilation, bronchodilatation
bronchoesophageal
    b. fistula
    b. muscle
bronchoesophageus

bronchoesophagoscopy
bronchogenic adenocarcinoma
bronchomediastinal trunk
bronchoplastic procedure
bronchoplasty
    balloon b.
bronchopleural
    b. fistula (BPF)
    b. leak squeak
bronchopleurocutaneous fistula
bronchopneumonia
    sequestration b.
bronchoprovocation test
bronchopulmonary
    b. dysplasia (BPD)
    b. fistula (BPF)
    b. foregut malformation
    b. segment
bronchorrhaphy
bronchoscope
    fiberoptic b. (FOB)
bronchoscope-guided intubation
bronchoscopic
    b. needle biopsy
    b. photodynamic therapy
bronchoscopy
    b. anesthetic technique
    fiberoptic b. (FOB)
    flexible fiberoptic b. (FFB)
    laser b.
    rigid b.
    ultrasound-guided b.
bronchospasm
    exercise-induced b. (EIB)
    induced b.
bronchospirography
bronchospirometry
bronchostomy
bronchotomy
bronchotracheal
bronchovesicular respiration
bronchus, *pl.* **bronchi**
    ectatic b.
    intermediate b.
    lobar b.
    right main b.
    segmental b.
    stem b.
Bronson foreign body removal
Brooke ileostomy
Brooks atlantoaxial subluxation tape repair technique
Brooks-Jenkins atlantoaxial fusion technique
Brooks-Seddon tendon transfer technique
Brooks-type fusion
Broomhead medial ankle approach
Brophy staphylorrhaphy

Broström-Gould ankle instability repair procedure
Broström lateral ankle instability procedure
Broviac catheter
brow
    b. fixation
    b. position
brow-anterior position
brow-down position
browlift
brown
    b. adipose tissue
    B. and Wickham pressure profile method
    b. atrophy
    B. dietary method for colon preparation
    B. endoscopic carpal tunnel release technique
    B. knee approach
    B. knee joint reconstruction
    B. lateral knee approach
Brown-Beard oculoplastic technique
brown-black lesion
brown-fat tumor
Browning vein
Brown-McHardy pneumatic mercury bougie dilation
Brown-Sharp gauge suture
brow-posterior position
brow-up position
Bruce bundle
Bruch membrane
Brudzinski sign
Brugada syndrome
Bruger
    cul-de-sac of B.
Bruhat
    B. laser fimbrioplasty
    B. neosalpingostomy technique
bruit
    continuous high-pitched b.
    peripheral b.
Brunner
    B. gland
    B. modified incision
    B. palmar incision
Brunn nest
Brunschwig pancreatoduodenectomy
Bruser
    B. knee approach
    B. lateral knee approach
    B. lateral knee technique
    B. skin incision
brush
    b. biopsy
    b. cytology
    b. technique filling

B

brush-border
  b.-b. membrane
  b.-b. membrane vesicle
brush-induced allodynia
brushing
  bronchial b.
bruxism
Bryan
  B. arthroplasty
  B. cervical disc system
Bryan-Morrey
  B.-M. elbow approach
  B.-M. extensive posterior
  approach
  B.-M. triceps-sparing humerus
  fracture repair technique
Bryant vascular repair
BSA
  body surface area
  broad-spectrum antibiotic
BSB
  body surface burned
BSER
  brainstem evoked response
BSO
  bilateral salpingo-oophorectomy
BTA
  botulinum toxin A
BTD
  bolus thermodilution
BTP
  breakthrough pain
bubble
  b. oxygenation
  b. ventriculography
bubbly bone lesion
bucca, *pl.* **buccae**
buccae (*pl. of* bucca)
buccal
  b. artery
  b. aspect
  b. branch
  b. cavity
  b. drug administration
  b. fat pad
  b. mucosal flap
  b. nerve
  b. ostectomy
  b. restoration
  b. smear
  b. space
  b. space abscess
  b. space infection
  b. surface
  b. transmucosal delivery
  b. vein
buccinator
  b. artery
  b. crest

  b. muscle
  b. nerve
  b. node
  b. plication
  b. space
buccolingual
  b. plane
  b. relation
bucconeural duct
buccoocclusal line angle
buccopharyngeal
  b. approach
  b. fascia
  b. space
Buck
  B. fascia
  B. spondylolisthesis repair
  method
bucket-handle
  b.-h. fracture
  b.-h. incision
  b.-h. tear
Buck-Gramcko
  B.-G. dorsal rotational advancement
  flap technique
  B.-G. pollicization
bucking
  coughing and b.
buckle
  b. fracture
  Katzin scleral b.
  Lincoff scleral b.
  scleral b.
buckling
  scleral b.
  Watzke scleral b.
Budd-Chiari
  B.-C. syndrome
  B.-C. syndrome with Behçet
  disease
  B.-C. syndrome without Behçet
  disease
Budin-Chandler femoral neck anteversion
  measurement method
Budinger blepharoplasty
Bugg-Boyd Achilles tendon repair
  technique
Buie position
built-in angulation
Buist intraabdominal pressure
  measurement method
bulb
  b. deformity
  duodenal b.
  jugular venous b.
  olfactory b.
  onion b.
  Rouget b.
  b. suction

bulbar
- b. cephalic pain tractotomy
- b. polio
- b. sheath fascia

bulbi (*pl. of* bulbus)

bulbocavernosus
- b. fat flap
- b. fat pad
- b. muscle

bulboid

bulbospongiosus muscle

bulbourethral gland

bulbourethralis

bulbous internal auditory canal

bulb-tip retrograde study

bulbus, *pl.* **bulbi**

bulge
- gastric b.

bulk
- tumor b.

bulkhead method

bulky adenopathy

bulla, *pl.* **bullae**
- ethmoid b.

bullae (*pl. of* bulla)

bulldog head

bullectomy
- transaxillary apical b.

bullet
- b. trajectory
- b. wound

bullous
- b. edema
- b. granulomatous inflammation
- b. skin lesion

bull's eye macular lesion

bumper fracture

BUN
- blood urea nitrogen
- bunion

bunching
- b. maneuver
- b. suture technique

Buncke microsurgical technique

bundle
- anterior ground b.
- anteromedial b.
- arcuate nerve fiber b.
- Arnold b.
- atrioventricular b.
- AV b.
- Bachmann b.
- b. bone
- b. branch block (BBB)
- b. branch reentrant tachycardia
- b. branch reentry
- Bruce b.
- cingulum b.
- coherent b.
- commissural b.
- fiber b.
- b. fiber
- fiberoptic b.
- Gierke respiratory b.
- Held b.
- Helweg b.
- His b.
- Hoche b.
- IG b.
- image guide b.
- inferior arcuate b.
- intercostal b.
- intermediate b.
- James b.
- Keith b.
- Kent b.
- Kent-His b.
- Killian b.
- Krause respiratory b.
- lateral ground b.
- LG b.
- light guide b.
- Lissauer b.
- Loewenthal b.
- maculopapillary b.
- Mahaim b.
- main b.
- Meynert retroflex b.
- microfilament b.
- Monakow b.
- neovascular b.
- nerve fiber b.
- neurovascular b.
- b. of His (BH, B-H, BOH)
- b. of Stanley Kent
- olfactory b.
- olivocochlear b.
- papillomacular nerve fiber b.
- paracentral nerve fiber b.
- Pick b.
- posterior longitudinal b.
- posterolateral b.
- precommissural b.
- predorsal b.
- principal fiber b.
- Rathke b.
- respiratory b.
- Schütz b.
- sensory nerve fiber b.
- solitary b.
- superior arcuate b.
- superior gluteal neurovascular b.
- Thorel b.
- Türck b.
- vascular b.
- Vicq d'Azyr b.

bundleof His

Bunge amputation

bunion
>b. deformity
>b. formation

bunionectomy
>Akin b.
>Austin b.
>chevron b.
>DuVries-Mann modified b.
>Hauser b.
>Joplin b.
>Keller b.
>Kreuscher b.
>Lapidus b.
>Ludloff b.
>Mayo-Heuter b.
>McBride b.
>Peabody-Mitchell b.
>Reverdin b.
>Reverdin-Laird b.
>Reverdin-McBride b.
>Silver b.
>tailor b.
>tricorrectional b.
>Wilson b.

bunk-bed fracture

Bunnell
>B. atraumatic technique
>B. modification
>B. modification of Steindler
> flexorplasty
>B. opponensplasty
>B. stitch
>B. suture technique
>B. tendon repair
>B. tendon transfer technique
>B. wire pull-out suture

Bunnell-Williams procedure

Bunyavirus infection

bupivacaine

buprenorphine narcotic analgesic therapy

bur, burr
>b. hole
>b. hole placement

Burch
>B. bladder suspension
>B. bladder suspension method
>B. bladder suspension
> procedure
>B. bladder suspension technique
>B. colposuspension
>B. colpourethropexy
>B. eye evisceration
>B. modification
>B. urethrovesical suspension

Burdach tract

burden
>tumor b.

Burger technique for scapulothoracic disarticulation

Burgess
>B. below-knee amputation
>B. method
>B. transtibial amputation
> technique

Burhenne biliary duct stone extraction

buried
>b. bumper syndrome
>b. flap
>b. mass far-and-near suture
> technique
>b. penis

Burkhalter
>B. modification of Stiles-Bunnell
> technique
>B. transfer technique

burn
>b. boutonnière deformity
>b. classification
>corneal alkali b.
>b. débridement
>first-degree b.
>B. Flight Team
>full-thickness b.
>b. injury
>irrigation b.
>b. pain
>partial-thickness b.
>plaster cast application b.
>radiation b.
>b. scar carcinoma
>second-degree b.
>b. shock
>B.'s space
>superficial b.
>third-degree b.

burned
>body surface b. (BSB)

Burnett syndrome

burn-induced muscle proteolysis

burning
>b. and itching
>b. dysesthesia
>b. feet syndrome
>b. mouth syndrome
>b. pain

burnout procedure

Burns-Haney incision

Burow
>B. triangle
>B. triangle advancement flap
>B. vein

BURP
>backward, upward, rightward pressure
>BURP maneuver

burr (*var. of* bur)

Burrows triple fixation limb salvage technique
bursa, *pl.* **bursae**
    Achilles b.
    b. Achillis
    acromial b.
    anserine b.
    anterior tibial b.
    bicipitoradial b.
    b. bicipitoradialis
    Boyer b.
    Brodie b.
    calcaneal b.
    Calori b.
    coracobrachial b.
    deep infrapatellar b.
    Fleischmann b.
    gluteofemoral b.
    iliac b.
    iliopectineal b.
    infrahyoid b.
    infrapatellar b.
    infraspinatus b.
    intermuscular gluteal b.
    intertendinous b.
    intrapatellar b.
    ischial b.
    laryngeal b.
    medial malleolar subcutaneous b.
    b. mucosa
    b. of Monro
    olecranon b.
    omental b.
    ovarian b.
    pharyngeal b.
    prepatellar b.
    radial b.
    retrocalcaneal b.
    retrohyoid b.
    retromammary b.
    subacromial b.
    subcoracoid b.
    subcutaneous acromial b.
    subcutaneous calcaneal b.
    subcutaneous infrapatellar b.
    subcutaneous olecranon b.
    subdeltoid b.
    subfascial prepatellar b.
    subhyoid b.
    sublingual b.
    subscapular b.
    subtendinous iliac b.
    subtendinous prepatellar b.
    suprapatellar b.
    synovial b.
    tibial intertendinous b.
    triceps b.
    trochanteric b.

    b. trochanterica
    trochlear synovial b.
    ulnar b.
bursae (*pl. of* bursa)
bursa-equivalent tissue
bursal
    b. flap
    b. projection
    b. sac
    b. tissue
bursectomy
burst
    b. fracture
    respiratory b.
    b. spike button
bursting dislocation
burst-type laceration
Burton line
Burwell-Scott modification of Watson-Jones incision
Buschke-Löwenstein
    B.-L. tumor
    B.-L. tumor operation
butamben
Butchart mesothelioma staging classification
Butler
    B. congenital varus correction procedure
    B. fifth toe operation
    B. procedure to correct overlapping toes
butterfly
    b. flap
    b. fracture
    b. fracture fragment
    b. patch
    b. pattern
buttocks pad
button
    b. abscess
    burst spike b.
    b. 1-step gastrostomy
    stoma b.
    suture b.
    b. suture technique
buttonhole
    b. approach
    b. deformity
    b. fracture
    b. iridectomy
    b. operation
    b. puncture technique for hemodialysis needle insertion
    b. skin incision
    b. suture technique
Buxton bolus suture technique
Buzzard patellar reflex maneuver

B

Buzzi artificial pupil operation
BVM
    bag-valve-mask
Bx
    biopsy
Byers hypospadias flap
bypass
    Alden loop gastric b.
    b. anesthesia
    aortobifemoral b.
    aortofemoral b.
    aortoiliac b.
    aortorenal b.
    Aria coronary b.
    atraumatic coronary artery b.
    axilloaxillary b.
    axillobifemoral b.
    axillofemoral b.
    axillounifemoral b.
    biliary enteric b.
    biliointestinal b. (BIB)
    biliopancreatic b.
    bowel b.
    cardiac b.
    cardiopulmonary b. (CPB)
    carotid artery b.
    carotid-subclavian artery b.
    cavoatrial b.
    cervical-to-MCA b.
    CFA-SFA b.
    conventional coronary artery b.
    coronary artery b. (CAB)
    dual-temperature cardiopulmonary b.
    end-to-end jejunoileal b.
    end-to-side jejunoileal b.
    exclusion b.
    extraanatomic b.
    extracorporeal venous b.
    extracranial-intracranial b.
    b. failure
    femoral-popliteal artery b.
    femoral-tibial-peroneal b.
    femorocaval b.
    femorodistal b.
    femorofemoral b.
    femoropopliteal b.
    full cardiopulmonary b.
    gastric b.
    gastric loop b.
    b. graft catheterization
    Greenville gastric b.
    Griffen Roux-en-Y b.
    Hallberg biliointestinal b.
    hand-assisted laparoscopic gastric b.
    hepatorenal b.
    ileojejunal b.
    iliocaval b.
    iliofemoral b.
    iliopopliteal b.

infrainguinal b.
infrapopliteal b.
in situ b.
jejunal-ileal b. (JIB)
jejunoileal b. (JIB)
laparoscopic gastric b.
laparoscopic mini gastric b.
left atrium to femoral artery
  circulatory b.
Litwak aortic b.
long-limb gastric b.
long-limb gastric artery b.
loop gastric b.
lower extremity b.
lymphaticovenous b.
b. method
minimally invasive direct coronary
  artery b. (MIDCAB)
nonanatomic renal b.
obturator b.
off-pump coronary artery b.
  (OPCAB)
open gastric b.
b. operation
operative biliary b.
palliative b.
pancreatic b.
partial cardiopulmonary b.
partial ileal b. (PIB)
Payne-DeWind jejunoileal b.
Payne morbid obesity jejunoileal b.
petrous to supraclinoid b.
plantar artery b.
primary antecubital jump b.
  (PAJB)
b. procedure
robot-enhanced Dresden technique
  coronary artery b. (REDTCAB)
robotically assisted vision-enhanced
  coronary artery b. (RAVECAB)
Roux-en-Y biliary b.
Roux-en-Y gastric b.
saphenous ICA b.
saphenous vein b. (SVB)
Scopinaro pancreaticobiliary b.
Scott jejunoileal b.
short-limb gastric b.
Silastic ring vertical-banded gastric
  b. (SRVGB)
simple b.
splanchnorenal b.
splenorenal b.
STA – MCA b.
standard gastric b.
subclavian-subclavian b.
superficial temporal artery to middle
  cerebral artery b.
b. surgery
tarsal artery b.

b. technique
thoracofemoral b.
total endoscopic coronary artery b.
b. tract
transected vertical gastric b.
venovenous b. (VVB)
venovenous extracorporeal b.

vertical gastric b.
very long-limb Roux gastric b.
Byron
   B. Smith ectropion operation
   B. Smith lazy-T correction
Bywaters lesion
Byzantine arch palate

B

C

carbon
  C fibers
  C graft
  C sliding osteotomy

CA

cancer
carcinoma

Ca

calcium

CA19-9

cancer antigen 19-9

CAB

coronary artery bypass

CABG

coronary artery bypass graft
  redo CABG

cable

FireWire c.
c. wire suture technique

Cabot-Nesbit orchiopexy
Cabot trumpet valve
cachexia

cancer c.
muscle c.

CACI

computer-assisted controlled
  infusion

CACT

celite-activated clotting time

CAD

coronary artery disease

cadaver

c. donor
c. renal preservation

cadaveric

c. donor
c. donor hepatectomy
c. hand transplant
c. whole organ transplant

caecum (*var. of* cecum)
caffeine-halothane contracture test (CHCT)
cage

thoracic c.

Cairns

C. maneuver
C. operation
C. trabeculectomy

Cajal
cake kidney
Calandriello orthopedic procedure
calcaneal, calcanean

c. apophysitis
c. arterial network

c. artery
c. avulsion fracture
c. bone
c. bursa
c. displaced fracture
c. exostectomy
c. fracture reduction
c. inclination angle
c. L osteotomy
c. process
c. region
c. spur syndrome
c. stance position
c. sulcus
c. tendon
c. tenodesis
c. tuber
c. tubercle

calcaneal-second metatarsal angle inclination angle
calcanean (*var. of* calcaneal)
calcanei (*pl. of* calcaneus)
calcaneoastragaloid
calcaneocavovarus deformity
calcaneocavus deformity
calcaneocuboid articulation
calcaneofibular
calcaneonavicular bar resection
calcaneoscaphoid
calcaneotibial fusion
calcaneovalgus deformity
calcaneovarus deformity
calcaneum (*var. of* calcaneus)
calcaneus, calcaneum, *pl.* **calcanei**
calcar
calcareous

c. artery
c. infiltration
c. metastasis

calcarina

arteria c.

calcarine artery
calces (*pl. of* calx)
calcific aortic stenosis
calcification

breast c.
clustered c.
focal c.
intratumoral c.
c. line
linear c.
multiple c.
subependymal brain c.
c. zone

calcified
- c. gallbladder
- c. granulomatous inflammation
- c. lesion
- c. liver metastasis
- c. renal mass

calcifying metastasis
calciotraumatic line
calcipexy
calciphylaxis
calcitonin
calcitriol supplementation
calcium (Ca)
- c. carbonate supplementation
- c. pyrophosphate deposition disease (CPDD, CPPD)
- c. sensor

calcium-bearing crystalloid solution
calcium-sensing receptor
calculi (*pl. of* calculus)
calculous
- c. biliary disease
- c. cholecystitis
- c. formation
- c. gallbladder

calculus, *pl.* **calculi**
- alvine c.
- apatite c.
- bile duct c.
- biliary c.
- bladder c.
- blood c.
- branched c.
- calyceal diverticular c.
- cat's-eye c.
- cerebral c.
- cholesterol c.
- combination c.
- common duct c.
- coral c.
- cystine c.
- decubitus c.
- dendritic c.
- ductal c.
- encysted c.
- fibrin c.
- gallbladder c.
- gastric c.
- hard c.
- hemic c.
- hepatic duct c.
- impacted c.
- infection c.
- intestinal c.
- matrix c.
- c. migration
- mulberry c.
- nephritic c.
- oxalate c.

- pancreatic c.
- pleural c.
- pocketed c.
- preputial c.
- primary renal c.
- prostatic c.
- renal c.
- secondary renal c.
- staghorn c.
- struvite c.
- urethral c.
- urinary c.
- vesical c.
- weddellite c.
- whewellite c.

Caldwell-Coleman flatfoot technique
Caldwell-Luc
- C.-L. incision
- C.-L. operation
- C.-L. sinus approach
- C.-L. sinus window procedure

Caldwell-Moloy pelvis type classification
Caldwell projection
calf, *pl.* **calves**
- c. bone
- c. inflate delay

calf-bone (*var. of* calf bone)
Calhoun-Hagler lens extraction operation
caliber
- airway c.

calibrated electrical stimulation
calibration
- c. curve
- oscillometric c.
- c. overshoot
- oxygen analyzer c.

caliceal (*var. of* calyceal)
- c. diverticulum

calicectasis (*var. of* caliectasis)
calicectomy, calycectomy
calices
caliciform, calyciform
calicine, calycine
calicoplasty (*var. of* calioplasty)
calicotomy, calicectomy, caliotomy
caliectasis, pyelocaliectasis, calicectasis
caliectomy
caligation
calioplasty, calicoplasty
caliorrhaphy
caliotomy (*var. of* calicotomy)
calix (*var. of* calyx)
- major c.

Callahan
- C. cataract operation
- C. enterolateral hip approach
- C. extension
- C. extension of cervical injury
- C. posterior spinal fusion technique

C. root canal filling method
C. silicone tube blepharoplasty
operation
C. silicone tube blepharoplasty
operation
Callander amputation
Callender cell-type classification
callosal disconnection syndrome
callosomarginal artery
callosotomy
corpus c.
callus
c. formation
fracture c.
irritation c.
c. response
Calori bursa
caloric
c. balance
c. expenditure
c. irrigation
calorimetry
indirect c.
Calot triangle
CALT
conjunctiva-associated lymphoid tissue
calvaria, *pl.* **calvariae**
calvariae (*pl. of* calvaria)
calvarial free bone graft
calves (*pl. of* calf)
calx, *pl.* **calces**
calyceal, caliceal
c. abnormality
c. diverticular calculus
c. extension
c. fistula
c. fornix
c. infundibulum
c. leak
c. nephrostolithotomy
calycectomy
calyces (*pl. of* calyx)
calyciform (*var. of* caliciform)
calycine (*var. of* calicine)
calycle, calyculus
calyculus (*var. of* calycle)
calyx, calix, *pl.* **calyces**
minor c.
c. puncture
CAM
chorioallantoic membrane
complementary and alternative
medicine
contralateral axillary metastasis
cystic adenomatoid malformation
Cambridge pancreatitis classification
cameral fistula
camera port
Cameron femoral component removal

Camey
C. enterocystoplasty
C. enterocystoplasty urinary
diversion
C. I, II detubalarized neobladder
operation
C. ileocystoplasty
C. total gastrectomy procedure
CAM-ICU
Confusion Assessment Method for
Intensive Care Unit
Camitz
C. palmaris longus abductorplasty
C. palmaris longus tendon
reconstruction technique
Campaign
Surviving Sepsis C.
Campbell
C. interpositional arthroplasty
C. onlay bone graft
C. opening-wedge thoracostomy
technique
C. osteotomy
C. posterior shoulder approach
C. posterolateral approach
C. resection arthroplasty
C. triceps reflection
**Campbell-Akbarnia bone graft of radius
procedure**
**Campbell-Goldthwait distal realignment
osteotomy of patella procedure**
Camper
C. chiasm
C. fascia
C. ligament
C. line
C. plane
Camp-Gianturco radiography method
Campodonico
C. canal
C. pterygium operation
campotomy
camptomelic syndrome (CS)
Campylobacter **infection**
*Campylobacter***-like**
C.-l. organism (CLO)
C.-l. organism biopsy
Can
cancer
Canadian
C. Cardiovascular Society
classification (CCSC)
C. Infectious Disease Society
canal
abdominal c.
accessory palatine c.
accessory root c.
acoustic c.
additional c.

C

canal (*continued*)
  adductor c.
  Alcock c.
  alimentary c.
  alveolar c.
  anal c.
  anterior condylar c.
  anterior semicircular c.
  anterior vertical c.
  antropyloric c.
  apical c.
  Arnold c.
  atrioventricular c. (AVC)
  auditory c.
  auxiliary c.
  basipharyngeal c.
  bayonet c.
  bayonet-curved c.
  Bernard c.
  Bichat c.
  birth c.
  blunderbuss apical c.
  bony semicircular c.
  Böttcher c.
  branching c.
  Braune c.
  Breschet c.
  bulbous internal auditory c.
  Campodonico c.
  caroticoclinoid c.
  caroticotympanic c.
  carotid c.
  cartilage c.
  caudal c.
  central c.
  cervical c.
  cervicoaxillary c.
  ciliary c.
  Cloquet c.
  collateral pulp c.
  common c.
  condylar c.
  cortical bone primary c.
  Cotunnius c.
  cranial c.
  craniopharyngeal c.
  crural c.
  C-shaped c.
  c. curvature
  curved c.
  c. débridement
  defalcated root c.
  deferent c.
  dehiscent mandibular c.
  dental c.
  dentinal c.
  dilacerated c.
  diploic c.
  Dorello c.

Dupuytren c.
ear c.
endocervical c.
ethmoid c.
external auditory c.
facial c.
fallopian c.
femoral c.
Ferrein c.
filling c.
Fontana c.
furcation c.
galactophorous c.
Gartner c.
gastric c.
gubernacular c.
Guyon c.
Hannover c.
haversian c.
Hensen c.
Hirschfeld c.
His c.
horizontal c.
Hovius c.
Hoyer c.
Huguier c.
humeral c.
Hunter c.
hyaloid c.
hypoglossal c.
identifying c.
incisal c.
incisive c.
infraorbital c.
inguinal c.
c. innominate osteotomy
inoperable c.
interdental c.
interfacial c.
internal auditory c.
intramedullary c.
c. irrigation
Kovalevsky c.
lacrimal c.
Lambert c.
large c.
lateral c.
Lauth c.
locating c.
longitudinal c.
Löwenberg c.
lumbar c.
lumbosacral c.
lymphatic c.
mandibular c.
maxillary c.
medullary c.
mental c.
mesiobuccal c.

musculotubal c.
nasal c.
nasolacrimal c.
neural c.
neurenteric c.
Nuck c.
nutrient c.
c. obturation
obturator c.
c. of Arantius
c. of Cuvier
c. of Hering
c. of Stilling
c. of Vesalius
optic c.
orbital c.
overfilled c.
palatine c.
palatomaxillary c.
palatovaginal c.
pancreaticobiliary c.
partial atrioventricular c.
parturient c.
pelvic c.
perforating c.
perivascular c.
persistent common atrioventricular c.
Petit c.
pharyngeal c.
pleuroperitoneal c.
portal c.
posterior vertical c.
pterygoid c.
pterygopalatine c.
pudendal c.
pulmoaortic c.
pulp c.
pyloric c.
radicular c.
c. resonance response
Rivinus c.
root c.
ruffed c.
sacral c.
Santorini c.
Schlemm c.
scleral c.
semicircular c.
sickle-shaped c.
Sondermann c.
sphenopalatine c.
spinal c.
straight c.
subsartorial c.
Sucquet c.
Sucquet-Hoyer c.
supplementary c.
supraciliary c.
supraoptic c.

supraorbital c.
talar c.
tarsal c.
temporal c.
tensor tympani c.
Tourtual c.
tympanic c.
type I–IV c.
uniting c.
urogenital c.
uterovaginal c.
van Horne c.
Velpeau c.
ventricular c.
Verneuil c.
vertebral c.
vertical c.
vesicourethral c.
vestibular c.
vidian c.
Volkmann c.
vomerine c.
vomerobasilar c.
vomerorostral c.
vomerovaginal c.
c. wall-up technique
Walther c.
Wirsung c.
zipped c.
Zuckerkandl perforating c.
zygomaticofacial c.
zygomaticotemporal c.

Canale
   C. distal humerus fracture pinning
     technique
   C. osteotomy
canalicular
   c. duct
   c. laceration
   c. sphincter
canaliculodacryocystostomy
canaliculodacryorhinostomy
   Barrie-Jones c.
canaliculorhinostomy
canaliculus
   auricular c.
   biliary c.
   lacrimal c.
   mastoid c.
   tympanic c.
   c. vein
   vestibular c.
canalis
canalith
   free-floating c.
   c. repositioning procedure
canalization
canaloplasty
cancellectomy

cancellous
> c. and cortical bone graft
> c. chip bone graft
> c. insert graft
> c. tissue

cancer (CA)
> American Joint Committee on C. (AJCC)
> ampullary c.
> anal c.
> c. antigen 19-9 (CA19-9)
> appendiceal c.
> biliary tract c.
> c. body
> Borrmann type I–IV gastric c.
> breast c.
> c. cachexia
> cardia c.
> clinically node-negative breast c.
> colloid c.
> colon c.
> colorectal c. (CRC)
> digestive glandular c.
> ductal c.
> early gastric c. (EGC)
> endobronchial c.
> endometrial c.
> esophageal c.
> esophagogastric c.
> European Organization for Research and Treatment of C. (EORTC)
> extrahepatic bile duct c.
> familial breast c.
> familial colon c. (FCC)
> gallbladder c.
> gastric c.
> c. genetics
> C. Genetics Network
> glandular c.
> hard palate c.
> hepatocellular c.
> hereditary breast c.
> hereditary nonpolyposis colon c. (HNPCC)
> hereditary nonpolyposis colorectal c. (HNPCC)
> high-risk papillary c.
> intraductal c.
> intrathoracic esophageal c.
> c. invasion
> invasive breast c.
> invasive ductal c.
> islet cell c.
> c. juice
> c. lesion
> life-threatening c.
> localized prostate c.
> low rectal c.
> low-risk papillary c.

> lung c.
> Merkel cell c.
> metastatic colorectal c.
> nasal cavity c.
> neuroendocrine c.
> node-positive breast c.
> nonpalpable invasive breast c.
> obstructing colorectal c.
> obstructive esophagogastric c.
> ovarian c.
> c. pain
> pancreas c.
> pancreatic head c.
> papillary c.
> penile c.
> perforated c.
> periampullary c.
> peritoneal c.
> postgastrectomy c.
> primary c.
> prostate c.
> proximal gastric c.
> QUART procedure for breast c.
> rectal c.
> rectum c.
> resectable periampullary c.
> skin c.
> soft palate c.
> c. status
> subcardiac c.
> C. Surveillance Program
> c. susceptibility syndrome
> suture line c.
> thyroid c.
> Union Internationale Contre le C. (UICC)
> unresectable periampullary c.
> urologic system c.
> Whitmore-Jewett classification for prostate c.
> W-J classification for staging of prostate c.
> young-onset c.

cancerization
> field c.

cancer-related pain
Candela lithotripsy
Candida **infection**
candidal infection
candidate
> early extubation c.

candidemia
canine
> c. fossa
> c. teeth

cannabidiol
cannabinoid receptor
cannabis-based medicinal extracts
Cannon point

cannula obstruction
cannulated nail
cannulation, cannulization
    arterial c.
    bile duct c.
    biliary c.
    ductal c.
    endoscopic retrograde c.
    endoscopic transpapillary c.
    ERCP c.
    ex vivo c.
    intravenous c.
    c. of biliary tree
    pedicle c.
    percutaneous arterial c.
    peripheral venous c.
    postsphincterotomy ERCP c.
    retrograde c.
    selective ductal c.
    transpapillary c.
    tubal c.
    unilateral pedicle c.
    vascular c.
    venous c.
cannulization (*var. of* cannulation)
canonical
    c. correlation
    c. univariate parameter
canthal
canthectomy
canthi (*pl. of* canthus)
cantholysis
canthomeatal line
canthopexy
canthoplasty
    Agnew c.
    Ammon c.
    Blaskovics c.
canthorrhaphy
    Elschnig c.
    Fuchs c.
canthotomy
    external c.
    lateral c. (LC)
canthus, *pl.* **canthi**
    external c.
    internal c.
    lateral c.
    medial c.
cantilevered bone graft
Cantlie line
Cantor tube
Cantrell pentalogy
Cantwell-Ransley
    C.-R. epispadias repair
    C.-R. hypospadias repair procedure
    C.-R. urethroplasty
cap
    corneal c.

    duodenal c.
    fibrous c.
    metanephric c.
    phrygian c.
CAP
    capsule
capacity
    antioxidant reserve c.
    decreased functional residual c.
    demand minimum functional c.
    diminished functional residual c.
    exercise c.
    forced expiratory c. (FEC)
    functional residual c. (FRC)
    knot holding c. (KHC)
    maximum breathing c. (MBC)
    single-breath diffusing c.
    treadmill exercise c.
    vital c.
CAPD
    continuous ambulatory peritoneal
    dialysis
Capello acetabular reconstruction
  technique
Capener lateral rhachotomy
Cape Town injection sclerotherapy
  technique
capillaroscopy
    nail fold c.
capillary
    c. angioma
    c. arteriole
    c. dilation
    c. drainage
    c. endothelium
    c. fracture
    c. hemangioma
    c. hyperfiltration
    c. leak syndrome
    c. malformation
    c. permeability
    c. vein
    c. wedge pressure
capillus
capita (*pl. of* caput)
capital
    c. femoral epiphysis
    c. fragment
    c. operation
capitate
    c. bone
    c. fracture
capitation
capitatum
capitellar fracture
capitellocondylar total elbow
  arthroplasty
capitellum
capitis (*gen. of* caput)

C

capitonnage
    c. suture
    c. suture technique
capitopedal
capitular
    c. epiphysis
    c. joint
capitulum
capnograph
capnography
    spectral edge frequency c.
capnometry
    volumetric c.
capping technique
caprolactam suture
Caprosyn monofilament suture
capsaicin analogue
capsicum plaster
capstan knot
capsula, *pl.* **capsulae**
capsulae (*pl. of* capsula)
capsular
    c. branch
    c. dissection
    c. exfoliation syndrome
    c. fixation
    c. flap pyeloplasty
    c. imbrication
    c. incision
    c. interposition arthroplasty
    c. invasion
    c. ligament
    c. shift procedure
    c. space
    c. support tissue
    c. tear
capsule
    adipose c.
    adrenal c.
    articular c.
    atrabiliary c.
    Bonnet c.
    cricothyroid articular c.
    Crosby c.
    Crosby-Kugler biopsy c.
    external c.
    extreme c.
    fatty renal c.
    fibrous articular c.
    c. flap technique
    c. forceps technique
    Gerota c.
    Glisson c.
    glissonian c.
    glomerular c.
    hepatic c.
    joint c.
    liver c.
    morphine extended-release c.

    Müller c.
    pancreatic c.
    renal c.
    suprarenal c.
    Tenon c.
    tumor c.
capsulectomy
capsulitis
    adhesive c.
    glenohumeral adhesive c.
capsulodesis
    Blatt c.
capsuloplasty
    Zancolli c.
capsulorrhaphy
    Boyd-Sisk posterior c.
    duToit-Roux staple c.
    medial c.
    pants-over-vest c.
    posterior c.
    Putti-Platt shoulder c.
    Rockwood posterior c.
    Roux-duToit staple c.
    staple c.
capsulotomy
    anterior c.
    Castroviejo c.
    Curtis PIP joint c.
    Darling c.
    dorsal transverse c.
    dorsolateral and medial c.
    posterior c.
    renal c.
    triangular c.
    T-shaped c.
    Vannas c.
    Verhoeff-Chandler c.
capture
    c. cross-section
    pacemaker c.
Capuron point
caput, *gen.* **capitis,** *pl.* **capita**
    c. medusae
    splenius capitis
carbamazepine
carbon (C)
    c. dioxide (bicarb, CO_2)
    c. dioxide concentration
    c. dioxide dissociation curve
    c. dioxide fixation
    c. dioxide laser plaque ablation
    c. dioxide narcosis
    c. dioxide pressure
    c. dioxide response
    c. gelatin mass
    c. monoxide (CO)
carbonaceous sputum
carbonate (CO_3^{2-})
carbonization

carbuncle
    kidney c.
carcinoembryonic antigen (CEA)
carcinogenesis
    foreign body c.
carcinoid
    goblet cell c.
    nonappendiceal c.
    c. syndrome
    c. tumor
    c. valve disease
carcinoma (CA), *pl.* **carcinomas,**
  carcinomata
    abdominal c.
    acinic cell c.
    acinous cell c.
    adenocystic c.
    adenoid cystic c.
    adenoid squamous cell c.
    adenosquamous c.
    adnexal c.
    adrenal c.
    adrenocortical c.
    aldosterone-producing c.
    alveolar cell c.
    ameloblastic c.
    ampullary c.
    anaplastic c.
    anorectal c.
    apocrine c.
    basal cell c.
    basosquamous cell c.
    benign-acting renal cell c.
    betel c.
    bile duct c.
    bilharzial c.
    biliary c.
    bladder c.
    Borrmann type I-IV gastric c.
    breast c.
    bronchial c.
    bronchioloalveolar c.
    bronchoalveolar c.
    burn scar c.
    cecal c.
    cerebriform c.
    cervical c.
    chimney sweep's c.
    cholangitis c.
    choroid plexus c.
    clay pipe c.
    clear cell hepatocellular c.
    colloid c.
    colon c.
    colonic c.
    colorectal c. (CRC)
    columnar cuff c.
    corpus c.
    cortisol-producing c.

    cribriform c.
    cutaneous metastatic breast c.
    cylindrical c.
    dendritic c.
    differentiated thyroid c.
    disseminated c.
    ductal c.
    Dukes classification of c.
    dye worker's c.
    eccrine c.
    Edmondson grading system for
      hepatocellular c.
    embryonal cell c.
    encephaloid gastric c.
    c. en cuirasse
    endometrial c.
    epidermoid c.
    esophageal c.
    ethmoid sinus c.
    excavated gastric c.
    exophytic c.
    extrahepatic abdominal c.
    fallopian tube c.
    false cord c.
    familial medullary thyroid c.
    follicular c.
    follicular thyroid c.
    gallbladder c.
    gastric stump c.
    gastrointestinal c.
    gelatinous c.
    genital c.
    glandular c.
    glottic c.
    granulosa cell c.
    gynecologic c.
    hepatic cell c.
    hepatocellular c. (HCC)
    hereditary nonpolyposis colon c.
      (HNPCC)
    hereditary renal c.
    hilar c.
    hypernephroid c.
    infantile embryonal c.
    infiltrating ductal c.
    infiltrating lobular c.
    infiltrative c.
    inflammatory breast c.
    c. in situ (CIS)
    insular c.
    intraductal c.
    intraepidermal c.
    intraepithelial nonkeratinizing c.
    invasive breast c.
    invasive ductal c.
    invasive lobular c.
    invasive signet ring cell c.
    Japanese Classification for Gastric
      C. (JCGC)

C

carcinoma (*continued*)
    juvenile embryonal c.
    Kulchitsky cell c.
    large cell c.
    laryngeal c.
    leptomeningeal c.
    lobular c.
    lung c.
    maxillary sinus c.
    medullary c.
    medullary thyroid c.
    meibomian gland c.
    melanotic c.
    meningeal c.
    Merkel cell c.
    metastatic colorectal c.
    metastatic prostatic c.
    metastatic renal cell c.
    microinvasive c.
    micropapillary c.
    microscopic multifocal medullary c.
    microtrabecular hepatocellular c.
    morpheaform basal cell c.
    mucoepidermal c.
    mucoepidermoid c.
    napkin-ring c.
    nasopharyngeal c. (NPC)
    neuroendocrine skin c.
    oat cell c.
    c. of uncertain primary site
    orofacial c.
    oropharyngeal c.
    ovarian c.
    Paget c.
    pancreatic c.
    papillary gastric c.
    papillary thyroid c.
    parathyroid c.
    parotid c.
    penile c.
    periampullary c.
    pharyngeal wall c.
    polypoid superficial gastric c.
    prickle cell c.
    primary bile duct c.
    primary intraosseous c.
    prostatic c.
    pure insular c.
    radiation-induced c.
    rectal c.
    rectosigmoid c.
    renal cell c.
    renal pelvis c.
    resectable c.
    residual ductal c.
    salivary duct c.
    salivary gland c.
    scar c.
    schistosomal bladder c.

    schneiderian c.
    sigmoid colon c.
    signet-ring cell c.
    sinonasal c.
    small-cell lung c. (SCLC)
    small round cell c.
    spindle cell c.
    splenic flexure c.
    sporadic renal cell c.
    squamous cell c. (SCC)
    stage B, C c.
    c. stage irresectable
    string cell c.
    swamp c.
    terminal duct c.
    testicular c.
    thymic c.
    thyroglossal duct c.
    thyroid c.
    transitional cell c.
    tuberous sclerosis-associated renal cell c.
    tubular c.
    undifferentiated squamous cell c.
    urachal c.
    ureteral c.
    urethral c.
    urothelial c.
    uterine papillary serous c.
    vaginal c.
    vulvar c.
    vulvovaginal c.
    wolffian duct c.
    yolk sac c.
carcinomas (*pl. of* carcinoma)
carcinomata (*pl. of* carcinoma)
carcinomatosis
    diffuse c.
    miliary c.
    peritoneal c.
carcinosarcoma
card
    Memorial Pain Assessment C. (MPAC)
cardia
    achalasia of c.
    c. cancer
    gastric c.
cardiac
    c. anesthesia
    C. Anesthesia Risk Evaluation (CARE)
    c. anesthetic
    c. anomaly
    c. arrest
    c. bypass
    c. catheterization
    c. compression
    c. decompression

c. defibrillation
c. dilation
c. edema
c. event
c. examination
c. fibrillation
c. fibrous skeleton
c. herniation
c. impression
c. index (CI)
c. injury
c. inward rectifier K+ channel
c. irradiation
c. lymphatic ring
c. mass
c. massage
c. metastasis
c. muscle wrap
c. nerve
c. output (Q̊)
c. patch
c. perforation
c. plexus
c. position
c. pump mechanism
c. resuscitation
c. retransplantation
c. rhabdomyoma
c. rhythm management device
c. rupture
c. segment
c. surgery
c. surgical recovery unit
c. symphysis
c. transplant
c. tumor
c. tumor plop
c. uncoupling
c. valvular malformation
c. vein

cardiac-allograft vasculopathy
cardiacum
    antrum c.
    ostium c.
    segmentum c.
cardiacus
cardiae
    sphincter constrictor c.
cardiectomy
cardinal
    c. ligament
    c. point
    c. position
    c. suture
cardioesophageal relaxation
Cardioflon suture
cardiogenic shock

cardiohepatic angle
cardiologist
    interventional c.
cardiomyopathy
    ischemic c.
    underlying c.
cardiomyoplasty
    dynamic c.
cardiomyotomy
    Heller c.
    laparoscopic c.
    stomach c.
    videolaparoscopic c.
Cardionyl suture
cardioomentopexy
cardiopericardiopexy
    Beck I c.
cardiopexy
cardiophrenic angle mass
cardioplasty
    Belsey Mark IV c.
cardioplegia
cardioplegic solution
cardiopressor reflex
cardioprotective effect
cardiopulmonary
    c. bypass (CPB)
    c. complication
    c. manifestation
    C. Research Institute
    c. resuscitation (CPR)
    c. risk index
cardiorespiratory
    c. complication
    c. endurance (CRE)
cardiorrhaphy
cardiothoracic surgery (CTS)
cardiotomy
cardiotoxic
    c. effect
    c. myolysis
cardiovagal function
cardiovalvotomy, cardiovalvulotomy
cardiovalvulotomy (*var. of* cardiovalvotomy)
cardiovascular
    c. adverse effect
    c. anesthesia
    c. complication
    c. disease (CVD)
    c. imaging technique
    c. malformation
    c. patch graft
    c. pressure
    c. stability
    c. surgery
cardiovasculorenal
cardioversion
cardiovert

C

care
  medical c.
  monitored anesthesia c. (MAC)
  palliative c.
  respiratory c.
  Tactical Combat Casualty C.
    (TCCC)
  tertiary c.
  trauma c.
caries classification
carina, *pl.* **carinae**
  splayed c.
carinae (*pl. of* carina)
carinal resection
carinate abdomen
carinatum
  pectus c.
carious
  c. pulp exposure
  c. restoration margin
**Carlo Traverso post-trabeculectomy
maneuver**
C-arm fluoroscopy
**Carmody-Batson zygoma and zygomatic
arch fracture reduction**
Carnesale
  C. acetabular extensile approach
  C. extremity amputation technique
  C. hip approach
**Carnesale-Stewart-Barnes hip dislocation
classification**
Caroli
  C. syndrome
  C. type I distal bile duct stricture
Carolinas
  C. Laparoscopic Advanced Surgery
    Program (CLASP)
  C. Laparoscopic Advanced Surgery
    Program minimal accessory surgery
    procedure
**Caroli-Sarles bile duct stricture
classification**
caroticoclinoid
  c. canal
  c. foramen
  c. ligament
caroticotympanic
  c. artery
  c. canal
  c. nerve
caroticum
caroticus
carotid
  c. ablative procedure
  c. angioplasty
  c. angioplasty with stenting
  c. arterial blood flow
  c. artery atherosclerotic stenosis
  c. artery bifurcation

  c. artery bypass
  c. artery compression
  c. artery disease
  c. artery dissection
  c. artery occlusion
  c. artery stenting
  c. artery stump pressure
  c. atherosclerosis
  c. body
  c. body tumor
  c. canal
  c. circulation
  c. clamping
  c. duplex ultrasonography
  c. ejection time
  c. endarterectomy (CEA)
  external c.
  c. foramen
  c. ganglion
  c. groove
  c. injury
  c. plaque
  c. preservation
  c. preservation technique
  c. sheath
  c. sinus
  c. sinus branch
  c. siphon
  c. space
  c. stenting
  c. sulcus
  c. surgery
  c. transposition
  c. triangle
  c. tubercle
  c. venous plexus
carotid-basilar anastomosis
carotid-cavernous sinus fistula
carotid-dural fistula
carotid-subclavian artery bypass
carotid-vertebral
  c.-v. anastomosis
  c.-v. vein bypass graft
carotidynia
carpal
  c. artery
  c. bone stress fracture
  c. boss
  c. compression test
  c. region
  c. synovectomy
  c. tunnel syndrome (CTS)
carpectomy
  distal-row c.
  Omer-Capen c.
  proximal-row c.
Carpentier
  C. anuloplasty
  C. tricuspid valvoplasty

Carpentier-Edwards
  C.-E. stented bovine pericardial valve
  C.-E. stented porcine xenograft valve
carpet lesion
carpetlike polyposis
carpi (*pl. of* carpus)
carpocarpal
carpometacarpal (CMC)
  c. arthroplasty
  c. articulation
  c. fracture-dislocation
  c. joint dislocation
  c. joint fracture
carpometacarpeae
  articulationes c.
carpopedal
Carpue rhinoplasty method
carpus, *pl.* **carpi**
carrageen, carragheen
carrageenan, carrageenin
carrageenin (*var. of* carrageenan)
carragheen (*var. of* carrageen)
Carrel
  C. experimental coronary artery bypass operation
  C. patch
  C. suture technique
Carrell
  C. distal fibula resection
  C. fibular substitution technique
carrier
  c. flap
  c. fluid
  c. gas composition
  mutation c.
  c. status
  suture c.
Carroll arthroplasty
Carstan reverse wedge osteotomy
Cartam-Treander reverse wedge osteotomy
Carter operation
cartilage
  alar c.
  anular c.
  arthrodial c.
  articular c.
  arytenoid c.
  auricular c.
  basilar c.
  branchial c.
  c. canal
  connecting c.
  corniculate c.
  costal c.
  cricoid c.
  cuneiform c.

  diarthrodial c.
  ensiform c.
  epiglottic c.
  falciform c.
  c. flap
  c. graft
  hypsiloid c.
  c. inflammation
  interosseous c.
  intervertebral c.
  intraarticular c.
  intrathyroid c.
  investing c.
  Jacobson c.
  Luschka c.
  mandibular c.
  c. matrix
  meatal c.
  Meckel c.
  Meyer c.
  Morgagni c.
  c. overgrowth
  pyramidal-shaped c.
  quadrangular c.
  Reichert c.
  c. repair
  Santorini c.
  Seiler c.
  semilunar c.
  sesamoid c.
  sternal c.
  sternum c.
  supraarytenoid c.
  thyroid c.
  tracheal c.
  triangular c.
  triquetrous c.
  triticeal c.
  uniting c.
  vomeronasal c.
  Weitbrecht c.
  Wrisberg c.
  xiphoid c.
  Y c.
cartilagines (*pl. of* cartilago)
cartilagineus
  vomer c.
cartilaginous
  c. defect
  c. growth plate disorder
  c. loose body
  c. part of skeletal system
  c. septum
  c. tissue
cartilago, *pl.* **cartilagines**
cartwheel fracture
caruncle
  Morgagni c.
  Santorini major c.

caruncle (*continued*)
 Santorini minor c.
 urethral c.
caruncula, *pl.* **carunculae**
 hymenal c.
 sublingual c.
carunculae (*pl. of* caruncula, caruncle)
caryothecae
 cisterna c.
CAS
 computer-assisted surgery
Casanellas lacrimal operation
cascade
 coagulation c.
 inflammatory c.
case
 clean c.
 clean-contaminated c.
 dirty c.
 pump c.
caseated tissue
caseating granulomatous inflammation
caseation
 c. necrosis
 tuberculous c.
case-by-case approach
caseous
 c. abscess
 c. inflammation
Casey operation
Casoni test
Caspari transglenoid repair
CASS
 computer-assisted stereotactic surgery
Casselberry position
Casser perforated muscle
cast
 c. application
 c. immobilization
 c. removal
Castaneda tetralogy of Fallot repair procedure
Castellani point
Castle femoral resection procedure
Castleman disease
castrate
castration
 female c.
 functional c.
 male c.
 parasitic c.
Castroviejo
 C. capsulotomy
 C. corneal transplantation operation
 C. iridectomy
 C. keratectomy
 C. minikeratoplasty
 C. radial iridotomy

Castroviejo-Scheie cyclodiathermy operation
catabolic condition
cataract
 c. aspiration
 congenital c.
 c. extraction
 c. extraction operation
 flap operation c.
 c. formation
 hard c.
 irradiation c.
 c. irradiation
 c. mask ring
 c. procedure
 radiation c.
 reduplication c.
 ring-form congenital c.
 ring-shaped c.
 Soemmerring ring c.
 soft c.
 c. surgery
catarrhal
 c. inflammation
 c. marginal ulceration
catastrophe
 intraabdominal c.
catastrophic
 c. cognition
 c. complication
 c. event
 c. illness
catastrophizing subscale
CAT-CAM
 contoured adduction
 trochanteric-controlled alignment method
catecholamine-resistant hypotension
caterpillar flap
catgut suture
cath
 catheter
 catheterization
 catheterize
catheter (cath)
 c. ablation
 adherent clot c.
 Advantiv Safety I.V. c.
 antibiotic-impregnated c.
 c. balloon valvoplasty (CBV)
 Broviac c.
 chronic dialysis c.
 continuous peripheral nerve c.
 c. dilation
 c. drainage
 c. embolectomy
 c. embolism
 end-hole c.

endotracheal ventilation c.
epidural c.
c. exchange
c. fixation
Fogarty embolectomy c.
c. fragment
Groshong c.
Hemo-Cath pheresis c.
Hickman c.
Hohn c.
c. insertion
c. instability
c. introduction method
c. kinking
c. knotting
c. knotting and entrapment
Kumar cholangiography c.
lumbar c.
lumbar epidural c.
Mahurkar c.
c. malposition
c. manipulation
c. mapping
multiport epidural c.
c. obstruction
passive safety intravenous c.
c. patency
percutaneous transhepatic c.
perineural c.
peripherally inserted central c.
 (PICC)
Pioneer c.
popliteal c.
c. position
pulmonary artery c.
Quinton dialysis c.
c. sepsis
SG c.
single-port epidural c.
c. site
c. specimen
stimulating c.
surgically implanted c.
Swan-Ganz c.
sympathetic-chain c.
Tenckhoff peritoneal
 dialysis c.
Tesio c.
thoracic epidural c.
c. tip placement
c. toe
torque tube c.
triple-lumen c.
c. tunnel
tunneled epidural c.
c. tunnel infection
van Andel c.
c. whip
whistle-tip c.

catheter-based
 c.-b. ablation
 c.-b. intervention
catheter-directed
 c.-d. fenestration
 c.-d. interventional procedure
 c.-d. thrombolysis
catheter-guided
 c.-g. biopsy
 c.-g. endoscopic intubation
**catheter-induced pulmonary artery
 hemorrhage**
catheterizable stoma
catheterization (cath)
 antegrade c.
 arterial c.
 bile duct c.
 bladder c.
 bypass graft c.
 cardiac c.
 central venous c.
 chronic c.
 clean intermittent c.
 combined heart c.
 coronary sinus c.
 cystic duct c.
 diagnostic cardiac c.
 fallopian tube c.
 in-and-out c.
 intermittent c.
 interventional cardiac c.
 Judkins-Sones technique of
  cardiac c.
 left heart c.
 long-term epidural c.
 percutaneous transhepatic
  cardiac c.
 portal vein c.
 pulmonary artery c.
 retrograde c.
 right heart c.
 Seldinger cystic duct c.
 selective c.
 subclavian vein c.
 c. technique
 thoracic epidural c.
 transfemoral venous c.
 transhepatic c.
 transnasal bile duct c.
 transpapillary c.
 transseptal left heart c.
 transvaginal fallopian tube c.
 transvaginal tubal c.
 umbilical artery c.
 umbilical vein c.
 ureteral c.
 urinary c.
catheterize (cath)
catheter-related infection

catheter-securing technique
catholysis
cation exchange
cat's eye
cat's-eye calculus
Cattell operation
Cattell-Warren pancreaticojejunostomy
Catterall of Perthe disease classification
cauda
    c. epididymis
    c. equina compression
    c. equina syndrome
caudad
caudal
    c. anesthesia
    c. angulation
    c. block
    c. canal
    c. corner
    c. direction
    c. dysplasia sequence
    c. epidural anesthetic technique
    c. epidural injection
    c. fragment
    kiddie c.
    c. lamina resection
    c. ligament
    c. pancreatic artery
    c. pancreatojejunostomy
    c. retinaculum
    c. sac
    c. translation
    c. transtentorial herniation
    c. transverse fissure
    c. vertebra
caudal-cranial rotation
caudalis
    trigeminal nucleus c.
caudate
    c. body
    c. branch
    c. hepatectomy
    c. lobe
    c. lobectomy
    c. process
caudocephalad
causalgia
    genitofemoral c.
cause
    cholestatic c.
    definitive c.
    idiopathic c.
    pathologic c.
    underlying c.
cause-effect relationship
cause-specific mortality
cauterant
cauterization
    bipolar c.

    Bovie c.
    phenol c.
    Scheie scleral c.
    unipolar c.
cauterize
cautery
    c. conization
    Gonin retinal c.
    hook c.
    c. incision
    insulated c.
    looped c.
    monopolar c.
    c. operation
    pure cutting c.
    snare c.
    wet field c.
cava (*pl. of* cavum)
caval
    c. drainage
    c. fold
    c. insertion
CAVD
    complete atrioventricular dissociation
cave
    C. hip approach
    C. knee approach
    Meckel c.
    Prévention du Risque d'Embolie
      Pulmonaire par Interruption C.
      (PREPIC)
    trigeminal c.
caverna
cavernosa
cavernosal alpha blockade technique
cavernous
    c. angioma
    c. body
    c. groove
    c. hemangioma
    c. malformation
    c. nerve
    c. nerve-sparing prostatectomy
    c. plexus
    c. respiration
    c. sinus fistula
    c. sinus syndrome
    c. venous sinus
Cave-Rowe shoulder dislocation
  technique
CAVH
    continuous arteriovenous hemofiltration
cavitary
    c. lung lesion
    c. small-bowel lesion
cavitas
cavitating
    c. inflammation
    c. metastasis

cavitation
  collapse c.
  pulmonary c.
  stable c.
  transient c.
Cavitron ultrasound aspiration
cavity (cav)
  abdominal c.
  abdominopelvic c.
  c. access
  access c.
  acetabular c.
  alveolar c.
  amniotic c.
  articular c.
  artificial classification c.
  axial surface c.
  biopsy c.
  blastocystic c.
  body c.
  buccal c.
  chorionic c.
  c. classification
  complex c.
  compound c.
  cotyloid c.
  cranial c.
  C. Creation System
  cystic c.
  c. débridement
  dental c.
  distal c.
  distal occlusal c.
  endodontic c.
  endolymphatic c.
  endometrial c.
  epidural c.
  exocelomic c.
  fissure c.
  frontal sinus c.
  gingival c.
  glenoid c.
  greater peritoneal c.
  idiopathic bone c.
  incisal c.
  inferior laryngeal c.
  inflammatory c.
  infraglottic c.
  intermediate laryngeal c.
  intracranial c.
  intraperitoneal c.
  joint c.
  labial c.
  laryngeal c.
  laser c.
  lesser peritoneal c.
  c. line angle
  lingual c.
  c. lining

  c. lining agent
  lung c.
  c. margin
  marrow c.
  mastoid c.
  maxillary sinus c.
  Meckel c.
  medullary c.
  miniature uterine c.
  nasal c.
  nephrotomic c.
  nonseptate c.
  occlusal c.
  open c.
  optic papilla c.
  oral c.
  orbital c.
  pelvic c.
  perilymphatic c.
  peritoneal c.
  pharyngonasal c.
  pit and fissure c.
  pleural c.
  postexcision c.
  c. preparation
  c. preparation base
  prepared c.
  c. primer
  proximal c.
  pulmonary c.
  pulp c.
  residual cystic c.
  retroperitoneal c.
  Retzius c.
  saclike c.
  c. seal
  seroma c.
  sinonasal c.
  sinus c.
  smooth surface c.
  Stafne idiopathic bone c.
  subarachnoid c.
  subdural c.
  subglottic c.
  superior laryngeal c.
  synovial c.
  syringohydromyelic c.
  c. test
  thoracic c.
  c. toilet
  trigeminal c.
  tympanic c.
  uterine c.
  vitreous c.
  c. wall
  wound c.
cavoatrial
  c. bypass
  c. shunt

C

cavohepatic junction
cavopulmonary anastomosis
cavotomy
    infrahepatic c.
cavovarus deformity
CAVU
    continuous arteriovenous ultrafiltration
cavum, *pl.* **cava**
    inferior vena cava (IVC)
    infrahepatic inferior vena cava
    infrarenal cava
    retrohepatic inferior vena cava
    c. septum pellucidum
    Spencer plication of vena cava
    superior vena cava (SVC)
    suprahepatic inferior vena cava
    suprahepatic vena cava
cavus
    c. deformity
    talipes c.
CAWO
    closing abductory wedge osteotomy
Cawthorne
    C. destruction
    C. labyrinth fenestration
Cawthorne-Day labyrinthectomy
 procedure
CBD
    common bile duct
CBF
    cerebral blood flow
CBT
    cognitive-behavioral therapy
CCAM
    congenital cystic adenomatoid
     malformation
CCM
    critical care medicine
CCS
    Clinical Classification System
CCSC
    Canadian Cardiovascular Society
     classification
CCSF
    carotid-cavernous sinus fistula
CCSG
    Children's Cancer Study Group
C-D
    Cotrel-Dubousset
     C-D screw modification
C:D
    cup to disc ratio
CDBR
    computerized diaphragmatic breathing
     retraining
CDCR
    conjunctivodacryocystorhinostomy
CDH
    congenital diaphragmatic hernia

CDS
    cardiovascular surgery
    controlled disc stimulation
    cul-de-sac
CEA
    carcinoembryonic antigen
    carotid endarterectomy
     CEA level
     serum CEA
ceanothus extract
CEAP
    clinical manifestations, etiologic factors,
     anatomic involvement,
     pathophysiologic features
ceca (*pl. of* cecum)
cecal
    c. appendix
    c. artery
    c. bascule
    c. carcinoma
    c. colonoscopy
    c. deformity
    c. distention
    c. diverticulitis
    c. flap
    c. fold
    c. foramen
    c. hernia
    c. imbrication procedure
    c. intussusception
    c. ligation
    c. ligation and puncture
    c. recess
    c. serosa
    c. volvulus
cecectomy
Cecil
    C. hypospadias repair procedure
    C. urethroplasty
cecocolostomy
cecocystoplasty
cecofixation
cecoileostomy
cecopexy
    laparoscopic c.
cecoplication
cecoproctostomy
cecorectal anastomosis
cecorrhaphy
cecosigmoidostomy
cecostomy
    percutaneous catheter c.
    tube c.
cecotomy
cecoureterocele
cecum, caecum, *pl.* **ceca**
Cedars-Sinai corneal topography
 classification
ceiling analgesia

celecoxib

Celermajer cardiovascular profiling method

Celestin tube carcinoma palliation procedure

celiac, coeliac
c. alcohol ablation
c. arterial system
c. artery
c. artery aneurysm
c. artery compression syndrome
c. axis
c. axis compression syndrome
c. band syndrome
c. branch
c. dimple
c. ganglion
c. gland
c. infantilism
c. lymph node metastasis
c. nervous plexus
c. nodal involvement
c. ostium
c. plexus block
c. plexus block anesthetic technique
c. plexus reflex
c. rickets
c. trunk
c. trunk bleeding
c. tumor
c. vessel

celiacography

celiacomesenteric artery

celiectomy

celiocentesis

celioenterotomy

celiogastrostomy

celiogastrotomy

celiohysterectomy

celiohysterotomy

celioma

celiomyomectomy

celiomyomotomy

celioparacentesis

celiorrhaphy

celiosalpingectomy

celiosalpingotomy

celioscopy

celiotomy
damage-control c.
exploratory c.
formal c.
c. incision
mandatory c.
negative c.
staging c.
vaginal c.

celite-activated clotting time (CACT)

cell
absorptive c.
Claudius c.
c. collection
Deiters c.
enterochromaffinlike c.
ependymal c.
epithelial c.
epitympanic c.
ethmoid c.
fasciculata c.
follicular c.
glial c.
gut epithelial c.
Hensen c.
human vascular c.
hypotympanic c.
inflammation c.
inflammatory c.
irradiated melanoma c.
islet c.
Ito c.'s
Kupffer c. (KC)
lymphocyte c.
malignant c.
mastoid c.
c. membrane
mesothelial c.
c. migration
multipotential stem c.
c. oxygenation
packed red blood c.'s (PRBC)
paranasal c.
parenchymal c.
petrous apex c.
pharyngeal c.
pheochrome c.
photosensitive c.
pit c.
pituitary tumor c.
pulmonary epithelial c.
retinal pigment epithelial c.
rod c.
c. salvage system
Schwann c.
stem c.
T c.
tumor c.
umbilical cord blood stem c.'s
c. web
white c.

cell-based assay

cell-cell adhesion

CellCept

cell-extracellular matrix adhesion

cellophane tape method

cellula, *pl.* **cellulae**

cellulae (*pl. of* cellula)

cellular
  c. biology
  c. cooperation
  c. damage
  c. debris
  c. hypoxia
  c. immunity
  c. infiltration
  c. migration
  c. nidus
  c. polyp
  c. proliferation
  c. xenograft rejection
  c. xenotransplantation
cellularity
  high c.
cellulitis
  orbital c.
  vaginal cuff c.
cellulocutaneous flap
celomic epithelium carcinoma of ovary
celotomy
Celsus-Hotz entropion operation
Celsus spasmodic entropion operation
cement
  c. base
  c. disease
  c. interface
  c. line
  c. removal
  c. substance
  c. technique
cemental
  c. lesion
  c. line
  c. repair
cementation
  final c.
  trial c.
cement-bone interface
cemented total hip arthroplasty
cementification
cementing line
cementless
  c. technique
  c. total hip arthroplasty
cementoid tissue
cementoma
cementum
  c. fracture
  c. pain
center
  ambulatory surgery c.
  Centers for Disease Control HIV infection classification
  limbic c.
  MGH Pain C.
  tertiary trauma c.

  trauma c.
  urban trauma c.
centesis
central
  c. ablative procedure
  c. anesthetic technique
  c. anticholinergic syndrome
  c. approach
  c. bearing point
  c. block
  c. bone
  c. canal
  c. carbon dioxide ventilatory response
  c. chemoreflex loop
  c. cone technique reduction
  c. cord syndrome
  c. core disease
  c. dislocation
  c. duct resection
  c. excitatory state
  c. extensor mechanism
  c. fibroelastic core
  c. fibrous body
  c. fixation
  c. fracture
  c. fusion
  c. heel pad syndrome
  c. hepatectomy
  c. hepatic gunshot wound
  c. herniation
  c. hyperalimentation
  c. illumination
  c. incisor teeth
  c. iridectomy
  c. landmark
  c. lesion
  c. line infection
  c. neck dissection
  c. nervous system (CNS)
  c. nervous system disease
  c. nervous system malformation
  c. nervous system manifestation
  c. nervous system tuberculosis
  c. neuraxial blockade
  c. neuropathic pain
  c. obesity
  c. pain
  c. palmar space
  c. perineum tendon
  c. physiolysis
  c. pontine myelinolysis
  c. posterior-anterior pressure
  c. poststroke pain (CPSP)
  c. ray amputation
  c. renosplenic shunt
  c. respiration
  c. retinal artery
  c. sensitization

c. slip-sparing technique
c. stellate laceration
c. sulcal artery
c. systemic-to-pulmonary shunt
c. tegmental tract
c. tendon
c. tendon diaphragm
c. vein
c. venous access
c. venous access device (CVAD)
c. venous alimentation
c. venous cannulation anesthetic technique
c. venous catheterization
c. venous hypercapnia
c. venous pressure (CVP)
c. venous pressure line
c. venous pressure monitoring
c. vision
c. yellow point
c. zone inflammation
centralis
centralization
Bayne-Klug c.
Bora c.
Manske-McCarroll-Swanson c.
tendon c.
centration
centric
c. fusion
c. jaw relation
c. occluding relation
c. occluding relation record
point c.
c. position
c. relation occlusion (CRO)
centriciput
centrifugal
c. nerve
c. pump
centrifugalization
centrifugation
centrifuged
centrilobular
c. lesion
c. necrosis
c. pancreatitis
centriole
distal c.
proximal c.
centripetal nerve
centrolateral nucleus
centroneuroaxis anesthesia
centrum
c. ossificationis
c. ossificationis primarium
c. ossificationis secundarium
c. ossificationis secundum

cephalad
c. corner
c. direction
c. fragment
c. translation
cephalalgia
coital c.
cephalic
c. arterial ramus
c. index
c. tetanus
c. triangle
c. vein
c. vein graft
cephalization
cephalocaudal axis
cephalocele
occipital c.
oral c.
cephalocentesis
cephalodactyly
cephalomedullary nail fracture
cephalometric
c. correction
c. landmark
cephalopelvic disproportion
cephalopharyngeus
cephalorrhachidian index
cephalothoracic
cephalotrigonal technique
ceramic restoration
ceramometal restoration
ceratectomy
ceratocricoid
c. ligament
c. muscle
ceratocricoideum
ligamentum c.
ceratocricoideus
ceratopharyngeus
cerclage
elective c.
emergent c.
McDonald c.
c. operation
Shirodkar cervical c.
c. wire fixation
cerebellar
c. artery
c. ectopia
c. hematoma
c. hemisphere
c. hemorrhage
c. vein
cerebellomedullary
c. cistern
c. malformation syndrome
cerebellopontile (*var. of* cerebellopontine)

C

cerebellopontine, cerebellopontile
    c. angle approach
    c. angle cistern
    c. angle syndrome
cerebellorubral tract
cerebellothalamic tract
cerebral
    c. abscess
    c. angioma
    c. aqueduct compression
    c. arteriovenous malformation
    c. artery
    c. autoregulation
    c. blood
    c. blood flow (CBF)
    c. calculus
    c. circulation
    c. circulation time
    c. cortex
    c. death
    c. decompression
    c. decortication
    c. edema
    c. event
    c. fornix
    c. hemicorticectomy
    c. hemisphere
    c. hemorrhage
    c. hernia
    c. herniation
    c. index
    c. injury
    c. lesion
    c. metabolic rate
    c. metastasis
    c. oximetric desaturation
    c. oximetry
    c. palsy pathological
     fracture
    c. perfusion
    c. perfusion pressure
    c. preconditioning
    c. protection
    c. protective therapy
    c. radiation necrosis
    c. respiration
    c. revascularization
    c. sinus
    c. spinal fluid drainage
    c. state index
    c. sulcus
    c. vascular malformation
    c. vasodilatory effect
    c. vein
cerebral-sacral loop
cerebration
cerebri
    pseudotumor c.
cerebriform carcinoma

cerebrospinal
    c. fluid (CSF)
    c. fluid-brain barrier
    c. fluid fistula
    c. fluid outflow
    c. fluid pressure
    c. fluid velocity
    c. index
cerebrotendinous xanthomatosis
cerebrotomy
cerebrovascular
    c. accident (CVA)
    c. complication
    c. disease
    c. event
    c. malformation
    c. resistance
cerebrovenous disease
cerebrum
cerecloth
cereoli
certified
    c. registered nurse anesthetist
     (CRNA)
    C. Surgical Technologist (CST)
    C. Surgical Technologist, First
     Assist (CSTFA)
cervical
    c. acceleration-deceleration
     syndrome
    c. adenocarcinoma
    c. adenopathy
    c. amputation
    c. anastomosis
    c. anesthesia
    c. anomaly
    c. approach
    c. aspiration
    c. branch
    c. canal
    c. carcinoma
    c. carcinoma stimulation
    c. compression syndrome
    c. condyloma
    c. cone biopsy
    c. conization
    c. corpectomy
    c. decompression surgery
    c. dilation
    c. discectomy
    c. disc excision
    c. disc surgery
    c. diverticulum
    c. dystonia
    c. esophagogastric anastomosis
    c. esophagogastric anastomotic leak
    c. esophagogastrostomy
    c. esophagoplasty
    c. esophagostomy

c. esophagotomy
c. esophagus
c. extension strength
c. facet syndrome
c. fascia
c. fistula
c. flap
c. fusion syndrome
c. ganglion
c. ganglionectomy
c. general rotation
c. gland
c. immobilization
c. incision
c. infection
c. inflammation
c. injury
c. insemination
c. instability
c. interbody fusion
c. laceration
c. leakage
c. lesion
c. ligament
c. line
c. loop
c. lymphadenopathy
c. manipulation
c. medial branch block
c. metastasis
c. midline disc herniation
c. nerve root injection
c. node dissection
c. os
c. osteotomy
c. perivascular sympathectomy
c. pleura
c. plexus
c. plexus block
c. plexus block anesthetic
  technique
c. position
c. rib
c. rotator muscle
c. screw fixation
c. screw insertion technique
c. segment
c. sinus
c. soft tissue
c. space
c. spine fracture
c. spine internal fixation
c. spine kyphotic deformity
c. spine laminectomy
c. spine posterior fusion
c. spine screw-plate fixation
c. spine stabilization
c. spine stabilization procedure
c. splanchnic nerve

c. spondylitic myelopathy
c. spondylotic myelopathy fusion
  technique
c. spondylotic myelopathy
  vertebrectomy
c. stenosis
c. stump
c. suture
c. syringomyelia
c. thymectomy
c. transformation zone
c. triangle
c. tumor
c. ulcer
c. ultrasound
c. vein
c. vertebra
c. vessel compression
cervicalis
  ansa c.
  c. ascendens
cervicalium
cervical-to-MCA bypass
cervicectomy
cervices (*pl. of* cervix)
cervicis (*pl. of* cervix)
cervicoaxillary
  c. canal
  c. sheath
cervicobrachial
cervicofacial
cervicogenic headache
cervicomedullary
  c. deformity
  c. junction compression
cervicooccipital
cervicoplasty
cervicothoracic
  c. approach
  c. ganglion
  c. junction stabilization
  c. junction surgery
  c. orthosis (CTO)
  c. pedicle anatomy
  c. sympathectomy
  c. transition
cervicothoracicum
cervicotomy
cervicotrochanteric displaced fracture
cervicovaginal
  c. artery
  c. fistula
  c. infection
cervicovaginalis
cervicovesical
cervix, *pl.* **cervicis, cervices**
  implant c.
  semispinalis cervicis
  c. vesicae urinariae

C

cesarean
    c. delivery
    c. hysterectomy
    c. operation
    c. resection
    c. section (C-section)
    c. section incision
cesium irradiation
CFA
    common femoral artery
CFA-SFA
    common femoral artery-superficial
      femoral artery
      CFA-SFA bypass
C-fiber
C-form osteotomy
CGS
    clinical grading scale
CHA
    common hepatic artery
    controlled hypotensive anesthesia
CHADD
    controlled heat-aided drug delivery
Chadwick-Bentley epiphysial injury
 prognosis classification
Chadwick sign
chain
        lymphatic c.
        obturator lymphatic c.
        recurrent nerve lymphatic c.
    c. suture technique
chain-of-lakes
    c.-o.-l. deformity
    c.-o.-l. filling defect
    c.-o.-l. sign
challenge
        methacholine bronchoprovocation c.
Chamberlain
    C. mediastinoscopy
    C. mediastinoscopy procedure
2-chamber longitudinal (2C-L)
chamber rupture
Chambers osteotomy
4-chamber transverse (4C-T)
5-chamber transverse (5C-T)
chamfer preparation
Chance
    C. fracture thoracolumbar
      spine
    C. vertebral fracture
chancre
        hard c.
        mixed c.
        monorecidive c.
    c. redux
        soft c.
chancriform
chancroid
chandelier sign

Chandler
    C. hip fusion
    C. iridectomy
    C. vitreous operation
Chandler-Verhoeff
    C.-V. lens extraction
    C.-V. vitreous operation
change
    aging degenerative c.
    degenerative c.
    diffuse c.
    emphysematous c.
    fibrocystic c.
    fractional area c. (FAC)
    hemodynamic c.
    Hürthle cell c.
    ischemic mesenteric c.
    metabolic c.
    mitral valve prolapse, aortic
      anomalies, skeletal changes, skin
      c.'s (MASS)
    morphologic c.
    motor c.
    multifocal c.
    muscular c.
    nail c.
    neurocognitive c.
    onion bulb c.'s
    parenchymal c.
    physiologic c.
    c. point
    postradiation c.
    postsurgical motor c.
    postthoracotomy c.
    sepsis-induced metabolic c.
    supraesophageal reflux c.'s
    surgical c.
Chang-Miltner incision
Chang needle
channel
    c. activity
    c. and core biopsy
    cardiac inward rectifier K+ c.
    c. diagnosis
    intramammary lymphatic c.
    ligand-gated cation c.
    ligand-gated ion c.
    lymphatic c.
    N-type voltage-sensitive
      calcium c.
    open venous c.
    c. shoulder pin technique
    sympathetic efferent output c.
    venous c.
    voltage-gated ion c.
Chaput
    C. anal operation
    C. fracture
    C. tibial operation

characteristic
  clinical c.
  heterogeneity c.
  histologic c.
  pathologic c.
  c. radiation
Charcot
  C. triad
  C. triangle
charged-particle irradiation
Charles
  C. lensectomy
  C. lymphedema debulking
    procedure
  C. operation
Charnley
  C. compression
  C. compression arthrodesis
  C. compression-type knee fusion
  C. incision
  C. total hip arthroplasty
Charrière catheter size scale
Charters
char-zone depth
chasm
Chassaignac
  C. space
  C. tubercle
Chassar
  C. Moir pubovaginal sling procedure
  C. Moir-Sims urinary fistula repair
    procedure
Chauffard point
chauffeur's fracture
Chaussier line
Chaves-Rapp muscle transfer technique
Chayes lost tooth replacement method
CHCT
  caffeine-halothane contracture test
Cheatle
  C. slit
  C. syndrome
Cheatle-Henry hernia
checklist
  Non-Communicating Children's Pain
    C. (NCCPC)
  C. of Nonverbal Pain Indicators
    (CNPI)
  Rotterdam Symptom C.
  Symptom C. 90 (SCL90)
checkrein deformity
cheek
  c. advancement flap
  c. bone
  c. muscle
  c. rotation flap
cheesy necrosis
cheilectomy, chilectomy
  Garceau c.

  Mann-Coughlin-DuVries c.
  Sage-Clark c.
cheilion
cheiloangioscopy, chiloangioscopy
cheiloplasty, chiloplasty
  Bernard-Burlow c.
cheilorrhaphy, chilorrhaphy
cheilostomatoplasty, chilostomatoplasty
cheilotomy, chilotomy
cheiroplasty, chiroplasty
chemexfoliation
chemical
  c. arachnoiditis
  c. disinfection
  c. enzymatic wound débridement
  c. exchange
  c. exposure
  c. hemostasis
  c. hypophysectomy
  c. litholysis
  c. matrixectomy
  c. peel
  c. peritonitis
  c. pneumonitis
  c. rhizolysis
  c. sedation
  c. splanchnicectomy
  c. sympathectomy
  c. thrombectomy
  c. tourniquet
  c. vapor sterilization
chemicocautery
chemiluminescence, chemoluminescence
chemiluminescent
chemo
  chemotherapy
chemoactivation
chemoattraction
  fibroblast c.
chemocautery
chemocoagulation
chemodectoma
chemoembolization
  arterial c.
  intraarterial c.
  transarterial c. (TACE)
chemoluminescence (*var. of*
  chemiluminescence)
chemolysis
  intrarenal c.
chemoneurolysis
  glycerol c.
  percutaneous retrogasserian glycerol
    c.
chemonucleolysis
  chymopapain c.
  double-needle c.
chemopallidectomy
chemopallidothalamectomy

chemopallidotomy
chemoprevention
  c. agent
  medical c.
chemopreventive agent
chemoprophylaxis
chemoradiation
  neoadjuvant c.
chemoradiotherapy
  c. effect
  preoperative c.
chemoreceptor trigger zone
chemoreflex
chemosensitive
chemosensitization
chemosterilization
chemostimulation
chemosurgery
chemosurgical gingivectomy
chemotactic property
chemotaxis assay
chemothalamectomy
chemothalamotomy
chemotherapeutic
  c. scheme
  c. treatment
chemotherapist
chemotherapy (chemo)
  adjunctive c.
  adjuvant c.
  combination c.
  concurrent c.
  induction c.
  infusional c.
  initial systemic c.
  intraarterial c.
  intraperitoneal hyperthermic c.
  intravesical c.
  postoperative systemic c.
  preoperative induction c.
  preoperative systemic c.
  c. protocol
  second-line c.
  systemic c.
chemotherapy-associated steatohepatitis
CHEOPS
  Children's Hospital of Eastern Ontario
  Pain Scale
Cherney
  C. lower transverse abdominal
    incision
  C. suture technique
cherry angioma
chessboard graft
chest
  c. anomaly
  c. binder
  c. compression
  c. computed tomography

  c. deformity
  c. examination
  flail c.
  flat c.
  c. index
  c. lesion
  c. physical therapy
  pneumonectomy c.
  c. port
  c. reopening
  stove-in c.
  c. tube drainage (CTD)
  c. tube output (CTO)
  c. wall
  c. wall compliance
  c. wall fixation
  c. wall invasion
  c. wall irradiation
  c. wall reconstruction
  c. wall rigidity
  c. wall stabilization
  c. x-ray (CXR)
Chester-Winter urinary stress
  incontinence repair procedure
chevron
  c. bunionectomy
  c. hallux valgus correction
  c. incision
  c. laceration
  c. osteotomy
  c. technique
chevron-shaped incision
chevron-type transmalleolar
  osteotomy
chewing method
chew-in technique
Cheyne antiseptic operation
Cheyne-Stokes respiration
CHF
  congestive heart failure
CHI
  closed head injury
Chiari
  C. anomaly
  C. I–III malformation
  C. II syndrome
  C. innominate osteotomy
  C. pelvis osteotomy
    technique
Chiari-Salter-Steel pelvic osteotomy
chiasm, chiasma, (Xa) *pl.* **chiasmata**
  Camper c.
  c. formation
chiasmal
  c. compression
  c. lesion
  c. metastasis
chiasmapexy
chiasmata (Xta) (*pl. of* chiasm, chiasma)

chiasmatic
    c. cistern
    c. cisterna
    c. groove
    c. sulcus
chiasmatis
Chicago human chromosome classification
chicken fat clot
Chiene incision
child, *pl.* **children**
    Children's Cancer Study Group
        (CCSG)
    C. classification of cirrhosis
    children's coma scale
    C. esophageal varix classification
    Faces Rating Scale for Children
    C. hepatic dysfunction classification
    C. hepatic risk criteria classification
    Children's Hospital of Eastern
        Ontario Pain Scale (CHEOPS)
    C. liver disease classification
    C. operation
    C. pancreatoduodenostomy
    C. radical pancreatectomy
    Children's Revised Impact of Event
        Scale (CRIES)
childbirth
    Kitzinger method of c.
childhood thyroid irradiation
Child-Pugh
    C.-P. chronic liver disease score
    C.-P. liver disease classification
children (*pl. of* child)
Childress ankle fixation technique
Childs-Phillips bowel plication
Child-Turcotte hepatic surgery
  classification
chilectomy (*var. of* cheilectomy)
chiloangioscopy (*var. of* cheiloangioscopy)
chiloplasty (*var. of* cheiloplasty)
chilorrhaphy (*var. of* cheilorrhaphy)
chilostomatoplasty (*var. of*
  cheilostomatoplasty)
chilotomy (*var. of* cheilotomy)
chimera
    radiation c.
chimerism
chimney sweep's carcinoma
chin
    c. augmentation
    double c.
    c. elevation
    c. muscle
    c. position
Chinese
    C. fingertrap suture
    C. radial forearm flap
chip
    bone c.

    c. fracture
    c. graft
    C. scale
CHIP
    Coping with Health, Injuries, and
        Problems
chiral asymmetry
chirality
chiroplasty (*var. of* cheiroplasty)
chiropractic treatment of fracture
chisel fracture
chlamydial infection
Chlamydia trachomatis **infection**
chloramine T technique
ChloraPrep skin preparation
chlorhexidine gluconate skin
  preparation
chlorine (Cl)
chloroform
4-chloro-m-cresol test
2-chloroprocaine
chloroprocaine-related neurotoxicity
Cho
    C. anterior cruciate ligament
        reconstruction
    C. tendon technique
choana, *pl.* **choanae**
choanae (*pl. of* choana)
chocolate cyst
cholangeitis (*var. of* cholangitis)
cholangiectasis
cholangiocarcinoma
    hilar c.
    hilar bile duct c.
    intrahepatic c.
    perihilar c.
cholangioenterostomy
cholangiofibroma
cholangiofibrosis
cholangiogastrostomy
cholangiogram
    common duct c.
    false-negative c.
    intraoperative c. (IOC)
    preoperative retrograde c.
    retrograde c.
cholangiographic
    c. interpretation
    c. technique
cholangiography
    completion c.
    drip infusion c.
    endoscopic retrograde c.
    infusion c.
    intraoperative dynamic c.
    magnetic resonance imaging c.
    MRI c.
    operative c.
    percutaneous transhepatic c.

cholangiohepatitis
    Oriental c.
    recurrent pyogenic c.
cholangiole
cholangioma
cholangiopancreatography
    endoscopic retrograde c. (ERCP)
    magnetic resonance c. (MRCP)
cholangiopancreatoscopy
    peroral c. (PCPS)
cholangiopathy
cholangioplasty
cholangioscopy
    3-dimensional virtual c.
    intraductal c.
    percutaneous transhepatic c.
    peroral c. (PCS)
cholangiostomy
cholangiotomy
cholangitis, cholangeitis
    c. carcinoma
    primary sclerosing c. (PSC)
cholecyst
cholecystectasia
cholecystectomy
    combined laparoscopic splenectomy and c.
    laparoscopic c. (lap chole)
    laparoscopic laser c.
    laser laparoscopic c.
    microlaparoscopic c.
    minilaparoscopic c.
    needlescopic laparoscopic c.
    open c.
    percutaneous c.
    prophylactic c.
    retrograde c.
    surgical c.
    transcylindrical c.
    c. treatment
    2-trocar laparoscopic c.
    3-trocar technique c.
cholecystenteric fistula
cholecystenteroanastomosis
cholecystenterorrhaphy
cholecystenterostomy
cholecystenterotomy
cholecystic
cholecystis
cholecystitis
    acalculous c.
    acute acalculous c. (AAC)
    acute calculous c.
    asymptomatic c.
    calculous c.
    chronic c.
    emphysematous c.
    erythromycin-induced c.
    follicular c.
    gangrenous c.
    gaseous c.
    perforated c.
    scleroatrophic c.
    suppurative c.
    typhoidal c.
    uncomplicated acute c.
    xanthogranulomatous c.
cholecystobiliary fistulation
cholecystocholangiography
cholecystocholedochal fistula
cholecystocholedocholithiasis
cholecystocolic fistula
cholecystocolonic fistula
cholecystocolostomy
cholecystoduodenal
    c. fistula
    c. ligament
cholecystoduodenocolic
    c. fistula
    c. fold
cholecystoduodenostomy
cholecystoendoprosthesis
    endoscopic retrograde c.
cholecystoenterostomy
    direct c.
cholecystogastrostomy
cholecystoileostomy
cholecystojejunostomy
cholecystokinin secretion
cholecystolithiasis
cholecystolithotomy
    percutaneous c.
cholecystolithotripsy
cholecystomy
cholecystopaque
cholecystopexy
    Czerny c.
cholecystorrhaphy
cholecystoscopy
    percutaneous transhepatic c.
cholecystostomy
    percutaneous c.
    surgical c.
    c. tube
cholecystotomy, cholecystomy
    laparoscopic c.
    transpapillary endoscopic c.
choledochal
    c. basal pressure
    c. cyst
    c. cyst disease
    c. region
    c. sphincter
choledochal-colonic fistula
choledochectomy
choledochendysis
choledochocele

choledochocholedochostomy side-to-side anastomosis
choledochocolonic fistula
choledochoduodenal
    c. fistula
    c. fistulotomy
    c. junction
    c. junctional stenosis
choledochoduodenostomy
choledochoenteric fistula
choledochoenterostomy
choledochofiberoscopy
    T-tube tract c.
choledochogastrostomy
choledochohepatostomy
choledochoileostomy
choledochojejunostomy (CDJ)
    Allen c.
    end-to-side c.
    laparoscopic Roux-en-Y c.
    loop c.
    retrocolic end-to-side c.
    Roux-en-Y c.
choledocholith
choledocholithiasis
choledocholithotomy
choledocholithotripsy
choledochopancreatic ductal junction
choledochoplasty
choledochorrhaphy
choledochoscopy
    Berci-Shore c.
    cystic duct c.
    jejunostomy tract c.
    operative c.
    postoperative c.
    transcystic c.
    T-tube tract c.
choledochostomy
choledochotomy
    c. incision
    laparoscopic common bile duct exploration c.
    longitudinal c.
choledochous
choledochus
cholelith, chololith
cholelithiasis, chololithiasis
cholelitholysis
cholelithotomy
cholelithotripsy, cholelithotrity
cholelithotrity (*var. of* cholelithotripsy)
cholescintigraphy
cholestasis
cholestatic
    c. cause
    c. cirrhosis
    c. jaundice

cholesteatoma
    pars flaccida c.
    c. pearl
cholesterol
    c. calculus
    c. embolus
    c. saturation index
    c. solitaire
    c. stone
cholicele
cholinergic
    c. blockade
    c. mechanism
    c. tract
chololith (*var. of* cholelith)
chololithiasis (*var. of* cholelithiasis)
chondral
    c. edge
    c. fracture
    c. fragment
chondrectomy
chondrification
chondritis
    xiphisternal junction c.
chondrocostal
chondrodermatitis
    nodular c.
chondroepiphysis
chondroglossus muscle
chondrolysis
    posttraumatic c.
chondromalacia patellae (CMP, CP)
chondromyofibroma
chondromyxofibroma
chondromyxoma
chondroosseous
chondroosteodystrophy
chondropharyngeus
chondrophyte
chondroplasty
    abrasion c.
    arthroscopic abrasion c.
chondroporosis
chondrosarcoma
chondrosteoma
chondrosternal
chondrosternoplasty
chondrotomy
chondroxiphoid ligament
chop amputation
Chopart
    C. amputation
    C. ankle dislocation
    C. articulation
chorda, *pl.* **chordae**
    chordae tendineae (CT)
    chordae tendineae rupture

C

chorda (*continued*)
    c. tympani
    c. tympani nerve
chordae (*pl. of* chorda)
chordal
    c. rupture
    c. shortening
chordee removal
chord incision
chordoblastoma
chordotomy
chorioadenoma
chorioallantoic membrane
chorioamnionic infection
chorioangioma
chorioblastoma
choriocapillaris
choriocarcinoma
choriocele
chorioepithelioma
chorioma
chorion
chorionic
    c. cavity
    c. sac
    c. villus biopsy
chorioretinitis
choristoblastoma
choristoma nest
choroid
    c. plexus
    c. plexus carcinoma
    c. plexus papilloma
    c. point
    c. vein
choroidal
    c. artery
    c. hemangioma
    c. hemorrhage
    c. infiltration
    c. lesion
    c. metastasis
    c. neovascularization
    c. neovascular membrane
    c. ring
    c. rupture
choroidectomy
choroiditis
choroidocapillaris
Chow endoscopic carpal tunnel release technique
CHPP
    continuous hyperthermic peritoneal perfusion
Chrisman-Snook
    C.-S. ankle ligament reconstruction
    C.-S. ankle technique
    C.-S. lateral ankle reconstruction procedure

Christmas
    C. disease
    C. tree deformity
chromaffin
    c. body
    c. tissue
chromated catgut suture
chromatic lens aberration
chromatin condensation
chromatinic body
chromatography
    gas c.
chromic
    c. blue dyed suture
    c. catgut suture
    c. collagen suture
    c. gut suture
    c. suture
chromicized catgut suture
chromocystoscopy
chromohydrotubation
chromopertubation (CPT)
chromoscopy
chromotubation
chronic
    c. allograft rejection
    c. anoplasty treatment
    c. anticoagulation therapy
    c. appendicitis
    c. atrial fibrillation
    c. catheterization
    c. cholecystitis
    c. course
    c. daily headache
    c. dialysis catheter
    c. digestive bleeding
    c. Epstein-Barr virus infection
    c. extrinsic alveolitis
    c. graft-versus-host disease
    c. granular myringitis
    c. hemolysis
    c. hyperparathyroid state
    c. hyperventilation syndrome
    c. inflammatory demyelinating polyradiculoneuropathy (CIDP)
    c. intestinal failure
    c. intestinal pseudoobstruction syndrome
    c. jejunal inflammation
    c. liver disease
    c. mesenteric ischemia
    c. motor disturbance
    c. multisystem disorder
    c. nonmalignant
    c. nonmalignant pain (CNMP)
    c. nonprogressive headache
    c. nonterminal pain

c. obstructive airways disease (COAD)
c. obstructive pulmonary dysfunction
c. opioid analgesic therapy (COAT)
c. pain disorder
c. pancreatitis
c. paroxysmal hemicrania (CPH)
c. postsurgical pain (CPSP)
c. presentation
c. progressive headache
c. prostatitis/chronic pelvic pain syndrome, types IIIA and IIIB (CP/CPPS)
c. reflux symptom
c. renal failure
c. sinusitis
c. stenosis
c. subareolar abscess
c. subcutaneous infusion
c. subdural hematoma
c. thrombosis
c. transplant rejection
c. ulcerative colitis (CUC)
c. upper airways obstruction
c. venous insufficiency (CVI)
c. widespread pain

chronicity
chronification
chronotropic insufficiency
Chuinard-Peterson ankle fusion
chylangioma
chyle

c. cistern
c. cyst
c. fistula
c. leak
c. vessel

chylifera
chyliform ascites
chylocyst
chyloma
chylopericardium
chyloperitoneum
chylosus
chylothorax
chylous

c. ascites
c. ascitic fluid
c. effusion
c. hydrotherapy
c. leak
c. leakage

chyme, chymus
chymopapain chemonucleolysis
chymus (*var. of* chyme)
CI

cardiac index
normal CI
supranormal CI

Cibis

C. liquid silicone retinal detachment procedure
C. retinal detachment operation

cicatrectomy
cicatrices (*pl. of* cicatrix)
cicatriceum
cicatricial

c. entropion
c. kidney
c. mass
c. obliteration
c. stricture
c. tissue

cicatricotomy, cicatrisotomy
cicatrisotomy (*var. of* cicatricotomy)
cicatrix, *pl.* **cicatrices**
cicatrizant
cicatrization
CIDP

chronic inflammatory demyelinating polyradiculoneuropathy

Cierny-Mader single-stage osteomyelitis repair technique
ciliarotomy
ciliary

c. artery
c. beat frequency
c. body
c. body band
c. canal
c. ganglion
c. ganglion root
c. injection
c. ligament
c. nerve
c. procedure
c. process
c. ring
c. vein
c. zone
c. zonule

ciliectomy
ciliodestructive surgery
cilioretinal artery
ciliotomy
ciliovitrectomy block
cilostazol
Cimino-Brescia arteriovenous fistula
Cimino fistula
cinacalcet
cinching operation
Cincinnati

C. incision
C. pelvic osteotomy technique

Cinderella hypothesis
cineangiography

biplane c.

cinedefecography

C

cine-esophagoscopy
cinefluoroscopic method
cinefluoroscopy
    valve c.
cinegastroscopy
cinerei
    arteria tuberis c.
cinereum
    artery of tuber c.
cine view
cingulate
    c. cortex
    c. herniation
    c. sulcus
cingulectomy (*var. of* cingulotomy)
cingulotomy, cingulectomy,
  cingulumotomy
    rostral c.
cingulum bundle
cingulumotomy (*var. of*
  cingulotomy)
CIPN
    critical illness polyneuropathy
CIPNM
    critical illness polyneuropathy and
    myopathy
circinate exudate
circle
    c. absorption anesthesia
    arterial cerebral c.
    articular vascular c.
    Bain c.
    c. breathing system
    closed c.
    c. dissipation
    Huguier c.
    c. loop biliary drainage
    Pagenstecher c.
    pediatric c.
    semiclosed c.
    c. straight cutting
    c. system
    c. system test
    vascular c.
    c. wire nephrostomy
circuit
    ancillary c.
    anesthesia breathing c.
    anesthetic c.
    Bain c.
    breathing c.
    extracorporeal cardiopulmonary c.
    feedback reduction c. (FRC)
    heparin-bonded cardiopulmonary
     bypass c.
    heparin-coated c.
    low-flow c.
    low-prime c.
    ventilation c.

circuitry
    intrinsic c.
circular
    c. anastomosis
    c. cherry-red lesion
    c. fold
    c. griseotomy
    c. incision
    c. myotomy
    c. open amputation
    c. pharyngeal muscle
    c. suture
    c. suture technique
    c. venous sinus
circulating
    c. air pocket
    c. blood
    c. hormone
circulation
    abdominal c.
    airway, breathing, c. (ABC)
    allantoic c.
    c. aneurysm
    arterial c.
    assisted c.
    bile acid c.
    bronchial c.
    carotid c.
    cerebral c.
    collateral abdominal c.
    collateral arterial c.
    collateral mesenteric c.
    compensatory c.
    conjunctival c.
    coronary collateral c.
    cutaneous collateral c.
    derivative c.
    ductal-dependent pulmonary c.
    enterohepatic c.
    episcleral c.
    extracorporeal c. (ECC)
    extracranial carotid c.
    femoral c.
    fetal c.
    fetoplacental c.
    hepatic c.
    hyperdynamic c.
    hypophysial portal c.
    hypothalamic-hypophysial portal c.
    intracranial c.
    left dominant coronary c.
    mesenteric c.
    perichondral c.
    peripheral c.
    persistent fetal c.
    placental c.
    portal-collateral c.
    portal-hypophysial c.
    portosystemic collateral c.

posterior fossa c.
pulmonary c.
c. rate
retinal c.
sludging of c.
spinal cord c.
splanchnic c.
submucosal collateral c.
systemic venous c.
thalamic c.
thebesian c.
c. time
umbilical c.
uteroplacental c.
venous c.
c. volume
circulator fold
circulatory
    c. arrest
    c. arrest anesthetic technique
    c. arrest procedure
    c. decompensation
    c. overload
    c. steal
circuli (*pl. of* circulus)
circulus, *pl.* **circuli**
    c. venous
circumalveolar fixation
circumanal gland
circumareolar
    c. incision
    c. mastopexy
    c. quadrant
circumaxillary
circumbulbar
circumcise
circumcision
    pharaonic c.
    Sunna c.
    c. suture technique
circumcisional suture
circumcorneal injection
circumcostal gastropexy
circumduction maneuver
circumference
    fetal head c.
    lung-to-head c.
circumferentia
circumferential
    c. esophageal reconstruction
    c. esophagomyotomy
    c. fibrocartilage
    c. fracture
    c. implantation
    c. incision
    c. mesorectal excision
    c. mobilization
    c. mucosal dissection
    c. strip

c. venolysis
c. wire-loop fixation
circumferentially ligated
circumflex
    c. femoral artery
    c. humeral artery
    c. iliac artery
    c. nerve
    c. scapular artery
    c. vein
circumflexus
circumintestinal
circumlental space
circumlimbal incision
circumlinear incision
circummandibular fixation
circummesencephalic cistern
circumocular
circumorbital
circumrenal
circumscribed
    c. inflammation
    c. mass
circumscribing incision
circumumbilical
    c. incision
    c. pyloromyotomy
circumvallate papilla
circumvascular
circumzygomatic fixation
cirrhosis
    alcoholic c.
    autoimmune c.
    biliary c.
    Child classification of c.
    cholestatic c.
    cryptogenic c.
    end-stage c.
    nonalcoholic c.
    primary biliary c.
    viral c.
cirrhotic
    c. liver
    c. liver parenchyma
    c. liver remnant
cirsectomy
cirsodesis
cirsotomy
CIS
    carcinoma in situ
cisatracurium
CISC
    clean intermittent self-catheterization
CISH
    classic intrafascial Semm hysterectomy
cistern
    basal c.
    cerebellomedullary c.
    cerebellopontine angle c.

C

cistern (*continued*)
    chiasmatic c.
    chyle c.
    circummesencephalic c.
    interpeduncular c.
    lumbar c.
    mesencephalic c.
    Pecquet c.
    perimesencephalic c.
    pontine c.
    prepontine c.
    quadrigeminal c.
    Stookey-Scarff opening from third
      ventricular to prechiasmal and
      interpeduncular c.
    subarachnoid c.
    suprasellar subarachnoid c.
    sylvian c.
cisterna, *pl.* cisternae
    ambient c.
    c. caryothecae
    chiasmatic c.
    cylindrical confronting c.
    c. magna
    perinuclear c.
    subsarcolemma c.
    terminal c.
cisternae (*pl. of* cisterna)
cisternal
    c. herniation
    c. puncture
citrate
    c. intoxication
    oral transmucosal fentanyl c.
    c. toxicity
Civinini
    C. ligament
    C. process
CKC
    cold knife cone
    cold knife conization
2C-L
    2-chamber longitudinal
Cl
    chlorine
Clado
    C. anastomosis
    C. band
    C. ligament
    C. point
Clagett
    C. closure
    C. empyema technique
    C. operation
Clagett-Barrett esophagogastrostomy
Clairmont approach
clam
    c. enterocystoplasty
    c. ileocystoplasty

clamp
    air detector c.
    Block-Potts bowel c.
    bone-holding c.
    Cooley c.
    c. crushing technique
    intracorporeal c.
    Kocher c.
    Kumar cholangiography c.
    Satinsky c.
clamp-and-sew technique
clamping
    aortic c.
    blind c.
    carotid c.
    portal triad c.
    selective vascular c. (SVC)
clamshell
    c. closure
    c. incision
    c. technique
    c. thoracotomy
Clancy
    C. cruciate ligament reconstruction
    C. ligament technique
    C. patellar tendon graft
    C. peroneal tenodesis procedure
CLAP
    contact laser ablation of prostate
Clapton line
Clark
    C. level
    C. transfer technique
Clark-Southwick-Odgen odontoid fracture
modification
CLASP
    Carolinas Laparoscopic Advanced
    Surgery Program
      CLASP minimal access surgery
      procedure
clasped thumb deformity
classic
    c. abdominal Semm hysterectomy
    c. DSRS technique
    c. intrafascial Semm hysterectomy
    (CISH)
    c. multiple organ failure syndrome
classical
    c. cesarean section
    c. Judd-Mayo overlap midline
    incisional hernioplasty
    c. subtotal resection
    c. transverse incision
classification
    Acosta endometriosis c.
    acromioclavicular injury c.
    Aitken epiphysial fracture c.
    AJCC TNM tumor c.
    Allman acromioclavicular injury c.

Alonso-Lej choledochal cyst c.
American Association for Surgery
of Trauma Organ Injury Scale c.
American Heart Association c.
American Society of
Anesthesiologists c.
American Society of
Anesthesiologists Physical Status
C. (ASAPSC)
Anderson-D'Alonzo odontoid
fracture c.
Anderson modification of
Berndt-Harty osteochondral talar
lesion c.
Angle malocclusion c.
Ann Arbor Hodgkin disease c.
AO c.
Arbeitsgemeinschaft für
Osteosynthesefragen c.
Arneth polymorphonuclear
neutrophil c.
Ashhurst-Bromer ankle fracture c.
Astler-Coller (A, B1, B2, C1, C2)
colorectal carcinoma c.
Astler-Coller modification of
Dukes c.
Bado Monteggia fracture c.
Bailyn c.
Banff renal allograft rejection c.
Bauer-Jackson traumatic chondral
lesion c.
Baume dental c.
bellows c.
Bennett c.
Bergey bacteria c.
Berndt-Harty osteochondral talar
lesion c.
Binet system of leukemia c.
BI-RADS abnormal mammogram
management c.
Bishop c.
Bismuth benign bile duct
stricture c.
Bismuth bile duct stricture (type
I-V) c.
Bismuth-Strasberg biliary injury
(type A-E) c.
Black carious lesion c.
bladder carcinoma c.
Borrmann gastric cancer
(type I–IV) c.
Bosniak renal cystic disease c.
Boyd c.
Boyd-Griffin trochanteric fracture c.
Breslow melanoma thickness c.
Broders index of malignant
tumor c.
burn c.
Butchart mesothelioma staging c.

Caldwell-Moloy pelvis type c.
Callender cell-type c.
Cambridge pancreatitis c.
Canadian Cardiovascular Society c.
(CCSC)
caries c.
Carnesale-Stewart-Barnes hip
dislocation c.
Caroli-Sarles bile duct stricture c.
Catterall of Perthe disease c.
cavity c.
Cedars-Sinai corneal topography c.
Centers for Disease Control HIV
infection c.
Chadwick-Bentley epiphysial injury
prognosis c.
Chicago human chromosome c.
Child esophageal varix c.
Child hepatic dysfunction c.
Child hepatic risk criteria c.
Child liver disease c.
Child-Pugh liver disease c.
Child-Turcotte hepatic surgery c.
clean-contaminated operative
wound c.
clean operative wound c.
cleft palate c.
clinical pathologic c.
Codman postoperative death c.
Cohen-Rentrop cardiac collateral
blood flow c.
Colonna hip fracture c.
Colton olecranon fracture c.
contaminated operative wound c.
Cori glycogen storage disease c.
Correa gastritis c.
Couinaud liver anatomy c.
Croften eosinophilic lung disease c.
Crowe hip dysplasia c.
Cummer partial denture c.
Cutler breast cancer c.
Dagradi esophageal variceal c.
Danis-Weber ankle injury c.
DeBakey aortic dissection c.
DeLee pediatric fracture c.
Denis Browne spinal fracture c.
denture c.
Denver human mitotic
chromosome c.
Dexter-Grossman aortic
regurgitation c.
Diamond c.
Dias-Tachdijian physical injury c.
dichotomous c.
Dickhaut-DeLee discoid meniscus c.
dirty operative wound c.
Dripps operative risk c.
Duane exodeviation c.
Dubin-Amelar varicocele c.

C

classification (*continued*)

Dukes colorectal carcinoma c.
Eckert-Davis peroneal tendon subluxation c.
Edmondson-Steiner hepatocellular carcinoma c.
Ellis tooth fracture c.
Enneking benign tumor c.
Epstein hip dislocation c.
Epstein-Thomas c.
Essex-Lopresti calcaneal fracture c.
Evans intertrochanteric fracture c.
FAB acute leukemia c.
Fielding femoral fracture c.
Fielding-Magliato subtrochanteric fracture c.
Flatt upper extremity congenital anomaly c.
Foucher epiphysial injury c.
fracture c.
Fränkel neurologic deficit c.
Frantz-O'Rahilly limb defect c.
Fredrickson hyperlipoproteinemia c.
Fredrickson-Levy-Lees hyperlipoproteinemia c.
Freeman calcaneal fracture c.
French-American-British acute leukemia c.
Frykman distal radius fracture c.
Frykman radial fracture c.
functional capacity c.
Garden femoral neck fracture c.
Gartland humeral supracondylar fracture c.
Gartland Universal radial fracture c.
gastric mucosal pattern c.
Geenen-Hogan unexplained biliary symptoms c.
Gell and Coombs drug allergy c.
Goldman diagnostic discrepancy c.
Grantham femur fracture c.
Greenfield spinocerebellar ataxia c.
Gustilo-Anderson open fracture c.
Gustilo puncture wound c.
Haggitt colorectal polyp and invasive carcinoma c.
Hannover chronic rejection c.
Hansen fracture c.
Hara gallbladder inflammation c.
Hardcastle tarsometatarsal joint injury c.
Hawkins talar fracture c.
Henderson functional results c.
hepatitis activity index c.
Herring lateral pillar radiographic c.
Hinchey diverticulitis grade c.
HIV c.
Hohl-Luck tibial plateau fracture c.
Hohl tibial condylar fracture c.

Holdsworth spinal fracture c.
House-Brackmann facial nerve injury c.
Hughston knee injury c.
human immunodeficiency virus c.
Hunt and Kosnik cerebral aneurysm c.
Ideberg glenoid fracture c.
immunologic c.
Insall patellar injury c.
International Cancer of Cervix C.
International Federation of Gynecology and Obstetrics c.
Isaacson gastric lymphoma c.
Jackson and Parker Hodgkin disease c.
Jansky blood type c.
Japanese cancer c.
Jeffery radial fracture c.
Jensen trochanteric fracture c.
Jewett and Whitmore prostate cancer c.
Johner-Wruhs tibial fracture c.
Jones-Barnes-Lloyd-Roberts c.
Kajava supernumerary breast tissue c.
Kalamchi avascular necrosis c.
Karnofsky performance rating scale c.
Kasugai pancreatitis c.
Kauffman-White Salmonella serotype c.
Keil tumor cell c.
Keith-Wagener retinal changes c.
Kelami penile curvature c.
Kellam-Waddel tibial plafond fracture c.
Kennedy partially edentulous c.
Kernohan system of glioma c.
KESS constipation scoring system c.
Key-Conwell pelvic fracture c.
Kiel c.
Kilfoyle humeral medial condylar fracture c.
Killip-Kimball heart failure c.
Killip myocardial infarct c.
Knowles-Eccersley-Scott Symptom constipation scoring system c.
Kocher humerus fracture c.
Kyle-Gustilo femoral fracture c.
Kyle-Gustilo-Premer dynamic hip screw fixation c.
Lancefield hemolytic Streptococcus c.
Lanza scale for drug-induced mucosal damage c.
Lauge-Hansen ankle fracture c.
Lauren gastric carcinoma c.
Le Fort facial fracture c.

Leishman hypertensive retinopathy c.
Lennert non-Hodgkin lymphoma c.
Letournel-Judet acetabular fracture c.
Leung thumb loss c.
Levine-Harvey cardiac auscultation c.
Lindell blanisotropic media c.
Lloyd-Roberts-Catteral-Salamon bone
  dysplasia c.
Loesche periodontal disease c.
Lown arrhythmia c.
Lukes and Butler Hodgkin
  disease c.
Lukes-Collins lymphoma c.
MacCallan trachoma c.
Macewen avascular necrosis c.
MacNicol-Voutsinas posterior tibial
  tear c.
malignant tumor c.
Mallampati pharyngeal visibility c.
Marseille pancreatitis c.
Mason radial head fracture c.
Mast-Spieghel-Pappas long bone
  fracture c.
Mathews olecranon fracture c.
Mayo carpal instability c.
Mayo rheumatoid elbow c.
McNeer gastric carcinoma c.
Melone distal radius fracture c.
Meyers-McKeever tibial fracture c.
microinvasive carcinoma c.
Milch condylar fracture c.
Milch elbow fracture c.
Milch humeral fracture c.
Ming gastric carcinoma c.
Minnesota EKG c.
Moore tibial plateau fracture c.
morphologic c.
Moss blood group c.
Mueller femoral supracondylar
  fracture c.
Mueller tibial fracture c.
multiaxial c.
Munro and Parker laparoscopic
  hysterectomy c.
Nalebuff swan-neck deformity c.
Neer femur fracture c.
Neer shoulder fracture c.
Newman radial neck and head
  fracture c.
New York Heart Association heart
  disease c.
Nicoll spinal fracture c.
Niemeier gallbladder perforation c.
Nyhus inguinal hernia c.
Ogden epiphysial fracture c.
Ogden knee dislocation c.
O'Rahilly limb deficiency c.
ordinal c.
Orthopaedic Trauma Association c.

Outerbridge chondral knee
  lesion c.
Paley fibular hemimelia c.
Papavasiliou olecranon fracture c.
Pap smear c.
Paris endoscopic superficial
  neoplastic lesion c.
Pauwels femoral neck fracture c.
Pell-Gregory tooth position c.
Pennal pelvic fracture c.
Pipkin femoral fracture c.
Pipkin posterior hip dislocation c.
Pipkin subclassification of
  Epstein-Thomas c.
Poland epiphysial fracture c.
Poland physical injury c.
Potter polycystic kidney c.
Pugh-Child bleeding esophageal
  varices grading scale c.
Pugh liver disease c.
Pulec and Freedman congenital ear
  abnormality c.
Quénu-Küss tarsometatarsal injury c.
Quinby pelvic fracture c.
Rai leukemia c.
Ranawat pneumatoid spondylitis c.
Ranson acute pancreatitis c.
Rappaport lymphoma c.
Rastelli ventricular septal defect c.
Rentrop cardiac collateral
  circulation c.
Riseborough-Radin intercondylar
  fracture c.
risk c.
Rockwood acromioclavicular
  injury c.
Rockwood clavicular fracture c.
Rosenthal nail injury c.
round-robin c.
Rowe calcaneal fracture c.
Rowe-Lowell hip dislocation c.
Rowe-Lowell system for
  fracture-dislocation c.
Ruedi-Allgower pilon fracture c.
Runyon nontuberculous
  mycobacteria c.
Russe c.
Russell-Taylor hip fracture c.
Rüter c.
Rutkow-Robbins-Gilbert inguinal
  hernia c.
Rutledge extended hysterectomy c.
Rye Hodgkin disease c.
Sage-Salvatore acromioclavicular
  joint injury c.
Saha shoulder muscle c.
Sakellarides calcaneal fracture c.
Salter epiphysial fracture c.
Salter-Harris epiphysial fracture c.

C

classification (*continued*)

Santiani-Stone pancreas head gunshot c.
Sassouni skeletal facial c.
Savary-Miller endoscopic reflux esophagitis c.
SBR breast cancer c.
scalar c.
Scarff-Bloom-Richardson breast cancer c.
Schatzker tibial plateau fracture c.
Scheie hypertensive retinopathy c.
Schuknecht age-related hearing loss c.
Seattle graft-versus-host disease c.
Seddon nerve injury c.
Seinsheimer femoral fracture c.
Severin radiographic residual hip dysplasia c.
Shaffer-Weiss central retinal vein occlusion c.
Shaher-Puddu coronary arterial anatomy c.
Shelton femoral fracture c.
Singh osteoporosis c.
Siurala gastritis c.
Skinner partially edentulous c.
Snyder SLAP lesion c.
Solcia gastric dysplasia c.
Sonnenberg c.
Sorbie calcaneal fracture c.
Spaulding sterilization of medical devices c.
Speed radial head fracture c.
Spetzler-Martin arteriovenous malformation c.
Stark cleft lip/palate c.
Steinbrocker arthritis functional c.
Stewart-Way bile duct injury c.
Strasberg laparoscopic biliary tract injury c.
Stulberg Legg-Calvé-Perthes disease c.
Suda papilla type I–III c.
Sunderland nerve injury c.
Swanson congenital limb anomalies c.
Sydney system gastritis c.
Tachdjian pediatric ankle fracture c.
Tessier facial cleft c.
Thomas body mass index and diastolic blood pressure c.
Thompson-Epstein femoral fracture c.
three-color concept of wound c.
Thrombolysis in Myocardial Infarction c.
Tile pelvic injury c.
TIMI c.

TNM c.
tongue thrust c.
Torg metatarsal fracture c.
Torode-Zieg pediatric pelvic fracture c.
Toronto pelvic fracture c.
Tronzo intertrochanteric fracture c.
Tscherne-Gotzen tibial fracture and soft tissue damage c.
Tscherne soft tissue injury in closed fracture c.
tumor, node, metastasis c.
UICC tumor c.
Veau congenital malformation of lip and palate c.
Venn-Watson polydactyly c.
Visick dysphagia c.
Vostal radial fracture c.
Wagner diabetic foot disease c.
Walter Reed HIV infection c.
Warren-Marshall gastritis c.
Wassel thumb duplication c.
Watanabe discoid meniscus c.
Watson-Jones tibial tubercle avulsion fracture c.
Weber-Danis ankle injury c.
Weber physical injury c.
Weiland osteomyelitis c.
Weissman intraoperative therapeutic intensity score c.
White diabetes mellitus in pregnancy c.
Whitehead gastritis c.
Whitmore-Jewett prostate cancer c.
WHO gastric carcinoma c.
Wiberg patellar c.
Wilkins radial fracture c.
Winquist femoral shaft fracture c.
Winquist-Hansen femoral fracture c.
Winter spastic hemiplegic cerebral palsy c.
Wolfe mammogram c.
World Health Organization c.
Yacoub and Radley-Smith congenital heart disease c.
Young pelvic fracture c.
Zickel fracture c.
Zlotsky-Ballard acromioclavicular injury c.
Zollinger hernia c.

claudication
neurogenic intermittent c.
Claudius
C. cell
C. fossa
claustral
claustrum
clavi (*pl. of* clavus)
clavicectomy

clavicle excision
clavicula
clavicular
    c. birth fracture
    c. branch
    c. epiphysis
    c. facet
    c. fracture aneurysm
    c. head
    c. incision
claviculectomy
claviculus
clavipectoral fascia
clavipectoralis
clavus, *pl.* clavi
clawfoot
claw hand
clawhand, claw hand
    Volkmann c.
clawing
clawtoe
clay
    c. pipe carcinoma
    c. shoveler's fracture
Clayton
    C. first metatarsophalangeal joint
      fusion procedure
    C. forefoot arthroplasty
    C. procedure with panmetatarsal
      head resection
CLE
    continuous lumbar epidural
clean
    c. case
    c. field
    c. intermittent catheterization
    c. intermittent self-catheterization
    c. operation
    c. operative wound classification
clean-catch collection method
clean-contaminated
    c.-c. case
    c.-c. field
    c.-c. operation
    c.-c. operative wound classification
    c.-c. surgery
cleaning solution
cleansing
    bowel c.
clear
    c. cell hepatocellular carcinoma
    c. cell hidradenoma
    c. effluent
    c. fluid
    c. liquid diet
    c. otorrhea
clearance
    elimination c.
    lactate c.

    mucociliary c.
    oncologic c.
    perfusion-limited c.
    c. technique
Cleasby iridectomy
cleavage
    c. fracture
    c. lesion
    c. line
    c. plane
cleft
    anal c.
    c. closure
    corneal c.
    facial c.
    c. hand deformity
    intradiscal c.
    Larrey c.
    c. lip
    c. lip deformity
    natal c.
    c. nose
    oblique facial c.
    c. palate
    c. palate classification
    pudendal c.
    residual c.
    soft palate c.
    subdural c.
    urogenital c.
cleidocostal
cleidocranial
cleidoepitrochlearis
cleidomastoideus
cleido-occipitalis
cleidotomy
Cleveland
    C. Clinic weighted scale
    C. procedure
Cleveland-Bosworth-Thompson technique
click
    dural c.
    sternal c.
clidal
clidocostal
clidocranial
clinch knot
clinic
    dialysis c.
    outpatient dialysis c.
clinical
    c. acute pancreatitis
    c. characteristic
    C. Classification System (CCS)
    c. correlation
    c. defect
    c. deterioration
    c. diagnosis
    c. encephalopathy

C

clinical (*continued*)
    c. evaluation
    c. evidence
    c. examination
    c. followup
    c. geneticist
    c. grading scale (CGS)
    c. implication
    c. improvement
    c. indication
    c. intestinal transplant
    c. jaundice
    c. manifestation
    c. manifestations, etiologic factors,
      anatomic involvement,
      pathophysiologic features (CEAP)
    c. outcome
    c. parameter
    c. pathologic classification
    c. pathology
    c. picture
    c. presentation
    c. principle
    c. problem
    c. response
    c. spectroscopy
    c. suspicion
    c. syndrome
clinically
    c. node-negative breast cancer
    c. severe obesity (CSO)
    c. silent rhabdomyoma
clinician
    nonsurgical c.
    surgical c.
clinicopathologic, clinicopathological
    c. correlation
    c. data
    c. factor
    c. feature
clinicopathological (*var. of*
  clinicopathologic)
Clinitron air-fluidized therapy
clinoidectomy
    anterior extradural c.
    extradural c.
clinoid process
clip
    c. application
    c. graft
    Hem-o-Lok c.
    c. migration
    c. occlusion
    c. placement
    c. technique
    titanium c.
clip-induced bile duct stricture
clitoral recession
clitoridectomy

clitorides (*pl. of* clitoris)
clitoris, *pl.* **clitorides**
    corpus clitoridis
    crus clitoridis
clitoroplasty
clitorovaginoplasty
clival
clivus
    Blumenbach c.
    c. canal line
    c. metastasis
    c. syndrome
CLO
    Campylobacter-like organism
    CLO biopsy
cloaca, *pl.* **cloacae**
cloacae (*pl. of* cloaca)
cloacal
    c. formation
    c. malformation
    c. membrane
clock
    around the c. (ATC)
clockwise
    c. direction
    c. rotation
clodronate
clomiphene fetal malformation
clonal
    c. deletion
    c. expansion
clonidine
C-loop intraocular lens
Cloquet
    C. canal
    C. canal remnant
    C. fascia
    C. hernia
    C. ligament
    C. node
    C. pseudoganglion
    C. septum
close
    c. margin
    c. monitoring
    c. proximity
closed
    c. anesthesia system
    c. approach
    c. break fracture
    c. chest commissurotomy
    c. chest thoracostomy
    c. circle
    c. circuit anesthesia
    c. circuit anesthetic technique
    c. circuit method
    c. dislocation
    c. flap amputation
    c. gloving technique

c. head injury (CHI)
c. hemorrhoidectomy
c. intramedullary osteotomy
c. irrigation
c. laparoscopy
c. loop automated delivery
c. loop intestinal obstruction
c. manipulative maneuver
c. nail
c. patch test
c. pericystectomy
c. pinning
c. reduction
c. reduction and percutaneous
   fixation (CRPF)
c. reduction/chemical splinting
c. skull fracture
c. soft tissue injury
c. space infection
c. suction drainage
c. surgery
c. system pars plana vitrectomy
c. transventricular mitral
   commissurotomy
c. tubule fixation technique
c. vascular loop
c. wedge osteotomy

closed-circuit anesthesia machine
closed-loop
c.-l. control
c.-l. system

closing
c. abductory wedge osteotomy
   (CAWO)
c. base wedge
c. base wedge osteotomy
c. pressure
c. ring of Winkler-Waldeyer

clostridial
c. infection
c. myonecrosis

closure
abdominal wall c.
abdominal wound c.
aponeurotic c.
auditory c.
Barsky cleft c.
Clagett c.
clamshell c.
cleft c.
colostomy c.
compression skull-cap c.
crowfoot c.
crural c.
delayed primary c.
direct c.
double-umbrella c.
end stoma c.
epiphysial c.

exstrophy c.
fascial c.
flask c.
floor-of-mouth c.
Fontan fenestration c.
forced eye c.
general c.
glottic c.
Graham c.
Hartmann c.
ileostomy c.
incision c.
King ASD umbrella c.
laparoscopic c.
latex c.
layered c.
2-layer latex c.
Marlex c.
mastectomy c.
maxillary antrum c.
midline aponeurotic c.
muscularis tunnel c.
nonoperative c.
nonprosthetic c.
c. of fistula
omental patch c.
palatopharyngeal c.
pancreatic stump c.
parietal peritoneal c.
percutaneous patent ductus
   arteriosus c.
premature airway c.
premature ductus arteriosus c.
c. pressure
primary c.
primary wound c.
c. principle
retainer c.
scalloped c.
scalp c.
secondary c.
shoelace fasciotomy c.
single-layer continuous c.
sinus c.
skin c.
Smead-Jones c.
spontaneous fistula c.
stoma c.
surgical c.
suture c.
sutureless colostomy c.
tertiary wound c.
transcatheter c.
transcatheter device c.
transmural c.
umbrella c.
vacuum-assisted c. (VAC)
vacuum-assisted wound c. (VAWC)
velopharyngeal c.

closure (*continued*)
    ventricular septal defect c.
    visual c.
    von Langenbeck palatal c.
    V-to-Y c.
    watertight c.
    wound c.

clot
    afferent c.
    agonal c.
    antemortem c.
    autologous c.
    black blood c.
    blood c.
    chicken fat c.
    c. colic
    currant jelly c.
    distal c.
    evacuating c.
    exogenous fibrin c.
    c. extension
    external c.
    c. formation
    fresh blood c.
    friable c.
    heart c.
    internal c.
    laminated c.
    marantic c.
    organized c.
    passive c.
    plastic c.
    postmortem c.
    c. propagation
    proximal c.
    c. regression
    c. retraction
    c. retraction coagulation panel
    retraction of c.
    Schede c.
    sentinel blood c.
    c. size
    spider-web c.
    stratified c.
    washed c.

clothespin H spinal fusion
clot-induced urinary tract obstruction
clotting
    abnormal c.
    c. abnormality
    c. factor (CF)
    graft c.
    c. mechanism
    c. parameter
    c. time coagulation panel
cloudy
    c. ascites
    c. fluid

cloverleaf
    c. condylar plate fixation
    c. skull
    c. skull deformity
    c. skull syndrome
Cloward
    C. anterior cervical discectomy and fusion technique
    C. anterior spinal fusion
    C. back fusion
    C. cervical disc approach
    C. cervical spine fusion operation
    C. cervical spine fusion procedure
    C. fusion discectomy
clubbed
    c. nail
    c. penis
clubbing
    nail c.
clubfoot deformity
cluneal
clunium
    crena c.
cluster
    c. headache
    c. operation
    c. reduction
    repetitive c.
    c. tic syndrome
clustered calcification
clysis
CMAP
    compound muscle action potential
Cmax
    maximal drug concentration
CMC
    carpometacarpal
CMI
    chronic mesenteric ischemia
CMTC
    cutis marmorata telangiectatica congenita
CMV
    continuous mandatory ventilation
    controlled mechanical ventilation
    cytomegalovirus
        CMV colitis
        CMV infection
        CMV prophylaxis
CMV-associated ulceration
CMV-induced esophageal ulceration
CMV-positive donor
CNAP
    continuous negative airway pressure
CN1–CN12
    cranial nerve 1–12
cnemial
cnemis

CNMP
   chronic nonmalignant pain
CNPI
   Checklist of Nonverbal Pain Indicators
CNS
   central nervous system
CO
   carbon monoxide
   cardiac output
Co
   coccygeal
   coenzyme
CO_2
   bicarbonate
   carbon dioxide
      arterial partial pressure of CO_2
        ($PaCO2$, $PaCO_2$)
      CO_2 elimination
      CO_2 inhalation test
      CO_2 pneumoperitoneum
CO_3^{2-}
   carbonate
COAD
   chronic obstructive airways disease
coadjuvant treatment
coagsc
   coagulation screen
coagula (*pl. of* coagulum)
coagulate
coagulating
   c. diathermy
   c. factor
coagulation
   argon beam c.
   argon beam plasma c. (ABPC)
   bipolar c.
   blood c.
   Bovie c.
   c. cascade
   cold c.
   c. defect
   diffuse intravascular c. (DIC)
   c. disorder
   disseminated intravascular c. (DIC)
   electric c.
   endoscopic microwave c.
   endovascular c.
   exogenous anticoagulant c.
   c. factor
   c. factor assay
   c. factor transfusion
   fibrinolysin c.
   free-beam c.
   heater-probe c.
   infrared c.
   intravascular c.
   laser c.
   light c.
   low-current monopolar c.

Meyer-Schwickerath light c.
   microwave c.
   monopolar c.
   multipolar c.
   c. necrosis
   c. pathway
   plasmin c.
   c. profile
   c. screen
   sepsis-induced disseminated
      intravascular c.
   tissue c.
coagulative
   c. laser therapy
   c. myocytolysis
coagulator
   suction c.
coagulopathic disorder
coagulopathy
   dilutional c.
   hypothermia-induced c.
   hypothermia-related c.
   uremia-related c.
coagulum, *pl.* **coagula**
   c. formation
   c. pyelolithotomy
Coakley suture technique
coalesce
coal-mining lensectomy
coapt
coaptation
   end-to-side nerve c.
   nerve c.
   c. site
   c. suture technique
   urethral c.
coarctate
coarctation
   c. of aorta
   c. of pulmonary artery
   postductal c.
   c. repair
   c. syndrome
coarctectomy
coarctotomy
coarticulation
   anticipatory c.
   backward c.
   forward c.
coat
   muscular c.
   seromuscular c.
COAT
   chronic opioid analgesic therapy
coated
   c. polyester suture
   c. Vicryl Rapide suture
   c. Vicryl suture
Coats white ring

coaxial
- c. illumination
- c. pressure

cobalamin

cobalt-60 moving strip technique

cobalt therapy

cobbler's suture technique

cobblestone appearance

Cobb scoliosis measuring technique

cobra-head anastomosis

cocaine anesthesia

cocaine-induced respiratory failure

cocainization

coccidian body

Coccidioides **infection**

coccygeal
- c. body
- c. cornu
- c. dimple
- c. fistula
- c. foveola
- c. ganglion
- c. gland
- c. horn
- c. joint
- c. muscle
- c. nerve
- c. plexus
- c. vertebra
- c. whorl

coccygectomy
- Lougheed-White c.

coccygeum
- cornu c.
- corpus c.
- glomus c.

coccygeus muscle

coccygotomy

coccyx fracture

cochlea

cochlear
- c. duct
- c. ganglion
- c. lesion
- c. nerve
- c. stimulator

cochleariform process

cochleosacculotomy

cochleostomy

cochleovestibular
- c. approach
- c. neurectomy

Cochrane
- C. Bone, Joint, and Muscle Trauma Group
- C. Musculoskeletal Injuries Group

cocked-half flap

Cocke maxillectomy

Cockett
- C. perforator
- C. varicose vein procedure

Cockroft-Gault glomerular filtration rate formula

cocktail
- lytic c.

cock-up deformity

code
- CPT c.

codfish deformity

Codivilla tendon lengthening technique

Codman
- C. incision
- C. postoperative death classification
- C. saber-cut shoulder approach

coefficient
- blood-gas partition c.
- octanol/water c.
- oil-gas partition c.

coeliac (*var. of* celiac)

coeluted

coenzyme
- ameliorating myocardial stunning liposomal c.

coexistence

coexisting anomalies

coffee-grounds
- c.-g. emesis
- c.-g. vomitus

Coffey
- C. incision
- C. ureterointestinal anastomosis
- C. ureterosigmoid transplant technique
- C. uterine suspension

Coffey-Witzel jejunostomy technique

Cofield rotator cuff reconstruction technique

Cogan syndrome

cognition
- catastrophic c.
- dysfunctional c.

cognitive
- c. anxiety subscale
- c. disruption
- c. dysfunction
- C. Errors Questionnaire
- c. intervention
- C. Risk Profile for Pain (CRPP)

cognitive-attitudinal factor inquiry

cognitive-behavioral therapy (CBT)

cogwheel respiration

Cohen
- C. antireflux procedure
- C. crosstrigonal reimplantation
- C. crosstrigonal technique

Cohen-Rentrop cardiac collateral blood flow classification

coherent bundle
coil
    asymmetric gradient c.
coiled
    c. intracranial aneurysm
    c. spring appearance
    c. spring sign
coiling
    endovascular c.
coil-shaped varix
coin
    c. biopsy
    fracture en c.
    c. lesion
coincidence correction
coinduction of anesthesia
coital cephalalgia
Coiter muscle
Colcher-Sussman
    C.-S. x-ray pelvimetry method
    C.-S. x-ray pelvimetry technique
cold
    c. abscess
    c. allodynia
    c. application
    c. autoimmune hemolytic anemia
    c. coagulation
    c. cone biopsy
    c. conization
    c. cup biopsy
    c. defect
    c. erythema
    c. exposure
    c. forceps ablation
    c. gangrene
    c. gas sterilization
    c. gas sterilized
    c. ischemia time
    c. knife cone (CKC)
    c. knife cone aspiration
    c. knife conization (CKC)
    c. knife method
    c. lesion
    c. light source
    c. nodule
    c. pressor test (CPT)
    c. pressor testing maneuver
    c. restraint stress
    c. saline-induced paresthesia technique
    c. snare ablation
    c. snare excision
    c. soak solution
    c. spot
    c. vein graft solution
cold-cup resection
cold-knife endoureterotomy
Cole
    C. intubation procedure

C. orthopaedic surgical technique
C. osteotomy
C. sign
C. tendon fixation
colectasia
colectomy
    abdominal c.
    Aylett total c.
    hand-assisted laparoscopic c.
    laparoscopic c.
    laparoscopic-assisted c.
    laparoscopic-assisted transverse c.
    left c.
    open c.
    partial c.
    Paul-Mikulicz sigmoid c.
    prophylactic c.
    restorative c.
    segmental c.
    1-stage left c.
    subtotal c.
    telerobotic-assisted laparoscopic c.
    total c. (TC)
    total abdominal c. (TAC)
    transverse c.
Coleman
    C. flatfoot technique
    C. plasty
coleocele
coleoptosis
coleotomy
coli
    adenomatous polyposis c. (APC)
    teniae c.
colic
    abdominal c.
    appendiceal c.
    appendicular c.
    c. a.'s
    bile duct c.
    biliary c.
    bilious c.
    clot c.
    common duct c.
    Devonshire c.
    episodic c.
    c. epithelium
    esophageal c.
    flatulent c.
    c. flexure
    gallbladder c.
    gallstone c.
    hepatic c.
    hysteric c.
    c. impression
    infantile c.
    intestinal c.
    kidney c.
    lead c.

colic (*continued*)
    mucous c.
    nephritic c.
    c. omentum
    painter's c.
    pancreatic c.
    c. patch
    c. patch esophagoplasty
    c. plexus
    psychogenic c.
    renal c.
    saturnine c.
    spasmodic c.
    c. sphincter
    ureteral c.
    ureteric c.
    c. vein
    vermicular c.
colicky pain
coliform urinary infection
coliplication
colipuncture
colitides (*pl. of* colitis)
colitis, *pl.* **colitides**
    amebic c.
    chronic ulcerative c.
      (CUC)
    CMV c.
    c. cystica profunda
    cytomegalovirus c.
    granulomatous c.
    indeterminate c.
    ischemic c.
    c. perineal complication
    pseudomembranous c.
    radiation-induced c.
    ulcerative c.
colla (*pl. of* collum)
collagen
    c. absorbable suture
    c. accumulation
    c. deposition
    c. injection
    c. production
    c. synthesis
collagenase level
collagenous
    c. sprue
    c. tissue
    c. trabecular ring
collapse
    abrupt hemodynamic c.
    bone graft c.
    c. cavitation
    dynamic tracheal c.
    hemodynamic c.
    lobar c.
collapsible venous reservoir
  bag

collar
    c. bone
    c. incision
collar-bone appearance
collar-button
    c.-b. abscess
    c.-b. ulceration
collar-buttonlike ulcer
collateral
    c. abdominal circulation
    c. arterial circulation
    c. digital artery
    c. ligament
    c. ligament rupture
    c. meridian therapy
    c. mesenteric
      circulation
    portal c.
    portal-systemic c.
    pulmonary c.
    c. pulp canal
    c. respiration
    c. vein
    venous c.
    c. vessel
collateralization
    ventilation c.
collecting duct
collection
    abdominal air c.
    abdominal fluid c.
    air c.
    arterial blood c.
    cell c.
    duodenal fluid c.
    encysted intraabdominal c.
    expired air c.
    extraaxial fluid c.
    extracerebral fluid c.
    extralymphatic c.
    fluid c.
    gas c.
    globular c.
    gravitational particle c.
    infected c.
    intraglandular fluid c.
    isokinetic c.
    pancreatic fluid c.
    pelvic c.
    periarticular fluid c.
    pericholecystic fluid c.
    perinephric fluid c.
    pleural fluid c.
    posttraumatic subcapsular hepatic
     fluid c.
    pus c.
    quantitative stool c.
    saccular c.
    urine specimen c.

Colles
C. fascia
C. fracture
C. ligament
C. space
colliculectomy
colliculi (*pl. of* colliculus)
colliculitis
colliculus, *pl.* **colliculi**
facial c.
seminal c.
Collier tract
collimator
high-resolution parallel hole c.
Collin-Beard orbicularis-levator fixation
Collis
C. antireflux operation
C. broken femoral stem technique
C. gastroplasty
C. gastroplasty procedure
C. thoracoabdominal repair
Collis-Dubrul femoral stem removal
Collis-Nissen
C.-N. esophageal lengthening
  procedure
C.-N. fundoplication
C.-N. fundoplication method
C.-N. fundoplication procedure
C.-N. fundoplication technique
C.-N. gastroplasty
collodion, collodium
flexible c.
hemostatic c.
c. membrane
styptic c.
collodium (*var. of* collodion)
colloid
c. body
c. cancer
c. carcinoma
c. cyst
c. formation
c. goiter
c. material
c. osmotic pressure
c. solution
c. theory of narcosis
colloidal osmotic pressure
collum, *pl.* **colla**
coloanal
c. anastomosis
c. resection
coloboma anomaly
colobronchial fistula
colocentesis
colocholecystostomy
colocolic
c. anastomosis
c. intussusception

colocolonic anastomosis
colocolostomy
colocutaneous fistula
colocystoplasty
seromuscular c.
coloendoanal anastomosis
cologastrocutaneous fistula
colography (*var. of* colonography)
colohepatopexy
coloileal fistula
cololysis
colon
c. and rectal surgery
ascending c.
c. cancer
c. carcinoma
c. conduit
descending c.
distended c.
c. epithelium
c. flexure
giant c.
haustration of c.
iliac c.
c. incarceration
lead-pipe c.
c. neoplasm
normal c.
c. obstruction
c. perforation
c. polyp
c. preparation
c. problem
c. procedure
pulled-down c.
rectosigmoid c.
c. resection
sigmoid c.
spastic c.
spike-burst on electromyogram of c.
transverse c.
c. tumor
colonic
c. abscess
c. adenocarcinoma
c. adenoma
c. air
c. carcinoma
c. dilation
c. distention
c. diverticular hemorrhage
c. esophagoplasty
c. explosion
c. fistula
c. foreign body
c. inertia
c. infiltration
c. intussusception
c. J-pouch

C

colonic (*continued*)
  c. J-pouch construction
  c. lavage
  c. lavage solution
  c. lesion identification
  c. loop
  c. mass
  c. mesenteric plexus
  c. metastasis
  c. mobilization
  c. mucosal line
  c. needle decompression
  c. neoplasia
  c. obstruction
  c. patch
  c. perforation
  c. pouch
  c. pouch anal anastomosis
  c. pseudoobstruction
  c. resection
  c. tattooing
  c. vascular lesion
  c. volvulus
colonization
  concomitant c.
  c. infection
colonizing organism
Colonna
  C. hip fracture classification
  C. trochanteric arthroplasty
Colonna-Ralston
  C.-R. ankle approach
  C.-R. incision
  C.-R. medial approach
colonography, colography
colonoscopic
  c. appendectomy
  c. biopsy
  c. examination
  c. polypectomy
  c. removal
colonoscopy, coloscopy
  cecal c.
  complete c.
  c. complication
  diagnostic c.
  emergency c.
  high-magnification c.
  incomplete c.
  pediatric c.
  c. per rectum
  c. per stoma
  real-time c.
  c. screening
  splenic flexure c.
  stomal c.
  tandem c.
  therapeutic c.
  total c.

upper endoscopy and c.
virtual c.
colonoscopy-related
  c.-r. emphysema
  c.-r. incarceration
colony
  c. culture
  c. formation
colopexostomy
colopexotomy
colopexy
coloplasty
  c. pouch
  c. procedure
coloplication
coloproctostomy
coloptosia (*var. of* coloptosis)
coloptosis, coloptosia
colopuncture
color
  c. aberration
  c. duplex ultrasonography
  c. imaging
  c. saturation
colorectal
  c. adenocarcinoma
  c. adenoma
  c. anastomosis
  c. biopsy
  c. bleeding
  c. cancer (CRC)
  c. cancer endoscopy
  c. cancer resection
  c. carcinoma (CRC)
  c. disease
  c. disorder
  c. distention pain
  c. duplication
  c. fistula
  c. hemorrhage
  c. metastasis
  c. mucosa
  c. operation
  c. pathology
  c. physiology
  c. polyp
  c. primary
  c. primary tumor
  c. segment
  c. septum
  c. specimen
  c. surgeon
  c. surgery
colorectostomy
Colored Visual Analogue Scale (CVAS)
colorrhaphy
coloscopy (*var. of* colonoscopy)
colosigmoidostomy
colosigmoid resection

colostogram
colostomy
> blowhole decompressing c.
> c. bridge
> c. closure
> continent c.
> decompression c.
> descending loop c.
> Devine c.
> diverting loop c.
> diverting proximal c.
> diverting transverse c.
> divided-stoma c.
> double-barrel c.
> dry c.
> end c.
> end-loop c.
> end-sigmoid c.
> exteriorization c.
> fecal diversion c.
> Hartmann c.
> ileoascending c.
> ileosigmoid c.
> ileotransverse c.
> initial c.
> juxtaanal c.
> Lazaro da Silva technique c.
> loop c.
> loop transverse c.
> Mikulicz c.
> permanent end c.
> c. pyloric autotransplantation
> resective c.
> sigmoid end c.
> sigmoid loop rod c.
> c. soiling
> c. takedown
> temporary diverting c.
> temporary end c.
> terminal c.
> transverse c.
> transverse loop rod c.
> Turnbull c.
> wet c.

colotomy
colovaginal fistula
colovesical fistula
colpectomy
> skinning c.

colpocleisis
> Latzko partial c.
> Le Fort partial c.
> Zimmerman c.

colpocystoplasty
colpocystotomy
colpocystoureterotomy
colpocystourethropexy
colpohysterectomy
colpohysteropexy

colpohysterotomy
colpomicroscopy
colpomyomectomy
colpoperineopexy
> abdominal-sacral c.

colpoperineoplasty
colpoperineorrhaphy
colpopexy
colpoplasty
colpopoiesis
colporectopexy
colporrhaphy
> Goffe c.
> posterior c.

colposcopic diagnosis
colposcopy
> digital imaging c.
> estrogen-assisted c.

colpostenotomy
colposuspension
> Burch c.
> laparoscopic needle c.
> laparoscopic retropubic c.

colpotomy incision
colpoureterotomy
colpourethrocystopexy
> retropubic c.

colpourethropexy
> Burch c.

Coltart
> C. calcaneotibial fusion
> C. fracture technique

Colton olecranon fracture classification
Columbia University selection factors for LVAD implantation
columellar
> c. reconstruction
> c. repair

column
> anal c.
> anterior c.
> Bertin c.
> lateral c.
> posterior c.
> rectal c.
> renal c.
> rugal c.
> spinal c.
> vaginal c.
> variceal c.
> vertebral c.

columnar
> c. cuff carcinoma
> c. epithelium
> c. metaplasia

columnar-lined esophagus
coma
> c. aberration
> acute hepatic c.

157

coma (*continued*)
    alcoholic c.
    apoplectic c.
    barbiturate c.
    c. dé passé
    diabetic c.
    electrolyte imbalance c.
    c. grade
    hepatic c.
    hyperosmolar diabetic c.
    hyperosmolar hyperglycemic
      nonketotic c. (HHNKC)
    insulin c.
    irreversible c.
    Kussmaul c.
    metabolic c.
    myxedema c.
    c. scale
    thyrotoxic c.
    trance c.
    uremic c.
    c. vigil
Comberg foreign body operation
combination
    c. calculus
    c. chemotherapy
    c. fracture
    c. of isotonics therapeutic exercise
      technique
    c. restoration
    c. skin
    c. surgery
combined
    c. analysis
    c. anterior and posterior approach
    c. cavus deformity
    c. chemoradiation therapy
    c. defect
    c. epidural and general anesthesia
    c. flexion-distraction injury and
      burst fracture
    c. gastrointestinal resection
    c. heart catheterization
    c. hiatal hernia
    c. injuries
    c. laparoscopic and thoracoscopic
      approach
    c. laparoscopic splenectomy and
      cholecystectomy
    c. low cervical and transthoracic
      approach
    c. method
    c. neurosurgical-external sinus
      approach
    c. organ resection
    c. presigmoid-transtransversarium
      intradural approach
    c. radial-ulnar-humeral fracture
    c. spinal-epidural (CSE)

    c. spinal-epidural anesthesia
      (CSEA)
    c. spinal-epidural anesthetic
      technique
    c. system disease (CSD)
    c. transsylvian and middle fossa
      approach
    c. ureterolysis
Combitube
    C. airway device
    C. esophagotracheal
      airway
comblike septum
comb sign
Combunox
combustion
    surgical drape c.
come-and-go anesthesia
comedo, *pl.* **comedos, comedones**
    c. extraction
    c. subtype
comedocarcinoma of breast
comedones (*pl. of* comedo)
comedos (*pl. of* comedo)
comitans, *pl.* **comitantes**
    c. vein
    vena c.
comitantes (*pl. of* comitans)
commando
    C. radical glossectomy
    C. radical glossectomy
      procedure
commensal organism
comminuted
    c. intraarticular fracture
    c. orbital fracture
    c. skull fracture
comminution
commissura, *pl.* **commissurae**
commissurae (*pl. of* commissura)
commissural
    c. bundle
    c. fusion
    c. lip pit
    c. myelorrhaphy
    c. myelotomy
commissure
    anterior commissure-posterior c.
      (AC-PC)
    anterior labial c.
    posterior labial c.
    c. reconstruction
commissurotomy
    balloon mitral c.
    Brockenbrough transseptal c.
    closed chest c.
    closed transventricular mitral c.
    mitral balloon c.
    percutaneous mitral balloon c.

percutaneous transatrial mitral c.
percutaneous transvenous mitral c.
transventricular mitral valve c.

committee
　c. for classification of chronic pain
　Hospital Infection Control Practices
　　Advisory C. (HICPAC)
　National Blood Resource Education
　　C.

common
　c. annular ring
　c. annular tendon
　c. basal vein
　c. bile duct (CBD)
　c. bile duct exploration
　c. bile duct ligation
　c. bile duct stone
　c. canal
　c. carotid plexus
　c. cavity phenomenon
　c. duct calculus
　c. duct cholangiogram
　c. duct colic
　c. duct obstruction
　c. dural sac
　c. extensor tendon
　c. facial vein
　c. femoral artery (CFA)
　c. femoral artery-superficial femoral
　　artery (CFA-SFA)
　c. flexor sheath
　c. hepatic artery (CHA)
　c. hepatic duct
　c. iliac artery
　c. interosseous artery
　c. mode rejection ratio
　c. palmar digital artery
　c. peroneal artery
　c. peroneal nerve
　c. peroneal nerve syndrome
　c. plantar digital artery
　c. tendinous ring
communicans, *pl.* **communicantes**
　gray rami communicantes
　rami c.
communicantes (*pl. of* communicans)
communicating
　c. artery
　c. branch
　c. fistula
　c. hematoma
　c. nerve
communication
　cystobiliary c.
　microfistulous c.
communis
　tendo carcaneus c.
community-acquired infection
commutator

comorbid medical problem
compact
　c. bone
　c. substance
companion
　c. artery
　c. lymph node
comparative radiographic examination
comparison operation
compartment
　c. compression syndrome
　extraaxial c.
　extracellular c.
　extravascular c.
　c. procedure
compartmental
　c. pressure
　c. radioimmunoglobulin therapy
　c. volume
compartmentalization
4-compartment fascial decompression
compensation
　c. reaction
compensatory
　c. antiinflammatory response
　　syndrome (CARS)
　c. basilar osteotomy
　c. blood supply
　c. circulation
　c. deformity
　c. head posture
　c. regeneration
　c. wedge
competence, competency
　oral c.
　valvular c.
competency (*var. of* competence)
competing messages integration
compilation autogenous vein graft
complementary
　c. and alternative medicine
　c. balloon angioplasty
　c. therapy
　c. treatment
complement fixation
complement-induced lung injury
complete
　c. adrenalectomy
　c. anterior dislocation
　c. atrioventricular dissociation
　　(CAVD)
　c. AV dissociation
　c. axillary dissection
　c. bilateral deformities
　c. blockage
　c. circumferential mesorectal
　　excision
　c. colonoscopy
　c. common peroneal nerve lesion

C

complete (*continued*)
    c. cytoreduction
    c. duplication
    c. fistula
    c. fracture
    c. hemostasis
    c. hernia
    c. inferior dislocation
    c. integration
    c. internal hemipelvectomy
    c. iridectomy
    c. laparoscopic distal pancreatectomy
    c. lateral hemilaminectomy
    c. left bundle branch block
    c. mesh excision
    c. motor paraplegia
    c. obstruction
    c. posterior dislocation
    c. pulpectomy
    c. pulpotomy
    c. resection
    c. right bundle branch block
    c. rupture
    c. skin-sparing mastectomy
    c. sphincter relaxation
    c. sternotomy
    c. superior dislocation
    c. surgical exploration
    c. thymectomy
    c. thyroidectomy
    c. wrap Nissen operation
completion
    c. cholangiography
    c. thyroidectomy
complex
    c. adrenal endocrine disorder
    c. anorectal fistula
    c. aortic disease
    areolar c.
    c. cavity
    c. chest mass
    disordered hip c.
    c. dissection
    dorsal venous c.
    epispadias-exstrophy c.
    exstrophy-epispadias c.
    factor Xase c.
    fibrocystic c.
    c. fracture
    fusion c.
    Ghon c.
    c. gonadal endocrine disorder
    growth plate c.
    c. hepaticojejunostomy
    internal hemorrhoidal c.
    c. intracranial aneurysm
    juxtaglomerular c.
    c. left ventricular outflow tract
      obstruction

limb-body wall c.
major histocompatibility c. (MHC)
Mycobacterium avium c. (MAC)
ostiomeatal c.
c. pituitary endocrine disorder
plasmin inhibitor c.
pterygoid venous c.
c. regional pain type I, II
    syndrome (CRPS)
c. signal transduction
sling-ring c.
c. syndactyly repair
c. thyroid endocrine disorder
triangular fibrocartilage c. (TFCC)
triarticular c.
tuberous sclerosis c.
vertebral subluxation c.
compliance
    chest wall c.
    dynamic c.
    pulmonary c.
    compliance, rate, oxygenation,
      pressure (CROP)
    static c.
compliant bowel
complicated
    c. diverticular disease
    c. fracture
complication
    abdominal c.
    anastomotic c.
    bacterial c.
    benign pneumatic colonoscopy c.
    cardiopulmonary c.
    cardiorespiratory c.
    cardiovascular c.
    catastrophic c.
    cerebrovascular c.
    colitis perineal c.
    colonoscopy c.
    concomitant obesity c.
    deep abdominal c.
    delayed c.
    diabetic c.
    disease-related c.
    embolic c.
    endoscopy c.
    extraabdominal infective c.
    extraintestinal c.
    feeding c.
    gastroduodenal c.
    gastrointestinal c.
    gonadal c.
    hematologic c.
    hemorrhagic c.
    hepatic c.
    immunologic c.
    infectious c.
    infective extraabdominal c.

intraoperative c.
late c.
life-threatening c.
metabolic c.
neurologic c.
neurovascular c.
nonfatal c.
nonimmunologic c.
noninfective extraabdominal c.
obstetric c.
operative site c.
opportunistic c.
oral c.
pancreatic c.
perioperative c.
postbiopsy vascular c.
postoperative respiratory c.
postsplenectomy c.
pregnancy c.
pulmonary c.
c. rate
recurrent thromboembolic c.
renal c.
respiratory c.
sclerotherapy c.
septic c.
stomal c.
surgery c.
thromboembolic c.
thrombotic c.
trocar wound site c.
urologic c.
vascular c.
venous-related c.
wound c.

component
affective c.
allogenic blood c.
discriminative c.
dominant c.
extensive intraductal c.
intraductal c.
monoclonal c.
nonseminomatous c.
trabecular arachnoid c.

composite
c. flap
c. free tissue transfer
c. joint
c. pelvic resection
c. pelvic resection method
c. pelvic resection procedure
c. pelvic resection technique
c. resin restoration
c. rib graft
c. skin graft
c. tissue transplant

composition
carrier gas c.

compound
c. aneurysm
c. cavity
c. comminuted fracture
c. cyst
c. dislocation
c. flap
c. joint
c. muscle action potential (CMAP)
c. restoration
c. skull fracture
c. suture
c. suture technique

compressed
c. body
c. fracture

compressible cavernous body

compression
c. anesthesia
anterior cord c.
anterior-posterior c.
anteroposterior c.
c. arthrodesis
axial c.
balloon c.
c. bandage
c. bone conduction
brainstem c.
c. button gastrojejunostomy
cardiac c.
carotid artery c.
cauda equina c.
cerebral aqueduct c.
cervical vessel c.
cervicomedullary junction c.
Charnley c.
chest c.
chiasmal c.
continuous c.
cord c.
c. cough
c. cyanosis
c. device
direct c.
disc c.
duodenal c.
duplex-guided c.
dynamic c.
early supraclavicular c.
elastic c.
esophageal c.
c. extension
external pneumatic calf c.
extrinsic bladder c.
c. fracture
gastric c.
gentle c.
head c.
image c.

compression (*continued*)
    c. injury
    c. instrumentation posterior
      construct
    interfragmentary c.
    intermittent pneumatic calf c.
    intrinsic c.
    ischemic c.
    lateral c.
    limbal c.
    lower plexus c.
    mechanical variceal c.
    median nerve c.
    c. molding
    napkin-ring c.
    nerve root c.
    optic chiasm c.
    optic tract c.
    c. overload
    c. paralysis
    percutaneous balloon c.
    c. plate fixation
    c. plating
    pneumatic c.
    prechiasmal c.
    progressive c.
    c. rod treatment
    root c.
    c. skull-cap closure
    spinal cord c.
    spot c.
    static c.
    c. strain
    supraclavicular c.
    suprascapular nerve c.
    c. switch
    c. syndrome
    c. technique
    c. test
    c. testing
    thecal sac c.
    thoracic outlet c.
    tissue c.
    tracheal c.
    ultrasound-guided c.
    uterine c.
    variable-release c.
    vascular c.
    venous c.
    vertebral c.
    vertical c.
    c. wiring
compression-evoked allodynia
compressor naris muscle
compromise
    airway c.
    hemodynamic c.
    organ c.
    renal c.

    respiratory c.
    visual c.
compromised systolic function
computed
    c. tomographic hepatic angiography
    c. tomography (CT)
    c. tomography arterial portography
      (CTAP)
    c. tomography discography
    c. tomography-guided biopsy
    c. tomography-guided localization
      using platinum microcoils
    c. tomography-guided selective
      drainage
    c. tomography scan
    c. tomography severity index (CTSI)
computer-assisted
    c.-a. anesthesia
    c.-a. assessment
    c.-a. continuous infusion anesthetic
      technique
    c.-a. controlled infusion (CACI)
    c.-a. design-controlled alignment
      method
    c.-a. instrumentation
    c.-a. stereotactic surgery (CASS)
    c.-a. surgery (CAS)
    c.-a. treatment
computer-controlled
    c.-c. drug administration anesthetic
      technique
    c.-c. infusion anesthetic technique
computer-enhanced instrumentation
computerized
    c. diaphragmatic breathing retraining
      (CDBR)
    c. electronic endoscopy
    c. image guidance
    c. thermal stimulator
concatenation
concave abdomen
concealed
    c. bypass tract
    c. hemorrhage
    c. hernia
    c. penis
    c. umbilical stoma
concentrate
    plasma product c.
    platelet c.
concentration
    alveolar c.
    ambient oxygen c.
    approximate lethal c.
    bactericidal c.
    bilirubin c.
    blood alcohol c. (BAC)
    carbon dioxide c.
    end-tidal nitrogen c.

end-tidal oxygen c.
hazardous c.
hydrogen ion c. (pH)
inspiratory vapor c.
lethal c.
mass c. (masc, massc)
maximal drug c. (Cmax)
maximum permissible c.
minimal alveolar c. (MAC)
minimal anesthetic c. (MAC)
minimal bactericidal c.
minimum alveolar c.
1-minimum alveolar c. (1-MAC)
minimum alveolar anesthetic c.
minimum bactericidal c.
minimum detectable c.
minimum effective c. (MEC)
minimum effective analgesic c.
minimum lethal c.
minimum local analgesic c. (MLAC)
nitrogen c.
oxygen c.
c. performance test
plasma endotoxin c.
plasma gastrin c.
plasma iron c.
plasma norepinephrine c.
plasma renin c.
plasma urea c.
predialysis plasma phosphate c.
prick-test c.
c. procedure
radioactive c.
renal vein renin c.
serum bactericidal c.
serum bilirubin c.
serum calcium c.
serum lithium c.
steroid c.
subanesthetic c.
substance c.
target plasma c.
thyroid hormone serum c.
time of maximum c. (Tmax)
c. times time
total L-chain c.
total protein c.
concentration-effect relation
concentric
  c. exercise
  c. hernia
  c. lesion
  c. mastopexy
  c. reduction
concept
  c. formation
  three-color c.
concertinalike fashion
concha

nasal c.
sphenoidal c.
concha-mastoid suture
conchoidal
concomitant
  c. acidosis
  c. administration
  c. antireflux surgery
  c. bleeding
  c. colonization
  c. hepatectomy
  c. median sternotomy
  c. medication
  c. obesity complication
  c. spinal cord injury
  c. therapy
concordance
  ventriculoarterial c.
concordant pain
Concorde position
concurrent
  c. chemotherapy
  c. DVT
  c. hepatic laceration
  c. medical condition
concussion
  brain c.
  spinal cord c.
condensation
  amalgam c.
  chromatin c.
  filling material c.
  gold foil c.
  heavy c.
  lateral c.
  porcelain c.
  pressure c.
  resin c.
  spatulation c.
  vibration c.
  warm c.
  whipping c.
condenser point
condition
  catabolic c.
  concurrent medical c.
  fibrocystic c.
  gastrointestinal c.
  genetic c.
  medical systemic c.
  predisposing c.
  premalignant c.
  systemic c.
  tumorlike bone c.
conditioning
  interceptive c.
  operant c.
  c. program
  c. therapy

C

conductance
  skin c.
conduction
  c. analgesia
  c. anesthesia
  compression bone c.
  osteotympanic bone c.
conductivity
  tissue c.
conduit
  antirefluxing colonic c.
  aortic c.
  biliary c.
  Bricker c.
  colon c.
  cutaneous appendiceal c.
  ileal c.
  ileocolic c.
  intestinal c.
  jejunal c.
  Koch c.
  Mitrofanoff c.
  Rastelli c.
  respiratory syncytial virus c.
  urinary c.
condylar
  c. articulation
  c. canal
  c. emissary vein
  c. femoral fracture
  c. guidance inclination
  c. hinge position
  c. implant arthroplasty
  c. process
  c. process fracture
  c. screw fixation
condylarthrosis
condyle
  c. cord
  c. dissection
  c. head
  lateral c.
  mandibular c.
  medial c.
  occipital c.
  c. resection
condylectomy
  DuVries plantar c.
  mandibular c.
  plantar c.
condylion
condylocephalic nail
condyloideum
condyloid process
condyloma, *pl.* **condylomas, condylomata**
  c. acuminatum
  anal c.
  cervical c.
  flat c.

genital c.
giant c.
perianal c.
c. planus
pointed c.
vaginal c.
venereal c.
condylomas (*pl. of* condyloma)
condylomata (*pl. of* condyloma)
condylomatous
condylotomy
condylus
cone
  c. biopsy
  cold knife c. (CKC)
coned-down view
configuration
  stellate c.
  V-shaped c.
  Y c.
confirmation
  histopathologic c.
  intraoperative c.
  tissue c.
confirmatory
  c. axillary dissection
  c. bupivacaine block
  c. incision
confluence
  hepatic venous c.
  vein c.
  venous c.
confluent inflammation
conformal radiation therapy
confrontation
  c. method
  c. testing
  c. visual field test
Confusion Assessment Method for Intensive Care Unit (CAM-ICU)
congenita
  arthrogryposis multiplex c. (AMC)
  cutis marmorata telangiectatica c. (CMTC)
congenital
  c. above-elbow amputation
  c. adrenal hyperplasia
  c. aspiration pneumonia
  c. below-elbow amputation
  c. brain malformation
  c. cataract
  c. central hypoventilation syndrome
  c. cerebral aneurysm
  c. cervical instability
  c. choledochal cyst
  c. conotruncal anomaly
  c. cystic adenomatoid malformation (CCAM)

c. cystic dilation
c. cystic duct stenosis
c. depigmentation
c. diaphragmatic hernia (CDH)
c. diverticulum
c. duplication
c. esotropia
c. eventration
c. fracture
c. goiter
c. heart malformation
c. hernia
c. hip dislocation
c. HIV infection
c. hyperinsulinism
c. lens dislocation
c. lesion
c. long QT syndrome
c. nasal mass
c. postural deformity
c. pulmonary airway
   malformation
c. pulmonary arteriovenous fistula
c. pulmonary venolobar syndrome
c. pyloric membrane
c. pyloric stenosis
c. renal mass
c. ring
c. ring syndrome
c. scapular elevation
c. splenomegaly
c. stippled epiphysis
c. tracheobiliary fistula
c. urethroperineal fistula
c. vascular malformation
congenitally altered anatomy
congestion
   brain c.
   flap c.
   hepatic c.
   sinusoidal c.
   splanchnic c.
congestive
   c. heart disease
   c. heart failure (CHF)
   c. hepatomegaly
conglomerate mass
conglutinant
conglutination
congruent affect
coniotomy
conization
   cautery c.
   cervical c.
   cold c.
   cold knife c. (CKC)
   hot knife c.
   laser cervical c.
   LEEP c.

loop diathermy cervical c.
loop electrosurgical excision
   procedure c.
conjoined
   c. anastomosis
   c. nerve-root anomaly
   c. tendon
conjoint tendon
conjugate
   c. axis
   c. foramen
   c. point
conjugation bridge
conjunctiva, *pl.* **conjunctivae**
**conjunctiva-associated lymphoid tissue
   (CALT)**
conjunctivae (*pl. of* conjunctiva)
conjunctival
   c. angioma
   c. circulation
   c. cul-de-sac
   c. exudate
   c. flap
   c. fornix
   c. hemorrhage
   c. incision
   c. injection
   c. laceration
   c. limbus
   c. melanotic lesion
   c. membrane
   c. patch graft
   c. ring
   c. sac
conjunctiva-Müller muscle excision
conjunctiviplasty (*var. of* conjunctivoplasty)
conjunctivitis
conjunctivodacryocystorhinostomy (CDCR)
   Lester-Jones c.
conjunctivodacryocystostomy
conjunctivoplasty, conjunctiviplasty
conjunctivorhinostomy
conjunctivo-Tenon flap
conjunctivus
Conn
   C. operation
   C. primary hyperaldosteronism
connecting cartilage
connection
   atriopulmonary c.
connective
   c. tissue
   c. tissue activating peptide
   c. tissue augmentation
   c. tissue disease
   c. tissue disorder
   c. tissue graft
   c. tissue manipulation
   c. tissue massage

connective (*continued*)
    c. tissue membrane
    c. tissue plasticity
Connell
    C. incision
    C. stitch
    C. suture
    C. suture technique
Connolly
    C. bone regeneration technique
    C. procedure
conoid
    c. process
    c. tubercle
conotruncal anomaly
Conradi line
Conrad orbital blowout fracture operation
consciousness
conscious sedation
consecutive
    c. amputation
    c. aneurysm
    c. dislocation
consent
    informed c.
consequence
    familial c.
    psychologic c.
    social c.
conservation
    perioperative blood c.
    splenic c.
    c. surgery
conservative
    c. resection
    c. surgery
    c. surgical treatment
    c. therapy
consideration
    anesthetic c.
    oncologic c.
    technical c.
consolability
    face, leg, activity, cry, c. (FLACC)
consonant position
consortial approach
constant
    c. flow insufflation
    c. vacuum
constipation
    functional c.
    idiopathic c.
constrained
    c. ankle arthroplasty
    c. reconstruction
    c. shoulder arthroplasty
constricting lesion

constriction
    duodenopyloric c.
    esophageal c.
    pyloric c.
    c. ring
constrictive pericarditis
constrictor
    inferior pharyngeal c.
construct
    AO dynamic compression plate c.
    compression instrumentation posterior c.
    double-rod c.
    hook-rod c.
    iliosacral and iliac fixation c.
    pedicle screw c.
    segmental compression c.
    TSRH double-rod c.
    Wiltse system double-rod c.
    Wiltse system H c.
    Wiltse system single-rod c.
construction
    Abbe vaginal c.
    absolute c.
    colonic J-pouch c.
    exocentric c.
    ileal reservoir c.
    ileostomy c.
    J-pouch c.
    loop ileostomy c.
    McIndoe-Hayes c.
    pelvic ileal reservoir c.
    single denture c.
    sphincteric c.
    stent c.
    tandem c.
    Thiersch-Duplay urethral c.
    U pouch c.
    vaginal c.
consultation for low back pain
consumption
    oxygen c. (VO_2)
    peak exercise oxygen c.
    splanchnic oxygen c.
consumptive thrombohemorrhagic disorder
contact
    c. activation product
    c. area point
    c. diode laser tonsillectomy
    c. dissolution therapy
    grid c.
    c. illumination
    c. laser ablation
    c. laser ablation of prostate (CLAP)
    c. laser vaporization
    c. manipulation
    c. metastasis
    c. method

contained rupture
contaminant
    wound c.
contaminated
    c. field
    c. operative wound
      classification
contamination
    bacterial c.
    fecal c.
    gas c.
    graft c.
    gross c.
    gross fecal c.
    gross wound c.
    hub c.
    intraoperative c.
    metastatic c.
    microbial c.
content
    abdominal c.
    bile-stained cyst c.
    cyst c.
    gastrointestinal c.
    intestinal c.'s
    intraabdominal c.
    luminal c.'s
    mixed venous
      oxygen c.
    platelet nucleotide c.
    protein c.
    tissue water c.
context-sensitive
    c.-s. decrement time
    c.-s. half-life
    c.-s. half-time
contiguity
    solution of c.
    spatial c.
contiguous loop
contiguum
    per c.
continence
    anal c.
    short-term total c.
    sphincteric c.
    total c.
continent
    c. colostomy
    c. cutaneous appendicocystostomy
    c. ileal pouch
    c. ileostomy
    c. urinary pouch
continua (*pl. of* continuum)
continuity
    bilioenteric c.
    bowel c.
    digestive c.
    gastrointestinal c.

    gut c.
    solution of c.
continuous
    c. ambulatory peritoneal dialysis
      (CAPD)
    c. arteriovenous hemofiltration
      (CAVH)
    c. arteriovenous ultrafiltration
      (CAVU)
    c. atrial fibrillation (CAF)
    c. bladder irrigation (CBI)
    c. catheter drainage
    c. compression
    c. distending airway pressure
      (CDAP)
    c. endothelium
    c. endotoxin apheresis
    c. epidural anesthesia
    c. flow ventilation
    c. gastric decompression
    c. gum technique
    c. hemofiltration
    c. high-pitched bruit
    c. hyperthermic peritoneal perfusion
      (CHPP)
    c. infusion anesthetic technique
    c. intramucosal PCO_2 measurement
    c. intraoperative spirometry
    c. locked stitch
    c. loop wiring
    c. lumbar epidural (CLE)
    c. lumbar peridural anesthesia
    c. mandatory ventilation (CMV)
    c. medical treatment
    c. negative airway pressure (CNAP)
    c. negative pressure
    c. NG suction
    c. on-line recording
    c. peripheral nerve block
    c. peripheral nerve catheter
    c. popliteal sciatic nerve block
    c. positive airway pressure (CPAP)
    c. positive pressure breathing
      (CPPB)
    c. positive pressure ventilation
      (CPPV)
    c. postoperative closed lavage
    c. pullthrough technique
    c. renal replacement therapy
      (CRRT)
    c. sanguineous perfusion
    c. spinal anesthesia
    c. spinal anesthetic technique
    c. subcutaneous insulin injection
    c. suture technique
    c. sympathetic spinal blockade
    c. venovenous hemodialysis
      (CVVHD)
    c. venovenous hemofiltration

C

continuous (*continued*)
    c. wave Doppler
    c. wave laser ablation
    c. wave technique
continuum, *pl.* **continua**
    acrodermatitis continua
    hemicrania continua
    per c.
contour
    breast c.
    corneal c.
    intonation c.
    c. line
    lobulated c.
    restoration c.
    c. restoration
    rounded c.
contoured
    c. adduction trochanteric-controlled
      alignment method (CAT-CAM)
    c. anterior spinal plate technique
contouring
    3-dimensional c.
contraangle
contraaperture
contraceptive method
contracted
    c. kidney
    c. pelvis
contractile
    c. motility
    c. ring
    c. ring dysphagia
contractility
    myocardial c.
contraction
    anal canal rhythmic c.
    angiotensin II-induced
      vascular c.
    c. fasciculation
    muscular c.
    propagating clustered c.
    c. wave
contract-relax technique
contracture
    Dupuytren c.
    functional c.
    Volkmann ischemic c.
contraindication
contralateral
    c. axillary metastasis
    c. carotid artery occlusion
    c. groin exploration
    c. ischemia
    c. microaldosteronoma
    c. mobile cord
    c. parathyroid gland
    c. sheath
    c. side

    c. site
    c. weakness
contralaterally
contrast
    c. bath
    blood oxygenation level-
      dependent c.
    c. enema
    c. injection
    intravenous c.
    I.V. c.
    c. material
    c. material instillation
    c. medium
    c. nephropathy
    c. study
    c. venography
    c. visualization
contrast-enhanced
    c.-e. computed tomography
    c.-e. CT
    c.-e. CT scan
    c.-e. CT scanning
    c.-e. ultrasonography
contrast-induced nephropathy
contrecoup fracture
control
    automatic muscle relaxation c.
    closed-loop c.
    damage c.
    endoscopic c.
    exsanguination tourniquet c.
    extrahepatic c.
    fluoroscopic c.
    hemorrhage c.
    inflow c.
    intrahepatic c.
    monitored anesthesia c. (MAC)
    nonpain symptom c.
    c. of ventilation
    outflow c.
    peripheral artery c.
    Pringle vascular c.
    pronation c.
    proximal vascular c.
    Study of the Efficacy of
      Nosocomial Infection C. (SENIC)
    tourniquet c.
    vascular c.
    x-ray c.
controlled
    c. diagnostic block
    c. diaphragmatic respiration
    c. disc stimulation
    c. expansion
    c. fistula
    c. heat-aided drug delivery
      (CHADD)
    c. hypotension

c. hypotensive anesthesia (CHA)
c. mechanical ventilation (CMV)
c. release anesthetic technique
c. reperfusion
c. rotational osteotomy
c. ventilation
c. water-added technique
controller
AESOP robotic voice-activated camera c.
oxygen-ratio monitoring c.
control-mode ventilation
contusion
brain c.
corneal c.
lung c.
myocardial c.
pulmonary c.
conus elasticus
convalescence
short-term c.
convection
hemodiafiltration c.
convenience
c. jaw relation
c. point
conventional
c. aortic aneurysmectomy
c. coronary artery bypass
c. distal pancreatectomy
c. endarterectomy
c. method
c. operation
c. pancreatoduodenectomy
c. parameter
c. procedure
c. surgery
c. suturing
c. technique
c. thoracoplasty
c. video trainer
convergence
c. facilitation
c. point
c. position
c. projection
convergent beam irradiation
converse
scalping flap of C.
conversion
above-knee amputation c.
c. disorder
extraglandular c.
pressure c.
converter
convex
c. condylar implant arthroplasty
c. fusion
c. nail

convexoconcave
convoluted seminiferous tubule
convulsion
ether c.
convulsive therapy
Conyers technique
cooled-knife method
Cooley
C. clamp
C. U suture
cooling
active core c.
c. blanket
external c.
passive tissue c.
topical c.
whole-body c.
Coonrad-Morrey total elbow arthroplasty
Coonrad total elbow arthroplasty
Coonse-Adams
C.-A. knee approach
C.-A. V-Y quadriceps turndown knee technique
Cooper
C. fascia
C. hernia
C. inguinal hernia operation
C. ligament
C. lung volume reduction
C. syndrome
cooperation
cellular c.
coordination
hand-eye c.
co-oximetry
Copeland
C. arthroscopic rotator cuff repair technique
C. retinoscopy
Copeland-Howard scapulothoracic fusion
Cope transseptal left atrium catheterization technique
coping
passive pain c.
C. Strategies Questionnaire (CSQ)
C. with Health, Injuries, and Problems (CHIP)
C. with Health Injuries and Problems Scale
copious
c. irrigation
c. peritoneal lavage
copper-wire
c.-w. arteriole
c.-w. artery
c.-w. reflex
coproporphyria
hereditary c.

C

copular point
copulating pouch
cor
    c. bovinum
    c. pulmonale
coracoacromial ligament
coracoaxillary fascia
coracobrachial
    c. bursa
    c. muscle
coracobrachialis muscle
coracoclavicular
    c. articulation
    c. ligament
    c. screw fixation
    c. space
    c. suture fixation
    c. technique
coracoclaviculare
coracohumeral ligament
coracoid
    c. fracture
    c. infraclavicular brachial plexus
    block
    c. process
coral calculus
Corbin rhinoplasty technique
cord
    anterior c.
    c. compression
    condyle c.
    contralateral mobile c.
    false vocal c.
    Ferrein c.
    gangliated c.
    genital c.
    germinal c.
    gonadal c.
    lateral c.
    nephrogenetic c.
    oblique c.
    c. paralysis
    presentation of c.
    rete c.
    spermatic c.
    spinal c.
    splenic c.
    c. structure
    tendinous c.
    testicular c.
    testis c.
    tethered spinal c.
    c. traction syndrome
    true vocal c.
    umbilical c.
    vocal c.
    Weitbrecht c.
    Willis c.
cordate pelvis, cordiform pelvis

cordectomy
cordiform pelvis
cordis
cordopexy
cordotomy
    anterolateral c.
    dorsal c.
    open surgical c.
    percutaneous c.
    posterior column c.
    spinothalamic c.
    stereotactic c.
core
    c. body temperature
    central fibroelastic c.
    c. drilling procedure
    c. hypothermia
    c. needle biopsy
    c. vitrectomy
corectomy
coreoplasty
    Franceschetti c.
corepexy
corepraxy
    Franceschetti c.
Cori glycogen storage disease
  classification
corium
corkscrew
    c. appearance
    c. maneuver
Cormack and Lehane laryngeal view
  scoring system
corn
    hard c.
    soft c.
    web c.
cornea
    anterior c.
    c. guttate lesion
corneal
    c. abrasion
    c. abscess
    c. abscission
    c. alkali burn
    c. anesthesia
    c. apex
    c. arcus
    c. astigmatism
    c. blood staining
    c. cap
    c. cleft
    c. contour
    c. contusion
    c. curvature
    c. dendrite
    c. diameter
    c. distortion
    c. dystrophy

c. ectasia
c. edema
c. endothelium
c. epithelium
c. erosion
c. facet
c. filament
c. fissure
c. fistula
c. flap
c. foreign body
c. full-thickness
c. graft operation
c. graft step
c. guttering
c. incision
c. inlay
c. iron line
c. laceration
c. lamella
c. lamellar groove
c. leakage
c. lens
c. light reflex
c. limbus
c. luster
c. marginal furrow
c. meridian
c. mushroom
c. nebula
c. neovascularization
c. nerve
c. perforation
c. protrusion
c. punctate lesion
c. reflection
c. rejection
c. scarring
c. spot
c. staining test
c. stria
c. substance
c. surgery
c. thinning
c. tissue
c. transplant
c. trauma
c. trephination
c. ulceration
c. velum

corneoscleral
c. incision
c. laceration

corner
caudal c.
cephalad c.
c. fracture
c. stitch

cornered

3-cornered
3-c. bone
3-c. therapy

4-corner midcarpal fusion

corniculate
c. cartilage
c. process
c. tubercle

corniculum laryngis

cornification disorder

cornu, *pl.* **cornua**
coccygeal c.
c. coccygeum
cornua of hyoid bone
styloid c.

cornua (*pl. of* cornu)

cornual anastomosis

cornucopia
sinusoidal endothelium c.

corona, *pl.* **coronae**

coronae (*pl. of* corona)

coronal
c. angulation
c. oblique projection
c. plane
c. plane correction
c. plane deformity
c. plane deformity sagittal translation
c. pulp tissue
c. reconstruction
c. section
c. split fracture
c. suture

coronalis

coronary
c. angioplasty versus excisional atherectomy
c. artery angioplasty
c. artery anomaly
c. artery bypass (CAB)
c. artery bypass graft (CABG)
c. artery disease (CAD)
c. artery dissection
c. artery ectasia
c. artery fistula
c. artery revascularization procedure
c. artery-right ventricular fistula
c. balloon angioplasty
c. bifurcation
c. button suture technique
c. bypass procedure
c. collateral circulation
c. endarterectomy
c. flow reserve technique
c. node
c. perfusion pressure
c. plexus
c. revascularization

C

coronary (*continued*)
- c. ring
- c. rotational ablation
- c. rotational atherectomy
- c. sinus
- c. sinus catheterization
- c. sinus perfusion system
- c. sulcus
- c. syndrome
- c. thrombolysis
- c. vein
- c. vein ligation
- c. venous pressure
- c. vessel anatomy

coronoid
- c. line
- c. process
- c. process fracture

coronoidectomy
coronoideus
- processus c.

coronoradicular stabilization
coroplasty
coroscopy
corotomy
corpectomy
- anterior c.
- cervical c.
- median c.
- c. model
- vertebral body c.

corpora (*pl. of* corpus)
corporal biopsy
Corporation
- Spinal Dynamics C.

corporeal
- c. aspiration
- c. reconstruction
- c. rotation procedure
- c. sacrospinous
  suspension

corporectomy
corporoplasty
- Essed-Schroeder c.
- incisional c.
- modified Essed-Schroeder c.

corporotomy
corpus, *pl.* **corpora**
- c. callosotomy
- c. carcinoma
- c. clitoridis
- c. coccygeum
- c. epididymis
- c. luteum
- c. luteum cyst
- c. luteum hematoma
- c. luteus

Correa gastritis classification
corrected sternal position

correction
- adaptive c.
- Allen c.
- Allison GE reflux c.
- anterior c.
- anteroposterior c.
- aphakic c.
- astigmatism c.
- attenuation c.
- Beckenbaugh c.
- Berke-Motais upper eyelid
  ptosis c.
- Bonferroni c.
- Bowman ptosis c.
- Byron Smith lazy-T c.
- cephalometric c.
- chevron hallux valgus c.
- coincidence c.
- coronal plane c.
- cubitus varus c.
- dioptric c.
- epicanthal c.
- Fergus lid ptosis c.
- frontal plane c.
- Gillies scar c.
- Glenn congenital cyanotic heart
  disease c.
- hallux varus c.
- heparinase c.
- Hotz-Anagnostakis entropion c.
- Johnson-Spiegl hallux varus c.
- King curve posterior c.
- Küstner uterine inversion c.
- kyphosis c.
- Mules eyelid ptosis c.
- occlusal c.
- oligosegmental c.
- operative c.
- optic c.
- phalangeal malunion c.
- protamine c.
- rotational c.
- Roveda epicanthus and
  blepharophimosis c.
- Ruiz-Mora c.
- scatter c.
- scoliosis c.
- secondary ptosis c.
- skeletal c.
- Smith-Gibson tetralogy of
  Fallot c.
- spectacle c.
- speech c.
- Steel c.
- surgical c.

corrective therapy
correlation
- canonical c.
- clinical c.

clinicopathologic c.
negative c.
positive c.
semilinear canonical c.
c. time
Correra line
corresponding point
corridor
c. incision
c. procedure
Corrigan respiration
corrosion preparation
corrugator
c. cutis muscle
c. supercilii muscle
corset suspension
cortex, *pl.* **cortices**
adrenal c.
anterior c.
anterolateral prefrontal c.
aspiration of c.
association c.
cerebral c.
cingulate c.
ovarian c.
renal c.
rostral anterior cingulate c.
somatosensory c.
suprarenal c.
vertebral body anterior c.
cortical
c. activation
c. arch of kidney
c. area
c. artery
c. atrophy
c. biopsy
c. bone
c. bone graft
c. bone primary canal
c. destruction
c. dysplasia
c. fracture
c. fragment
c. hamartoma
c. implantation
c. incision
c. lateralization
c. lesion
c. mass
c. perforation
c. respiration
c. ring sign
c. stimulation
c. strut graft
c. substance
c. tuber
corticalosteotomy
corticectomy

cortices (*pl. of* cortex)
corticoadenoma
corticobulbar tract
corticocancellous bone graft
corticoid injection
corticomedullary demarcation
corticopontine tract
corticospinal
c. axon
c. tract
corticosteroid
depot c.
c. efficacy
corticotomy
DeBastiani c.
percutaneous c.
Corti organ
cortisol-producing carcinoma
Cortrosyn stimulation test
**Cosgrove mitral valve
  replacement**
cosmesis
cosmetic
c. evaluation
c. outcome
c. problem
c. result
c. score
c. surgery
costa, *pl.* **costae**
costae fluctuantes
costae (*pl. of* costa)
costal
c. angle
c. cartilage
c. facet
c. groove
c. margin
c. notch
c. pit
c. pleura
c. process
c. respiration
c. surface
c. tuberosity
costectomy
cost-effective alternative
Costen syndrome
costicartilage
costiform
costoaxillary vein
costocentral
costocervical
c. artery
c. trunk
costochondral
c. articulation
c. joint
c. junction

C

costoclavicular
    c. compression syndrome
    c. ligament
    c. line
    c. maneuver
    c. space
costocolic ligament
costocoracoid
costodiaphragmatic recess
costoinferior
costomediastinal
    c. recess
    c. sinus
costophrenic septal line
costoscapular
costoscapularis
costosternal
costosternoplasty
costosuperior
costotomy
costotransversarium
    ligamentum c.
costotransverse
    c. foramen
    c. joint
    c. ligament
costotransversectomy
    c. approach
    Seddon dorsal spine c.
    c. technique
costoversion thoracoplasty
costovertebral joint
costoxiphoid ligament
cot
    finger c.
cotransplantation
Cotrel-Dubousset (C-D)
    C.-D. fixation
Cotte
    C. presacral neurectomy
    C. presacral neurotomy for
      dysmenorrhea operation
Cotting toenail operation
cotton
    C. ankle fracture
    C. cartilage graft
    c. dressing
    C. lung volume reduction
    c. nonabsorbable suture
cotton-loader position
cotton-wool
    c.-w. exudate
    c.-w. patch
    c.-w. separation
    c.-w. sign
cottony Dacron hollow
  suture
Cotunnius
    C. aqueduct

    C. canal
    C. space
cotyloid
    c. cavity
    c. joint
    c. ligament
cough
    compression c.
    extrapulmonary c.
    c. fracture
    c. pressure transmission ratio
    c. trick
coughing
    c. and bucking
    expulsive c.
Couinaud
    C. liver anatomy classification
    C. nomenclature
Coumadin
coumadinization
coumarin necrosis
Councilman lesion
counseling
    vocational c.
Counsellor-Davis artificial vagina
  operation
Counsellor-Flor
    C.-F. modification
    C.-F. modification of McIndoe
      vaginoplasty technique
count
    blood cell c.
    ex vivo c.
    pitted erythrocyte c.
    posttetanic c.
counterbalance
counterclockwise
    c. derotation
    c. direction
    c. rotation
countercurrent
    c. extraction
    c. heat exchanger
    c. mechanism
counterincision
counterirritation
counteropening
counterpressure
    Michaelson c.
counterpulsation
    balloon c.
    enhanced external c. (EECP)
    intraaortic balloon c. (IABCP)
    intraarterial c.
    percutaneous intraaortic
      balloon c.
counterpuncture
countersinking osteotomy
counterstimulation

countertraction
coup injury
coupling
>EEG phase c.
course
>chronic c.
>intrahepatic c.
>postoperative c.
Courvoisier
>C. gastroenterostomy
>C. incision
>C. sign
Couvelaire
>C. ileourethral anastomosis
>C. incision
Coventry
>C. distal femoral osteotomy
>C. vagal osteotomy
cove plane
Cowden disease
Cowen-Loftus toe-phalanx
transplant
cow face
cowl muscle
Cowper
>C. gland
>C. ligament
COX-2
>cyclooxygenase-2
>COX-2 inhibitor
coxa, *pl.* **coxae**
coxae (*pl. of* coxa)
coxal bone
Cox maze III for atrial fibrillation
procedure
coxofemoral articulation
coxsackievirus A, B virus
Cozen-Brockway
>C.-B. postaxial polydactyly
>technique
>C.-B. Z-plasty
CPAP
>continuous positive airway pressure
CPB
>cardiopulmonary bypass
CP/CPPS
>chronic prostatitis/chronic pelvic pain
>syndrome, types IIIA and IIIB
CPDD
>calcium pyrophosphate deposition
>disease
CPH
>chronic paroxysmal hemicrania
C-plasty
CPPB
>continuous positive pressure breathing
CPPD
>calcium pyrophosphate deposition
>disease

CPPV
>continuous positive pressure ventilation
CPR
>cardiopulmonary resuscitation
>over-the-head CPR
CPS
>cumulative pain score
CPSP
>central poststroke pain
>chronic postsurgical pain
CPT
>chromopertubation
>cold pressor test
>current perception threshold
>*Current Procedural Terminology*
>CPT code
Cracchiolo
>C. forefoot arthroplasty
>C. hallux limitus implant
>arthroplasty procedure
Cragg endoluminal graft
cramp
>abdominal c.
Crampton
>C. line
>C. orthostatics test
crania (*pl. of* cranium)
craniad
cranial
>c. base
>c. bone
>c. canal
>c. cavity
>c. duplication
>c. epidural space
>c. extension
>c. fontanelle
>c. fossa
>c. fracture
>c. index
>c. insufflation
>c. irradiation
>c. nerve (CN1–CN12)
>c. nerve dissection
>c. nerve manipulation
>c. nerve rhizotomy
>c. nerve rootlet
>c. osteopetrosis
>c. osteosynthesis
>c. pin
>c. section
>c. suture
>c. vault
>c. venous sinus
craniamphitomy
craniectomy
>endoscopic strip c.
>keyhole-shaped c.
>linear c.

C

craniectomy (*continued*)
    partial-thickness c.
    retromastoid suboccipital c.
    strip c.
cranio-aural
craniocele
craniocerebral
craniocervical flexion test
craniofacial
    c. anomaly
    c. axis
    c. deformity
    c. en bloc resection
    c. fixation
    c. malformation
    c. myalgia
    c. notch
    c. osteotomy
    c. pain
    c. reconstruction
    c. reconstructive surgery
    c. suspension wiring
craniomeningocele
craniometric point
cranioorbital surgery
craniopathy
craniopharyngeal
    c. canal
    c. duct
craniopharyngioma
    ectopic c.
cranioplasty
    aluminum c.
    hydroxyapatite
      cement c.
    metallic c.
    tantalum c.
craniopuncture
craniorrhachidian
craniosacral
    c. outflow
    c. technique
    c. therapy
cranioscopy
craniosinus fistula
craniospinal
    c. irradiation
    c. space
craniosynostosis
craniotomy
    attached c.
    awake c.
    bifrontal c.
    c. defect
    detached c.
    endoscopic frontal c.
    frontal c.
    frontotemporal c.
    left frontal c.

    open stereotactic c.
    osteoplastic c.
    pterional c.
    right temporoparietal c.
    stereotactic c.
    subtemporal c.
    supratentorial c.
    Yasargil c.
craniotonoscopy
craniotrypesis
craniotympanic
cranium, *pl.* **crania**
crash technique
crassum
    intestinum c.
crater formation
Crawford
    C. epidural needle
    C. eyelid tarsofrontalis sling
    C. graft inclusion technique
    C. incision
    C. ptosis correction method
Crawford-Adams cup arthroplasty
Crawford-Marxen-Osterfeld staged talipes
  equinovarus repair technique
craze line
CRC
    colorectal cancer
    colorectal carcinoma
    CRC resection
    sporadic CRC
CRE
    cardiorespiratory endurance
cream, creme
    imiquimod 5% c.
crease
    digital flexion c.
    flexion c.
    inframammary c.
    midline abdominal c.
    palmar c.
    skin c.
    torso c.
    c. wound
creation
    kyphosis c.
    lordosis c.
    McIndoe vaginal c.
    Politano-Leadbetter tunnel c.
    tunnel c.
Credé
Creech
    C. aortoiliac graft
    C. endoaneurysmorrhaphy
      technique
creeping fat
Crego
    C. femoral osteotomy
    C. tendon transfer technique

cremasteric
    c. fascia
    c. muscle
    c. reflex
    c. vein
creme (*var. of* cream)
crena clunium
Creola body
crescent
    articular c.
    c. body
    c. corneal graft
    glomerular c.
    c. mastopexy
    c. operation
    sublingual c.
crescentic
    c. calcaneal osteotomy
    c. osteotomy
    c. rupture
Crespo operation
crest
    articular c.
    buccinator c.
    deltoid c.
    endoalveolar c.
    ethmoidal c.
    external occipital c.
    falciform c.
    frontal c.
    iliac c.
    infratemporal c.
    inguinal c.
    intermediate sacral c.
    internal occipital c.
    interosseous c.
    intertrochanteric c.
    interureteric c.
    lacrimal c.
    nasal c.
    obturator c.
    pubic c.
    sacral c.
    supinator c.
    supraventricular c.
    terminal c.
    tibial c.
    trochanteric c.
    urethral c.
    vestibular c.
cribriform
    c. area
    c. carcinoma
    c. fascia
    c. plate
    c. subtype
cribrosus
    status c.
cribrous lamina

cribrum
cricoarytenoid
    c. joint
    c. ligament
    c. muscle
cricoesophageal tendon
cricohyoidepiglottopexy
cricoid
    c. cartilage
    c. myotomy
    c. pressure
    c. pressure anesthetic technique
    c. ring
    stenotic c.
    c. yoke
cricomyotomy
cricopharyngeal
    c. dilation
    c. myotomy
cricopharyngeus muscle
cricothyroid
    c. artery
    c. articular capsule
    c. articulation
    c. joint
    c. ligament
    c. membrane
    c. muscle
cricothyroidotomy (*var. of* cricothyrotomy)
cricothyrotomy, cricothyroidotomy
    scalpel c.
    wire-guided c.
cricotracheal
    c. ligament
    c. membrane
    c. resection (CTR)
cricotracheotomy
cricovocal membrane
CRIES
    Children's Revised Impact of Event Scale
Crile-Matas regional anesthesia
criminal nerve of Grassi
crises (*pl. of* crisis)
crisis, *pl.* **crises**
    pheochromocytoma c.
    pulmonary hypertensive c. (PHTC)
crisscrossing abdominal wall incisions
crista, *pl.* **cristae**
    c. galli
cristae (*pl. of* crista)
crit
    hematocrit
Critchett corneal staphyloma operation
criteria (*pl. of* criterion)
critical
    c. care anesthesiology
    c. care medicine (CCM)
    c. closing pressure

C

critical (*continued*)
    c. illness polyneuropathy (CIPN)
    c. illness polyneuropathy and
      myopathy (CIPNM)
    c. illumination
    c. mass
CRN
    cerebral radiation necrosis
CRNA
    certified registered nurse anesthetist
CRO
    centric relation occlusion
**Crock anterior cervical spine encircling
operation**
**Croften eosinophilic lung disease
classification**
Crohn
    C. disease
    C. tag
Cronkhite-Canada syndrome
CROP
    compliance, rate, oxygenation, pressure
Crosby
    C. capsule
    C. lung volume reduction
Crosby-Kugler
    C.-K. biopsy capsule
    C.-K. capsule for biopsy
cross (X)
    c. flap
    c. infection
    c. section
crossarch fulcrum line
cross-arm (*var. of* crossarm)
crossarm, cross-arm
    c. flap
cross-bar (*var. of* crossbar)
crossbar, cross-bar
    c. stomach deformity
cross-bracing, crossbracing
crossbracing (*var. of* cross-bracing)
cross-clamping, crossclamping
    aortic c.-c.
    infrarenal aortic c.-c.
    thoracic aortic c.-c. (TAC)
crossclamping (*var. of* cross-clamping)
crosscompression
    neurovascular c.
Crosseal human fibrin sealant
crossed (X-ed)
    c. anesthesia
    c. extension reflex
    c. extensor reflex
    c. fixation
    c. pyramidal tract
cross-facial, crossfacial
    c.-f. nerve graft
    c.-f. nerve graft anastomosis
    c.-f. technique

crossfacial (*var. of* cross-facial)
cross-finger flap
cross-hatch (*var. of* crosshatch)
crosshatch, cross-hatch
    c. incision
cross-leg (*var. of* crossleg)
crossleg, cross-leg
    c. flap
crosslink plate size
cross-lip (*var. of* crosslip)
crosslip, cross-lip
    c. pedicle flap
cross-modality matching
crossover
    femorofemoral c.
    FF c.
    c. toe deformity
crosspin
cross-polarization photography
crossreact
crossreactivity
cross-section
    capture c.-s.
cross-sectional
    c.-s. area
    c.-s. method
    c.-s. projection
crosstable lateral projection
cross-tolerance, crosstolerance
crosstolerance (*var. of* cross-tolerance)
crosstrigonal repair
cross-tunneling, crosstunneling
    c.-t. incision
crosstunneling (*var. of* cross-tunneling)
crossvector A scan
crotaphion
croup
    postextubation c.
    postintubation c.
croupous
    c. inflammation
    c. membrane
Crouzon
    C. disease
    C. syndrome
crowded carpal sign
Crowe
    C. hip dysplasia classification
    C. pilot point
crowfoot closure
crowing inspiration
crown
    c. angulation
    c. fracture
    c. inclination
    c. restoration
    C. suture technique
crown-contouring method
crown-root fracture

Crozat orthodontic therapy
CRPF
closed reduction and percutaneous fixation
CRPP
Cognitive Risk Profile for Pain
CRPS
complex regional pain type I, II syndrome
crucial
c. anastomosis
c. incision
cruciate
c. anastomosis
c. eminence
c. incision
c. ligament reconstruction
c. muscle
cruciform
c. eminence
c. ligament
c. suture technique
crunch-stick anastomosis
cruor
crura (*pl. of* crus)
crural
c. arch
c. area
c. canal
c. closure
c. fascia
c. fossa
c. hernia
c. repair
c. ring
c. septum
c. sheath
crurotomy
crus, *pl.* **crura**
c. clitoridis
lateral c.
medial c.
c. muscle
crush
c. fracture
c. injury
c. preparation
c. syndrome
crushed
c. eggshell fracture
c. tissue
crushing
c. anastomosis
c. technique
crusotomy
Crutchfield closed cervical spine fracture-dislocation technique
Cruveilhier
C. fascia

C. fossa
C. plexus
C. ulcer
Cruveilhier-Baumgarten anomaly
cryoablation
argon gas c.
encircling c.
laparoscopically guided c.
liquid nitrogen c.
c. probe
cryoanalgesia
cryoanesthesia
cryoapplication
cryoassisted resection
cryocautery
cryocoagulation
cryoconization
cryoelectron microscopy
cryoextraction operation
cryogenic
c. ablation
c. neuroablation
cryohypophysectomy
CryoLife
cryolysis
cryopallidectomy
cryopexy
barrage c.
double freeze-thaw c.
cryoprecipitate
cryopreservation
cryopreserved
c. aortic homograft
c. extrapelvic ovarian transplant
c. heart-valve allograft
c. tissue bank
cryoprostatectomy
cryopulvinectomy
cryoretinopexy
cryoscopy
cryostat
c. section
c. tissue section
cryosurgery
cryosurgical
c. ablation
c. technique
cryothalamectomy
cryotherapy operation
crypt
c. abscess
anal c.
c. atrophy
enamel c.
c. epithelium
ileal c.
Lieberkühn c.
Morgagni c.
tonsillar c.

crypta, *pl.* **cryptae**
cryptae (*pl. of* crypta)
cryptectomy
cryptococcal infection
Cryptococcus **infection**
cryptogenic
    c. cirrhosis
    c. infection
cryptoglandular
    c. disease
    c. infection
cryptorchidectomy
cryptorchidopexy
cryptorchid testis
cryptorchism
cryptosis
cryptosporidial infection
crystalline lens equator
crystallized trypsin
crystalloid
    c. cardioplegic solution
    Reinke c.
Csapody orbital repair
CSEA
    combined spinal-epidural anesthesia
    CSEA technique
C-section
    lower uterine segment transverse
      C-s.
    LUST C-s.
CSF
    cerebrospinal fluid
    blood-tinged CSF
    CSF pressure
C-shaped
    C-s. canal
    C-s. scalp flap
CSO
    clinically severe obesity
CSQ
    Coping Strategies Questionnaire
CST
    Certified Surgical Technologist
CSTFA
    Certified Surgical Technologist, First
    Assist
4C-T
    4-chamber transverse
5C-T
    5-chamber transverse
CT
    circulation time
    computed tomography
      appendiceal CT
      contrast-enhanced CT
      CT epidurography
      helical CT
      CT portography
      CT scan

      CT scan-guided needle aspiration
      CT scanning
      thin-section CT
      CT volumetry
      CT with hepatic arterial injection
CTAP
    computed tomography arterial
      portography
CTD
    chest tube drainage
    mediastinal CTD
CT-directed needle aspiration
CT-guided
    CT-g. fine-needle aspiration
    CT-g. liver biopsy
    CT-g. needle aspiration biopsy
    CT-g. selective drainage
    CT-g. stereotactic evacuation
CTL
    cytotoxic T-lymphocyte
    CTL immunity
    CTL immunity against melanoma
CTL-inducing peptide antigen
CT–1 needle suture
CT–2 needle suture
CTO
    cervicothoracic orthosis
    chest tube output
CT-proven necrosis
CTS
    cardiothoracic surgery
    carpal tunnel syndrome
CTSI
    computed tomography severity index
Cubbins
    C. arthroplasty
    C. incision
    C. open reduction
    C. shoulder approach
    C. shoulder dislocation technique
cubital tunnel syndrome
cubiti (*pl. of* cubitus)
cubitus, *pl.* **cubiti**
    c. valgus
    c. valgus deformity
    c. varus correction
cuboid bone
CUC
    chronic ulcerative colitis
cuff
    c. abscess
    aortic c.
    denuded rectal c.
    distal vein c.
    c. filling
    gastric c.
    c. laceration
    c. leak
    c. malfunction

massive c. (MaC)
Miller c.
musculotendinous c.
neoatrial c.
oscillometric blood pressure c.
rectal muscle c.
c. resection
rotator c.
suprahepatic c.
c. suspension
c. tear arthropathy
c. tear arthroplasty
vaginal c.
vein c.
4-cuff technique segmental pressure measurement
Cuignet retinoscopy method
cuirasse
carcinoma en c.
cuirass ventilation
cul-de-sac
conjunctival c.-d.-s.
c.-d.-s. fluid
glaucomatous c.-d.-s.
greater c.-d.-s.
Gruber c.-d.-s.
lesser c.-d.-s.
c.-d.-s. mass
ocular c.-d.-s.
c.-d.-s. of Bruger
c.-d.-s. of Douglas
ophthalmic c.-d.-s.
optic c.-d.-s.
rectouterine c.-d.-s.
c.-d.-s. restoration
culdoplasty
Halban c.
Marion-Moschcowitz c.
McCall c.
culdoscopy
culdotomy
Cullen sign
culprit
c. lesion
c. lesion angioplasty
Culp spiral flap pyeloplasty
culture
bronchoalveolar lavage c.
colony c.
fibroblast c.
c. medium
pus c.
sputum c.
cultured
c. epithelial autograft
c. human skin equivalent
Cummer partial denture classification
cumulative
c. operative morbidity

c. operative mortality
c. pain score (CPS)
c. score
c. trauma disorder
cuneiform
c. bone
c. cartilage
c. osteotomy
c. tubercle
cuneocerebellar tract
cuneonavicular
cunnus
cup
c. insemination
optic c.
c. to disc ratio (C:D)
cup-and-ball osteotomy
cup-and-cone method
cup-cement interface
cupola (*var. of* cupula)
cup-patch ileocystoplasty technique
Cüppers
C. euthyscopy method
C. method of pleoptics
cupping
cupula, cupola, *pl.* **cupulae**
pleural c.
cupulae (*pl. of* cupula)
cupular blind sac
cupulolithiasis
curability
curage
curare
curarization
curative
c. intent
c. potential
c. procedure
c. radical total gastrectomy
c. resection
c. sphincter-saving operation
curative-intent
c.-i. operation
c.-i. procedure
c.-i. surgery
curb tenotomy
curettage, curettement
dilatation and c. (D&C)
dilation and c. (D&C)
endocervical c.
endometrial c.
fractional dilation and c.
periapical c.
soft-tissue c.
suction c.
curettement (*var. of* curettage)
curioscopy
curlicue ureter
currant jelly clot

C

current
  amplitude-summation interferential c.
  demarcation c.
  Limoge c.
  membrane c.
  c. perception threshold (CPT)
  C. Procedural Terminology (CPT)
  saturation c.
curse
  Ondine c.
Curth-Maklin cornification disorder
Curtin
  C. incision
  C. plantar fibromatosis excision
Curtis
  C. flexion contracture release
    technique
  C. PIP joint capsulotomy
Curtis-Fisher knee technique
curtsy
  laparoscopic c.
curvatura
curvature, curvatura
  c. aberration
  anterior corneal c.
  canal c.
  corneal c.
  greater c.
  lesser c.
curve
  accommodation c.
  area under c. (AUC)
  articulation c.
  calibration c.
  carbon dioxide dissociation c.
  discrimination c.
  displacement c.
  dissociation c.
  dose-effect c.
  dose-response c.
  elimination c.
  Frank-Starling c.
  hemoglobin-oxygen dissociation c.
  indicator-dilution c.
  interpolated c.
  intracardiac pressure c.
  load-deflection c.
  load-deformation c.
  load-displacement c.
  oxygen dissociation c.
  oxygen-hemoglobin dissociation c.
  oxyhemoglobin dissociation c.
  pressure-natriuresis c.
  pressure-volume c.
  strength-duration c.
  survival c.
  time-concentration c.
  Traube-Hering c.
  whole-body titration c.

curved
  c. approach
  c. canal
  c. end-to-end anastomosis
  c. flank position
  c. incision
  c. radiolucent line
curved-needle surgeon's knot
curvilinear incision
Cushing
  C. adrenal hyperplasia
  C. pituitary operation
  C. pressure response
  C. reflex
  C. suture
  C. suture technique
  C. syndrome
cushioning suture technique
Cusick blepharoptosis operation
Cusick-Sarrail ptosis operation
cusp
  c. fenestration
  c. plane
  c. restoration
  valve c.
cusp-fossa relation
cuspid-molar position
Custodis
  C. nondraining procedure
  C. suture
cut
  c. end
  c. point
  sector c.
  semilunate c.
  c. surface
**Cutalon nylon polyamide surgical
  suture**
cut-and-sew technique
cutaneobiliary fistula
cutaneomucosal
cutaneomucous muscle
cutaneomucouveal syndrome
cutaneous
  c. analgesic effect
  c. appendiceal conduit
  c. bacterial infection
  c. burn injury
  c. cervical nerve
  c. collateral circulation
  c. examination
  c. forearm flap
  c. gangrene
  c. gland
  c. graft-versus-host disease
  c. graft-versus-host reaction
  c. heat loss
  c. hemorrhoid
  c. ileocystostomy

c. innervation
c. lesion
c. loop ureterostomy
c. malformation
c. manifestation
c. melanoma
c. metastasis
c. metastatic breast carcinoma
c. muscle
c. perception
c. stimulation
c. stria
c. suture technique
c. tissue
c. vesicostomy
c. viral infection
cutaneus
nodulus c.
cutback anoplasty
cutback-type vaginoplasty
cutdown
c. access
c. incision
c. technique
venous c.
cuticular
c. membrane
c. stitch
c. suture technique
cuticularization
cutin
cutis
c. anserina
c. graft
c. marmorata telangiectatica
congenita (CMTC)
Cutler
C. breast cancer classification
C. ophthalmic operation
Cutler-Beard
C.-B. bridge flap
C.-B. eyelid repair
cutoff
anesthetic c.
cutpoint
cutter
suture c.
valve c.
cutting
circle straight c.
c. needle biopsy
section c.
ultrasonic c.
Cuvier
canal of C.
CVA
cerebrovascular accident
CVAD
central venous access device

CVAS
Colored Visual Analogue Scale
CVD
cardiovascular disease
CVI
chronic venous insufficiency
CVP
central venous pressure
intraoperative CVP
CVP line
CVVHD
continuous venovenous hemodialysis
CXR
chest x-ray
cyanosis
compression c.
shunt c.
cyanotic induration
Cybex dynamometer
cyclarthrodial
cyclarthrosis
cycle
healing c.
cyclectomy
cyclic, cyclical
c. ether
c. fasting motility
c. pain
c. respiration
c. vertigo
cyclical (*var. of* cyclic)
cyclicotomy
cyclitic membrane
cyclocryopexy
cyclodestructive procedure
cyclodialysis
Barkan double c.
cyclodiathermy operation
cycloelectrolysis
cyclooxygenase-2 (COX-2)
cyclopentolate
cyclophotocoagulation
Nd:YAG c.
transpupillary c.
cycloplegia
cyclopropane
cyclops
c. formation
c. procedure
cycloscopy
cyclotomy
cylicotomy
cylinder
hilar c.
c. retinoscopy
cylindrical
c. carcinoma
c. confronting cisterna
c. osteotomy

C

cylindroadenoma
cylindroid aneurysm
cylindroma
cylindromatous lesion
cylindrosarcoma
cyma line
Cymbalta
Cyrano de Bergerac nose
 deformity
cyst
    air c.
    amebic c.
    anterior c.
    arachnoid c.
    c. aspiration
    Baker c.
    benign liver c.
    benign subcutaneous c.
    blue dome breast c.
    branchial c.
    branchial cleft c.
    branchiogenous c.
    breast c.
    chocolate c.
    choledochal c.
    chyle c.
    colloid c.
    compound c.
    congenital choledochal c.
    c. content
    corpus luteum c.
    daughter c.
    dermoid c.
    double unilateral c.'s
    duplication c.
    echinococcal liver c.
    echinococcus c.
    enteric c.
    enterogenous c.
    epidermal inclusion c.
    epidermoid c.
    epithelial c.
    c. fenestration
    follicular c.
    foregut c.
    ganglion c.
    gastric duplication c.
    granddaughter c.
    hepatic parasitic c.
    hydatid liver c.
    hyperplastic c.
    intraluminal c.
    involution c.
    laryngeal c.
    liver c.
    mesenteric c.
    milk-filled c.
    mother c.
    multilocular c.

    myoid c.
    nabothian c.
    nonparasitic liver c.
    omental c.
    ovarian dermoid c.
    pancreatic c.
    parasitic c.
    perforated c.
    pilonidal c.
    posterior c.
    preauricular c.
    primordial c.
    Rathke pouch c.
    renal c.
    residual c.
    retention c.
    sacrococcygeal c.
    Sampson c.
    sebaceous c.
    simple c.
    simple liver c.
    splenic c.
    subcutaneous c.
    sublingual c.
    theca lutein c.
    thymic c.
    thyroglossal duct c.
    thyroid c.
    Tornwaldt c.
    unilateral c.
    unilocular c.
    vitellointestinal c.
    c. wall
    wolffian c.
    young c.
cystadenocarcinoma
    bile duct c.
    mucinous c.
    papillary c.
    pseudomucinous c.
    serous c.
cystadenofibroma
cystadenoma
    biliary c.
    ductal c.
    duct-ectatic mucinous c.
    hyperplastic c.
    mucinous c.
    mucous c.
    thyroid c.
cystectomy
    Bartholin c.
    ovarian c.
    partial c.
    pilonidal c.
    radical c.
    salvage c.
    total c.
    vulvovaginal c.

cystenterostomy
    direct c.
    endoscopic c.
cystic
    c. acute inflammation
    c. adenocarcinoma
    c. adenomatoid malformation (CAM)
    c. artery
    c. bone lesion
    c. cavity
    c. chronic inflammation
    c. dilation
    c. duct
    c. duct catheterization
    c. duct choledochoscopy
    c. duct-infundibulum junction
    c. duct marking technique
    c. duct stump leak
    c. echinococcosis
    c. granulomatous inflammation
    c. hidradenoma
    c. kidney
    c. kidney disease
    c. lymphangioma
    c. lymphoepithelial AIDS-related lesion
    c. mass
    c. medial necrosis
    c. metastasis
    c. neoplasia
    c. neoplasm
    c. node
    c. polyp
    c. puncture
    c. structure
cystica
    arteria c.
cysticercal infection
cystici
cysticolithectomy
cysticolithotripsy
cysticorrhaphy
cysticotomy
cysticus
    ductus c.
cystidoceliotomy
cystidolaparotomy
cystidotrachelotomy
cystine calculus
cystis
cystitis
    interstitial c.
    schistosomal c.
cystoadenoma
cystobiliary communication

cystocarcinoma
cystocele repair
cystochromoscopy
cystocolostomy
cystodiaphanoscopy
cystoduodenal ligament
cystoduodenostomy
    endoscopic c.
    pancreatic c.
cystoenterocele
cystoenterostomy
    pancreatic c.
cystoepithelioma
cystofibroma
cystogastric fistula
cystogastrostomy
    endoscopic c.
    pancreatic c.
    surgical c.
cystography
cystoid body
cystojejunostomy
    Roux-en-Y c.
cystolith
cystolithectomy
cystolithiasis
cystolithic
cystolitholapaxy
cystolithotomy
cystolysis
cystoma
cystometrography (*var. of* cystometry)
cystometry, cystometrography
cystopanendoscopy
cystopericystectomy
    total closed c.
    total open c.
cystopexy
cystoplasty
    augmentation c.
    Gil-Vernet ileocecal c.
    human lyophilized dura c.
    ileocecal c.
    nonsecretory sigmoid c.
    sigmoid c.
cystoproctostomy
cystoprostatectomy
cystoprostatourethrectomy
cystoprostatovesiculectomy
cystorectostomy
cystorrhaphy
cystosarcoma phyllodes
cystoscopic electrohydraulic lithotripsy
cystoscopy
    percutaneous fetal c.
    steerable c.
    virtual c.
cystostomy
    trocar c.

C

cystotomy
    suprapubic c.
cystotrachelotomy
cystourethrocele
cystourethrography
cystourethropexy
    obturator shelf c.
    Pereyra-Raz c.
    vaginal c.
cystourethroplasty
    Kropp c.
    Leadbetter c.
cystourethroscopy
    dynamic c.
cytobrush biopsy
cytochrome
    myocardial c.
cytoid body
cytokeratin immunostain
cytokine
    inflammatory c.
    c. network
    c. production
    c. receptor inhibitor
cytologic
    c. abnormality
    c. biopsy
    c. diagnosis
    c. evaluation
    c. examination
    c. feature
    c. result
    c. specimen
    c. study
    c. washing
cytological assessment
cytology
    abnormal c.
    aspiration biopsy c. (ABC)
    brush c.
    endometrial c.
    endoscopic brush c.
    endoscopic fine-needle aspiration c.
    endoscopic ultrasonography-guided c.

    equivocal pancreatic c.
    EUS-guided c.
    c. examination
    exfoliative c.
    fine-needle aspiration c.
    gastric c.
    guided needle aspiration c.
    intraoperative touch prep c.
    needle aspiration c.
    negative c.
    negative peritoneal c.
    nipple aspiration c.
    oral cavity c.
    peritoneal c.
    positive c.
    positive peritoneal c.
    salvage c.
    c. sample
    c. specimen
cytomegalovirus (CMV)
    c. colitis
    c. infection
    c. prophylaxis
cytomegalovirus-positive donor
cytometric bead array
cytoplasm
cytoplasmic membrane
cytopreparation
cytoreduction
    complete c.
    optimal c.
cytoreductive surgery
cytotoxic
    c. T-lymphocyte (CTL)
    c. T-lymphocyte immunity
cytotoxicity
Czermak pterygium operation
Czerny
    C. cholecystopexy
    C. suture
    C. suture technique
Czerny-Lembert
    C.-L. suture
    C.-L. suture technique

2D

2D transit time

3D

3-dimensional
3D computer reconstruction
3D transesophageal
echocardiography
3D ultrasound probe
3D visualization

D

D line
D point

D1

limited gastric cancer lymph node
dissection

D2

extended gastric cancer lymph node
dissection
D2 dissection
D2 lymphadenectomy

D3

superextended gastric cancer lymph
node dissection

da

d. Vinci robot
d. Vinci robotic telemanipulation
system

daclizumab

Dacron

D. bolstered suture
D. exoskeleton
D. suture
D. traction suture

dacryoadenectomy operation
dacryocyst
dacryocystectomy operation
dacryocystocele
dacryocystoethmoidostomy
dacryocystorhinostomy

Mosher d.
Mosher-Toti d.
Polyak endonasal d.

dacryocystorhinotomy operation
dacryocystostomy

Ammon d.
d. operation

dacryon
dacryorhinocystostomy
dacryorhinocystotomy
dacryostenosis
dacryostomy

Arroyo d.
Arruga d.
Blaskovics d.
Dupuy-Dutemps d.

Gutzeit d.
Rowinski d.

dactyledema
dactylitis
dactylomegaly
dactyloscopy
dactylospasm
dacuronium
Dafilon suture
dagger sign
Dagradi esophageal variceal
classification
Dagrofil suture
Dale-Laidlaw clotting time method
Dalgleish eyelid reconstruction
Dallas operation
Dalrymple sign
damage

anterior cervical surgery vocal
cord d.
cellular d.
d. control
end-organ d.
endothelial d.
irradiation d.
liver d.
nervous d.
obturator nerve d.
postsurgical nervous d.
projection fiber d.
radiation d.
soft tissue d.
subretinal d.
sun and chemical
combination d.
thermal injury-induced lung d.
tourniquet-related nerve d.
vocal cord d.

damage-control celiotomy
damaged parenchyma
Damian graft procedure
Damus-Kaye-Stansel (DKS)

D.-K.-S. pulmonary artery to
ascending aorta anastomosis
procedure
D.-K.-S. pulmonary artery to
ascending aorta anastomotic
operation

Dana

D. operation
D. posterior rhizotomy

DANA

designed after natural anatomy

Dana-Farber Cancer Institute
Dance sign

D

Dandy
- D. cerebrospinal fluid leak maneuver
- D. myocutaneous scalp flap
- D. retroganglial neurotomy
- D. third ventriculostomy
- D. trigeminal rhizotomy

Dandy-Walker
- D.-W. deformity
- D.-W. malformation
- D.-W. syndrome

Danforth fetal operation

danger space

Daniel iliac bone graft

Danielson posterior annuloplasty method

Danis-Weber
- D.-W. ankle injury classification
- D.-W. fracture

Dardik umbilical graft

dark-field
- d.-f. examination
- d.-f. illumination
- d.-f. microscopy

dark-ground illumination

Darling capsulotomy

Darrach
- D. distal ulna resection
- D. extensor carpi ulnaris tendesis procedure

Darrach-McLaughlin shoulder technique

darting incision

dartos
- d. fascia
- d. muscle
- d. pouch procedure

Das
- D. Gupta scapular excision
- D. Gupta scapulectomy
- D. Gupta transbronchial needle aspiration procedure

dashboard
- d. dislocation
- d. fracture

Daubenton
- D. angle
- D. line
- D. plane

d'Aubigné
- d. femoral reconstruction
- d. resection reconstruction

daughter cyst

Davey-Rorabeck-Fowler decompression technique

David Letterman sign

Daviel extracapsular cataract extraction

Davis
- D. drainage technique
- D. fusion
- D. intubated ureterostomy
- D. intubated ureterotomy
- D. muscle-pedicle graft

Davis-Geck (DG)
- D.-G. blepharoplasty
- D.-G. Softgut suture
- D.-G. suture

Davis-Kitlowski otoplasty procedure

Davydov vaginoplasty procedure

DAWG
- demucosalized augmentation with gastric segment
- DAWG procedure

Dawson criteria

day
- d. care surgical unit (DCSU)
- postoperative d. (POD)
- posttransplant d.

day-case operation

DBM
- demineralized bone matrix

D&C
- dilatation and curettage
- dilation and curettage

DCD
- donation after cardiac death

DCIS
- ductal carcinoma in situ
- focal DCIS
- multifocal extensive DCIS
- residual DCIS

DCR
- dacryocystorhinostomy

DCS
- dorsal column stimulation
- dorsal cord stimulation

DCSU
- day care surgical unit

DCT
- deceleration time

D-D anastomosis

DDA
- dorsal digital artery

DDx
- differential diagnosis

de
- d. Grandmont operation
- d. Mussy point
- d. novo lesion
- d. novo needle-knife technique
- d. Quervain fracture
- d. Quervain stenosing tenosynovitis release
- d. Quervain syndrome
- d. Quervain tenosynovitis
- d. Vincentiis goniotomy

deactivation
- trigger point d.

dead
>d. space
>d. space obliteration
>d. space to tidal volume ratio
>d. tract

deafferentation
>d. pain
>d. pain syndrome
>spinal d.

deairing procedure
Dean and Webb titration
dearterialization
>hepatic d.

death
>apoptotic endothelial cell d.
>brain d.
>cerebral d.
>donation after cardiac d. (DCD)
>intraoperative d.
>noncancer d.
>perioperative d.
>postoperative d.
>thymic d.
>trauma-related d.
>tumor-related d.
>vascular disease d.

Deaver incision
DeBakey
>D. aortic dissection classification
>D. type I aortic dissection
>D. VAD
>D. woven polyester graft

DeBakey-Creech aneurysm repair
DeBakey-type
>D.-t. aortic dissection
>D.-t. noncrushing grasper

DeBastiani corticotomy
debilitated patient
debility
debouch
débouchement
Debove membrane
debridement
>mechanical d.

débridement
>d. arthroplasty
>arthroscopy and d.
>autolytic d.
>burn d.
>canal d.
>cavity d.
>chemical enzymatic wound d.
>diagnostic arthroscopy and d.
>enzymatic d.
>exploration and d.
>operative d.
>root canal d.
>surgical d.
>tangential d.

debris
>cellular d.
>valve d.

debt
>oxygen d.

debubbling procedure
debulking
>d. of tumor
>d. operation
>ovarian carcinoma d.
>d. procedure
>d. surgery
>surgical d.

decalcification
decannulation
>accidental d.

decapsulation
>partial laparoscopic d.

decayed, extracted, filled
deceleration time (DCT)
deception
>pain d.

decerebration
>bloodless d.

decerebrize
dechondrification
decidua
decidual membrane
deciduous
decimal reduction time
declamping
>d. phenomenon
>d. shock

declination angle
décollement
>d. hemicolectomy
>d. maneuver

decompensated liver disease
decompensation
>circulatory d.
>hepatic d.
>d. injury
>respiratory d.
>vascular d.

decompress
decompression
>abdominal d.
>anterior retroperitoneal d.
>bone graft d.
>cardiac d.
>cerebral d.
>colonic needle d.
>d. colostomy
>4-compartment fascial d.
>continuous gastric d.
>endoscopic biliary d.
>extensive posterior d.
>fascial d.
>d. fasciotomy

D

decompression (*continued*)
    gaseous d.
    gastric d.
    d. incision
    internal d.
    d. jejunostomy
    d. laminectomy
    laser disc d. (LDD)
    microvascular d. (MVD)
    nasogastric d.
    nerve d.
    Ogura orbital d.
    orbital d.
    paraclavicular thoracic outlet d.
    percutaneous disc d.
    pericardial d.
    portal d.
    posterior fossa d.
    retroperitoneal d.
    d. rhachotomy
    Rowbotham orbital d.
    selective portal d.
    spinal d.
    suboccipital d.
    subtemporal d.
    surgical portal d.
    d. technique
    thoracic outlet d.
    transduodenal endoscopic d.
    trigeminal d.
    tube d.
    variceal d.
    vein d.
    vertebral body d.
decompressive
    d. laminectomy
    d. neurosurgery
    d. surgery
deconditioned exercise response
deconditioning
    postoperative d.
decontamination
    selective bowel d.
deconvolution
decortication
    arterial d.
    cerebral d.
    laparoscopic cyst d.
    renal cyst d.
    reversible d.
    d. technique
decrease
    hypoxic ventilatory d.
decreased
    d. afterload
    d. alveolar ventilation
    d. functional residual capacity
    d. preload
    d. respiration

decubital gangrene
decubitus
    d. calculus
    d. position
    d. view
decussation
    dorsal tegmental d.
    Forel d.
    fountain d.
    Held d.
    Meynert d.
    motor d.
    oculomotor d.
    optic d.
    pyramidal d.
    rubrospinal d.
    tectospinal d.
    ventral tegmental d.
    Wernekinck d.
dedolation
deendothelialization
deendothelialized
deep
    d. abdominal complication
    d. anal sphincter
    d. anterior neck
    d. anterior wall
    d. articular aorta
    d. articulation test
    d. auricular artery
    d. brachial artery
    d. brain stimulation (DBS)
    d. cardiac plexus
    d. cervical artery
    d. cervical fascia
    d. cervical vein
    d. chest therapy
    d. circumflex iliac artery-iliac crest flap
    d. circumflex inguinal artery
    d. crural arch
    d. delayed infection
    d. Doppler velocity interrogation
    d. epigastric artery
    d. extubation in tonsil position
    d. femoral artery
    d. forearm
    d. gastric-longitudinal (DG-L)
    d. gastric-transverse (DG-T)
    d. gastric transverse (DG-T)
    d. hypothermia
    d. hypothermia and circulatory arrest (DHCA)
    d. hypothermic circulatory arrest (DHCA)
    d. iliac dissection
    d. inferior epigastric perforator flap (DIEP)
    d. infrapatellar bursa

d. inguinal ring
d. interloop abscess
d. lamina
d. liver tract
d. lymphatic vessel
d. orbit
d. palmar arch
d. palmar branch
d. penis
d. perineal pouch
d. perineal space
d. peroneal nerve
d. peroneal nerve block
d. petrosal nerve
d. plantar branch
d. postanal anorectal space
d. profunda brachial artery
d. stitch
d. temporal artery
d. temporal nerve
d. tissue massage (DTM)
d. tumor
d. vein thrombosis (DVT)
d. venous thrombosis (DVT)
d. venous thrombosis prophylaxis
d. venous thrombus
d. volatile anesthesia
d. wound infection
deep-breathing exercise
deepicardialization
deepithelialization, deepithelization
deepithelialized, deepithelized
d. rectus abdominis muscle (DRAM)
d. rectus abdominis muscle flap
deepithelization (*var. of* deepithelialization)
deepithelized (*var. of* deepithelialized)
deep-seated fungal infection
defalcated root canal
Defares rebreathing method
defasciculating dose
defeat
mental d.
defecation
d. score
sense of d.
defecography
defect
aponeurotic d.
atrial septal d. (ASD)
atrioventricular canal d.
atrioventricular septal d. (AVSD)
bandeau d.
cartilaginous d.
chain-of-lakes filling d.
clinical d.
coagulation d.

cold d.
combined d.
craniotomy d.
dentinoenamel d.
diaphragmatic d.
direct d.
fascial d.
filling d.
frondlike filling d.
hernia d.
hot d.
iatrogenic hernia d.
indirect d.
mass d.
medial direct d.
napkin-ring d.
neural tube d.
oromandibular d.
osteoarticular d.
osteochondral d.
parasternal d.
parietal d.
perineal d.
peritoneal d.
pinpoint gastric mucosal d.
postinfarction ventricular septal d.
postinjury immunologic d.
postresection d.
Rastelli classification (A–C) of atrioventricular septal d.
repairable parietal d.
septal d.
slitlike d.
surgical d.
tumor d.
ventilation d.
ventilation/perfusion d.
ventricular septal d. (VSD)
ventricular septal wound d.
defense
antioxidant d.
thermoregulatory d.
deferens
vas d.
deferent
d. canal
d. duct
deferentectomy
deferential
d. artery
d. plexus
deferentialis
arteria d.
deferentis
ampulla ductus d.
deferentitis
deferoxamine
deferred shock, delayed shock

D

defibrillation
  cardiac d.
  d. shock
  d. threshold
defibrillator
  automatic external d. (AED)
defibrillatory shock
deficiency
  protein C d.
  pseudocholinesterase d.
  pyruvate kinase d.
deficit
  base d.
  delayed ischemic neurological d.
  neurologic d.
  neuropsychological d.
  normal base d.
  reversible ischemic neurologic d.
    (RIND)
  transient neurologic d.
  transient profound neurologic d.
defined sterilization
definitive
  d. cause
  d. local therapy
  d. method
  d. resection
  d. stabilization
  d. surgery
  d. tracheostomy
  d. treatment
deflation
  targeted lobar d.
deformation
deformity
  abduction d.
  acetabular protrusio d.
  acquired d.
  adduction d.
  adduction-internal rotation d.
  adductovarus d.
  Åkerlund d.
  d. analysis
  Andy Gump d.
  angel-wing d.
  d. angle
  angular d.
  angulation d.
  apple-peel d.
  Arnold-Chiari d.
  back-knee d.
  batwing d.
  bell-clapper d.
  bifid thumb d.
  bird-beak d.
  bony d.
  boutonnière d.
  bowing d.
  bowleg d.

bulb d.
bunion d.
burn boutonnière d.
buttonhole d.
calcaneocavovarus d.
calcaneocavus d.
calcaneovalgus d.
calcaneovarus d.
cavovarus d.
cavus d.
cecal d.
cervical spine kyphotic d.
cervicomedullary d.
chain-of-lakes d.
checkrein d.
chest d.
Christmas tree d.
clasped thumb d.
cleft hand d.
cleft lip d.
cloverleaf skull d.
clubfoot d.
cock-up d.
codfish d.
combined cavus d.
compensatory d.
complete bilateral deformities
congenital postural d.
coronal plane d.
craniofacial d.
crossbar stomach d.
crossover toe d.
cubitus valgus d.
Cyrano de Bergerac nose d.
Dandy-Walker d.
dentofacial d.
duodenal bulb d.
elevatus d.
equinovalgus d.
equinus d.
Erlenmeyer flask d.
eversion-external rotation d.
extension d.
facial d.
finger d.
fishtail d.
fixed d.
flat back d.
flexion d.
flexion-internal rotation d.
foot d.
funnel chest d.
garden spade d.
genu valgum d.
genu varum d.
gibbous d.
gingival d.
gooseneck d.
gross d.

Haglund d.
hallux valgus d.
hammertoe d.
hand d.
hatchet-head d.
Hill-Sachs d.
hindbrain d.
hindfoot d.
hip d.
hockey-stick d.
hook-nail d.
hourglass d.
humpback d.
hyperextension d.
internal rotation d.
intrinsic minus d.
intrinsic plus d.
joint d.
J-sella d.
keyhole d.
Kirner d.
kleeblatschädel d.
Klippel-Feil d.
knock-knee d.
kyphotic d.
lanceolate d.
limb d.
lobster-claw d.
lumbar spine kyphotic d.
Madelung d.
mallet finger d.
mallet toe d.
Michel d.
Mondini d.
nasal d.
opera-glass d.
parachute d.
pectus carinatum d.
pectus excavatum d.
pencil-in-cup d.
penile d.
percutaneous compression
  device-toe d.
pes planus d.
phrygian cap d.
pigeon-breast d.
ping-pong ball d.
1-plane d.
2-plane d.
3-plane d.
plantar flexion-inversion d.
posttraumatic spinal d.
postural d.
protrusio d.
pseudoboutonnière d.
rat-tail d.
recurvatum angulation d.
rotational d.
round back d.

round shoulder d.
sabre-shin d.
saddle-nose d.
sagittal d.
scoliotic d.
shepherd's crook d.
shoulder d.
silver-fork d.
skeletal d.
skull d.
spastic thumb-in-palm d.
spinal coronal plane d.
spine d.
spinning-top d.
splayfoot d.
splenic vein d.
split-hand d.
split-nail d.
spondylitic d.
Sprengel d.
S-shaped d.
stomach d.
subcondylar d.
supination d.
swan-neck finger d.
talipes cavus d.
thoracic spine kyphotic d.
thoracic spine scoliotic d.
thumb d.
thumb-in-palm d.
trefoil d.
triphalangeal thumb d.
turned-up pulp d.
ulnar deviation d.
ulnar drift d.
valgus d.
varus hindfoot d.
Velpeau d.
volar angulation d.
Volkmann clawhand d.
whistling d.
Whitehead d.
windblown d.
windsock d.
windswept d.
winged scapula d.
wrist d.
Zancolli procedure for
  clawhand d.
zig-zag compensatory d.
Z-type d.
deformity-instability
  spinal d.-i.
defunctionalization
defunctioning loop ileostomy
Dega pelvic osteotomy
degasified distilled water
degenerated fibroadenolipoma
degenerating otoconia

D

degeneration
    aberrant third nerve d.
    age-related macular d. (ARMD)
    intervertebral disc d.
    malignant d.
degenerative
    d. change
    d. discogenic endplate disease
    d. encephalopathy
    d. inflammation
    d. mitral valve insufficiency
degloving procedure
degradation
    anesthetic d.
    heme d.
    intracellular protein d.
    d. product
    protein d.
degrade
degree of inspiration
270-degree laparoscopic posterior fundoplasty
dehiscence
    abdominal incision d.
    anastomotic d.
    myofascial d.
    Roux limb stump d.
    scar d.
    staple line d.
    stump d.
    suture line d.
    total d.
    uterine d.
    wound d.
dehiscent mandibular canal
dehydration
    d. fever
    hyperosmolar d.
dehydrogenation
Deisting prostatic dilation technique
Deiter operation
deiterospinal tract
Deiters cell
Dejerine-Roussy syndrome
Deklene
    D. II cardiovascular suture
    D. polypropylene suture
Deknatel silk suture
delay
    calf inflate d.
    fixation d.
    d. line
delayed
    d. complication
    d. cutaneous hypersensitivity
    d. direct coloanal anastomosis
    d. expansion
    d. femoral osteotomy

    d. flap
    d. fracture union
    d. gastric emptying
    d. graft
    d. hemolytic reaction
    d. hyperacute transplant rejection
    d. ischemic neurological deficit
    d. massive hemorrhage
    d. onset muscle soreness (DOMS)
    d. open reduction
    d. pericardial tamponade
    d. pneumothorax
    d. primary closure
    d. primary repair
    d. primary suture technique
    d. pulmonary toxicity syndrome
    d. resuscitation
    d. urination
DeLee
    D. fetal positioning maneuver
    D. pediatric fracture classification
deletion
    clonal d.
deliberate
    d. hypotension
    d. hypotension anesthetic technique
delimiting keratotomy
delineating
delirium
    emergence d.
    postoperative d.
delivery
    buccal transmucosal d.
    cesarean d.
    closed loop automated d.
    controlled heat-aided drug d. (CHADD)
    epidural d.
    laser-assisted drug d.
    spinal d.
    tissue oxygen d.
    transmucosal d.
    vacuum extractor d.
Dellepiane hysterectomy
Deller modification
Delorme
    D. rectal prolapse repair
    D. rectal prolapse repair procedure
    D. thoracoplasty
delphian node
delta
    d. fibers
    portal d.
delta-shaped anastomosis
deltoid
    d. branch
    d. crest
    d. eminence

d. flap
d. muscle
deltoid-splitting
d.-s. incision
d.-s. shoulder approach
deltopectoral
d. approach
d. fascia
d. flap
d. groove
d. incision
d. sulcus
Del Toro hematopoietic stem cell transplant
deltoscapular flap
demand
d. minimum functional capacity
myocardial oxygen d.
demand-adapted administration anesthetic technique
demarcation
corticomedullary d.
d. current
d. potential
dementia
Pain Assessment in Advanced D. (PAINAD)
demineralization
bony d.
demineralized bone matrix (DBM)
demonstration
angiographic d.
Demours membrane
demucosalized
d. augmentation
d. augmentation with gastric segment (DAWG)
demyelinating lesion
demyelination, demyelinization
autoimmune d.
axonal d.
intramedullary d.
demyelinization (*var. of* demyelination)
DeMyer system of cerebral malformation
dendriform
dendrite
corneal d.
dendritic
d. calculus
d. carcinoma
d. lesion
dendrocytoma
denervate
denervation
d. disease
d. dysesthesia
extrinsic d.
facet d.
flank bulge post d.

d. hypersensitivity
Krause d.
law of d.
d. of pancreas
d. potential
preganglionic sympathetic d.
radiofrequency d.
sinoaortic d.
sympathetic d.
dengue hemorrhagic fever infection
Denham external fixation
Denis
D. Browne spinal fracture classification
D. Browne urethroplasty technique
denitrogenation
sympathetic d.
Denker sinus operation
Dennie line
Dennie-Morgan line
Dennis-Brooke ileostomy
Dennis left atrium cannulation technique
Dennis-Varco pancreatoduodenostomy
Denonvilliers
D. aponeurosis
D. fascia
D. ligament
D. space
dens, *pl.* **dentes**
d. anterior screw fixation
facet (of atlas) for d.
d. fracture
pit of atlas for d.
dense
d. adhesion
d. body
d. brain mass
d. nature
density
functional capillary d.
lymphatic microvessel d.
microvessel d.
raspberrylike d.
vapor d.
density-dependent repair
dental
d. anatomy
d. anesthesia
d. anomaly
d. anxiety
d. arch expansion
d. articulation
d. canal
d. cavity
d. fenestration
d. fistula
d. implant
d. index
d. infection

D

dental (*continued*)
    d. mycotic abdominal aneurysm
    d. nerve
    d. polyp
    d. prosthetic laboratory procedure
    d. psychosedation
    d. pulp extirpation
    d. puncture
    d. restoration
    d. sac
    d. sinus tract
    d. surgery
    d. trephination
    d. tubercle
    d. wedge
dentate
    d. fracture
    d. line
    d. margin
    d. suture
dentatectomy
dentatothalamic tract
dentes (*pl. of* dens)
denticulate ligament
dentin, dentine
    d. crystal alteration
    d. pain
dentinal canal
dentine (*var. of* dentin)
dentinoenamel
    d. defect
    d. membrane
dentoalveolar joint
dentofacial
    d. anomaly
    d. deformity
    d. surgery
denture
    d. classification
    d. foundation
    d. foundation area
    d. foundation surface
    d. space
denudation
    endothelial d.
    interdental d.
denuded
    d. bowel
    d. connective tissue
    d. furcation
    d. rectal cuff
Denver human mitotic chromosome classification
Denys-Drash syndrome
deoxyribonucleic acid (DNA)
Depage incision
Depage-Janeway
    D.-J. gastrostomy
    D.-J. gastrotomy

DePalma modified patellar technique
Department of Veterans Affairs pulmonary risk index
dependency
    preload d.
    ventilator d.
dependent drainage
depigmentation
    congenital d.
depigmented lesion
depilation
deplasmolysis
depletion
    intravascular volume d.
    pretransplant lymphoid d.
deployment
    stent d.
DepoDur
depolarization
    d. block
    primary afferent d.
depolarizing
    d. block
    d. blockade
    d. relaxant
Depo-Medrol
deposition
    abdominal iron d.
    collagen d.
depot
    d. corticosteroid
    d. formulation
depressant
depressed
    d. lesion
    d. side
    d. skull fracture
    d. type
depression
    d. fracture
    Hamilton Rating Scale for D.
    induced ventilatory d.
    inspiratory rib cage d.
    major d.
    respiratory d.
    twitch d.
    ventilatory d.
depression-related amotivation
deprivation amblyopia
depth
    anesthetic d.
    char-zone d.
    d. electrode
    indicator of anesthetic d.
    d. of anesthesia
    d. of anesthesia monitoring
    d. of insertion (DOI)
    d. pulse technique

derby
  D. fascia lata eyelid sling operation
  d. hat fracture
derivation
derivative
  d. circulation
  Thrombate III blood product d.
dermabrasion
  laser d.
  mechanical d.
DermaGlide oculoplastic suture
dermal
  d. fasciectomy
  d. fat free flap
  d. fat free tissue transfer
  d. fat graft
  d. fat pedicle flap
  d. fibroblast
  d. injection
  d. lesion
  d. loss
  d. lymphatics
  d. pouch
  d. pouch reconstruction
  d. route of injection
  d. scar
  d. sinus tract
  d. suture
  d. suture technique
  d. wound separation
Dermalene polyethylene suture
Dermalon cuticular suture
dermatitis
  intertriginous d.
  irritant d.
  perianal d.
dermatoalloplasty
dermatoautoplasty
dermatocele
dermatofibroma
dermatofibrosarcoma
dermatoheteroplasty
dermatohomoplasty
dermatologic
  d. disorder
  d. problem
dermatolysis
dermatomal
  d. distribution
  d. level of analgesia
  d. mapping
dermatome
  d. mapping
  sensory d.
  trigeminal d.
dermatomyoma
dermatophyte fungal infection
dermatoplasty
dermatoscopy

dermatoses (*pl. of* dermatosis)
dermatosis, *pl.* **dermatoses**
dermatoxenoplasty
dermis
  human fibroblast-derived d.
    (HFDD)
  d. patch graft
dermodesis
  resection d.
dermoepidermic graft
dermoid cyst
dermoidectomy
dermolipoma
dermolysis
dermoplasty
dermovascular
derotation
  counterclockwise d.
derotational osteotomy
desaturation
  apnea-induced hemoglobin d.
  arterial oxygen d.
  cerebral oximetric d.
  jugular bulb oxyhemoglobin d.
  oxygen d.
  red d.
Desault wrist dislocation
Descemet
  D. membrane
  D. membrane detachment
descending
  d. anterior branch
  d. aortic aneurysm
  d. artery of knee
  d. colon
  d. genicular artery
  d. genicular vein
  d. loop colostomy
  d. mesocolon
  d. nerve
  d. pain pathway
  d. palatine artery
  d. posterior branch
  d. scapular artery
  d. technique
Descot fracture
**Descriptor Differential Scale of Pain
  Intensity**
desensitization with towel rubbing
desflurane
desiccation
  electrosurgical d.
  mucous d.
design
  prodrug d.
designated blood donation
**designed after natural anatomy
  (DANA)**
Desjardins point

D

Desmarres
>   D. operation
>   D. pterygium procedure

desmocytoma

desmoid lesion

desmoplastic
>   d. medulloblastoma
>   d. trichilemmoma

desmopressin

desmotomy

destruction
>   bone d.
>   bony element d.
>   bony necrosis and d.
>   Cawthorne d.
>   cortical d.
>   moth-eaten bone d.
>   mucosal d.
>   neutrophil-dependent tissue d.
>   parenchymal d.
>   progressive parenchymal d.

destructive bone lesion

desyndactylization
>   Weinstock d.

detached
>   d. cranial section
>   d. craniotomy

detachment
>   Descemet membrane d.
>   exudative retinal d.
>   traction d.

detection
>   pancreatic fungal d.
>   sentinel lymph node d.
>   (SLND)
>   d. threshold

detector response

deterioration
>   aortic wall d.
>   clinical d.
>   microarchitectural d.

determinant
>   prognostic d.

determination
>   dye dilution d.
>   Fick d.
>   myeloperoxidase d.

detoxification
>   rapid opiate d.

detritus
>   tissue d.

detrusor
>   d. areflexia
>   d. instability
>   d. muscle
>   d. pressure
>   d. stability

devascularization
>   gastric d.

>   intraoperative complete liver d.
>   paraesophagogastric d.

devascularized parathyroid remnant

DeVega tricuspid valve anuloplasty

development
>   discontinuation-emergent symptom d.
>   pouch d.
>   sternal d.

developmental
>   d. coordination disorder
>   d. landmark
>   d. line
>   d. retardation

Deventer pelvis

Deverle fixation

deviant articulation

deviated septum

deviation to right

device
>   band-assist d.
>   bioartificial liver d.
>   bipolar ablation d.
>   biventricular assist d. (biVAD)
>   cardiac rhythm management d.
>   central venous access d. (CVAD)
>   Combitube airway d.
>   compression d.
>   internal microinfusion d.
>   interspinous process compression d.
>   intrauterine d. (IUD)
>   left ventricular assist d. (LVAD)
>   left ventricular assistive d. (LVAD)
>   plate-guided distraction d.
>   right ventricular assistive d.
>   (RVAD)
>   SonoPrep therapeutic ultrasound d.
>   staple-line reinforcement d.
>   d. therapy
>   vascular closure d.
>   ventricular assist d. (VAD)

Devine
>   D. antral exclusion
>   D. colostomy
>   D. hypospadias repair

devitalization
>   pulp d.

devitalized
>   d. bone graft
>   d. tissue

devitalize the tracheal mucosa

devolvulization
>   endoscopic d.

Devonshire colic

Dewar
>   D. posterior cervical fixation
>   procedure
>   D. posterior cervical fusion
>   D. posterior cervical fusion
>   technique

Dewar-Barrington
    D.-B. arthroplasty
    D.-B. clavicular dislocation
      technique
Dewar-Harris shoulder technique
DeWecker glaucoma operation
dewy appearance
dexiocardia (*var. of* dextrocardia)
dexmedetomidine
Dexon
    D. absorbable synthetic polyglycolic
      acid suture
    D. II suture
    D. mesh splenorrhaphy
    D. Plus suture
    D. suture
Dexter-Grossman aortic regurgitation
  classification
dextran reaction
dextrocardia, dexiocardia
    d. with situs inversus
dextrogyration
dextromethorphan
dextrorotation
dextrotorsion
dextroversion
Deyerle femoral fracture technique
DFI
    disease-free interval
DFS
    disease-free survival
DG
    Davis-Geck
      DG suture
DG-L
    deep gastric-longitudinal
DG-T
    deep gastric-transverse
    deep gastric transverse
DHCA
    deep hypothermia and circulatory
      arrest
    deep hypothermic circulatory arrest
diabetes
    frank d.
    d. mellitus
    posttransplant d.
diabetic
    d. coma
    d. complication
    d. foot
    d. gangrene
    d. ketoacidosis (DKA)
    d. neuropathic ulcer
    d. neuropathy
    d. patient
    d. peripheral nephropathy
    d. pseudotabes
    d. puncture

    d. retinal treatment
    d. retinopathy
diacele
diacetylcholine
diacondylar fracture
diagnoses (*pl. of* diagnosis)
diagnosis (Dx), *pl.* **diagnoses**
    anatomic d.
    channel d.
    clinical d.
    colposcopic d.
    cytologic d.
    differential d. (DDx)
    frozen section d.
    genetic d.
    histologic d.
    histopathologic d.
    microscopic d.
    noninvasive d.
    nonoperative d.
    operative d.
    pathologic d.
    postoperative d.
    preoperative d.
    presumptive d.
    surgical d.
diagnostic
    d. accuracy
    d. and operative arthroscopy
    D. and Statistical Manual of Mental
      Disorders, 4th Edition (DSM-IV)
    d. anesthesia
    d. arthroscopy and débridement
    d. arthroscopy, operative arthroscopy,
      possible operative arthrotomy
    d. articulation test
    d. aspiration
    d. biopsy
    d. block
    d. cardiac catheterization
    d. colonoscopy
    d. dilemma
    d. endoscopy
    d. fiberoptic stomatoscopy
    d. finding
    d. IGBB
    d. imaging evaluation
    d. investigation
    d. laparoscopy
    d. modality
    d. peritoneal lavage (DPL)
    d. procedure
    d. program
    d. radiation
    d. small-bowel series
    d. step
    d. study
    d. surgical therapy
    d. technique

D

diagnostic (*continued*)
    d. tube
    d. value
    d. workup
diagonal section
dial
    d. pelvic osteotomy
    d. periacetabular osteotomy
dialectical behavioral therapy
dialysate preparation module
dialysis
    d. access surgery
    arteriovenous d.
    d. clinic
    continuous ambulatory peritoneal d.
      (CAPD)
    d. disequilibrium syndrome
    d. encephalopathy syndrome
    extracorporeal d.
    d. fistula
    inpatient d.
    maintenance d.
    d. membrane
    outpatient d.
    peritoneal d.
    postoperative d.
    d. treatment
dialysis-dependent patient
dialytic ultrafiltration
dialyzer membrane
diameter
    biparietal d. (BPD)
    corneal d.
    end-diastolic d. (EDD)
    end-systolic d. (ESD)
    maximal rectal d.
    rectal d.
diametric pelvic fracture
diamond
    d. anastomosis
    D. classification
    d. ejection murmur
    d. inlay bone graft
Diamond-Gould
    D.-G. reduction syndactylia
    D.-G. syndactyly operation
diamond-shaped incision
Dianoux sclerotomy
diaphoresis
diaphragm
    bare area d.
    central tendon d.
    d. eventration
    d. injury
    d. laceration
    laryngeal d.
    myopectineal d.
    pelvic d.
    d. perforation

    respiratory d.
    sternal part of d.
    urogenital d.
diaphragma, *pl.* **diaphragmata**
diaphragmata (*pl. of* diaphragma)
diaphragmatic
    d. anomaly
    d. crural repair
    d. defect
    d. elevation
    d. eventration
    d. hernia
    d. herniation
    d. injury
    d. laceration
    d. node
    d. pleura
    d. reflection
    d. respiration
    d. rupture
    d. surface
diaphragmatic-abdominal respiration
diaphyseal (*var. of* diaphysial)
diaphysial, diaphyseal
    d. fracture
    d. osteotomy
diaphyses (*pl. of* diaphysis)
diaphysis, *pl.* **diaphyses**
    femoral d.
diarrhea
    intractable d.
    secretory d.
diarthric
diarthrodial
    d. cartilage
    d. joint
diarthrosis
diarticular
diary
    electronic chronic pain d.
    pain d.
Dias-Giegerich
    D.-G. fracture technique
    D.-G. open reduction
Dias-Tachdijian physical injury classification
diastasis
    ankle mortise d.
    d. fibula
    iris d.
    palpable rib d.
    pubic d.
    rectus d.
    rib d.
    sutural d.
    tibiofibular d.
diastatic skull fracture
diastolic
    d. blood pressure
    d. filling pressure

d. hypertension
d. pressure-time index
d. pressure-volume relation
d. relaxation
d. suction
diathermic
d. fistulotomy
d. loop biopsy
d. resection
d. therapy
diathermocoagulation
diathermy
coagulating d.
d. dissection
electrocoagulation d.
d. hemorrhoidectomy
medical d.
monopolar d.
d. operation
d. puncture
short wave d.
surgical d.
diatomaceous earth
Dibbell cleft lip-nasal reconstruction
DIC
disseminated intravascular coagulation
dichotomization
dichotomous classification
dichotomy
**Dickey rectus muscle blepharoptosis
  operation**
Dickhaut-DeLee
D.-D. classification of discoid
  meniscus
D.-D. discoid meniscus classification
Dickinson
D. approach
D. calcaneal bursitis technique
**Dickinson-Coutts-Woodward-Handler
  osteotomy**
Dickson
D. geometric osteotomy
D. transplant technique
**Dickson-Diveley total joint replacement
  procedure**
**Dickson-Wright fascial transplant
  operation**
dicondylar fracture
Didiee projection
Dieffenbach
D. operation
D. sliding flap method
**Dieffenbach-Duplay hypospadias
  technique**
DIEP
deep inferior epigastric perforator flap
die punch fracture
dieresis
dieretic

diet
advance to regular d.
clear liquid d.
regular d.
diethyl ether
Dieulafoy
D. lesion
D. vascular malformation
D. vascular malformation of
  stomach
Dieulafoy-like lesion
difference
alveolar-arterial pressure d.
  $(p(A\text{-}a)O_2)$
alveolar end-capillary d.
morphological d.
differential
d. blood pressure
d. diagnosis (DDx)
d. nerve block
d. relaxation
d. spinal anesthesia
d. spinal block
d. spinal block anesthetic technique
d. ureteral catheterization test
d. variable reluctance transducer
differentiated thyroid carcinoma
differentiation failure
difficult
d. airway algorithm
d. ventilation
diffuse
d. abdominal pain
d. abdominal tenderness
d. abscess
d. acute inflammation
d. air space disease
d. aneurysm
d. breast involvement
d. carcinomatosis
d. change
d. chronic inflammation
d. colloid goiter
d. esophageal spasm (DES)
d. fatty infiltration
d. fibroma
d. fusiform dilation
d. GI hamartoma
d. GI polyposis
d. hemorrhagic pancreatitis
d. idiopathic skeletal hyperostosis
  (DISH)
d. idiopathic skeletal hyperostosis
  syndrome
d. illumination
d. intravascular coagulation
d. lobular fibrosis
d. lymphatic tissue
d. metastasis

D

diffuse (*continued*)
    d. microcalcification
    d. microvascular thrombosis
    d. mucosal polyposis
    d. multinodular goiter
    d. necrosis
    d. papillomatosis
    d. peritonitis
    d. plane
    d. pulmonary alveolar hemorrhage
    d. reflection
    d. toxic nonnodular goiter
    d. transmural ganglioneuromatosis
    d. tumor
    d. ulceration
    d. ulcerative lesion
    d. variety
    d. vasculitis
diffusely tender abdomen
diffusion
    d. anoxia
    exchange d.
    d. hypoxia
    d. respiration
    d. root canal filling method
digastric
    d. branch
    d. fossa
    d. groove
    d. line
    d. muscle
    d. muscle flap
    d. space
    d. triangle
digestive
    d. apparatus
    d. bleeding
    d. continuity
    d. glandular cancer
    d. manifestation
    d. system
    d. system vascular disease
    d. tract
    d. tract malignancy
    d. tube
digital
    d. artery protection
    d. beam attenuation
    d. block
    d. block anesthesia
    d. collateral artery
    d. dilation
    d. dissection
    d. divulsion
    d. extensor mechanism
    d. extensor tendon
    d. flap
    d. flexion crease
    d. furrow

    d. imaging colposcopy
    d. mammography
    d. manipulation
    d. nail
    d. pad
    d. pressure
    d. pulp
    d. rectal evacuation
    d. rectal examination
    d. retinacular ligament
    d. subtraction echocardiography
    (DSE)
    d. templating
    d. vein
digitalis effect
digitalization
digitally guided biopsy
digitate impression
digitation
digiti (*pl. of* digitus)
digitoclasy
digitorum
Digit Symbol Substitution Test
digitus, *pl.* **digiti**
dilacerated canal
dilaceration
    sharp d.
dilatable lesion
dilatation (*var. of* dilation)
    d. and curettage (D&C)
    d. and evacuation (D&E)
    aneurysmal d.
    Loreta outlet of stomach d.
    percutaneous transhepatic balloon d.
    (PTBD)
    prestenotic d.
dilatator (*var. of* dilator)
dilated loop of bowel
dilating window
dilation (dil, dilat), dilatation
    achalasia balloon d.
    anal d.
    d. and curettage (D&C)
    d. and evacuation (D&E)
    aneurysmal d.
    balloon d.
    bile duct d.
    biliary d.
    blind d.
    bootstrap d.
    bowel d.
    Brown-McHardy pneumatic mercury
    bougie d.
    capillary d.
    cardiac d.
    catheter d.
    cervical d.
    colonic d.
    congenital cystic d.

cricopharyngeal d.
cystic d.
diffuse fusiform d.
digital d.
ductal d.
ectatic d.
Eder-Puestow d.
endoscopic papillary
  balloon d.
endoscopic retrograde
  balloon d.
episcleral vascular d.
esophageal d.
extrahepatic biliary cystic d.
ex vacuo d.
finger d.
Frank technique of d.
fusiform d.
gaseous d.
gastric d.
Grüntzig balloon d.
hepatic web d.
homatropine d.
hydrostatic balloon d.
idiopathic d.
inadequate d.
intrahepatic biliary cystic d.
intrahepatic ductal d.
intraoperative d.
junctional d.
lag d.
d. lag
Lord d.
Loreta outlet of stomach d.
mechanical ureteral d.
medical d.
mucosal vascular d.
pancreatic duct d.
percutaneous balloon d.
percutaneous transhepatic balloon d.
  (PTBD)
percutaneous stricture d.
periportal sinusoidal d.
peroral esophageal d.
pneumatic d.
pneumatic bag esophageal d.
pneumatic balloon catheter d.
pneumostatic d.
postoperative ductal d.
poststenotic d.
pouch d.
prestenotic d.
progressive d.
pupil d.
pupillary d.
pyloric d.
reactive d.
rectal d.
secondary arrest of d.

segmental d.
serial d.
submucosal vascular d.
d. therapy
through-the-scope balloon d.
tract d.
transurethral balloon d.
TTS balloon d.
urethral d.
ventricular d.
Virchow-Robin space d.
wire-guided d.
Wirsung d.

dilator, dilatator
  d. muscle
  d. placement
  d. placement failure
dilator-and-sheath technique
dilemma
  diagnostic d.
Dillwyn-Evans
  D.-E. osteotomy
  D.-E. relapsed club foot resection
dilution
  tracer d.
dilutional coagulopathy
dilution-filtration technique
dimenhydrinate
dimension
  X, Y d.
2-dimensional (2D)
  2-d. monitoring
3-dimensional (3D)
  3-d. contouring
  3-d. grid electrode
  3-d. projection reconstruction
    imaging
  3-d. stereography
  3-d. videoscopy
  3-d. virtual cholangioscopy
4-dimensional (4D)
diminished functional residual capacity
Dimon-Hughston
  D.-H. fracture fixation
  D.-H. intertrochanteric hip fracture
    reduction technique
  D.-H. intertrochanteric osteotomy
dimorphism
  gender d.
dimple
  celiac d.
  coccygeal d.
dinitrogen monoxide
dioptric
  d. aberration
  d. correction
dioxide
  arterial carbon d.
  carbon d. (bicarb, CO_2)

D

dioxide (*continued*)
    end-tidal carbon d. (ETCO$_2$)
    intraabdominally insufflated
      carbon d.
    partial pressure of arterial carbon d.
      (PaCO$_2$)
    partial pressure of carbon d.
      (PCO$_2$)
    partial pressure of intramuscular
      carbon d.
    partial pressure of mesenteric
      venous carbon d.

DIP
    distal interphalangeal
    DIP fusion

diphosphate
    adenosine d.

diphtheritic membrane

DIPI
    direct intraperitoneal insemination

diplegia
    spastic d.

diploë

diploic
    d. artery
    d. canal
    d. vein

dipole

Diprivan anesthetic technique

direct
    d. acrylic restoration
    d. brain stimulation
    d. cardiac puncture
    d. cautery puncture
    d. cholecystoenterostomy
    d. closure
    d. composite resin restoration
    d. compression
    d. current electrocoagulation
    d. current shock ablation
    d. cystenterostomy
    d. defect
    d. electrical nerve stimulation
    d. embolectomy
    d. flap
    d. fluoroscopic visualization
    d. fracture
    d. gold restoration
    d. hemoperfusion
    d. histologic investigation
    d. illumination
    d. immunofluorescence test
    d. inguinal hernia
    d. insertion technique
    d. intraperitoneal insemination (DIPI)
    d. laparoscopic vision
    d. laryngoscopy
    d. ligation
    d. manipulation

    d. mechanical ventricular actuation
    d. method
    d. method for making inlays
    d. muscle lysis
    d. needle puncture
    d. neural stimulation
    d. obturator nerve block
    d. ophthalmoscopy
    d. percutaneous endoscopic
      jejunostomy (DPEJ)
    d. percutaneous endoscopic
      jejunostomy tube
    d. pressure
    d. pyramidal tract
    d. respiration
    d. SSPCS
    d. suturing
    d. thrombin inhibitor
    d. transfusion
    d. vein anesthesia

direct/indirect technique

direction
    antegrade d.
    anterograde d.
    caudal d.
    cephalad d.
    clockwise d.
    counterclockwise d.
    flow d.
    line of d.
    pelvic d.
    phase-encoding d.
    principal visual d.
    retrograde d.
    visual d.
    Z d.

directional coronary atherectomy

directive
    advance d.

direct-vision
    d.-v. internal urethrotomy
    d.-v. liver biopsy

dirty
    d. case
    d. field
    d. operative wound classification
    d. surgery

disarticular amputation

disarticulation
    Batch-Spittler-McFaddin knee d.
    Boyd hip d.
    Burger technique for scapulothoracic
      d.
    elbow d.
    hip d.
    joint d.
    Lisfranc d.
    Mazet d.
    metatarsophalangeal joint d.

sacroiliac d.
scapulothoracic d.
shoulder d.
wrist d.
disassociation
disc, disk
acromioclavicular d.
artificial d.
d. compression
d. diffusion method
d. drusen hemorrhage
d. excision
extruded d.
d. extrusion
d. fragment
free fragment d.
herniated d.
d. herniation
intercalated d.
interpubic d.
d. lesion
mandibular d.
d. neovascularization
optic d.
d. oxygenation
d. plication
d. pressure
protruded d.
ruptured d.
sacrococcygeal d.
d. sensitivity method
d. space
d. space infection
d. space narrowing
d. spacer
d. space saline acceptance test
sternoclavicular d.
temporomandibular articular d.
discectomy, diskectomy
anterior d.
automated percutaneous d. (APD)
Barrios lumbar d.
cervical d.
Cloward fusion d.
laminotomy and d.
lumbar d.
microlumbar d. (MLD)
microsurgical d. (MSD)
partial d.
percutaneous lumbar d.
Robinson anterior cervical d.
Smith-Robinson anterior cervical d.
thoracic d.
thoracoscopic d.
transthoracic d.
Williams d.
discharge
breast d.
d. letter

pathologic breast d.
physiologic breast d.
same-day d.
spontaneous nipple d.
disci (*pl. of* discus)
discission
Moncrieff d.
disclosing solution
discogenic pain
discography, diskography
computed tomography d.
provocative d.
discography-provoked pain response
discoid skin lesion
disconnection
portal azygos d.
d. syndrome
disconnect wedge
discontinuation-emergent symptom development
discontinuous
d. endothelium
d. neck dissection
d. sterilization
discotomy, diskotomy
discrete
d. bleeding source
d. lesion
d. mass
d. stenosis
d. tumor
discrimination
d. curve
d. loss
d. score
discriminative component
discus, *pl.* **disci**
excavatio disci
disease
abdominal hydatid d.
Abrami d.
acid peptic d.
acute graft-versus-host d.
adaptation d.
adhesive d.
adult familial hyaline membrane d.
adult polycystic liver d.
advanced d.
air space d.
alcoholic liver d. (ALD)
amyloid oral cavity d.
aneurysmal d.
antiglomerular basement membrane antibody d.
aortic aneurysmal d.
aortic arch d.
aortic atheromatous d.
aortic occlusive d.
aortic valve d.

D

disease (*continued*)
aortoiliac occlusive d. (AIOD)
Arbuthnot Lane d.
arterial occlusive d. (AOD)
asymptomatic d.
atherosclerotic carotid artery d. (ACAD)
atherosclerotic heart d. (ASHD)
autosomal dominant polycystic kidney d. (ADPKD)
Behçet d.
benign inflammatory d.
Berger d.
biliary tract d.
bilobar d.
bone d.
Bright d.
Budd-Chiari syndrome with Behçet d.
Budd-Chiari syndrome without Behçet d.
calcium pyrophosphate deposition d. (CPDD, CPPD)
calculous biliary d.
carcinoid valve d.
cardiovascular d. (CVD)
carotid artery d.
Castleman d.
cement d.
central core d.
central nervous system d.
cerebrovascular d.
cerebrovenous d.
choledochal cyst d.
Christmas d.
chronic graft-versus-host d.
chronic liver d.
chronic obstructive airways d. (COAD)
colorectal d.
combined system d.
complex aortic d.
complicated diverticular d.
congestive heart d.
connective tissue d.
coronary artery d. (CAD)
Cowden d.
Crohn d.
Crouzon d.
cryptoglandular d.
cutaneous graft-versus-host d.
cystic kidney d.
decompensated liver d.
degenerative discogenic endplate d.
denervation d.
diffuse air space d.
digestive system vascular d.
distant nodal d.
diverticular d.

donor-transmitted d.
early-onset graft-versus-host d.
echinococcal cyst d.
Economo d.
elevator d.
endogenous d.
endomyocardial d.
end-stage liver d.
endstage renal d. (ESRD)
eosinophilic endomyocardial d.
eventration d.
exanthematous d.
exogenous d.
exophytic joint d.
extensive-stage d.
extraabdominal d.
extracapsular d.
extracranial carotid artery d.
extracranial carotid occlusive d.
extracranial occlusive vascular d.
extrahepatic nodal d.
extramammary Paget d.
extranodal d.
extraorbital d.
extrapyramidal d.
exudative papulosquamous d.
eye d.
familial multigland d.
femoropopliteal occlusive d.
fibrocystic d.
Fournier d.
fracture d.
gallstone d.
gastroesophageal reflux d. (GERD)
Gaucher d.
glomerular basement membrane d.
graft-versus-host d. (GVHD)
Graves d.
gross cystic d.
gross residual d. (R2)
hard metal d.
hard pad d.
hepatic d.
hepatic venous web d.
heritable connective tissue d.
Hirschsprung d.
Hodgkin d.
humeroperoneal neuromuscular d.
Huntington d.
hyaline membrane d.
hydatid d.
hyperacute graft-versus-host d.
idiopathic eczematous d.
idiopathic peptic ulcer d.
immunoproliferative small intestine d. (IPSID)
inclusion body d.
inflammatory bowel d.
inflammatory vascular d.

infrainguinal d.
interfacetal d.
intraabdominal d.
in-transit d.
intraperitoneal endometrial
  metastatic d.
intrathoracic d.
irresectable d.
ischemic aortic d.
ischemic heart d.
Jackson and Parker classification of
  Hodgkin d.
Jeune d.
Kashin-Beck d.
Killip classification of heart d.
Lafora body d.
late-onset d.
late-stage d.
Leri-Weill d.
lichenoid graft-versus-host d.
liver d.
localization of d.
locally advanced d.
lower extremity occlusive d.
lower extremity vascular
  occlusive d.
lung d.
lupus-associated valve d.
lysosomal storage d.
malignant neoplastic d.
malignant pancreatic d.
Marion d.
Meige d.
Ménétrier d.
Ménière d.
mesenteric nodal d.
metastatic d.
microcystic d.
micrometastatic peritoneal d.
microscopic d.
Milroy d.
minimal-change d. (MCD)
mixed connective tissue d. (MCTD)
Model for End-Stage Liver D.
  (MELD)
Mondor d.
multicentric d.
multifocal extensive d.
multigland d.
multiglandular d.
multilevel atherosclerotic arterial
  occlusive d.
multiple hydatid d.
neurologic d.
nil d.
nodal d.
node-negative d.
node-positive d.
nonalcoholic fatty liver d.

noncirrhotic metabolic liver d.
nonfamilial multiglandular d.
nonmalignant d.
no residual d. (R0)
obstructive lung d.
occlusive carotid artery d.
occlusive coronary artery d.
occult extrahepatic d.
occult hepatic d.
occult irresectable d.
occult systemic d.
omental nodal d.
Ormond d.
osteoarthritis d.
Paget extramammary d.
pancreatic d.
Parkinson d.
pediatric end-stage liver d. (PELD)
pelvic adhesive d.
pelvic inflammatory d. (PID)
peptic ulcer d. (PUD)
perianal Crohn d.
periodontal d. (PERIO)
peripheral arterial aneurysmal d.
peripheral vascular d. (PVD)
peritoneal d.
Peyronie d.
Plummer d.
polycystic kidney d. (PKD)
popliteal artery occlusive d. (PAOD)
posttransplant lymphoproliferative d.
  (PTLD)
preeclamptic liver d.
Preiser d.
progressive d.
pulmonary valve d.
radiation-induced d.
radiation lung d.
Recklinghausen type I d.
d. recurrence rate
recurrent thromboembolic d.
reflux d.
d. regression
Reiter d.
renal artery occlusive d.
renal artery stenotic d.
renal vascular d.
resectable hepatic d.
residual d. (R1)
sclerodermoid graft-versus-host d.
short-segment d.
sickle cell d.
single hydatid d.
sinonasal d.
sixth venereal d.
space-occupying d.
sporadic multigland d.
d. stage
Steinert d.

D

disease (*continued*)
    stenotic d.
    supraesophageal reflux d.
    surgical pancreatic d.
    symptomatic abdominal
      aneurysm d.
    systemic d.
    systemic vascular d.
    Takayasu d.
    thin basement membrane d.
    thoracic aortic d.
    thromboembolic d. (TED)
    thrombotic d.
    thyroid d.
    tricuspid valve d.
    unanticipated hepatic d.
    undifferentiated connective
      tissue d.
    unilobar d.
    unresectable extrahepatic d.
    upper tract d.
    urinary tract d.
    valvular aortic d.
    valvular heart d.
    van Buren d.
    vascular d.
    vasculo-Behçet d.
    venereal d.
    venous stasis d.
    venous web d.
    vertebral artery d.
    vibration d.
    von Economo d.
    von Hippel-Lindau d.
    Winiwarter-Buerger d.
disease-associated mortality
disease-based approach
disease-free
    d.-f. interval (DFI)
    d.-f. patient
    d.-f. survival (DFS)
disease-modifying antirheumatoid drug (DMARD)
disease-related complication
dish face
DISH
    diffuse idiopathic skeletal hyperostosis
    DISH syndrome
dishpan fracture
disinfecting solution
disinfection
    chemical d.
    high-level d.
    root canal d.
    spray-wipe-spray d.
    surface d.
    thermal d.
disintegration
    endoscopic stone d.

    myofilament d.
    d. rate
disinvagination
disjoined pyeloplasty
disk (*var. of* disc)
diskectomy (*var. of* discectomy)
diskography (*var. of* discography)
diskotomy (*var. of* discotomy)
dislocation
    acromioclavicular joint d.
    ankle d.
    antenatal d.
    anterior complete d.
    anterior hip d.
    anterior-inferior d.
    anterior shoulder d.
    anterolateral d.
    atlantoaxial d. (AAD)
    atlantooccipital joint d.
    atypical d.
    Bankart shoulder d.
    bayonet d.
    Bell-Dally cervical d.
    Bennett d.
    bilateral interfacetal d.
    boutonnière hand d.
    bursting d.
    carpometacarpal joint d.
    central d.
    Chopart ankle d.
    closed d.
    complete anterior d.
    complete inferior d.
    complete posterior d.
    complete superior d.
    compound d.
    congenital hip d.
    congenital lens d.
    consecutive d.
    d. contour abnormality
    dashboard d.
    Desault wrist d.
    divergent elbow d.
    dorsal perilunate d.
    dorsal transscaphoid perilunar d.
    dysplasia d.
    elbow d.
    facet d.
    fracture d.
    d. fracture
    frank d.
    gamekeeper's thumb d.
    glenohumeral joint d.
    habitual d.
    Hill-Sachs shoulder d.
    hip d.
    incomplete d.
    inferior complete closed d.
    inferior complete compound d.

interphalangeal joint d.
intraocular lens d.
isolated d.
Kienböck d.
knee d.
lens d.
Lisfranc d.
lumbosacral d.
lunate d.
luxatio erecta shoulder d.
mandibular d.
metatarsophalangeal joint d.
midcarpal d.
milkmaid's elbow d.
Monteggia d.
Nélaton ankle d.
occipitoatlantal d.
Otto pelvis d.
Palmer transscaphoid perilunar d.
panclavicular d.
parachute jumper's d.
partial d.
patellar intraarticular d.
pathologic d.
perilunar transscaphoid d.
perilunate carpal d.
peroneal d.
phalangeal d.
posterior hip d.
posterior shoulder d.
posteromedial d.
prenatal d.
primitive d.
proximal tibiofibular joint d.
radial head d.
radiocarpal d.
recent d.
recurrent patellar d.
retrosternal d.
rotational d.
sacroiliac d.
scapholunate d.
shoulder d.
Smith d.
spontaneous hyperemic d.
sternoclavicular joint d.
subastragalar d.
subcoracoid shoulder d.
subglenoid shoulder d.
subtalar d.
superior d.
swivel d.
talar d.
tarsal d.
tarsometatarsal d.
temporomandibular joint d.
teratologic d.
tibialis posterior d.
tibiofibular joint d.

transscaphoid perilunate d.
traumatic atlantooccipital d.
triquetrolunate d.
unilateral interfacetal d.
unreduced d.
volar semilunar wrist d.
wrist d.
dislodged tube
dislodgement (*var. of* dislodgment)
dislodgment, dislodgement
stent d.
dismantling
dismembered
d. anastomosis
d. pyeloplasty
d. reimplanted appendicocystostomy
disobliteration
disodium
fospropofol d.
disorder
accommodation d.
acquired cornification d.
affective d.
anorectal d.
anxiety d.
arterial d.
articulation d.
autoimmune connective tissue d.
benign esophageal d.
bipolar d.
bipolar affective d.
blood coagulation d.
borderline personality d.
cartilaginous growth plate d.
chronic multisystem d.
chronic pain d.
coagulation d.
coagulopathic d.
colorectal d.
complex adrenal endocrine d.
complex gonadal endocrine d.
complex pituitary endocrine d.
complex thyroid endocrine d.
connective tissue d.
consumptive thrombohemorrhagic d.
conversion d.
cornification d.
cumulative trauma d.
Curth-Maklin cornification d.
dermatologic d.
developmental coordination d.
ejaculation d.
elimination d.
endocrine d.
endonasal d.
esophageal d.
evacuation d.
experimental d.
functional sleep d.

D

disorder (*continued*)
  gamma loop d.
  generalized anxiety d. (GAD)
  gonadal endocrine d.
  gynecologic d.
  hematologic d.
  hemidysplasia cornification d.
  immune-mediated coagulation d.
  intestinal ischemic d.
  keratitis-deafness-cornification d.
  lymphoproliferative d.
  lysosomal enzyme d.
  mastication d.
  metabolic d.
  mitral valve d.
  mixed connective tissue d.
  motility d.
  motor d.
  movement d.
  multisystem d.
  musculoskeletal d.
  myeloproliferative d.
  myogenous temporomandibular d.
  nail d.
  neurologic d.
  ocular motility d.
  organic articulation d.
  pituitary endocrine d.
  posttransplant lymphoproliferative d.
    (PTLD)
  posttraumatic stress d. (PTSD)
  somatization d.
  substance abuse d.
  temporomandibular d.
  temporomandibular muscle d.
    (TMD)
  thrombogenic d.
  thyroid endocrine d.
  unilateral hemidysplasia
    cornification d.
  unipolar d.
  urinary tract d.
  voice d.
  whiplash-associated d. (WAD)
disordered hip complex
disordering
  membrane d.
disparate point
displaced fracture
displacement
  d. analysis
  anterior d.
  d. curve
  hilar d.
  d. implantation
  d. osteotomy
  port d.
  d. threshold
  water d.

display
  graphical anesthesia drug d.
  vibrotactile d.
disposition kinetics
disproportion
  cephalopelvic d.
disruption
  anastomotic d.
  cognitive d.
  internal disc d.
  pancreatic ductal d.
  vessel d.
  wound d.
dissected tissue arm
dissecting
  d. aneurysm
  d. intramural hematoma
  d. sealer
dissection
  acute aortic d.
  aortic d.
  arterial wall d.
  axillary lymph node d. (ALND)
  axillary node d. (AND)
  balloon d.
  bilateral neck d.
  blind d.
  blunt d.
  blunt and sharp d.
  bone d.
  bone-ligament d.
  bony d.
  capsular d.
  carotid artery d.
  central neck d.
  cervical node d.
  circumferential mucosal d.
  complete axillary d.
  complex d.
  condyle d.
  confirmatory axillary d.
  coronary artery d.
  cranial nerve d.
  D2 d.
  DeBakey-type aortic d.
  DeBakey type I aortic d.
  deep iliac d.
  diathermy d.
  digital d.
  discontinuous neck d.
  elective lymph node d. (ELND)
  elective neck d. (END)
  en bloc d.
  endoscopic d.
  endoscopic submucosal d. (ESD)
  epiphenomena of d.
  esophageal d.
  extended gastric cancer lymph node
    d. (D2)

extensive lymph node d.
extracapsular d.
extrahepatic d.
extraperitoneal endoscopic pelvic
  lymph node d.
field d.
2-field d.
3-field d.
field of d.
finger fracture d.
fingertip d.
flank d.
Freer d.
full axillary d.
functional lymph node d.
functional neck d. (FND)
gauze d.
gentle blunt d.
groin d.
hard palate d.
hydraulic d.
iliac artery d.
incisural d.
inguinal canal d.
inguinal-femoral node d.
in situ d.
intracapsular d.
intradural d.
intramural air d.
intraparenchymal digital d.
jugular vein d.
laparoscopic pelvic lymph node d.
lateral cervical node d.
lateroaortic lymph node d.
limited gastric cancer lymph node
  d. (D1)
limited obturator node d.
lymphatic d.
lymph node d. (LND)
d. margin
mastoscopic axillary lymph
  node d.
medial d.
mediastinal lymph node d.
mesoesophageal d.
modified radical neck d.
muscle d.
nasal d.
neck d.
nerve-sparing d.
node d.
d. of aorta
Pack-Ehrlich deep iliac d.
paraaortic lymph node d.
parenchymal d.
parotid d.
partial zonal d.
pelvic lymph node d. (PLND)
pelvic node d.

periadventitial d.
periesophageal lymph node d.
perirectal pelvic d.
plane of d.
postradical neck d.
precise d.
radical axillary d.
radical lymph node d.
radical mediastinal d.
radical neck d. (RND)
retrogastric d.
retroperitoneal lymph node d.
  (RLND)
retroperitoneal pelvic lymph node d.
  (RPLND)
scissors d.
selective inguinal node d.
sharp d.
sharp and blunt d.
soft tissue d.
spermatic cord d.
spiral d.
sponge d.
spontaneous coronary artery d.
Stanford (type A, B) aortic d.
subligamentous d.
submucosal d.
subperiosteal d.
subtemporal d.
suction d.
superextended gastric cancer lymph
  node d. (D3)
suprahyoid neck d.
supraomohyoid neck d.
sylvian d.
symptomatic traumatic d.
systemic d.
Taussig-Morton node d.
2-team d.
therapeutic d.
therapeutic lymph node d.
  (TLND)
thoracic aortic d.
tissue d.
tongue-jaw-neck d.
transthoracic d.
traumatic internal carotid artery d.
d. tubercle
ultrasonic d.
vein-sparing d.
vertebral d.
water d.

disseminated
  d. asymptomatic unilateral
    neovascularization
  d. carcinoma
  d. inflammation
  d. intravascular coagulation (DIC)
  d. neonatal hemangiomatosis

D

dissemination
  hematologic d.
  intraperitoneal d.
  neoplastic d.
  peritoneal d.
Disse space
dissipation
  circle d.
dissociable tetrameric hemoglobin
dissociated
  d. anesthesia
  d. position
dissociation, disassociation
  d., analgesia, immobility, and
    tension scale
  atrial d.
  atrioventricular d.
  AV d.
  complete atrioventricular d. (CAVD)
  complete AV d.
  d. curve
  electromechanical d. (EMD)
  electromyocardial d.
  hypnotic d.
  incomplete atrioventricular d.
  incomplete AV d.
  interference d.
  intracavitary pressure-electrogram d.
  isorhythmic d.
  longitudinal d.
  lunotriquetral d.
  microbic d.
  d. movement
  radioulnar d.
  scapholunate d.
  scapulothoracic d.
  sleep d.
  syringomyelic d.
  tabetic d.
dissociative anesthesia
distal
  d. anastomosis
  d. aortic perfusion
  d. atresia
  d. biceps brachii tendon rupture
  d. bile duct
  d. bile duct stricture
  d. bleeding
  d. catheter lengthening
  d. cavity
  d. centriole
  d. clavicular excision
  d. clot
  d. ectasia
  d. esophageal diverticulum
  d. esophageal ring
  d. esophagectomy
  d. extension restoration
  d. femoral epiphysial fracture

  d. femoropopliteal bypass graft
  d. fragment
  d. humeral epiphysis
  d. humeral fracture
  d. interphalangeal (DIP)
  d. interphalangeal fusion
  d. interphalangeal joint approach
  d. laparoscopic pancreatectomy
  d. ligation
  d. limb
  d. metaphysis
  d. metastasis
  d. nail matrix
  d. nerve graft
  d. neurolysis
  d. occlusal
  d. occlusal cavity
  d. pancreas
  d. pancreatectomy
  d. pancreaticojejunostomy
  d. phalanx
  d. portion
  d. radial fracture
  d. radioulnar joint
  d. radioulnar joint stabilization
  d. radius-ulnar joint
  d. remnant
  d. shave section
  d. splenoadrenal shunt
  d. splenorenal shunt (DSRS)
  d. splenorenal shunt technique
  d. stump
  d. tibiofibular fusion
  d. tumor
  d. ureterectomy
  d. vein cuff
  d. vertebral artery reconstruction
  d. visceral perfusion
  d. with excision of ulcer
    gastrectomy
distal-row carpectomy
distance
  interincisor d.
  skin-epidural d.
  skin-to-tumor d.
  thyromental d.
  tube-carina d.
  tube-patient d.
  tube-to-film d.
distant
  d. flap
  d. metastasis
  d. nodal disease
  d. recurrence
  d. recurrence-free survival (DRFS)
distantial aberration
distended
  d. abdomen
  d. afferent loop

d. colon
d. gallbladder
distension (*var. of* distention)
distention, distension
abdominal d.
bladder d.
cecal d.
colonic d.
gallbladder d.
gaseous d.
gastric d.
liver d.
postprandial d.
progressive abdominal d.
proximal bowel d.
rectal d.
vessel d.
distilled water
distoangular position
distobuccal line angle
distobuccoocclusal point angle
distolabial line angle
distolabioincisal point angle
distolingual line angle
distolinguoincisal point angle
distoocclusal point angle
distortion
d. aberration
corneal d.
pincushion d.
distraction
d. arthroplasty
bone d.
muscle d.
d. of fracture
d. osteogenesis
d. technique
distraction/compression scoliosis treatment
distractive extension
distractor
femur d.
hip d.
plate-guided d.
tibial d.
distress
D. Risk Assessment Method
(DRAM)
D. Scale for Ventilated Newborn
Infants (DSVNI)
distribution
dermatomal d.
lesion d.
loop d.
d. pattern
pattern of d.
stocking-glove pain d.
ventilation/perfusion d.
disturbance
acid-base d.

chronic motor d.
hemodynamic d.
interdigestive motility d.
microcirculatory d.
motility d.
motor d.
postsurgical d.
sensitive visceral postsurgical d.
upper small-bowel motor d.
visceral postsurgical d.
diuresis
balanced salt solution volume d.
diuretic therapy
diurnal
d. enuresis
d. intraocular pressure measurement
divergent
d. elbow dislocation
d. ray projection
diversified chiropractic technique
diversion
biliopancreatic d.
Camey enterocystoplasty urinary d.
Duke pouch cutaneous urinary d.
fecal d.
Gil-Vernet ileocecal cystoplasty
urinary d.
ileal conduit urinary d.
ileocolic pouch urinary d.
Indiana continent reservoir urinary
d.
Koch pouch cutaneous urinary d.
laparoscopic biliopancreatic d.
Mainz II pouch continent urinary d.
Mainz pouch cutaneous urinary d.
Mainz pouch I continent urinary d.
orthotopic urinary d.
pancreaticojejunal d.
simple d.
Studer reservoir urinary d.
temporary fecal d.
ureterointestinal urinary d.
urinary d.
diversionary ileostomy
diverticula (*pl. of* diverticulum)
diverticular
d. disease
d. hemorrhage
d. hernia
diverticularization
diverticulation abnormality
diverticulectomy
bladder d.
endocavitary bladder d.
esophageal d.
Harrington esophageal d.
Meckel d.
d. of hypopharynx
open d.

diverticulectomy (*continued*)
    pharyngoesophageal d.
    urethral d.
    vesical d.
    d. with myotomy
diverticulitis
    cecal d.
diverticulopexy
diverticulotomy
    Dohlman endoscopic stapling d.
    stapling d.
diverticulum, *pl.* **diverticula**
    acquired d.
    caliceal d.
    cervical d.
    congenital d.
    distal esophageal d.
    esophageal d.
    extraluminal d.
    false d.
    intraluminal duodenal d.
    large intestine d.
    Meckel d.
    midesophageal traction d.
    periampullary duodenal d.
    pharyngoesophageal d.
    pulsion d.
    traction d.
    true d.
    Zenker d.
    Zuckerkandl d.
diverting
    d. loop colostomy
    d. loop ileostomy
    d. proximal colostomy
    d. stoma
    d. transverse colostomy
divided
    doubly ligated and d.
    d. respiration
divided-stoma colostomy
division
    anterior primary d.
    Ball anal sensory nerve d.
    d. I–IV lesion
    intrahepatic vascular d.
    maturation d.
    posterior primary d.
    puborectalis d.
    reduction d.
    Stoffel spastic paralysis motor nerve
      d.
    vascular ring d.
divulse
divulsion
    digital d.
Dix-Hallpike benign positional vertigo
  maneuver
Dixon

DKA
    diabetic ketoacidosis
DKS
    Damus-Kaye-Stansel
      DKS pulmonary artery to ascending
        aorta anastomosis procedure
      DKS pulmonary artery to ascending
        aorta anastomotic operation
D-loop transposition of great arteries
DMARD
    disease-modifying antirheumatoid drug
DMD
    Descemet membrane detachment
DMFC
    demand minimum functional capacity
DN4
    neuropathic pain diagnostic
      questionnaire
DNAP
    dynamic negative airway pressure
DNA
    deoxyribonucleic acid
      DNA ploidy abnormality
dobutamine stress echocardiography
Döderlein
    D. roll-flap hysterectomy
    D. vaginal hysterectomy method
Dodge area-length method
DOE
    dyspnea on exertion
dog-ear repair
dog-leg fracture
Dohlman
    D. endoscopic stapling
      diverticulotomy
    D. pharyngeal pouch repair
      procedure
DOI
    depth of insertion
dolasetron mesylate
Dolenc cavernous sinus exploration
  technique
dolens
    phlegmasia alba d.
    phlegmasia cerulea d.
dolichocephalic head
dolichoectatic artery
dolichopellic pelvis
doll's
    d. eye maneuver
    d. head maneuver
    d. head phenomenon
Doll trochanteric reattachment
  technique
dolorosa
    anesthesia d.
domain
    abdominal d.
D'ombrain operation

dome
    d. excursion
    d. fracture
    d. osteotomy
dome-shaped osteotomy
dominant
    d. component
    d. gland
    d. mass
domino
    d. procedure
    d. transplant
DOMS
    delayed onset muscle soreness
Donald-Fothergill uterine suspension
donation
    d. after cardiac death (DCD)
    autologous blood d. (ABD)
    blood d.
    designated blood d.
    organ d.
Donders
    D. line
    space of D.
donor
    altruistic d.
    bacteremic d.
    d. button technique
    cadaver d.
    cadaveric d.
    CMV-positive d.
    cytomegalovirus-positive d.
    extended criteria d. (ECD)
    d. hepatectomy
    d. iliac Y graft
    d. kidney
    living lung d.
    living-related d. (LRD)
    living relative d.
    nonheart-beating d. (NHBD)
    organ d.
    d. pancreatectomy
    d. pool
    subhuman primate d.
    d. tissue
donor-specific bone marrow augmentation
donor-transmitted disease
donut (*var. of* doughnut)
dopamine receptor
dopaminergic
    d. medication
    d. tract
Doppler
    D. auto-correlation technique
    D. color flow
    D. color flow imaging
    continuous wave D.
    D. duplex ultrasonography
    endoscopic color D.

    D. flow probe examination
    D. interrogation
    D. method
    precordial D.
    D. pressure gradient
    D. pulse evaluation
    D. signal
    D. study
    D. tissue imaging (DTI)
    transcranial D. (TCD)
    D. ultrasound
    D. ultrasound segmental blood
        pressure testing
dopplergram
Doppler-guided artery ligation
  hemorrhoidectomy
Dor
    D. anterior fundoplication
    D. fundoplication method
    D. fundoplication procedure
    D. fundoplication technique
Dorello canal
Dormia noose
Dorrance push-back cleft palate
  procedure
dorsa (*pl. of* dorsum)
dorsabdominal
dorsal
    d. aspect
    d. branch
    d. closing wedge osteotomy
    d. column stimulation (DCS)
    d. column tractotomy
    d. cordotomy
    d. cord stimulation (DCS)
    d. cross-finger flap
    d. decubitus position
    d. digital artery (DDA)
    d. elevated position
    d. enteric fistula
    d. excision
    d. expansion
    d. finger approach
    d. fissure
    d. horn
    d. induction
    d. inertia position
    d. intercalary segmental instability
    d. interosseous artery
    d. interosseous nerve
    d. linear incision
    d. lithotomy
    d. lithotomy position
    d. longitudinal incision
    d. lumbotomy incision
    d. midline approach
    d. pancreatic artery
    d. penis
    d. perilunate dislocation

D

dorsal (*continued*)
    d. plate
    d. point
    d. proximal metatarsal osteotomy
    d. radius tubercle
    d. rami nerve
    d. recumbent position
    d. rhizotomy
    d. rigid position
    d. root
    d. root entry zone (DREZ)
    d. root entry zone lesion
    d. root entry zone lesioning
     procedure
    d. root ganglion
    d. root ganglionectomy
    d. rotation flap
    d. sacrococcygeal muscle
    d. scapular artery
    d. scapular nerve
    d. spine
    d. supine position
    d. surface
    d. sympathectomy
    d. synovectomy
    d. talonavicular bone
    d. tegmental decussation
    d. tenosynovectomy
    d. thoracic artery
    d. thyroid mobilization
    d. tissue
    d. translation
    d. transposition flap
    d. transscaphoid perilunar dislocation
    d. transverse capsulotomy
    d. transverse incision
    d. vein patch graft
    d. venous complex
    d. venous plexus
    d. vertebra
    d. V osteotomy
    d. wire-loop fixation
dorsalis pedis (DP)
dorsalward approach
dorsiflexion of ankle
dorsiflexory wedge osteotomy
dorsiscapular
dorsispinal vein
dorsocephalad
dorsolateral
    d. and medial capsulotomy
    d. approach
    d. incision
    d. tract
dorsolumbar
dorsomedial
    d. approach
    d. incision
dorsopancreaticus

dorsoplantar
    d. approach
    d. projection
dorsoradial approach
dorsorostral approach
dorsosacral position
dorsoulnar approach
dorsoventrad
dorsum, *pl.* **dorsa**
    d. ephippii
dose
    body mass-dependent d.
    defasciculating d.
    d. escalation
    fixed d.
    fixed subcutaneous d.
    physiologic d.
    preoperative d.
    priming d.
    subcatastrophic d.
    subcutaneous d.
    subparalyzing d.
    tissue tolerance d.
dose-effect curve
dose-related effect
dose-response curve
dosing
    around-the-clock d.
    ATC d.
dot-and-blot hemorrhage
dot-blot technique
dot hemorrhage
Dotter-Judkins superselective
    visceralangiography technique
Dotter percutaneous recanalization of
    arterial occlusion technique
Doubilet sphincterotomy
double
    d. adenomas
    d. aortic arch
    d. bubble sign
    d. chin
    d. decidual sac
    d. enterostomy
    d. exposure
    d. extra stimulus
    d. fracture
    d. freeze-thaw cryopexy
    d. graft
    d. halo sign
    d. incision
    d. jaw surgery
    d. lateral advancement flap
    d. Maddox rod test
    d. osteotomy
    d. pedicle TRAM flap
    d. pyloroplasty
    d. right-angle suture
    d. ring

d. simultaneous stimulation
d. stapling technique (DST)
d. unilateral cysts
double-armed
d.-a. suture technique
d.-a. wire suture
double-balloon
d.-b. enteroscopy
d.-b. technique
d.-b. valvoplasty
d.-b. valvotomy
double-barrel
d.-b. colostomy
d.-b. ileostomy
d.-b. stoma
double-burst
d.-b. stimulation
d.-b. transmission
double-button suture technique
double-contrast
d.-c. barium enema examination
d.-c. enema
d.-c. visualization
double-density sign
double-doughnut approach
double-dummy technique
double-exposed rib
double-folded cup-patch ileocystoplasty technique
double-freeze technique
double-incision fasciotomy
double-inlet ventricle anomaly
double-loop
d.-l. hernia
d.-l. pouch
double-looped semitendinosus technique
double-lumen
d.-l. endotracheal tube
d.-l. intubation
double-lung transplant
double-needle
d.-n. chemonucleolysis
d.-n. technique
double-papilla pedicle graft
double-point threshold
double-puncture laparoscopy
double-rod
d.-r. construct
d.-r. technique
double-running penetrating keratoplasty suture
double-sealant technique
double-seton modified surgical approach
double-skin mastopexy
double-stapled
d.-s. ileoanal reservoir method
d.-s. ileoanal reservoir procedure
d.-s. ileoanal reservoir technique
double-staple technique

double-stick technique
double-tube technique
double-umbrella closure
double-volume exchange transfusion
double-wire technique
double-wrap graciloplasty
doubly
d. ligated
d. ligated and divided
d. sutured
doughnut, donut
d. mastopexy
d. ring
doughy
d. abdomen
d. mass
Douglas
D. abscess
D. bag collection method
D. bag technique
cul-de-sac of D.
D. fold
D. line
D. pouch
D. sieve skin graft
douloureux
tic d.
dowel
d. bone graft
d. spinal fusion
d. technique
doweling spondylolisthesis technique
downregulate
downstream
d. sampling method
d. signaling
d. venous pressure
downward
d. drainage
d. retraction
doxapram
Doyen vaginal hysterectomy
Doyle operation
DP
dorsalis pedis
DPEJ
direct percutaneous endoscopic jejunostomy
DPEJ tube
DPL
diagnostic peritoneal lavage
DR
diabetic retinopathy
dorsal root
dragon worm infection
drain
Blake d.
gastric d.
Jackson-Pratt d.

D

drain (*continued*)
  JP d.
  d. site evisceration
  transcystic d.
  d. volume
drainable ostomy pouch
drainage
  abdominal d.
  aberrant lymphatic d.
  bile tract d.
  biliary d.
  bladder d.
  capillary d.
  catheter d.
  caval d.
  cerebral spinal fluid d.
  chest tube d. (CTD)
  circle loop biliary d.
  closed suction d.
  computed tomography-guided
    selective d.
  continuous catheter d.
  CT-guided selective d.
  dependent d.
  downward d.
  endoscopic biliary d.
  endoscopic nasobiliary catheter d.
  endoscopic pancreatic d.
  endoscopic transpapillary cyst d.
  endosonography-guided d.
  enteric d.
  external bile d.
  external bile tract d.
  external biliary d.
  external ventricular d.
  extrapetrosal d.
  fluid d.
  free-flowing d.
  d. gastrostomy
  hematoma d.
  d. implant
  incision and d. (I&D)
  internal d.
  kinetic venous d.
  Laroyenne pelvic suppuration d.
  lymphatic d.
  lymphocele d.
  Molteno d.
  nephrostomy d.
  open d.
  operative d.
  paranasal sinus d.
  d. pattern
  pattern of d.
  percutaneous abscess d. (PAD)
  percutaneous catheter d.
  percutaneous external d. (PED)
  percutaneous transhepatic biliary d.
    (PTBD)

  peripancreatic abdominal d.
  peritoneal d.
  portal d.
  postoperative irrigation-suction d.
  postural d.
  pseudocyst d.
  sclerotomy with d.
  simple external d.
  spinal fluid d.
  stereotactic catheter d.
  suction d.
  systemic d.
  thorascopic d.
  tidal d.
  transampullary d.
  transcystic d.
  transpapillary d.
  T-tube d.
  venous d.
  video thoracoscopic d.
  Wangensteen d.
  wound d.
draining abscess
drain-trap stomach
Drake tandem clipping technique
DRAM
  deepithelialized rectus abdominis
    muscle
  Distress Risk Assessment Method
    DRAM flap
draped
  prepped and d.
draping
  preparation and d.
drawer sign
drawing
  pain d.
draw-over vaporizer
dressing
  cotton d.
  hydrophobic d.
  island wound d.
  occlusive surgical glue d.
  paraffin gauze d.
  d. therapy
  transparent adhesive d.
  wound d.
DREZ
  dorsal root entry zone
    DREZ ankle joint arthroscopy
      procedure
    DREZ lesion
    DREZ lesioning procedure
    DREZ modification of Eriksson
      ankle joint arthroscopy technique
DRFS
  distant recurrence-free survival
drift
  laparoscopic d.

drilling technique
drip
    d. infusion
    d. infusion cholangiography
    intravenous d.
    d. transfusion
Dripps-American Surgical Association
score
Dripps operative risk classification
drip-tube feeding
drive
    exploratory d.
    hypercapnic d.
    respiratory d.
driver
    laparoscopic needle d.
drop
    flow-dependent pressure d.
    d. metastasis
droperidol
droplet infection
drop-lock ring
dropped peristalsis
drug
    d. administration
    antiepileptic d.
    antifibrinolytic d.
    antiretroviral d.
    disease-modifying antirheumatoid d.
      (DMARD)
    gastroprotective d.
    glutamatergic d.
    d. infusion
    neuromuscular blocking d.
      (NMBD)
    nonsteroidal antiinflammatory d.
      (NSAID)
    platelet-inhibiting d.
    d. resistance
    second-line d.
    d. synergy
drug-drug interaction
drug-seeking behavior
drum membrane
Drummond interspinous wiring
technique
Drummond-Morison omentofixation
drunken sailor effect
drusen
dry
    d. abscess
    d. amputation
    d. colostomy
    d. field technique
    d. gangrene
    d. heat oven sterilization
    d. hernia
    d. mucous membranes
    d. needling

DSE
    digital subtraction echocardiography
    dobutamine stress echocardiography
DSM-IV
    Diagnostic and Statistical Manual of
      Mental Disorders, 4th Edition
DSRS
    distal splenorenal shunt
      DSRS technique
DST
    double stapling technique
DSVNI
    Distress Scale for Ventilated Newborn
    Infants
DTI
    Doppler tissue imaging
DTM
    deep tissue massage
du
    d. meridian
    d. qi sensation
dual
    d. compression scoliosis treatment
    d. impression technique
    d. onlay cortical bone graft
    d. percutaneous endoscopic
      gastrostomy (DPEG)
    d. therapy
dual-action analgesia
dual-delivery platform
dual-temperature cardiopulmonary bypass
Duane
    D. anomaly
    D. exodeviation classification
Dubin-Amelar varicocele classification
Dubowitz
    D. evaluation
    D. examination
Duckett tubularized neourethra
procedure
duct
    aberrant bile d.
    accessory pancreatic d.
    anomalous junction of
      pancreatobiliary d. (AJPBD)
    Arantius d.
    Bartholin d.
    Bernard d.
    bile d.
    biliary d.
    Blasius d.
    bucconeural d.
    canalicular d.
    d. cell adenocarcinoma
    cochlear d.
    collecting d.
    common bile d. (CBD)
    common hepatic d.
    craniopharyngeal d.

D

duct (*continued*)
  cystic d.
  deferent d.
  distal bile d.
  d. ectasia
  efferent d.
  ejaculatory d.
  endolymphatic d.
  excretory d.
  extrahepatic bile d.
  frontonasal d.
  galactophorous d.
  gall d.
  Gartner d.
  genital d.
  hemithoracic d.
  Hensen d.
  hepatic d. (HD)
  hepatocystic d.
  Hoffmann d.
  hypophysial d.
  incisive d.
  inferior lacrimal d.
  d. injury
  intrahepatic bile d.
  jugular d.
  lactiferous d.
  lymphatic d.
  main pancreatic d. (MPD)
  mamillary d.
  mammary d.
  mesonephric d.
  metanephric d.
  milk d.
  minor sublingual d.
  Müller d.
  nasofrontal d.
  d. of Luschka
  pancreatic d.
  papillary d.
  paramesonephric d.
  paraurethral d.
  parotid d.
  Pecquet d.
  perilymphatic d.
  periotic d.
  pronephric d.
  prostatic d.
  right lymphatic d.
  Rivinus d.
  salivary d.
  Santorini d.
  Schüller d.
  secretory d.
  segmental d.
  semicircular d.
  seminal d.
  spermatic d.
  Stensen d.

  d. stone
  striated d.
  subclavian d.
  sublingual d.
  submandibular d.
  submaxillary d.
  sudoriferous d.
  superior lacrimal d.
  sweat d.
  d. system
  testicular d.
  thoracic d.
  thymic d.
  thyroglossal d.
  thyrolingual d.
  uniting d.
  utriculosaccular d.
  d. wall
  Walther d.
  Wharton d.
  wide-mouthed cystic d.
  Wirsung d.
  wolffian d.
ductal
  d. adenoma
  d. calculus
  d. cancer
  d. cannulation
  d. carcinoma
  d. carcinoma in situ (DCIS)
  d. cystadenoma
  d. dilation
  d. ectasia
  d. hyperplasia
  d. obstruction
  d. proliferation
  d. system
  d. system perforation
ductal-dependent
  d.-d. lesion
  d.-d. pulmonary circulation
ductectasia
duct-ectatic mucinous cystadenoma
ductless gland
ductography
ductopenic rejection
ductoscopy
duct-to-duct (D-D)
  d.-t.-d. anastomosis
duct-to-mucosa
  d.-t.-m. anastomosis
  d.-t.-m. pancreaticojejunostomy
  d.-t.-m. technique
ductule
  aberrant d.
  biliary d.
  efferent d.
  inferior aberrant d.
  interlobular d.

pancreatic d.
prostatic d.
superior aberrant d.
transected d.
ductuli (*pl. of* ductulus)
ductulus, *pl.* **ductuli**
ductus, *pl.* **ductus**
    d. arteriosus
    d. cysticus
    d. ejaculatorius
    d. hemithoracicus
Duddell membrane
Dufourmentel pilonidal cyst and sinus
  closure technique
Duhamel
    D. abdominoperineal pullthrough
      procedure
    D. colon operation
    D. laparoscopic pull-through
Dührssen
    D. incision
    D. vaginofixation
Duke
    D. bleeding time
    D. pouch cutaneous urinary
      diversion
Duke-Elder strabismus operation
Dukes
    D. classification of carcinoma
    D. colorectal carcinoma classification
    D. procedure
    D. stage
duloxetine HCl
Dulox suture
dumbbell
    d. mass
    d. tumor
dumbbelling
    d. of tumor
    d. of veins
dumping
    d. stomach
    d. syndrome
Dunbar syndrome
Duncan-Lovell modification
Duncan position
dunk
dunked
dunking technique
Dunn
    D. acromioclavicular joint technique
    D. biopsy
    D. osteotomy
Dunn-Brittain foot stabilization technique
Dunn-Hess trochanteric osteotomy
Dunnington lateral rectus recession
duodenal (D, duod)
    d. adenocarcinoma
    d. adenoma

d. ampulla
d. atresia
d. bulb
d. bulb deformity
d. cap
d. compression
d. content examination
d. diverticularization procedure
d. duplication
d. endoscopic polypectomy
d. fistula
d. flap
d. fluid collection
d. foreign body
d. fossa
d. gland
d. hematoma
d. hernia
d. ileus
d. impression
d. loop
d. mass
d. metastasis
d. migrating activity
d. papilla
d. passage
d. perforation
d. recess
d. scarring
d. seromyectomy
d. sphincter
d. stump
d. stump leak
d. switch
d. tumor
d. ulcer
d. ulceration
d. web
duodenectomy
    pylorus-preserving total d.
duodenobiliary pressure gradient
duodenocaval fistula
duodenocholecystostomy
duodenocholedochotomy
duodenocolic fistula
duodenocystostomy
duodenoduodenostomy
duodenoenterocutaneous fistula
duodenoenterostomy
duodenogastroscopy
    retrograde d.
duodenoileostomy
    antecolic d.
    d. ileoileostomy
duodenojejunal
    d. angle
    d. flexure
    d. fold
    d. fossa

D

duodenojejunal (*continued*)
    d. hernia
    d. junction
    d. motor recording
    d. recess
    d. sphincter
duodenojejunostomy
    suprapapillary Roux-en-Y d.
duodenolysis
duodenomesocolic fold
duodenopancreatic resection
duodenopyloric constriction
duodenorenal ligament
duodenorrhaphy
duodenoscopy
duodenostomy
    Witzel d.
duodenotomy
    transverse d.
duodenum
duodenum-preserving resection
DuoDerm
Duplay I, II hypospadias repair technique
duplex
    d. arterial mapping
    d. ultrasonography
duplex-guided compression
duplication
    alimentary tract d.
    d. anomaly
    colorectal d.
    complete d.
    congenital d.
    cranial d.
    d. cyst
    duodenal d.
    esophageal d.
    fetal d.
    gallbladder d.
    gastric d.
    incomplete d.
    Marks-Bayne technique for thumb d.
    partial d.
    renal d.
    symmetric thumb d.
    thumb d.
    trunk d.
    tubular colonic d.
    ureteral d.
    Wassel thumb d.
Dupuy-Dutemps
    D.-D. dacryocystorhinostomy dye test
    D.-D. dacryostomy
    D.-D. lower lid blepharoplasty
Dupuytren
    D. canal

    D. contracture
    D. fracture
    D. suture technique
dural
    d. arteriovenous fistula
    d. arteriovenous malformation
    d. cavernous sinus fistula
    d. click
    d. ectasia
    d. incision
    d. nerve root
    d. patch reconstruction
    d. puncture
    d. puncture headache
    d. rent
    d. repair
    d. ring
    d. shunt syndrome
    d. venous sinus
dura mater
Duran aortic vegetation approach
duraplasty
duration
    d. tetany
    d. time
Duret
    D. hemorrhage
    D. lesion
Durham
    D. flatfoot operation
    D. plasty
Durkan carpal compression test
Durr
    D. nonpenetrating keratoplasty
    D. operation
dusky stoma
dust-borne infection
Dutcher body
duToit-Roux
    d.-R. arthroplasty
    d.-R. staple capsulorrhaphy
Duval
    D. pancreaticojejunostomy
    D. pancreaticojejunostomy procedure
Duverger-Velter operation
Duverney
    D. fissure
    D. fracture
    D. gland
    D. muscle
DuVries
    D. deltoid ligament reconstruction technique
    D. hammertoe repair
    D. incision
    D. plantar condylectomy
    D. plantar fasciotomy approach
DuVries-Mann modified bunionectomy

DVC
dorsal venous complex
DVRT
differential variable reluctance
transducer
DVT
deep vein thrombosis
deep venous thrombosis
concurrent DVT
DVT prevention
DVT prophylaxis
dwarfism
achondroplastic d.
dwarf pelvis
DWM
Dandy-Walker malformation
DWS
Dandy-Walker syndrome
Dwyer
D. clawfoot operation
D. incision
D. orthopaedic procedure
D. osteotomy
Dx
diagnosis
dye
d. dilution cardiac output technique
d. dilution determination
d. dilution method
d. exclusion test
d. injection
d. reduction spot test
d. scattering method
d. sham intrarenal lesion
d. worker's carcinoma
2-dye method
dynamic
d. bolus tracking technique
d. cardiomyoplasty
d. closure pressure
d. compliance
d. compression
d. compression plate fixation
d. condylar screw fixation
d. cystourethroscopy
d. end-tidal forcing
d. fluorescence video endoscopy
d. graciloplasty
d. image
d. lumbar stabilization
d. negative airway pressure (DNAP)
d. relation
d. relaxation
d. repair
d. storage allocation
d. tracheal collapse
d. traction method
dynamometer
Cybex d.

dynamometry
isometric force d.
dysarthric lesion
dysautonomia
familial d.
dyscinesia (*var. of* dyskinesia)
dyscrasic fracture
dysejaculation
dysesthesia
burning d.
denervation d.
dysesthetic pain
dysfuncation
inflammation-induced postoperative
gastrointestinal tract d.
dysfunction
acquired neurologic d.
bladder d.
bone marrow d.
chronic obstructive pulmonary d.
cognitive d.
ejaculatory d.
end-organ d.
endothelial cell d.
erectile d. (ED)
esophageal body motor d.
extensor mechanism d.
gastrointestinal tract d.
hepatic d.
hepatocellular synthetic d.
ileostomy d.
late graft d.
multiorgan system d.
multiple organ d. (MOD)
myofascial d.
neurogenic bladder d.
neuromotor d.
obstructive pulmonary d.
organ d.
pancreatic d.
pelvic floor d.
postanesthetic central nervous
system d.
postgastrectomy d.
postoperative cognitive d. (POCD)
postoperative gastrointestinal tract d.
(PGID)
postoperative renal d.
proximal myofascial d.
pulmonary d.
renal d.
sacroiliac joint d.
significant organ d.
small nerve fiber d.
sphincter of Oddi d.
surfactant d.
swallowing d.
vascular d.
vocal d.

D

dysfunctional cognition
dysgenesia (*var. of* dysgenesis)
dysgenesis, dysgenesia
dysgnathic anomaly
dyskinesia, dyskinesis, dyscinesia
    biliary d.
    extrapyramidal d.
    levodopa-induced d.
    retrolisthesis positional d.
dyskinesis (*var. of* dyskinesia)
dysmenorrheal membrane
dysmotility
    esophageal d.
dysmyelination
dysosteogenesis
dysostosis
dyspepsia
    flatulent d.
    postcholecystectomy flatulent d.
dysphagia, dysphagy
    benign d.
    contractile ring d.
    long-term d.
    postoperative d.
    postvagotomy d.
    recurrent d.
dysphagy (*var. of* dysphagia)
dysphasia
    expressive d.
dysphoric
    d. mood state
    d. patient mood
dyspigmentation
dysplasia
    asphyxiating thoracic d.
    bronchopulmonary d. (BPD)
    cortical d.
    d. dislocation
    fibromuscular d. (FMD)
    focal cortical d.
    high-grade d. (HGD)
    low-grade d.
    oculoauriculovertebral d. (OAVD)
dysplasia-associated
    d.-a. lesion
    d.-a. mass
dysplasminogenemia
dysplastic epithelium

dyspnea
    exertional d.
    expiratory d.
    1-flight exertional d.
    2-flight exertional d.
    d. on exertion (DOE)
dysraphia (*var. of* dysraphism)
dysraphic malformation
dysraphism, dysraphia
    occult spinal d.
    spinal d.
dysreflexia
    autonomic d.
dysregulation
    autonomic d.
    emotional d.
    microcirculatory d.
    neurogenic d.
    sensory d.
dysrhythmia
    atrial d.
    supraventricular d.
    ventricular d.
dysrhythmogenicity
dysthymia
dystonia
    cervical d.
    muscle d.
    posttraumatic cervical d.
dystonic
    d. pain
    d. tic
dystrophia (*var. of* dystrophy)
dystrophic nail
dystrophy, dystrophia
    Becker muscular d.
    corneal d.
    Emery-Dreifuss muscular d.
    facioscapulohumeral
     muscular d.
    muscular d. (MD)
    myotonic d.
    oculopharyngeal muscular d.
    reflex sympathetic d. (RSD)
    sympathic d.
dysuria, dysury
dysuric
dysury (*var. of* dysuria)

E

E point

EA

electroacupuncture
electroanesthesia
epidural anesthesia

Eagle-Barrett syndrome
Eagle syndrome
Eagleton operation
EAL

endoscopic aspiration
lumpectomy

ear

e. anesthesia
e. bone
e. canal
e. cartilage inflammation
external e.
surfer's e.

earlobe adipose tissue
early

e. active treatment
e. cancer lesion
e. enteral feeding
e. extubation
e. extubation candidate
e. gastric cancer
e. graft thrombosis
e. infection rate
e. oversewing
e. postoperative period
e. supraclavicular compression
e. thoracoscopic repair
e. thrombectomy
e. unequivocal shock

early-onset graft-versus-host disease
earth

diatomaceous e.

easily reducible hernia
EAST

elevated arm stress test

Eastern Cooperative Oncology Group (ECOG)
Eastwood anesthesia technique
Eaton

E. closed reduction
E. implant arthroplasty
E. volar plate arthroplasty

Eaton-Lambert syndrome
Eaton-Littler

E.-L. carpometacarpal thumb repair
technique
E.-L. ligament reconstruction

Eaton-Malerich

E.-M. fracture-dislocation operation

E.-M. fracture-dislocation
technique
E.-M. reduction

Ebbehoj penile straightening-reinforcing procedure
Eberle contracture release technique
Ebner

imbrication line of von E.
E. line
E. reticulum

EBNS

endoscopic bladder neck suspension

ebonation
EBP

epidural blood patch

ébranlement
Ebstein

E. anomaly
E. cardiac anomaly
E. congenital anomaly
E. malformation

eburnation
EBV

Epstein-Barr virus
EBV infection

ECA

external carotid artery

ECA-PCA

external carotid artery-posterior cerebral
artery
ECA-PCA bypass surgery

ecarin
ecarin-based test
ECBP

extracorporeal bypass pump

ECC

endocervical curettage
extracorporeal circulation

ECCE

extracapsular cataract extraction

eccentric

e. exercise
e. fixation
e. hypertrophy
e. interocclusal record
e. jaw position
e. jaw relation
e. ledge
e. maxillomandibular record
e. narrowing
e. occlusion

eccentricity index
ecchondrosis
ecchymosed
ecchymosis

E

ecchymotic
    e. mark
    e. mask
ECCO₂R
    extracorporeal carbon dioxide
    removal
eccrine
    e. carcinoma
    e. sweat gland
ECD
    extended criteria donor
ECF-A
    eosinophilic chemotactic factor of
    anaphylaxis
ECFV
    extracellular fluid volume
ECG
    electrocardiogram
    electrocardiography
echinococcal
    e. cyst disease
    e. liver abscess
    e. liver cyst
echinococcosis
    alveolar e.
    cystic e.
echinococcotomy
echinococcus cyst
echo
    echocardiogram
    echocardiography
    e. formation
    e. imaging
    inconsequential e.
    e. sign
    specular e.
    e. zone
echocardiogram (echo)
    intraoperative multiplane
    transesophageal e.
echocardiographic assessment
echocardiography (echo)
    digital subtraction e. (DSE)
    dobutamine stress e. (DSE)
    3D transesophageal e.
    epicardial e.
    perioperative e.
    transesophageal e. (TEE)
    transesophageal color Doppler e.
    transthoracic e.
echodense
    e. mass
    e. structure
echodensity
echoduodenoscopy
echogenic
    e. liver
    e. plaque
    e. tissue

echographic layer
echolucency
echolucent plaque
echopenic liver metastasis
echothiophate
echovirus infection
EC-IC
    extracranial-intracranial
Ecker fissure
Ecker-Lotke-Glazer
    E.-L.-G. patellar tendon repair
    E.-L.-G. tendon reconstruction
    technique
Eckert-Davis peroneal tendon subluxation
classification
Eck fistula
Eckhout vertical gastroplasty
eclipse
    e. amblyopia
    e. phase
ECLP
    extracorporeal liver perfusion
ECLS
    extracorporeal life support
ECMO
    extracorporeal membrane oxygenation
ECoG
    electrocorticography
    ECoG monitoring
    ECoG performance status scale
ECOG
    Eastern Cooperative Oncology Group
Economo disease
ECPL
    endocavitary pelvic lymphadenectomy
ECRB
    extensor carpi radialis brevis
ECRL
    extensor carpi radialis longus
E2CS
    Edinburgh 2 Coma Scale
ECS
    elective cosmetic surgery
    electrocerebral silence
ECST
    European Carotid Surgery Trial
ectal origin
ectasia, ectasis
    alveolar e.
    aortoannular e.
    artery e.
    corneal e.
    coronary artery e.
    distal e.
    duct e.
    ductal e.
    dural e.
    gastric antral vascular e. (GAVE)
    iris e.

mammary duct e.
papillary e.
scleral e.
senile e.
vascular e.

ectasis (*var. of* ectasia)
ectatic
    e. aneurysm
    e. bronchus
    e. carotid artery
    e. dilation
    e. emphysema
    e. vascular lesion
    e. vessel
ectocolostomy
ectoderm
ectodermal
ectopia, ectopy
    cerebellar e.
    gallbladder e.
    macular e.
    renal e.
    testicular e.
    ureteral e.
ectopic
    e. ACTH syndrome
    e. activity
    e. anus
    e. atrial tachycardia
    e. bone
    e. craniopharyngioma
    e. cutaneous schistosomiasis
    e. endometrial tissue
    e. eruption
    e. eyelash
    e. focus
    e. gastric mucosa
    e. hyperparathyroidism
    e. impulse
    e. kidney
    e. pancreas
    e. parathormone production
    e. parathyroid adenoma
    e. pregnancy
    e. rhythm
    e. sebaceous gland
    e. spleen
    e. ureter
    e. ureterocele
    e. varix
ectopy (*var. of* ectopia)
ectoscopy
ectosteal
ectostosis
ectothrix infection
ECTR
    endoscopic carpal tunnel release
ectropion, ectropium
ectropium (*var. of* ectropion)

ECU
    extensor carpi ulnaris
    extracorporeal ultrafiltration
eczematoid pruritic plaque
eczematous
    e. lesion
    e. patch
    e. polymorphous light eruption
    e. reaction
ED
    erectile dysfunction
EDB
    extensor digitorum brevis
EDD
    end-diastolic diameter
Edebohls
    E. incision
    E. position
edema
    antral e.
    brain e.
    bullous e.
    cardiac e.
    cerebral e.
    corneal e.
    endothelial cell e.
    hemodynamic pulmonary e.
    hemorrhagic e.
    ileocecal e.
    laryngeal e.
    lower extremity e.
    lymphatic e.
    massive pulmonary hemorrhagic e.
    negative pressure pulmonary e.
    nephrotic e.
    neurogenic pulmonary e. (NPE)
    pericholecystic e.
    peripheral extremity e.
    postobstructive pulmonary e.
    pulmonary e.
    reexpansion pulmonary e. (REPE)
    retroarytenoidal e.
    stasis e.
    subglottic e.
    supraglottic e.
    transient e.
    unilateral supraglottic e.
    visceral e.
edematous
    e. bowel
    e. bowel wall
    e. mesentery
Eden-Hybbinette
    E.-H. anterior glenoid bone block
      procedure
    E.-H. arthroplasty
Eden-Lange trapezius procedure
Eden-Lawson hysterectomy
edentulous space

E

Eder-Puestow dilation
edge
    anastomotic e.
    chondral e.
    inferior e.
    lateral e.
    shelving e.
    superior e.
edge-detection method
edge-to-edge suture technique
Edinburgh 2 Coma Scale (E2CS)
Edinger-Westphal nucleus
edition
    Diagnostic and Statistical Manual of
      Mental Disorders, 4th E.
      (DSM-IV)
EDL
    extensor digitorum longus
Edlan-Mejchar mucogingival subperiosteal
  vestibule extension operation
Edmondson grading system for
  hepatocellular carcinoma
Edmondson-Steiner hepatocellular
  carcinoma classification
Edmonton
    E. Staging System for Cancer Pain
    E. Symptom Assessment Schedule
EDR
    extreme drug resistance
edrophonium
EDT
    emergency department thoracotomy
Edwards
    E. septectomy
    E. transposing atrial septum
      procedure
Edwards-Tapp arterial graft
EEA
    end-to-end anastomosis
      EEA stapler
EEG
    electroencephalogram
    electroencephalography
      EEG monitor
      EEG phase coupling
      EEG silence
EEG-based anesthesia monitor
EELV
    end-expiratory lung volume
EEV
    encircling endocardial ventriculotomy
effect
    adverse e.
    amnestic e.
    analgesic e.
    anorexigenic e.
    antiangiogenic e.
    anticoagulant e.
    Bernoulli e.

    biologic e.
    Bohr e.
    cardioprotective e.
    cardiotoxic e.
    cardiovascular adverse e.
    cerebral vasodilatory e.
    chemoradiotherapy e.
    cutaneous analgesic e.
    digitalis e.
    dose-related e.
    drunken sailor e.
    esophageal e.
    Hawthorne e.
    hepatotoxic e.
    hypnotic e.
    hypothermic e.
    immunomodulating e.
    motilin e.
    negative e.
    oxygen e.
    e. parameter
    pulmonary e.
    reverse steal e.
    second gas e.
    sedative e.
    stimulating e.
    synergistic e.
    therapeutic e.
effective
    e. function
    e. renal blood flow
    e. renal plasma flow
    e. setting expansion
effector
    e. operation
    e. organ
    e. pathway
effect-site decrement time
efferens
    vas e.
efferent
    e. duct
    e. ductule
    e. glomerular arteriole
    e. limb
    e. limb syndrome
    e. loop
    e. nerve activity
    PJA e.
    e. sympathetic response
    e. vasodilation
efficacy
    corticosteroid e.
    medication e.
    therapeutic e.
Effler-Groves
    E.-G. mode
    E.-G. mode of Allison antireflux
      procedure

Effler hiatal hernia repair
effluent
> clear e.

effort thrombosis
effusion
> chylous e.
> exudative pleural e.
> pericardial e.
> pleural e.
> subdural e.

Eftekhar broken femoral stem technique
EG/BUS
> external genitalia, Bartholin, urethral,
> Skene

EGD
> esophagogastroduodenoscopy

EGF
> epidermal growth factor
>> salivary EGF
>> serum EGF
>> urinary EGF

egg
> e. activation
> e. membrane

Egger line
Eggers
> E. neurectomy
> E. tendon transfer technique

Eggleston rapid digitalization method
eggshell nail
Eglis gland
EHF
> electrohydraulic fragmentation

EHL
> extensor hallucis longus

Ehlers-Danlos syndrome
EHPVO
> extrahepatic portal vein obstruction

Ehrenritter ganglion
Ehrlich inner body
Ehrlich-Türck line
EIA
> exercise-induced asthma
> external iliac artery

Eicken hypopharyngoscopy method
eighth cranial nerve
EIS
> endoscopic injection sclerotherapy

Eisenberger technique
ejaculation
> e. disorder
> retrograde e.

ejaculatorius
> ductus e.

ejaculatory
> e. duct
> e. dysfunction

ejection
> e. murmur

> e. phase
> e. phase index
> e. rate
> e. shell image
> e. time

ejection-fraction image
Ejrup collateral circulation maneuver
Ekehorn
> E. rectal prolapse repair
> E. rectopexy

EKG
> electrocardiogram
> electrocardiography

elastance
> airway e.

elastic
> e. band fixation
> e. band ligation
> e. barrier
> e. compression
> e. fiber fragmentation
> e. lamella
> e. recoil
> e. recoil pressure
> e. tissue
> e. vascular loop

elasticus
> conus e.

elastofibroma
elastolysis
> generalized e.

elastomeric pump
Elaut triangle
elbow
> e. approach
> e. arthroplasty
> e. disarticulation
> e. dislocation
> e. extensor tendon
> e. fracture
> tennis e.

ELCA
> excimer laser coronary angioplasty

elderly
> Pain Assessment for the Dementing
> E. (PADE)

elective
> e. aneurysmectomy
> e. cerclage
> e. cosmetic surgery (ECS)
> e. dilatational tracheostomy
> e. hernia repair
> e. herniorrhaphy
> e. laparotomy
> e. lymphadenectomy
> e. lymph node dissection (ELND)
> e. neck dissection (END)
> e. oral tracheal intubation
> e. procedure

E

elective (*continued*)
  e. sigmoid resection
  e. surgery
  e. surgical procedure
electric
  e. anesthesia
  e. aversion therapy
  e. coagulation
  e. differential therapy
  e. induction
  e. stimulation
electrical
  e. activation abnormality
  e. catheter ablation
  e. fulguration
  e. heart position
  e. nerve stimulation
  e. stimulation therapy
  e. stimulator waveform
  e. surface stimulation
electroacupoint stimulation
electroacupuncture (EA)
electroanalgesia
electroanesthesia (EA)
electrobioscopy
electrocardiogram (ECG, EKG)
electrocardiography
  (ECG, EKG)
electrocauterization
electrocautery
  bipolar e.
  bleeding controlled with e.
  hook e.
  low-current e.
  monopolar e.
  multipolar e.
  needlepoint e.
  e. resection
electrocerebral silence (ECS)
electrocholecystectomy
electrocoagulation
  bipolar e.
  e. diathermy
  direct current e.
  endoscopic e.
  monopolar e.
  multipolar e.
  e. necrosis
  pinpoint e.
  radiofrequency e.
  snare e.
  transendoscopic e.
electrocorticography (ECoG)
  awake intraoperative e.
electrode
  depth e.
  3-dimensional grid e.
  grid e.
  e. impedance

  e. migration
  multiple array radiofrequency
    needle e.
  e. placement
  e. potential
  e. response time
  surface e.
electrodesiccated bleeding point
electrodesiccation
electrode-skin interface
electrodiagnostic testing
electrodiaphake
electrodispersive skin patch
electroejaculation
  rectal probe e.
electroencephalogram (EEG)
electroencephalography
  (EECG, EEG)
electroepilation
electroexcision
electrofulguration
electrogalvanic stimulation
electrogastroenterostomy
electrogenesis
electrogram
  atrial e.
electrohemostasis
electrohydraulic
  e. fragmentation (EHF)
  e. lithotripsy
  e. shock wave lithotripsy (ESWL)
electrolaryngogram
electrolysis
electrolyte
  e. abnormality
  e. flush solution
  e. imbalance
  e. imbalance coma
electrolytic solution
electromagnetic
  e. field (EMF)
  e. interference (EMI)
  e. radiation exposure
  e. signal
  e. system
  e. tracking
electromechanical dissociation (EMD)
electromyocardial dissociation
electromyogram (EMG)
  surface e.
electromyographic study
electromyography (EMG)
  laryngeal e.
electron (e, E)
  intraoperative radiotherapy with
    electrons
  e. microscopy (EM, EMC,
    E-MICR)
electronarcosis

electroneurolysis
electronic
    e. bone stimulation
    e. chronic pain diary
    e. magnification
    e. momentary assessment
    e. nose
    e. prescription-monitoring program
    (ePMP)
electroparacentesis
electrophoresis
    hemoglobin e.
    protein e.
electrophrenic respiration
electrophysiologic (EP)
    e. function
    e. monitoring
electrophysiological stimulation
electrophysiology (EP)
    flickering blockade e.
    North American Society of Pacing
    and E. (NASPE)
    patch clamp e.
    e. study
electropuncture
electroresection
electroscission
electrosection
electrosterilization
    root canal e.
electrosurgery unit (ESU)
electrosurgical
    e. desiccation
    e. fulguration
    e. snare polypectomy
**electrotherapeutic sleep
 therapy**
electrotherm
electrotomy
element
    glandular e.
elementary
    e. fracture
    e. lesion
**elephant trunk aortic graft
 technique**
elevated
    e. arm stress test
    (EAST)
    e. hemidiaphragm
    e. lesion
elevation
    e. angle
    blanched cutaneous e.
    chin e.
    congenital scapular e.
    diaphragmatic e.
    flap e.
    Gillies fractured zygoma e.

    e. of extremity
    e. paresis
    periosteal e.
    scapular e.
    ST segment e.
    unilateral diaphragmatic e.
elevator
    e. disease
    e. esophagus
    e. extraction
    femoral e.
    e. muscle
elevatus
    e. deformity
    metatarsus primus e.
eleventh
    e. cranial nerve
    e. rib flank incision
    e. rib transperitoneal
    incision
elimination
    e. clearance
    CO_2 e.
    e. curve
    e. disorder
    e. half-life
    Hoffman e.
    nonpulmonary route of e.
    e. pocket
    e. procedure
    pulmonary carbon dioxide e.
    ($VECO_2$)
    e. reaction
Elizabethtown osteotomy
Elliot
    E. position
    E. sclerocornea
    trephination
ellipsoid
    e. joint
    e. method
ellipsoidal joint
elliptical
    e. anastomosis
    e. biopsy
    e. excision technique
    e. recess
    e. uterine incision
elliptocytosis
    hereditary e.
Ellis
    E. skin traction technique
    E. tooth fracture classification
**Ellis-Jones peroneal tendon
 technique**
Ellison
    E. iliotibial band transfer for ACL
    repair technique
    E. lateral knee reconstruction

E

Elmslie-Trillat
      E.-T. patellar procedure
      E.-T. patellar realignment method
ELND
      elective lymph node dissection
Eloesser thoracostomy flap
Elsberg incision
Elschnig
      E. blepharorrhaphy
      E. body
      E. canthorrhaphy
      E. canthorrhaphy operation
      E. central iridectomy
      E. keratoplasty
Ely protruding ear corrective operation
embedded toenail
embolectomy
      arterial e.
      balloon e.
      catheter e.
      direct e.
      femoral e.
      pulmonary e.
emboli (*pl. of* embolus)
embolic
      e. complication
      e. gangrene
emboliform
embolism
      air e.
      amniotic fluid e.
      atheroma e.
      autologous blood clot pulmonary e.
      catheter e.
      gas e.
      paradoxical e.
      pulmonary e. (PE)
      transfusion-related air e.
      tumor e.
      vascular air e.
      venous air e. (VAE)
embolization
      accelerated arteriolar gas e.
      angiographic e.
      arterial e.
      hepatic artery e. (HAE)
      particulate e.
      portal vein e.
      pulmonary e.
      renal arterial e.
      selective arterial e.
      subselective e.
      superselective microcoil e.
      symptomatic e.
      venous e.
embolotherapy
embolus, *pl.* **emboli**
      air e.
      cholesterol e.

fatal air e.
hemodynamically significant air e.
e. migration
paradoxical e.
embouchement
embrasure space
embryectomy
embryo
      e. biopsy
      e. encapsulation
      e. reduction
embryonal
      e. cell carcinoma
      e. sarcoma
      e. tumor
embryonic
      e. fixation syndrome
      e. neural tube
      e. sac
embryotomy
EMD
      electromechanical dissociation
emedullate
Emend
emergence
      e. agitation
      anesthetic e.
      e. delirium
      metachronous e.
      synchronous e.
emergency
      access e.
      e. airway management
      e. appendectomy
      e. colonoscopy
      e. department resuscitation
      e. department thoracotomy (EDT)
      e. indication
      e. laparotomy
      e. medicine
      e. operation
      e. procedure
      e. room (ER)
      e. room thoracotomy
      e. SSPCS
      e. surgery
      surgical e.
      e. tracheal intubation
      e. tracheostomy
      e. ventilation
emergent
      e. appendectomy
      e. cerclage
      e. endoscopic sclerotherapy
      e. herniorrhaphy
      e. intubation
      e. operation
      e. surgery
Emery-Dreifuss muscular dystrophy

emesis
    coffee-grounds e.
EMF
    electromagnetic field
EMG
    electromyogram
    electromyography
        EMG biofeedback
EMI
    electromagnetic interference
        EMI scan
eminence
    arcuate e.
    cruciate e.
    cruciform e.
    deltoid e.
    frontal e.
    genital e.
    hypothenar e.
    ileocecal e.
    iliopectineal e.
    iliopubic e.
    intercondylar e.
    intertubercular e.
    orbital e.
    parietal e.
    pyramidal e. (PE)
    thenar e.
    thyroid e.
eminentia, *pl.* **eminentiae**
eminentiae (*pl. of* eminentia)
emissarium
emissary
    e. sphenoidal foramen
    e. vein
emission
    gas e.
    e. line
EMLA
    eutectic mixture of local anesthetics
Emmet
    E. operation
    E. suture technique
Emmon osteotomy
EMMV
    extended mandatory minute
    ventilation
Emory Pain Estimate Model
    (EPEM)
emotional
    e. dysregulation
    e. support system
emphysema
    colonoscopy-related e.
    ectatic e.
    endoscopy-related e.
    nonbullous e.
    postlaparoscopic subcutaneous e.
    subcutaneous e.

    subgaleal e.
    surgical e.
emphysematous
    e. change
    e. cholecystitis
    e. gangrene
empiric therapy
emprosthotonos position
empty
    e. gestational sac
    e. sella
emptying
    delayed gastric e.
    gastric e.
empyema
    bilious e.
    parapneumonic e.
    pleural e.
    postpneumonectomy
        tuberculous e.
    tuberculous e.
empyemic
EMR
    endoscopic mucosal resection
emulsion
    perfluorocarbon e.
en
    e. bloc
    e. bloc celiac axis resection
    e. bloc dissection
    e. bloc distal pancreatectomy
    e. bloc excision
    e. bloc lymphadenopathy
    e. bloc no-touch technique
    e. bloc removal
    e. bloc vein resection
    e. face position
enamel
    e. crypt
    e. excrescence
    e. fracture
    e. knot
    e. membrane
    e. projection
    e. rod inclination
    e. sac
enameloplasty
enantiomer
enarthrodial joint
enarthrosis
encapsulated
    e. brain abscess
    e. breast implant
encapsulation
    embryo e.
    peritoneal e.
    tumor e.
encasement
encatarrhaphy, enkatarrhaphy

encephalemia
encephali
    arachnoidea mater e.
    arachnoid mater e.
encephalitis
encephalization
encephalocele
encephaloid gastric carcinoma
encephaloma
encephalomeningocele
encephalomyelitis
    experimental allergic e.
encephalomyelocele
encephalopathia (*var. of* encephalopathy)
encephalopathy, encephalopathia
    clinical e.
    degenerative e.
    hepatic e.
    ischemic e.
    portal-systemic e. (PSE)
    progressive e.
    refractory e.
    traumatic progressive e.
encephaloscopy
encephalotomy
enchondral
enchondroma of bone
enchondrosarcoma
encircling
    e. cryoablation
    e. endocardial ventriculotomy (EEV)
    e. explant
encroachment
encrustation
    bile e.
encysted
    e. calculus
    e. hernia
    e. intraabdominal collection
end
    blind e.
    e. colostomy
    cut e.
    e. exhalation
    e. expiration
    e. expiratory
    e. ileostomy
    e. inspiration
    e. point
    proximal e.
    stapled blind e.
    e. stoma
    e. stoma closure
    e. tube
    upper e.
END
    elective neck dissection
endarterectomy
    aortoiliac e.

    blunt eversion carotid e.
    carotid e. (CEA)
    conventional e.
    coronary e.
    eversion carotid e.
    femoral e.
    gas e.
    open e.
    surgical e.
    transaortic e.
    transaortic mesenteric e.
    visceral vessel e.
endaural mastoid incision
end-diastolic
    e.-d. cross-sectional area
    e.-d. diameter (EDD)
    e.-d. left ventricular pressure
endemic fungal infection
Ender femoral fracture technique
end-expiratory
    e.-e. intragastric pressure
    e.-e. lung volume (EELV)
    e.-e. phase
endgut
end-hole catheter
end-inspiratory volume
Endius posterior keyhole pedicle screw
  approach
endless-loop tachycardia
endloop
    e. ileocolostomy
    e. ileostomy
    e. stoma
end-loop colostomy
endoabdominal fascia
endoalveolar crest
endoanal
    e. anastomosis
    e. mucosectomy
    e. ultrasonography
endoaneurysmoplasty
endoaneurysmorrhaphy
    Matas e.
    ventricular e.
endoauscultation
endobrachyesophagus
endobronchial
    e. blocker
    e. brachytherapy
    e. cancer
    e. fistula
    e. intubation
    e. intubation anesthetic
      technique
    e. spill
    e. tree
    e. tuberculosis
endocapsular
endocardiac, endocardial

endocardial (*var. of* endocardiac)
    e. flow
    e. mapping
    e. murmur
    e. resection
    e. stain
    e. thickening
endocarditic
endocarditis
    prosthetic valve e. (PVE)
endocardium
EndoCatch bag
endocavitary
    e. bladder diverticulectomy
    e. pelvic lymphadenectomy (ECPL)
    e. radiation therapy
endoceliac
endocervical
    e. canal
    e. curettage (ECC)
    e. mucosa
    e. polyp
    e. sampling
endocervix
endochondral bone
endocolitis
endocolpitis
endocranial
endocranium
endocrine
    e. adenomatosis
    e. disorder
    e. fracture
    e. gland
    e. imaging
    e. insufficiency
    e. pancreas
    e. screening
    e. surgeon
    e. surgery
    e. toxicity
    e. tumor
endocrinology
endocrinopathy
    multiple e.
    opiate-induced e.
endocryopexy
endocryoretinopexy
endocyst
endocytosis
endodermal sinus
endodiathermy
endodontia (*var. of* endodontics)
endodontic
    e. armamentarium
    e. cavity
    e. irrigation
    e. surgery
    e. technique

endodontics, endodontia, endodontology
    pedodontic e.
    1-sitting e.
    surgical e.
endodontist
endodontium
endodontologist
endodontology (*var. of* endodontics)
endofaradism
endofluoroscopic technique
endofluoroscopy
    flexible e.
    percutaneous e.
    rigid e.
endogalvanism
endogastric
endogenic (*var. of* endogenous)
endogenous, endogenic
    e. algogenic agent
    e. aneurysm
    e. AV fistula
    e. disease
    e. event-related potential
    e. fiber
    e. flora
    e. infection
    e. lipid pneumonia
    e. microflora
    e. opiate receptor
    e. opioid
    e. opioid peptide (EOP)
    e. opioid system
    e. protection
    e. pyrogen
    e. smile
    e. steroid
    e. uveitis
endoglobar
endograft
    aortic e.
endoherniotomy
endoillumination
Endoknot suture
endolacrimal procedure
endolaryngeal
endoleak
    proximal e.
    retrograde collateral e.
    type II e.
endoligature
endolith
Endoloop suture
endoluminal
    e. excision
    e. repair
    e. stenting
    e. technology
    e. therapy
endolymph

E

endolymphatic
 e. cavity
 e. duct
 e. fluid
 e. hydrops
 e. sac
 e. space
endolymphaticus
endolymphic
endometria (*pl. of* endometrium)
endometrial
 e. ablation
 e. adenocarcinoma
 e. atrophy
 e. biopsy
 e. cancer
 e. carcinoma
 e. cavity
 e. chemical shift imaging
 e. curettage
 e. cytology
 e. island
 e. jet washing
 e. morphology
 e. polyp
 e. receptor
 e. resection
 e. sampling
 e. shedding
 e. spiral artery
 e. thickness
 e. tuberculosis
endometric epithelium
endometrioid
endometrioma
endometriosis
endometriotic focus
endometritis
endometrium, *pl.* **endometria**
endometropic
endomyocardial
 e. biopsy
 e. disease
endonasal disorder
endoneurium
endoneurolysis
endoosseous (*var. of*
 endosseous)
endopelvic fascia
endophlebectomy
endophotocoagulation
 argon laser e.
endophthalmitis
 phacoanaphylactic e.
endophytic
endoplasmic reticulum
endoprostheses (*pl. of* endoprosthesis)
endoprosthesis, *pl.* **endoprostheses**
endopyelotomy

endopyeloureterotomy
 percutaneous e.
endorectal
 e. coil magnetic resonance imaging
 e. flap
 e. ileal pouch
 e. ileal pullthrough
 e. ileoanal pullthrough
 e. ileoanal pullthrough method
 e. ileoanal pullthrough procedure
 e. ileoanal pullthrough technique
end-organ
 e.-o. damage
 e.-o. dysfunction
 e.-o. failure
endoribonuclease
endorphin
endorrhachis
endoscope-assisted technique
endoscope-body position relationship
endoscope impaction
endoscopic
 e. adrenalectomy
 e. ampullary stenting
 e. anterior cruciate ligament
  reconstruction
 e. approach
 e. aspiration lumpectomy (EAL)
 e. band ligation
 e. biliary decompression
 e. biliary drainage
 e. biliary stent placement
 e. biopsy site
 e. bladder neck suspension (EBNS)
 e. breast augmentation
 e. brush cytology
 e. cardiac surgery
 e. carpal tunnel release (ECTR)
 e. color Doppler
 e. color Doppler assessment
 e. condylectomy and costochondral
  graft reconstruction
 e. control
 e. cystenterostomy
 e. cystoduodenostomy
 e. cystogastrostomy
 e. devolvulization
 e. dissection
 e. electrocoagulation
 e. electrohydraulic lithotripsy
 e. esophageal ultrasound
 e. esophagectomy
 e. esophagogastric variceal
  ligation
 e. ethmoidectomy
 e. examination
 e. extraction
 e. extraction of pancreatic duct
  stone

e. finding
e. fine-needle aspiration cytology
e. fine-needle puncture
e. fistulotomy
e. frontal craniotomy
e. fulguration
e. fundoplication
e. gastrocnemius release
e. gastrostomy
e. healing
e. hemostasis
e. hemostatic therapy
e. incision
e. India ink injection
e. injection sclerotherapy (EIS)
e. injection therapy
e. jejunostomy
e. laser therapy
e. light source
e. management
e. mastopexy
e. microwave coagulation
e. mitral valve repair
e. mucosal ablation
e. mucosal resection (EMR)
e. mucosal resection method
e. mucosal resection procedure
e. mucosal resection technique
e. mucosectomy
e. nasobiliary catheter drainage
e. optical urethrotomy
e. pancreatic drainage
e. pancreatic duct sphincterotomy
e. pancreatic stenting
e. pancreatic therapy
e. papillary balloon dilation
e. papillotomy
e. papillotomy and stenting
e. parathyroidectomy
e. photodynamic therapy
e. photography
e. plantar fasciotomy
e. pulsed dye laser lithotripsy
e. radial artery harvesting
e. reflectance
e. reflectance spectrophotometry
e. removal
e. retroflexion
e. retrograde balloon dilation
e. retrograde biliary stenting
e. retrograde cannulation
e. retrograde cholangiography
e. retrograde
  cholangiopancreatography (ERCP)
e. retrograde cholecystoendoprosthesis
e. retrograde sclerotherapy
e. route
e. sessile polypectomy
e. sigmoidopexy

e. sinus surgery (ESS)
e. small-bowel biopsy
e. snare resection
e. sphenoidal biopsy
e. sphincterectomy
e. sphincterotomy
e. spinal fusion
e. stent exchange
e. stone disintegration
e. stricturotomy
e. strip craniectomy
e. submucosal dissection
e. surveillance
e. sympathectomy
e. technology
e. transesophageal fine-needle
  aspiration
e. transpapillary cannulation
e. transpapillary cyst drainage
e. treatment
e. ultrasonographic imaging
e. ultrasonography (EUS)
e. ultrasonography-guided cytology
e. ultrasound (EUS)
e. ultrasound evaluation
e. variceal sclerotherapy (EVS)
e. vertical ramus osteotomy
e. video-assisted surgery
e. video image
e. visualization

endoscopically
e. normal patient
e. performed longitudinal
  incision

**endoscopic-assisted microsurgical
  technique**
endoscopic-controlled lithotripsy
endoscopist
endoscopy
  advanced therapeutic e.
  American Society for
    Gastrointestinal E. (ASGE)
  anal e.
  biliary e.
  colorectal cancer e.
  e. complication
  computerized electronic e.
  diagnostic e.
  dynamic fluorescence video e.
  fiberoptic intraosseous e.
  flexible fiberoptic e.
  flexible fiberoptic nasopharyngeal e.
  fluorescent electronic e.
  gastrointestinal e.
  high-altitude e.
  high-magnification e.
  intestinal e.
  intragastric provocation under e.
  intralacrimal e.

E

endoscopy (*continued*)
    intraoperative biliary e.
    intraventricular e.
    laser-assisted spinal e.
      (LASE)
    lumbar epidural e.
    lung-imaging fluorescent e.
    nasal e.
    outpatient e.
    pancreatic e.
    pancreaticobiliary e.
    pediatric e.
    percutaneous e.
    peripartum e.
    peroral e.
    postsurgical e.
    primary diagnostic e.
    e. procedure
    sinus e.
    small intestinal e.
    e. suite
    surveillance e.
    therapeutic upper e.
    transesophageal e.
    transnasal e.
    transoral e.
    UGI e.
    ultrahigh-magnification e.
    upper alimentary e.
    upper gastrointestinal e.
    upper intestinal e.
    virtual e.
endoscopy-related emphysema
endosellar structure
endoskeleton
endosonography-guided
  drainage
endosonoscopy
endosseous, endoosseous
endosteal, endosseous
    e. implant arm
    e. surface
    e. vessel
endosteum
endostitis
endostoma
endothelia (*pl. of* endothelium)
endothelial
    e. barrier
    e. bleb
    e. cell basement membrane
    e. cell dysfunction
    e. cell edema
    e. damage
    e. denudation
    e. injury
    e. lysis
    e. tube
endothelial-dependent relaxation

endothelin
    e. A, B receptor
    e. plasma level
endotheliochorial placenta
endothelio-endothelial placenta
endothelioma
endotheliosis
endothelium, *pl.* **endothelia**
    capillary e.
    continuous e.
    corneal e.
    discontinuous e.
    fenestrated e.
    gastrointestinal e.
    sinusoidal e.
    vascular e.
endothelium-dependent fibrinolysis
endothelium-derived hyperpolarizing
  factor
endothelium-mediated relaxation
endothoracic fascia
endothorax
    tension e.
endothrix infection
endothyropexy
endotoxemia
    systemic e.
endotoxic
    e. exposure
    e. shock
endotoxicosis
endotoxin
    bacterial e.
    e. hyporesponsiveness
    e. shock
endotracheal
    e. anesthesia
    e. aspirate
    e. induction
    e. insufflation
    e. intubation
    e. suctioning
    e. tube placement
    e. ventilation catheter
endotrachelitis
endoultrasonography
endoureterotomy
    cold-knife e.
endourological
    e. cold knife incision
    e. therapy
endourologic laser surgery
endourology
endovaginal
    e. finding
    e. imaging
endovascular
    e. aneurysm
    e. aneurysm repair

e. approach
e. balloon occlusion
e. coagulation
e. coiling
e. graft insertion
e. graft treatment
e. intervention
e. repair
e. stent graft
e. stenting
e. stenting technique
e. surgery
e. technology
e. therapy

endovasculitis
hemorrhagic e.

endovenosum
septum e.

endovenous septum, septum endovenosum
endoventricular circular patch plasty
endplate compression fracture
endplate-muscular block
endpoint
e. measurement
primary e.
resuscitation e.
resuscitative e.
therapeutic e.

end-sigmoid colostomy
end-stage
e.-s. cirrhosis
e.-s. intestinal failure
e.-s. liver disease
e.-s. lymphangiomyomatosis
e.-s. reflux nephropathy

endstage renal disease (ESRD)
end-systolic
e.-s. area (ESA)
e.-s. cross-sectional area
e.-s. diameter (ESD)
e.-s. left ventricular pressure
e.-s. pressure-length relationship (ESPLR)
e.-s. pressure-volume relation
e.-s. stress-dimension relation
e.-s. wall thickness (ESWT)

end-tidal
e.-t. carbon dioxide (ETCO$_2$)
e.-t. carbon dioxide pressure (PETCO$_2$)
e.-t. nitrogen concentration
e.-t. oxygen concentration

end-to-back bowel anastomosis
end-to-end
e.-t.-e. anastomosis (EEA)
e.-t.-e. ductal repair
e.-t.-e. enterostomy
e.-t.-e. esophagogastrostomy
e.-t.-e. esophagojejunostomy

e.-t.-e. ileoanal anastomosis
e.-t.-e. ileoanal anastomosis without mucosal resection
e.-t.-e. intussuscepted pancreaticojejunostomy
e.-t.-e. invaginating
e.-t.-e. inverting pancreaticojejunostomy
e.-t.-e. jejunoileal bypass
e.-t.-e. reconstruction
e.-t.-e. reconstruction method
e.-t.-e. reconstruction procedure
e.-t.-e. reconstruction technique
e.-t.-e. repair
e.-t.-e. splenoadrenal anastomosis
e.-t.-e. suture
e.-t.-e. tendon repair

end-to-side
e.-t.-s. anastomosis (ESA)
e.-t.-s. arteriotomy
e.-t.-s. choledochojejunostomy
e.-t.-s. esophagogastrostomy
e.-t.-s. esophagojejunostomy
e.-t.-s. jejunoileal bypass
e.-t.-s. nerve coaptation
e.-t.-s. portocaval shunt
e.-t.-s. reimplantation
e.-t.-s. repair
e.-t.-s. splenorenal shunt
e.-t.-s. suture
e.-t.-s. vasoepididymostomy technique

endurance
cardiorespiratory e.
e. exercise

end-viewing sector
end-weave anastomosis
enema
air e.
air-contrast barium e. (ACBE)
antegrade continence e. (ACE)
barium e. (BaE)
contrast e.
double-contrast e.
Hypaque e.
water-soluble contrast e.

energy
e. expenditure
hepatic intracellular e.

enervation
enflurane
engaged head
engineering
Englisch sinus
English
E. position
E. rhinoplasty

engorged
engorgement
engraftment

E

engulf
enhanced external counterpulsation
(EECP)
enhancing
    e. brain lesion
    e. ring
enkatarrhaphy (*var. of* encatarrhaphy)
enlarged
    e. parathyroid gland
    e. spleen
enlargement
    asymmetric parathyroid e.
    mediastinal e.
Enneking
    E. benign tumor classification
    E. resection arthrodesis
ensiform
    e. appendix
    e. cartilage
    e. process
ensisternum cartilage
entangling technique
enteral
    e. alimentation
    e. feeding
    e. nutrition
enterelcosis
enteric
    e. cyst
    e. drainage
    e. fistula
    e. infection
    e. intussusception
    e. nervous system
    e. organism
    e. plexus
enteric-drained pancreas graft
entericus
    plexus (nervosus) e.
enteritis
    radiation e.
    regional e.
enteroanastomosis
enterocele sac
enterocentesis
enterocholecystostomy
enterocholecystotomy
enterochromaffinlike cell
enterocleisis
    omental e.
enterocolic fistula
enterocolitis
    necrotizing e. (NEC)
    recurrent e.
enterocolostomy
enterocutaneous fistula
enterocystoplasty
    Camey e.
    clam e.

    seromuscular e.
    sigmoid e.
enteroenteral fistula
enteroenteric fistula
enteroenterostomy
    2-layer e.
enterogenital fistula
enterogenous cyst
enterohepatic circulation
enterohepatopexy
enterolith
enterolithiasis
enterolithotomy
enterolysis
enteropathy
    radiation e.
enteropeptidase
enteroperitoneal abscess
enteropexy
enteroplasty
    serial transverse e. (STEP)
enterorenal
enterorrhagia
enterorrhaphy
enteroscopy
    double-balloon e.
    intraoperative e.
    push e.
    push-type e.
    Roux-en-Y limb e.
    transgastrostomic e.
    (TGE)
    video small-bowel e.
enterostomal therapy
enterostomy
    double e.
    end-to-end e.
    percutaneous e.
    Stamm e.
    Witzel e.
enterotomy
    antimesenteric e.
    inadvertent e.
    longitudinal e.
    occult e.
enterourethral fistula
enterourethrostomy
enterovaginal fistula
enterovesical fistula
enteroviral infection
enthesis
enthesitis
enthesopathy
entity
    pathologic e.
entocranial
entocranium
entomion
entoptoscopy

entrainment
    air e.
entrapment
    catheter knotting and e.
    lateral canal e.
    leaflet e.
    peroneal nerve e.
    popliteal artery e.
    e. sack
    scapula e.
    e. syndrome
entrapped
    e. gland
    e. nerve
entropion, entropium
    cicatricial e.
entropionize
entropium (*var. of* entropion)
entropy
    approximate e.
    e. monitor
    response e.
    spectral e.
    state e.
entry
    air e.
    implant e.
    e. phenomenon
    e. point
    e. site
    e. zone
    e. zone lesion
enucleate
enucleation
    eye e.
    Foix e.
    leiomyoma e.
    e. method
    e. procedure
    Suarez-Villafranca e.
    surgical e.
    e. technique
enuresis
    diurnal e.
    nocturnal e.
envelope
    axillary e.
    breast skin e.
    e. flap
    peritoneal e.
    soft-tissue e.
enveloping scar tissue
environment
    e. modification
    moist wound e.
environmental mycobacterial infection
enzymatic, enzymic
    e. débridement
    e. zonulolysis

enzyme
    e. induction
    pancreatic e.
enzymic (*var. of* enzymatic)
EOA
    esophageal obturator airway
EOM
    extraocular movement
    extraocular muscle
EOP
    endogenous opioid peptide
EORTC
    European Organization for Research
    and Treatment of Cancer
eosin
eosinophilic
    e. chemotactic factor of anaphylaxis
    (ECF-A)
    e. endomyocardial disease
    e. fibrohistiocytic lesion
EP
    electrophysiologic
    electrophysiology
epactal bone
epaulet flap
epauxesiectomy
epaxial
EPB
    extensor pollicis brevis
EPEM
    Emory Pain Estimate Model
ependymal cell
ependymoastrocytoma
ependymoblastoma
ependymoma
    anaplastic e.
EPH
    episodic paroxysmal hemicrania
ephaptic sprouting
ephippii
    dorsum e.
epiaortic imaging technique
epicanthal
    e. correction
    e. fold
epicardial
    e. echocardiography
    e. fat pad
    e. monitoring
epicondylalgia
epicondylar avulsion fracture
epicondyle
epicondylectomy
epicondylian
epicondylic
epicondylitis
    lateral e.
epicondylus
epicoracoid

E

epicranial
- e. aponeurosis
- e. muscle

epicranium

epicranius muscle

epicritic pain

epicystotomy

epidemiologic study

epidermal, epidermatic, epidermic
- e. flap
- e. graft
- e. growth factor (EGF)
- e. inclusion cyst
- e. necrolysis
- e. ridge

epidermalization, epidermization

epidermatic (*var. of* epidermal)

epidermatoplasty

epidermic (*var. of* epidermal)

epidermidis
- *Staphylococcus e.*

epidermization

epidermoid
- e. carcinoma
- e. cyst
- e. resection

epidermoidoma
- black e.
- incisural e.
- intradural e.
- prepontine white e.
- white e.

epidermolysis

epididymal
- e. sperm
- e. sperm aspiration (ESA)

epididymectomy

epididymidectomy

epididymides (*pl. of* epididymis)

epididymis, *pl.* **epididymides**
- cauda e.
- corpus e.
- e. lesion
- lobule of e.

epididymisoplasty

epididymitis

epididymoorchitis

epididymoplasty

epididymotomy

epididymovasectomy

epididymovasostomy

epidural
- e. abscess
- e. abscess evacuation
- e. administration
- e. analgesia
- e. anesthesia (EA)
- e. anesthetic
- e. block
- e. blood patch (EBP)
- e. blood patch anesthetic technique
- e. catheter
- e. catheter placement
- e. cavity
- continuous lumbar e. (CLE)
- e. delivery
- e. electrode array
- e. extramedullary lesion
- e. fibrosis
- e. hematoma
- e. hemorrhage
- e. neural blockade
- e. neuroplasty
- e. opioid
- e. opioid infusion
- e. pressure waveform (EPWF)
- e. procedure
- e. space
- e. space infection
- e. steroid injection (ESI)
- e. stimulation test
- e. top-up
- e. tumor evacuation
- walking e.

epidurogram

epidurography
- CT e.

epiduroscopy

epifascicular epineurotomy

epifluorescent microscopy

epigastric
- e. angle
- e. artery
- e. fold
- e. fossa
- e. fullness
- e. hernia
- e. incision
- e. pain
- e. region
- e. sinus
- e. vein

epigastrium

epigastrius

epigastrocele

epigastrorrhaphy

epiglottic, epiglottidean
- e. cartilage
- e. reconstruction

epiglottidean (*var. of* epiglottic)

epiglottis

epiglottoplasty

epignathus teratoma

epihyal ligament

epihyoid

epiillumination

epikeratophakic keratoplasty

epikeratoplasty
> tectonic e.

epilation
epilepidoma
epilepsia
epilepsy
> extratemporal e.
> intractable e.
> e. surgery

epilepticus
> status e.

epileptogenic process
epimorphic regeneration
epimysiotomy
epinephrine-anesthetic mixture
epinephros
epineural
> e. repair
> e. suture technique

epineurectomy
> interfascicular e.

epineurial neurorrhaphy
epineurolysis
> volar e.

epineurotomy
> anterior e.
> epifascicular e.
> interfascicular e.
> local e.

epipapillary membrane
epipharynx
epiphenomena of dissection
epiphrenal (*var. of* epiphrenic)
epiphrenic, epiphrenal
epiphyseal (*var. of* epiphysial)
epiphyseolysis (*var. of* epiphysiolysis)
epiphyses (*pl. of* epiphysis)
epiphysial, epiphyseal
> e. bar resection
> e. closure
> e. growth plate fracture
> e. line
> e. plate injury
> e. ring
> e. slip fracture
> e. tibial fracture

epiphysial-metaphysial osteotomy
epiphysiodesis
> open bone graft e.
> screw e.

epiphysiolysis, epiphyseolysis
> femoral e.
> proximal femoral e.

epiphysis, *pl.* **epiphyses**
> atavistic e.
> ball-and-socket e.
> balloon e.
> capital femoral e.
> capitular e.

> clavicular e.
> congenital stippled e.
> distal humeral e.
> femoral e.
> humeral e.
> iliac e.
> ossifying e.
> pressure e.
> ring e.
> slipped capital femoral e.
> stippled e.
> tibial e.
> traction e.

epiphyte
epiplocele
epiploectomy
epiploic
> e. appendage
> e. appendicitis
> e. appendix
> e. branch
> e. foramen of Winslow

epiploica
epiplomerocele
epiplomphalocele
epiplopexy
epiplosarcomphalocele
epiploscheocele
epipteric bone
epiretinal membrane
episcleral
> e. circulation
> e. explant
> e. ganglion
> e. space
> e. tissue
> e. vascular dilation

episioperineoplasty
episioperineorrhaphy
episioplasty
episiorrhaphy
episiotomy
> median e.
> mediolateral e.
> e. repair
> ruptured e.
> e. scar

episode
> bleeding e.
> thrombotic e.

episodic
> e. colic
> e. hypoxemia
> e. pain
> e. paroxysmal hemicrania
> (EPH)

epispadias-exstrophy complex
epispadias repair
epispinal

E

epistasis
epistaxis (EPIS)
episternal bone
episternum
epistropheus
epitarsus
epithelia (*pl. of* epithelium)
epithelial
    e. barrier
    e. basement membrane
    e. breakdown
    e. cell
    e. cyst
    e. hemangioendothelioma
    e. inlay
    e. invagination
    e. migration
epithelialization technique
epithelioserosa
epithelium, *pl.* **epithelia**
    Barrett e.
    bile duct e.
    biliary e.
    colic e.
    colon e.
    columnar e.
    corneal e.
    crypt e.
    dysplastic e.
    endometric e.
    esophageal e.
    external dental e.
    external enamel e.
    follicular e.
    gastric e.
    germinal e.
    glandular e.
    gut e.
    junctional e.
    metaplastic e.
    pseudostratified e.
    pseudostratified ciliated e.
    pyramidal e.
    regenerated esophageal e.
    salivary e.
    salmon-pink e.
    squamous e.
    stratified e.
    surface e.
    transitional e.
    villous e.
epithelization
epithesis
epitrochlea
epitrochlear
epituberculous infiltration
epitympanic
    e. cell
    e. recess

EPL
    extensor pollicis longus
Epley benign positional vertigo
  maneuver
épluchage
ePMP
    electronic prescription-monitoring
     program
epoophorectomy
epoophoron
Eppright dial osteotomy
Epstein-Barr
    E.-B. virus (EBV)
    E.-B. virus infection
Epstein hip dislocation
  classification
Epstein-Thomas classification
eptifibatide
epulofibroma
EPWF
    epidural pressure waveform
equal sagittal flap
equation
    alveolar gas e.
    Bohr e.
    Harris-Benedict basal energy
     expenditure e.
    Henderson-Hasselbalch e.
equator
    anatomic e.
    crystalline lens e.
    eyeball e.
    geometric e.
    lens e.
equatorial plane
equilibrating operation
equilibration
    mandibular e.
    occlusal e.
equilibrium
    acid-base e.
    sedimentation e.
equinovalgus deformity
equinovarus
    talipes e.
equinus
    e. deformity
    e. position
equipotent
equivalence, equivalency
    e. point
    e. relation
equivalency (*var. of*
  equivalence)
equivalent
    cultured human skin e.
    human skin e. (HSE)
    e. refracting plane
    ventilation e.

equivocal
    e. finding
    e. pancreatic cytology
ER
    emergency room
    extended release
      Opana ER
      ER thoracotomy
eradication
    e. therapy
    variceal e.
Erb point
ERCP
    endoscopic retrograde
      cholangiopancreatography
      ERCP cannulation
      postoperative ERCP
      preoperative ERCP
ERCP-guided biopsy
ERCP-induced splenic rupture
Erdheim cystic medial necrosis
erectile dysfunction
erect illumination
erection
    intraoperative penile e.
    penile e.
    pharmacologically induced e.
    reflex e.
    reflexogenic e.
erector
    e. spinae muscles
    e. spinae tendon
erector-spinal reflex
ergonovine provocation test
Erickson-Leider-Brown 2-level spinal
  burst fracture repair technique
erigentes
    nervi e.
Eriksson
    E. brachial block technique
    E. ligament technique
Eriksson-Drez intraarticular ACL repair
Erlangen pull-type sphincterotomy
Erlenmeyer flask deformity
erosion
    band e.
    corneal e.
    implant e.
    infraspinatus insertion e.
    limiting plate e.
    recurrent corneal e.
    skin e.
    tumor e.
    wedge-shaped e.
erosive inflammation
erroneous projection
eruption
    ectopic e.
    eczematous polymorphous light e.

erythema nodosum-like e.
    surgical e.
erysipelas
    surgical e.
erysipelas-like skin lesion
erysipeloid
erysiphake technique
erythema
    cold e.
    necrolytic migratory e.
    e. nodosum-like eruption
    periwound e.
erythroblastoma
erythrocyte
    e. mass
    e. membrane
erythrocytolysis
erythrodermatous lesion
erythrolysis
erythromelalgia
erythromycin-induced cholecystitis
erythropoietin therapy
ESA
    end-systolic area
    end-to-side anastomosis
    epididymal sperm aspiration
escalation
    dose e.
    opioid e.
Escapini cataract operation
escharectomy
eschar excision
escharotomy
ESD
    endoscopic submucosal dissection
    end-systolic diameter
ESI
    epidural steroid injection
Esmarch bandage
Esmarch-Rizzoli ankylosed
  temporomaxillary articulation operation
esmolol hydrochloride
esodic nerve
esophageal
    e. A, B ring
    e. achalasia
    e. adenocarcinoma
    e. artery
    e. atresia
    e. banding technique
    e. band ligation
    e. biopsy
    e. body motor dysfunction
    e. branch
    e. cancer
    e. carcinoma
    e. colic
    e. compression
    e. constriction

E

esophageal (*continued*)
  e. contractile ring
  e. contraction ring
  e. dilation
  e. dilation treatment
  e. disorder
  e. dissection
  e. diverticulectomy
  e. diverticulum
  e. duplication
  e. dysmotility
  e. ectopic sebaceous gland
  e. effect
  e. epithelium
  e. fistula
  e. foreign body
  e. fungal infection
  e. gap
  e. hernia
  e. heterotopic pancreas
  e. hiatus
  e. impression
  e. inflammation
  e. injury
  e. instrumentation
  e. intubation
  e. leak
  e. lengthening
  e. Lewy body
  e. manometry
  e. mass
  e. measurement
  e. mobilization
  e. mucosal ring
  e. mucosa metaplasia
  e. muscular ring
  e. myotomy
  e. obstruction
  e. obturator airway (EOA)
  e. perforation
  e. peristaltic pressure
  e. pH
  e. pH monitoring
  e. photodynamic therapy
  e. plexus
  e. pressure
  e. remnant
  e. resection
  e. rupture
  e. shortening
  e. sling procedure
  e. spasm
  e. sphincter
  e. sphincter pressure
  e. sphincter relaxation
  e. stenosis
  e. stent
  e. stricture
  e. suture line

  e. tear
  e. transection
  e. tumor
  e. ulceration
  e. variceal bleeding
  e. variceal sclerotherapy (EVS)
  e. varix
  e. vein
  e. web
esophageal-jejunal anastomosis
esophagectasia (*var. of* esophagectasis)
esophagectasis, esophagectasia
esophagectomy
  distal e.
  endoscopic e.
  3-incision e.
  Ivor Lewis e.
  Ivor Lewis 2-stage subtotal e.
  laparoscopic e.
  laparoscopic-assisted e.
  laparoscopic transhiatal e.
  Lewis-Tanner e.
  mediastinoscopy-assisted
    transhiatal e.
  minimally invasive e.
  near-total e.
  open e.
  split-sternum e.
  subtotal e.
  thoracoabdominal e.
  thoracoscopic-assisted e.
  total endoscopic e.
  total laparoscopic e.
  total thoracic e.
  transhiatal e.
  transhiatal blunt e.
  transthoracic e.
  video-assisted transsternal
    radical e.
  e. with thoracotomy
esophageus
  hiatus e.
esophagi (*pl. of* esophagus)
esophagitis
  pill-induced e.
  reflux e.
esophagobronchial fistula
esophagocardiomyotomy
  Heller e.
esophagocardioplasty
esophagocolic anastomosis
esophagocutaneous fistula
esophagodiverticulostomy
esophagoduodenostomy
esophagoenterostomy
esophagogastrectomy
  Ivor Lewis e.
  McKeown e.
  thoracoabdominal e.

esophagogastric
  e. anastomosis
  e. cancer
  e. fat pad
  e. fundoplasty
  e. intubation
  e. junction
  e. orifice
  e. resection
  e. variceal bleeding
  e. vestibule
esophagogastroanastomosis
esophagogastroduodenoscopy (EGD)
  pediatric e.
esophagogastromyotomy
esophagogastropexy
esophagogastroplasty
  Grondahl-Finney e.
esophagogastroscopy
  Abbott e.
  intrathoracic e.
  Johnson e.
  Thal e.
  Woodward e.
esophagogastrostomy
  Abbott e.
  cervical e.
  Clagett-Barrett e.
  end-to-end e.
  end-to-side e.
  intrathoracic e.
  Johnson e.
  Thal e.
  thoracic e.
  Woodward e.
esophagogram (*var. of* esophagram)
esophagojejunostomy
  end-to-end e.
  end-to-side e.
  loop e.
  mechanical e.
  mediastinal e.
  Roux-en-Y e.
  Schlatter total gastrectomy with
    side-to-side e.
  stapled e.
  transhiatal e.
esophagomediastinal fistula
esophagomyotomy
  circumferential e.
  Heller e.
  Heller-Nissen thorascopic e.
  laparoscopic e.
  modified Heller e.
  open e.
  thoracic short e.
  thoracoscopic e.
esophagoplasty
  balloon e.

behind-sternum column e.
Belsey e.
cervical e.
colic patch e.
colonic e.
gastric patch e.
gastric tube e.
Grondahl e.
Grondahl-Finney e.
intrathoracic e.
laparoscopic e.
patch e.
pectoralis myocutaneous e.
pediatric e.
posterior mediastinal e.
reverse gastric tube e.
single-step e.
subtotal e.
esophagopleural fistula
esophagoplication
esophagoproximal gastrectomy
esophagopulmonary fistula
esophagorespiratory fistula
esophagoscopy
  fiberoptic e.
esophagostomy
  cervical e.
  palliative e.
esophagotomy
  cervical e.
esophagotracheal
  e. airway
  e. fistula
esophagram, esophagogram
  barium e.
  water-soluble contrast e.
esophagus, *pl.* **esophagi**
  anterior e.
  Barrett e.
  cervical e.
  columnar-lined e.
  elevator e.
  native e.
  nutcracker e.
  proximal e.
  supradiaphragmatic pouch of e.
  e. temperature
  thoracic e.
esotropia (ESO, ET, ST)
  congenital e.
ESPLR
  end-systolic pressure-length
  relationship
Espocan epidural needle
ESRD
  endstage renal disease
ESS
  endoscopic sinus surgery
Essed-Schroeder corporoplasty

E

essential
  e. brown induration
  e. brown induration of lung
  e. hypertension
  e. tremor
Esser
  E. inlay skin graft
  E. inlay skin graft operation
Essex-Lopresti
  E.-L. axial fixation technique
  E.-L. calcaneal fracture
    classification
  E.-L. calcaneal fracture technique
  E.-L. joint depression fracture
  E.-L. open reduction
esterase-metabolized opioid
ester local anesthetic
Estersohn osteotomy
Estes
  E. ovarian transfer procedure
  E. ovary implantation
esthetic, aesthetic
  e. procedure
  e. restoration
  e. rhinoplasty
  e. septorhinoplasty
esthetics, aesthetics
  gingival tissue e.
estimated
  e. blood volume
  e. Fick method
  e. time of ovulation
Estlander
  E. lip reconstruction flap
  E. operation
Estlander-Abbe lip reconstruction
  flap
estrogen-assisted colposcopy
estrogen receptor localization
ESU
  electrosurgery unit
ESWL
  extracorporeal shock wave lithotripsy
ESWT
  end-systolic wall thickness
  extracorporeal shock wave treatment
ETCO$_2$
  end-tidal carbon dioxide
ethanol (EtOH)
  e. ablation
  e. injection
  e. injection therapy
  e. sclerotherapy
ethanol-induced tumor necrosis
ether
  e. convulsion
  cyclic e.
  diethyl e.
  methyl-*tert*-butyl e. (MTBE)

ether-a-go-go gene
etherization
Ethibond
  E. polybutilate-coated polyester
    suture
  E. suture
Ethicon
  E. micropoint suture
  E. Sabreloc suture
  E. silk suture
Ethiflex retention suture
Ethilon nylon suture
ethmocranial
ethmofrontal
ethmoid
  e. bone
  e. bulla
  e. canal
  e. cell
  e. exenteration
  e. fistula
  e. registration point
  e. sinus carcinoma
ethmoidal
  e. approach
  e. artery
  e. crest
  e. foramen
  e. groove
  e. infundibulum
  e. labyrinth
  e. lacrimal fistula
  e. nerve
  e. notch
  e. osteotomy
  e. plate
  e. vein
ethmoidectomy
  anterior e.
  endoscopic e.
  external e.
  internal e.
  intranasal e.
  partial e.
  total e.
  transantral e.
ethmoidolacrimal suture
ethmoidomaxillary suture
ethmolacrimal
ethmomaxillary
ethmonasal
ethmopalatal
ethmosphenoid
ethmoturbinal
ethmovomerine
ethylene
  e. oxide (ETO)
  e. oxide sterilization
etiologic factors

etiology
    infectious e.
    malignant e.
etiopathology
ETO
    ethylene oxide
    ETO sterilization
EtOH
    ethanol
etoricoxib
Eu
    euryon
EUA
    examination under anesthesia
eucupine
eugnathic anomaly
EUPF
    extended uvulopalatal flap
euplastic
eupnea
European
    E. Carotid Surgery Trial (ECST)
    E. Organization for Research and
      Treatment of Cancer (EORTC)
    E. System for Cardiac Operative
      Risk Evaluation (euroSCORE)
euroSCORE
    European System for Cardiac
    Operative Risk Evaluation
euryon (Eu)
EUS
    endoscopic esophageal ultrasound
    endoscopic ultrasonography
    endoscopic ultrasound
EUS-guided
    E.-g. cytology
    E.-g. fine-needle aspiration
eustachian
    e. tube
    e. tube orifice
**eutectic mixture of local anesthetics
(EMLA)**
euthyroid sick syndrome
euthyscopy
euvolemia
euvolemic
evacuating clot
evacuation
    CT-guided stereotactic e.
    digital rectal e.
    dilatation and e. (D&E)
    dilation and e. (D&E)
    e. disorder
    epidural abscess e.
    epidural tumor e.
    fimbrial e.
    fluid e.
    hematobilia e.
    hematoma e.

    pericardial cavity e.
    e. procedure
    rectal e.
    e. score
    stool e.
    transsphenoidal e.
evagination
    optic e.
evaluation
    angiographic e.
    anthropometric e.
    baseline capacity e.
    Cardiac Anesthesia Risk E.
      (CARE)
    clinical e.
    cosmetic e.
    cytologic e.
    diagnostic imaging e.
    Doppler pulse e.
    Dubowitz e.
    endoscopic ultrasound e.
    European System for Cardiac
      Operative Risk E. (euroSCORE)
    followup e.
    functional capacity e. (FCE)
    genitourinary e.
    Gibson Approach to Functional
      Capacity E. (GAPP FCE)
    hearing aid e. (HAE)
    hormonal e.
    infertility e.
    job capacity e. (JCE)
    laparoscopic e.
    mammographic e.
    manometric e.
    medical care e.
    mental status e.
    metabolic e.
    neurodiagnostic e.
    neurological e.
    neuroradiologic e.
    noninvasive e.
    pedicle e.
    physical capacity e.
    postoperative followup e.
    preoperative staging e.
    presurgical medical e.
    pretransplant e.
    pretreatment e.
    e. protocol
    quantitative e.
    radiographic e.
    radiologic e.
    roentgenographic e.
    serial radiographic e.
    sexual e.
    Smith physical capacity e.
    staging e.
    static e.

E

evaluation (*continued*)
    status e.
    stent e.
    stroboscopic e.
    sudomotor e.
    urologic e.
    uterine e.
    videoscopic e.
    videourodynamic e.
    visual function e.
    wake-up e.
Evans
    E. ankle instability procedure
    E. ankle reconstruction technique
    E. ankle tenodesis reconstruction
    E. anterior calcaneal osteotomy
    E. intertrochanteric fracture
      classification
even-echo rephasing
event
    acute cardiac e.
    adverse e.
    anatomic e.
    cardiac e.
    catastrophic e.
    cerebral e.
    cerebrovascular e.
    fatal cardiac e.
    neuroelectric e.
    noxious e.
    precipitating noxious e.
    sentinel e.
    serious adverse e.
      (SAE)
    soft e.
    subdiaphragmatic e.
    thromboembolic e.
    thrombotic e.
eventration
    acquired e.
    congenital e.
    diaphragm e.
    diaphragmatic e.
    e. disease
    pericardial e.
Everard Williams retropubic
  cystourethropexy suspension procedure
everolimus
Eversbusch eyelid ptosis operation
eversion
    e. carotid endarterectomy
    e. operation
    e. orchiopexy
    e. osteotomy
    e. technique
eversion-external
    e.-e. rotation
    e.-e. rotation deformity
evert

everting
    e. interrupted suture technique
    e. mattress suture
evidement
evidence
    biochemical e.
    clinical e.
    macroscopic e.
    radiologic e.
    sonographic e.
evidence-based
    e.-b. medicine
    e.-b. surgery
eviration
evisceration
    abdominal e.
    Burch eye e.
    drain site e.
    e. operation
    small-bowel e.
    total abdominal e. (TAE)
    upper abdominal e.
evisceroneurotomy
evoked
    e. external urethral sphincter
      potential monitoring
    e. potential technique
    e. twitch
evolution
    lesion e.
    e. time
evolving myocardial infarction
EVS
    endoscopic variceal sclerotherapy
    esophageal variceal sclerotherapy
evulsion
Ewald
    E. capitellocondylar total elbow
      arthroplasty
    E. tube
Ewald-Walker kinematic knee
  arthroplasty
Ewing sarcoma operation
ex
    e. situ
    e. situ bench surgery
    e. situ hepatectomy
    e. situ-in situ hepatectomy
    e. situ-in situ liver resection
    e. situ-in situ technique
    e. situ-in vivo procedure
    e. utero intrapartum treatment
      (EXIT)
    e. utero intrapartum treatment
      procedure
    e. vacuo dilation
    e. vivo
    e. vivo cannulation
    e. vivo count

e. vivo fertilization
e. vivo gene therapy
e. vivo marrow treatment
e. vivo perfusion
e. vivo resection
e. vivo technique
exacerbated
exacerbation of pain
exaggerated sniffing position
exam (*var. of* examination)
examination, exam
abdominal e.
arthroscopic e.
Ballard e.
barium enema e.
bench e.
bile fluid e.
bimanual pelvic e.
bone marrow e.
cardiac e.
chest e.
clinical e.
colonoscopic e.
comparative radiographic e.
cutaneous e.
cytologic e.
cytology e.
dark-field e.
digital rectal e.
Doppler flow probe e.
double-contrast barium enema e.
Dubowitz e.
duodenal content e.
endoscopic e.
eye e.
fiberoptic e.
flashlight e.
followup e.
full-body cutaneous e.
full-spine radiographic e.
funduscopic e.
gastric residue e.
gray-scale e.
hand-held Doppler flow
  probe e.
histologic e.
histopathologic e.
history and physical e.
immunofluorescent e.
laparoscopic e.
laparoscopic ultrasound e.
limited e.
LUS e.
mediastinoscopic e.
mental status e.
motor e.
needle electrode e.
neonate e.
nerve conduction velocity e.

neurologic e.
neuroophthalmologic e.
neurophysiologic e.
neurotologic e.
newborn e.
ophthalmic e.
oral peripheral e.
palpatory e.
parasternal e.
pathologic e.
pathology e.
pelvic e.
pericardial fluid e.
peripheral e.
peritoneal fluid e.
physical e.
pleural fluid e.
postmortem e.
proctoscopic e.
radiographic e.
radiologic e.
rectal e.
rectovaginal e.
reflex e.
retinal e.
self-breast e.
sensory e.
serologic e.
soft x-ray e.
speculum e.
sterile vaginal e.
suboptimal e.
supraclavicular e.
suprasternal e.
synovial fluid e.
systemic e.
tangent screen e.
tender point e.
thermographic e.
transvaginal ultrasonographic e.
ultrasonographic e.
ultrasound e.
e. under anesthesia (EUA)
vaginal e.
Wood light e.
exanthem (*var. of* exanthema)
exanthema, exanthem
exanthematous
e. disease
e. fever
e. inflammation
exanthesis arthrosia
excavated
e. gastric carcinoma
e. lesion
excavatio disci
excavation
atrophic e.
glaucomatous e.

E

251

excavation (*continued*)
    physiologic e.
    retinal e.
excavatum
    pectus e.
excementosis
    extension e.
    intraepithelial e.
    pronglike e.
    ultraterminal e.
excess
    e. androgen
    mandibular e.
    marginal e.
    maxillary e.
    morbidity e.
    e. mucus
    vertical maxillary e.
excessive
    e. bleeding
    e. blood loss
    e. callus formation
    e. fatigue
    e. heat production
    e. lacrimation
    e. lip support
    e. spacing
    e. straining
    e. tearing
    e. weight loss
exchange
    air e.
    air-fluid e.
    blood gas e.
    catheter e.
    cation e.
    chemical e.
    e. diffusion
    endoscopic stent e.
    fetal-maternal e.
    fiberoptic-assisted coaxial
      endotracheal tube e.
    fluid-gas e.
    gas e.
    gas-fluid e.
    inadequate gas e.
    lens e.
    multiple inert gas e.
    plasma e.
    pulmonary gas e.
    respiratory e.
    e. technique
    e. transfusion
    wire-guided balloon-assisted
      endoscopic biliary stent e.
exchanger
    countercurrent heat e.
excimer
    e. laser ablation

    e. laser coronary angioplasty
      (ELCA)
    e. laser photorefractive keratectomy
    e. vascular recanalization
excipient
excised specimen
excision
    abdominoperineal e.
    alar wedge e.
    Arlt-Jaesche e.
    e. arthroplasty
    Bartlett nail fold e.
    e. biopsy
    bone cyst e.
    Bose nail fold e.
    Bowman pupil e.
    cervical disc e.
    circumferential mesorectal e.
    clavicle e.
    cold snare e.
    complete circumferential
      mesorectal e.
    complete mesh e.
    conjunctiva-Müller muscle e.
    Curtin plantar fibromatosis e.
    Das Gupta scapular e.
    disc e.
    distal clavicular e.
    dorsal e.
    en bloc e.
    endoluminal e.
    eschar e.
    extended mesorectal e.
    extratemporal e.
    Ferciot e.
    Ferciot-Thomson e.
    Flatt e.
    funicular e.
    fusiform e.
    goiter e.
    Heisrath tarsus and conjunctiva e.
    hemivertebral e.
    hemorrhoid e.
    Hochenegg rectal e.
    incomplete e.
    interdental e.
    intralesional e.
    laser hemorrhoid e.
    local e.
    marginal e.
    mass e.
    McKeever-Buck fragment e.
    meniscal e.
    mesorectal e.
    microlumbar disc e.
    operative e.
    partial mesh e.
    pentagonal block e.
    radical compartmental e.

rectal e.
retropulsed bone e.
ruptured disc e.
sentinel node e.
sheet mesh e.
Stewart distal clavicular e.
subperichondrial e.
superficial e.
surgical e. (SE)
tangential e.
Thompson e.
thymus gland e.
total mesenteric e. (TME)
total mesorectal e. (TME)
transanal e.
transoral odontoid e.
ulnar head e.
wedge e.
wide local e. (WLE)
Williams microlumbar
  disc e.

excisional
e. arthrodesis
e. atherectomy
e. biopsy
e. biopsy method
e. biopsy procedure
e. biopsy site
e. biopsy technique
e. cardiac surgery
e. removal
excision-curettage technique
excitability
neuronal e.
e. test
excitation
nicotinic e.
excitatory
e. junction potential
e. neuromediator
e. postsynaptic potential
e. synapse
e. synaptic signaling
e. synaptic transmission
excited skin syndrome
excitement phase
exciting eye
excitoreflex nerve
excitor nerve
exclave
exclusion
antral e.
e. bypass
Devine antral e.
hepatic vascular e.
intermittent vascular e.
partial hepatic vascular e.
subtotal gastric e.
total hepatic venous e.

total vascular e.
vascular e.
excoriate
excoriation
neurotic e.
excrement
excrementitious
excrescence
bony e.
enamel e.
Lambl e.
wartlike e.
excrete
excretion
urinary calcium e.
excretory
e. duct
e. urogram
excursion
dome e.
insertional e.
lateral e.
protrusive e.
range of e.
respiratory e.
retrusive e.
tendon e.
excystation
execution time
exemia
exencephalia (*var. of* exencephaly)
exencephalic, exencephalous
exencephalocele
exencephalous (*var. of* exencephalic)
exencephaly, exencephalia
exenteration
anterior pelvic e.
ethmoid e.
Iliff e.
orbital e.
pelvic e.
petrous pyramid e.
posterior pelvic e.
supralevator pelvic e.
total pelvic e. (TPE)
exercise
aerobic e.
e. capacity
concentric e.
deep-breathing e.
eccentric e.
endurance e.
e. hyperemia blood flow
e. imaging
e. index
e. intolerance
e. ischemia
neuromuscular proprioception e.
e. oximetry

E

exercise (*continued*)
    e. physiology
    plyometric e.
    specific adjuvant e.
    strengthening e.
    stretching e.
    e. study
    e. therapy
    treadmill e.
exercise-associated acute renal failure
exercise-based rehabilitation
exercise-induced
    e.-i. arrhythmia
    e.-i. asthma (EIA)
    e.-i. bronchospasm (EIB)
    e.-i. incontinence
    e.-i. silent myocardial ischemia
    e.-i. ventricular tachycardia
exeresis
    palliative e.
exergonic reaction
exertion
    dyspnea on e. (DOE)
    perceived e.
    rated perceived e.
    rating of perceived e.
exertional
    e. amblyopia
    e. anterior compartment syndrome
    e. deep posterior compartment syndrome
    e. dyspnea
    e. rhabdomyolysis
exfoliant
exfoliate
exfoliation
    lamellar e.
    e. syndrome
    true e.
exfoliative cytology
exhalation
    end e.
exhaled oxygen tension
exhaustion
    e. atrophy
    nervous e.
    neuroendocrine e.
    ovarian follicle e.
    postactivation e.
    e. state
exhilarant
exit
    e. access
    e. block
    e. block murmur
    e. point
    e. pupil
    e. site

    e. site infection
    e. wound
EXIT
    ex utero intrapartum treatment
    EXIT procedure
Exner plexus
exocardia
exocardial murmur
exoccipital bone
exocelomic
    e. cavity
    e. membrane
exocentric construction
exocervix
exocranial orifice
exocrine
    e. pancreas
    e. pancreatic insufficiency
exocrinopathic process
exocytosis
exodic nerve
exodontia
exodontics
exodontist
exodontology
exogamy
exogenous
    e. aneurysm
    e. anticoagulant coagulation
    e. disease
    e. fiber
    e. fibrin clot
    e. flora
    e. hormone
    e. infection
    e. reconstruction
    e. smile
    e. substance
    e. tumor
exognathia
exognathion
exophoria
exophoric
exophthalmic
exophthalmogenic
exophthalmometric
exophthalmometry
exophthalmos, exophthalmus
    recurrent e.
exophthalmos-producing substance
exophthalmus (*var. of* exophthalmos)
exophytic
    e. carcinoma
    e. growth
    e. gut mass
    e. joint disease
exoplant
    scleral e.
exopneumopexy

exoserosis
exoskeletal
exoskeleton
    Dacron e.
exosmosis
exostectomy, exostosectomy
    calcaneal e.
exostosectomy (*var. of* exostectomy)
exostosis
    external auditory e. (EAE)
    hereditary multiple exostoses
    multiple exostoses
exothermic
exotropia
    X-pattern e.
exotropic
expandable
expanded plasma
expander
    tissue e.
expanding retroperitoneal hematoma
expansible
expansile
    e. abdominal mass
    e. unilocular well-demarcated bone
      lesion
expansion
    e. and activator therapy
    clonal e.
    controlled e.
    delayed e.
    dental arch e.
    dorsal e.
    effective setting e.
    external tissue e.
    field e.
    hygroscopic e.
    infarct e.
    intravascular volume e.
    investment e.
    lateral extensor e.
    linear thermal e.
    lung e.
    maxillary e.
    membrane e.
    mesangial matrix e.
    monoclonal e.
    e. of the arch
    palatal e.
    perceptual e.
    plasma volume e.
    rapid maxillary e.
    repeated tissue e.
    secondary e.
    setting e.
    slow maxillary e.
    stent e.
    thermal coefficient e.
    tissue e.

    volume e.
    wax e.
expansive laminoplasty
expectancy
    life e.
expectant management
expectorate
expectoration
    prune-juice e.
expenditure
    caloric e.
    energy e.
    resting energy e.
experimental
    e. allergic encephalomyelitis
    e. disorder
    e. method
    e. neurasthenia
    e. pain
    e. pathology
    e. threshold
expiration
    assisted e.
    end e.
expiratory
    e. computed tomography
    e. dyspnea
    end e.
    e. flow rate
    e. grunt
    e. murmur
    e. nitrogen
    e. positive airway pressure
    e. prolongation
    e. reserve volume
    e. residual volume
    e. retard
    e. rhonchi
    e. valve
    e. wheezing
expired
    e. air
    e. air collection
explant
    encircling e.
    episcleral e.
    Molteno episcleral e.
    posterior e.
    segmental e.
    sponge e.
explantation
explanted heart
explicit memory
exploding head syndrome
exploration
    abdominal e.
    e. and débridement
    bilateral neck e.
    bile duct e.

E

exploration (*continued*)
    common bile duct e.
    complete surgical e.
    contralateral groin e.
    formal surgical e.
    groin e.
    laparoscopically guided transcystic e.
    laparoscopic common bile duct e.
    laparoscopic transcystic common bile
      duct e. (LTCBDE)
    laparoscopic transcystic duct e.
    macroscopic e.
    neck e.
    open common bile duct e.
    petrous pyramid air cell e.
    remedial inguinal e.
    routine bilateral neck e.
    routine unilateral e.
    sclerotomy with e.
    standard neck e.
    unilateral neck e.

exploratory
    e. celiotomy
    e. drive
    e. laparotomy (ex lap)
    e. operation
    e. puncture
    e. stroke
    e. surgery

explosion
    colonic e.
    e. fracture
    e. injury

explosive doubling time
exponential phase
exposed pulp
exposure
    Abbott-Gill epiphysial plate e.
    accidental pulp e.
    aerosolized pollutant e.
    allergen e.
    anesthetic gas e.
    anterior surgical e.
    bone e.
    bony e.
    carious pulp e.
    chemical e.
    cold e.
    double e.
    electromagnetic radiation e.
    endotoxic e.
    extradural e.
    extrapharyngeal e.
    graded e.
    heat e.
    Henry posterior interosseous
      nerve e.
    imaginal e.
    incident e.

    industrial e.
    in utero e.
    e. keratopathy
    Kocher-Langenbeck e.
    light e.
    mechanical pulp e.
    methamphetamine e.
    midline e.
    noise e.
    occupational toxin e.
    operative e.
    operator e.
    prenatal diethylstilbestrol e.
    prior drug e.
    radiation e.
    repeated e.
    subclavian vessel e.
    subperiosteal e.
    sun e.
    surgical pulp e.
    thoracolumbar junction surgical e.
    thoracolumbar spine anterior e.
    toxin e.
    transpalatal e.
    transperitoneal e.
    upper cervical spine anterior e.
    vertebral e.
    vessel e.

expressed skull fracture
expression
    facial e.
    intragraft e.
    pain e.

expressive dysphasia
expressivity
expressor loop
expulsion
    graft e.

expulsive
    e. coughing
    e. hemorrhage
    e. pain

exquisitely tender abdomen
exquisite pain
exsanguinate
exsanguinating hemorrhage
exsanguination
    fetal e.
    e. protocol
    e. tourniquet control
    e. transfusion

exsanguine
exsanguinotransfusion
exsect
exsection
exsiccant
exsiccate
exsiccation fever
exstrophy closure

exstrophy-epispadias complex
extended
- e. criteria donor (ECD)
- e. end-to-end anastomosis
- e. gastric cancer lymph node dissection (D2)
- e. iliofemoral approach
- e. jargon paraphasia
- e. left hepatectomy
- e. left subcostal incision
- e. mandatory minute ventilation (EMMV)
- e. maxillotomy
- e. mesorectal excision
- e. myotomy
- e. pancreatoduodenectomy
- e. pelvic lymphadenectomy
- e. pyelotomy
- e. radical mastectomy
- e. release (ER, XR)
- e. resection
- e. right hemicolectomy
- e. right hepatectomy
- e. Ross procedure
- e. shoulder flap
- e. subfrontal approach
- e. uvulopalatal flap (EUPF)

extensibility
- penile e.

extensible
extension
- atlantooccipital e.
- attached gingiva e.
- e. base
- e. block splinting method
- e. bridge
- Callahan e.
- calyceal e.
- clot e.
- compression e.
- cranial e.
- e. deformity
- distractive e.
- e. excementosis
- extranodal tumor e.
- extrapancreatic e.
- extrascleral e.
- femoral-trunk e.
- e. fiber
- fingerlike e.
- flexion, abduction, external rotation, e. (fabere)
- flexion, adduction, internal rotation, e. (FADIR, fadire)
- flexion and e.
- e. form
- e. for prevention
- full e.
- groove e.

- hip e.
- infarct e.
- e. injury
- e. injury posterior atlantoaxial arthrodesis
- e. instability
- internal rotation in e.
- intrasellar e.
- knee e.
- local tumor e.
- lumbar e.
- e. malposition
- orbital e.
- e. osteotomy
- paraplegia in e.
- radiolucent operating room table e.
- e. restriction
- ridge e.
- e. stent graft
- subependymal e.
- e. teardrop fracture
- thrombus e.

extension-type cervical spine injury
extensive
- e. approach
- e. bilateral pneumonia
- e. intraductal component
- e. lymph node dissection
- e. posterior approach
- e. posterior decompression

extensive-stage disease
extensor
- e. carpi radialis brevis (ECRB)
- e. carpi radialis brevis muscle
- e. carpi radialis brevis tendon
- e. carpi radialis longus (ECRL)
- e. carpi radialis longus flap
- e. carpi radialis longus muscle
- e. carpi radialis longus tendon
- e. carpi ulnaris (ECU)
- e. carpi ulnaris muscle
- e. carpi ulnaris tendon
- e. digiti minimi muscle
- e. digiti minimi tendon
- e. digitorum brevis (EDB)
- e. digitorum brevis muscle
- e. digitorum brevis tendon
- e. digitorum communis tendon
- e. digitorum longus (EDL)
- e. digitorum longus muscle
- e. digitorum longus tendon
- e. digitorum tendon
- e. hallucis
- e. hallucis brevis muscle
- e. hallucis longus (EHL)
- e. hallucis longus muscle
- e. hallucis longus strength
- e. hallucis longus tendon
- e. hood mechanism

E

extensor (*continued*)
   e. indicis muscle
   e. indicis proprius tendon
   knee e.
   e. lengthening
   e. mechanism dysfunction
   e. pollicis brevis (EPB)
   e. pollicis brevis muscle
   e. pollicis brevis tendon
   e. pollicis longus (EPL)
   e. pollicis longus muscle
   e. pollicis longus tendon
   radial wrist e.
   e. retinaculum
   e. surface
   e. tendon injury
   e. tendon repair
   e. tenodesis
   e. tenotomy
   e. tetanus
   e. thrust reflex
   toe e.
   wrist e.
exteriorization colostomy
exteriorize
exteriorized
   e. stuttering
   e. uterine repair
externa
   otitis e.
external
   e. absorption
   e. acoustic foramen
   e. acoustic meatus
    artery
   e. arcuate fiber
   e. auditory canal
   e. auditory exostosis
   e. auditory larynx
   e. auditory meatus
   e. beam irradiation
   e. bevel incision
   e. bile drainage
   e. bile leak
   e. bile tract drainage
   e. biliary drainage
   e. biliary fistula
   e. biliary lavage
   e. bleeding
   e. bracing
   e. branch
   e. branch of superior laryngeal
    nerve
   e. canthotomy
   e. canthus
   e. capsule
   e. cardiac massage
   e. carotid
   e. carotid artery (ECA)

   e. carotid artery-posterior cerebral
    artery (ECA-PCA)
   e. carotid plexus
   e. clot
   e. cooling
   e. cuneate nucleus
   e. dental epithelium
   e. direct pressure
   e. ear
   e. elastic lamina
   e. enamel epithelium
   e. ethmoidectomy
   e. female genital organ
   e. fetal monitoring
   e. geniculate body
   e. genitalia
   e. genitalia, Bartholin, urethral,
    Skene (EG/BUS)
   e. grid
   e. hemipelvectomy
   e. hemorrhage
   e. hemorrhoid
   e. hordeolum
   e. iliac artery (EIA)
   e. iliac plexus
   e. ilium
   e. ilium movement
   e. inguinal ring
   e. ligament
   e. male genital organ
   e. mammary artery
   e. maxillary artery
   e. maxillary plexus
   e. nasal nerve
   e. nose
   e. oblique
   e. oblique aponeurosis
   e. oblique fascia
   e. oblique line
   e. oblique reflex
   e. oblique ridge
   e. occipital crest
   e. orbital fracture
   e. os
   e. pancreatic fistula
   e. pin fixation
   e. pneumatic calf compression
   posteroinferior e.
   e. pudendal artery
   e. rectal sphincter
   e. respiration
   e. rotation
   e. rotation-abduction stress test
   e. rotation-recurvatum test
   e. rotator
   e. route
   e. saphenous nerve
   e. scanning
   e. shock wave lithotripsy

e. spermatic artery
e. spermatic fascia
e. spermatic nerve
e. sphincterotomy
e. spinal fixation
e. stimulus
e. support
e. surface
e. swelling
e. tissue expansion
e. to internal rotation ratio
e. transcutaneous pacing
e. trauma
e. urethral orifice
e. urethral sphincter
e. urethrotomy
e. vacuum therapy
e. ventricular drainage
e. x-ray therapy
external-coil electrical stimulation
external/internal rotation
externalization
externalized catheter system
externally
e. releasable knot
e. rotated
externum
externus
exteroceptive
extinction
e. phenomenon
sensory e.
visual e.
extinguishing
extirpate
extirpation
Amreich vaginal e.
dental pulp e.
nodal e.
pulp e.
Rubbrecht e.
sac e.
surgical e.
extorsion
extortor
extraabdominal
e. anastomosis
e. anastomotic healing
e. disease
e. infective complication
e. injury
e. operation
e. position
e. site
extra 1 acupoint
extraalveolar
extraanatomic
e. bypass

e. bypass method
e. bypass procedure
e. bypass technique
extraanatomical renal revascularization technique
extraarachnoid injection
extraarticular
e. ankylosis
e. arthrodesis
e. augmentation
e. graft
e. hip fusion
e. pain syndrome
e. procedure
e. reconstruction
e. resection
e. structure
e. subtalar fusion
e. subtalar joint
e. technique
e. tissue
e. tuberculosis
extraaxial
e. compartment
e. fluid collection
extrabuccal
extrabursal approach
extracaliceal
extracanthic
extracapillary crescent formation
extracapsular
e. ankylosis
e. aphakia
e. approach
e. arterial ring
e. cataract extraction (ECCE)
e. cataract extraction operation
e. disease
e. dissection
e. fracture
e. metastasis
e. tissue
extracardiac
e. mass
e. murmur
extracavitary approach
extracellular
e. compartment
e. fluid
e. fluid volume (ECFV)
e. granule
e. ground substance
e. mass
e. matrix
e. matrix remodeling
e. matrix system
e. plasma
e. space
e. toxin

E

extracellular (*continued*)
    e. volume
    e. water
extracellularlike calcium-free solution
extracerebral fluid collection
extrachorial placenta
extrachromic suture
extrachromosomal
extraciliary fiber
extracolonic
extraconal fat reticulum
extracoronal
    e. retention
    e. splinting
extracoronary
extracorporeal
    e. anastomosis
    e. bypass pump (ECBP)
    e. carbon dioxide removal
    (ECCO$_2$R)
    e. cardiopulmonary circuit
    e. circulation (ECC)
    e. dialysis
    e. exchange hypothermia
    e. heart
    e. irradiation
    e. jamming knot
    e. life support (ECLS)
    e. liver perfusion (ECLP)
    e. membrane oxygenation (ECMO)
    e. method
    e. partial nephrectomy
    e. piezoelectric shock wave
    lithotripsy
    e. procedure
    e. renal preservation
    e. repair
    e. shock wave lithotripsy (ESWL)
    e. shock wave treatment (ESWT)
    e. surgery
    e. technique
    e. ultrafiltration (ECU)
    e. venous bypass
extracranial
    e. carotid artery disease
    e. carotid circulation
    e. carotid occlusive disease
    e. cerebral vasculature
    e. mass lesion
    e. occlusive vascular disease
extracranial-intracranial (EC-IC)
    e.-i. bypass
    e.-i. bypass surgery
extract
    adipose tissue e.
    adrenocortical e.
    aqueous e.
    cannabis-based medicinal e.'s
    ceanothus e.

    lyophilized e.
    pancreatic e.
    parathyroid e.
    phenol-preserved e.
    Rauwolfia e.
    venom e.
    whole-body e.
extraction
    allograft e.
    Arroyo cataract e.
    Arruga cataract e.
    bag e.
    Baker pyridine e.
    e. balloon technique
    breech e.
    Burhenne biliary duct stone e.
    cataract e.
    Chandler-Verhoeff lens e.
    comedo e.
    countercurrent e.
    Daviel extracapsular cataract e.
    elevator e.
    endoscopic e.
    extracapsular cataract e. (ECCE)
    first-pass e.
    e. flap
    forceps e.
    foreign body e.
    Graefe cataract e.
    harpoon e.
    Himly cataract e.
    e. incision
    intracapsular cataract e.
    intraocular cataract e.
    lactate e.
    laparoscopic stone e.
    liquid e.
    magnetic e.
    manual e.
    Marshall-Taylor vacuum e.
    Mauksch-Maumenee-Goldberg
    cataract e.
    Maumenee-Goldberg cataract e.
    menstrual e.
    micro liquid e.
    e. of bile duct stone
    e. of pancreatic stone
    Pagenstecher intracapsular cataract e.
    partial breech e.
    planned extracapsular cataract e.
    podalic e.
    progressive e.
    rubber-band e.
    serial e.
    e. site
    solvent e.
    e. space
    splanchnic oxygen e.
    spontaneous breech e.

stone e.
systemic oxygen e.
tooth e.
total breech e.
vacuum e.
Wilmer lens e.
extractor
acetabular cup e.
intramedullary nail e.
extracystic
extradental projection
extradural
e. abscess
e. anesthesia
e. anesthetic technique
e. block
e. clinoidectomy
e. cortical stimulation
e. exposure
e. granulation
e. hematoma
e. hematorrhachis
e. hemorrhage
e. phase
e. space
e. vertebral artery
extraembryonic mesoderm
extraepiphysial
extrafascial hysterectomy
extragenital
extraglandular conversion
extraglomerular mesangium
extragonadal
extrahepatic
e. abdominal carcinoma
e. access
e. bile duct
e. bile duct cancer
e. bile duct obstruction
e. biliary atresia
e. biliary cystic dilation
e. biliary obstruction
e. biliary tree
e. control
e. dissection
e. lesion
e. metastasis
e. nodal disease
e. portal vein obstruction
e. portal venous hypertension
e. stone
e. tumor
e. tumor site
extraintestinal complication
extrajection
extralaryngeal approach
extraligamentous
extralobar sequestration
extraluminal

e. diverticulum
e. gas
e. hemorrhage
extralymphatic
e. collection
e. metastasis
extramammary Paget disease
extramaxillary anchorage
extramedullary
e. alignment
e. alignment arch
e. involvement
e. mass
e. myelopoiesis
e. segment
e. toxicity
extramucosal
e. mass
e. pyloromyotomy
e. stitch
extramural
e. lesion
e. upper airway obstruction
extraneous movement
extranodal
e. disease
e. site
e. tumor extension
extraoctave fracture
extraocular
e. movement (EOM)
e. muscle (EOM)
e. muscle involvement
e. muscles of Tillaux
extraoral
e. anchorage
e. radiographic examination profile
extraorbital disease
extraovular
extrapancreatic
e. extension
e. nerve plexus
extrapapillary
extraperineal
extraperiosteal
extraperitoneal
e. approach
e. carbon dioxide insufflation
e. cesarean section
e. CO_2 insufflation
e. endoscopic hernia repair
e. endoscopic pelvic lymph node
dissection
e. fascia
e. ileostomy
e. laparoscopic bladder neck
suspension
e. laparoscopic herniorrhaphy
e. laparoscopic nephrectomy

E

extraperitoneal (*continued*)
    e. location
    e. space
    e. tissue
    totally e.
extrapetrosal drainage
extrapharyngeal
    e. approach
    e. exposure
extraplacental
extrapleural
    e. air
    e. anastomosis
    e. apicolysis
    e. approach
    e. pneumothorax
    e. space
extrapolate
extrapolation
extraprostatic
extrapsychic
extrapulmonary
    e. cough
    e. *Pneumocystis carinii* infection
    e. site
    e. tuberculosis
extrapyramidal
    e. disease
    e. dyskinesia
    e. function assessment
    e. nucleus
    e. pathway
    e. reaction
    e. sign
    e. syndrome
    e. tract
extrarectus
extrarenal
    e. mass
    e. renal pelvis
extraretinal
extrasaccular hernia
extrascleral extension
extrasensory
extraskeletal
extrasphincteric anal fistula
extraspinal osteoid osteoma
extrastimulus test
extratemporal
    e. epilepsy
    e. excision
extratesticular lesion
extrathalamic lesion
extrathoracic
    e. metastasis
    e. position
    e. tuberculosis

extrathyroid
    e. invasion
    e. spread
extratracheal
extrauterine pelvic mass
extravaginal testicular torsion
extravasate
extravasated urine
extravasation
    e. extremity
    e. extrusion
    e. feces
    fluid e.
    e. gas
    e. injury
    e. irrigation solution
    liver dome stent exit site e.
    e. phenomenon
    urinary e.
extravascular
    e. compartment
    e. fluid balance
    e. granulomatous feature
    e. lung water
    e. mass
    e. space
extraventricular
extraversion, extroversion
    urinary e.
extravesical
    e. anastomosis
    e. infrasphincteric ectopic ureter
    e. Lich approach
    e. ureteral reimplantation technique
    e. ureterolysis
extreme
    e. capsule
    e. drug resistance (EDR)
    e. hearing loss
    e. lateral transcondylar approach
    e. somatosensory evoked potential
extremis
    in e.
extremital
extremitas
extremity, extremitas
    e. abnormality
    acromial e.
    e. amputation
    anterior e.
    elevation of e.
    extravasation e.
    flaccid e.
    e. injury
    e. ischemia

left lower e. (LLE)
left upper e. (LUE)
e. lesion
lower e.
e. malformation
e. melanoma
e. mobilization technique
e. preservation
right lower e. (RLE)
right upper e. (RUE)
upper e.

extrinsic
e. allergic alveolitis
e. asthma
e. bladder compression
e. denervation
e. entrapment test
e. environmental staining
e. esophageal impression
e. lesion
e. mass
e. mechanism
e. muscle
e. muscle strength
e. nerve
e. network of lymphatics
e. pathway
e. semiconductor
e. sphincter

extrodactyly
extroversion (*var. of*
extraversion)
extruded
e. disc
e. disc fragment
e. teeth
extrusion
bone graft e.
disc e.
extravasation e.
implant e.
oocyte e.
placental e.
sealer e.
tube e.
wire e.
extubate
extubation
e. anesthetic technique
early e.
postoperative e.
tracheal e.
exuberant granulation tissue
exudate
acute inflammatory e.
circinate e.
conjunctival e.
cotton-wool e.

fatty e.
fibrinous e.
fluffy cotton-wool e.
foaming e.
gingival e.
hard e.
inflammatory e.
mucopurulent e.
pharyngeal e.
purulent e.
retinal e.
sanguineous e.
serous e.
soft e.
suppurative e.
waxy e.
exudation
aqueous e.
fibrinous e.
gingival e.
proteinaceous aqueous e.
purulent e.
exudative
e. ascites
e. eye
e. granulomatous
inflammation
e. papulosquamous disease
e. pleural effusion
e. retinal detachment
e. tuberculosis
e. vitreoretinopathy
e. zone
exude
exumbilication
eye
cat's e.
e. disease
e. enucleation
e. examination
exciting e.
exudative e.
e. irrigating solution
e. muscle surgery
owl's e.
pineal e.
e. point
e. rotation
stony-hard e.
e. tumor
e. tumor localization
web e.
eyeball
e. compression reflex
e. equator
eyebrow
e. fixation
e. laceration

E

eye-closure reflex
eye-ear plane
eyelash
    ectopic e.
    e. reflex
eyelid
    e. crease suture

e. fusion
e. molluscum contagiosum infection
e. surgery
e. tumor
upper e.
eyelid-closure reflex
Eyler flexorplasty

F
   French
   French scale
FAB
   French-American-British
      FAB acute leukemia classification
      FAB staging
fabellae
faber
   flexion, abduction, external rotation
   flexion in abduction and external rotation
fabere
   flexion, abduction, external rotation,
    extension
      fabere sign
Fabricius ship
FAC
   fractional area change
face
      cow f.
      dish f.
      f. form
      inferior f.
      f., leg, activity, cry, consolability
      (FLACC)
      f. line
      F.'s Pain Scale
      F.'s Rating Scale for Children
      superior f.
      f. to face venacavaplasty
face-down position
face-lift (*var. of* facelift)
facelift, face-lift
      lunchtime f.
facet, facette
      f. anomaly
      articular f.
      clavicular f.
      corneal f.
      costal f.
      f. denervation
      f. dislocation
      f. excision technique
      f. fracture stabilization wiring
      f. fusion
      f. imbrication
      inferior costal f.
      f. joint
      f. joint injection
      f. joint preparation
      f. joint syndrome
      f. (of atlas) for dens
      f. pain
      perched f.
      f. plane

      f. rhizotomy
      f. subluxation stabilization wiring
      superior costal f.
      transverse costal f.
      f. tropism
facetectomy
      O'Donoghue f.
      partial f.
face-to-pubes fetal position
facette (*var. of* facet)
facetted corneal scar
facial
      F. Action Coding System (FACS)
      f. angiofibroma
      f. angle
      f. artery
      f. axis
      f. bipartition
      f. bone
      f. butt joint preparation
      f. canal
      f. cleft
      f. colliculus
      f. deformity
      f. excursion measurement
      f. expression
      flashlamp f.
      f. foundation
      f. fracture
      f. height
      f. index
      f. laser resurfacing
      f. muscle
      f. nerve
      f. nerve-preserving parotidectomy
      f. nerve root
      f. osteosynthesis
      f. pain
      f. plane
      f. plexus
      f. profile
      f. reanimation
      f. restoration
      f. root
      transverse f.
      f. triangle
      f. vein
facies
      acromial articular f.
      Potter f.
facilitated angioplasty
facilitating restoration
facilitation
      convergence f.
      neuromuscular f.

F

facilitation (*continued*)
    postactivation f.
    posttetanic f.
    proprioceptive neuromuscular f.
    spatial f.
    Wedensky f.
facioplasty
facioscapulohumeral muscular dystrophy
faciotelencephalic malformation
FACS
    Facial Action Coding System
    Fellow of American College of Surgeons
factitious hyperthyroidism
factor
    brain-derived neurotrophic f.
    clinicopathologic f.
    clotting f.
    coagulating f.
    coagulation f.
    endothelium-derived hyperpolarizing f.
    epidermal growth f. (EGF)
    growth f.
    gut proliferative f.
    neurotrophic f.
    pathophysiologic f.
    patient-dependent f.
    perioperative risk f.
    plasmatic coagulation f.
    platelet activating f.
    platelet-derived growth f. (PDGF)
    predisposing f.
    preoperative f.
    prognostic f.
    proliferative f.
    recombinant activated coagulation f. VII
    recombinant activated f. VII (rFVIIa)
    recombinant f. VIIa
    f. replacement therapy
    risk f.
    technical f.
    thromboembolic risk f.
    vascular-endothelial growth f. (VEGF)
    f. V Leiden mutation
    von Willebrand f. (vWF)
    f. Xase complex
faculty
    fusion f.
fade
    tetanic f.
Faden
    F. esotropia repair operation
    F. esotropia repair procedure
    F. suture

fadir
    flexion in adduction and internal rotation
fadire
    flexion, adduction, internal rotation, extension
Fahey
    F. hip arthrotomy approach
    F. technique
Fahey-O'Brien unicameral bone cyst subtotal resection and grafting technique
failed
    f. airway
    f. anesthesia
    f. back surgery syndrome (FBSS)
    f. femoral osteotomy
    f. intubation
    f. procedure
    f. spinal
    f. surgery
fail-safe valve
failure
    acute circulatory f.
    acute respiratory f.
    f. analysis
    anastomotic f.
    bone marrow f.
    bypass f.
    chronic intestinal f.
    chronic renal f.
    cocaine-induced respiratory f.
    congestive heart f. (CHF)
    differentiation f.
    dilator placement f.
    end-organ f.
    end-stage intestinal f.
    exercise-associated acute renal f.
    fulminant hepatic f. (FHF)
    functional intestinal f.
    graft f.
    Harrington rod instrumentation f.
    heart f.
    hepatic f.
    hepatorenal f.
    implant f.
    implantation f.
    infrainguinal arterial reconstruction graft f.
    instrumentation f.
    intestinal f.
    intubation f.
    irradiation f.
    late graft f.
    late-onset hepatic f.
    late wound f.
    liver f.
    microcirculatory f.

multiorgan f. (MOF)
multiorgan system f. (MOSF)
multiple organ f. (MOF)
multiple organ system f. (MOSF)
multiple system organ f. (MSOF)
multisystem f.
multisystem organ f. (MSOF)
neurologic f.
pacemaker f.
postburn bone marrow f.
postoperative hepatic f.
postoperative liver f.
posttraumatic renal f.
pouch f.
progressive liver f.
progressive respiratory f.
pump f.
renal f.
respiratory f.
sclerotherapy f.
surgeon-dependent technique f.
surgical f.
suture f.
technical f.
tissue f.
f. to awaken
f. to rescue
wound f.

Fairbanks-Sever brachial plexus repair procedure
Fairbanks uvulopalatopharyngoplasty technique
falcate
falces (*pl. of* falx)
falciform
f. cartilage
f. crest
f. ligament
f. margin
f. process
f. retinal fold
Falconer lobectomy
Falk-Shukuris operation
Falk vesicovaginal fistula technique
falling hematocrit
fallopian
f. canal
f. hiatus
f. ligament
f. tube
f. tube carcinoma
f. tube catheterization
f. tube mass
f. tube metastasis
Fallot
simple tetralogy of F.
tetralogy of F. (TET, TOF)
untreated tetralogy of F.

false
f. aneurysm
f. channel formation
f. cord carcinoma
f. diverticulum
f. knot
f. membrane
f. negative
f. passage
f. pelvis
f. positive
f. projection
f. rib
f. suture
f. vertebra
f. vocal cord
false-negative
f.-n. cholangiogram
f.-n. result
false-positive
f.-p. interpretation
f.-p. result
falx, *pl.* **falces**
familial
f. adenomatous polyposis (FAP)
f. aortic ectasia syndrome
f. atypical mole and melanoma (FAM-M)
f. atypical multiple-mole melanoma (FAMMM)
f. atypical multiple mole melanoma syndrome
f. breast cancer
f. cardiac myxoma syndrome
f. cholestasis syndrome
f. colon cancer (FCC)
f. consequence
f. dysautonomia
f. exudative vitreoretinopathy
f. hemiplegic migraine
f. HPT
f. hypocalciuric hypercalcemia
f. indication
f. juvenile polyposis (FJP)
f. Mediterranean fever
f. medullary thyroid carcinoma
f. multigland disease
f. osteochondrodystrophy
f. paroxysmal rhabdomyolysis
f. polyposis syndrome
f. visceral myopathy
FAM-M
familial atypical mole and melanoma
FAM-M syndrome
FAMMM
familial atypical multiple-mole melanoma
FAMM syndrome
fan beam projection

F

Fanconi anemia
Fanta cataract operation
fan-type retractor
FAP
    familial adenomatous polyposis
far
    f. lateral inferior suboccipital
      approach
    f. point
Farabeuf
    F. amputation
    F. ischiopubiotomy
    F. triangle
Faraday
far-and-near suture technique
Farmer
    F. in utero myelomeningocele repair
      operation
    F. technique
Farre white line
FARS
    Fatal Accident Reporting System
Fasanella operation
Fasanella-Servat
    F.-S. blepharoptosis repair
      procedure
    F.-S. ptosis operation
fascia, pl. fasciae, fascias
    Abernethy f.
    alar f.
    anal f.
    antebrachial f.
    anterior rectus f.
    axillary f.
    brachial f.
    broad f.
    buccopharyngeal f.
    Buck f.
    bulbar sheath f.
    Camper f.
    cervical f.
    clavipectoral f.
    Cloquet f.
    Colles f.
    Cooper f.
    coracoaxillary f.
    cremasteric f.
    cribriform f.
    crural f.
    Cruveilhier f.
    dartos f.
    deep cervical f.
    deltopectoral f.
    Denonvilliers f.
    endoabdominal f.
    endopelvic f.
    endothoracic f.
    external oblique f.
    external spermatic f.

extraperitoneal f.
fusion f.
geniohyoid f.
Gerota f.
gluteal f.
Godman f.
Hesselbach f.
iliac f.
f. iliaca block
f. iliaca compartment
    blockade
iliopectineal f.
incised f.
infundibuliform f.
intercolumnar f.
internal spermatic f.
investing f.
lacrimal f.
f. lata
lumbodorsal f.
masseteric f.
middle cervical f.
muscular f.
nuchal f.
obturator f.
f. of abdomen
orbital f.
palpebral f.
pancreatic f.
parietal pelvic f.
parotid f.
parotideomasseteric f.
pectineal f.
pectoral f.
pectoralis f.
pelvic f.
perirenal f.
pharyngobasilar f.
phrenicopleural f.
popliteal f.
Porter f.
prepubic f.
presacral f.
pretracheal f.
prevertebral f.
prevesical f.
psoas f.
rectal f.
rectovesical f.
renal f.
retrosacral f.
retrovisceral f.
salpingopharyngeal f.
scalene f.
Scarpa f.
Sibson f.
subcutaneous f.
subperitoneal f.
superficial inguinal f.

superior f.
temporal f.
Thompson f.
thoracolumbar f.
Toldt f.
transversalis f.
transverse f.
Treitz f.
triangular f.
Tyrrell f.
umbilical prevesical f.
umbilicovesical f.
visceral pelvic f.
Zuckerkandl f.
fasciae (*pl. of* fascia)
fascial
f. arthroplasty
f. bridge
f. closure
f. decompression
f. defect
f. flap
f. graft
f. hernia
f. layer
f. plane
f. shutter mechanism
f. sling approach
f. sling procedure
f. space
f. space infection
f. stranding
f. wrapping
f. zipper
fasciaplasty, fascioplasty
fascias (*pl. of* fascia)
fascia-splitting incision
fascicular
f. graft
f. repair
fasciculata cell
fasciculation
benign f.
contraction f.
malignant f.
f. potential
tongue f.
fasciculi (*pl. of* fasciculus)
fasciculus (fasc), *pl.* **fasciculi**
wedge-shaped f.
fasciectomy
dermal f.
limited f.
partial f.
radical palmar f.
fasciitis, fascitis
necrotizing f.
plantar f.
fasciitis-panniculitis syndrome

fasciocutaneous
f. free flap
f. island flap
fasciodesis
fasciola
fascioplasty (*var. of* fasciaplasty)
fasciorrhaphy
fascioscapulohumeral
fasciotomy
decompression f.
double-incision f.
endoscopic plantar f.
percutaneous plantar f.
plantar f.
prophylactic f.
Rorabeck f.
single-incision f.
Skoog f.
subcutaneous f.
Yount f.
fascitis (*var. of* fasciitis)
fashion
concertina-like f.
isolated f.
perpendicular f.
standard f.
Z f.
FAST
focused abdominal sonography for trauma
focused assessment with sonography for trauma
fast-flush test
fastigiobulbar tract
fasting
preoperative f.
f. recording
fast-pathway radiofrequency ablation
fast-track
f.-t. anesthesia
f.-t. cardiac anesthesia
f.-t. surgery
fat
abdominal f.
anterior mediastinal f.
body f.
f. body
f. cell space
creeping f.
f. flap
f. globule
f. graft
herniated preperitoneal f.
f. herniation
f. line
f. necrosis
f. pad
f. pad sign
periesophageal f.

F

fat (*continued*)
    f. plane
    preperitoneal f.
    properitoneal f.
    total body f.
fatal
    F. Accident Reporting System
    (FARS)
    f. air embolus
    f. cardiac event
fat-density line
fat-free mass (FFM)
fatigability
    muscle f.
fatigue
    excessive f.
    f. fracture
    implant f.
    postoperative f.
    suture f.
fat-suppression technique
fatty
    f. apron
    f. ascites
    f. exudate
    f. hernia
    f. infiltration
    f. prostatic tissue
    f. renal capsule
fauces, *pl.* **fauces**
faucial branch
faulty
    f. contact point
    f. restoration
Favaloro saphenous vein bypass graft
FBSS
    failed back surgery syndrome
FCC
    familial colon cancer
FCE
    functional capacity evaluation
FDA
    Food and Drug Administration
        FDA Anesthesia Apparatus Checkout
        Recommendations
FDPCA
    fixed-dose patient-controlled
    analgesia
Feagin shoulder dislocation test
fear
    f. avoidance
    F. Avoidance Beliefs Questionnaire
    pain-related f.
    f. subscale
fear-related activity avoidance
feather-edged proximal finishing line
featural surgery

feature
    clinical manifestations, etiologic
        factors, anatomic involvement,
        pathophysiologic f.'s (CEAP)
    clinicopathologic f.
    cytologic f.
    extravascular granulomatous f.
    histopathologic f.
    immunohistochemical f.
    preoperative f.
    tumor f.
febrile morbidity
FEC
    forced expiratory capacity
fecal
    f. abscess
    f. contamination
    f. diversion
    f. diversion colostomy
    f. fistula
    f. impaction
    f. incontinence
    f. load
    f. loading
    f. occult blood testing
    (FOBT)
    f. soiling
    f. stream
fecalith
    appendiceal f.
fecaloma
    stercoral f.
fecaluria
feces
    extravasation f.
fecundity rate
feedback
    hypothalamic f.
    f. reduction circuit (FRC)
feeder-frond ablative photocoagulation technique
feeding
    f. complication
    drip-tube f.
    early enteral f.
    enteral f.
    gastrostomy f.
    f. gastrostomy
    jejunostomy elemental diet f.
    jejunostomy tube f.
    oral f.
    postoperative regimen for oral early
        f. (PROEF)
    postpyloric f.
    tube f.
    f. tube placement
feet (*pl. of* foot)
Feiss line
Feist-Mankin position

Fellow of American College of Surgeons (FACS)
felon infection
Felson
    silhouette sign of F.
feltwork
Felty syndrome
fem
    femoral
female
    f. castration
    f. gonad
    f. prostate
    f. urethra
    f. urethral syndrome
fem-fem
    femoral-femoral
    femorofemoral
feminization syndrome
feminizing genitoplasty
femoral (fem)
    f. arch
    f. artery
    f. artery aneurysm
    f. artery approach
    f. canal
    f. circulation
    f. cortical ring allograft
    f. diaphysial fracture
    f. diaphysis
    f. elevator
    f. embolectomy
    f. endarterectomy
    f. epiphysial fracture
    f. epiphysiolysis
    f. epiphysis
    f. fossa
    f. head
    f. head line
    f. hernia
    f. 3-in-1 technique
    f. intertrochanteric fracture
    f. metaphysis
    f. muscle
    f. nailing
    f. neck fracture
    f. neck fracture reduction
    f. nerve
    f. nerve block (FNB)
    f. nerve traction test
    f. osteotomy
    f. plexus
    f. prosthesis
    f. prosthesis fixation
    f. puncture
    f. region
    f. resection
    f. ring
    f. septum

    f. shaft
    f. shaft fracture
    f. sheath
    f. stem removal
    f. supracondylar fracture
    f. triangle
    f. vein
femoral-femoral (fem-fem)
femoral-popliteal (fem-pop)
    f.-p. artery bypass
femoral-tibial-peroneal bypass
femoral-trunk extension
femoris
    f. rectus
    f. rectus muscle
    rectus f. (muscle)
femorocaval bypass
femorodistal
    f. bypass
    f. reconstructive surgery
femorofemoral (fem-fem)
    f. bypass
    f. crossover
femoroischial transplant
femoropopliteal (fem-pop)
    f. bypass
    f. bypass graft
    f. occlusive disease
    f. vein
femorotibial
fem-pop
    femoral-popliteal
    femoropopliteal
femur distractor
fender fracture
fenestra, *pl.* **fenestrae**
fenestrae (*pl. of* fenestra)
fenestrated
    f. endothelium
    f. Fontan operation
    f. membrane
    f. sheath
fenestration
    alveolar plate f.
    aortopulmonary f.
    apical f.
    atrophic f.
    baffle f.
    catheter-directed f.
    Cawthorne labyrinth f.
    cusp f.
    cyst f.
    dental f.
    intercellular f.
    laparoscopic f.
    Lempert f.
    f. operation
    tracheal f.
fenoldopam

F

fentanyl
    f. buccal tablet
    OraVescent f.
Fenton vaginoplasty
Fentora
Ferciot excision
Ferciot-Thomson excision
Fergus lid ptosis correction
Ferguson
    F. hemorrhoidectomy
    F. scoliosis measuring method
Fergusson incision
Ferkel torticollis technique
fermentation
    mixed acid f.
Fernandez
    F. extensile anterior approach
    F. osteotomy
Ferrein
    F. canal
    F. cord
    F. foramen
    F. ligament
    F. pyramid
ferromagnetic microembolization treatment
Ferry line
fertility
fertilization
    f. age
    ex vivo f.
    in vitro f. (IVF)
    in vivo f.
FESS
    functional endoscopic sinus surgery
festination
FET
    forced expiratory time
fetal
    f. acoustic stimulation test
    f. aspiration syndrome
    f. body movement
    f. bone fracture
    f. cardiac anomaly
    f. cell transplant
    f. chest anomaly
    f. circulation
    f. cystic adenomatoid malformation
    f. drug therapy
    f. duplication
    f. exsanguination
    f. gastrointestinal anomaly
    f. growth retardation
    f. head
    f. head circumference
    f. head position
    f. head to abdominal circumference ratio
    f. heart rate

    f. heart rate monitoring
    f. hemorrhage
    f. infection
    f. intracranial anatomy
    f. intrahepatic vein
    f. liver biopsy
    f. liver transplant
    f. lymphoid tissue
    f. malpresentation
    f. membrane
    f. reduction
    f. rejection
    f. scalp oxygenation
    f. skin biopsy
    f. surgery
    f. thymus transplant
    f. tissue sampling
    f. tissue transplant
    f. urogenital tract
    f. vascular anomaly
fetalis
    hydrops f.
    placenta f.
fetal-maternal
    f.-m. exchange
    f.-m. hemorrhage (FMH)
fetation
fetoplacental circulation
fetoscopy
FEV
    forced expiratory volume
FEV1
    forced expiratory volume in 1 second
fever
    dehydration f.
    exanthematous f.
    exsiccation f.
    familial Mediterranean f.
    fracture f.
    inundation f.
    Mediterranean exanthematous f.
    syphilitic f.
FF
    femorofemoral
    FF crossover
FFG
    free fat graft
FFM
    fat-free mass
FFP
    fresh frozen plasma
FGF
    fresh gas flow
FHF
    fulminant hepatic failure
fiber, fibra, fibre
    accelerator f.
    anastomotic f.
    association f.

B f.'s
f. bundle
bundle f.
f. bundle volume (FBV)
C f.'s
delta fibers
endogenous f.
exogenous f.
extension f.
external arcuate f.
extraciliary f.
Gerdy f.
intercolumnar f.
intercrural f.
mature collagen f.
Nélaton f.
osteogenetic f.
parasympathetic f.
postganglionic parasympathetic f.
postganglionic sympathetic f.
preganglionic parasympathetic f.
preganglionic sympathetic f.
projection f.
pupillodilator f.
rod f.
Rosenthal f.
Sappey f.
secretomotor parasympathetic f.
Sharpey f.
skinned muscle f.
sympathetic f.
f. tip modification
zonular f.
fiberglass graft
fiberoptic
f. bronchoscope (FOB)
f. bronchoscopy (FOB)
f. bronchoscopy anesthetic technique
f. bundle
f. endoscopy anesthetic technique
f. esophagoscopy
f. examination
f. injection sclerotherapy (FIS)
f. intraosseous endoscopy
f. intubation
f. intubation method
f. intubation procedure
f. laryngoscopy
f. panendoscopy
f. sigmoidoscopy
f. stomatoscopy
f. tracheal intubation anesthetic technique
fiberoptic-assisted coaxial endotracheal tube exchange
fiberotomy
fiber-splitting incision
fibra, *pl.* **fibrae**
fibrae zonulares

fibrae (*pl. of* fibra)
fibre (*var. of* fiber)
fibrillary astrocyte, fibrous astrocyte
fibrillation
atrial f.(Afib)
cardiac f.
chronic atrial f.
continuous atrial f.
idiopathic ventricular f.
lone atrial f.
paroxysmal atrial f. (PAF)
f. potential
refractory atrial f.
f. rhythm
synchronized f.
f. threshold
ventricular tachycardia/ventricular f.
fibrillation-flutter, fibrilloflutter
atrial f.-f. (AFF)
fibrilloflutter (*var. of* fibrillation-flutter)
fibrillogranuloma
fibrin
f. calculus
f. degradation product
f. glue
f. peel
f. polymerization
postvitrectomy f.
f. sealant
fibrinogen
fibrinogenolysis
fibrinoid necrotizing inflammation
fibrinolysin coagulation
fibrinolysis
endothelium-dependent f.
primary f.
fibrinopeptide A
fibrinopurulent inflammation
fibrinoscopy
fibrinous
f. adhesion
f. exudate
f. exudation
f. inflammation
fibroadenolipoma
degenerated f.
fibroadenoma
giant f.
fibroadipose tissue
fibroangioma
fibroblast
f. chemoattraction
f. culture
dermal f.
harvested f.
keloid f.
f. migration
f. proliferation
wound f.

F

fibroblastic tissue
fibroblastoma
fibrocalcification
fibrocalcific lesion
fibrocarcinoma
fibrocartilage
    basilar f.
    circumferential f.
    interarticular f.
    semilunar f.
    stratiform f.
fibrocartilaginous
fibrocaseous inflammation
fibrocementoma
fibrochondroma
fibrocystic
    f. breast syndrome
    f. change
    f. complex
    f. condition
    f. disease
fibrocystoma
fibrodentinoma
fibroelastic tissue
fibroelastoma
fibroenchondroma
fibroepithelioma
fibrofascial compartment
  syndrome
fibrofatty breast tissue
fibrofolliculoma
fibrogliosis
fibrogranuloma
fibrohemangioma
fibrohistiocytic lesion
fibrohistiocytoma
fibroid
    f. adenoma
    f. inflammation
fibroidectomy
fibrokeratoma
fibroleiomyoma
fibrolipoma
fibroliposarcoma
fibroma
    ameloblastic f.
    breast f.
    diffuse f.
    ossifying f.
    psammomatoid ossifying f.
    ungual f.
fibromectomy
fibromus
fibromuscular dysplasia (FMD)
fibromusculoelastic lesion
fibromyalgia trigger point
fibromyectomy
fibromyoma
    uterine f.

fibroneuroma
fibronodular hyperplasia
fibroosseous
    f. lesion
    f. ring of Lacroix
fibroplasia
    progressive f.
fibroplate
fibroproliferative membrane
fibrosa (var. of fibrous)
fibrosarcoma
fibroscopy
fibrosis
    diffuse lobular f.
    epidural f.
    hepatic f.
    idiopathic pulmonary f. (IPF)
    interstitial pulmonary f. (IPF)
    periductal f.
    periesophageal f.
    pulmonary f.
    retroperitoneal f.
fibrosum
fibrothorax
fibrotic
    f. nub
    f. reaction
    f. tissue
    f. wall
fibrotomy
fibrous, fibrosa
    f. adhesion
    f. articular capsule
    f. bone lesion
    f. cap
    f. connective tissue
    f. ingrowth
    f. integration
    f. joint
    f. loose body
    f. obliteration
    f. polypoid lesion
    f. repair
    f. ring
    f. scar
    f. scar tissue
    f. skeleton
    f. tendon sheath
    f. union
fibula
    diastasis f.
fibular
    f. flap
    f. fracture
    f. head
    f. metaphysis
    f. ostectomy
    f. sesamoidectomy
    f. strut graft

fibularis
  f. brevis muscle
  f. longus muscle
  f. longus tendon
  f. tertius muscle
  f. tertius tendon
fibulectomy
  partial f.
fibulocalcaneal ligament
Ficat hip procedure
Fick
  F. cardiac output measurement
  F. cardiac output technique
  F. determination
  F. oxygen extraction method
  F. position
  F. principle
field
  f. anesthesia machine
  f. block
  f. block anesthesia
  bloodless f.
  f. cancerization
  clean f.
  clean-contaminated f.
  contaminated f.
  dirty f.
  f. dissection
  electromagnetic f.
  f. expansion
  infected f.
  f. lymphadenectomy
  f. method
  f. of dissection
  operative f.
  pulsed electromagnetic f.
    (PEMF)
  surgical f.
2-field
  2-f. dissection
  2-f. lymphadenectomy
3-field
  3-f. dissection
  3-f. lymphadenectomy
Fielding
  F. femoral fracture
    classification
  F. membrane
  F. modification
  F. modification of Gallie
    atlantoaxial instability spine fusion
    technique
Fielding-Magliato subtrochanteric fracture
  classification
fierce cellular rejection
fifth
  f. cranial nerve
  f. metatarsal base fracture
fighter's fracture

FIGO
  International Federation of Gynecology
    and Obstetrics
    FIGO classification staging
figure-of-8
  f.-o.-8 preparation
  f.-o.-8 stitch
  f.-o.-8 suture
  f.-o.-8 suture technique
figure-of-4 position
fila (*pl. of* filum)
filament
  corneal f.
  f. suture
filar mass
Filatov
  F. keratoplasty
  F. penetrating keratoplasty
  F. tubed flap
Filatov-Gillies
  F.-G. tubed flap
  F.-G. tubed pedicle
Filatov-Marzinkowsky operation
fill breast implant
filled
  decayed, extracted, f.
filler graft
filleted graft
fillet local flap graft
filling
  bead technique f.
  brush technique f.
  f. canal
  cuff f.
  f. defect
  f. first technique
  flow technique f.
  f. material condensation
  nature root canal f.
  postresection f.
  pressure technique f.
  f. procedure
  root canal f.
film
  abdominal f.
  f. identification
  f. oxygenation
  plain abdominal f.
filmy adhesion
filopressure
filter
  f. placement
  reflection f.
  f. tilt
filtered-back projection
filtered radioisotope
filtering
  f. operation
  f. procedure

F

FilterWire
filtration
    f. angle
    fluid f.
    gel f.
    glass-wool f.
    glomerular f.
    f. method
    rate of fluid f.
    spontaneous ascites f.
    f. surgery
filtration-slit membrane
filtrum
filum, *pl.* **fila**
fimbria, *pl.* **fimbriae**
    ovarian f.
fimbriae (*pl. of* fimbria)
fimbrial evacuation
fimbriated fold
fimbriectomy
fimbrioplasty
    Bruhat laser f.
final
    f. cementation
    f. growth
    f. outcome
finding
    barium enema f.
    diagnostic f.
    endoscopic f.
    endovaginal f.
    equivocal f.
    histologic liver biopsy f.
    intraoperative ultrasound f.
    irresectable f.
    mammographic f.
    manometric f.
    operative f.
    physical f.
    prognostic f.
    suspicious f.
    ultrasonic endovaginal f.
fine
    f. chromic suture
    f. manipulation
    f. silk suture
fine-needle
    f.-n. aspiration (FNA)
    f.-n. aspiration biopsy
    f.-n. aspiration cytology
finger
    f. cot
    f. deformity
    f. dilation
    f. flap
    f. fracture
    f. fracture dissection
    f. fracture technique
    f. indicator

    f. joint arthroplasty
    mallet f.
    F. Oscillation Test
    ring f.
    swan-neck f.
    f. web
finger-fillet flap
fingerlike extension
fingerprint line
fingertip
    f. amputation
    f. dissection
fingertrap
    f. suspension
    f. suture
Finkelstein tendinitis maneuver
Fink inferior oblique recession
Finney
    F. gastroenterostomy
    F. operation
    F. pyloroplasty
    F. stricturoplasty
Finochietto-Billroth I gastrectomy
  technique
fire
    airway f.
    nosocomial f.
    surgical f.
    f. triangle
firm
    f. lesion
    f. mass
    f. texture
first
    f. arch syndrome
    f. carpometacarpal joint fracture
    f. cranial nerve
    f. cuneiform bone
    f. intention
    f. line screening technique
    f. metacarpal artery
    f. parallel pelvic plane
    f. ray surgery
    f. rib resection via subclavicular
      approach
      technique
    f. stage repair
    f. twitch height (T1)
    f. web space
first-degree
    f.-d. burn
    f.-d. hemorrhoid
    f.-d. radiation injury
    f.-d. tuberculum
first-grade fusion
first-pass
    f.-p. extraction
    f.-p. technique
first-set graft rejection

FIS

    fiberoptic injection sclerotherapy

Fischer projection

Fish cuneiform osteotomy technique

Fisher advancement flap

fisherman's knot

fish-eye sign

Fishgold line

fishmouth

    f. amputation
    f. anastomosis
    f. fracture
    f. incision

fishtail

    f. deformity
    f. flap

fissura, *pl.* **fissurae**

fissurae (*pl. of* fissura)

fissure

    abdominal f.
    anal f.
    auricular f.
    azygos f.
    caudal transverse f.
    f. cavity
    corneal f.
    dorsal f.
    Duverney f.
    Ecker f.
    glaserian f.
    horizontal f.
    inferior accessory f.
    inferior orbital f.
    major f.
    minor f.
    oral f.
    orbital f.
    palpebral f.
    petrooccipital f.
    petrosquamous f.
    petrotympanic f.
    portal f.
    pterygoid f.
    pterygomaxillary f.
    rectal f.
    right sagittal f.
    Rolando f.
    sagittal f.
    Santorini f.
    sphenoidal f.
    sphenomaxillary f.
    sphenopetrosal f.
    squamotympanic f.
    superior orbital f.
    sylvian f.
    tympanomastoid f.
    tympanosquamous f.
    umbilical f.
    vestibular f.

fissured fracture

fistula, *pl.* **fistulae, fistulas**

    abdominal wall f.
    alveolar f.
    amphibolic f.
    anal f.
    anastomotic f.
    anorectal f.
    antecubital arteriovenous f.
    aortocaval f.
    aortoduodenal f.
    aortoenteric f.
    aortoesophageal f.
    aortogastric f.
    aortograft duodenal f.
    aortosigmoid f.
    arterial-arterial f.
    arterial-enteric f.
    arterial-portal f.
    arteriobiliary f.
    arterioportal f.
    arterioportobiliary f.
    arteriosinusoidal penile f.
    arteriovenous f. (AVF)
    arteriovenous subclavian f.
    aural f.
    AV f.
    benign duodenocolic f.
    biliary f.
    biliary-bronchial f.
    biliary-cutaneous f.
    biliary-duodenal f.
    biliary-enteric f.
    biliocystic f.
    biliopleural f.
    bladder f.
    blind f.
    Blom-Singer tracheoesophageal f.
    bowel f.
    BP f.
    brachioaxillary bridge graft f.
    brachiosubclavian bridge graft f.
    branchial f.
    Brescia-Cimino AV f.
    bronchobiliary f.
    bronchoesophageal f.
    bronchopleural f. (BPF)
    bronchopleurocutaneous f.
    bronchopulmonary f. (BPF)
    calyceal f.
    cameral f.
    carotid-cavernous sinus f.
    carotid-dural f.
    cavernous sinus f.
    cerebrospinal fluid f.
    cervical f.
    cervicovaginal f.
    cholecystenteric f.
    cholecystocholedochal f.

F

fistula (*continued*)
   cholecystocolic f.
   cholecystocolonic f.
   cholecystoduodenal f.
   cholecystoduodenocolic f.
   choledochal-colonic f.
   choledochocolonic f.
   choledochoduodenal f.
   choledochoenteric f.
   chyle f.
   Cimino f.
   Cimino-Brescia arteriovenous f.
   closure of f.
   coccygeal f.
   colobronchial f.
   colocutaneous f.
   cologastrocutaneous f.
   coloileal f.
   colonic f.
   colorectal f.
   colovaginal f.
   colovesical f.
   communicating f.
   complete f.
   complex anorectal f.
   congenital pulmonary
     arteriovenous f.
   congenital tracheobiliary f.
   congenital urethroperineal f.
   controlled f.
   corneal f.
   coronary artery f.
   coronary artery-right ventricular f.
   craniosinus f.
   cutaneobiliary f.
   cystogastric f.
   dental f.
   dialysis f.
   dorsal enteric f.
   duodenal f.
   duodenocaval f.
   duodenocolic f.
   duodenoenterocutaneous f.
   dural arteriovenous f.
   dural cavernous sinus f.
   Eck f.
   endobronchial f.
   endogenous AV f.
   enteric f.
   enterocolic f.
   enterocutaneous f.
   enteroenteral f.
   enteroenteric f.
   enterogenital f.
   enterourethral f.
   enterovaginal f.
   enterovesical f.
   esophageal f.
   esophagobronchial f.

   esophagocutaneous f.
   esophagomediastinal f.
   esophagopleural f.
   esophagopulmonary f.
   esophagorespiratory f.
   esophagotracheal f.
   ethmoid f.
   ethmoidal lacrimal f.
   external biliary f.
   external pancreatic f.
   extrasphincteric anal f.
   fecal f.
   forearm graft arteriovenous f.
   gastric f.
   gastrocolic f.
   gastrocutaneous f.
   gastroduodenal f.
   gastroenteric f.
   gastrogastric f.
   gastrointestinal f.
   gastrointestinal-cutaneous f.
   gastrojejunocolic f.
   gastropleural f.
   genitourinary f.
   gingival f.
   graft-enteric f.
   Gratz f.
   Gross tracheoesophageal f.
   hepatic artery-portal vein f.
   hepatopleural f.
   hepatoportal biliary f.
   horseshoe f.
   H-type tracheoesophageal f.
   iatrogenic arteriovenous f.
   ileoduodenal f.
   ileosigmoid f.
   ileovesical f.
   f. in ano
   incomplete f.
   inflammatory f.
   internal lacrimal f.
   intersphincteric anal f.
   intestinal f.
   intracranial arteriovenous f.
   intrahepatic arterioportal f.
   intrahepatic AV f.
   intrahepatic spontaneous
     arterioportal f.
   intralabyrinthine f.
   intraocular f.
   jejunocolic f.
   labyrinthine f.
   lacrimal f.
   lacteal f.
   lactiferous duct f.
   mammary f.
   Mann-Bollman f.
   mesenteric arteriovenous f.
   metroperitoneal f.

mucous f.
oroantral f.
orocutaneous f.
orofacial f.
oronasal f.
pancreatic f.
pancreatic-cutaneous f.
pancreaticopleural f.
pararectal f.
parietal f.
perianal f.
perilymph f.
perilymphatic f.
perineal urinary f.
perineovaginal f.
peristomal f.
pharyngocutaneous f.
pilonidal f.
pleurobiliary f.
pleuroesophageal f.
postbiopsy renal AV f.
postoperative pleurobiliary f.
postradiation f.
posttraumatic pancreatic-cutaneous f.
pouch-vaginal f.
preauricular f.
primary arteriovenous f.
pseudocystobiliary f.
pulmonary arteriovenous f. (PAVF)
radiculomedullary f.
rectal f.
rectolabial f.
rectoscrotal f.
rectourethral f.
rectourinary f.
rectovaginal f.
rectovesical f.
rectovestibular f.
rectovulvar f.
renal f.
renogastric f.
respiratory-esophageal f.
retroperitoneal f.
reverse Eck f.
salivary f.
scleral f.
sigmoid cutaneous f.
sigmoidovesical f.
solitary pulmonary arteriovenous f.
spermatic f.
spinal dural arteriovenous f.
splanchnic AV f.
splenic AV f.
splenobronchial f.
stercoral f.
subclavian arteriovenous f.
submental f.
suprasphincteric f.
sylvian f.

synovial f.
systemic arteriovenous f.
TE f.
f. test
thigh graft arteriovenous f.
Thiry f.
Thiry-Vella f.
thoracic duct f.
thromboembolic f.
thyroglossal f.
tracheobiliary f.
tracheobronchoesophageal f.
tracheocutaneous f.
tracheoesophageal f. (TEF)
transsphincteric anal f.
traumatic f.
ulcerogenic f.
umbilical f.
urachal f.
ureteral f.
ureterocolic f.
ureterocutaneous f.
ureteroperitoneal f.
ureterouterine f.
ureterovaginal f.
urethrocavernous f.
urethroperineal f.
urethrorectal f.
urethrovaginal f.
urinary f.
urinary-rectal f.
urinary-umbilical f.
urinary-vaginal f.
urogenital f.
uteroperitoneal f.
vaginal f.
vasocutaneous f.
Vella f.
venobiliary f.
vesical f.
vesicoacetabular f.
vesicocolic f.
vesicocutaneous f.
vesicoenteric f.
vesicointestinal f.
vesicoovarian f.
vesicorectal f.
vesicosalpingovaginal f.
vesicouterine f.
vesicovaginal f.
vesicovaginorectal f.
vitelline f.
fistulae (*pl. of* fistula)
fistular formation
fistulas (*pl. of* fistula)
fistulation, fistulization
artificial f.
cholecystobiliary f.
spreading f.

F

fistulectomy
    scleral f.
fistulization (*var. of* fistulation)
fistulizing surgery
fistuloenterostomy
fistulography
fistulotomy
    anal f.
    choledochoduodenal f.
    diathermic f.
    endoscopic f.
    laying-open f.
    Parks method of anal f.
    Parks staged f.
fistulous tract
fitness for general anesthesia
fitting
fixation
    acromioclavicular pin f.
    adjunctive screw f.
    alcohol f.
    anatomic porous replacement f.
    angled blade plate f.
    anomalous f.
    f. anomaly
    anterior internal f.
    anterior metallic f.
    anterior plate f.
    anterior screw f.
    anterior spinal f.
    AO external f.
    AO rigid f.
    AO spinal internal f.
    APR cement f.
    Association for the Study of
      Internal F. (ASIF)
    atlantoaxial rotatory f. (AARF)
    autotrophic f.
    axial f.
    axis f.
    bar bolt f.
    Barr open reduction and
      internal f.
    Barr tibial fracture f.
    f. base
    bicortical screw f.
    bifocal f.
    bifoveal f.
    binocular f.
    biologic f.
    biphase pin f.
    blade plate f.
    bolt f.
    bone ingrowth f.
    bridge plate f.
    brow f.
    capsular f.
    carbon dioxide f.
    catheter f.

central f.
cerclage wire f.
cervical screw f.
cervical spine internal f.
cervical spine screw-plate f.
chest wall f.
circumalveolar f.
circumferential wire-loop f.
circummandibular f.
circumzygomatic f.
closed reduction and percutaneous f.
  (CRPF)
cloverleaf condylar plate f.
Cole tendon f.
Collin-Beard orbicularis-levator f.
complement f.
compression plate f.
condylar screw f.
coracoclavicular screw f.
coracoclavicular suture f.
Cotrel-Dubousset f.
craniofacial f.
crossed f.
f. delay
Denham external f.
dens anterior screw f.
Deverle f.
Dimon-Hughston fracture f.
dorsal wire-loop f.
dynamic compression plate f.
dynamic condylar screw f.
eccentric f.
elastic band f.
external pin f.
external spinal f.
eyebrow f.
femoral prosthesis f.
flexion f.
formalin f.
fracture f.
Galveston pelvic f.
Gouffon pin f.
graft f.
greenstick f.
Guyton-Noyes f.
Hackethal intramedullary bouquet f.
half-pin f.
hook f.
hook-plate f.
iliac f.
Ilizarov external f.
ingrowth f.
interference fit f.
intermaxillary f.
internal spinal f.
interosseous wire f.
intestinal f.
intramedullary bouquet f.
intramedullary rod f.

intraosseous f.
Kavanaugh-Brower-Mann f.
Kirschner pin f.
Kirschner wire f.
Kronner external f.
Kyle internal f.
lag screw f.
line of f.
loop f.
lumbar pedicle f.
lumbar spine segmental f.
lumbar spine transpedicular f.
Luque-Galveston f.
Luque loop f.
Luque rod f.
Magerl posterior cervical screw f.
mandibular f.
mandibulomaxillary f. (MMF)
Matta-Saucedo f.
maxillomandibular f. (MMF)
McKeever medullary clavicle f.
medial malleolus f.
medullary clavicle f.
medullary nail f.
mesh f.
metallic rod f.
microwave f.
monocular f.
multiple-point sacral f.
nail plate f.
nasomandibular f.
near f.
neutralization plate f.
Nichols sacrospinous f.
f. object
occipitocervical f.
odontoid fracture internal f.
odontoid screw f.
open reduction and internal f.
  (ORIF)
osseous f.
pedicle screw-rod f.
pedicular f.
pelvic f.
percutaneous f.
phalangeal fracture f.
Phemister acromioclavicular pin f.
pin f.
pin-and-plaster f.
plate f.
plate-screw f.
4-point f.
f. point
porous ingrowth f.
posterior cervical f.
posterior screw f.
posterior segmental f.
prophylactic skeletal f.
provisional f.

pubic f.
f. reflex
restorative f.
rigid internal f.
rigid plate f.
rod sleeve f.
role f.
rotatory f.
sacral pedicle screw f.
sacral spine f.
sacroiliac extension f.
sacroiliac flexion f.
sacrospinous ligament vaginal f.
sacrum fusion screw f.
Schneider f.
scoliotic curve f.
screw f.
screw-and-plate f.
screw-and-wire f.
secondary f.
segmental f.
skeletal f.
spinal f.
split f.
spring f.
standard formalin f.
staple f.
static f.
Steinmann pin f.
strut plate f.
sublaminar f.
sulcus f.
suture f.
f. suture technique
tack f.
f. target
f. technique
tension band f.
tibial fracture f.
transarticular wire f.
transcapitellar wire f.
transiliac rod f.
transodontoid screw f.
transpedicular screw-rod f.
transverse f.
TSRH rod f.
tunnel and sling f.
vaginal f.
white f.
wire-loop f.
fixator
  f. interne
  f. muscle
fixed
  f. deformity
  f. dose
  f. drain pipe urethra
  f. hiatal hernia
  f. lung

F

fixed (*continued*)
    f. maintainer space
    f. point
    f. subcutaneous dose
fixed-dose
    f.-d. analysis
    f.-d. patient-controlled analgesia
    (FDPCA)
fixture
    implant f.
FJP
    familial juvenile polyposis
flabby abdomen
FLACC
    face, leg, activity, cry, consolability
flaccida
    pars f.
flaccid extremity
flag flap
flail
    f. chest
    f. knee
Flajani
    F. iridectomy
    F. operation
flame hemorrhage
flame-shaped hemorrhage
flammable anesthetic
flank
    f. approach
    f. bone
    f. bulge post denervation
    f. dissection
    f. gunshot wound
    f. incision
    f. incisional hernia
    f. mass
    f. position
flap
    Abbe f.
    Abbe-Estlander f.
    Abbe-Estlander vascularized lip f.
    Abbe lip-switch f.
    abdominal fasciocutaneous f.
    access f.
    advancement f.
    advancement of rectal f.
    anconeus muscle f.
    anoplasty f.
    anterior helical rim free f.
    aponeurotic f.
    apron f.
    arm f.
    arterial f.
    arterialized f.
    artery island f.
    Atasoy-Kleinert hand advancement f.
    Atasoy palmar f.
    Atasoy triangular advancement f.

Atasoy-type f.
Atasoy volar V-Y f.
axial flag f.
axial pattern scalp f.
axillary f.
Baner f.
bicoronal scalp f.
bilateral V-Y Kutler f.
bilobed skin f.
bilobed transposition f.
bipedicle dorsal f.
bladder f.
Bland onlay f.
Blaskovics eyelid f.
Boari bladder f.
Boari-Ockerblad ureteral f.
bone f.
brachioradialis f.
breast f.
bridge pedicle f.
buccal mucosal f.
bulbocavernosus fat f.
buried f.
Burow triangle advancement f.
bursal f.
butterfly f.
Byers hypospadias f.
carrier f.
cartilage f.
caterpillar f.
cecal f.
cellulocutaneous f.
cervical f.
cheek advancement f.
cheek rotation f.
Chinese radial forearm f.
cocked-half f.
composite f.
compound f.
f. congestion
conjunctival f.
conjunctivo-Tenon f.
corneal f.
cross f.
crossarm f.
cross-finger f.
crossleg f.
crosslip pedicle f.
C-shaped scalp f.
cutaneous forearm f.
Cutler-Beard bridge f.
Dandy myocutaneous scalp f.
deep circumflex iliac artery-iliac
   crest f.
deep inferior epigastric perforator f.
   (DIEP)
deepithelialized rectus abdominis
   muscle f.
delayed f.

deltoid f.
deltopectoral f.
deltoscapular f.
dermal fat free f.
dermal fat pedicle f.
digastric muscle f.
digital f.
direct f.
distant f.
dorsal cross-finger f.
dorsal rotation f.
dorsal transposition f.
double lateral advancement f.
double pedicle TRAM f.
DRAM f.
duodenal f.
f. elevation
Eloesser thoracostomy f.
endorectal f.
envelope f.
epaulet f.
epidermal f.
equal sagittal f.
Estlander-Abbe lip reconstruction f.
Estlander lip reconstruction f.
extended shoulder f.
extended uvulopalatal f. (EUPF)
extensor carpi radialis longus f.
extraction f.
fascial f.
fasciocutaneous free f.
fasciocutaneous island f.
fat f.
fibular f.
Filatov-Gillies tubed f.
Filatov tubed f.
finger f.
finger-fillet f.
Fisher advancement f.
fishtail f.
flag f.
flat f.
foot first-web f.
foramen ovale f.
forearm f.
forehead f.
foreskin f.
forked f.
fornix-based f.
free bone f.
free fasciocutaneous f.
free fibular harvest f.
free latissimus dorsi f.
free microsurgical f.
free radial forearm f.
free skin f.
free temporal f.
French f.
Fujimori gate f.'s

full-thickness periodontal f.
fusiform f.
galeal f.
gastrocnemius sliding f.
Gilbert scapular f.
Gillies fan f.
gingival f.
glabellar bilobed f.
glabellar rotation f.
gluteal free f.
gluteus maximus f.
gracilis muscle f.
gracilis myocutaneous f.
f. graft
groin f.
Gunderson conjunctival f.
hemipulp f.
hemitongue f.
hinged corneal f.
horizontal f.
horseshoe-shaped f.
House rotational f.
Hughes tarsoconjunctival f.
hypogastric f.
ideal f.
iliac crest free f.
iliac crest osseous f.
iliac crest osteocutaneous f.
iliac crest osteomuscular f.
iliac osteocutaneous free f.
iliofemoral pedicle f.
immediate f.
Indian forehead nasal
  reconstruction f.
inferior f.
intercostal f.
intercostal muscle f.
interdigitating skin f.
internal oblique osteomuscular f.
interpolated f.
interpolation f.
intimal f.
intraoral f.
inverted skin f.
I-shaped scalp f.
island pedicle scalp f.
island skin f.
Italian inner arm nose
  reconstruction f.
jejunal free f.
jump f.
Karapandzic lip reconstruction f.
Karydakis pilonidal sinus f.
Koerner canal wall-down
  mestoidectomy f.
Kutler digital f.
Kutler double lateral advancement f.
Kutler V-Y f.
lateral cartilage f.

F

flap (*continued*)

latissimus dorsi island f.
latissimus dorsi muscle f.
latissimus dorsi musculocutaneous f.
latissimus dorsi myocutaneous f.
latissimus-scapular muscle f.
latissimus-serratus muscle f.
limbal-based f.
Limberg pilonidal disease f.
lined f.
lingual tongue f.
Linton perforator interruption f.
lip switch f.
liver f.
local muscle f.
local skin f.
lower trapezius f.
lumbrical muscle f.
major myocutaneous f.
maple leaf f.
Martius bulbocavernosus fat f.
masseter muscle f.
Mathieu island onlay f.
McCraw gracilis myocutaneous f.
McFarlane skin f.
McGregor temporal z-plasty
  eyelid f.
medial f.
melolabial f.
f. meniscal tear
mesiolabial bilobed transposition f.
microsurgical free f.
microvascular free f.
midline forehead f.
Moberg advancement f.
modified f.
modified dorsalis pedis myofascial f.
Morrison neurovascular free f.
mucoperichondrial f.
mucoperiosteal periodontal f.
mucoperiosteal sliding f.
mucosal advancement f.
mucosal periodontal f.
multistaged carrier f.
muscle f.
muscle-periosteal f.
musculocutaneous free f.
musculotendinous f.
Mustardé rotational cheek f.
myocutaneous f.
myodermal f.
myofascial f.
Nakajima cheiloplasty fan f.
nasolabial rotation f.
neck f.
f. necrosis
necrotic f.
neurocutaneous island f.
neurovascular free f.

neurovascular island pedicle f.
nutrient f.
oblique f.
Ockerblad-Boari ureteral f.
omental f.
omocervical f.
onlay island f.
open f.
opening f.
f. operation
f. operation cataract
Oriental V-Y f.
osseous f.
osteocutaneous f.
osteomuscular f.
osteomusculocutaneous f.
osteomyocutaneous f.
osteoperiosteal f.
osteoplastic f.
osteoplastic bone f.
palatal f.
palatine f.
palmar advancement f.
palmar cross-finger f.
parabiotic f.
paraexstrophy skin f.
parascapular f.
parasitic f.
partial-thickness f.
pectoralis major muscle f.
pectoralis major myocutaneous f.
  (PMMCF, PMMF)
pectoralis myocutaneous f.
pectoralis myofascial f.
pedicled myocutaneous f.
pedicle groin f.
peg f.
penile island f.
perforator f.
pericardial f.
pericoronal f.
pericranial temporalis f.
perineal f.
periodontal f.
periosteal f.
permanent pedicle f.
peroneal island f.
pharyngeal f.
f. physiology
platysma myocutaneous f.
Pontén fasciocutaneous f.
postangioplasty intimal f.
posterior f.
puborectalis fasciocutaneous f.
pulp f.
racket-shaped f.
radial-based f.
radial forearm f.
random cutaneous f.

random pattern f.
rectal f.
rectus abdominis free f. (RAFF)
rectus abdominis muscle f.
rectus abdominis
  musculocutaneous f.
rectus abdominis myocutaneous f.
  (RAMCF)
rectus femoris f.
rectus femoris fasciocutaneous f.
rectus femoris musculocutaneous f.
regional f.
remote pedicle f.
retinal f.
retroauricular free f.
reversal pedicle f.
reverse cross-finger f.
reverse forearm island f.
rhomboid transposition f.
rope f.
rotation f.
rotational f.
rotator f.
Rubens breast f.
saphenous f.
scalping f.
scalp sickle f.
scapular f.
Scardino vertical pyeloplasty f.
scleral f.
segmented f.
semilunar f.
serratus anterior muscle f.
shoulder f.
sickle f.
simple periodontal f.
single pedicle TRAM f.
skate flaps
skew f.
skin f.
sliding f.
soft tissue f.
Sorrin periodontal abscess f.
split-thickness periodontal f.
3-square f.
Steichen neurovascular free f.
stepladder f.
subcutaneous f.
superior f.
supramalleolar f.
supraorbital pericranial f.
supraperiosteal f.
surgical f.
Tait vaginal f.
tarsoconjunctival f.
f. technique
temporal f.
temporalis fascia f.
temporalis fascial f.

temporalis muscle f.
temporoparietal fascial f.
tendon f.
tensor fascia lata muscle f.
Tenzel rotational cheek f.
thenar f.
thoracoacromial f.
thoracoepigastric f.
tongue f.
f. tracheostomy
TRAM f.
transposition f.
transverse rectus abdominis
  muscle f.
trapezius f.
triangular advancement f.
triceps f.
Truc f.
tubed groin f.
tubed pedicle f.
tubularized cecal f.
tumbler f.
tummy tuck f.
turned-down tendon f.
turnover f.
tympanomeatal f.
umbilical f.
unipedicled f.
unipedicle transverse rectus
  abdominus f.
unrepositioned f.
upper trapezius f.
Urbaniak neurovascular free f.
Urbaniak scapular f.
U-shaped scalp f.
uvulopalatal f. (UPF)
van Lint f.
vascularized free f.
vascularized pericranial f.
ventrum penis f.
vertical f.
vesical f.
f. viability
visor f.
volar V-Y f.
von Langenbeck bipedicle
  mucoperiosteal f.
von Langenbeck pedicle f.
V-Y advancement f.
V-Y Kutler f.
waltzed f.
Warren vaginal anal incontinence f.
web space f.
Webster 3D-degree f.
Wei composite maxillary defect
  reconstruction f.
Widman gingival f.
winged V double f.
wraparound neurovascular free f.

F

flap (*continued*)
> Y-V rotational f.
> Zimany bilobed f.

flapping valve syndrome
flap-valve mechanism
4-flap Z-plasty
flash
> f. photolysis
> f. sterilization

flashback protocol
flashlamp facial
flashlight examination
flashpoint
flask closure
flat
> f. abdomen
> f. back deformity
> f. chest
> f. condyloma
> f. depressed lesion
> f. elevated lesion
> f. flap
> f. pelvis

flatfoot
> peroneal spastic f.

Flatt
> F. excision
> F. hand surgery technique
> F. upper extremity congenital anomaly classification

flattened duodenal fold
flatulence
flatulent
> f. colic
> f. dyspepsia

flatus tube insertion
Flechsig tract
Fleischmann bursa
Fleischner line
Fletcher rule of irradiation tolerance
flexed
> f. incision
> f. position

flexibility
Flexiblade laryngoscope
flexible
> f. collodion
> f. endofluoroscopy
> f. endoscopic surgery
> f. fiberoptic bronchoscopy
> f. fiberoptic endoscopy
> f. fiberoptic myeloscopy
> f. fiberoptic nasopharyngeal endoscopy
> f. hinge suspension
> f. laparoscopy
> f. lightwand-guided intubation
> f. nephroscopy
> f. sigmoidoscopy
> f. ureteropyeloscopy

flexion
> flexion, abduction, external rotation (faber)
> flexion, abduction, external rotation, extension (fabere)
> flexion, adduction, internal rotation, extension (fadire)
> f. and extension
> f. compression spine injury stabilization
> f. crease
> f. deformity
> f. fixation
> f. in abduction and external rotation (faber)
> f. in adduction and internal rotation (fadir)
> neck f.
> f. osteotomy
> f. teardrop fracture

flexion-extension
> f.-e. arc
> f.-e. axis
> f.-e. injury
> f.-e. maneuver
> f.-e. plane
> f.-e. reflex

flexion-internal
> f.-i. rotation
> f.-i. rotation deformity

flexion-inversion
> plantar f.-i.

flexion-rotation-drawer knee instability test
Flexon temporary cardiac pacing lead
flexor
> f. carpi radialis tendon
> f. digitorum longus tendon
> f. digitorum profundus tendon
> f. digitorum superficialis tendon
> f. hallucis brevis muscle
> f. hallucis brevis tendon
> f. hallucis longus muscle
> f. hallucis longus tendon
> f. pollicis longus abductorplasty
> f. pollicis longus tendon
> f. sheath
> f. tendon anastomosis
> f. tendon laceration
> f. tendon repair
> f. tendon rupture
> f. tenosynovectomy

flexorplasty
> Bunnell modification of Steindler f.
> Eyler f.
> Steindler f.

flexor-pronator
    f.-p. origin
    f.-p. origin release
flexura, *pl.* **flexurae**
flexurae (*pl. of* flexura)
flexural
flexure
    anorectal f.
    colic f.
    colon f.
    duodenojejunal f.
    fluctuant f.
    hepatic f.
    iliac f.
    inferior f.
    lumbar f.
    perineal f.
    right colic f.
    sigmoid f.
    splenic f.
    superior f.
flicker fusion
flicker-fusion
    f.-f. stimulus
    f.-f. threshold
flickering
    f. blockade
    f. blockade electrophysiology
Flick-Gould osteoarthritis dissecans of ankle repair technique
flight
1-flight exertional dyspnea
2-flight exertional dyspnea
flip-flap
    Mathieu-Horton-Devine f.-f.
    f.-f. procedure
    f.-f. technique
floating
    f. forehead operation
    f. gallbladder
    f. kidney
    f. liver
    f. organ
    f. rib
    f. spleen
floccillation
floccular fossa
flocculation
flocculonodular arteriovenous malformation
floor
    f. fracture
    rectal f.
floor-of-mouth
    f.-o.-m. closure
    f.-o.-m. lesion
floppy
    f. Nissen fundoplication
    f. Nissen fundoplication method

    f. Nissen fundoplication procedure
    f. Nissen fundoplication technique
    f. valve syndrome
floppy-type Nissen fundoplication
flora
    aerobic f.
    bacterial f.
    endogenous f.
    exogenous f.
    GI tract f.
    intestinal f.
    skin f.
florid
    f. duct lesion
    f. hyperplasia
flotation rate
flow
    anastomotic f.
    blood f.
    carotid arterial blood f.
    cerebral blood f. (CBF)
    f. convergence method
    f. detection technique
    f. direction
    Doppler color f.
    effective renal blood f.
    effective renal plasma f.
    endocardial f.
    exercise hyperemia blood f.
    free f.
    fresh gas f. (FGF)
    hepatofugal f.
    hepatopetal f.
    f. interruption technique
    intraluminal f.
    f. mapping technique
    microcirculatory f.
    nonpulsatile f.
    f. pattern
    peak expiratory f.
    plug f.
    pulsatile f.
    regional cerebral blood f. (rCBF)
    rotational blood f.
    f. technique filling
    tracheal blood f.
    tricuspid valve f.
    xenon-enhanced cerebral blood f.
flow-dependent
    f.-d. oxygen
    f.-d. pressure drop
flower
    F. bone
    F. dental index
flowmetry
    fluorescein f.
    laser Doppler f. (LDF)
    scanning laser Doppler f.
flow-over vaporizer

F

flow-volume loop
fluctuans
    myotonia f.
fluctuant
    f. abscess
    f. flexure
    f. mass
fluctuantes
    costae f.
fluctuation test
fluffy cotton-wool exudate
fluid
    ascitic f.
    f. aspiration
    bloody peritoneal f.
    body f.
    f. bolus
    carrier f.
    cerebrospinal f. (CSF)
    chylous ascitic f.
    clear f.
    cloudy f.
    f. collection
    cul-de-sac f.
    f. drainage
    endolymphatic f.
    f. evacuation
    extracellular f.
    f. extravasation
    f. filtration
    free peritoneal f.
    infused f.
    interstitial f.
    intracellular f.
    f. loading anesthetic technique
    loculation of f.
    maintenance f.
    f. management
    motor oil peritoneal f.
    oxygen-carrying resuscitative f.
    pancreatic f.
    perilymphatic f.
    peritoneal cavity f.
    pleural f.
    prostatic f.
    prune-juice peritoneal f.
    f. replacement
    respiratory tract f.
    f. resuscitation
    resuscitative f.
    scolicidal f.
    seminal f.
    serosal f.
    serosanguineous f.
    f. shift
    subphrenic f.
    supraphysiologic f.
    synovial f.
    turbid peritoneal f.

    f. warmer
    wound f.
fluid-attenuated
fluid-filled sac
fluid-gas exchange
fluke
    tissue f.
fluorescein
    f. angiography
    f. flowmetry
    f. fundus angioscopy
    f. instillation test
    f. string test
fluorescence
    f. intensity
    f. microscopy
    f. spectrophotometry
fluorescent
    f. electronic endoscopy
    f. optode technology
fluoride-induced nephrotoxicity
fluorinated hydrocarbon
fluorodeoxyglucose-positron
fluoroscopic
    f. control
    f. guidance
    f. insertion
    f. method
    f. placement
    f. pushing technique
    f. visualization
fluoroscopically
    f. guided corticosteroid injection
    f. guided low-volume peritendinous
      corticosteroid injection
fluoroscopy
    f. beam
    biplanar f.
    biplane f.
    C-arm f.
    lateral f.
    2-plane f.
    portable C-arm image intensifier f.
    rapid scan f.
flush
    f. aortogram
    f. method
flush-and-bathe technique
flushing
    postprandial f.
    f. technique
    vasoactive instability and f.
fluxmetry
    laser Doppler f.
Flynn femoral neck fracture reduction
FMD
    fibromuscular dysplasia
FMH
    fetal-maternal hemorrhage

FMIA
    Frankfort mandibular incisor angle
FMIV
    forced mandatory intermittent
      ventilation
fMRI
    functional magnetic resonance imaging
FNA
    fine-needle aspiration
      FNA biopsy
      follicular FNA
      Hürthle FNA
      indeterminate FNA
      nondiagnostic FNA
      percutaneous FNA
      FNA sample
      FNA specimen
      suspicious FNA
FNB
    femoral nerve block
FND
    functional neck dissection
FNH
    focal nodular hyperplasia
foaming exudate
FOB
    fiberoptic bronchoscope
    fiberoptic bronchoscopy
FOBT
    fecal occult blood testing
focal
    f. bleeding point
    f. calcification
    f. cortical dysplasia
    f. DCIS
    f. fatty infiltration
    f. granulomatous inflammation
    f. hemorrhage
    f. illumination
    f. image point
    f. infection
    f. neuropathy
    f. nodular hyperplasia (FNH)
    f. parenchymal brain lesion
    f. peritonitis
    f. plane
    f. segmental glomerulosclerosis
      (FSGS)
    f. splenic lesion
    f. tumor
foci (*pl. of* focus)
focus, *pl.* **foci**
    ectopic f.
    endometriotic f.
    hemorrhage f.
    image-space f.
    f. localization
    necrotic f.
    object-space f.

    f. of tumor
    residual f.
    septic f.
focused
    f. abdominal sonography
    f. abdominal sonography for trauma
      (FAST)
    f. assessment with sonography for
      trauma (FAST)
    f. radiation therapy
Foerster operation
Fogarty embolectomy catheter
fogging retinoscopy
Foix enucleation
folate-targeted imaging
fold
    adipose f.
    alar f.
    amniotic f.
    anterior axillary f.
    aryepiglottic f.
    axillary f.
    Bartlett nail f.
    caval f.
    cecal f.
    cholecystoduodenocolic f.
    circular f.
    circulator f.
    Douglas f.
    duodenojejunal f.
    duodenomesocolic f.
    epicanthal f.
    epigastric f.
    falciform retinal f.
    fimbriated f.
    flattened duodenal f.
    gastric f.
    gastropancreatic f.
    glossoepiglottic f.
    glossopalatine f.
    Guérin f.
    Hasner f.
    haustral f.
    hepatopancreatic f.
    Houston f.
    ileocecal f.
    incudal f.
    inferior duodenal f.
    inferior rectal f.
    inferior transverse rectal f.
    inframammary f.
    inguinal aponeurotic f.
    interureteric f.
    Kerckring f.
    labioscrotal f.
    lacrimal f.
    lateral glossoepiglottic f.
    lateral nail f.
    longitudinal f.

F

fold (*continued*)
 malar f.
 mallear f.
 median glossoepiglottic f.
 mucobuccal f.
 nail f.
 nasojugal f.
 Nélaton f.
 f. of laryngeal nerve
 palatoglossal f.
 palatopharyngeal f.
 palmate f.
 palpebronasal f.
 Passavant f.
 pharyngoepiglottic f.
 pleuroperitoneal f.
 presplenic f.
 rectal f.
 rectouterine f.
 rectovesical f.
 retinal f.
 right umbilical f.
 sacrogenital f.
 sacrouterine f.
 sacrovaginal f.
 sacrovesical f.
 salpingopalatine f.
 salpingopharyngeal f.
 sigmoid f.
 spiral f.
 sublingual f.
 superior duodenal f.
 superior rectal f.
 synovial f.
 tarsal f.
 tonsillar f.
 transverse palatine f.
 transverse rectal f.
 transverse vesical f.
 Treves f.
 triangular f.
 ungual labia f.
 urachal f.
 ureteric f.
 uterosacral f.
 uterovesical f.
 vascular f.
 Vater f.
 ventricular f.
 vestibular f.
 vocal f.
folding
 f. larynx
 skin f.
Foley
 F. operation
 F. Y-plasty pyeloplasty
 F. Y-V plasty
foliate papilla

follicle maturation stimulation
follicular
 f. carcinoma
 f. cell
 f. cholecystitis
 f. cyst
 f. epithelium
 f. FNA
 f. hematoma
 f. inflammation
 f. lesion
 f. neoplasm
 f. proliferation
 f. thyroid carcinoma
folliculi (*pl. of* folliculus)
folliculoma
folliculus, *pl.* **folliculi**
follow-up (*var. of* followup)
followup, follow-up
 clinical f.
 f. data
 f. evaluation
 f. examination
 long-term f.
 f. time
fondaparinux
Fones
Fontan
 F. atriopulmonary anastomosis
 F. fenestration closure
 F. modification of Norwood heart
  procedure
 F. operation
 F. repair
 F. revision
Fontana
 F. canal
 F. space
 space of F.
Fontan-Baudet tricuspid atresia repair
 procedure
fontanelle
 anterior f.
 anterolateral f.
 bregmatic f.
 cranial f.
 occipital f.
 posterior f.
Fontan-Kreutzer atriopulmonary
 anastomosis procedure
fonticuli (*pl. of* fonticulus)
fonticulus, *pl.* **fonticuli**
food
 F. and Drug Administration (FDA)
 f. bolus impaction
foot, *pl.* **feet**
 f. deformity
 diabetic f.
 f. first-web flap

goose f.
f. rotation
forage
f. core biopsy
f. procedure
foramen, *pl.* **foramina**
acoustic f.
anterior condyloid f.
aortic f.
blind f.
caroticoclinoid f.
carotid f.
cecal f.
f. compression test
conjugate f.
costotransverse f.
emissary sphenoidal f.
ethmoidal f.
external acoustic f.
Ferrein f.
frontal f.
great f.
Huschke f.
Hyrtl f.
incisive f.
inferior dental f.
infraorbital f.
internal auditory f.
internal neurocranial f.
intervertebral f.
jugular f.
lacerated f.
Luschka f.
Magendie f.
f. magnum
f. magnum line
malar f.
mandibular f.
mastoid f.
mental f.
Monro f.
Morgagni f.
nasal f.
foramina nervosa
nutrient f.
obturator f.
oculomotor f.
optic f.
f. ovale flap
palatine f.
papillary f.
parietal f.
petrosal f.
pleuroperitoneal f.
posterior condyloid f.
round f.
sacral f.
solitary f.
sphenoid emissary f.

sphenopalatine f.
sphenotic f.
stylomastoid f.
supraorbital f.
transverse f.
venous f.
vertebral f.
vertebroarterial f.
Vesalius f.
zygomaticofacial f.
zygomaticoorbital f.
zygomaticotemporal f.
foramina (*pl. of* foramen)
foraminal
f. approach
f. compression test
f. herniation
f. node
foraminalis
nodus lymphoideus f.
foraminotomy
Forane
Forbes modification of Phemister graft technique
force
f. application
f. feedback system
scar f.
f. translation
traumatic shear f.
forcé
redressement f.
force-couple splint reduction
forced
f. air warming
f. alimentation
f. duction test
f. expiratory capacity (FEC)
f. expiratory spirogram
f. expiratory time (FET)
f. expiratory volume (FEV)
f. expiratory volume in 1 second (FEV$_1$)
f. eye closure
f. generation test
f. mandatory intermittent ventilation (FMIV)
f. respiration
force-frequency relation
force-length relation
forceps
f. extraction
guidewire dilating f.
f. maneuver
f. removal
f. rotation
suture clip f.
suture tag f.
suture tying platform f.

F

force-velocity-length relation
force-velocity relation
force-velocity-volume relation
forcing
    dynamic end-tidal f.
forcipate
forcipressure
fore-and-aft suture technique
forearm
    f. amputation
    deep f.
    f. flap
    f. fracture
    f. graft
    f. graft arteriovenous
     fistula
    f. ischemic exercise test
    f. plethysmography
    superficial f.
    f. supination test
forebrain
forefoot arthroplasty
foregut
    f. cyst
    f. malformation
forehead
    f. flap
    f. reflectance oximetry
forehead-nose position
foreign
    f. body
    f. body aspiration
    f. body carcinogenesis
    f. body extraction
    f. body infection
    f. body loop
    f. body management
    f. body reaction
    f. body removal
    f. body response
    f. body retrieval
    f. body sclerotomy
    f. body trauma
    f. body tumorigenesis
foreign-body fibroblastic
  response
forekidney
Forel decussation
forequarter amputation
foreskin
    f. flap
    f. restoration
Forest I, II lesion
forestomach
forked flap
form
    extension f.
    face f.
    Pelvic Pain Assessment f.

    Quality of Well-Being Scale
     Self-Administered f.
    QWB-SA f.
formal
    f. celiotomy
    f. hemipelvectomy
    f. hepatic resection
    f. laparotomy
    f. method
    f. surgical exploration
formaldehyde catgut suture
formalin fixation
formatio, *pl.* **formationes**
formation
    abscess f.
    adhesion f.
    anastomotic stricture f.
    anterior synechia f.
    antiantibody f.
    antibody f.
    ascites f.
    aspergilloma f.
    balloon-cell f.
    blood vessel f.
    bone f.
    branching tubule f.
    bunion f.
    calculous f.
    callus f.
    cataract f.
    chiasma f.
    cloacal f.
    clot f.
    coagulum f.
    colloid f.
    colony f.
    concept f.
    crater f.
    cyclops f.
    echo f.
    excessive callus f.
    extra-capillary crescent f.
    false channel f.
    fistular f.
    gallstone f.
    Gothic arch f.
    granuloma f.
    hematoma f.
    hemostatic plug f.
    heterotopic bone f.
    hypertrophic scar f.
    identity f.
    ileostomy f.
    image f.
    impulse f.
    inflammatory pseudotumor f.
    intramembranous f.
    keloid f.
    kerion f.

ketone body f.
lappet f.
localized plaque f.
mesencephalic reticular f.
micelle f.
midbrain reticular f.
neocartilage f.
neointima f.
osteophyte f.
pancreatic fistula f.
pannus f.
paramedian pontine reticular f.
periosteal new bone f.
plaque f.
pontine paramedian reticular f.
posterior synechia f.
procallus f.
pseudoaneurysm f.
pseudotumor f.
reaction f.
reticular f.
root f.
rouleaux f.
sac f.
scar f.
somite f.
spur f.
star f.
stone granuloma f.
stricture f.
struvite crystal f.
symptom f.
synechia f.
thrombin f.
trellis f.
tumor f.
twin f.
web f.
formationes (*pl. of* formatio)
formication
formocresol pulpotomy
formula, *pl.* **formulas, formulae**
Cockroft-Gault glomerular filtration rate f.
formulae (*pl. of* formula)
formulas (*pl. of* formula)
formulation
depot f.
fornices (*pl. of* fornix)
fornix, *pl.* **fornices**
anterior vaginal f.
f. approach
calyceal f.
cerebral f.
conjunctival f.
pharyngeal f.
posterior vaginal f.
f. reformation
vaginal f.

fornix-based flap
fortification
fortified topical preparation
forward
f. coarticulation
f. head posture
f. traction test
f. triangle method
f. triangle technique
Fosnaugh nail biopsy
fospropofol disodium
fossa, *pl.* **fossae**
anterior cranial f.
axillary f.
Bichat f.
Biesiadecki f.
Broesike f.
canine f.
Claudius f.
cranial f.
crural f.
Cruveilhier f.
digastric f.
duodenal f.
duodenojejunal f.
epigastric f.
femoral f.
floccular f.
gallbladder f.
Gerdy hyoid f.
glenoid f.
greater supraclavicular f.
Gruber-Landzert f.
hepatorenal f.
hyoid f.
hypophysial f.
iliac f.
iliacosubfascial f.
f. iliacosubfascialis
iliopectineal f.
incisive f.
inferior duodenal f.
infraclavicular f.
infraduodenal f.
infraspinous f.
infratemporal f.
inguinal f.
intercondylar f.
intrabulbar f.
ischioanal f.
ischiorectal f.
Jobert de Lamballe f.
Jonnesco f.
jugular f.
juxtaauricular f.
lacrimal sac f.
Landzert f.
lesser supraclavicular f.
Malgaigne f.

F

fossa (*continued*)
    mandibular f.
    mastoid f.
    Merkel f.
    mesentericoparietal f.
    Mohrenheim f.
    Morgagni f.
    mylohyoid f.
    f. of Luschka
    omoclavicular f.
    paraduodenal f.
    parajejunal f.
    pararectal f.
    paravesical f.
    pericecal f.
    petrosal f.
    piriform f.
    pituitary f.
    popliteal f.
    posterior cranial f.
    preauricular f.
    pterygoid f.
    pterygomaxillary f.
    pterygopalatine f.
    retroduodenal f.
    retromandibular f.
    retromolar f.
    Rosenmüller f.
    scaphoid f.
    sigmoid f.
    sphenomaxillary f.
    splenic f.
    subarcuate f.
    subcecal f.
    subinguinal f.
    sublingual f.
    submandibular f.
    submaxillary f.
    subscapular f.
    superior duodenal f.
    supramastoid f.
    supraspinous f.
    supratonsillar f.
    supravesical f.
    temporal f.
    tonsillar f.
    Treitz f.
    triangular f.
    trochlear f.
    umbilical f.
    Velpeau f.
    vermian f.
    Waldeyer f.
    zygomatic f.
fossae (*pl. of* fossa)
fossula, *pl.* **fossulae**
    petrosal f.
fossulae (*pl. of* fossula)
fossulate

Foster suture
Fothergill
    F. prolapsed uterus suspension
    operation
    F. stitch
    F. suture
Fothergill-Donald operation
Fothergill-Hunter uterine prolapse repair
FotoFacial
Foucher epiphysial injury classification
foundation
    anhydrous facial f.
    denture f.
    facial f.
    level f.
    f. surface
fountain decussation
Fournier
    F. disease
    F. gangrene
    syphiloma of F.
fourth
    f. carpometacarpal joint fracture
    f. cranial nerve
    f. lumbar nerve
    f. parallel pelvic plane
fourth-degree radiation injury
fovea, *pl.* **foveae**
    Morgagni f.
    pterygoid f.
    trochlear f.
foveae (*pl. of* fovea)
foveola, *pl.* **foveolae**
    coccygeal f.
foveolae (*pl. of* foveola)
foveolar
Fowler-Philip
    F.-P. incision
    F.-P. retrocalcaneal exostosis
    approach
Fowler-Stephens
    F.-S. orchiopexy
    F.-S. spermatic vessel division
    procedure
    F.-S. spermatic vessel ligation
    maneuver
Fowles
    F. dislocation technique
    F. open reduction
Fox-Blazina pes anserinus transfer procedure
Fox operation
Fr
    French
    French scale
fraction
    alveolar dead-space f.
    right ventricular ejection f.
    (RVEF)

fractional
  f. area change (FAC)
  f. dilation and curettage
  f. epidural anesthesia
  f. spinal anesthesia
  f. sterilization
fractionated
  f. external beam irradiation
  f. radiation therapy
fractionation
  indicator f.
  f. protocol
fracture
  abduction-external rotation f.
  acetabular rim f.
  acute f.
  agenetic f.
  alveolar process f.
  alveolar socket wall f.
  anatomic f.
  Anderson-Hutchins unstable tibial
    shaft f.
  angulated f.
  angulation f.
  ankle mortise f.
  anterior column f.
  anterolateral compression f.
  apex f.
  apophysial f.
  arch f.
  articular mass separation f.
  articular pillar f.
  Atkin epiphysial f.
  atlantal f.
  atlas-axis combination f.
  atrophic f.
  avulsion stress f.
  axial loading f.
  axis f.
  axis-atlas combination f.
  backfire f.
  banana f.
  f. band
  Bankart f.
  Barton f.
  Barton-Smith f.
  basal neck f.
  basal skull f.
  baseball finger f.
  basilar femoral neck f.
  basilar skull f.
  beak f.
  f. bed
  bedroom f.
  Bennett comminuted f.
  bicondylar T-shaped f.
  bicondylar Y-shaped f.
  bicycle spoke f.
  bimalleolar ankle f.

  birth f.
  f. blister
  blow-in f.
  blow-out f.
  boot-top f.
  Bosworth f.
  both-bone f.
  both-column f.
  bowing f.
  boxer's f.
  f. bracing
  bronchial f.
  bucket-handle f.
  buckle f.
  bumper f.
  bunk-bed f.
  burst f.
  butterfly f.
  buttonhole f.
  calcaneal avulsion f.
  calcaneal displaced f.
  f. callus
  capillary f.
  capitate f.
  capitellar f.
  carpal bone stress f.
  carpometacarpal joint f.
  cartwheel f.
  cementum f.
  central f.
  cephalomedullary nail f.
  cerebral palsy pathological f.
  cervical spine f.
  cervicotrochanteric displaced f.
  Chance vertebral f.
  Chaput f.
  chauffeur's f.
  chip f.
  chiropractic treatment of f.
  chisel f.
  chondral f.
  circumferential f.
  f. classification
  clavicular birth f.
  clay shoveler's f.
  cleavage f.
  closed break f.
  closed skull f.
  coccyx f.
  Colles f.
  combination f.
  combined flexion-distraction injury
    and burst f.
  combined radial-ulnar-humeral f.
  comminuted intraarticular f.
  comminuted orbital f.
  comminuted skull f.
  complete f.
  complex f.

F

fracture (*continued*)

complicated f.
compound comminuted f.
compound skull f.
compressed f.
compression f.
condylar femoral f.
condylar process f.
congenital f.
contrecoup f.
coracoid f.
corner f.
coronal split f.
coronoid process f.
cortical f.
Cotton ankle f.
cough f.
cranial f.
crown f.
crown-root f.
crush f.
crushed eggshell f.
Danis-Weber f.
dashboard f.
dens f.
dentate f.
depressed skull f.
depression f.
de Quervain f.
derby hat f.
Descot f.
diacondylar f.
diametric pelvic f.
diaphysial f.
diastatic skull f.
dicondylar f.
die punch f.
direct f.
f. disease
dishpan f.
f. dislocation
dislocation f.
displaced f.
distal femoral epiphysial f.
distal humeral f.
distal radial f.
distraction of f.
dog-leg f.
dome f.
double f.
Dupuytren f.
Duverney f.
dyscrasic f.
elbow f.
elementary f.
enamel f.
f. en coin
endocrine f.
endplate compression f.

f. en rave
epicondylar avulsion f.
epiphysial growth plate f.
epiphysial slip f.
epiphysial tibial f.
Essex-Lopresti joint depression f.
explosion f.
expressed skull f.
extension teardrop f.
external orbital f.
extracapsular f.
extraoctave f.
facial f.
fatigue f.
femoral diaphysial f.
femoral epiphysial f.
femoral intertrochanteric f.
femoral neck f.
femoral shaft f.
femoral supracondylar f.
fender f.
fetal bone f.
f. fever
fibular f.
fifth metatarsal base f.
fighter's f.
finger f.
first carpometacarpal joint f.
fishmouth f.
fissured f.
f. fixation
flexion teardrop f.
floor f.
forearm f.
fourth carpometacarpal joint f.
f. fragment
frontal sinus f.
Gaenslen f.
Galeazzi f.
f. gap
Garden femoral neck f.
glenoid rim f.
Gosselin f.
greater trochanteric femoral f.
greater tuberosity f.
greenstick f.
growing f.
growth plate f.
Guérin f.
gunshot f.
Gustilo-Anderson open clavicular f.
gutter f.
Hahn-Steinthal f.
hairline f.
hamate tail f.
hangman f.
head-splitting humeral f.
healed f.
healing f.

f. healing
hemicondylar f.
Henderson f.
Hermodsson f.
hickory-stick f.
high-energy f.
Hill-Sachs f.
hip f.
hockey-stick f.
Hoffa f.
Holstein-Lewis f.
hoop stress f.
horizontal maxillary f.
humeral head-splitting f.
humeral physial f.
humeral shaft f.
humeral supracondylar f.
Hutchinson f.
hyoid bone f.
ice skater's f.
iliofemoral wing f.
impacted f.
implant f.
impression f.
incomplete compound f.
indirect f.
inflammatory f.
infraction f.
insufficiency f.
intercondylar femoral f.
intercondylar humeral f.
intercondylar tibial f.
internal fixation f.
interperiosteal f.
intertrochanteric femoral f.
intertrochanteric 4-part f.
intraarticular proximal tibial f.
intracapsular f.
intraoperative f.
intrauterine f.
inverted-Y f.
ipsilateral acetabular f.
ipsilateral femoral neck f.
ipsilateral femoral shaft f.
ipsilateral pelvic f.
ipsilateral tibial f.
irreducible f.
Jefferson f.
joint depression f.
Jones f.
juxtacortical f.
knee f.
Kocher f.
Kocher-Lorenz f.
laminar f.
lap seatbelt f.
laryngeal cartilage f.
lateral condylar humeral f.
lateral mass f.

Laugier f.
lead-pipe f.
Le Fort I–III f.
Le Fort fibular f.
Le Fort mandibular f.
Le Fort-Wagstaffe f.
lesser trochanter f.
f. line
linear skull f.
Lisfranc f.
loading f.
long bone f.
longitudinal f.
loose f.
lorry driver's f.
low-energy f.
lower extremity f.
low lumbar spine f.
lumbar spine burst f.
lumbosacral junction f.
Maisonneuve fibular f.
malar f.
Malgaigne pelvic f.
malleolar f.
mallet f.
malunited calcaneus f.
malunited forearm f.
malunited radial f.
mandibular body f.
mandibular condyle f.
mandibular ramus f.
mandibular symphysis f.
march f.
marginal ridge f.
maternal f.
maxillary f.
maxillofacial f.
mesiodistal f.
metacarpal neck f.
metaphysial tibial f.
metatarsal f.
midface f.
midfoot f.
midshaft f.
Milkman f.
minimally displaced f.
missed f.
Moberg-Gedda f.
molar tooth f.
monomalleolar ankle f.
Monteggia forearm f.
Montercaux f.
Moore f.
Mouchet f.
multangular ridge f.
multilevel f.
multiple f.
multiray f.
nasal f.

F

fracture (*continued*)
    nasoorbital f.
    navicular f.
    naviculocapitate f.
    neck f.
    neoplastic f.
    neurogenic f.
    neuropathic f.
    nightstick f.
    nonarticular distal radial f.
    noncontiguous f.
    nondisplaced f.
    nonphysial f.
    nonrotational burst f.
    nonunion f.
    nonunited f.
    nutcracker f.
    oblique f.
    obturator avulsion f.
    occipital condyle f.
    occult f.
    odontoid condyle f.
    odontoid neck f.
    olecranon f.
    open-book f.
    open-break f.
    open skull f.
    open type I, II, III, IIIA, IIIB, IIIC f.
    orbital blow-out f.
    orbital floor f.
    orbital rim f.
    orbital wall f.
    osteochrondral slice f.
    osteoporotic f.
    outlet strut f.
    pacemaker lead f.
    Pais f.
    paratrooper's f.
    1-part f.
    2-part f.
    3-part f.
    4-part f.
    patellar sleeve f.
    pathological f.
    Pauwels f.
    pedicle f.
    pelvic avulsion f.
    pelvic ring f.
    pelvic straddle f.
    pelvic type A, B, C f.
    pelvic type I, II AP compression f.
    pelvic type I, II lateral compression f.
    penetrating f.
    penile f.
    periarticular f.
    periprosthetic f.
    peritrochanteric f.

    petrous pyramid f.
    phalangeal diaphysial f.
    physial f.
    Piedmont f.
    pillion f.
    pillow f.
    pilon ankle f.
    ping-pong f.
    pisiform f.
    plafond f.
    plaque f.
    plastic bowing f.
    pond f.
    porcelain f.
    Posada f.
    posterior arch f.
    posterior column f.
    posterior element f.
    posterior ring f.
    posterior wall f.
    postirradiation f.
    postoperative f.
    Pott f.
    Pott ankle f.
    pronation-abduction f.
    pronation-eversion f.
    proximal femoral f.
    proximal humeral f.
    proximal tibial metaphysial f.
    pyramidal f.
    radial head f.
    radial neck f.
    radial styloid f.
    f. reduction
    f. repair
    reverse Barton f.
    reverse Colles f.
    reverse Monteggia f.
    rib f.
    ring f.
    ring-disrupting f.
    Rolando f.
    roof f.
    root f.
    rotation f.
    rotational burst f.
    sacral f.
    sacroiliac f.
    sacrum f.
    sagittal slice f.
    Salter I–VI f.
    Salter-Harris f.
    scaphoid f.
    scotty dog f.
    seatbelt f.
    secondary f.
    segmental f.
    Segond f.
    sentinel spinous process f.

SER type I–IV f.
shaft f.
shear f.
Shepherd f.
short oblique f.
sideswipe elbow f.
simple skull f.
single f.
f. site (FS)
skier's f.
Skillern f.
skull f. (SF)
sleeve f.
slice f.
slot f.
Smith f.
spinal compression f.
spine f.
spinous process f.
spiral oblique f.
splintered f.
split f.
split-heel f.
splitting f.
spontaneous f.
sprain f.
sprinter's f.
f. stabilization
stable burst f.
stairstep f.
stellate skull f.
Stieda f.
straddle f.
stress f.
strut f.
subcapital f.
subperiosteal f.
subtrochanteric femoral f.
supination-adduction f.
supination-eversion f.
supination-external rotation type
  I–IV f.
supraclavicular f.
supracondylar humeral f.
supracondylar Y-shaped f.
surgical neck f.
suture f.
T f.
talar avulsion f.
talar neck f.
talar osteochondral f.
tarsal bone f.
T condylar f.
teacup f.
teardrop f.
temporal bone f.
tension f.
testis f.
thoracic spine f.

thoracolumbar burst f.
thoracolumbar spine f.
through-and-through f.
thrower's f.
tibial bending f.
tibial condyle f.
tibial diaphysial f.
tibial open f.
tibial plafond f.
tibial plateau f.
tibial shaft f.
tibial triplane f.
tibial tuberosity f.
Tillaux f.
Tillaux-Chaput f.
Tillaux-Kleiger f.
toddler's f.
tongue f.
tooth f.
torsional f.
torus f.
trabecular bone f.
tracheal f.
traction f.
trampoline f.
transcaphoid f.
transcapitate f.
transcervical femoral f.
transchondral f.
transcondylar f.
transepiphysial f.
transhamate f.
transiliac f.
translational f.
transsacral f.
transscaphoid dislocation f.
transtriquetral f.
transverse comminuted f.
transverse facial f.
transversely oriented endplate
  compression f.
transverse maxillary f.
transverse process f.
trapezium f.
traumatic f.
trimalleolar ankle f.
triplane tibial f.
tripod f.
triquetral f.
trophic f.
tuft f.
type I, II, III, IIIA, IIIB, IIIC
  open f.
ulnar f.
uncinate process f.
uncomminuted f.
undisplaced f.
unicondylar f.
unimalleolar f.

F

fracture *(continued)*
 unstable f.
 ununited f.
 Vancouver f.
 vertebral body f.
 vertebral compression f.
 vertebral stable burst f.
 vertebral wedge compression f.
 vertebra plana f.
 vertical shear f.
 vertical tooth f.
 Volkmann f.
 wagon-wheel f.
 Wagstaffe f.
 Walther f.
 wedge compression f.
 wedge-shaped uncomminuted tibial
  plateau f.
 willow f.
 Wilson f.
 Y f.
 Y-T f.
 zygomatic arch f.
 zygomatic-maxillary complex f.
 zygomaticomaxillary f.
fracture-dislocation
 atlantoaxial f.-d.
 Bennett f.-d.
 carpometacarpal f.-d.
 Galeazzi f.-d.
 Lisfranc f.-d.
 pedicolaminar f.-d.
 perilunate f.-d.
 posterior f.-d.
 f.-d. reduction
 tarsometatarsal f.-d.
 thoracolumbar spine f.-d.
 tibial plateau f.-d.
 transcapitate f.-d.
 transhamate f.-d.
 transtriquetral f.-d.
 unstable f.-d.
 volar plate arthroplasty technique
  f.-d.
fragment
 articular f.
 avascular f.
 avulsed f.
 bone f.
 bony f.
 butterfly fracture f.
 capital f.
 catheter f.
 caudal f.
 cephalad f.
 chondral f.
 cortical f.
 disc f.
 distal f.

 f. E
 extruded disc f.
 fracture f.
 free f.
 free disc f.
 free-floating cartilaginous f.
 hinged f.
 hypervascular f.
 loose f.
 metallic f.
 osteochondral f.
 placental f.
 residual f.
 retained placental f.
 sternal f.
 trapdoor f.
 tuberosity f.
fragmentation
 elastic fiber f.
 electrohydraulic f. (EHF)
 graft f.
 laser-induced f.
 stone f.
 ultrasonic f.
Fraley syndrome
frame application
frame-based stereotaxis
frameless
 f. stereotactic guidance
 f. stereotactic surgery
 f. stereotaxis
framework
 implant f.
Franceschetti
 F. coreoplasty
 F. corepraxy
 F. deviation operation
 F. keratoplasty operation
 F. pupil deviation operation
 F. syndrome
frank
 f. diabetes
 f. dislocation
 f. hemorrhage
 f. intrabiliary rupture
 f. necrosis
 F. nonsurgical perineal
  autodilation
 f. perforation
 F. permanent gastrotomy
  technique
 f. pus
 f. rigors
 F. technique of dilation
Fränkel
 F. neurologic deficit classification
 F. white line
Frankenhäuser ganglion
Franke tabes operation

Frankfort
- F. horizontal light line
- F. horizontal plane
- F. mandibular incisor angle (FMIA)
- F. mandibular plane angle

Frank-Starling
- F.-S. curve
- F.-S. relation

Frantz-O'Rahilly limb defect classification

frappage therapy

Fraser syndrome

Fraunfelder no-touch intraocular malignant melanoma technique

Fraunhofer line

Frazier
- F. incision
- F. suction

Frazier-Spiller
- F.-S. operation
- F.-S. rhizotomy

FRC
- functional residual capacity

freckle
- Hutchinson f.

Fredet-Ramstedt
- F.-R. extramucosal longitudinal myotomy procedure
- F.-R. pyloromyotomy

Fredrickson hyperlipoproteinemia classification

Fredrickson-Levy-Lees hyperlipoproteinemia classification

free
- f. air
- f. bone flap
- f. disc fragment
- f. fasciocutaneous flap
- f. fat graft (FFG)
- f. fibular harvest flap
- f. flap transfer
- f. flow
- f. fragment
- f. fragment disc
- f. fragment herniation
- f. gastric margin
- f. hepatic venous pressure
- f. latissimus dorsi flap
- f. ligature suture technique
- f. microsurgical flap
- f. node
- f. peritoneal fluid
- f. radial forearm flap
- f. radical scavenger
- f. rupture
- f. skin flap
- f. temporal flap
- f. tenia
- f. tenotomy
- f. tissue transfer

free-beam coagulation

Freebody-Bendall-Taylor transperitoneal lumbar fusion technique

free-floating
- f.-f. canalith
- f.-f. cartilaginous fragment
- f.-f. particle

free-flowing drainage

freehand
- f. method
- f. suturing technique

Freeman calcaneal fracture classification

Freer dissection

free-root insertion technique

freeway space

freezing
- gastric f.
- f. point

frena (*pl. of* frenum)

frenal

French (F, Fr)
- F. cardiac surgery risk score
- F. energetic acupuncture
- F. flap
- F. fracture technique
- F. lateral closing wedge osteotomy
- F. method
- F. plane
- F. position
- F. scale (F, Fr)
- F. supracondylar fracture operation

French-American-British (FAB)
- F.-A.-B. acute leukemia classification
- F.-A.-B. staging

frenectomy

frenoplasty

frenotomy

frenula (*pl. of* frenulum)

frenulectomy

frenuloplasty

frenulum, *pl.* **frenula**
- lingual f.
- synovial frenula

frenum, *pl.* **frena**
- Morgagni f.
- synovial f.

Frenzel middle ear pressure maneuver

frequency
- ciliary beat f.
- median f.
- f. modulation
- respiratory f.
- wavelength f.

frequency-difference interferential current therapy

frequency-duration index

F

fresh
- f. blood clot
- f. extrapelvic ovarian transplant
- f. frozen plasma (FFP)
- f. gas flow (FGF)
- f. tissue allocation
- f. wound

Fresnel membrane
freta (*pl. of* fretum)
fretum, *pl.* **freta**
Freund
- F. anomaly
- F. thorax resection

Frey
- F. pancreatic head resection and lateral pancreaticojejunostomy procedure
- F. pancreaticojejunostomy
- F. syndrome

friable clot
Friberg microsurgical agglutination test
Fricke reconstructive blepharoplasty
friction
- intraabdominal f.
- f. knot

Friede full-thickness eye wall resection
Friedenwald eyelid ptosis operation
Friedenwald-Guyton blepharoptosis operation
Friedewald approximation
Fried-Hendel tendon technique
fringe
- Richard f.
- synovial f.

frogleg
- f. lateral projection
- f. position

Froimson
- F. bicipital groove keyhole technique
- F. tendon interposition thumb procedure

Froimson-Oh upper limb tendon interposition repair
frondlike filling defect
frons
frontal
- f. abscess
- f. arteriovenous malformation
- f. artery
- f. bone
- f. border
- f. branch
- f. cortical approach
- f. craniotomy
- f. crest
- f. eminence
- f. foramen
- f. gyrectomy

- f. lobotomy
- f. margin
- f. notch
- f. plane
- f. plane correction
- f. projection
- f. recess
- f. section
- f. sinus
- f. sinus cavity
- f. sinus fracture
- f. sinus mucocele
- f. sinus septoplasty
- f. squama
- f. suture
- f. triangle
- f. tuber
- f. vein
- f. x-ray
- f. x-ray view

frontalis
- f. muscle
- f. sling procedure
- f. sling technique

frontalium
frontoanterior fetal position
frontoethmoidal
- f. mucocele
- f. suture

frontoethmoidalis
- sutura f.

frontoethmoidectomy
frontolacrimalis
- sutura f.

frontolateral laryngectomy
frontomalar
frontomaxillaris
- sutura f.

frontomaxillary suture
frontonasal
- f. duct
- f. suture

frontonasalis
- sutura f.

frontonasomaxillary osteotomy
frontooccipital
frontoorbital osteotomy
frontoparietal
- f. arteriovenous malformation
- f. suture

frontopontine tract
frontoposterior fetal position
frontosphenoidal process
frontosphenoid suture
frontotemporal
- f. approach
- f. craniotomy
- f. tract

frontotransverse fetal position

frontozygomatic suture
Froriep induration
Frost
    F. ingrown nail procedure
    F. stitch
    F. suture
    F. suture technique
frosted liver
Frost-Lang implantation of metal ball in Tenon capsule operation
Frouin
frown incision
frozen
    f. section
    f. section analysis
    f. section diagnosis
    f. section method
fructose infusion
Frykman
    F. distal radius fracture classification
    F. radial fracture classification
FSGS
    focal segmental glomerulosclerosis
Fuchs
    F. canthorrhaphy
    F. iris bombé transfixation
    F. position
fugax
    proctalgia f.
Fuhrman nuclear grading system
Fujimori gate flaps
Fukala lens removal
fulcrum line
Fulford subtalar arthrodesis procedure
fulgurant
fulgurating
fulguration (fulg), direct fulguration, indirect fulguration
    electrical f.
    electrosurgical f.
    endoscopic f.
    nephroscopic f.
full
    f. axillary dissection
    f. cardiopulmonary bypass
    f. cast restoration
    f. diagnostic laparoscopy
    f. extension
    f. mastopexy
    f. shoulder preparation
full-body cutaneous examination
fullness
    epigastric f.
full-spine radiographic examination
full-stomach precautions
full-thickness
    f.-t. burn
    corneal f.-t.
    f.-t. periodontal flap

    f.-t. rectal aspiration
    f.-t. wound
fulminant
    f. hepatic failure (FHF)
    f. hepatitis
    f. hyperpyrexia
functio laesa
function
    atrioventricular nodal f.
    autonomous f.
    bowel f.
    cardiovagal f.
    compromised systolic f.
    effective f.
    electrophysiologic f.
    gait f.
    graft f.
    hemodynamic f.
    hepatocellular f.
    homeostatic f.
    liver f.
    mucociliary f.
    neorectal f.
    neurologic f.
    preoperative liver f.
    pulmonary f.
    renal f.
    sinuatrial nodal f.
functional
    f. activation PET scanning
    f. capacities assessment
    f. capacity classification
    f. capacity evaluation
    f. capillary density
    f. castration
    f. constipation
    f. contracture
    f. electrical stimulation
    f. endoscopic sinus surgery (FESS)
    f. intestinal failure
    f. lymph node dissection
    f. magnetic resonance imaging (fMRI)
    f. neck dissection (FND)
    f. neuromuscular stimulation
    f. orthodontic therapy
    f. outcome
    f. parenchyma
    f. prepubertal castration syndrome
    f. problem
    f. renal tissue
    f. repair
    f. residual capacity (FRC)
    f. sleep disorder
    f. sphincter
    f. stereotactic neurosurgery
    f. technique
    f. veloplasty
functioning allograft

F

fundal plication
fundament
fundectomy
fundi (*pl. of* fundus)
fundic
    f. patch
    f. wrap
fundiform ligament
fundoplasty
    anterior f.
    Belsey IV f.
    270-degree laparoscopic posterior f.
    esophagogastric f.
    Gomez f.
    Hill f.
    laparoscopic esophagogastric f.
    Nissen f.
    posterior f.
    Thal f.
    Thal-Nissen f.
    Toupet f.
fundoplication
    Belsey Mark IV f.
    Belsey partial f.
    Belsey 2/3 wrap f.
    bolstering partial posterior f.
    Collis-Nissen f.
    Dor anterior f.
    endoscopic f.
    floppy Nissen f.
    floppy-type Nissen f.
    Guarner wrap f.
    Heller myotomy with Dor f.
    Heller plus Nissen f.
    herniated f.
    high-resistance f.
    Hill gastropexy f.
    Hunter technique for Toupet f.
    intrathoracic Nissen f.
    laparoscopic anterior partial f.
    laparoscopic esophagogastroplasty
      with Nissen f.
    laparoscopic Nissen f. (lap Nissen)
    laparoscopic Nissen and Toupet f.
    low-resistance f.
    microlaparoscopic Nissen f.
    modified Belsey f.
    Nissen f.
    Nissen-Rossetti f.
    open f.
    open Nissen f.
    redo f.
    Rossetti-Hell modification of
      Nissen f.
    Rossetti modification of
      Nissen f.
    slipped Nissen f.
    Thal f.
    total f.

    Toupet hemifundoplication f.
    transthoracic Nissen f.
    twisted f.
    uncut Collis-Nissen f.
    videoscopic f.
fundus, *pl.* **fundi**
    f. gland
    f. microscopy
    f. rotation gastroplasty
funduscopic examination
fundusectomy
fungal
    f. antibody
    f. organism
    f. overgrowth
    f. pancreatic infection
    f. pathogen
    f. sinusitis
    f. species
    f. superinfection
fungating
    f. mass
    f. sore
    f. tumor
fungemia
fungi (*pl. of* fungus)
fungous infection
fungus, *pl.* **fungi**
    pancreatic f.
funic reduction
funicular
    f. excision
    f. graft
    f. inguinal hernia
    f. process
funiculi (*pl. of* funiculus)
funiculopexy
funiculus, *pl.* **funiculi**
funnel
    f. chest deformity
    f. stitch
funnelization of metaphysis
funnel-shaped pelvis
furcalis
    nervus f.
furcal nerve
furcation
    f. canal
    denuded f.
    invaded f.
    root f.
Furlow-Fisher
    F.-F. modification
    F.-F. modification of Virag 1
      erectile failure microsurgical
      operation
Furlow palatal lengthening procedure
Furniss anastomosis
furrier's suture technique

furrow
> corneal marginal f.
> digital f.
> mentolabial f.

furrowing

fusca lamina

fusiform
> f. aneurysm
> f. dilation
> f. excision
> f. flap

fusing point

fusion
> Adkins spinal f.
> Albee spinal f.
> amplitude of f.
> Anderson ankle f.
> ankle f.
> anterior cervical discectomy and f. (ACDF)
> anterior lumbar vertebral interbody f.
> anterior spinal f. (ASF)
> f. area
> atlantoaxial f.
> atlantooccipital f.
> autograft f.
> Bailey-Badgley cervical spine f.
> binaural f.
> binocular f.
> Blair f.
> Bosworth spinal f.
> Bradford f.
> Brooks-type f.
> calcaneotibial f.
> central f.
> centric f.
> cervical interbody f.
> cervical spine posterior f.
> Chandler hip f.
> Charnley compression-type knee f.
> Chuinard-Peterson ankle f.
> clothespin H spinal f.
> Cloward anterior spinal f.
> Cloward back f.
> Coltart calcaneotibial f.
> commissural f.
> f. complex
> convex f.
> Copeland-Howard scapulothoracic f.
> 4-corner midcarpal f.
> Davis f.
> Dewar posterior cervical f.
> DIP f.
> distal interphalangeal f.
> distal tibiofibular f.
> dowel spinal f.
> endoscopic spinal f.
> extraarticular hip f.

> extraarticular subtalar f.
> eyelid f.
> facet f.
> f. faculty
> f. fascia
> first-grade f.
> flicker f.
> Gallie spinal f.
> Gallie subtalar ankle f.
> Glissane ankle f.
> f. grade
> Hall facet f.
> Harris-Smith cervical f.
> Henry-Geist spinal f.
> H-graft f.
> Hibbs-Jones spinal f.
> hip f.
> Horwitz-Adams ankle f.
> f. implantation
> f. in situ
> in situ spinal f.
> interbody spinal f.
> interfacet wiring and f.
> intertransverse f.
> intraarticular hip f.
> intraarticular knee f.
> joint f.
> Kellogg-Speed lumbar spinal f.
> King intraarticular hip f.
> knee f.
> labial f.
> Langenskiöld f.
> lateral f.
> long-segment spinal f.
> lower cervical spine f.
> lumbar interbody f.
> lumbar spinal f.
> lumbar spine f.
> lumbar vertebral interbody f.
> lumbosacral f.
> lunotriquetral f.
> Michaelson vertebral f.
> midcarpal f.
> motor f.
> müllerian duct f.
> naviculocuneiform f.
> f. nonunion rate
> occipitocervical f.
> pantalar f.
> partial wrist f.
> f. peptide
> peripheral f.
> posterior cervical f.
> posterior interbody lumbar spinal f.
> posterior-lateral lumbar spinal f.
> posterior lumbar interbody f. (PLIF)
> posterior spinal f.
> posterolateral interbody f. (PLIF)
> posterolateral lumbosacral f.

F

fusion (*continued*)
  radiolunate f.
  radioscaphoid f.
  f. reflex
  robertsonian f.
  Robinson cervical spine f.
  root f.
  sacral spine f.
  scaphocapitate f.
  scaphotrapeziotrapezoidal f.
  scapulothoracic f.
  second-grade f.
  selective thoracic spine f.
  sensory f.
  short-segment spinal f.
  Simmons cervical spine f.
  single-level spinal f.
  Smith-Petersen sacroiliac joint f.
  Smith-Robinson anterior f.
  Smith-Robinson cervical f.
  Smith-Robinson interbody f.
  Soren ankle f.
  spinal f.
  splenogonadal f.
  2-stage hip f.
  Stamm procedure for intraarticular
    hip f.
  f. stiffness

  symmetric vertebral f.
  talocalcaneal f.
  talonavicular f.
  f. technique
  third-grade f.
  thoracic facet f.
  thoracic spinal f.
  tibiofibular f.
  tibiotalar f.
  tibiotalocalcaneal f.
  tissue f.
  total wrist f.
  trapeziometacarpal f.
  triscaphe f.
  upper cervical spine f.
  urethrohymenal f.
  vertebral f.
  vertebral interbody f.
  Watson scaphotrapeziotrapezoidal f.
  f. welding
  White posterior ankle f.
  whole-arm f.
  Wilson ankle f.
  Wiltberger posterior interbody f.
  Wiltse bilateral lateral f.
  Winter convex f.
fusion-free position
Futcher line

G
  gastric
    G syndrome
    G tube
GA
  general anesthesia
gabapentin
Gabitril
GAD
  generalized anxiety disorder
Gaenslen
    G. fracture
    G. split-heel incision
    G. split-heel technique
Gail
    G. model
    G. model of breast cancer risk
      prediction
Gaillard-Arlt suture
Gaines and Ford technique for determining adequate lengthening of tendo Achillis
gait
    antalgic g.
    g. function
    vaulting g.
galactocele
galactography
galactophorous
    g. canal
    g. duct
galea
galeal flap
Galeati gland
galeatomy
Galeazzi
    G. fracture
    G. fracture-dislocation
    G. patellar operation
Galen
    G. anastomosis
    G. nerve
galenic
    g. preparation
    g. venous malformation
gallamine triethiodide
gallbladder
    g. agenesis
    body of g.
    calcified g.
    calculous g.
    g. calculus
    g. cancer
    g. carcinoma
    g. colic

    distended g.
    g. distention
    g. duplication
    g. ectopia
    g. ejection rate
    floating g.
    g. fossa
    g. neck
    g. perforation
    g. plate
    porcelain g.
    g. removal
    stasis g.
    g. wall abscess
gallbladder-vena cava line
gall duct
galli
    crista g.
Gallie
    G. ankle arthrodesis
    G. ankle arthrodesis
      procedure
    G. atlantoaxial fusion wiring
      technique
    G. spinal fusion
    G. subtalar ankle fusion
    G. transplant
gallstone
    g. colic
    g. disease
    g. formation
    g. ileus
    Mercedes-Benz sign for g.'s
    g. migration
    g. pancreatitis
    silent g.
    symptomatic g.'s
GALT
  gastrointestinal-associated lymphoid
    tissue
  gut-associated lymphoid
    tissue
galvanic stimulation
galvanocautery
galvanosurgery
Galveston
    G. pelvic fixation
    G. spinopelvic reconstruction
      technique
Gambee
    G. suture
    G. suture technique
Gambee-type suture
gamekeeper's thumb
  dislocation

G

gamete
  g. intrafallopian tube transfer (GIFT)
  g. manipulation
  g. micromanipulation
Gamgee tissue
gamma
  g. irradiation
  g. loop disorder
  g. probe localization
  g. thalamotomy
gamma-amino butyric acid receptor
gammagraphy
gamma-probe radiolocalization
Gamna-Gandy body
ganglia (*pl. of* ganglion)
ganglial tissue
gangliated
  g. cord
  g. nerve
gangliectomy
gangliocytoma
ganglioglioma
gangliolysis
  percutaneous radiofrequency g.
ganglioma
  intracerebral g.
ganglion, *pl.* **ganglia, ganglions**
  aberrant g.
  Acrel g.
  Andersch g.
  aorticorenal g.
  Arnold g.
  Auerbach g.
  auricular g.
  basal g.
  g. blockage
  g. blocker
  Bock g.
  carotid g.
  celiac g.
  cervical g.
  cervicothoracic g.
  ciliary g.
  coccygeal g.
  cochlear g.
  g. cyst
  dorsal root g.
  Ehrenritter g.
  episcleral g.
  Frankenhäuser g.
  gasserian g.
  geniculate g.
  glossopharyngeal g.
  hypogastric g.
  g. impar block
  inferior cervical g.
  inferior mesenteric g.
  intermediate g.

  intervertebral g.
  intracranial g.
  jugular g.
  lacrimal g.
  Laumonier g.
  Lee g.
  Lobstein g.
  Ludwig g.
  lumbar g.
  Meckel g.
  mesenteric g.
  middle cervical ganglia
  nasociliary g.
  nodose g.
  oculomotor g.
  optic g.
  otic g.
  parasympathetic g.
  paravertebral g.
  pelvic g.
  petrosal g.
  petrous g.
  phrenic g.
  ganglia plexuum autonomicorum
  prevertebral g.
  pterygopalatine g.
  Remak g.
  renal g.
  Ribes g.
  sacral g.
  Scarpa g.
  Schacher g.
  semilunar g.
  Soemmerring g.
  solar g.
  sphenopalatine g.
  spinal g.
  spiral g.
  splanchnic g.
  stellate g.
  sublingual g.
  submandibular g.
  submaxillary g.
  superior g.
  superior cervical g.
  superior mesenteric g.
  thoracic g.
  trigeminal g.
  vertebral g.
  vestibular g.
  Vieussens g.
  Walther g.
ganglionated bowel
ganglionectomy
  cervical g.
  dorsal root g.
  Meckel sphenopalatine g.
  sphenopalatine g.
  superior cervical g.

ganglioneuroblastoma
ganglioneuroma
ganglioneuromatosis
    diffuse transmural g.
ganglionic
    g. blockade
    g. branch
ganglionostomy
ganglions (*pl. of* ganglion)
gangrene
    appendiceal g.
    arteriosclerotic g.
    bacterial synergistic g.
    cold g.
    cutaneous g.
    decubital g.
    diabetic g.
    dry g.
    embolic g.
    emphysematous g.
    Fournier g.
    gas g.
    hemorrhagic g.
    hot g.
    Meleney g.
    moist g.
    nosocomial g.
    Pott g.
    pressure g.
    primary g.
    progressive bacterial
     synergistic g.
    secondary g.
    static g.
    thrombotic g.
    traumatic g.
    venous g.
    wet g.
    white g.
gangrenosum
    pyoderma g.
gangrenous
    g. appendicitis
    g. cholecystitis
    g. granulomatous inflammation
    g. hernia
Ganley forefoot osseous reconstruction
  technique
Ganoderma lucidum
gantry rotation
Ganzfeld stimulation
gap
    Bochdalek g.
    esophageal g.
    fracture g.
    interincisor g.
GAPP FCE
    Gibson Approach to Functional
    Capacity Evaluation

Garceau
    G. cheilectomy
    G. tendon technique
garden
    G. femoral neck fracture
    G. femoral neck fracture
     classification
    g. spade deformity
Gardner
    G. meningocele repair
    G. operation
    G. syndrome
Garré
    sclerosing osteomyelitis of G.
Garrett orientation line
Gartland
    G. forefoot reconstruction
     procedure
    G. humeral supracondylar fracture
     classification
    G. Universal radial fracture
     classification
Gartner
    G. canal
    G. duct
Gärtner method
gas
    g. abscess
    anesthetic g.
    g. anesthetic
    arterial blood g. (ABG)
    blood g.
    g. chromatography
    g. chromatography-mass spectrometry
     (GC-MS)
    g. clearance method
    g. collection
    g. contamination
    g. density line
    g. embolism
    g. emission
    g. endarterectomy
    g. exchange
    extraluminal g.
    extravasation g.
    g. gangrene
    g. incontinence
    inspired g.
    g. insufflation
    laparoscopic g.
    nonanesthetic g.
    serial blood g.
    g. sterilization
    g. trapping
    venous blood g.
    volume of alveolar g.
     (V_A)
    xenon g.
gas-bloat syndrome

G

gaseous
- g. cholecystitis
- g. decompression
- g. dilation
- g. distention
- g. laparoscopy
- g. laparoscopy method
- g. laparoscopy procedure
- g. laparoscopy technique

gas-fluid exchange

gas-forming
- g.-f. liver abscess
- g.-f. pyogenic liver infection

Gaskell bridge

gasless
- g. endoscopic thyroidectomy
- g. laparoscopic approach
- g. laparoscopic hysterectomy
- g. laparoscopy
- g. laparoscopy method
- g. laparoscopy procedure
- g. laparoscopy technique

gas-producing streptococcal infection

gasserectomy

gasserian
- g. ganglion
- g. ganglion block
- g. ganglion blockade

gastrectasia (*var. of* gastrectasis)

gastrectasis, gastrectasia

gastrectomy
- Billroth I, II g.
- Billroth I partial g.
- curative radical total g.
- distal with excision of ulcer g.
- esophagoproximal g.
- hand-assisted laparoscopic g.
- high subtotal g.
- Hofmeister g.
- Horsley g.
- Japanese standard g.
- Japanese-style g.
- laparoscopic-assisted distal g.
- laparoscopic-assisted subtotal g.
- laparoscopic remnant g.
- laparoscopic total g.
- limited g.
- near-total g.
- palliative total g.
- pancreatic-preserving total g.
- partial g.
- Pólya g.
- proximal g.
- pylorus-preserving g. (PPG)
- radical total g.
- segmental g.
- sleeve g.
- g. specimen
- standard D1 g.

standardized curative radical total g.
subtotal g.
total g.
video-assisted g.

gastric (G)
- g. accommodation test
- g. adenocarcinoma
- g. angioma
- g. antral vascular ectasia (GAVE)
- g. antrum
- g. area
- g. arteriovenous malformation
- g. artery
- g. atony
- g. atrophy
- g. balloon implantation
- g. band
- g. bed
- g. bed metastasis
- g. branch
- g. bulge
- g. bypass
- g. bypass procedure (GBP)
- g. bypass surgery
- g. calculus
- g. canal
- g. cancer
- g. cardia
- g. chloric acid
- g. coin removal
- g. compression
- g. cuff
- g. cytology
- g. decompression
- g. devascularization
- g. dilation
- g. distention
- g. drain
- g. drainage procedure
- g. duplication
- g. duplication cyst
- g. electrical stimulation
- g. emptying
- g. emptying procedure (GEP)
- g. epithelial cell infiltration
- g. epithelium
- g. fistula
- g. fluid aspiration
- g. fold
- g. foreign body
- g. freezing
- g. fundus wrap
- g. gland
- g. hemorrhage
- g. hernia
- g. impression
- g. infection
- g. inhibitory peptide
- g. insufflation

g. leiomyoma resection
g. loop bypass
g. malignancy
g. MALT lymphoma
g. margin
g. mass
g. mucosa
g. mucosal barrier
g. mucosal hypercapnia
g. mucosal pattern classification
g. mucosal pH
g. non-Hodgkin lymphoma
g. outlet obstruction (GOO)
g. pacemaker region
g. partitioning procedure
g. patch esophagoplasty
g. perforation
g. perforation peritonitis
g. pit
g. polypectomy
g. pouch
g. pressure
g. protection agent
g. pullthrough procedure
g. pull-up
g. pullup procedure
g. reduction surgery
g. reflux
g. remnant
g. residue examination
g. rupture
g. segment
g. serosa
g. stapling
g. stromal tumor
g. stump carcinoma
g. tonometry
g. tube (GT, G tube)
g. tube esophagoplasty
g. tubulization
g. ulcer
g. ulceration
g. vagotomy
g. valve tightening
g. valve tightening method
g. valve tightening procedure
g. valve tightening technique
g. variceal bleeding
g. vein
g. vessel
g. volvulus
g. wall
g. wrap
gastric-longitudinal
deep g.-l. (DG-L)
gastric-transverse
deep g.-t. (DG-T)
gastricus
gastrinoma triangle

gastrin secretion
gastritis
alkaline reflux g. (ARG)
phlegmonous g.
gastroanastomosis
gastrocardiac
gastrocele
gastrocnemius
Baker tongue in groove slide lengthening of distal aponeurosis of g.
Silfverskiöld transplantation of heads of origin of g.
Silver and Simon modification of Silfverskiöld procedure with selective neurectomy of g.
g. sliding flap
gastrocolic
g. fistula
g. ligament
g. omentum
g. reflux
g. vein
gastrocolostomy
gastrocutaneous fistula
gastrocystoplasty
gastrodiaphragmatic ligament
gastroduodenal
g. anastomosis
g. artery (GDA)
g. complication
g. fistula
g. mucosa
g. mucosal protection
g. orifice
gastroduodenopancreatectomy
gastroduodenoscopy
gastroduodenostomy
Billroth I g.
Jaboulay g.
vagotomy and antrectomy with g.
gastroendoscopy
gastroenteric fistula
gastroenteroanastomosis
gastroenterocolostomy
gastroenterologist
gastroenteropancreatic (GEP)
gastroenteroplasty
gastroenteroptosis
gastroenterostomy
Balfour g.
Billroth I, II g.
Braun-Jaboulay g.
Courvoisier g.
Finney g.
Heineke-Mikulicz g.
Hofmeister g.
g. intussusception
laparoscopic g.

G

gastroenterostomy (*continued*)
    percutaneous g. (PGE)
    Pólya g.
    prophylactic g.
    Roux g.
    Roux-en-Y g.
    Schoemaker g.
    short limb Roux-en-Y g.
    side-to-side g.
    g. stoma
    truncal vagotomy and g.
    von Haberer g.
    Wölfler g.
gastroenterotomy
gastroepiploic
    g. arcade
    g. artery (GEA)
    g. artery graft
    g. vein
    g. vessel
gastroesophageal (GE)
    g. hernia
    g. junction (GEJ)
    g. reflux
    g. reflux disease (GERD)
    g. variceal plexus
    g. vestibule
gastroesophagostomy
gastrogastric fistula
gastrogastrostomy
gastrogavage
gastrohepatic
    g. ligament
    g. omentum
gastroileac augmentation
gastroileostomy
gastrointestinal (GI)
    g. anastomosis (GIA)
    g. anomaly
    g. bleeding
    g. carcinoma
    g. complication
    g. condition
    g. content
    g. continuity
    g. endoscopy
    g. endothelium
    g. fistula
    g. infection
    g. lesion
    g. malignancy
    g. metastasis
    g. pop-off silk suture
    g. problem
    G. Quality of Life Index (GIQLI)
    g. resection
    g. stoma
    g. stricture
    g. stromal tumor (GIST)

    g. surgery
    g. surgical gut suture
    g. surgical linen suture
    g. surgical silk suture
    g. tract
    g. tract dysfunction
    g. ulceration
    upper g. (UGI)
gastrointestinal-associated lymphoid tissue (GALT)
gastrointestinal-cutaneous fistula
gastrojejunal
    g. anastomosis
    g. loop obstruction syndrome
    g. reconstruction
gastrojejunocolic fistula
gastrojejunostomy (GJ)
    antecolic long-loop isoperistaltic g.
    Billroth II g.
    compression button g.
    loop g.
    partial inferior retrocolic end-to-side g.
    partial superior retrocolic end-to-side g.
    percutaneous endoscopic g. (PEG-J)
    prophylactic g.
    retrocolic end-to-side g.
    Roux-en-Y g.
    total retrocolic end-to-side g.
    g. tube
gastrolavage
gastrolienal ligament
gastrolith
gastrolithiasis
gastrolysis
gastronesteostomy
gastroomental
    g. artery
    g. node
gastropancreatic
    g. fold
    g. vagovagal reflex
gastroparesis
    postsurgical g.
    postvagotomy g.
gastropathy
    indomethacin-induced g.
gastropexy
    anterior g.
    Belsey Mark IV g.
    belt loop g.
    Boerema anterior g.
    circumcostal g.
    Hill posterior g.
    incisional g.
    laparoscopic-assisted g.
    percutaneous anterior g.
    posterior diaphragmatic g.

T-fastener g.
T-tack g.
gastrophrenic
  g. anchorage
  g. ligament
gastrophrenicum
gastroplasty
  adjustable ring g.
  Albert-Lembert g.
  banded g.
  Collis g.
  Collis-Nissen g.
  Eckhout vertical g.
  fundus rotation g.
  Gomez horizontal g.
  greater curvature banded g.
  hand-assisted laparoscopic
    vertical-banded g.
  horizontal g.
  Kuzmak g.
  laparoscopic g.
  layer-to-layer g.
  Mason morbid obesity vertical
    banded g.
  Mason vertical banded g.
  McLean banded g.
  open vertical banded g.
  silicone elastomer ring vertical g.
    (SRVG)
  Stamm g.
  tubular vertical g.
  unbanded g.
  V-banded g.
  vertical adjustable banded g.
  vertical banded g. (VBG)
  vertical ring g. (VRG)
  vertical silastic ring g.
  V-Y g.
gastropleural fistula
gastroplication
gastropneumonic
gastroprotective drug
gastroptosia (*var. of* gastroptosis)
gastroptosis, gastroptosia
gastroptyxis
gastropulmonary
gastropylorectomy
gastropyloric
gastrorrhagia
gastrorrhaphy
gastrorrhexis
gastroschisis hernia
gastroscope
  Benedict blind perforating g.
gastroscopic
gastroscopy
  high-magnification g.
  infrared transillumination g.
gastrosphincteric pressure gradient

gastrosplenic
  g. ligament
  g. omentum
gastrosplenicum
gastrostaxis
gastrostenosis
gastrostogavage
gastrostolavage
gastrostomy
  Beck g.
  Beck-Carrel-Jianu g.
  button 1-step g.
  Depage-Janeway g.
  drainage g.
  dual percutaneous endoscopic g.
  endoscopic g.
  g. feeding
  feeding g.
  Gauderer-Ponsky-Izant percutaneous
    endoscopic g.
  Glassman g.
  Janeway g.
  Kader g.
  Kader-Senn g.
  laparoscopic g.
  Olympus g.
  palliative g.
  Partipilo g.
  percutaneous endoscopic g. (PEG)
  radiologic percutaneous g. (RPG)
  Russell percutaneous endoscopic g.
  g. scarring
  Spivack g.
  Ssabanejew-Frank g.
  Stamm g.
  surgical g.
  tube g.
  g. tube (GT, G tube)
  ultrasound-assisted percutaneous
    endoscopic g.
  venting percutaneous g. (VPG)
  Witzel g.
gastrotomy
  anterior g.
  Depage-Janeway g.
gastrulation
GAT
  Goldmann applanation tonometer
gate
  spinal g.
gate-control
  g.-c. hypothesis
  g.-c. theory
gated technique
Gatellier-Chastang
  G.-C. ankle approach
  G.-C. incision
  G.-C. posterolateral approach
Gaucher disease

G

Gauderer-Ponsky-Izant percutaneous endoscopic gastrostomy
Gauderer-Ponsky percutaneous endoscopic operation
Gaur retroperitoneal balloon distention technique
gaussian line
gauze dissection
gavage
Gavard muscle
GAVE
    gastric antral vascular ectasia
Gay gland
Gaynor-Hart position
GBP
    gastric bypass procedure
GC-MS
    gas chromatography-mass spectrometry
GCS
    Glasgow coma scale
    Glasgow coma score
GDA
    gastroduodenal artery
GE
    gastroesophageal
        GE junction
GEA
    gastroepiploic artery
        GEA graft
Geenen-Hogan unexplained biliary symptoms classification
Geenen sphincterotomy
GEJ
    gastroesophageal junction
gel
    g. filtration
    ketamine g.
gelatin
    g. compression body
    modified fluid g.
gelatinous
    g. acute inflammation
    g. ascites
    g. carcinoma
    g. infiltration
gelation
Gelfoam particles transarterial embolization treatment
Gell and Coombs drug allergy classification
gelling phenomenon
Gelpi-Lowry hysterectomy
Gély
    G. suture
    G. suture technique
gemination
gemistocyte
gemistocytoma

gender dimorphism
gene
    ether-a-go-go g.
    g. replacement therapy
    g. silencing
    g. transfer therapy
general
    g. adaptation reaction
    g. anesthesia
    g. anesthetic
    g. anesthetic technique
    g. bloodletting
    g. closure
    g. closure suture
    g. endotracheal anesthesia
    g. laparoscopic surgical procedure
    g. radiation
    g. surgeon
    g. thoracic surgery
    g. thrust manipulation
generales termini
generalized
    g. anxiety disorder (GAD)
    g. cortical hyperostosis
    g. elastolysis
    g. peritonitis
genetic
    g. abnormality
    g. anomaly
    g. condition
    g. diagnosis
    g. lesion
    g. marker
    g. testing
geneticist
    clinical g.
genetics
    cancer g.
    molecular g.
genial tubercle
genicular
    g. anastomosis
    g. artery
geniculate
    g. body
    g. ganglion
    g. neuralgia
geniculocalcarine
    g. radiation
    g. tract
geniculotemporal tract
geniculum
genioglossal muscle
genioglossus
geniohyoglossus
geniohyoid
    g. fascia

g. muscle
g. space
geniohyoideus
genion
genioplasty
augmentation g.
genital
g. branch
g. carcinoma
g. condyloma
g. cord
g. duct
g. eminence
g. gland
g. infection
g. organ
g. papulosquamous lesion
g. reconstruction
g. swelling
g. tract
g. tract trauma
g. tract tumor
g. tubercle
g. ulcer
g. ulceration
genitalia
ambiguous external g.
external g.
indifferent g.
genitocrural nerve
genitofemoral
g. causalgia
g. nerve
g. nerve block
g. neurectomy
genitoinguinal ligament
genitoplasty
feminizing g.
masculinizing g.
genitourinary (GU)
g. anomaly
g. apparatus
g. evaluation
g. fistula
g. infection
g. tract
Gennari
line of G.
gentle
g. blunt dissection
g. compression
g. traction
genu, *pl.* **genua**
g. valgum
g. valgum deformity
g. varum
g. varum deformity
genua (*pl. of* genu)
genual

genucubital position
genufacial position
genupectoral position
geographic stippling
geometric
g. equator
g. supracondylar extension
osteotomy
George line
GEP
gastric emptying procedure
gastroenteropancreatic
GEPA
gastroepiploic artery
GER
gastroesophageal reflux
Gerbert-Mellilo hallux Z-osteotomy method
Gerbert osteotomy
Gerbode anuloplasty
GERD
gastroesophageal reflux disease
Gerdy
G. fiber
G. hyoid fossa
G. tubercle
geriatric
g. anesthesia
g. injury
Gerlach
G. tonsil
G. valve
G. valvula
germ
g. line
g. tube
g. tube test
German method
germinal
g. cord
g. epithelium
g. matrix
g. matrix hemorrhage
g. membrane
germinoma
Gerota
G. capsule
G. fascia
gestant anomaly
gestational sac
Ghon
G. complex
G. primary lesion
GI
gastrointestinal
GI oncology
GI pop-off silk suture
GI tract
GI tract flora

G

315

GIA
gastrointestinal anastomosis
Giannestras
G. modification of Lapidus hallux valgus technique
G. oblique metatarsal osteotomy
giant
g. cell arteritis
g. cell astrocytoma
g. cell lesion
g. colon
g. condyloma
g. fibroadenoma
g. prosthetic reinforce
g. prosthetic reinforcement of visceral sac (GPRVS)
Giardia infection
Gibbon hernia
gibbous deformity
Gibson
G. Approach to Functional Capacity Evaluation (GAPP FCE)
G. long vertical relaxing incision
G. posterior hip approach
G. suture technique
Gibson-Piggott osteotomy
Gibson-type incision
Giemsa-stained section
Gierke respiratory bundle
Gifford delimiting keratotomy
GIFT
gamete intrafallopian tube transfer
gift wrap suture technique
Gigli lateral os pubis section
Gilbert scapular flap
Gilbert-Tamai-Weiland free fibular bone transfer technique
Gilchrist urinary diversion procedure
Giliberty bipolar femoral head
Gill
G. laminectomy
G. laminectomy procedure
G. lesion
G. massive sliding graft
G. sliding graft technique
Gilles soft palate reconstruction
Gilliam-Doleris
G.-D. operation
G.-D. uterine suspension
Gilliam operation
Gillies
G. bone graft
G. fan flap
G. fractured zygoma elevation
G. horizontal dermal suture
G. scar correction
Gillies-Millard cocked-hat thumb reconstruction technique

Gill-Jonas modification of Norwood hypoplastic left heart procedure
Gill-Manning-White spondylolisthesis technique
Gillquist procedure
Gil-Vernet
G.-V. anti-vesicoureteral reflux technique
G.-V. ileocecal cystoplasty
G.-V. ileocecal cystoplasty urinary diversion
G.-V. ileocecocystoplasty procedure
G.-V. ureterocystoneostomy
Gimbernat ligament
gingiva, *pl.* **gingivae**
gingivae (*pl. of* gingiva)
gingival
g. anatomy
g. artery
g. augmentation
g. cavity
g. cavity wall
g. deformity
g. exudate
g. exudation
g. finishing line
g. fistula
g. flap
g. hemorrhage
g. inflammation
g. point
g. position
g. space
g. stimulation
g. tissue
g. tissue esthetics
g. zone
gingivectomy
chemosurgical g.
Ochsenbein g.
gingivolabial groove
gingivoplasty
ginglymoarthrodial
ginglymoid joint
ginglymus
helicoid g.
lateral g.
Giordano suburethral sling operation
GIQLI
Gastrointestinal Quality of Life Index
GIQLI score
Girard keratoprosthesis operation
girdle
g. anesthesia
pelvic g.
shoulder g.
thoracic g.

Girdlestone
  G. arthroplasty of hip resection
  G. laminectomy
  G. orthopedic procedure
Girdlestone-Taylor muscle transfer clawtoe repair procedure
Gironcoli hernia
girth
  abdominal g.
GIST
  gastrointestinal stromal
  tumor
Gittes
  G. endoscopic bladder neck
  suspension
  G. endoscopic bladder neck
  suspension procedure
  G. genitourinary technique
  G. urethrocystopexy
Gittes-Loughlin
  G.-L. bladder neck suspension
  G.-L. needle bladder suspension
  procedure
GJ
  gastrojejunostomy
  GJ tube
Gl
  glabella
glabella (Gl)
glabellar
  g. bilobed flap
  g. exposure osteotomy
  g. rotation flap
  g. tapping
gladiate
gladiolus
glancing wound
gland
  abnormally hyperplastic g.
  abnormal parathyroid g.
  accessory parotid g.
  accessory suprarenal g.
  accessory thyroid g.
  acid g.
  acinous g.
  admaxillary g.
  adrenal g.
  aggregate g.
  agminate g.
  Albarran g.
  anterior lingual g.
  apical g.
  apocrine g.
  g. appearance
  areolar g.
  arteriococcygeal g.
  arytenoid g.
  Aselli g.
  axillary sweat g.

Bartholin g.
Bauhin g.
Blandin g.
Blandin-Nuhn g.
Boerhaave g.
Bowman g.
brachial g.
bronchial g.
Brunner g.
bulbourethral g.
celiac g.
cervical g.
circumanal g.
coccygeal g.
contralateral parathyroid g.
Cowper g.
cutaneous g.
dominant g.
ductless g.
duodenal g.
Duverney g.
eccrine sweat g.
ectopic sebaceous g.
Eglis g.
endocrine g.
enlarged parathyroid g.
entrapped g.
esophageal ectopic sebaceous g.
fundus g.
Galeati g.
gastric g.
Gay g.
genital g.
Gley g.
greater vestibular g.
Guérin g.
Havers g.
hematopoietic g.
hypercellular g.
hyperplastic g.
inferior g.
inguinal g.
intestinal g.
ipsilateral g.
Knoll g.
labial g.
lactiferous g.
laryngeal g.
lesser vestibular g.
Lieberkühn g.
lingual g.
Littré g.
Luschka g.
lymph g.
mammary g.
master g.
Meibom g.
meibomian g.
Méry g.

G

gland (*continued*)
   mesenteric g.
   milk g.
   Moll g.
   Montgomery g.
   mucilaginous g.
   muciparous g.
   mucous g.
   nondominant g.
   Nuhn g.
   odoriferous g.
   oil g.
   palatine g.
   parathyroid g.
   paraurethral g.
   parotid g.
   peptic g.
   perspiratory g.
   Peyer g.
   pharyngeal g.
   pineal g.
   pituitary g.
   Poirier g.
   prehyoid g.
   preputial g.
   prostate g.
   pyloric g.
   remnant g.
   g. removal
   retrosternal g.
   Rivinus g.
   Rosenmüller g.
   salivary g. (SG)
   sebaceous g. (SG)
   seminal g.
   seromucous g.
   serous g.
   sexual g.
   g. size
   Skene g.
   solitary g.
   subinguinal salivary g.
   sublingual g.
   submandibular g. (SMG)
   substernal g.
   sudoriferous g.
   supernumerary g.
   suprahyoid g.
   suprarenal g.
   synovial g.
   target g.
   tarsal g.
   thymus g.
   thyroid g.
   tracheal g.
   trachoma g.
   Tyson g.
   urethral g.
   uterine g.

   vaginal g.
   vesical g.
   vestibular g.
   g. volume
   von Ebner g.
   vulvovaginal g.
   Waldeyer g.
   Wasmann g.
   Wepfer g.
   Wölfler g.
   Zeis g.
4-gland
   4-g. hyperplasia
   4-g. parathyroid visualization
glandes (*pl. of* glans)
glandula, *pl.* **glandulae**
   g. atrabiliaris
   glandulae tubariae
glandulae (*pl. of* glandula)
glandular
   g. branch
   g. cancer
   g. carcinoma
   g. element
   g. epithelium
   g. substance
   g. tissue
glandulectomy
glandulopexy
glans, *pl.* **glandes**
   g. penis
glansplasty
   meatal advancement and g.
    (MAGPI)
glanuloplasty
Glanzmann thrombasthenia
glaserian fissure
Glasgow
   G. coma scale (GCS)
   G. coma score (GCS)
   G. Outcome Scale
    (GOS)
   G. Outcome Score (GOS)
glass-bead retention method
Glassman gastrostomy
glass-rod
   g.-r. negative phenomenon
   g.-r. positive phenomenon
glass-wool filtration
glassy membrane
glaucoma
   g. surgery
   uncontrollable g.
glaucomatous
   g. cul-de-sac
   g. excavation
   g. ring
Gleason score
Gleich osteotomy

Glenn
    G. anastomosis
    G. congenital cyanotic heart disease correction
    G. shunt
    G. superior vena cava to right pulmonary artery anastomosis procedure

Glenn-Anderson
    G.-A. perioscrotal transposition repair technique
    G.-A. ureteroneocystostomy

glenohumeral
    g. adhesive capsulitis
    g. articulation
    g. dislocation repair
    g. joint
    g. joint dislocation

glenoid
    g. cavity
    g. fossa
    g. osteotomy
    g. point
    g. rim fracture
    g. surface

glenoplasty
    posterior g.
    Scott posterior g.

Gley gland
glial
    g. cell
    g. ring
    g. tumor

GlideScope Cobalt video laryngoscope
gliding-hole-first technique
gliding joint
glioblastoma
glioma
    low-grade g.
    malignant g.
    mixed malignant g.
    g. sarcomatosum

glioma-polyposis
gliomatous
glioneuroma
gliosarcoma
gliosis
gliotic membrane
Glissane ankle fusion
Glisson
    G. capsule
    G. sphincter

glissonian
    g. capsule
    g. pedicle
    g. sheath

global
    g. hemostasis
    g. hypoperfusion

    g. pain assessment (GPA)
    g. pain intensity
    G. Severity Index (GSI)

globi (*pl. of* globus)
globular collection
globule
    fat g.

globulin
    antilymphocyte g.

globus, *pl.* **globi**
    g. hystericus
    g. sensation

glomangioma
glomangiomatous osseous malformation syndrome
glomangiosarcoma
glomangiosis
    pulmonary g.

glomectomy
glomerular, glomerulose
    g. basement membrane disease
    g. capillary pressure
    g. capsule
    g. crescent
    g. extracellular matrix
    g. filtration
    g. filtration rate
    g. hyperfiltration
    g. macrophage infiltration
    g. neutrophil infiltration
    g. tip lesion
    g. ultrafiltration

glomerulation
glomeruli (*pl. of* glomerulus)
glomerulitis
glomerulonephritides (*pl. of* glomerulonephritis)
glomerulonephritis, *pl.* **glomerulonephritides**
    membranoproliferative g.

glomerulosa
glomerulosclerosis
    focal segmental g. (FSGS)

glomerulose (*var. of* glomerular)
glomerulus, *pl.* **glomeruli**
glomus
    g. arteriovenous malformation
    g. body
    g. coccygeum
    g. tumor

glossectomy, glossosteresis
    Commando radical g.
    partial g.
    radical g.
    subtotal g.
    total g.

glossocinesthetic
glossodynia
glossoepiglottic fold

G

glossopalatine
- g. fold
- g. muscle

glossopharyngeal
- g. ganglion
- g. nerve
- g. nerve block
- g. nerve root
- g. neuralgia

glossopharyngeus
glossoplasty
glossorrhaphy
glossoscopy
glossosteresis (*var. of* glossectomy)
glossotomy
- labiomandibular g.
- median labiomandibular g.

glottic
- g. carcinoma
- g. closure
- g. insufficiency
- g. stenosis

glottidis
- rima g.

glottidospasm (*var. of* laryngospasm)
glove anesthesia
gloved-fist technique
Glover suture technique
glucagonlike peptide 1
glucagonoma syndrome
Gluck incision
glucocorticoid-producing adrenal adenoma
glucocorticoid receptor
glucose oxidase method
glucuronidation
glue
- fibrin g.
- g. patch
- g. patch leak

glue-in suture
glutamatergic
- g. drug
- g. neurotransmission
- g. release
- g. transmission

glutamate toxicity
glutamic-oxaloacetic transaminase
glutamic pyruvic transaminase
glutaraldehyde sterilization
glutathione modification
gluteal
- g. fascia
- g. free flap
- g. hernia
- g. line
- g. region

gluteofemoral bursa
gluteoinguinal

gluteus
- g. maximus flap
- g. maximus muscle
- g. medius
- g. medius muscle
- g. minimus muscle

glycerin (*var. of* glycerol)
- g. method

glycerol, glycerin
- g. chemoneurolysis
- g. rhizotomy

glycine receptor
glycogen
- g. infiltration
- g. synthase kinase

glycol
- polyethylene g.

glycopyrrolate
glycosis
- anaerobic g.

Glypressin
gnathic index
gnathoplasty
gnathoschisis
goblet
- g. cell carcinoid
- g. incision

Godman fascia
Goebel-Frangenheim-Stoeckel urethrovesical technique
Goebel-Stoeckel-Frangenheim urethrovesical suspension procedure
Goethe bone
Goffe colporrhaphy
goiter
- aberrant g.
- colloid g.
- congenital g.
- diffuse colloid g.
- diffuse multinodular g.
- diffuse toxic nonnodular g.
- g. excision
- multinodular g.
- g. recurrence
- toxic multinodular g.

goitrous thyroid
gold (Au)
- g. foil condensation
- g. plate technique
- g. ring
- g. seed implantation technique
- g. weight and wire spring facial paralysis reanimation operation

Goldberg clavicle fracture repair technique
Goldblatt
- G. kidney
- G. phenomenon

Golden closing wedge osteotomy

Goldman
- G. cardiac risk index
- G. classification operative risk
- G. diagnostic discrepancy classification

Goldmann
- G. applanation tonometer (GAT)
- G. perimeter

Goldmann-Larson
- G.-L. foreign body
- G.-L. foreign body operation

Goldner-Clippinger multangular bone excision technique

Goldner-Hayes clubfoot release procedure

Goldner thumb reconstruction

Goldsmith operation

Goldstein spinal fusion technique

Goldthwait-Hauser orthopedic procedure

golf-hole ureteral orifice

Golgi membrane

Goligher extraperitoneal ileostomy

Gomco
- G. circumcision technique
- G. suction

Gomez
- G. fundoplasty
- G. horizontal gastroplasty

Gomez-Marquez lacrimal operation

Gomori

gomphosis

GON
- greater occipital nerve
- GON block

gonad
- female g.
- male g.

gonadal
- g. artery
- g. branch
- g. complication
- g. cord
- g. endocrine disorder
- g. vein

gonadectomy

gonadoblastoma

gonadopathy

gonadotrophic

gonaduct

gonangiectomy

gonatocele

gonecyst, gonecystis

gonecystis (*var. of* gonecyst)

gonecystolith

Gonin retinal cautery

gonioma

goniometer

goniometry

goniophotocoagulation

gonioplasty

gonioscopy
- indentation g.

goniotomy
- de Vincentiis g.
- g. operation

gonocele

gonococcal (GC)
- g. arthritis
- g. infection
- g. perihepatitis

Gonzalez-Ulloa
- G.-U. body lift operation
- G.-U. facelifting operation

GOO
- gastric outlet obstruction

Goodall-Power uterine prolapse repair

Goodsall anal fistula rule

Goodwin
- G. cup-patch principle
- G. orthotopic ileal neobladder technique

Goodwin-Hohenfellner ureteric reimplantation technique

Goodwin-Scott plastic reconstruction of prepuce technique

goose foot

gooseneck deformity

Gordon
- G. approach
- G. elementary body
- G. joint injection technique

Gordon-Broström technique

Gordon-Taylor
- G.-T. hindquarter amputation
- G.-T. hip disarticulation technique

Gore-Tex suture

Gorlin-Chaudhry-Moss syndrome

GOS
- Glasgow Outcome Scale
- Glasgow Outcome Score

gossamer silk suture

Gosselin fracture

Gothic arch formation

Gouffon pin fixation

Gould
- G. ankle procedure
- G. suture
- G. suture technique

Gowen decompression tube

Gowers tract

Goyrand hernia

GPA
- global pain assessment

GPN
- glossopharyngeal nerve
- glossopharyngeal neuralgia

G

GPRVS
  giant prosthetic reinforcement of
  visceral sac
    Stoppa GPRVS
grabbing technique
gracilis
  g. flap technique
  g. muscle flap
  g. myocutaneous flap
  g. neosphincter
  g. procedure
  g. tendon
graciloplasty
  double-wrap g.
  dynamic g.
gradation
  Levine 1–6 cardiac murmur g.
grade
  coma g.
  fusion g.
  g. I, II oscillation
  g. 1–5 mobilization
  nuclear g.
  SBR breast cancer g.
  Scarff-Bloom-Richardson breast
    cancer g.
  tumor g.
graded
  g. exposure
  g. spinal anesthesia
gradient
  alveolar-arterial oxygen g. ((A-a)O$_2$)
  alveolocapillary partial pressure g.
  aortic pressure g.
  aortic valve g.
  biliary-duodenal pressure g.
  Doppler pressure g.
  duodenobiliary pressure g.
  gastrosphincteric pressure g.
  intracavitary pressure g.
  g. method
  mitral valve g.
  peak systolic g.
  peak transaortic valve g.
  pressure g.
  pullback pressure g.
  pulmonary valve g.
  temperature g.
  transaortic valve g.
  transcapillary hydrostatic pressure g.
  transmural hydrostatic pressure g.
  transvalvular g.
  transvalvular pressure g.
gradient-echo
gradient-reversal fat suppression method
grading
  acinic cell tumor g.
  histomorphologic g.
  tumor g.

Gradle keratoplasty
graduated tenotomy
Graefe cataract extraction
graft
  accordion g.
  acetabular augmentation g.
  adipodermal g.
  adipose g.
  adrenal medulla g.
  advancement flap g.
  allogenic bone g.
  allogenic fetal g.
  allogenous bone g.
  anastomosed g.
  g. anastomosis
  aortofemoral bypass g. (AFBG)
  g. area
  g. atrophy
  augmentation g.
  autogeneic g.
  autogenous bone g.
  axillobifemoral bypass g.
  g. bed
  Berens g.
  bifurcated vascular g.
  bifurcation g.
  bilateral myocutaneous g.
  Björk-Shiley g.
  Blair-Brown skin g.
  bone autogenous g.
  bone chip g.
  bone graft substitute g.
  bone marrow g.
  bone peg g.
  bone-retinaculum-bone autograft g.
  bone-tendon-bone g.
  bone-to-bone g.
  Bonfiglio bone g.
  Boplant g.
  brachiosubclavian bridge g.
  branched vascular g.
  Braun-Wangensteen g.
  brephoplastic g.
  Brescia-Cimino g.
  bridge g.
  C g.
  calvarial free bone g.
  Campbell onlay bone g.
  cancellous and cortical bone g.
  cancellous chip bone g.
  cancellous insert g.
  cantilevered bone g.
  cardiovascular patch g.
  carotid-vertebral vein bypass g.
  cartilage g.
  cephalic vein g.
  chessboard g.
  chip g.
  Clancy patellar tendon g.

clip g.
g. clotting
compilation autogenous vein g.
composite rib g.
composite skin g.
conjunctival patch g.
connective tissue g.
g. contamination
coronary artery bypass g. (CABG)
cortical bone g.
cortical strut g.
corticocancellous bone g.
Cotton cartilage g.
Cragg endoluminal g.
Creech aortoiliac g.
crescent corneal g.
cross-facial nerve g.
cutis g.
Daniel iliac bone g.
Dardik umbilical g.
Davis muscle-pedicle g.
DeBakey woven polyester g.
delayed g.
dermal fat g.
dermis patch g.
dermoepidermic g.
devitalized bone g.
diamond inlay bone g.
distal femoropopliteal bypass g.
distal nerve g.
donor iliac Y g.
dorsal vein patch g.
double g.
double-papilla pedicle g.
Douglas sieve skin g.
dowel bone g.
dual onlay cortical bone g.
Edwards-Tapp arterial g.
endovascular stent g.
enteric-drained pancreas g.
epidermal g.
Esser inlay skin g.
g. expulsion
extension stent g.
extraarticular g.
g. failure
fascial g.
fascicular g.
fat g.
Favaloro saphenous vein bypass g.
femoropopliteal bypass g.
fiberglass g.
fibular strut g.
filler g.
filleted g.
fillet local flap g.
g. fixation
flap g.
forearm g.

g. fragmentation
free fat g. (FFG)
g. function
funicular g.
gastroepiploic artery g.
Gillies bone g.
Gill massive sliding g.
H g.
Haldeman bone g.
Hancock pericardial valve g.
Hancock vascular g.
Harris superior acetabular g.
g. harvest
Henderson onlay bone g.
Henry bone g.
heterodermic g.
heterogeneous g.
heterologous g.
heteroplastic g.
heterospecific g.
heterotopic g.
Hey-Groves-Kirk bone g.
H-graft bone g.
HLA-identical kidney g.
Hoaglund bone g.
homogeneous g.
homologous g.
homoplastic g.
Horton-Devine dermal g.
Huntington bone g.
HUV bypass g.
hyperplastic g.
IEA g.
IMA g.
g. impingement
implantation g.
infarcted g.
infected g.
g. infection
inferior epigastric artery g.
infrarenal g.
infusion g.
inlay bone g.
insert g.
in situ saphenous vein g.
interbody bone g.
intercalary g.
internal mammary g.
internal mammary artery g.
interposition saphenous vein g.
interspecific g.
g. interstice
intracranial-extracranial nerve g.
intracranial-intratemporal nerve g.
intramedullary g.
island g.
isogeneic g.
isologous g.
isoplastic g.

G

graft (*continued*)
Judet vascularized bone g.
jump g.
kebab emulsion surface g.
keystone g.
Kiel heterogeneous bone g.
Kimura cartilage g.
Koenig coronary artery g.
Krause-Wolfe full-thickness skin g.
Kutler V-Y flap g.
Langenskiöld bone g.
Lee anterosuperior iliac spine g.
Lee bone g.
ligament g.
g. limb
g. limb thrombosis
load-bearing g.
loop forearm g.
g. loss
lyophilized bone g.
mandrel g.
Marquez-Gomez conjunctival g.
Massie sliding g.
matchstick g.
Matti-Russe bone g.
McFarland bone g.
McMaster bone g.
medullary bone g.
mesenteric bypass g.
Meyers quadratus muscle-pedicle
   bone g.
g. migration
Millesi interfascicular g.
Millesi nerve g.
mitral valve homograft g.
morcellized bone g.
mucoperiosteal periodontal g.
mucosal periodontal g.
mucous membrane g.
Mueller patellar tendon g.
multivisceral g.
mushroom corneal g.
myocutaneous g.
nerve g.
neuromuscular pedicle g.
neurovascular island g.
Nicoll cancellous bone g.
Nicoll cancellous insert g.
nonisometric g.
g. occlusion
Ollier thick split free g.
Ollier-Thiersch split-thickness skin g.
orthotopic g.
osteoarticular g.
osteocartilaginous g.
osteochondral g.
osteoperiosteal bone g.
Ostrup vascularized rib g.
Overton dowel g.

Palma crossover saphenous
   vein g.
papillary pedicle g.
Papineau bone g.
paraffin g.
particulate cancellous bone g.
g. patency
pattern-cut corneal g.
pedicle fat g.
peg bone g.
Phemister onlay bone g.
pie-crusting skin g.
pigskin g.
pinch skin g.
g. placement
polytetrafluoroethylene g.
portacaval H g.
postage stamp skin g.
posterior cartilage g.
powdered bone g.
preclotted g.
g. preparation
prophylactic bone g.
prosthetic arterial g.
proud g.
punch g.
Rastelli pericardial roll g.
reduced-size g.
g. rejection
reoperative coronary artery bypass
   g. (rCABG)
Reverdin epidermal free g.
reversed left saphenous vein
   bypass g.
rigid g.
roof-patch g.
Ryerson bone g.
sandwiched iliac bone g.
saphenous vein bypass g.
saphenous vein patch g.
scotty dog g.
seamless g.
Seddon nerve g.
segmental tendon g.
g. sepsis
Sheen tip g.
shish kebab g.
sieve g.
g. site
skin g.
skip g.
sleeve g.
sliding inlay bone g.
Soto-Hall bone g.
g. spatulation
Speed osteotomy g.
spiral vein g.
split-thickness skin g.
spreader g.

Stark iliac bone to mandibular
  body g.
stent g.
stentless composite g.
straight g.
g. strength
g. structure
strut g.
supraceliac aortic origin g.
g. surveillance
g. survival
syngeneic g.
Taylor-Townsend-Corlett iliac crest
  bone g.
tendon g.
Thiersch-Duplay tube g.
Thiersch medium split free g.
Thiersch split-thickness skin g.
Thiersch thin split free g.
Thomas extrapolated bar g.
thrombosed g.
g. thrombosis
transplanted stamp g.
g. treatment
tubed free skin g.
tube flap g.
Tudor-Thomas corneal g.
tumbler g.
tunnel g.
upper arm straight g.
vascularized bone g.
g. vasculopathy
vein g.
venous interposition g.
g. versus host (GVH)
wedge g.
g. weight
Weiland iliac crest bone g.
white g.
Whitecloud-LaRocca fibular
  strut g.
whole lobar g.
Wilson bone g.
Wilson-Jacobs patellar g.
Windsor-Insall-Vince bone g.
Wolfe-Kawamoto bone g.
Wolfe-Krause full-thickness fat-free
  skin g.
xenogeneic g.
xenograft g.
Y g.
zooplastic g.
Z-plasty local flap g.
graftectomy
graft-enteric fistula
graft-host interface
grafting
off-pump coronary
  bypass g.

graft-versus-host (GVH)
g.-v.-h. disease (GVHD)
g.-v.-h. disease reaction
Graham
G. closure
G. plication
gram-negative
g.-n. aerobe
g.-n. aerobic organism
g.-n. microorganism
g.-n. pneumonia
g.-n. sepsis
gram-positive
g.-p. bacterial infection
g.-p. microorganism
g.-p. sepsis
Gram stain morphology
granddaughter cyst
Granger
G. line
G. method
G. projection
granisetron
granny knot
Grantham femur fracture classification
Grant-Small-Lehman supracondylar
extension osteotomy
Grant-Ward head and neck operation
granular
g. appearance
g. kidney
g. pit
g. respiration
granulation
arachnoid g.
extradural g.
pacchionian g.
g. phase
red g.
g. stenosis
g. tissue
toxic g.
granule
extracellular g.
membrane-coating g.
rod g.
seminal g.
granuloma, *pl.* **granulomata**
g. formation
infectious g.
inflammatory g.
pyogenic g.
sterile g.
Teflon g.
vocal process g.
granulomata (*pl. of* granuloma)
granulomatous
g. bacterial infection
g. colitis

G

granulomatous (*continued*)
    g. fungal infection
    g. inflammation
    g. mastitis
    g. tissue
granulosa cell carcinoma
graphical anesthesia drug display
Graphic Rating Scale (GRS)
grasper
    DeBakey-type noncrushing g.
grasping technique
grasp reflex
Grassi
    criminal nerve of G.
Gratiolet radiation
grattage
Gratz fistula
Graves
    G. disease
    G. epiphora operation
    G. technique
gravidarum
    nasal granuloma g.
gravidity
gravis
    myasthenia g.
gravitation abscess
gravitational
    g. line
    g. particle collection
gravity (g)
    intensity-weighted center of g.
    g. line
    g. method
    g. method of Stimson
gray
    g. hepatization
    g. induration
    g. infiltration
    g. line
    g. patch
    g. platelet syndrome
    g. rami communicantes
    Grey Turner sign
gray-line incision
gray-scale examination
gray-white corneal scar
great
    g. anastomotic artery
    g. auricular nerve
    g. foramen
    G. Ormond Street tracheostomy
    g. pancreatic artery
    g. radicular artery
    g. saphenous vein
    g. superior pancreatic artery
    g. toe
greater
    g. cul-de-sac

    g. curvature
    g. curvature banded gastroplasty
    g. curve position
    g. multangular bone
    g. occipital nerve (GON)
    g. occipital nerve block
    g. omentectomy
    g. omentum
    g. palatine artery
    g. pelvis
    g. peritoneal cavity
    g. peritoneal sac
    g. rhomboid muscle
    g. ring
    g. saphenous phlebectomy
    g. sciatic notch
    g. supraclavicular fossa
    g. trochanter
    g. trochanteric femoral fracture
    g. tuberosity fracture
    g. vestibular gland
green
    G. and McDermott gastrocnemius lengthening at origin with/without neurectomy
    g. braided suture
    g. Mersilene suture
    g. monofilament polyglyconate suture
Greene spinal needle
Greenfield
    G. osteotomy
    G. spinocerebellar ataxia classification
Greenhow incision
Green-Reverdin osteotomy
greenstick
    g. dorsal proximal metatarsal osteotomy
    g. fixation
    g. fracture
Greenville gastric bypass
Green-Watermann osteotomy
Gregoir-Lich ureteroneocystostomy procedure
grenz ray therapy
Greulich-Pyle skeletal age estimation technique
Grice-Green subtalar extraarticular arthrodesis technique
Grice incision
grid
    g. contact
    g. electrode
    external g.
gridiron incision
Griffen Roux-en-Y bypass
Griffith incision
Grimsdale eye operation

griseotomy
    circular g.
Gristina-Webb total shoulder arthroplasty
Gritti-Stokes
    G.-S. amputation
    G.-S. knee amputation technique
gritty tumor
groin
    g. dissection
    g. exploration
    g. flap
    g. hernia
    g. mass
Grondahl esophagoplasty
Grondahl-Finney
    G.-F. esophagogastroplasty
    G.-F. esophagoplasty
groove
    alar g.
    alveololabial g.
    anterior auricular g.
    arterial g.
    auriculoventricular g.
    bicipital g.
    carotid g.
    cavernous g.
    chiasmatic g.
    corneal lamellar g.
    costal g.
    deltopectoral g.
    digastric g.
    ethmoidal g.
    g. extension
    gingivolabial g.
    inferior petrosal g.
    infraorbital g.
    intermuscular g.
    interosseous g.
    intertubercular g.
    intraorbital g.
    lateral bicipital g.
    Lucas g.
    median g.
    meningeal g.
    musculospiral g.
    mylohyoid g.
    nail g.
    nasolabial g.
    nasopharyngeal g.
    obturator g.
    occipital g.
    palatovaginal g.
    paraglenoid g.
    pectoral g.
    peroneal g.
    pharyngotympanic g.
    popliteal g.
    posterior auricular g.

    preauricular g.
    pterygopalatine g.
    Sibson g.
    skin g.
    spiral g.
    subclavian g.
    subcostal g.
    supraacetabular g.
    g. suture
    g. suture technique
    tracheoesophageal g.
    transverse anthelicine g.
    uncinate g.
    urethral g.
    venous g.
    vertebral g.
    vomerovaginal g.
grooved incision
Groshong catheter
gross
    g. contamination
    g. cystic disease
    g. deformity
    g. fecal contamination
    G. herniorrhaphy
    g. lesion
    g. manipulation
    g. residual disease (R2)
    G. tracheoesophageal fistula
    g. tumor volume (GTV)
    g. wound contamination
Grosse-Kempf tibial locked nailing technique
Grossmann retinal detachment operation
ground
    lateral g.
ground-glass
    g.-g. appearance
    g.-g. lesion
group
    g. A beta-hemolytic streptococcal infection
    g. A streptococcus infection
    Children's Cancer Study G. (CCSG)
    Cochrane Bone, Joint, and Muscle Trauma G.
    Cochrane Musculoskeletal Injuries G.
    Eastern Cooperative Oncology G. (ECOG)
    g. fascicular repair
    PREPIC study g.
    Prévention du Risque d'Embolie Pulmonaire par Interruption Cave study g.
    g. therapy
grouping
    tumor stage g.
Groves-Goldner proximal median-radial palsy technique

G

growing
 g. fracture
 g. point
growth
 g. acceleration
 g. arrest line
 exophytic g.
 g. factor
 final g.
 hamartomatous g.
 monoclonal g.
 oligoclonal g.
 g. plate abscess
 g. plate complex
 g. plate fracture
 polyclonal g.
 g. retardation
 tumor g.
 vasoinvasive g.
GRS
 Graphic Rating Scale
Gruber
 G. cul-de-sac
 G. ligament
 G. suture technique
Gruber-Landzert fossa
Gruca stabilization
grunt
 expiratory g.
grunting
 g. maneuver
 g. respiration
Grüntzig
 G. balloon dilation
 G. transaortic intraluminal
  angioplasty technique
Grynfeltt
 G. hernia
 G. triangle
GSI
 Global Severity Index
GSW
 gunshot wound
  single GSW
GTV
 gross tumor volume
GU
 genitourinary
guaiac-negative stool
guaiac-positive stool
guanethidine
 intravenous regional block with g.
guard
 hypoxic g.
guardian suture
guarding
 abdominal g.
 involuntary g.
 voluntary g.

Guarner wrap fundoplication
gubernacular canal
gubernaculum
 Hunter g.
Gubler line
Gudas
 G. scarf Z-plasty
 G. scarf Z-plasty osteotomy
Guéneau de Mussy point
Guérin
 G. fold
 G. fracture
 G. gland
 G. sinus
 valve of G.
Guhl ankle arthroscopy technique
guidance
 computerized image g.
 fluoroscopic g.
 frameless stereotactic g.
 g. image
 laparoscopic g.
 magnetic imaging g.
 g. method
 stereotactic g.
 ultrasound g.
 videolaparoscopic g.
guidance-cooperation model
guide
 image g. (IG)
 g. plane
 suture g.
 g. wire and mini-snare technique
 g. wire exchange technique
 g. wire manipulation
 g. wire perforation
 g. wire reflection
guided
 g. fine-needle aspiration
 g. imagery
 g. needle aspiration cytology
 g. transcutaneous biopsy
guidewire dilating forceps
guiding plane
guillotine
 g. amputation
 g. needle biopsy
guinea worm infection
**Guleke-Stookey lumbar fusion
 approach**
Guller sigmoid resection
gullet
gullwing incision
gum
 g. line
 g. resection
Gunderson conjunctival flap
Gunderson-Sosin modification
gunpowder lesion

gunshot
>g. fracture
>g. wound (GSW)

Gunston arthroplasty

Gurd
>G. distal clavicle open resection
>   procedure
>G. distal clavicle resection

Gussenbauer
>G. pancreatic cyst external drainage
>   operation
>G. suture
>G. suture technique

gustation

gustatory
>g. anesthesia
>g. nerve
>g. sweating

Gustilo-Anderson
>G.-A. open clavicular fracture
>G.-A. open fracture classification

Gustilo puncture wound classification

gut
>blind g.
>g. continuity
>g. epithelial cell
>g. epithelium
>g. lumen
>g. mucosal homeostasis
>g. mucosal weight
>g. proliferative factor
>g. suture

gut-associated lymphoid tissue (GALT)

gut-derived gram-negative aerobic organism

Guthrie muscle

gutter
>abdominal g.
>g. fracture
>left g.
>paracolic g.
>paravertebral g.
>g. wound

guttering
>corneal g.

Guttmann technique

Gutzeit dacryostomy

Guyon
>G. ankle amputation technique
>G. canal

guy suture technique

Guyton-Friedenwald suture technique

Guyton-Noyes fixation

Guyton ptosis operation

GVH
>graft versus host

GVHD
>graft-versus-host disease

GW
>gastric wrap
>gunshot wound

Gy
>Gray

gynandroblastoma

gynecoid pelvis

gynecologic, gynecological
>g. anesthesia
>g. carcinoma
>g. disorder
>g. laparoscopy
>g. malignancy
>g. pain
>g. surgeon
>g. tumor

gynecological (*var. of* gynecologic)

gynecomastia, gynecomasty
>mastectomy for g.

gynecomasty (*var. of* gynecomastia)

gynoplastics

gynoplasty

gyration

gyrectomy
>frontal g.
>postcentral g.
>precentral g.

gyri (*pl. of* gyrus)

gyrose

gyrus, *pl.* **gyri**
>precentral g.

G

H

H graft
H space

H2

histamine 2

habena, *pl.* **habenae**
habenae (*pl. of* habena)
habenula, *pl.* **habenulae**
habenulae (*pl. of* habenula)
habenular trigone
habenulointerpeduncular,
  habenulopeduncular
h. tract
habenulopeduncular (*var. of*
  habenulointerpeduncular)
Haber-Kraft osteotomy
habit
bowel h.'s (BH)
parafunctional h.
habitual
h. dislocation
h. temporomandibular joint luxation
habitus
body h.
Hackethal
H. intramedullary bouquet fixation
H. stacked nailing humeral shaft
technique
Haddad metatarsal osteotomy
Hadju-Cheney acroosteolysis syndrome
HAE
hepatic artery embolization
haemoglobin (*var. of* hemoglobin)
Haemostasis
International Society on Thrombosis
and H. (ISTH)
Haggitt colorectal polyp and invasive
  carcinoma classification
Haglund deformity
Hahn-Steinthal fracture
HAI
hepatic arterial infusion
hospital-acquired infection
Haight anastomosis
hair bulb incubation test
hairline
h. fracture
pubic h.
Hajek incision
Håkanson technique
Halban
H. culdoplasty
H. culdoplasty procedure
Haldeman bone graft
half-and-half nail

half-axial projection
half-body irradiation
half-hitch knot
half-life
context-sensitive h.-l.
elimination h.-l.
plasma h.-l.
HalfLytely
half-mouth technique
half-pin fixation
half-Pringle technique
half-time
context-sensitive h.-t.
h.-t. method
Hall
H. facet fusion
H. preformed metal crown technique
H. pterygium method
Hallberg biliointestinal bypass
Halle point
Haller
H. ansa
H. anulus
H. insula
H. membrane
H. rete
H. tripod
Hallermann-Streiff-François syndrome
Hallermann-Streiff syndrome
hallucal
halluces (*pl. of* hallucis, *pl. of* hallux)
hallus (*var. of* hallux)
hallux, hallus, *pl.* **halluces**
extensor hallucis
h. limitus (HL)
hallucis longus laceration
h. rigidus (HR)
h. valgus (HV)
h. valgus deformity
h. valgus procedure
h. varus correction
halogenated volatile anesthetic
halo sign
halothane
h. hepatitis (HH)
1-MAC h.
halothane-caffeine contracture test
HALS
hand-assisted laparoscopic surgery
Halsted
H. inguinal herniorrhaphy
H. ligament
H. mattress suture
H. operation
H. radical mastectomy

H

Halsted *(continued)*
    H. suture technique
    H. thoracic outlet maneuver
Halsted-Bassini
    H.-B. hernia repair
    H.-B. herniorrhaphy
hamartoblastoma
hamartoma
    benign vascular h.
    cortical h.
    diffuse GI h.
    plaquelike h.
    visceral h.
hamartomatous
    h. growth
    h. lesion
Hamas endoscopic facial rejuvenation technique
hamate
    h. bone
    h. tail fracture
hamatum
Hamazaki-Wesenberg body
Hamilton
    H. cardiac output method
    H. Rating Scale for Depression
hammertoe deformity
hammock
    omental h.
Hamou hysteroscopic endometrial ablation technique
Hampton
    H. air-contrast radiograph maneuver
    H. line
    H. operation
hamstring
    lateral h.
    h. ligament augmentation
    medial h.
    h. muscle
    h. tendon
hamular procedure
hamuli *(pl. of* hamulus*)*
hamulus, *pl.* **hamuli**
    pterygoid h.
Hancock
    H. pericardial valve graft
    H. vascular graft
hand
    h. amputation
    h. anomaly
    h. assist
    h. assisted
    h. deformity
    h. massage
    radial club h.
    h. ratio
    h. reconstruction
    h. ventilation

hand-assisted
    h.-a. laparoscopic colectomy
    h.-a. laparoscopic gastrectomy
    h.-a. laparoscopic gastric bypass
    h.-a. laparoscopic hemicolectomy
    h.-a. laparoscopic live-donor nephrectomy
    h.-a. laparoscopic surgery (HALS)
    h.-a. laparoscopic vertical-banded gastroplasty
    h.-a. laparoscopy
handed
1-handed knot
hand-eye coordination
handgun aspirator
hand-held Doppler flow probe examination
Handley
    H. carcinoma of breast operation
    H. incision
    H. lymphangioplasty
handling
    rough tissue h.
handmade anastomosis
handsewn anastomosis
hand-sutured ileoanal anastomosis
hanger
    yoke h.
hanging
    h. chain method
    h. hip operation
    h. toe operation
hangman fracture
hangnail
Hanhart syndrome
Hankin lung volume reduction
Hanley-McNeil area under ROC curve method
Hanley rectal bladder procedure
Hannington-Kiff sign
Hannover
    H. canal
    H. chronic rejection classification
Hansen fracture classification
Hantavirus infection
Hapsburg jaw
Hara
    H. gallbladder inflammation classification
    H. infiltration block
Harada-Ito excyclotorsion correction procedure
hard
    h. adhesion
    h. and soft tissue
    h. calculus
    h. callus stage
    h. cataract
    h. chancre
    h. corn

h. exudate
h. mass
h. metal disease
h. pad disease
h. palate
h. palate cancer
h. palate dissection
h. percussion
h. socket
h. sore
h. stool
h. tubercle
Hardcastle tarsometatarsal joint injury classification
hard-copy image
hardening solution
Hardinge
H. hip prosthesis measurement technique
H. lateral hip approach
hardness
indentation h.
hard-soft palate junction
harelip suture technique
Hark
Harmon
H. cervical approach
H. hip reconstruction
H. incision
H. modified posterolateral approach
H. shoulder approach
H. suppurative hip arthroplasty
H. transfer technique
harmonic
H. hemorrhoidectomy
H. Scalpel
h. suture
Harms-Dannheim trabeculotomy
Harper-Warren incision
harpoon extraction
Harrington
H. esophageal diverticulectomy
H. rod instrumentation failure
H. total hip arthroplasty
Harrington-Allison hiatal hernia repair
Harris
H. anterolateral ankle approach
H. femoral component removal
H. growth arrest line
H. lateral trigeminal neurolytic approach
H. superior acetabular graft
H. suture technique
H. 4-wire trochanter reattachment
Harris-Beath projection
Harris-Benedict basal energy expenditure equation
Harrison atrial end of ventriculoatrial shunt method

Harris-Smith cervical fusion
harsh respiration
Hartel trigeminal neuralgia alcohol injection technique
Harting body
Hartley-Dunhill subtotal thyroidectomy
Hartmann
H. closure
H. colostomy
H. neobladder
H. operation
H. perforated sigmoid diverticulitis resection
H. point
H. pouch
H. reconstruction technique
H. resection of intestine procedure
H. solution (lactated Ringer)
H. stump
Hartman solution (dentin desensitizer)
harvest
graft h.
organ h.
harvested fibroblast
harvesting
autograft h.
endoscopic radial artery h.
laparoscopic h.
Hasner
H. fold
H. injured eye operation
valve of H.
Hassab gastric variceal operation
Hassall body
Hassmann-Brunn-Neer elbow reconstruction technique
Hasson
H. open trocar technique
H. port
Hass procedure
Hastings
H. bipolar hemiarthroplasty
H. open reduction
Hatafuku fundus onlay patch esophageal repair
hatchet-head deformity
Hatle pressure half-time Doppler echocardiography method
Haultain
H. inverted uterus operation
H. uterine inversion repair procedure
Hauri penile revascularization technique
Hauser
H. bunionectomy
H. patellar realignment technique
H. patellar tendon procedure
haustra (*pl. of* haustrum)

H

haustral
h. fold
h. indentation
h. pouch
haustration of colon
haustrum, *pl.* haustra
Havers gland
haversian canal
Hawkins
H. inside-out nephrostomy technique
H. line
H. shoulder procedure
H. single-stick technique
H. talar fracture classification
Hawthorne effect
Hayes Martin incision
Hay lateral hip approach
hazardous concentration
Hb
hemoglobin
H2 blocker
HBO
hyperbaric oxygen
hyperbaric oxygenation
HBO therapy
HCC
hepatocellular carcinoma
HCl
hydrochloride
duloxetine HCI
oxymorphone HCI
HCO_3
bicarbonate
Hct
hematocrit
HCV
hepatitis C virus
HCV antibody
HDR
high-dose radiation
high dose rate
HDR intracavitary radiation therapy
He
helium
head
h. and neck cancer pain
breech h.
bulldog h.
h. circumference to abdominal circumference ratio
clavicular h.
h. compression
h. compression test
condyle h.
h. dependent position
h. distraction test
dolichocephalic h.
h. elevated position
engaged h.
femoral h.
fetal h.
fibular h.
Giliberty bipolar femoral h.
H. hip arthroplasty
hourglass h.
humeral h.
h. injury
lateral h.
H. line
mandibular h.
Matroc femoral h.
Medusa's h.
metatarsal h.
Morse h.
h. movement
oblique h.
optic nerve h.
pancreatic h.
H. paradoxical reflex
h. posture
radial h.
h. ring
short h.
sternocostal h.
superficial h.
terminal h.
h. tetanus
h. titubation
h. to body ratio
transverse h.
h. trauma
h. turn technique
ulnar h.
h. weaving
H. zone
headache
acute h.
acute recurrent h.
analgesic abuse h.
bilateral h.
brain tumor h.
cervicogenic h.
chronic daily h.
chronic nonprogressive h.
chronic progressive h.
cluster h.
dural puncture h.
holocranial h.
low-pressure h.
myogenic h.
occipital h.
postdural puncture h. (PDPH)
postural h.
primary h.

primary cough h.
primary exertional h.
primary stabbing h.
rebound h.
refractory h.
secondary h.
spinal h.
temporal h.
tension h.
tension-type h.
traction h.
visually triggered h.
warning h.

head-bobbing doll syndrome
head-down
    h.-d. tilt
    h.-d. tilt test
head-dropping test
head-injured patient
headless bone screw
head-splitting humeral fracture
head-tilt
    h.-t. method
    h.-t. test
head-turning reflex
head-up
    h.-u. preoxygenation
    h.-u. tilt
    h.-u. tilt position
    h.-u. tilt-table test
    h.-u. tilt test
healed
    h. fracture
    h. yellow atrophy
healing
    anastomotic h.
    h. by secondary intention
    h. cycle
    endoscopic h.
    extraabdominal anastomotic h.
    h. fracture
    fracture h.
    impaired h.
    intestinal anastomotic h.
    intestinal wound h.
    primary h.
    h. process
    h. retardation
    h. ridge
    secondary wound h.
    soft tissue h.
    tertiary h.
    wound h.
health
    International Classification of
    Functioning, Disability and H.
    National Survey on Drug Use and
    H. (NSDUH)
healthy tissue

Heaney
    H. suture
    H. suture ligature stitch
    H. total vascular isolation maneuver
    H. vaginal hysterectomy operation
    H. vaginal hysterectomy technique
hearing aid evaluation
heart
    h. and lung transplant
    h. anomaly
    h. clot
    explanted h.
    extracorporeal h.
    h. failure
    h. laser revascularization
    h. position
    h. rate
    h. rate lymphedema
    h. rate variability (HRV)
    H. Rhythm Society (HRS)
    h. sac
    h. synchronized ventilation
    h. transplant
    transverse section of h.
    h. valve leaflet
    h. valve replacement
heart-lung
    h.-l. preparation
    h.-l. resuscitation
heart-shaped pelvis
heat
    h. application
    h. balance
    h. exposure
    h. hyperalgesia
    local h.
    h. production temperature
    h. shock
heater-probe coagulation
Heaton hernia repair
heat-pain threshold
heavy
    h. condensation
    h. metal injection
    h. monofilament suture
    h. retention suture
    h. silk retention suture
    h. wire suture
heavy-gauge suture
heavy-ion irradiation
heel
    h. bone
    h. fat pad
    h. pad thickening
    h. tendon
heel-toe anastomosis
heel-to-ear maneuver
Heifetz nail matrix excision
  procedure

H

height
- anterior facial h. (AFH)
- block h.
- facial h.
- first twitch h. (T1)
- nasal h.
- orbital h.
- twitch h.

height-length index

Heimlich valve

Heineke-Mikulicz
- H.-M. gastroenterostomy
- H.-M. incision
- H.-M. pyloroplasty
- H.-M. stricturoplasty

Heineke pyloroplasty

Heine operation

Heinz body

Heinz-Ehrlich body

Heisrath tarsus and conjunctiva excision

Heister
- valve of H.

Helal flap arthroplasty

helcoma

helcoplasty

Held
- H. bundle
- H. decussation

helical
- h. axis of motion
- h. CT
- h. suture
- h. suture technique

helices (*pl. of* helix)

helicine artery

helicoid ginglymus

helicotrema

helium (He)
- h. dilution method
- h. equilibration time
- h. insufflation

helix, *pl.* **helices,** *pl.* **helixes**

helixes (*pl. of* helix)

helix-loop-helix structure

Heller
- H. cardiomyotomy
- H. esophagocardiomyotomy
- H. esophagomyotomy
- H. myotomy
- H. myotomy with Dor fundoplication
- H. plexus
- H. plus Nissen fundoplication

Heller-Belsey esophageal operation

Heller-Dor esophageal operation

Heller-Nissen thorascopic esophagomyotomy

Helmholtz line

helminthoma

helmintic infection

heloma

helotomy

helplessness subscale

Helweg bundle

hemal
- h. arch
- h. spine

hemangiectasia (*var. of* hemangiectasis)

hemangiectasis, hemangiectasia

hemangiectatic hypertrophy

hemangioameloblastoma

hemangioblastoma

hemangioendothelioblastoma

hemangioendothelioma
- epithelial h.
- kaposiform h.

hemangioendotheliosarcoma

hemangioepithelioma

hemangiofibroma
- juvenile h.

hemangiolipoma

hemangiolymphangioma

hemangioma, *pl.* **hemangiomata**
- capillary h.
- cavernous h.
- choroidal h.
- hepatic h.
- noninvoluting congenital h. (NICH)
- port-wine h.
- rapidly involuting congenital h. (RICH)
- vertebral h.

hemangiomata (*pl. of* hemangioma)

hemangioma-thrombocytopenia syndrome

hemangiomatosis
- disseminated neonatal h.

hemangiomatous tissue

hemangiopericytoma

hemangiosarcoma

hematencephalon

hemathorax (*var. of* hemothorax)

hematobilia (*var. of* hemobilia)
- h. evacuation

hematocele
- pelvic h.
- pudendal h.
- scrotal h.

hematocrit (crit, Hct)
- falling h.
- h. measurement

hematocystis

hematogenic
- h. metastasis
- h. metastasis
- h. micrometastasis

hematogenous mechanism

hematologic
    h. complication
    h. disorder
    h. dissemination
    h. workup
hematolymphangioma
hematolysis
hematoma
    acute subdural h.
    aneurysmal h.
    aortic intramural h.
    h. aspiration
    axillary h.
    basal ganglia h.
    bladder flap h.
    bowel wall h.
    cerebellar h.
    chronic subdural h.
    communicating h.
    corpus luteum h.
    dissecting intramural h.
    h. drainage
    duodenal h.
    epidural h.
    h. evacuation
    expanding retroperitoneal h.
    extradural h.
    follicular h.
    h. formation
    interhemispheric subdural h.
    interstitial loculated h.
    intracerebral h.
    intracranial h.
    intrahepatic h.
    intramural h.
    intraparenchymal h.
    isodense subdural h.
    mediastinal h.
    mesenteric h.
    nasopharyngeal h.
    orbital h.
    organized h.
    paraaortic h.
    parenchymatous h.
    perianal h.
    periaortic mediastinal h.
    pericardial h.
    peridiaphragmatic h.
    perigraft h.
    perinephric h.
    perirenal h.
    placental h.
    puerperal h.
    pulsatile h.
    rectus sheath h.
    renal h.
    retroperitoneal h.
    retropharyngeal h.
    retroplacental h.

    sciatic nerve palsy h.
    scrotal h.
    septal h.
    solid visceral h.
    spinal h.
    subcapsular renal h.
    subchorionic h.
    subcutaneous h.
    subdural h.
    subfascial h.
    subgaleal h.
    subgluteal h.
    sublingual h.
    submembranous placental h.
    submental h.
    subperiosteal h.
    subungual h.
    sylvian h.
    traumatic intracranial h.
    umbilical cord h.
    wound h.
    wrap h.
hematomphalocele
hematomyelia
hematomyelopore
hematopoietic (*var. of* hemopoietic)
    h. gland
    h. metastasis
    h. tissue
hematorrhachis, hemorrhachis
    extradural h.
    subdural h.
hematospermatocele
hematospermia
hematoxylin body
heme degradation
hemendothelioma
heme-negative stool
heme-positive stool
hemiacidrin irrigation
hemiacrosomia
hemianopia, hemianopsia,
  hemiopia
hemianopsia (*var. of* hemianopia)
    homonymous h.
hemiarthroplasty
    Bateman h.
    Hastings bipolar h.
    I-beam hip h.
    large humeral head h.
    McKeever and MacIntosh h.
    Neer h.
    prosthetic h.
    Smith-Petersen h.
hemiazygos vein
hemibody irradiation
hemic calculus
hemicentrum
hemicircular incision

H

337

hemicolectomy
    décollement h.
    extended right h.
    hand-assisted laparoscopic h.
    laparoscopic-assisted h.
    laparoscopic left h.
    left h.
    right h.
    standard right h.
    telerobotic-assisted right h.
hemicondylar fracture
hemicorporectomy
hemicorticectomy
    cerebral h.
hemicrania
    chronic paroxysmal h. (CPH)
    h. continua
    episodic paroxysmal h. (EPH)
    paroxysmal h.
hemicraniectomy
hemicraniosis
hemicraniotomy
hemidiaphragm
    elevated h.
    left h.
    right h.
    h. rupture
hemidouble stapling
hemi-double stapling method
hemidysplasia cornification disorder
hemielliptica
hemifacial
hemi-Fontan
    h.-F. operation
    h.-F. procedure
hemifundoplication
    laparoscopic posterior h.
    Toupet h.
hemigastrectomy
hemiglossal
hemiglossectomy
hemihepatectomy
hemihepatic
    h. ischemia
    h. vascular occlusion
hemihydranencephaly
hemi-Koch procedure
hemilaminectomy
    complete lateral h.
    lumbar h.
    partial h.
    unilateral h.
hemilaryngectomy
hemilingual
hemiliver
hemimandible reconstruction
hemimandibulectomy
hemimaxillectomy
hemimyelocele

heminephroureterectomy
hemiopia (*var. of* hemianopia)
hemiorchiectomy
hemipancreatectomy
hemipancreaticosplenectomy
hemipelvectomy
    complete internal h.
    external h.
    formal h.
    internal h.
    Jaboulay-Doyen-Winkleman h.
    partial internal h.
hemipelvis
hemiplegic migraine
hemipulp flap
hemiresection interposition arthroplasty
hemiscrotectomy
hemisection
    tooth h.
    triple h.
hemisectomy
hemisphere
    cerebellar h.
    cerebral h.
hemispherectomy
hemispheria (*pl. of* hemispherium)
hemispherica
hemispheric disconnection syndrome
hemispherium, *pl.* **hemispheria**
hemistrumectomy
hemithoracic duct
hemithoracicus
    ductus h.
hemithorax
hemithyroidectomy
hemitongue flap
hemivertebral excision
hemivulvectomy
hemoaccess
hemobilia, hematobilia
Hemo-Cath pheresis catheter
hemocholecyst
hemocholecystitis
hemochromatosis
hemochromogen
hemoclip-induced injury
hemocryoscopy
hemocytoblastoma
hemocytolysis
hemodiafiltration convection
hemodialysis
    anemia of h.
    continuous venovenous h. (CVVHD)
    h. treatment
hemodialysis-dependent patient
hemodilution
    acute isovolemic h.
    acute normovolemic h. (ANH)
    hypervolemic h.

isovolemic h.
normovolemic h.

hemodynamic
    h. aberration
    h. change
    h. collapse
    h. compromise
    h. disturbance
    h. function
    h. impairment
    h. instability
    h. intolerance
    h. maneuver
    h. monitoring
    h. perturbation
    h. pulmonary edema
    h. push
    h. response
    h. stability

hemodynamically
    h. significant air embolus
    h. stable

hemodynamics

hemofiltration
    arteriovenous h.
    continuous h.
    continuous arteriovenous h. (CAVH)
    continuous venovenous h.
    prophylactic h.
    h. therapy

hemoglobin (Hb, Hgb), haemoglobin
    dissociable tetrameric h.
    h. electrophoresis

hemoglobin-oxygen dissociation curve

hemoglobinuria
    paroxysmal nocturnal h.

Hemolink

hemolith

Hem-o-Lok clip

hemolymphangioma

hemolysis
    acid h.
    chronic h.
    suction-induced h.

hemolytic
    h. mechanism
    h. reaction
    h. uremic syndrome (HUS)

hemomediastinum

hemonephrosis

hemoperfusion
    direct h.
    hepatic venous isolation by direct
    h. (HVI-DHP)

hemopericardium

hemoperitoneum

hemophilic
    h. arthritis
    h. arthropathy

hemoplasty

hemopneumopericardium

hemopoietic, hematopoietic

Hemopure

hemopyelectasia (*var. of* hemopyelectasis)

hemopyelectasis, hemopyelectasia

hemorrhachis (*var. of* hematorrhachis)

hemorrhage
    abdominal h.
    accidental h.
    active h.
    adrenal h.
    alveolar h.
    anastomotic h.
    aneurysmal h.
    antepartum h.
    arachnoid h.
    arterial h.
    8-ball h.
    bilateral adrenal h.
    bladder h.
    blot h.
    brainstem h.
    catheter-induced pulmonary artery h.
    cerebellar h.
    cerebral h.
    choroidal h.
    colonic diverticular h.
    colorectal h.
    concealed h.
    conjunctival h.
    h. control
    delayed massive h.
    diffuse pulmonary alveolar h.
    disc drusen h.
    diverticular h.
    dot h.
    dot-and-blot h.
    Duret h.
    epidural h.
    expulsive h.
    exsanguinating h.
    external h.
    extradural h.
    extraluminal h.
    fetal h.
    fetal-maternal h. (FMH)
    flame h.
    flame-shaped h.
    focal h.
    h. focus
    frank h.
    gastric h.
    germinal matrix h.
    gingival h.
    hepatic h.
    Icelandic form of intracranial h.
    intermediate h.
    internal h.

H

hemorrhage (*continued*)
    intestinal h.
    intraabdominal arterial h.
    intraalveolar h.
    intracapsular h.
    intracerebral h. (ICH)
    intracranial h. (ICH)
    intrahepatic h.
    intraluminal h.
    intramural intestinal h.
    intraocular h.
    intraoperative h.
    intraparenchymal h.
    intrapartum h.
    intraperitoneal h.
    intraplaque h.
    intrathecal h.
    intraventricular h.
    laryngeal h.
    lobar h.
    lower gastrointestinal h.
    massive h.
    mediastinal h.
    mesencephalic h.
    nasal h.
    nasopharyngeal h.
    neonatal intracranial h.
    neonatal intraventricular h.
    nonaneurysmal perimesencephalic
      subarachnoid h.
    oropharyngeal h.
    pancreatitis-related h.
    parenchymatous intracerebral h.
    perianeurysmal h.
    perinephric space h.
    periventricular-intraventricular h.
    h. per rhexis
    petechial h.
    placental h.
    pontine h.
    postextraction h.
    postgastrectomy h.
    postoperative h.
    postpartum h.
    postpolypectomy h.
    posttraumatic h.
    posttreatment h.
    preplacental h.
    preretinal h.
    primary h.
    punctate h.
    refractory variceal h.
    renal cyst h.
    reperfusion-induced h.
    retinal h.
    retinopathy h.
    retrobulbar h.
    retroperitoneal h.
    retropharyngeal h.

    round h.
    salmon-patch h.
    scleral h.
    secondary h.
    signal h.
    slit h.
    splinter h.
    spontaneous renal h.
    sternocleidomastoid h.
    stigmata of recent h.
    stress ulcer h.
    subarachnoid h.
    subcapsular h.
    subchorial h.
    subchorionic h.
    subconjunctival h.
    subcortical h.
    subdural h.
    subependymal h.
    subepithelial h.
    subgaleal h.
    subhyaloid h.
    subintimal h.
    submucosal gastric h.
    subperiosteal h.
    subretinal h.
    suprachoroidal h.
    syringomyelic h.
    thalamic-subthalamic h.
    torrential h.
    transplacental h.
    trauma h.
    unavoidable h.
    uncontained h.
    uncontrolled h.
    upper gastrointestinal h.
    variceal h.
    venous h.
    vitreal h.
    vitreous breakthrough h.
    white-centered h.
    yellow-ochre h.
hemorrhagic
    h. angiomyolipoma
    h. ascites
    h. complication
    h. edema
    h. endovasculitis
    h. gangrene
    h. infarction
    h. inflammation
    h. lesion
    h. metastasis
    h. radiation injury
    h. shock
    h. stroke
    h. transformation
hemorrhoid
    cutaneous h.

h. excision
external h.
first-degree h.
internal h.
ligation of h.
Lord dilation of h.
mixed h.
mucocutaneous h.
necrotic h.
prolapsed h.
rubber-band ligation of h.
second-degree h.
strangulated h.
third-degree h.
thrombosed internal and external h.'s
hemorrhoidal
h. nerve
h. plexus
h. vein
h. zone
hemorrhoidectomy
ambulatory h.
anoderm-preserving h.
closed h.
diathermy h.
Doppler-guided artery ligation h.
Ferguson h.
Harmonic h.
laser h.
ligation h.
limited h.
Longo h.
Lord h.
Milligan-Morgan h.
modified Whitehead h.
nonmucosal h.
open h.
Parks h.
2-quadrant h.
3-quadrant h.
4-quadrant h.
radical h.
rubber-band h.
scissors-excision h.
semiopen h.
stapled h.
hemospermia
hemostasia (*var. of* hemostasis)
hemostasis, hemostasia
chemical h.
complete h.
endoscopic h.
global h.
immaculate h.
meticulous h.
meticulous surgical h.
proactive h.
hemostatic
h. activation

h. agent
h. collodion
h. plug formation
h. staple line
h. suture
h. suture technique
hemostat technique
hemostyptic
hemosuccus pancreatitis
hemotherapeutics (*var. of* hemotherapy)
hemotherapy, hemotherapeutics
hemothoraces (*pl. of* hemothorax)
hemothorax, hemathorax, *pl.*
hemothoraces
Henderson
H. fracture
H. functional results classification
H. onlay bone graft
H. posterolateral tibia approach
H. posteromedial knee approach
H. skin incision
Henderson-Hasselbalch equation
Hendler unitunnel ACL repair technique
Henke
H. space
H. triangle
Henle
H. body
H. elastic membrane
H. fenestrated membrane
H. loop
H. tubule
Hennemans size principle
Henning inside-to-outside meniscal repair technique
Henry
H. acromioclavicular technique
H. anterior strap approach
H. anterolateral approach
H. bone graft
H. extensile approach
H. femoral neck resection
H. incarcerated and strangulated femoral hernia operation
H. incision
H. posterior interosseous nerve approach
H. posterior interosseous nerve exposure
H. radial approach
H. splenectomy
Henry-Geist spinal fusion
Hensen
H. body
H. canal
H. cell
H. duct
H. plane
Hensing ligament

H

hepaplastin test
hepar lobatum
heparin
    h. cofactor II plasma level
    h. irrigation
    low-molecular weight h. (LMWH)
    h. neutralized thrombin time
heparinase correction
heparin-associated antiplatelet
  antibodies
heparin-binding protein
heparin-bonded cardiopulmonary bypass
  circuit
heparin-coated circuit
heparin-induced
    h.-i. lipolysis
    h.-i. thrombocytopenia (HIT)
    h.-i. thrombocytopenia and
      thrombosis syndrome (HITTS)
heparinization procedure
hepatectomize
hepatectomy
    cadaveric donor h.
    caudate h.
    central h.
    concomitant h.
    donor h.
    ex situ h.
    ex situ-in situ h.
    extended left h.
    extended right h.
    laparoscopic h.
    laparoscopic-assisted h.
    LCVP-aided h.
    LCVP-assisted h.
    left h.
    limited h.
    living donor partial h.
    local h.
    partial h.
    recipient h.
    regional h.
    right h.
    right lobe h.
    segmental h.
    simultaneous segmental h.
    standardized h.
    subsegmental h.
    subtotal h.
    total left h.
    triple lobe h.
    wedge h.
hepatic
    h. abscess
    h. adenoma
    h. allograft
    h. apoptosis
    h. arterial buffer response
    h. arterial infusion (HAI)

h. arterial therapy
h. artery
h. artery embolization (HAE)
h. artery-portal vein fistula
h. artery pseudoaneurysm
h. branch
h. candidal infection
h. capsule
h. cell carcinoma
h. circulation
h. colic
h. colorectal metastasis
h. coma
h. complication
h. congestion
h. dearterialization
h. decompensation
h. disease
h. duct
h. duct calculus
h. dysfunction
h. encephalopathy
h. failure
h. fibrosis
h. flexure
h. function reserve
h. fungal infection
h. gunshot wound
h. hemangioma
h. hemorrhage
h. hilum
h. hydrothorax
h. immunity
h. injury
h. intraarterial yttrium-90
  microspheres treatment
h. intracellular energy
h. intracellular energy status
h. ischemia
h. ischemic time
h. lobectomy
h. lobule
h. malignancy
h. margin
h. mass lesion
h. necrosis
h. neoplasia
h. neoplasm
h. outflow block
h. outflow tract
h. parasitic cyst
h. parenchyma
h. parenchymal transection
h. pedicle
h. perfusion
h. plexus
h. portal vein (HPV)
h. portojejunostomy
primary h.

h. regeneration
h. resection
h. resectional surgery
h. rupture
h. scintigraphy
h. segment
h. sinusoid
h. steatosis
h. subsegmentectomy
h. surface
h. territory
h. transplant
h. trauma
h. triad
h. tumor
h. vascular exclusion (HVE)
h. vascular isolation (HVI)
h. vascular isolation technique
h. venous confluence
h. venous isolation by direct
   hemoperfusion (HVI-DHP)
h. venous outflow obstruction
h. venous trunk
h. venous web disease
h. web
h. web dilation

hepaticocholangiojejunostomy,
  hepatocholangiojejunostomy
hepaticocutaneous jejunostomy
hepaticocystojejunostomy
hepaticodochotomy
hepaticoduodenostomy,
  hepatoduodenostomy
hepaticoenterostomy,
  hepatocholangioenterostomy
hepaticogastrostomy
hepaticojejunostomy, hepatojejunostomy

complex h.
Hepp-Couinaud h.
high h.
hilar h.
intracystic h.
laparoscopic h.
mucosa-to-mucosa Roux-en-Y h.
palliative h.
pediatric h.
peripheral h.
Roux-en-Y h.
side-to-side h.
simple h.
wide mucosa-to-mucosa Roux-en-Y
   h.

hepaticolithotomy
hepaticolithotripsy
hepaticoportoenterostomy
hepaticopulmonary (*var. of*
  hepatopneumonic)
hepaticostomy
hepaticotomy

hepatic-renal angle
hepatis
porta h.
hepatitides (*pl. of* hepatitis)
hepatitis, *pl.* **hepatitides**
h. activity index classification
h. A-E infection
anesthetic h.
autoimmune h.
h. C virus (HCV)
fulminant h.
halothane h.
peliosis h.
radiation h.
short incubation h.
hepatization
gray h.
red h.
yellow h.
hepatobiliary
h. imaging
h. iminodiacetic acid (HIDA)
h. manifestation
h. surgery
hepatoblastoma
unresectable h.
hepatocarcinoma
hepatocaval ligament
hepatocele
hepatocellular
h. acidosis
h. cancer
h. carcinoma
h. function
h. synthetic dysfunction
hepatocholangioenterostomy (*var. of*
  hepaticoenterostomy)
hepatocholangiojejunostomy (*var. of*
  hepaticocholangiojejunostomy)
hepatocholangitis
hepatocolic ligament
hepatocolicum
ligamentum h.
hepatocystic duct
hepatocyte
h. arrangement
h. transplant
hepatocytic necrosis
hepatoduodenal
h. ligament
h. reflection
hepatoduodenal-peritoneal reflection
hepatoduodenostomy (*var. of*
  hepaticoduodenostomy)
hepatoenteric
hepatoesophageal ligament
hepatoesophageum
ligament h.
hepatofugal flow

H

343

hepatogastric ligament
hepatogastricum
  ligament h.
hepatojejunal anastomosis
hepatojejunostomy (*var. of*
  hepaticojejunostomy)
hepatolith
hepatolithectomy
hepatolithiasis
  intrahepatic h.
hepatoma
hepatomegalia (*var. of* hepatomegaly)
hepatomegaly, hepatomegalia
  congestive h.
hepatomphalocele, hepatomphalos
hepatomphalos (*var. of* hepatomphalocele)
hepatonephoric syndrome
hepatonephric (*var. of* hepatorenal)
hepatonephromegaly
hepatopancreatic
  h. ampulla
  h. fold
  h. sphincter
hepatopathy
  radiation h.
hepatoperitonitis
hepatopetal flow
hepatopexy
hepatopleural fistula
hepatopneumonic, hepaticopulmonary,
  hepatopulmonary
hepatoportal biliary fistula
hepatoportoenterostomy
  Kasai-type h.
hepatoptosis
hepatopulmonary (*var. of*
  hepatopneumonic)
  h. movement
  h. transit
hepatorenal, hepatonephric
  h. angle
  h. bypass
  h. failure
  h. fossa
  h. ligament
  h. pouch
  h. recess
  h. syndrome
hepatorrhagia
hepatorrhaphy
hepatorrhexis
hepatoscopy
hepatosplenomesenteric trunk
hepatostomy
hepatotomy
hepatotoxemia
hepatotoxic effect
hepatotoxicity
  anesthetic h.

hepatotrophic nutrient
hepatovenous oxygen saturation
Hepp-Couinaud
  H.-C. biliary reconstruction
  technique
  H.-C. biliary tract procedure
  H.-C. hepaticojejunostomy
herald patch
herbal
  h. medicine
  h. therapy
Herbert scleral flap operation
hereditary
  h. breast cancer
  h. cancer syndrome
  h. coproporphyria
  h. elliptocytosis
  h. flat adenoma syndrome
  h. hemolytic anemia
  h. hemorhagic telangectasia
  h. malignancy
  h. multiple exostoses
  h. nonpolyposis colon cancer
  (HNPCC)
  h. nonpolyposis colon carcinoma
  (HNPCC)
  h. nonpolyposis colorectal cancer
  (HNPCC)
  h. nonpolyposis colorectal cancer
  syndrome
  h. predisposition
  h. renal carcinoma
  h. sensory and autonomic
  neuropathy (HSAN)
  h. spherocytosis
Hering
  canal of H.
  H. nerve
Hering-Breuer reflex
heritable connective tissue disease
Herman-Gartland osteotomy
Hermansky-Pudlak syndrome
Hermodsson
  H. fracture
  H. internal rotation technique
  H. tangential projection
hernia, *pl.* **hernias, herniae**
  abdominal incisional h.
  abdominal intercostal h.
  abdominal wall h.
  acquired h.
  amniotic h.
  antevesical h.
  axial hiatal h.
  Barth h.
  Béclard h.
  bilateral inguinal h.
  bilocular femoral h.
  Birkett h.

bladder h.
Bochdalek h.
broad ligament h.
cecal h.
cerebral h.
Cheatle-Henry h.
Cloquet h.
combined hiatal h.
complete h.
concealed h.
concentric h.
congenital h.
congenital diaphragmatic h. (CDH)
Cooper h.
crural h.
h. defect
diaphragmatic h.
direct inguinal h.
diverticular h.
double-loop h.
dry h.
duodenal h.
duodenojejunal h.
easily reducible h.
h. en bissac
encysted h.
epigastric h.
esophageal h.
extrasaccular h.
fascial h.
fatty h.
femoral h.
fixed hiatal h.
flank incisional h.
funicular inguinal h.
gangrenous h.
gastric h.
gastroesophageal h.
gastroschisis h.
Gibbon h.
Gironcoli h.
gluteal h.
Goyrand h.
groin h.
Grynfeltt h.
Hesselbach h.
Hey h.
hiatal h.
Holthouse h.
iliacosubfascial h.
incarcerated h.
incarcerated vesicoinguinal h.
h. incarceration
h. incision
incisional h.
incomplete h.
indirect inguinal h.
infantile h.
inferior ileocecal h.

inguinal h.
inguinocrural h.
inguinofemoral h.
inguinolabial h.
inguinoproperitoneal h.
inguinoscrotal h.
inguinosuperficial h.
h. in recto
intermuscular h.
internal h.
internal supravesical h.
interparietal h.
intersigmoid h.
interstitial h.
intraepiploic h.
intrailiac h.
intrapelvic h.
irreducible h.
ischiatic h.
Krönlein h.
labial h.
laparoscopic repair of paraesophageal
  h. (LRPH)
Larrey h.
Laugier h.
left inguinal h.
Lesgaft h.
lesser sac h.
levator h.
Littré h.
Littré-Richter h.
lower quadrant abdominal
  incisional h.
lumbar h.
Madden repair of incisional h.
Malgaigne h.
massive ventral h.
Maydl h.
meningeal h.
mesenteric h.
mesocolic h.
metachronous h.
h. metastasis
midline incisional h.
Morgagni h.
Morgagni-Larrey type h.
mucosal h.
multiorgan h.
muscle h.
nontraumatic h.
oblique h.
obturator h.
omental h.
omphalocele h.
orbital h.
ovarian h.
pannicular h.
pantaloon h.
paraduodenal h.

H

345

hernia (*continued*)

paraesophageal diaphragmatic h.
paraesophageal hiatal h.
parahiatal h.
paraileostomal h.
h. paralysis
paraperitoneal h.
parapubic h.
parasaccular h.
parastomal h.
paraumbilical h.
parietal h.
pectineal h.
pediatric h.
pericolostomy h.
perineal h.
peristomal h.
peritoneal h.
peritoneopericardial diaphragmatic h.
periumbilical h.
Peterson h.
Petit h.
pleuroperitoneal h.
port site h.
posterior vaginal h.
postoperative h.
posttraumatic diaphragmatic h.
h. pouch
primary indirect inguinal h.
properitoneal inguinal h.
psoas h.
pudendal h.
pulsion h.
rectal h.
recurrent incisional h.
reducible h.
h. repair
retroanastomotic h.
retrocecal h.
retrocolic h.
retrograde h.
retroperitoneal h.
retropubic h.
retrosternal h.
retrovesical h.
Richter h.
Rieux h.
right inguinal h.
Rokitansky h.
rolling hiatal h.
h. rupture
h. sac
sciatic h.
scrotal h.
secondary h.
Serafini h.
short esophagus type hiatal h.
sliding abdominal h.
sliding esophageal hiatal h.

sliding hiatal h.
slipped h.
spigelian h.
Spigelius h.
spontaneous lateral ventricle h.
spontaneous ventrolateral h.
sports h.
stoma h.
strangulated h.
strangulated incisional h.
strangulated paraesophageal h.
subpubic h.
subxiphoid h.
superior ileocecal h.
suprapubic h.
supravesical h.
synovial h.
thyroidal h.
tonsillar h.
transient hiatal h.
transmesenteric h.
transomental h.
traumatic h.
traumatic diaphragmatic h.
Treitz h.
trocar site h.
true h.
tunicary h.
umbilical h.
unilateral h.
uterine h.
h. uterus inguinale
vaginal h.
vaginolabial h.
Velpeau h.
ventral h.
ventral abdominal h.
ventral incisional h.
ventrolateral h.
vesicle h.
vesicoinguinal h.
vitreous h.
von Bergman h.
W h.
wound h.

herniae (*pl. of* hernia)
hernial
h. aneurysm
h. ring
hernias (*pl. of* hernia)
herniated
h. disc
h. fundoplication
h. preperitoneal fat
h. presacral fat pad
h. viscus
herniation
brain h.
cardiac h.

caudal transtentorial h.
central h.
cerebral h.
cervical midline disc h.
cingulate h.
cisternal h.
diaphragmatic h.
disc h.
fat h.
foraminal h.
free fragment h.
hindbrain h.
intercervical disc h.
intervertebral disc h.
lumbar disc h.
midline disc h.
nucleus pulposus h.
h. pit
posterolateral h.
rostral transtentorial h.
sphenoidal h.
subfalcial h.
synovial h.
tentorial h.
thoracic disc h.
tonsillar h.
transtentorial h.
traumatic cervical disc h.
uncal h.
ureteroneocystostomy h.
visceral h.
vitreous h.
hernioappendectomy
hernioenterotomy
hernioid
herniolaparotomy
hernioplasty
abdominal midline incisional h.
classical Judd-Mayo overlap midline
  incisional h.
incisional h.
Judd-Mayo overlap midline
  incisional h.
laparoscopic h.
Lichtenstein tension-free h.
massive incisional h.
mesh plug h.
midline incisional h.
modified Shouldice h.
modified TAPP h.
overlap midline incisional h.
prosthetic incisional h.
Shouldice h.
tension-free h.
transabdominal preperitoneal h.
herniopuncture
herniorrhaphy
anterior inguinal h.
Bassini inguinal h.

h. chronic inguinodynia
elective h.
emergent h.
extraperitoneal laparoscopic h.
Gross h.
Halsted-Bassini h.
Halsted inguinal h.
hiatal h.
Hill-type hiatus h.
inguinal h.
laparoscopic total extraperitoneal h.
Lichtenstein h.
Macewen h.
Madden incisional h.
McVay h.
mesh h.
modified Bassini h.
modified McVay h.
Ogilvie h.
open h.
pants-over-vest h.
polypropylene mesh h.
Ponka h.
primary inguinal h.
Shouldice h.
sutureless laparoscopic extraperitoneal
  inguinal h.
totally extraperitoneal inguinal h.
transabdominal laparoscopic h.
umbilical h.
ventral h.
vest-over-pants h.
herniotomy
Petit h.
herpes
h. epithelial tropic ulceration
h. simplex virus infection
h. zoster infection
h. zoster pain
herpetic infection
herpetoid lesion
Herring lateral pillar radiographic
  classification
hersage
hesitation phenomenon
Hespan
Hess
H. eyelid operation
H. ptosis operation
Hesselbach
H. fascia
H. hernia
H. ligament
H. triangle
hetastarch
heteroautoplasty
heterocheiral, heterochiral
heterochiral (*var. of* heterocheiral)
heterodermic graft

H

heterogeneity characteristic
heterogeneous
    h. attenuation
    h. gland size
    h. graft
    h. keratoplasty
heterograft
    autogenous fascial h.
heterokeratoplasty
heterolateral
heterologous
    h. graft
    h. insemination
heterolysis
heterophoric position
heteroplastic graft
heteroplastid
heteroplasty
heteroscopy
heterospecific graft
heterotopic
    h. bone formation
    h. gastric mucosa
    h. graft
    h. ossification prevention
    h. transplant
heterotransplantation
heterozygosis (*var. of* heterozygosity)
heterozygosity, heterozygosis
Heuser membrane
hexafluorobenzene
hexametazime (HMPAO)
hex procedure
hexylcaine
Hey-Groves
    H.-G. anterior cruciate ligament
    reconstruction technique
    H.-G. fascia lata ACL repair
    technique
Hey-Groves-Kirk bone graft
Hey hernia
Heyman-Herndon clubfoot procedure
Heyman-Herndon-Strong correction of
  metatarsus varus technique
HFDD
    human fibroblast-derived dermis
HFJV
    high-frequency jet ventilation
H-flap incision
HFOV
    high-frequency oscillation ventilation
    high-frequency oscillatory ventilation
HFPPV
    high-frequency positive-pressure
    ventilation
HFV
    high-frequency ventilation
Hgb
    hemoglobin

HGD
    high-grade dysplasia
H-graft
    H-g. bone graft
    H-g. fusion
    mesocaval H-g.
HHCA
    hypothermic hypokalemic cardioplegic
    arrest
HHNKC
    hyperosmolar hyperglycemic nonketotic
    coma
hiatal
    h. hernia
    h. herniorrhaphy
hiatopexy
hiatoplasty
    tension-free h.
hiatotomy
hiatus, *pl.* **hiatus**
    adductor h.
    aortic h.
    Breschet h.
    esophageal h.
    h. esophageus
    fallopian h.
    maxillary h.
    pleuroperitoneal h.
    sacral h.
    saphenous h.
    scalene h.
    Scarpa h.
    semilunar h.
Hibbs-Jones spinal fusion
Hibbs lumbar fusion procedure
hibernal epidemic viral infection
hibernation
    myocardial h.
hibernoma
Hibiclens
Hickman catheter
hickory-stick fracture
HICPAC
    Hospital Infection Control Practices
    Advisory Committee
HIDA
    hepatobiliary iminodiacetic acid
    HIDA scan
hidden
    h. layer
    h. nail skin
hidradenitis suppurativa
hidradenoma, hydradenoma
    clear cell h.
    cystic h.
    nodular h.
    papillary h.
    poroid h.
    solid h.

hidrocystoma
Hiff operation
Higgins cardiac surgery risk score
high
- h. attenuation
- h. blind tract
- h. blood pressure
- h. cellularity
- h. cervical anterior retropharyngeal approach
- h. dose rate (HDR)
- h. endothelial venule
- h. hepaticojejunostomy
- h. intraluminal pressure
- h. intrauterine insemination
- h. ligation
- h. lip line
- h. lithotomy
- h. neurological lesion
- h. predictive value
- h. pressure zone (HPZ)
- h. smile line
- h. spinal anesthesia
- h. subtotal gastrectomy
- h. sympathectomy
- h. threshold receptor
- h. tibial osteotomy (HTO)

high-affinity progestin receptor
high-altitude
- h.-a. endoscopy
- h.-a. simulation test

high-amplitude sucking technique
high-attenuation mass
high-capacity fluid warmer
high-dose
- h.-d. radiation (HDR)
- h.-d. radioiodine therapy
- h.-d. rate radiation test
- h.-d. rate radiation therapy
- h.-d. scan
- h.-d. thrombin time (HiTT)
- h.-d. thrombin time test

high-energy fracture
high-frequency
- h.-f. jet
- h.-f. jet ventilation (HFJV)
- h.-f. jet ventilator
- h.-f. oscillation
- h.-f. oscillation ventilation (HFOV)
- h.-f. oscillatory ventilation (HFOV)
- h.-f. percussive ventilation
- h.-f. positive pressure
- h.-f. positive-pressure ventilation (HFPPV)
- h.-f. positive-pressure ventilator
- h.-f. TENS
- h.-f. ventilation (HFV)

high-grade
- h.-g. astrocytoma
- h.-g. dysplasia (HGD)
- h.-g. MALT lymphoma
- h.-g. primary extremity liposarcoma
- h.-g. sarcoma
- h.-g. squamous intraepithelial lesion (HSIL)
- h.-g. stricture

high-intensity lesion
high-level disinfection
high-loop cutaneous ureterostomy
highly selective vagotomy (HSV)
high-magnification
- h.-m. colonoscopy
- h.-m. endoscopy
- h.-m. gastroscopy

Highmore
- H. abscess
- antrum of H.
- H. body

high-output ileostomy
high-resistance fundoplication
high-resolution
- h.-r. image
- h.-r. parallel hole collimator
- h.-r. ultrasonography

high-risk
- h.-r. angioplasty
- h.-r. papillary cancer
- h.-r. patient
- h.-r. recipient (HRR)

high-speed rotational atherectomy (HSRA)
high-tension suturing technique
high-voltage
- h.-v. pulsed galvanic stimulation
- h.-v. therapy

high-volume hospital
hila (*pl. of* hilum)
hilar
- h. bile duct cholangiocarcinoma
- h. biopsy
- h. carcinoma
- h. cholangiocarcinoma
- h. cylinder
- h. displacement
- h. hepaticojejunostomy
- h. mass
- h. plate
- h. region
- h. release
- h. structure scar tissue

Hilgenreiner horizontal Y line
Hilgenreiner-Perkins line
Hill
- H. antireflux operation
- H. antireflux procedure
- H. fundoplasty
- H. gastropexy fundoplication
- H. hiatus hernia repair

H

349

Hill (*continued*)
    H. median arcuate repair
    H. posterior gastropexy
Hillis-Müller maneuver
Hill-Nahai-Vasconez-Mathes tensor fasciae latae free flap technique
hillock
    seminal h.
Hill-Sachs
    H.-S. deformity
    H.-S. fracture
    H.-S. shoulder dislocation
    H.-S. shoulder lesion
Hill-type hiatus herniorrhaphy
HILP
    hyperthermic isolated limb perfusion
Hilton
    H. law
    H. nerve division ulcer pain relief method
    H. white line
hilum, *pl.* **hila**
    hepatic h.
    splenic h.
    h. stimulation
Himly
    H. artificial pupil
    H. cataract extraction
Hinchey diverticulitis grade classification
hindbrain
    h. deformity
    h. herniation
hindfoot
    h. amputation
    h. deformity
    varus h.
hindgut
hindquarter amputation
hinge
    h. joint
    h. osteotomy
    h. position
    soft tissue h.
hinge-axis point
hinged
    h. corneal flap
    h. fragment
Hinman
    H. stress incontinence procedure
    H. syndrome
Hinsberg labyrinth operation
hip
    h. arthroplasty
    h. bone
    h. deformity
    h. disarticulation
    h. dislocation

    h. distractor
    h. extension
    h. fracture
    h. fusion
    h. pinning
    h. positioner
    h. reduction
    h. replacement
    h. replacement surgery
    h. rotation
    transient osteoporosis of h.
Hippel operation
hippocampectomy
Hippocrates manipulation
Hippocratic anterior shoulder reduction maneuver
Hirano body
Hirayma osteotomy
Hirschberg strabismic eye deviation method
Hirschfeld canal
Hirschsprung disease
Hirst cystocele operation
hirudin
hirudinization
His
    angle of H.
    H. bundle
    H. bundle ablation
    H. bundle heart block
    bundle of H. (BH, B-H, BOH)
    H. canal
    H. line
    H. perivascular space
    H. plane
His-Purkinje tissue
histamine 2 (H2)
histangic (*var. of* histoangic)
histiocyte, histocyte
histiocytic tissue
histiocytoma
histiocytosis, histocytosis
histioma (*var. of* histoma)
histoangic, histangic
histocompatibility
histocyte (*var. of* histiocyte)
histocytosis (*var. of* histiocytosis)
histoid neoplasm
histologic, histological
    h. assessment
    h. characteristic
    h. diagnosis
    h. examination
    h. investigation
    h. lesion
    h. liver biopsy finding
    h. marker
    h. pattern
    h. result

h. study
h. tolerance
h. type
histological (*var. of* histologic)
histology
histolysis
histoma, histioma
histomorphologic grading
histonectomy
histopathologic
h. analysis
h. confirmation
h. data
h. diagnosis
h. examination
h. feature
h. information
h. validation
Histoplasma **infection**
history and physical examination
histotoxic anoxia
HIT
heparin-induced thrombocytopenia
immune-mediated HIT
Hitchcock biceps tendon technique
HiTT
high-dose thrombin time
HiTT test
HITTS
heparin-induced thrombocytopenia and
thrombosis syndrome
HIV
human immunodeficiency virus
HIV classification
HIV-1, -2 infection
HIV-related abdominal pain
HLA
human leukocyte antigen
HLA-identical kidney graft
HMPAO
hexametazime
HNPCC
hereditary nonpolyposis colon
cancer
hereditary nonpolyposis colon
carcinoma
hereditary nonpolyposis colorectal
cancer
HNPCC syndrome
HnTT
heparin neutralized thrombin time
Ho
holmium
Hoaglund bone graft
hobnailed appearance
hobnail liver
Hoche
H. bundle
H. tract

Hochenegg rectal excision
hockey-stick
h.-s. deformity
h.-s. fracture
hockey stick incision
Hodge plane
Hodgkin disease
Hodgson hypospadias repair technique
Hoffa
H. fat pad
H. fracture
Hoffman
H. elimination
H. jejunoplasty
Hoffmann
H. approach
H. duct
H. panmetatarsal head resection
**Hoffmann-Clayton panmetatarsal excision
procedure**
Hofmeister
H. anastomosis
H. gastrectomy
H. gastrectomy procedure
H. gastric resection technique
H. gastroenterostomy
H. operation
Hofmeister-Pólya anastomosis
Hogan operation
Hoguet
H. hernial sac conversion maneuver
H. inguinal hernia operation
H. pantaloon hernia repair
**Hohl-Luck tibial plateau fracture
classification**
**Hohl-Moore tibial plateau fracture
repair technique**
**Hohl tibial condylar fracture
classification**
Hohmann hallux osteotomy procedure
Hohn catheter
Hoke foot arthrodesis procedure
Hoke-Kite arthrodesis technique
Hoke-Miller pes planus procedure
Holdaway line
Holden line
holder
needle h.
purpose-made tube h.
suture h.
hold-relax
h.-r. method
h.-r. technique
Holdsworth spinal fracture classification
hole
bur h.
lag screw thread h.
h. preparation method
hole-in-1 technique

H

Hollander insulin-induced hypoglycemia test
Holl ligament
hollow
    h. bone
    Sebileau h.
    h. visceral injury
    h. visceral myopathy
    h. viscus
    h. viscus injury
    h. viscus myopathy
holmium (Ho)
    h.: yttrium-aluminum-garnet (Ho:YAG)
    h.: yttrium-aluminum-garnet laser angioplasty
holoacrania
holocord
holocranial headache
hologastroschisis
holoprosencephaly
holorachischisis
Holstein-Lewis fracture
Holth
    H. iridencleisis
    H. scleral punch operation
    H. sclerectomy
Holthouse hernia
Holzknecht space
Homans sign
homatropine dilation
homeostasis
    acid-base h.
    gut mucosal h.
    mucosal h.
    operational h.
homeostatic function
home parenteral nutrition
homocladic
homogeneity
    tissue h.
homogeneous
    h. ablation
    h. graft
homogenous
    h. keratoplasty
    h. radiation
    h. tooth transplant
homograft
    h. aortic valve replacement
    cryopreserved aortic h.
    homovital h.
    pulmonary h.
    h. reaction
    h. rejection
homokeratoplasty
homolateral
homologous
    artificial insemination h. (AIH)

    h. blood transfusion
    h. graft
homolysis
homomorphic
homonomous
homonomy
homonymous hemianopsia
homoplastic graft
homoplasty
homotopic transplant
homotransplant
homotransplantation
homotype
homotypic, homotypical
homotypical (*var. of* homotypic)
homovital homograft
homozygous achondroplasia
honeycombed appearance
honeycomb lesion
hood
    H. and Kirklin incision
    laminar flow h.
hook
    h. cautery
    h. electrocautery
    h. fixation
    suture pickup h.
hooked
    h. bone
    h. bundle of Russell
    h. intramedullary nail
    h. wire localization
hook-lying position
hook-nail deformity
hook-plate fixation
hook-rod construct
hoop stress fracture
Hopkins tetralogy of Fallot operation
Hoppenfeld-Deboer
    H.-D. orthopaedic approach
    H.-D. orthopaedic technique
Horay cataract operation
hordeolum
    external h.
Hori umbilicus reconstruction technique
horizontal
    h. angulation
    h. canal
    h. external rotation
    h. fissure
    h. flap
    h. gastroplasty
    h. incision
    h. mattress stitch
    h. mattress suture technique
    h. maxillary fracture
    h. osteotomy
    h. plane

h. position
h. projection
h. section
hormonal evaluation
hormone
adrenocorticotropic h. (ACTH)
anabolic h.
circulating h.
exogenous h.
intact parathyroid h. (iPTH)
parathyroid h. (PTH)
steroid h.
syndrome of inappropriate secretion
of antidiuretic h. (SIADH)
h. system
tropic h.
horn
coccygeal h.
dorsal h.
lesser h.
nail h.
sacral h.
superior h.
Horner
H. muscle
H. syndrome
hornification
hornpipe position
horripilation
horseshoe
h. abscess
h. fistula
h. incision
h. kidney
horseshoe-shaped
h.-s. flap
h.-s. incision
Horsley
H. anastomosis
H. gastrectomy
H. suture
horticulture therapy
Horton-Devine
H.-D. dermal graft
H.-D. hypospadias flip-flap procedure
Horwitz-Adams ankle fusion
hospital
H. Anxiety and Depression Scale
high-volume h.
Imperial College London H. (ICLH)
H. Infection Control Practices
Advisory Committee (HICPAC)
Massachusetts General H. (MGH)
h. monitoring
h. mortality
h. pneumoperitoneum
h. stay
Texas Scottish Rite H. (TSRH)
hospital-acquired infection (HAI)

host
graft versus h. (GVH)
reservoir h.
hostile abdomen
hot
h. abscess
h. axilla
h. axillary bed
h. biopsy
h. biopsy technique
h. defect
h. gangrene
h. knife conization
h. lesion
h. line
h. nodule
h. sentinel node
hot-dog ACL repair technique
hottest spot
**Hotz-Anagnostakis entropion
correction**
Hotz entropion operation
Houghton-Akroyd
H.-A. fracture technique
H.-A. open reduction
hour
postoperative h.
postprandial h.
hourglass
h. deformity
h. head
h. membrane
h. stomach
1-hour office pad test
House
H. advancement anoplasty
H. flap anoplasty
H. otosclerosis cochlear implant
technique
H. rotational flap
H. stapedectomy
H. upper limb reconstruction
**House-Brackmann facial nerve injury
classification**
Houston
H. fold
H. muscle
valve of H.
Hovius
H. canal
H. membrane
Howard
H. auditory neural prosthetic
implant method
H. differential ureteral catheterization
technique
H. test
Howell-Jolly body
Howland lock

H

Howorth
    H. approach
    H. hip procedure
Howship-Romberg sign
Ho:YAG
    holmium: yttrium-aluminum-garnet
    Ho:YAG laser
    Ho:YAG laser angioplasty
Hoyer
    H. anastomosis
    H. canal
HPT
    hyperparathyroidism
        familial HPT
        nonfamilial untreated HPT
        primary untreated HPT
        secondary HPT
        sporadic primary HPT
        symptomatic primary HPT
        untreated HPT
HPV
    hepatic portal vein
    human papillomavirus
    hypoxic pulmonary
        vasoconstriction
HPZ
    high pressure zone
        anal HPZ
HRS
    Heart Rhythm Society
    hepatorenal syndrome
HRV
    heart rate variability
HSAN
    hereditary sensory and autonomic
        neuropathy
HSE
    human skin equivalent
H-shaped
    H-s. capsular incision
    H-s. ileal pouch-anal anastomosis
HSIL
    high-grade squamous intraepithelial
        lesion
HSV
    highly selective vagotomy
HTN
    hypertension
HTO
    high tibial osteotomy
H-type tracheoesophageal fistula
hub contamination
Huber
    H. adductor digiti quinti
        opponensplasty
    H. needle
Hubscher adult flatfoot maneuver
Hudson line
Hudson-Stähli line

hue
    salmon-patch h.
Huebner recurrent artery
Hueck ligament
Hueter
    H. incision
    H. line
    H. stomach tube introduction
        maneuver
Hu-Friedy Perma Sharp suture
Huggins orchiectomy
Hughes
    H. colorectal operation
    H. modification
    H. modification of Burch
        colposuspension technique
    H. tarsoconjunctival flap
Hughston
    H. external rotation recurvatum test
    H. knee injury classification
    H. lateral knee instability procedure
Hughston-Degenhardt ACL reconstruction
Hughston-Hauser patellar dislocation
repair procedure
Hughston-Jacobson
    H.-J. lateral compartment
        reconstruction
    H.-J. tibial tunnel knee repair
        technique
Huguier
    H. canal
    H. circle
    H. sinus
Hui-Linscheid ulnotriquatral
augmentation tenodesis procedure
human
    h. bite infection
    h. fibroblast-derived dermis (HFDD)
    h. immunodeficiency virus (HIV)
    h. immunodeficiency virus
        classification
    h. leukocyte antigen (HLA)
    h. lung
    h. lyophilized dura cystoplasty
    h. ovum fertilization test
    h. papillomavirus (HPV)
    h. papillomavirus infection
    h. placental umbilical cord blood
    h. proteome
    h. skin equivalent (HSE)
    h. subject
    h. thrombin
    h. T-lymphotrophic virus
    h. umbilical vein (HUV)
    h. vascular cell
humeral
    h. approach
    h. artery
    h. articulation

h. canal
h. epiphysis
h. fracture malunion
h. head
h. head-splitting fracture
h. line
h. physial fracture
h. shaft fracture
h. supracondylar fracture
humeri (*pl. of* humerus)
humeroperoneal neuromuscular disease
humeroradial articulation
humeroscapular
humeroulnar articulation
humerus, *pl.* **humeri**
humidity
absolute h.
relative h.
Hummelsheim
H. transposition of vertical recti operation
H. transposition of vertical recti procedure
humor
aqueous h.
vitreous h.
humpback deformity
hump removal
hunger
bone h.
Hungerford-Krackow-Kenna knee arthroplasty
hungry bone syndrome
Hunt
H. and Kosnik cerebral aneurysm classification
H. cerebral aneurysm operation
Hunt-Early technique
Hunter
H. aneurysm ligation
H. canal
H. gubernaculum
H. line
H. technique for Toupet fundoplication
hunterian ligation
Hunter-Schreger line
Huntington
H. bone graft
H. disease
H. tibial technique
H. uterine inversion repair procedure
Hunt-Lawrence jejunal pouch
Hunt-Transley lid ptosis operation
Hürthle
H. cell change
H. fine-needle aspiration
H. FNA

HUS
hemolytic uremic syndrome
husband
artificial insemination h. (AIH)
Huschke foramen
Hustead epidural needle
Hutchinson
H. fracture
H. freckle
H. patch
Hutchison syndrome
Hutch ureteroneocystostomy
HUV
human umbilical vein
HUV bypass graft
HV
hallux valgus
hyperventilation
HVE
hepatic vascular exclusion
HVI
hepatic vascular isolation
HVI-DHP
hepatic venous isolation by direct hemoperfusion
hyaline
h. basement membrane
h. bodies
h. mass
h. membrane disease
h. membrane syndrome
hyalinization
hyalitis anterior membrane
hyalocapsular ligament
hyaloid
h. artery
h. body
h. canal
h. membrane
hyaloidotomy
hybridization-subtraction technique
hybrid myocardial revascularization
hybridoma technique
hydatid
h. cyst intrahepatic rupture
h. disease
h. liver cyst
h. material
hydatidocele
hydatidoma
hydatidosis
multiple hepatic h.
hydatidostomy
hydradenoma (*var. of* hidradenoma)
hydranencephaly
hydrate microcrystal theory of anesthesia
hydration
adequate h.
intravenous h.

H

hydration (*continued*)
    h. layer water
    maternal h.
    h. status
    h. therapy
    vigorous h.
hydraulic dissection
hydrencephalocele, hydrocephalocele,
  hydroencephalocele
hydrencephalomeningocele
hydrencephalus
hydroappendix
hydrocalycosis
hydrocarbon
    fluorinated h.
hydrocele
    postoperative h.
    h. sac
hydrocelectomy
hydrocephalic
hydrocephalocele (*var. of*
  hydrencephalocele)
hydrocephaloid
hydrocephalus, hydrocephaly
    normal-pressure h.
    obstructive h.
    postsubarachnoid hemorrhage h.
hydrocephaly (*var. of* hydrocephalus)
hydrochloride (HCl)
    esmolol h.
    intranasal hydromorphone h.
    nicardipine h.
hydrocholecystis
hydrocirsocele
hydrocolpocele, hydrocolpos
hydrocolpos (*var. of* hydrocolpocele)
hydrocystoma
hydrocytosis
hydrodelamination
hydrodelineation
hydrodissection
hydrodistended
hydroencephalocele (*var. of*
  hydrencephalocele)
hydroflotation
hydroflow technique
hydrogel reservoir
hydrogen (H)
    h. inhalation technique
    h. ion concentration (pH)
    power of h. (pH)
    h. washout blood flow method
hydrogenation
hydrogenolysis
hydrolysis
    intragastric h.
    h. of solution
    h. of surfactant
    urea h.

hydroma (*var. of* hygroma)
hydromeningocele
hydromyelia
hydromyelocele
hydromyelomeningocele
hydromyoma
hydronephrosis
hydronephrotic
hydroperitoneum, hydroperitonia
hydroperitonia (*var. of*
  hydroperitoneum)
hydropertubation
hydrophobic
    h. dressing
    h. topical medication
hydropneumoperitoneum
hydropneumothorax
hydrops
    endolymphatic h.
    h. fetalis
hydropyonephrosis
hydrorchis
hydrosarca
hydrosarcocele
hydrostatic
    h. balloon dilation
    h. pressure
hydrosyringomyelia
hydrotherapy
    chylous h.
hydrothorax
    hepatic h.
hydrotomy
hydrotubation
hydroureter
hydroxyapatite, hydroxylapatite
    h. arthropathy
    h. cement cranioplasty
hydroxyethyl starch
hydroxylapatite (*var. of* hydroxyapatite)
5-hydroxytryptamine type 3 (5-HT$_3$)
hyfrecation
hygroma, hydroma
    subdural h.
hygroscopic
    h. expansion
    h. technique
hyla
hylan G-F 20
hyloma
hymenal
    h. caruncula
    h. membrane
    h. ring
    h. syndrome
hymenectomy
hymenoplasty
hymenorrhaphy
hymenotomy

Hynes pharyngoplasty
hyoepiglottic ligament
hyoepiglotticum
    ligamentum h.
hyoepiglottidean
hyoglossal
    h. membrane
    h. muscle
hyoid
    h. apparatus
    h. bone
    h. bone fracture
    h. bone resection
    h. fossa
    h. muscle
    h. syndrome
hyoideus
    apparatus h.
hyopharyngeus
hyothyroid
hyothyroidea
Hypaque enema
hyparterial
hypaxial
hypencephalon
hyperactivity
    sympathetic h.
hyperacute
    h. graft-versus-host disease
    h. rejection
hyperaeration
hyperaesthesia (*var. of* hyperesthesia)
hyperaldosteronism
    Conn primary h.
hyperalgesia, hyperalgia
    barbiturate-related h.
    heat h.
    incision-induced h.
    mechanical h.
    opioid-induced h.
    secondary h.
    visceral h.
hyperalgia (*var. of* hyperalgesia)
hyperalimentation
    central h.
    intravenous h.
    parenteral h.
    peripheral h.
hyperbaric
    h. local anesthetic
    h. oxygen (HBO)
    h. oxygenation (HBO)
    h. oxygen therapy
    h. pressure
    h. spinal anesthesia
    h. tetracaine
hyperbilirubinemia
hypercalcemia
    familial hypocalciuric h.

    persistent h.
    recurrent h.
hypercapnia, hypercarbia
    central venous h.
    gastric mucosal h.
    permissive h.
    pneupreperitoneum-induced h.
    venous h.
hypercapnic
    h. drive
    h. ventilatory response
hypercarbia (*var. of* hypercapnia)
hypercellular gland
hyperchloremic metabolic acidosis
hypercoagulable state
hypercoagulation
hypercontractile external sphincter
  response
hyperdense brain lesion
hyperdeviation
hyperdistended abdomen
hyperdynamic
    h. circulation
    h. shock
hyperemia
    reactive h.
hyperemic
hyperesthesia, hyperaesthesia
hypereuryprosopic
hyperexplexia
hyperextension deformity
hyperextension-hyperflexion injury
hyperfibrinolysis
hyperfiltration
    capillary h.
    glomerular h.
    h. injury
    renal h.
hyperfractionated total body
  irradiation
hyperfractionation
hyperfunctioning
    h. adenoma
    h. nodule
hyperglycemia
    postprandial h.
    stress-induced h.
hyperhidrosis
    axillary h.
    palmar h.
hyperhydration
hyperhydropexis (*var. of* hyperhydropexy)
hyperhydropexy, hyperhydropexis
hyperimmunoglobulin M
  immunodeficiency
hyperinfection
hyperinflation
hyperinsulinemia, hyperinsulinism
    peripheral h.

H

hyperinsulinism (*var. of* hyperinsulinemia)
    congenital h.
hyperintense
    h. brain lesion
    h. image
hyperkeratotic lesion
hyperlactation
hyperlactemia
hypermetabolic
    h. response
    h. sepsis
hypermetabolism
hypermetropia
hypermobility
    thermal injury-induced vascular h.
hypernephroid carcinoma
hypernephroma
hyperorchidism
hyperosmolar
    h. dehydration
    h. diabetic coma
    h. hyperglycemic nonketotic coma
    (HHNKC)
hyperostosis
    diffuse idiopathic skeletal h. (DISH)
    generalized cortical h.
hyperoxic ventilation
hyperparathyroidism (HPT)
    ectopic h.
    neonatal severe h.
    primary h.
    sporadic primary h.
    untreated h.
hyperpathia
hyperphosphaturia
hyperpigmented lesion
hyperplasia
    adenomatous h.
    asymmetric h.
    atypical h.
    basal cell h.
    benign prostatic h. (BPH)
    congenital adrenal h.
    Cushing adrenal h.
    ductal h.
    fibronodular h.
    florid h.
    focal nodular h. (FNH)
    4-gland h.
    idiopathic cortical adrenal h.
    intimal h.
    intraductal h.
    lingual tonsil h. (LTH)
    lobular h.
    moderate h.
    multigland h.
    multiglandular parathyroid h.
    multiple gland h.
    neointimal h.

    papillary h.
    parathyroid h.
    polyclonal h.
    polypoid h.
    pseudointimal h.
    solid h.
    sporadic multigland h.
    sporadic multiple gland parathyroid
    h.
    squamous h.
    stent-induced intimal h.
    thyroid h.
hyperplastic
    h. cyst
    h. cystadenoma
    h. gland
    h. graft
    h. inflammation
    h. polyp
    h. tissue
    h. tumor
hyperpronation
hyperpyrexia
    fulminant h.
    malignant h.
hyperreflexic bladder
hyperresonant abdomen
hypersalivation
hypersecretory process
hypersensitive xiphoid syndrome
hypersensitivity
    h. angiitis
    delayed cutaneous h.
    denervation h.
    pain h.
    thermal h.
    visceral h.
hypersensitization
hyperspectral analysis
hypersplenism
    secondary h.
hypertelorism
hypertension (HTN)
    arterial h.
    diastolic h.
    essential h.
    extrahepatic portal venous h.
    idiopathic intracranial h.
    intraabdominal h.
    intrahepatic h.
    lithotripsy-induced h.
    malignant h.
    neurogenic h.
    pediatric portal h.
    portal h.
    primary pulmonary h. (PPH)
    pulmonary artery h. (PAH)
    recumbent h.
    renal h.

renovascular h. (RVH)
surgically corrected h.
unshuntable portal h.
hypertensive lower esophageal sphincter
hyperthermia
malignant h.
stress-induced h. (SIH)
h. therapy
whole-body h.
hyperthermic
h. isolated limb perfusion (HILP)
h. temperature
hyperthymization
hyperthyroidism
factitious h.
hypertonic
h. bladder
h. hyponatremia
h. lactated saline
h. saline resuscitation
hypertonic-hyperoncotic fluid resuscitation
hypertrophia (*var. of* hypertrophy)
hypertrophic
h. granulation tissue
h. pyloric stenosis
h. scar
h. scar formation
h. scarring
hypertrophy, hypertrophia
benign prostatic h. (BPH)
eccentric h.
hemangiectatic h.
hypervascular
h. fragment
h. tumor
hypervascularity
hyperventilation
alveolar h.
isocapnic h.
h. maneuver
h. syndrome
h. test
h. tetany
hypervolemia
hypervolemic hemodilution
hyphema
hypnosis anesthesia
hypnotherapy
hypnotic
h. dissociation
h. effect
intravenous h.
h. response
hypoactive bowel sounds
hypoaeration
hypoalgesia
somatic h.
hypobaria
hypobaric spinal anesthesia

hypocalcemia
postoperative h.
transient h.
hypocapnia, hypocarbia
hypocarbia (*var. of* hypocapnia)
hypocellular fibrous tissue
hypochondria (*pl. of* hypochondrium)
hypochondriaca
regio h.
hypochondriac region
hypochondrium, *pl.* **hypochondria**
hypochordal
hypocystotomy
hypodense brain lesion
hypoderm
hypodermatomy
hypodermic implantation
hypodermoclysis
hypoeccrisis
hypoechoic lesion
hypoesthesia
hypogastric
h. artery
h. artery ligation
h. flap
h. ganglion
h. nerve
h. plexus
h. plexus block anesthetic
technique
h. region
h. vein
hypogastricus
nervus h.
hypogastrium
hypogastrocele
hypogastroschisis
hypogenitalism
hypoglossal, hypoglossus
h. artery
h. canal
h. canal venous plexus
h. facial nerve anastomosis
h. facial transfer procedure
h. nerve
hypoglossis (*var. of* hypoglottis)
hypoglossus (*var. of* hypoglossal)
h. muscle
hypoglottis, hypoglossis
hypoglycemia
hypognathous
hypogonadism
opiate-induced h.
hypohyloma
hypolobulation
hypomelanotic macule
hyponatremia
hypertonic h.
hypotonic h.

H

hyponatremia (*continued*)
    hypovolemic h.
    isotonic h.
    spurious h.
hyponychium
hypooncotic plasma substitute
hypoparathyroidism
    permanent h.
hypoperfusion
    brainstem h.
    global h.
    regional h.
    splanchnic h.
    spreading h.
    systemic h.
    tissue h.
hypoperfusion-induced PGID
hypopharynx
    diverticulectomy of h.
hypophyseal (*var. of*
  hypophysial)
hypophysectomize
hypophysectomy
    chemical h.
    partial central h.
    total h.
    transsphenoidal h.
    unilateral h.
hypophyseoportal vein
hypophysial, hypophyseal
    h. artery
    h. duct
    h. fossa
    h. portal circulation
hypophysis
hypopigmentation
    postinflammatory h.
hypopituitarism
hypoplasia
    aortic h.
    pulmonary h.
hypoplastic
    h. left heart repair
    h. left heart syndrome
hyporesponsiveness
    endotoxin h.
hyposalivation
hyposcheotomy
hyposensitivity
    pain h.
hypospadiac
hypospadias
hyposplenism
hypostasis
    postmortem h.
    pulmonary h.
hypostatic abscess
hypostomia

hypotension
    catecholamine-resistant h.
    controlled h.
    deliberate h.
    induced h.
    intracranial h.
    orthostatic h.
    systemic h.
hypotensive
    h. anesthesia
    h. resuscitation
    h. surgery
hypothalamic
    h. activation
    h. feedback
hypothalamic-hypophysial-ovarian-endometrial axis
hypothalamic-hypophysial portal circulation
hypothalamic-pituitary-axis suppression
hypothalamohypophysial tract
hypothalamotomy
hypothenar
    h. eminence
    h. hammer syndrome
    h. muscle
    h. prominence
hypothermia
    accidental h.
    h. anesthetic technique
    core h.
    deep h.
    extracorporeal exchange h.
    inadvertent h.
    intraoperative core h.
    moderate resuscitative h.
    pediatric h.
    profound h.
    redistribution h.
    regional h.
    therapeutic h.
    total body h.
hypothermia-induced coagulopathy
hypothermia-related coagulopathy
hypothermic
    h. anesthesia
    h. circulatory arrest
    h. effect
    h. hepatic perfusion
    h. hypokalemic cardioplegic arrest (HHCA)
hypotheses (*pl. of* hypothesis)
hypothesis, *pl.* **hypotheses**
    Cinderella h.
    gate-control h.
hypotonia, hypotonus, hypotony
    skeletal muscle h.

hypotonic
    h. hyponatremia
    h. solution
hypotonus (*var. of* hypotonia)
hypotony (*var. of* hypotonia)
hypotympanic cell
hypotympanum
hypouresis
hypoventilation
    alveolar h.
    benzodiazepine-induced h.
    sedation-induced h.
hypovolemia
hypovolemic
    h. hyponatremia
    h. shock
hypoxemia
    episodic h.
    severe h.
    stagnant h.
hypoxia
    cellular h.
    diffusion h.
    hypoxic h.
    ischemic h.
    local h.
    stagnant h.
    tissue h.
    tumor h.
hypoxia-induced rhabdomyolysis
hypoxic
    h. brain insult
    h. guard
    h. hypoxia
    h. pulmonary vasoconstriction (HPV)
    h. ventilatory decrease
    h. ventilatory response
hypsibrachycephalic
hypsiconchous
hypsiloid
    h. angle
    h. cartilage
hypsistaphylia
hypsistenocephalic
Hyrtl
    H. anastomosis
    H. foramen
    H. loop
    H. sphincter
hysterectomy
    abdominal h.
    abdominovaginal h.
    Bonney abdominal h.
    cesarean h.
    classic abdominal Semm h.
    classic intrafascial Semm h. (CISH)
    Dellepiane h.
    Döderlein roll-flap h.

    Doyen vaginal h.
    Eden-Lawson h.
    extrafascial h.
    gasless laparoscopic h.
    Gelpi-Lowry h.
    intrapartum h.
    laparoscopically assisted vaginal h.
      (LAVH)
    laparoscopic-assisted vaginal h.
      (LAVH)
    laparoscopic Döderlein h.
    laparoscopic radical h.
    Latzko radical abdominal h.
    Mayo h.
    Meigs-Werthein h.
    modified radical h.
    obstetric h.
    paravaginal h.
    pelviscopic intrafascial h.
    prophylactic h.
    radical h.
    radical abdominal h.
    radical vaginal h.
    Reis-Wertheim vaginal h.
    Schauta radical vaginal h.
    subtotal h.
    supracervical h.
    TeLinde modified radical h.
    total h.
    total abdominal h. (TAH)
    vaginal h.
    Ward-Mayo vaginal h.
hysteresis
hysteric, hysterical
    h. anesthesia
    h. colic
    h. paralysis
hysterical (*var. of* hysteric)
hystericus
    globus h.
hysterocele
hysterocleisis
hysterocystocleisis
    Bozeman h.
hysterocystopexy
hysterolysis
hysteromyoma
hysteromyomectomy
hysteromyotomy
hystero-oophorectomy
hysteropexy
    abdominal h.
    Alexander-Adams h.
hysteroplasty
hysterorrhaphy
hysterosacropexy
hysterosalpingectomy
    laparoscopic h.

H

hysterosalpingo-oophorectomy
hysterosalpingostomy
hysteroscopic
  surgery
hysteroscopy
    laparoscopic-assisted
     vaginal h.

hysterotomy
    abdominal h.
    vaginal h.
hysterotrachelectomy
hysterotracheloplasty
hysterotrachelorrhaphy
hysterotrachelotomy

I&A
irrigation and aspiration
IA
inferior apical
IA segment
IAA
ileoanal anastomosis
IABCP
intraaortic balloon counterpulsation
IABP
intraaortic balloon pump
IAC
internal auditory canal
IAP
intraabdominal pressure
IAR
immediate asthmatic reaction
IAS
internal anal sphincter
IASP
International Association for the Study
of Pain
IASP classification of chronic pain
iatrogenic
i. arteriovenous fistula
i. bile duct injury
i. biliary stricture
i. bowel injury
i. colonic perforation
i. hernia defect
i. impotence
i. infection
i. tension pneumothorax
i. transmission
iatrotechnique
IB
inferior basal
IB segment
I-beam
I-b. hip hemiarthroplasty
I-b. hip operation
IBPB
interscalene brachial plexus block
IBR
immediate breast reconstruction
ibuprofen
oxycodone HCl and i.
IBW
ideal body weight
ICA
internal carotid artery
ICBN
intercostobrachial nerve
ICCE
intracapsular cataract extraction

ICDA
International Classification of Diseases,
Adapted for Use in the United
States
ice
i. application
i. point
i. skater's fracture
i. slush
ice-cold saline
**Icelandic form of intracranial
hemorrhage**
ICH
intracerebral hemorrhage
intracranial hemorrhage
icing liver
ICISS
International Classification of
Diseases-9 Version of Injury Severity
Score
ICLH
Imperial College London Hospital
ICLH double-cup arthroplasty
ICP
intracranial pressure
ICS
immotile cilia syndrome
ICSI
intracytoplasmic sperm injection
ictal abnormality
ICU
intensive care unit
ICU care priority
ICU sedation
I&D
incision and drainage
ideal
i. body weight (IBW)
i. flap
i. flow rate
i. solution
Ideberg glenoid fracture classification
identical point
identification
colonic lesion i.
film i.
lesion i.
nasal mucosal i.
i. phenomenon
radiofrequency i. (RFID)
identifying canal
identity formation
IDET
intradiscal electrothermal therapy
idiographic approach

idiopathic
    i. achalasia
    i. adult intussusception
    i. bone cavity
    i. brachial plexopathy
    i. brown induration
    i. cause
    i. constipation
    i. cortical adrenal hyperplasia
    i. dilation
    i. eczematous disease
    i. hypertrophic subaortic stenosis
    (IHSS)
    i. ileocecal intussusception
    i. intracranial hypertension (IIH)
    i. neck pain
    i. paroxysmal rhabdomyolysis
    i. peptic ulcer disease
    i. preretinal membrane
    i. pulmonary fibrosis (IPF)
    i. thrombocytopenic purpura (ITP)
    i. ventricular fibrillation
IDSA
    Infectious Disease Society of America
IEA
    inferior epigastric artery
    IEA graft
IG
    image guide
    intragastric
    IG bundle
IGBB
    diagnostic IGBB
IGBB
    image-guided breast biopsy
IGHL
    inferior glenohumeral ligament
ignition point
IGPA
    infragenicular popliteal artery
IGS
    image-guided surgery
IHP
    isolated hepatic perfusion
IHSS
    idiopathic hypertrophic subaortic
    stenosis
IIH
    idiopathic intracranial hypertension
IINB
    ilioinguinal-iliohypogastric nerve block
ileac
ileal
    i. artery
    i. biopsy
    i. bladder
    i. conduit
    i. conduit urinary diversion
    i. crypt

    i. inflammation
    i. inflow tract
    i. J-pouch
    i. loop
    i. neobladder urinary pouch
    i. outflow tract
    i. patch ureteroplasty
    i. perforation
    i. pouch-anal anastomosis (IPAA)
    i. pouch-distal rectal anastomosis
    i. pouch surgery
    i. resection
    i. reservoir construction
    i. small-bowel lymphangioma
    i. sphincter
    i. vein
    i. W-pouch
ileal-sigmoid anastomosis
ileectomy
ileitis
    backwash i.
    pouch i.
    terminal i.
ileoanal
    i. anastomosis (IAA)
    i. endorectal pull-through
    i. pouch
    i. pouch procedure
    i. pullthrough procedure
ileoascending colostomy
ileocecal
    i. cystoplasty
    i. edema
    i. eminence
    i. fat pad
    i. fold
    i. junction
    i. opening
    i. orifice
    i. ostium
    i. pouch
    i. recess
    i. region
    i. ureterocolostomy
    i. valve
ileocecocolic sphincter
ileocecocystoplasty bladder augmentation
ileocecostomy
ileocecum
ileocolectomy
ileocolic, ileocolonic
    i. artery
    i. conduit
    i. intussusception
    i. pouch
    i. pouch urinary diversion
    i. resection
    i. vein
ileocolonic resection

ileocolonoscopy
ileocolostomy
    endloop i.
    LeDuc-Camey i.
ileocystoplasty
    Camey i.
    clam i.
    LeDuc-Camey i.
ileocystostomy
    cutaneous i.
ileoduodenal fistula
ileoentectropy
ileogastrostomy
ileoileostomy
    duodenoileostomy i.
    laparoscopic duodenoileostomy i.
ileojejunal bypass
ileopexy
ileoproctostomy
ileorectal anastomosis (IRA)
ileorectostomy
ileorrhaphy
ileoscopy
ileosigmoid
    i. anastomosis (ISA)
    i. colostomy
    i. fistula
    i. knot
ileosigmoidostomy
ileostomy
    Bishop-Koop i.
    blowhole i.
    Brooke i.
    i. closure
    i. construction
    continent i.
    defunctioning loop i.
    Dennis-Brooke i.
    diversionary i.
    diverting loop i.
    double-barrel i.
    i. dysfunction
    end i.
    endloop i.
    extraperitoneal i.
    i. formation
    Goligher extraperitoneal i.
    high-output i.
    incontinent i.
    J-loop i.
    Koch continent i.
    Koch reservoir i.
    loop i.
    loop-end i.
    permanent loop i.
    pouched i.
    i. reversal
    split i.
    i. spout

    i. stenosis
    i. stoma
    temporary loop i.
    terminal i.
    Turnbull end-loop i.
ileotomy
ileotransverse
    i. colon anastomosis
    i. colostomy
ileotransversostomy
ileovesical
    i. anastomosis
    i. fistula
ileovesicostomy
    incontinent i.
ileum
    terminal i.
ileus
    adhesive i.
    duodenal i.
    gallstone i.
    meconium i.
    occlusive i.
    panenteric inflammatory i.
    paralytic i.
    persistent i.
    postoperative i.
    potential complications of
    postoperative i.
ilia (*pl. of* ilium)
iliac
    i. apophysis
    i. arterial tree
    i. artery
    i. artery aneurysm
    i. artery angioplasty
    i. artery dissection
    i. bone
    i. branch
    i. bursa
    i. buttressing procedure
    i. colon
    i. compression test
    i. crest
    i. crest biopsy
    i. crest bone aspiration
    i. crest bone graft stabilization
    i. crest free flap
    i. crest osseous flap
    i. crest osteocutaneous flap
    i. crest osteomuscular flap
    i. crest resection
    i. epiphysis
    i. fascia
    i. fixation
    i. flexure
    i. fossa
    i. muscle
    i. osteocutaneous free flap

iliac (*continued*)
    i. osteotomy
    i. plexus
    i. region
    i. roll
    i. spine
    i. steal
    i. tubercle
    i. vein
    i. wing resection
iliacosubfascial
    i. fossa
    i. hernia
iliacosubfascialis
    fossa i.
iliacus muscle
Iliff
    I. blepharoptosis
      approach
    I. exenteration
iliocaval bypass
iliococcygeal muscle
iliococcygeus
iliocolotomy
iliocostalis
iliocostal muscle
iliofemoral
    i. approach
    i. bypass
    i. flap artery
    i. pedicle flap
    i. wing fracture
iliohypogastric
    i. muscle
    i. nerve
    i. nerve block
    i. neurectomy
ilioinguinal
    i. acetabular approach
    i. incision
    i. nerve
    i. nerve block
    i. neurectomy
    i. ring
ilioinguinal-iliohypogastric nerve block (IINB)
iliolumbar
    i. artery
    i. ligament
ilioneoureterocystotomy
iliopectineal
    i. arch
    i. bursa
    i. eminence
    i. fascia
    i. fossa
    i. line
iliopelvic sphincter
iliopopliteal bypass

iliopsoas
    i. muscle
    i. ring
    i. tendon
iliopubic
    i. eminence
    i. tract
iliosacral and iliac fixation construct
iliosciatic
iliospinal
iliotibial
    i. band (ITB)
    i. band graft augmentation
    i. tract
iliotrochanteric
ilium, *pl.* **ilia**
    external i.
    internal-external i.
Ilizarov
    I. external fixation
    I. limb-lengthening method
    I. limb-lengthening technique
ILL
    intracorporeal laser lithotripsy
ill-defined mass
illness
    catastrophic i.
    life-threatening i.
    medical i.
illumination
    axial i.
    background i.
    central i.
    coaxial i.
    contact i.
    critical i.
    dark-field i.
    dark-ground i.
    diffuse i.
    direct i.
    erect i.
    focal i.
    Köhler i.
    lateral i.
    narrow-slit i.
    oblique i.
    slit i.
    vertical i.
ILMA
    intubating laryngeal mask airway
ILP
    isolated limb perfusion
IM
    intramuscular
IMA
    inferior mesenteric artery
    internal mammary artery
    internal maxillary artery
    IMA graft

IMAG
    internal mammary artery graft
image
    i. acquisition
    i. analysis
    axial spin-echo i.
    body i.
    i. compression
    dynamic i.
    ejection-fraction i.
    ejection shell i.
    endoscopic video i.
    i. formation
    i. formation principle
    guidance i.
    i. guide
    i. guide bundle
    hard-copy i.
    high-resolution i.
    hyperintense i.
    i. intensification
    i. interpretation
    multiplanar i.
    i. point
    point-counting i.
    radiographic i.
    real-time echo-planar i.
    real-time multiplanar i.
    i. registration
    sagittal spin-echo i.
    second-echo i.
    spin-echo i.
    static i.
    i. subtraction
    surface-projection rendering i.
    thin-section axial i.
    transmission i.
    T1-weighted spin-echo i.
    T2-weighted spin-echo i.
    ultrasound i.
    video i.
image-guided
    i.-g. breast biopsy (IGBB)
    i.-g. fine-needle aspiration biopsy
    i.-g. interactive neurosurgery
    i.-g. navigation
    i.-g. pancreatic core aspiration
    i.-g. stereotactic brain biopsy
    i.-g. surgery (IGS)
image-integrated surgery treatment
  planning
image-related screening technique
imagery
    guided i.
image-selected in vivo spectroscopy
image-space focus
imaginal exposure
imaging
    abdominal i.

    anatomic i.
    B-mode i.
    color i.
    3-dimensional projection
      reconstruction i.
    Doppler color flow i.
    Doppler tissue i. (DTI)
    echo i.
    endocrine i.
    endometrial chemical shift i.
    endorectal coil magnetic
      resonance i.
    endoscopic ultrasonographic i.
    endovaginal i.
    exercise i.
    folate-targeted i.
    functional magnetic resonance i.
      (fMRI)
    hepatobiliary i.
    intraoperative i.
    intravenous digital subtraction i.
    magnetic resonance i. (MRI)
    magnetic source i.
    i. method
    i. modality
    neuroelectric source i.
    neuromagnetic source i.
    noninvasive i.
    orthogonal polarization
      spectral i.
    pancreatic i.
    point i.
    power Doppler i.
    preoperative i.
    projection-reconstruction i.
    projection tract i.
    rapid bedside i.
    rotating frame i.
    sagittal plane i.
    serial i.
    sestamibi systemic i.
    i. strategy
    i. study
    i. technique
    time-of-flight echoplanar i.
    tissue Doppler i.
    transverse section i.
    tumor i.
    ultrafast magnetic resonance i.
      (UMRI)
    ventilation/perfusion i.
    xenon lung ventilation i.
Imanaga Billroth I reconstruction
  method
imbalance
    electrolyte i.
imbricate, imbricated
    i. suture technique
imbricated (*var. of* imbricate)

imbrication
  capsular i.
  facet i.
  i. line of Pickerill
  i. line of von Ebner
  MacNab line for facet i.
  medial capsular i.
  medialis obliquus i.
  retinal i.
imiquimod 5% cream
IML
  internal mammary lymphoscintigraphy
immaculate hemostasis
immediate
  i. amputation
  i. asthmatic reaction (IAR)
  i. breast reconstruction (IBR)
  i. extension technique
  i. flap
  i. postoperative period
  i. transfusion
immersion
  i. method
  i. microscopy
  i. technique
imminent cardiac arrest
immobilization
  cast i.
  cervical i.
  i. method
  postoperative i.
  rigid cervical i.
  Rowe-Zarins shoulder i.
  sling i.
  spica cast i.
  sternal-occipital-mandibular i. (SOMI)
  tooth i.
  Treponema pallidum i.
  Webril i.
immotile cilia syndrome (ICS)
immovable joint
IMMPACT
  Initiative on Methods, Measurement,
  and Pain Assessment in Clinical
  Trials
immune
  i. electron microscopy
  i. inflammation
  i. mechanism
  i. modulation
  i. response
  i. system anatomy
immune-mediated
  i.-m. coagulation disorder
  i.-m. heparin-induced
  thrombocytopenia
  i.-m. HIT
immunity
  cellular i.

CTL i.
cytotoxic T-lymphocyte i.
hepatic i.
immunochemiluminescent therapy
immunocompetent tissue therapy
immunocytoma
immunodeficiency
  hyperimmunoglobulin M i.
immunodeficient
immunodepression
immunodiffusion test
immunofluorescence
  i. microscopy
  i. test
immunofluorescent examination
immunohistochemical
  i. analysis
  i. feature
  i. marker
  i. stain
  i. staining
immunohistochemistry
immunoincompetent
immunologic, immunological
  i. classification
  i. complication
  i. impairment
  i. method of purging
immunological (*var. of* immunologic)
immunomodulating
  i. effect
  i. infection
immunomodulation
immunonutrition
immunoprecipitation
immunoproliferative
  i. lesion
  i. small intestine disease (IPSID)
immunoreactivity
immunoscintigraphy
immunostain
  cytokeratin i.
immunostaining
immunostimulation
immunosuppressed patient
immunosuppression
  pharmacologic i.
  short-term i.
  tacrolimus-based i.
immunosympathectomy
immunotherapy
  active specific i.
  systemic i.
impacted
  i. calculus
  i. fracture
impaction
  basket i.
  endoscope i.

fecal i.
food bolus i.
i. lesion
i. point
stool i.

impaired
    i. healing
    i. mobility
    i. oxygen utilization
    i. regeneration syndrome
impairment
    hemodynamic i.
    immunologic i.
impalement
    abdominal i.
    anorectal i.
impalpable testis
impar
    tuberculum i.
impatent
impedance
    electrode i.
    i. method
    pacemaker i.
    i. plethysmography
    i. pneumography
imperfecta
    lethal osteogenesis i.
    osteogenesis i.
    severe deforming osteogenesis i.
    Sillence type I-IV osteogenesis i.
imperforate anus
imperforation
Imperial
    I. College London Hospital (ICLH)
    I. College of London double-cup
    arthroplasty
impetiginization
impingement
    graft i.
    i. sign
implant
    i. abutment
    i. alloy aluminum
    i. arthroplasty
    i. biocompatibility
    breast i.
    i. cervix
    dental i.
    drainage i.
    encapsulated breast i.
    i. entry
    i. erosion
    i. extrusion
    i. failure
    i. fatigue
    fill breast i.
    i. fixture
    i. fracture

i. framework
i. gingival sulcus
i. infrastructure
i. installation
i. mesostructure
i. migration
i. model
i. neck
neoplastic port site i.
palatal i.
2-piece dental i.
i. placement
porous polyethylene i.
porous tantalum i.
prosthetic i.
i. reaction
i. removal
i. restoration
i. stage
i. structure
i. substructure interspace
i. superstructure neck
i. survival rate
titanium vocal fold medialization i.
implantable
    i. cardioverter-defibrillator/atrial
    tachycardia pacing
    i. gastric stimulation
    i. infusion port
    i. infusion system
    i. intrathecal pump
    i. pain modality
implantation
    i. bleeding
    circumferential i.
    Columbia University selection factors
    for LVAD i.
    cortical i.
    displacement i.
    Estes ovary i.
    i. failure
    fusion i.
    gastric balloon i.
    i. graft
    hypodermic i.
    interstitial i.
    in-the-bag i.
    intracavitary i.
    intraocular lens i.
    intrusive i.
    mesh i.
    i. metastasis
    metastatic i.
    needle tract i.
    nerve i.
    periosteal i.
    i. phase
    placental i.
    radioactive seed i.

implantation (*continued*)
    radon seed i.
    real-time 3D biplanar transperineal prostate i.
    i. response
    screw i.
    i. site
    stent i.
    subcutaneous i.
    subdural grid i.
    submuscular i.
    subpectoral i.
    superficial i.
    tension-free mesh i.
    i. test
    tubouterine i.
    ureter i.
    virtual i.
implant-bearing surface
implant-cement interface
implanted
    i. neural stimulator
    i. suture technique
implication
    clinical i.
    psychologic i.
implicit memory
implosive therapy
impotence, impotency
    iatrogenic i.
    vasculogenic i.
impotency (*var. of* impotence)
impregnation
impressio, *pl.* **impressiones**
impression, impressio
    cardiac i.
    colic i.
    digitate i.
    duodenal i.
    esophageal i.
    extrinsic esophageal i.
    i. fracture
    gastric i.
    i. preparation
    prepared cavity i.
    renal i.
    suprarenal i.
    surgical bone i.
    i. technique
    trigeminal i.
impressiones (*pl. of* impressio)
imprint
    tissue i.
improvement
    clinical i.
impulse
    ectopic i.
    i. formation

    mobilization with i.
    point of maximum i. (PMI)
Imre keratoplasty
Imrie prognostic scoring index
Imuran
imus
IMV
    inferior mesenteric vein
    intermittent mandatory ventilation
in
    i. extremis
    opting i.
    i. situ
    i. situ bypass
    i. situ dissection
    i. situ hypothermic perfusion
    i. situ photocoagulation
    i. situ pinning
    i. situ procedure
    i. situ reconstruction
    i. situ saphenous vein graft
    i. situ spinal fusion
    i. situ split liver procurement
    i. situ uterine repair
    i. utero exposure
    i. vitro contracture test (IVCT)
    i. vitro fertilization (IVF)
    i. vitro fertilization-embryo transfer
    i. vivo
    i. vivo duplex ultrasound
    i. vivo fertilization
    i. vivo optical spectroscopy
In
    inion
inactivation
    trigger-point i.
inadequate
    i. dilation
    i. gas exchange
    i. postoperative oxygenation
    i. postoperative ventilation
    i. surgery
    i. visualization
inadvertent
    i. endobronchial intubation
    i. enterotomy
    i. hypothermia
    i. laceration
    i. serosal tear
    i. trauma
    i. venous injury
in-and-out catheterization
inapparent infection
Inapsine
in-between size
3-in-1 block
incarcerated
    i. hernia

i. intussuscepted bowel
i. vesicoinguinal hernia
incarceration
    colon i.
    colonoscopy-related i.
    hernia i.
    iris i.
    penile i.
    retrograde i.
incarial bone
incarnant
incarnative
incentive spirometer
incidence
incident
    i. exposure
    i. pain
    i. point
incidental
    i. appendectomy
    i. parathyroidectomy
    i. rupture
    i. splenectomy
incidentaloma
    adrenal i.
    pancreatic i.
    periampullary i.
incineration
incisal
    i. canal
    i. cavity
    i. mandibular plane angle
    i. point
    i. preparation
incised
    i. fascia
    i. wound
incision
    abdominal wall i.
    abdominoinguinal i.
    abdominothoracic i.
    ab externo i.
    ab interno i.
    Abruzzini i.
    Agnew-Verhoeff i.
    alar i.
    Alexander i.
    i. aligner
    Amussat i.
    i. and drainage (I&D)
    angular i.
    anterior i.
    anterolateral thoracotomy i.
    anteromedial i.
    antimesenteric i.
    appendectomy i.
    apron flap i.
    apron skin i.
    arcuate i.

areolar i.
Auvray i.
axillary i.
backcut i.
Bacon-Babcock abdominal-anal i.
Banks-Laufman i.
Battle i.
battledore i.
Battle-Jalaguier-Kammerer i.
bayonet-type i.
Bergmann i.
Bergmann-Israel i.
Bevan abdominal i.
bicoronal i.
bifrontal i.
bikini skin i.
bilateral subcostal i.'s
bilateral transabdominal i.'s
bisubcostal i.
Blair i.
boutonnière i.
Brackin i.
breast i.
Brock i.
Brockman i.
Brunner modified i.
Brunner palmar i.
Bruser skin i.
bucket-handle i.
Burns-Haney i.
Burwell-Scott modification of
  Watson-Jones i.
buttonhole skin i.
Caldwell-Luc i.
capsular i.
cautery i.
celiotomy i.
cervical i.
cesarean section i.
Chang-Miltner i.
Charnley i.
Cherney lower transverse
  abdominal i.
chevron i.
chevron-shaped i.
Chiene i.
choledochotomy i.
chord i.
Cincinnati i.
circular i.
circumareolar i.
circumferential i.
circumlimbal i.
circumlinear i.
circumscribing i.
circumumbilical i.
clamshell i.
classical transverse i.
clavicular i.

incision (*continued*)
    i. closure
    Codman i.
    Coffey i.
    collar i.
    Colonna-Ralston i.
    colpotomy i.
    confirmatory i.
    conjunctival i.
    Connell i.
    corneal i.
    corneoscleral i.
    corridor i.
    cortical i.
    Courvoisier i.
    Couvelaire i.
    Crawford i.
    crisscrossing abdominal wall i.'s
    crosshatch i.
    cross-tunneling i.
    crucial i.
    cruciate i.
    Cubbins i.
    Curtin i.
    curved i.
    curvilinear i.
    cutdown i.
    darting i.
    Deaver i.
    decompression i.
    deltoid-splitting i.
    deltopectoral i.
    Depage i.
    diamond-shaped i.
    dorsal linear i.
    dorsal longitudinal i.
    dorsal lumbotomy i.
    dorsal transverse i.
    dorsolateral i.
    dorsomedial i.
    double i.
    Dührssen i.
    dural i.
    DuVries i.
    Dwyer i.
    Edebohls i.
    eleventh rib flank i.
    eleventh rib transperitoneal i.
    elliptical uterine i.
    Elsberg i.
    endaural mastoid i.
    endoscopic i.
    endoscopically performed
      longitudinal i.
    endourological cold knife i.
    epigastric i.
    extended left subcostal i.
    external bevel i.
    extraction i.

    fascia-splitting i.
    Fergusson i.
    fiber-splitting i.
    fishmouth i.
    flank i.
    flexed i.
    Fowler-Philip i.
    Frazier i.
    frown i.
    Gaenslen split-heel i.
    Gatellier-Chastang i.
    Gibson long vertical relaxing i.
    Gibson-type i.
    Gluck i.
    goblet i.
    gray-line i.
    Greenhow i.
    Grice i.
    gridiron i.
    Griffith i.
    grooved i.
    gullwing i.
    Hajek i.
    Handley i.
    Harmon i.
    Harper-Warren i.
    Hayes Martin i.
    Heineke-Mikulicz i.
    hemicircular i.
    Henderson skin i.
    Henry i.
    hernia i.
    H-flap i.
    hockey stick i.
    Hood and Kirklin i.
    horizontal i.
    horseshoe i.
    horseshoe-shaped i.
    H-shaped capsular i.
    Hueter i.
    ilioinguinal i.
    infraclavicular i.
    inframammary i.
    infraumbilical i.
    inguinal i.
    inner bevel i.
    intercartilaginous i.
    internal bevel i.
    intracapsular i.
    intraoral i.
    intraperitoneal i.
    inverse bevel i.
    inverted bevel i.
    inverted-U abdominal i.
    inverted-Y i.
    Jackson i.
    Jergesen i.
    Joel-Cohen abdominal wall i.
    J-shaped skin i.

Kammerer-Battle i.
Kehr i.
keyhole i.
Killian i.
Kocher i.
Koenig-Schaefer i.
Küstner i.
Lanz i.
laparotomy i.
LaRoque herniorrhaphy i.
lateral utility i.
lazy-C i.
lazy-H i.
lazy-S i.
lazy-Z i.
L-curved i.
Lempert i.
Lilienthal i.
limbal i.
i. line
linear i.
Linton i.
lip-splitting i.
Loeffler-Ballard i.
longitudinal i.
low-collar i.
lower uterine segment i.
low-segment transverse i.
low transverse i.
L-shaped capsular i.
Ludloff i.
Lynch i.
MacFee i.
Mackenrodt i.
Mallard i.
marginal i.
Martin i.
Mason i.
mastectomy i.
mastoid i.
Mayfield i.
Maylard i.
Mayo-Robson i.
McArthur i.
McBurney appendectomy i.
McLaughlin-Ryder i.
McVay i.
medial parapatellar i.
median sternotomy i.
Mexican hat i.
Meyer i.
midabdominal transverse i.
midaxillary line i.
midline lower abdominal i.
midline oblique i.
midline upper abdominal i.
Mikulicz i.
minilaparotomy i.
modified elliptical i.

modified Gibson i.
Morison i.
multiple-port i.
muscle-sparing i.
muscle-splitting i.
Nagamatsu i.
Nicola i.
nonrib-spreading thoracotomy i.
Ober i.
Ollier i.
omega-shaped i.
Orr i.
ovarian i.
overlapping i.
palmar i.
parainguinal i.
paramedial i.
paramedian i.
parapatellar i.
pararectus i.
parasagittal i.
parascapular i.
paraumbilical i.
paravaginal i.
Parker i.
Péan i.
perianal i.
periareolar i.
perilimbal i.
perineal i.
periscapular i.
peritoneal i.
periumbilical i.
Perthes i.
Pfannenstiel i.
Phemister i.
Picot i.
plantar longitudinal i.
plaque i.
popliteal i.
port i.
postauricular i.
posterior hemicircular i.
posterior transthoracic i.
posterolateral costotransversectomy i.
preauricular i.
precut i.
Pridie i.
proximal i.
Pulvertaft fishmouth i.
puncture i.
racket i.
racket-shaped i.
racquet i.
racquet-shaped i.
radial skin i.
recently healed surgical i.
rectus muscle-splitting i.
rectus sheath i.

incision (*continued*)
    recumbent i.
    relaxing i.
    relief i.
    relieving i.
    Rethi i.
    retroauricular i.
    retroperitoneal i.
    reverse bevel i.
    reverse-Y i.
    right-sided submandibular
      transverse i.
    rim i.
    Robertson i.
    Rockey-Davis i.
    Rodman i.
    Rollet i.
    Rosen i.
    Roux-en-Y jejunal loop i.
    Ruddy i.
    S i.
    saber-cut i.
    Salmon backcut i.
    Sanders i.
    Sanger i.
    scalp i.
    Schobinger i.
    Schuchardt relaxing i.
    scoring i.
    scratch-type i.
    Sellheim i.
    semiflexed i.
    semilunar i.
    serpentine i.
    S-flap i.
    Shambaugh i.
    shelving i.
    shoulder strap i.
    Simon i.
    single midline extraperitoneal i.
    Singleton i.
    skin crease i.
    skin knife i.
    skived i.
    Sloan i.
    smiling i.
    Smith-Petersen anterior hip
      joint i.
    spindle-shaped i.
    spiral i.
    split i.
    split-heel i.
    S-shaped i.
    stab skin i.
    stab wound i.
    standard clavicular i.
    standard Kocher i.
    standard retroperitoneal flank i.
    stellate i.

    steri-stripped i.
    sternal-splitting i.
    sternotomy i.
    Stewart i.
    stocking-seam i.
    straight i.
    subciliary i.
    subcostal flank i.
    subcostal transperitoneal i.
    subinguinal i.
    sublabial i.
    submammary i.
    subtrochanteric i.
    subumbilical i.
    supracervical i.
    suprapubic Pfannenstiel i.
    supraumbilical i.
    surgical i.
    Sutherland-Rowe i.
    Swan i.
    T i.
    tangential i.
    temporal i.
    tennis racquet i.
    Thomas-Warren i.
    thoracoabdominal i.
    thoracotomy i.
    transection i.
    transmeatal tympanoplasty i.
    transpubic i.
    transrectus i.
    transurethral laser i.
    transverse i.
    transverse fundal i.
    transverse mastectomy i.
    transverse skin i.
    trap i.
    trapdoor i.
    trapezoidal i.
    T-shaped i.
    umbilical skin-knife i.
    unilateral subcostal i.
    upper midline i.
    upright-Y i.
    U-shaped i.
    uterine i.
    vertical i.
    vertical midline i.
    vertical uterine i.
    volar midline oblique i.
    volar zig-zag finger i.
    von Noorden i.
    V-shaped i.
    Wagner skin i.
    Warren i.
    watchband i.
    Watson-Jones i.
    Weber-Fergusson i.
    web space i.

wedge i.
Weir i.
Westin-Hall i.
Whipple i.
Wilde i.
Willy Meyer
  mastectomy i.
W-shaped i.
xiphoid-to-pubis midline
  abdominal i.
xiphoid-to-umbilicus i.
Y i.
York-Mason i.
Y-shaped i.
Y-V plasty i.
Z i.
Z-flap i.
zig-zag finger i.
Z-plasty i.
Z-shaped i.
incisional
  i. biopsy
  i. corporoplasty
  i. gastropexy
  i. hernia
  i. hernioplasty
  i. infiltration
  i. metastasis
  i. pain
  i. scar
3-incision esophagectomy
incision-induced hyperalgesia
4-incision procedure
5-incision procedure
incisive
  i. canal
  i. duct
  i. foramen
  i. fossa
incisor point
incisura, *pl.* **incisurae**
  i. angularis
  i. mastoidea
incisurae (*pl. of* incisura)
incisural
  i. dissection
  i. epidermoidoma
  i. space
inciting pathology
inclination
  axial i.
  condylar guidance i.
  crown i.
  enamel rod i.
  lateral condylar i.
  lingual i.
  pelvic i.
inclinatio pelvis
inclinometer

1-inclinometer method
2-inclinometer method
inclusion
  i. body
  i. body disease
incompetence, incompetency
  primary vascular i.
  saphenofemoral i.
incompetency (*var. of* incompetence)
incompetent
  i. perforator
  i. sphincter
incomplete
  i. amputation
  i. atrioventricular dissociation
  i. AV dissociation
  i. colonoscopy
  i. compound fracture
  i. dislocation
  i. duplication
  i. excision
  i. fistula
  i. hernia
  i. polypectomy
  i. reduction
  i. regeneration
  i. relaxation
  i. right bundle branch block
  i. tumor resection
inconsequential echo
incontinence, incontinentia
  anal i.
  Blaivas classification of urinary i.
  exercise-induced i.
  fecal i.
  gas i.
  neurogenic i.
  overflow i.
  paradoxical i.
  passive i.
  postprostatectomy i.
  reflex i.
  stress urinary i.
  urge i.
  urinary i.
  urinary exertional i.
incontinent
  i. ileostomy
  i. ileovesicostomy
incontinentia (*var. of* incontinence)
incorporated
  meatal advancement and
    glansplasty i.
incorporation
  bone graft i.
increased
  i. lateral joint space
  i. pressure
  i. systemic vascular resistance

incremental
    i. blood sampling
    i. reactivation
    i. therapy
incretin
incrustation
    stent i.
incudal fold
incudes (*pl. of* incus)
incudomalleolar
    i. articulation
    i. joint
incudostapedial
incus, *pl.* **incudes**
indenization
indentation
    i. gonioscopy
    i. hardness
    haustral i.
    i. operation
    prominent i.
    i. tonometer
    i. tonometry
independent
    i. ambulation
    i. exercise program
indeterminate
    i. colitis
    i. FNA
index, *pl.* **indices**
    Abdominal Trauma I. (ATI)
    acute physiology prognostic
      scoring i.
    Addiction Severity I.
    A-line AEP i.
    A-line ARX i. (AAI)
    A-line auditory evoked potential i.
    A-line autoregressive i. (AAI)
    alveolar i.
    American Rheumatism Association i.
    American Urological Association
      symptom i.
    analgesic i.
    anesthetic i.
    ankle-brachial pressure i. (ABPI)
    Arthritis Helplessness I. (AHI)
    articulation i.
    ARX i.
    atherectomy i.
    atrial stasis i.
    auricular i.
    basilar i.
    biliary saturation i.
    bispectral i.
    body mass i. (BMI)
    Broders i.
    cardiac i. (CI)
    cardiopulmonary risk i.
    cephalic i.

    cephalorrhachidian i.
    cerebral i.
    cerebral state i.
    cerebrospinal i.
    chest i.
    cholesterol saturation i.
    computed tomography severity i.
      (CTSI)
    cranial i.
    dental i.
    Department of Veterans Affairs
      pulmonary risk i.
    diastolic pressure-time i.
    eccentricity i.
    ejection phase i.
    exercise i.
    facial i.
    Flower dental i.
    frequency-duration i.
    Gastrointestinal Quality of Life I.
      (GIQLI)
    Global Severity I. (GSI)
    gnathic i.
    Goldman cardiac risk i.
    height-length i.
    Imrie prognostic scoring i.
    irritation i.
    juxtaglomerular granulation i.
    length-breadth i.
    length-height i.
    limb salvage i.
    Mannheim peritonitis i.
    maturation i.
    mean shunt i.
    i. metacarpophalangeal joint
      reconstruction
    mitral valve closure i.
    Modified Pain Disability I.
      (MPDI)
    nasal i.
    Neck Disability I.
    i. of variability
    orbital i.
    orbitonasal i.
    Oswestry Disability I. (ODI)
    oxygenation i. (OI)
    oxygen saturation i.
    palatal i.
    palatomaxillary i.
    patient state i. (PSI)
    pectus i.
    penetrating abdominal trauma i.
      (PATI)
    penile-brachial pressure i. (PBPI)
    phosphate excretion i.
    physical therapy i.
    i. pollicization
    portal shunt i.
    portal-systemic encephalopathy i.

Present Pain I.
pressure-volume i.
PSE i.
pulmonary vascular resistance i.
(PVRI)
Quetelet body mass i.
Ranson prognostic scoring i.
rapid shallow breathing i.
i. ray amputation
recovery i.
relaxation time i.
renal resistive i.
right ventricular stroke work i.
(RVSWI)
risk i.
Röhrer i.
sacral i.
saturation i.
sedimentation i.
segmental pressure i.
Shoulder Pain and Disability I.
shunt i.
Singh osteoporosis i.
supranormal cardiac i.
systemic vascular resistance i.
systolic pressure time i.
(SPTI)
thoracic i.
transversovertical i.
venous-filling i.
ventilation i.
vertical i.
zygomaticoauricular i.

Indian
I. forehead flap method
I. forehead nasal reconstruction
flap
I. rhinoplasty

Indiana
I. continent reservoir urinary
diversion
I. urinary diversion pouch

India rubber suture
indication
clinical i.
emergency i.
familial i.
surgical i.

indicator
Checklist of Nonverbal Pain I.'s
(CNPI)
finger i.
i. fractionation
i. of anesthetic depth
prognostic i.
redox i.

indicator-dilution curve
indices (*pl. of* index)
indifferent genitalia

indirect
i. calorimetry
i. defect
i. fracture
i. hemagglutination test
i. hernial sac
i. inguinal hernia
i. laryngoscopy
i. manipulation
i. memory
i. obturator nerve block
i. ophthalmoscopy
i. portography
i. pulpal therapy
i. reduction
i. restorative method
i. technique
i. transfusion
i. triangulation

indiscriminate lesion
indocyanine
i. green clearance result
i. green indicator dilution technique
i. green retention test

indomethacin-induced gastropathy
induced
i. apnea
i. bronchospasm
i. hypotension
i. hypotension anesthetic technique
i. tension pneumothorax
i. ventilatory depression

induction
anesthetic i.
i. anesthetic technique
i. chemotherapy
dorsal i.
electric i.
endotracheal i.
enzyme i.
lysogenic i.
magnetic i.
menstrual cycle i.
neuromuscular system electric i.
i. of anesthesia
ovulation i.
pain i.
rapid sequence i. (RSI)
remission i.
single-breath i.
sputum i.
superovulation i.
i. therapy

induration
brawny i.
cyanotic i.
essential brown i.
Froriep i.
gray i.

induration (*continued*)
  idiopathic brown i.
  plastic i.
  red i.
industrial exposure
ineffective esophageal motility
inequality
  ventilation/perfusion i.
inertia
  colonic i.
inextensible
infancy
  persistent hyperinsulinemia and
    hyperglycemia of i.
infant
  Distress Scale for Ventilated
    Newborn Infants (DSVNI)
  i. respiratory distress syndrome
    (IRDS)
infantile
  i. articulation
  i. choriocarcinoma syndrome
  i. colic
  i. embryonal carcinoma
  i. hernia
  i. perseveration
infantilism
  celiac i.
infarct
  i. expansion
  i. extension
infarcted graft
infarction
  evolving myocardial i.
  hemorrhagic i.
  myocardial i. (MI)
  renal i.
  small-bowel i.
  subendocardial myocardial i. (SEMI)
  Thrombolysis in Myocardial I.
    (TIMI)
  ureteral i.
infarctive lesion
infected
  i. collection
  i. field
  i. graft
  i. necrosis
  i. pancreatic necrosis
  i. tract
infection
  abortive i.
  Absidia i.
  active systemic bacterial i.
  adenoviral i.
  adenovirus i.
  adnexal i.
  aerobic i.
  airborne i.

amebic i.
anaerobic ocular i.
antifungal esophageal i.
antifungal-resistant opportunistic i.
apical i.
Aspergillus i.
asymptomatic i.
atypical mycobacterial i.
bacterial i.
benign papillomavirus i.
beta hemolytic streptococcus i.
biliary tract i.
blood-borne i.
bloodstream i.
brain i.
buccal space i.
Bunyavirus i.
i. calculus
Campylobacter i.
Candida i.
candidal i.
catheter-related i.
catheter tunnel i.
central line i.
cervical i.
cervicovaginal i.
chlamydial i.
Chlamydia trachomatis i.
chorioamnionic i.
chronic Epstein-Barr virus i.
closed space i.
clostridial i.
CMV i.
Coccidioides i.
coliform urinary i.
colonization i.
community-acquired i.
congenital HIV i.
cross i.
cryptococcal i.
Cryptococcus i.
cryptogenic i.
cryptoglandular i.
cryptosporidial i.
cutaneous bacterial i.
cutaneous viral i.
cysticercal i.
cytomegalovirus i.
deep delayed i.
deep-seated fungal i.
deep wound i.
dengue hemorrhagic fever i.
dental i.
dermatophyte fungal i.
disc space i.
dragon worm i.
droplet i.
dust-borne i.
EBV i.

echovirus i.
ectothrix i.
endemic fungal i.
endogenous i.
endothrix i.
enteric i.
enteroviral i.
environmental mycobacterial i.
epidural space i.
Epstein-Barr virus i.
esophageal fungal i.
exit site i.
exogenous i.
extrapulmonary *Pneumocystis carinii* i.
eyelid molluscum contagiosum i.
fascial space i.
felon i.
fetal i.
focal i.
foreign body i.
fungal pancreatic i.
fungous i.
gas-forming pyogenic liver i.
gas-producing streptococcal i.
gastric i.
gastrointestinal i.
genital i.
genitourinary i.
Giardia i.
gonococcal i.
graft i.
gram-positive bacterial i.
granulomatous bacterial i.
granulomatous fungal i.
group A beta-hemolytic streptococcal i.
group A streptococcus i.
guinea worm i.
Hantavirus i.
helmintic i.
hepatic candidal i.
hepatic fungal i.
hepatitis A-E i.
herpes simplex virus i.
herpes zoster i.
herpetic i.
hibernal epidemic viral i.
Histoplasma i.
HIV-1, -2 i.
hospital-acquired i. (HAI)
human bite i.
human papillomavirus i.
iatrogenic i.
immunomodulating i.
inapparent i.
intestinal i.
intraabdominal i.
intraamniotic i.

intrauterine i.
invasive fungal i.
IUD-related i.
kala-azar i.
laryngeal i.
latent herpes simplex virus i.
line i.
liver cyst i.
local i.
lower genital tract i.
lower respiratory tract i.
MAC i.
MAI i.
mass i.
masticator space i.
maternal i.
Meleney i.
metasynchronous bacterial urinary tract i.
middle ear i.
mixed fungal/bacterial i.
mixed nail i.
monilial i.
Mucor i.
multiple hepatitis virus i.
musculoskeletal i.
mycobacterial i.
Mycobacterium avium complex i.
Mycobacterium avium-intracellulare i.
mycoplasma i.
mycotic i.
necrotizing i.
neisserial i.
nematode i.
neonatal i.
neutropenia-related bacterial i.
nondermatophyte fungal i.
nonopportunistic i.
nontuberculous mycobacterial i.
nosocomial i.
nosocomial fungal i.
odontogenic i.
opportunistic systemic fungal i.
oral i.
organ space i.
overwhelming postsplenectomy i.
pancreatic bacterial i.
papillomavirus i.
parainfluenza virus i.
parasitic i.
parastomal i.
paravaccinia virus i.
paronychial i.
pelvic i.
percutaneous bone marrow i.
perianal i.
periapical i.
perinatal i.
perineal i.

infection (*continued*)
  perioperative wound i.
  periorbital i.
  peripancreatic i.
  peristomal i.
  peritoneal fungal i.
  persistent tolerant i.
  pharyngeal gonococcal i.
  pin tract i.
  pneumococcal i.
  polymicrobial i.
  postoperative i.
  postpartum i.
  postsplenectomy i.
  i. prevention
  primary fungal i.
  primary herpes simplex i.
  protozoal i.
  Pseudomonas i.
  puerperal i.
  pulmonary bacterial i.
  pulmonary fungal i.
  pulmonary parenchymal i.
  pure fungal i.
  pyodermatous i.
  pyogenic spinal i.
  i. rate
  recurrent upper respiratory
    tract i.
  renal cyst i.
  renal fungal i.
  repeated respiratory i.
  reservoir of i.
  respiratory syncytial virus i.
  respiratory tract i.
  retroperitoneal i.
  retrovirus i.
  rhinocerebral i.
  Rhizopus i.
  rickettsial i.
  rotavirus i.
  Salinem i.
  salivary gland i.
  scalp i.
  secondary fungal i.
  serpent i.
  Shigella i.
  shunt i.
  skin i.
  spinal i.
  spirochetal i.
  spirochete i.
  staphylococcal i.
  streptococcal i.
  Streptococcus i.
  subclinical i.
  subcutaneous fungal i.
  subcutaneous necrotizing i.
  subperiosteal i.
  subumbilical i.
  superficial subumbilical i.
  suppurative i.
  surgical i.
  surgical site i. (SSI)
  sycosiform fungous i.
  symptomatic i.
  synchronous urinary tract i.
  systemic fungal i.
  tarsal joint i.
  temporal space i.
  terminal i.
  Torulopsis i.
  trematode i.
  Trichomonas i.
  tunnel i.
  ultralow anterior resection
    parastomal i.
  unusual opportunistic i.
  upper genital tract i.
  upper respiratory i. (URI)
  upper respiratory tract i.
  urinary tract i. (UTI)
  uterine i.
  vaccinia i.
  vaginal i.
  varicella i.
  varicella-zoster virus i.
  vertically acquired i.
  vesicular viral i.
  Vincent i.
  viral respiratory i.
  vulvar i.
  vulvovaginal premenarchal i.
  web space i.
  whipworm i.
  wound i.
  xenogeneic i.
  yeast i.
  zoonotic i.
infectious
  i. complication
  I. Disease Society of America
    (IDSA)
  i. etiology
  i. granuloma
  i. peritonitis
**infective extraabdominal
  complication**
inferior
  i. aberrant ductule
  i. accessory fissure
  i. alveolar artery
  i. alveolar nerve
  i. alveolar vein
  i. apical (IA)
  i. apical segment
  i. arcuate bundle
  i. articular pit

i. articular process
i. basal (IB)
i. basal segment
i. boundary
i. carotid artery
i. carotid triangle
i. cerebral artery
i. cervical ganglion
i. complete closed dislocation
i. complete compound dislocation
i. costal facet
i. costal pit
i. dental foramen
i. duodenal fold
i. duodenal fossa
i. duodenal recess
i. edge
i. epigastric artery (IEA)
i. epigastric artery graft
i. epigastric lamina
i. extradural approach
i. face
i. flap
i. flexure
i. fornix reformation
i. gland
i. glenohumeral ligament
  (IGHL)
i. gluteal artery
i. hemorrhoidal artery
i. hemorrhoidal nerve
i. hemorrhoidal plexus
i. hypogastric plexus
i. hypophysial artery
i. ileocecal hernia
i. ileocecal recess
i. iliac spine
i. internal parietal artery
i. interosseous vein
i. labial artery
i. lacrimal duct
i. lacrimal papilla
i. lacrimal punctum
i. laryngeal artery
i. laryngeal cavity
i. laryngeal nerve
i. laryngotomy
i. lateral genicular artery
i. lateral genicular vein
i. lingular segment
i. longitudinal sinus
i. meatal antrostomy
i. meatus
i. medial genicular artery
i. medial genicular vein
i. mediastinum
i. mesenteric artery
i. mesenteric ganglion
i. mesenteric lymph node
i. mesenteric plexus
i. mesenteric vein (IMV)
i. occipital triangle
i. omental recess
i. orbital fissure
i. palpebral nerve
i. pancreatic artery
i. pancreaticoduodenal artery
i. pancreatic vein
i. parietal lobe
i. pelvic aperture
i. petrosal groove
i. petrosal sinus
i. petrosal sulcus
i. pharyngeal constrictor
i. phrenic artery
i. pole
i. pubic ligament
i. pulmonary ligament
i. rectal artery
i. rectal fold
i. rectal nerve
i. rectal plexus
i. sagittal sinus
i. suprarenal artery
i. surface
i. tarsus
i. temporal branch
i. thoracic aperture
i. thoracic artery
i. thyroid artery
i. thyroid notch
i. thyroid plexus
i. thyroid tubercle
i. transvermian approach
i. transverse rectal fold
i. transverse scapular ligament
i. turbinate blade
i. ulnar collateral artery
i. vena cava (IVC)
i. vena cava balloon occlusion
i. vena cava ligation
i. vena cava occlusion
i. vena cava pressure
i. vena cava reconstruction
i. vertebral notch
i. vesical artery
i. vesical nerve
i. vesical plexus

inferioris
  vellus olivae i.
inferior-lateral endonasal transsphenoidal approach
inferolateral
inferomedial aspect
infertility evaluation
infestation
  noninvasive i.
infiltrate

infiltrating
    i. duct adenocarcinoma
    i. ductal carcinoma
    i. lobular carcinoma
infiltration
    adipose i.
    i. anesthesia
    i. anesthetic technique
    bacterial mucosal i.
    i. block
    bone marrow i.
    brachial plexus i.
    calcareous i.
    cellular i.
    choroidal i.
    colonic i.
    diffuse fatty i.
    epituberculous i.
    fatty i.
    focal fatty i.
    gastric epithelial cell i.
    gelatinous i.
    glomerular macrophage i.
    glomerular neutrophil i.
    glycogen i.
    gray i.
    incisional i.
    leukemic i.
    leukocyte i.
    leukocytic i.
    lipomatous i.
    local tissue i.
    lymphocytic i.
    lymphoid i.
    massive malignant i.
    mononuclear cell i.
    neutrophilic i.
    panmucosal inflammatory cell i.
    paraneural i.
    patchy i.
    peribronchiolar lymphocyte i.
    pericapsular fat i.
    perineural i.
    plasma cell portal i.
    root i.
    sanguineous i.
    tuberculous i.
    tumor i.
infiltrative carcinoma
inflamed synovial pouch
inflammable
inflammation
    active chronic i.
    acute and chronic i.
    acute hemorrhagic i.
    adhesive i.
    allergic i.
    alterative i.
    atrophic i.

blenorrhagic i.
bronchial i.
bullous granulomatous i.
calcified granulomatous i.
cartilage i.
caseating granulomatous i.
caseous i.
catarrhal i.
cavitating i.
i. cell
central zone i.
cervical i.
chronic jejunal i.
circumscribed i.
confluent i.
croupous i.
cystic acute i.
cystic chronic i.
cystic granulomatous i.
degenerative i.
diffuse acute i.
diffuse chronic i.
disseminated i.
ear cartilage i.
erosive i.
esophageal i.
exanthematous i.
exudative granulomatous i.
fibrinoid necrotizing i.
fibrinopurulent i.
fibrinous i.
fibrocaseous i.
fibroid i.
focal granulomatous i.
follicular i.
gangrenous granulomatous i.
gelatinous acute i.
gingival i.
granulomatous i.
hemorrhagic i.
hyperplastic i.
ileal i.
immune i.
interstitial i.
intralobular i.
ischemic ocular i.
localized i.
membranous acute i.
microbiliary i.
miliary granulomatous i.
mucosal i.
multifocal i.
myocardial i.
necrotic i.
necrotizing granulomatous i.
neutrophilic i.
nonnecrotizing granulomatous i.
obliterative i.
ocular i.

organizing i.
ossifying i.
pelvic i.
periodontal i.
perirectal i.
phlegmonous i.
portal eosinophilic i.
portal tract i.
prepatellar bursa i.
productive i.
proliferative i.
pseudomembranous acute i.
purulent i.
pustular i.
i. reaction
recurrent i.
retrodiscal temporomandibular joint
  pad i.
sanguineous i.
sclerosing i.
serofibrinous i.
serous acute i.
spinal i.
subacute i.
suppurative acute i.
suppurative chronic i.
suppurative granulomatous i.
transmural i.
transudative i.
traumatic i.
ulcerative i.
urate-associated i.
uremic i.
vaginal i.
vesicular acute i.
vesicular granulomatous i.
**inflammation-induced postoperative
gastrointestinal tract dysfuncation**
inflammatory
  i. abdominal aortic aneurysm
  i. arteritis
  i. bowel disease
  i. breast carcinoma
  i. cascade
  i. cavity
  i. cell
  i. cytokine
  i. exudate
  i. fistula
  i. fracture
  i. granuloma
  i. lesion
  i. mediator
  i. membrane
  i. pain
  i. perforation
  i. problem
  i. pseudotumor
  i. pseudotumor formation

  i. response
  i. rupture
  i. sinus tract
  i. vascular disease
inflammatory-associated stenosis
inflated lung
inflation
  balloon i.
  i. reflex
inflection, inflexion
  point of i.
inflexion (*var. of* inflection)
inflow
  arterial i.
  i. control
  i. occlusion
  portal i.
  i. tract
  i. vessel
influence reaction
infold
informal method
information
  anatomic imaging i.
  histopathologic i.
  prognostic i.
informed consent
infraauricular mass
infraclavicular
  i. brachial plexus block
  i. fossa
  i. incision
  i. node
  i. part of brachial plexus
  i. triangle
infraclinoid aneurysm
infracostal line
infracotyloid
infraction fracture
infradiaphragmatic
infraduodenal fossa
infragastric pancreatoscopy
**infragenicular popliteal artery
  (IGPA)**
infraglenoid tubercle
infraglottic
  i. cavity
  i. space
infrahepatic
  i. cavotomy
  i. inferior vena cava
infrahyoid
  i. bursa
  i. muscle
infrainguinal
  i. arterial reconstruction graft failure
  i. bypass
  i. disease
infralabyrinthine approach

inframammary
    i. approach
    i. crease
    i. fold
    i. incision
    i. region
inframandibular
inframarginal
inframaxillary
inframesocolic space
infraorbital
    i. anesthesia
    i. artery
    i. canal
    i. foramen
    i. groove
    i. injection
    i. nerve
    i. nerve block
    i. notch
    i. region
    i. space
    i. space abscess
    i. suture
    i. vein
infrapatellar
    i. bursa
    i. fat body
    i. tendon rupture
infrapopliteal
    i. bypass
    i. revascularization
    i. transluminal angioplasty
    i. vessel
infrared
    i. coagulation
    near i.
    i. photocoagulation
    i. spectroscopy
    i. therapy
    i. transillumination gastroscopy
infrarenal
    i. abdominal aorta
    i. aorta
    i. aortic aneurysm
    i. aortic cross-clamping
    i. aortic reconstruction
    i. cava
    i. endograft placement
    i. graft
    i. template procedure
infrascapular
    i. artery
    i. region
infraspinatus
    i. bursa
    i. insertion erosion
    i. muscle
infraspinous fossa

infrasplenic
infrasternal angle
infrastructure
    implant i.
infratemporal
    i. crest
    i. fossa
    i. fossa approach
    i. space
infratentorial
    i. arteriovenous malformation
    i. lesion
    i. structure
    i. supracerebellar approach
    i. tumor
infrathoracic
infratrochlearis
    nervus i.
infratrochlear nerve
infraumbilical
    i. incision
    i. omphalocele
    i. position
infraversion
infundibula (*pl. of* infundibulum)
infundibular wedge resection
infundibulectomy
    Brock i.
infundibuliform
    i. fascia
    i. sheath
infundibuloma
infundibuloovarian ligament
infundibulopelvic ligament
infundibulotomy
infundibulum, *pl.* **infundibula**
    calyceal i.
    ethmoidal i.
infused fluid
infusion
    analgesic i.
    i. cholangiography
    chronic subcutaneous i.
    computer-assisted controlled i.
      (CACI)
    drip i.
    drug i.
    epidural opioid i.
    fructose i.
    i. graft
    hepatic arterial i. (HAI)
    intravariceal i.
    lipid i.
    mesenteric vasodilator i.
    nerve block i.
    phentolamine i.
    i. port
    portal i.
    propofol i.

protracted venous i.
i. rate
steady-state i.
subcutaneous i.
target-controlled i. (TCI)
triple-lumen i.
vasodilator i.
infusional chemotherapy
Ingelman-Sundberg gracilis muscle
  vesicovaginal fistula repair procedure
ingested foreign body
Inglis-Cooper flexor slide technique
Inglis-Ranawat-Straub
  I.-R.-S. elbow synovectomy
  I.-R.-S. synovectomy and
    débridement of elbow technique
Inglis triaxial total elbow arthroplasty
Ingram bony bridge resection
Ingram-Canle-Beaty
  epiphysial-metaphysial osteotomy
Ingram-Withers-Speltz motor test
ingrowing toenail
ingrown nail
ingrowth
  fibrous i.
  i. fixation
  local i.
inguen
inguinal
  i. aponeurotic fold
  i. approach
  i. branch
  i. canal
  i. canal dissection
  i. crest
  i. field block
  i. fossa
  i. gland
  i. hernia
  i. herniorrhaphy
  i. incision
  i. ligament
  i. lymphadenectomy
  i. lymph node metastasis
  i. neuralgia
  i. neurectomy
  i. perivascular block
  i. plexus
  i. region
  i. ring
  i. triangle
  i. trigone
  i. vasal obstruction
inguinale
  hernia uterus i.
inguinal-femoral node dissection
inguinocrural hernia
inguinodynia
  herniorrhaphy chronic i.

mesh i.
post herniorrhaphy i.
inguinofemoral hernia
inguinolabial hernia
inguinoperitoneal
inguinoproperitoneal hernia
inguinoscrotal hernia
inguinosuperficial hernia
inhalant anesthesia
inhalation
  i. aerosol
  i. agent
  i. analgesia
  i. anesthetic technique
  i. mask anesthesia
  i. method
  i. pneumonia
  i. therapy
  i. tuberculosis
inhalational anesthesia
inhaled
  i. agent
  i. anesthetic
  i. nitrous oxide (INO)
inherent
  i. ischemia
  i. risk
inherited
  i. cancer syndrome
  i. neuropathy
inhibition
  muscle i.
  pyruvate dehydrogenase i.
inhibitor
  bivalent reversible direct thrombin i.
  COX-2 i.
  cytokine receptor i.
  direct thrombin i.
  monoamine reuptake i.
  phosphodiesterase III i.
  proton pump i. (PPI)
  renin-angiotensin i.
  selective serotonin reuptake i.
    (SSRI)
inhibitory
  i. nerve
  i. neuromodulator
  i. reflex
  i. role
inhibitory-excitatory mechanism
in-hospital mortality rate
inion (In)
initial
  i. colostomy
  i. consonant position
  i. manifestation
  i. necrosectomy
  i. operation
  i. preparation

initial (*continued*)
    i. primary pathogen
    i. resection
    i. screening procedure
    i. syphilitic lesion
    i. systemic chemotherapy
initialization
initiation
    tumor i.
Initiative on Methods, Measurement, and Pain Assessment in Clinical Trials (IMMPACT)
injected
injection
    air i.
    Aquavan i.
    block i.
    blood patch i.
    bolus i.
    caudal epidural i.
    cervical nerve root i.
    ciliary i.
    circumcorneal i.
    collagen i.
    conjunctival i.
    continuous subcutaneous insulin i.
    contrast i.
    corticoid i.
    CT with hepatic arterial i.
    dermal i.
    dermal route of i.
    dye i.
    endoscopic India ink i.
    epidural steroid i. (ESI)
    ethanol i.
    extraarachnoid i.
    facet joint i.
    fluoroscopically guided corticosteroid i.
    fluoroscopically guided low-volume peritendinous corticosteroid i.
    heavy metal i.
    infraorbital i.
    i. injury
    intraarticular i.
    intraarticular facet i.
    intracavernosal i.
    intracavernous i.
    intracordal silicone i.
    intracytoplasmic sperm i. (ICSI)
    intradermal i.
    intralesional i.
    intramuscular i.
    intraosseous i.
    intrapulpal i.
    intrasphincteric i.
    intratendinous i.
    intrathecal i.
    intratumoral i.

    intravariceal i.
    intravascular i.
    intravenous i.
    intraventricular i.
    intravitreal i.
    ipsilateral i.
    isotope i.
    local i.
    lumbar epidural steroid i. (LESI)
    lumbar facet i.
    lumbar nerve root i.
    i. mass
    mental block i.
    i. method
    morphine sulfate extended-release liposome i.
    nasopalatine i.
    nerve root sleeve i.
    i. of local anesthetic
    paracervical i.
    paramagnetic contrast i.
    paravariceal i.
    parenchymal route of i.
    percutaneous alcohol i.
    percutaneous ethanol i. (PEI)
    peribulbar i.
    periocular i.
    peroneal tendon sheath i.
    polymethylmethacrylate i.
    retrobulbar i.
    retrogasserian glycerol i.
    root i.
    route of i.
    saline i.
    i. sclerotherapy
    selective i.
    sensitizing i.
    sham i.
    i. site
    steroid i.
    i. study
    subarachnoid i.
    subconjunctival i.
    subcutaneous i.
    tangential colonic submucosal i.
    i. technique
    test i.
    test-dose i.
    therapeutic i.
    i. therapy
    trigger point i.
    ultrasonographically guided i.
    van Lint i.
    vocal cord i.
    i. volume
injury
    acceleration i.
    acceleration/deceleration i.
    acute lung i.

Ajmalin liver i.
anal sphincter i.
anterior abdominal i.
arterial i.
associated i.
axial compression i.
axillary vascular i.
axonal i.
bile duct i.
biliary i.
blast gut i.
blast lung i.
blunt carotid i.
blunt liver i.
blunt torso i.
bowel i.
brachial plexus traction i.
brain i.
burn i.
Callahan extension of cervical i.
cardiac i.
carotid i.
cerebral i.
cervical i.
closed head i. (CHI)
closed soft tissue i.
combined injuries
complement-induced lung i.
compression i.
concomitant spinal cord i.
coup i.
crush i.
cutaneous burn i.
decompensation i.
diaphragm i.
diaphragmatic i.
duct i.
endothelial i.
epiphysial plate i.
esophageal i.
explosion i.
extension i.
extension-type cervical spine i.
extensor tendon i.
extraabdominal i.
extravasation i.
extremity i.
first-degree radiation i.
flexion-extension i.
fourth-degree radiation i.
geriatric i.
head i.
hemoclip-induced i.
hemorrhagic radiation i.
hepatic i.
hollow visceral i.
hollow viscus i.
hyperextension-hyperflexion i.
hyperfiltration i.

iatrogenic bile duct i.
iatrogenic bowel i.
inadvertent venous i.
injection i.
innominate vascular i.
intestinal radiation i.
intraabdominal i.
intraoperative inadvertent venous i.
intrathoracic i.
I/R i.
irradiation i.
ischemia-reperfusion i.
ischemic liver i.
ischemic neuronal i.
ischemic reperfusion i.
isolated arterial i.
isolated liver i.
isolated venous i.
kneecapping i.
laryngeal nerve i.
lateral compression i.
left-sided i.
levator i.
liver i.
major vascular i.
manipulation-induced PGID i.
medication-induced i.
microwave radiation i.
mild traumatic brain i. (MTBI)
minor splenic i.
missile i.
needlestick i. (NSI)
nerve i.
neurologic i.
nonsevered i.
obstetric traction i.
obturator nerve i.
occult diaphragmatic i.
open head i.
organ-specific pattern of i.
osteochondral i.
pediatric i.
penetrating liver i.
penetrating thoracoabdominal i.
percutaneous i.
perigenicular vascular i.
peripheral nerve i.
peroneal nerve i.
i. prevention
pronation i.
pronation-abduction i.
pronation-eversion i.
pronation-eversion-external rotation i.
proximal subclavian i.
radiation i.
recurrent nerve i.
reperfusion i.
repetitive motion i.
retroclavicular i.

injury (*continued*)
    right-sided i.
    second-degree radiation i.
    severe traumatic brain i.
    I. Severity Score (ISS)
    soft tissue extremity i.
    solid organ i.
    sphincter i.
    spinal cord i. (SCI)
    splenic i.
    stretch i.
    subclavian i.
    suction i.
    supination i.
    supination-external rotation i.
    supination-inversion rotation i.
    supination-plantar flexion i.
    terror-induced multiple
      casualty i.
    thermal i.
    third-degree radiation i.
    thoracic inlet vascular i.
    thoracoabdominal i.
    torso i.
    tracheal i.
    transfusion-related acute lung i.
      (TRALI)
    transfusion-related lung i.
    translation i.
    traumatic brain i.
    trifurcation i.
    trocar i.
    trocar-related i.
    ureteral i.
    urinary tract i.
    valgus-external rotation i.
    vascular i.
    venous i.
    ventilator-induced lung i. (VILI)
    visceral i.
    viscus i.
    whiplash i.
    zygomatic i.
injury-prevention strategy
inlay
    i. bone graft
    corneal i.
    direct method for making
      inlays
    epithelial i.
    i. restoration
inlet
    i. allotransplantation
    i. patch mucosa
    i. port
    thoracic i.
in-line
    i.-l. intravenous fluid warming
    i.-l. perfusion

inner
    i. bevel incision
    i. cell mass
    i. ear tack procedure
    i. limiting membrane
    i. table
innervation
    cutaneous i.
    lumbar facet joint i.
    i. of head and neck
    parasympathetic i.
    i. problem
    sensory i.
    striated muscle i.
innominate
    i. artery
    i. artery compression syndrome
    i. artery reconstruction
    i. bone
    i. bone resection
    i. cardiac vein
    i. line
    i. osteotomy
    i. vascular injury
    i. vessel
innovative therapy
INO
    inhaled nitrous oxide
inoperable
    i. canal
    i. patient
inoscopy
inotrope
    i. resuscitation
    i. resuscitation technique
inotropic state
inotropism
inotropy
    negative i.
Inoue balloon mitral valvotomy
inpatient
    i. dialysis
    i. dialysis unit
input layer
inquiry
    cognitive-attitudinal factor i.
INR
    international normalized ratio
Insall
    I. anterior cruciate ligament
      reconstruction
    I. ligament reconstruction technique
    I. patella alta method
    I. patellar injury classification
    I. patellar instability repair
      procedure
Insall-Burstein-Freeman knee arthroplasty
inscription
    tendinous i.

insemination
    artificial intravaginal i.
    cervical i.
    cup i.
    direct intraperitoneal i. (DIPI)
    heterologous i.
    high intrauterine i.
    intrafollicular i.
    intratubal i.
    intrauterine i.
    Makler i.
    subzonal i. (SUZI)
    i. swim-up technique
    therapeutic i.
    washed intrauterine i.
insert graft
insertion
    anatomic i.
    anomalous i.
    anuloplasty band i.
    axillary i.
    biliary endoprosthesis i.
    blind i.
    buttonhole puncture technique for
      hemodialysis needle i.
    catheter i.
    caval i.
    depth of i. (DOI)
    endovascular graft i.
    flatus tube i.
    fluoroscopic i.
    jejunal tube i.
    J-tube i.
    i. loss
    marginal i.
    needle i.
    path of i.
    PEG tube i.
    percutaneous catheter i.
    percutaneous endoscopic gastrostomy
      tube i.
    percutaneous endoscopic tube i.
    percutaneous pin i.
    Pierrot-Murphy advancement i.
    i. point
    rerouting i.
    retrograde catheter i.
    route of i.
    screw i.
    subclavian central venous
      catheter i.
    i. technique
    tendinous i.
    tensor i.
    transjugular i.
    tube-over-needle airway i.
    velamentous i.
    wire i.
insertional excursion

inside-out technique
inside-to-outside technique
insidious onset of symptoms
inspiration
    crowing i.
    degree of i.
    end i.
    shallow i.
    suspended i.
    i. time
inspiratory
    i. bulbospinal neuron
    i. intercostal activity
    i. occlusion pressure
    i. positive airway pressure
    i. pressure support
    i. rib cage depression
    i. time
    i. to expiratory ratio
    i. vapor concentration
    i. warmer
inspiratory/expiratory
inspired
    i. air
    i. gas
    i. ventilation
inspissate
inspissated meconium
inspissation
instability
    atlantoaxial i. (AAI)
    catheter i.
    cervical i.
    congenital cervical i.
    detrusor i.
    dorsal intercalary segmental i.
    extension i.
    hemodynamic i.
    membrane i.
    1-plane i.
    sagittal plane i.
    spinal i.
installation
    implant i.
    i. method
in-stent restenosis
instillation
    contrast material i.
    lavage i.
    i. of anesthetic
    i. procedure
    i. therapy
institute
    Cardiopulmonary Research I.
    Dana-Farber Cancer I.
    National Cancer I. (NCI)
instrument
    i. migration
    multiple dimension i.

instrument (*continued*)
    Noncommunicative Patient's Pain
      Assessment I. (NOPPAIN)
    North American Spine Society
      Lumbar Spine Outcome
      Assessment I.
    i. recirculation
instrumental perforation
instrumentation
    computer-assisted i.
    computer-enhanced i.
    esophageal i.
    i. failure
    interspinous segmental spinal i.
      (ISSI)
    segmental spinal i. (SSI)
instrument-tract seeding
insufficiency
    adrenal i.
    aortic i.
    aortic valve i.
    atrioventricular valve i.
    chronic venous i. (CVI)
    chronotropic i.
    degenerative mitral valve i.
    endocrine i.
    exocrine pancreatic i.
    i. fracture
    glottic i.
    left ventricular i.
    mesenteric i.
    mitral valve i.
    pulmonary valve i.
    renal i.
    respiratory i.
    transverse plane motion i.
    tricuspid i.
    venous i.
insufficient airway maintenance
insufflate
insufflation
    air i.
    i. anesthesia
    i. anesthetic technique
    antegrade tracheal gas i.
    bidirectional tracheal gas i. (Bi-TGI)
    constant flow i.
    cranial i.
    endotracheal i.
    extraperitoneal carbon dioxide i.
    extraperitoneal CO_2 i.
    gas i.
    gastric i.
    helium i.
    intraperitoneal carbon dioxide i.
    intraperitoneal CO_2 i.
    i. of stomach
    perirenal i.
    peritoneal i.

    presacral i.
    i. pressure
    retroperitoneal gas i.
    Rubin tubal i.
    talc i.
    i. test set
    thoracoscopic talc i.
    tracheal gas i. (TGI)
    tubal i.
insula, *pl.* **insulae**
    Haller i.
    insulae pancreaticae
insulae (*pl. of* insula)
insular
    i. artery
    i. carcinoma
insulated
    i. cautery
    i. epidural needle
insulin
    i. coma
    i. coma treatment
    i. preparation
    i. resistance
    i. secretion
    i. shock therapy
insulinoma
    intrahepatic i.
    pancreatic i.
insult
    hypoxic brain i.
    macrotraumatic i.
    microtraumatic i.
intact
    i. gastric serosa
    i. membrane
    i. parathyroid hormone (iPTH)
integrated therapy
integration
    binaural i.
    body side i.
    competing messages i.
    complete i.
    fibrous i.
    large-scale i.
    medium-scale i.
    very large scale i.
integrity
    anatomic i.
    soft tissue i.
integument
integumentary barrier
intensification
    image i.
intensity
    Descriptor Differential Scale of
      Pain I.
    fluorescence i.
    global pain i.

intensity-encoded receptor
intensity-weighted center of gravity
intensive
 i. care unit (ICU)
 i. care unit jaundice
 i. care unit psychosis
intent
 curative i.
 palliative i.
intention
 first i.
 healing by secondary i.
 second i.
 secondary i.
 third i.
intentional
 i. rebreathing
 i. replantation
 i. rotation
 i. saccade
 i. tooth reimplantation
interaction
 additive i.
 antagonistic drug i.
 drug-drug i.
 synergistic i.
 synergistic drug i.
interactive volume rendering
interalveolar space
interarticular
 i. fibrocartilage
 i. joint
interarytenoid notch
interatrial septum
interaural attenuation
interbody
 i. bone graft
 i. spinal fusion
intercalary
 i. allograft procedure
 i. graft
 i. resection
intercalated disc
intercapillary
intercapitales
intercapitular vein
intercarotic, intercarotid
intercarotid (var. of intercarotic)
 i. nerve
intercarpal articulation
intercartilaginous incision
intercavernosus septum
intercavernous venous sinus
intercellular
 i. fenestration
 i. space
intercentral
interceptive conditioning
intercervical disc herniation

interchangeability
interchondral
 i. articulation
 i. ligament
interclavicular
 i. ligament
 i. notch
interclinoid ligament
intercoccygeal
intercolonoscopy
intercolumnar
 i. fascia
 i. fiber
intercondylar, intercondylic,
 intercondyloid
 i. eminence
 i. femoral fracture
 i. fossa
 i. humeral fracture
 i. line
 i. notch
 i. space
 i. tibial fracture
intercondylic (var. of intercondylar)
intercondyloid
intercoronary anastomosis
intercostal
 i. anesthesia
 i. artery
 i. bundle
 i. flap
 i. fossa block
 i. lymph node
 i. membrane
 i. muscle
 i. muscle flap
 i. muscle pedicle
 i. nerve
 i. nerve block
 i. nerve block anesthetic technique
 i. neuralgia
 i. space
 i. vein
 i. vessel
intercostalia
intercostobrachial nerve (ICBN)
intercostohumeral nerve
intercricothyrotomy
intercristal space
intercrural fiber
intercuspal position
intercuspation
intercutaneomucous
interdeferential
interdental
 i. canal
 i. denudation
 i. excision
 i. ligation

interdental (*continued*)
    i. papilla
    i. resection
    i. space
    i. tissue
interdigestive
    i. motility disturbance
    i. period
interdigit
interdigital
interdigitating skin flap
interdigitation
interdisciplinary pain management
interendognathic suture
interface
    bone-cement i.
    bone-implant i.
    cement i.
    cement-bone i.
    cup-cement i.
    electrode-skin i.
    graft-host i.
    implant-cement i.
    long-term bone-instrumentation i.
    pin-bone i.
    prosthesis i.
    prosthesis-cement i.
    soft tissue i.
interfacetal disease
interfacet wiring and fusion
interfacial canal
interfascial
    i. approach
    i. space
interfascicular
    i. epineurectomy
    i. epineurotomy
    i. fibrous tissue
interfemoral
interference
    i. dissociation
    electromagnetic i. (EMI)
    i. fit fixation
    i. modification
    pain i.
    i. screw technique
interferential
    i. current stimulation
    i. stimulator
    i. therapy
interferon therapy
interforniceal approach
interfoveolar ligament
interfragmentary compression
interfrontal
interganglionic rami
interglobular space of Owen
intergluteal
intergonial

interhemispheric
    i. approach
    i. propagation time
    i. subdural hematoma
interilioabdominal amputation
interincisor
    i. distance
    i. gap
interinnominoabdominal amputation
interischiadic
interlamellar space
interlesional therapy
interlobar
interlobular
    i. artery
    i. artery of kidney
    i. ductule
interlocking suture technique
intermaxilla
intermaxillary
    i. fixation
    i. relation
    i. suture
intermediary nerve
intermediate
    i. amputation
    i. anterior wall
    i. bronchus
    i. bundle
    i. cuneiform bone
    i. digastric tendon
    i. ganglion
    i. hemorrhage
    i. laryngeal cavity
    i. line
    i. mesoderm
    i. omohyoid tendon
    i. phalangectomy
    i. restoration
    i. sacral crest
    i. temporal artery
intermediate-risk patient
intermediolateral
intermesenteric
    i. abscess
    i. arterial anastomosis
    i. plexus
intermetacarpal articulation
intermetameric
intermittent
    i. acute porphyria
    i. apnea technique
    i. bolus technique
    i. catheterization
    i. demand ventilation
    i. inflow occlusion
    i. mandatory ventilation (IMV)
    i. pneumatic calf compression
    i. positive pressure (IPP)

i. positive pressure breathing (IPPB)
i. positive-pressure ventilation (IPPV)
i. self-obturation
i. sterilization
i. subclavian vein obstruction
i. vascular exclusion

intermodulation
intermuscular
i. gluteal bursa
i. groove
i. hernia
i. membrane
i. septum

internal
i. abdominal ring
i. anal sphincter (IAS)
i. auditory artery
i. auditory canal (IAC)
i. auditory foramen
i. auditory vein
i. bevel incision
i. branch
i. canthus
i. carotid artery (ICA)
i. carotid venous plexus
i. clot
i. decompression
i. disc disruption
i. drainage
i. ethmoidectomy
i. female genital organ
i. fixation, closed reduction
i. fixation fracture
i. hemipelvectomy
i. hemorrhage
i. hemorrhoid
i. hemorrhoidal complex
i. hernia
i. iliac artery
i. inguinal ring
i. jugular vein
i. jugular vein cannulation anesthetic technique
i. jugular vein catheterization anesthetic technique
i. jugular vein puncture anesthetic technique
i. lacrimal fistula
i. male genital organ
i. mammary artery (IMA)
i. mammary artery graft
i. mammary graft
i. mammary lymphoscintigraphy (IML)
i. mammary node
i. mammary node biopsy
i. mammary plexus
i. maxillary artery

i. maxillary plexus
i. maxillary vein
i. microinfusion device
i. neurocranial foramen
i. neurolysis
i. oblique aponeurosis
i. oblique line
i. oblique osteomuscular flap
i. occipital crest
i. pudendal artery
i. pudendal vein
i. radiation therapy
i. rectal artery
i. rectal nerve
i. reflection
i. respiration
i. rotation
i. rotation deformity
i. rotation in extension
i. rotator
i. spermatic artery
i. spermatic fascia
i. sphincterotomy
i. spinal fixation
i. spiral sulcus
i. supravesical hernia
i. surface
i. thoracic artery
i. thoracic lymphatic plexus
i. thoracic vein
i. urethral orifice
i. urethral sphincter
i. urethrotomy

internal-external
i.-e. ilium
i.-e. rotation

internasal suture
international
I. Association for the Study of Pain (IASP)
I. Cancer of Cervix Classification
I. Classification of Diseases, Adapted for Use in the United States (ICDA)
I. Classification of Diseases-9 Version of Injury Severity Score (ICISS)
I. Classification of Functioning, Disability and Health
I. Federation of Gynecology and Obstetrics (FIGO)
I. Federation of Gynecology and Obstetrics classification
I. Federation of Gynecology and Obstetrics staging
i. normalized ratio (INR)
I. Pelvic Pain Society (IPPS)
I. Society on Thrombosis and Haemostasis (ISTH)

interne
> fixator i.

internervous plane

internodal tract of Bachmann

internus

interocclusal rest space

interorbital

interosseal

interosseous
> i. border
> i. cartilage
> i. crest
> i. groove
> i. margin
> i. muscle
> i. nerve
> i. sacroiliac ligament
> i. wire fixation

interosseus

interpalpebral

interparietal
> i. bone
> i. hernia
> i. suture

interpediculate

interpeduncular
> i. cistern
> i. fossa lesion

interpelviabdominal amputation

interperiosteal fracture

interphalangeal
> i. amputation
> i. articulation
> i. collateral ligament
> distal i. (DIP)
> i. joint dislocation

interpleural
> i. administration
> i. analgesia
> i. anesthesia
> i. anesthetic technique
> i. application
> i. block

interpolated
> i. curve
> i. flap

interpolation
> i. flap
> i. technique

interposing

interposition
> jejunal i.
> i. membrane
> i. mesocaval shunt
> Portmann posterior crus of
>   stapes i.
> i. saphenous vein graft
> soft tissue i.
> tissue i.

interpositional
> i. elbow arthroplasty
> i. shoulder arthroplasty

interpretation
> cholangiographic i.
> false-positive i.
> image i.
> intraoperative i.
> mirror-image i.
> i. variability

interprismatic space

interproximal
> i. reduction
> i. space

interpubic disc

interpulmonary septum

interradicular
> i. alveoloplasty
> i. lesion
> i. septum
> i. space

interrater reliability

interrenal

interrogation
> deep Doppler velocity i.
> Doppler i.
> stereoscopic i.

interrupted
> i. aortic arch
> i. corner stitch
> i. pledgeted suture
> i. respiration
> i. stitch
> i. suture technique

interruption
> sympathetic i.

interscalene
> i. approach
> i. blockade
> i. block anesthetic technique
> i. brachial plexus block
>   (IBPB)
> i. triangle

interscapular amputation

interscapulum

intersection syndrome

intersegmental rotation

intersheath space

intersigmoid
> i. hernia
> i. recess

interspace
> implant substructure i.

interspecific graft

intersphincteric
> i. abscess
> i. anal fistula
> i. anorectal space
> i. proctectomy

interspinal
    i. line
    i. muscle
    i. plane
interspinous
    i. ligament
    i. process compression device
    i. segmental spinal instrumentation
      (ISSI)
    i. wiring
interstice
    graft i.
interstimulus interval
interstitial
    i. brachytherapy
    i. cystitis
    i. fluid
    i. hernia
    i. implantation
    i. inflammation
    i. irradiation
    i. loculated hematoma
    i. neovascularization
    i. nephritis
    i. photodynamic therapy
    i. pressure
    i. pulmonary fibrosis (IPF)
    i. radiation therapy
    i. rejection
    i. space
    i. tissue
intertendinous bursa
intertransverse
    i. fusion
    i. ligament
    i. muscle
intertriginous dermatitis
intertrigo with ulceration
intertroch
    intertrochanteric
intertrochanteric
    i. crest
    i. femoral fracture
    i. line
    i. 4-part fracture
    i. varus osteotomy
intertubercular
    i. eminence
    i. groove
    i. line
    i. plane
    i. sheath
    i. sulcus
interureteric
    i. crest
    i. fold
intervaginal space
interval
    i. appendectomy

    disease-free i. (DFI)
    interstimulus i.
    i. operation
    pacemaker escape i.
    rupture-delivery i.
interval-strength relation
intervascular
intervening connective tissue
intervention
    angiographic i.
    catheter-based i.
    cognitive i.
    endovascular i.
    medical i.
    neurosurgical i.
    operative i.
    primary i.
    prophylactic angiographic i.
    surgical i.
interventional
    i. cardiac catheterization
    i. cardiologist
    i. neuroradiology
    i. option
    i. procedure
    i. radiologist
    i. radiology
    i. technique
    i. therapy
interventricular
    i. septal rupture
    i. septum
intervertebral
    i. cartilage
    i. disc blockade
    i. disc degeneration
    i. disc herniation
    i. foramen
    i. ganglion
    i. notch
    i. symphysis
    i. vein
interview
    structured pain i. (SPI)
intervolar plate ligament
intestina (*pl. of* intestinum)
intestinal
    i. allograft
    i. anastomosis
    i. anastomotic healing
    i. anastomotic leakage
    i. angina
    i. arterial arcade
    i. artery
    i. atresia
    i. biopsy
    i. bypass procedure
    i. calculus
    i. colic

intestinal (*continued*)
- i. conduit
- i. contents
- i. decompression tube
- i. endoscopy
- i. failure
- i. fistula
- i. fixation
- i. flora
- i. gland
- i. hemorrhage
- i. infection
- i. ischemic disorder
- i. loop
- i. malrotation
- i. obstruction
- i. perforation
- i. permeability
- i. pneumatosis
- i. radiation injury
- i. resection
- i. rotation
- i. stoma
- i. surgery
- i. tract
- i. transplant
- i. trunk
- i. ulceration
- i. vein
- i. villous atrophy
- i. villus
- i. web
- i. wound healing

intestine
- large i.
- small i.

intestinum, *pl.* **intestina**
- i. crassum

in-the-bag implantation

intima

intimal
- i. flap
- i. hyperplasia
- i. thrombosis

intolerance
- exercise i.
- hemodynamic i.
- organ-induced i.

intonation contour

intortor

intoxication
- i. amaurosis
- citrate i.

intraabdominal
- i. abscess
- i. adhesion
- i. arterial hemorrhage
- i. bleeding
- i. catastrophe

- i. content
- i. disease
- i. friction
- i. hypertension
- i. infection
- i. injury
- i. lesion
- i. mass
- i. organ
- i. pressure (IAP)
- i. sepsis
- i. spillage
- i. surgery
- i. tip

intraabdominally insufflated carbon dioxide

intraadenoidal

intraalveolar hemorrhage

intraamniotic infection

intraanal pressure

intraaortic
- i. balloon counterpulsation (IABCP)
- i. balloon pump (IABP)

intraarterial
- i. chemoembolization
- i. chemotherapy
- i. counterpulsation
- i. therapy

intraarticular
- i. anesthetic technique
- i. cartilage
- i. facet injection
- i. hip fusion
- i. injection
- i. knee fusion
- i. loose body
- i. osteotomy
- i. procedure
- i. proximal tibial fracture
- i. reconstruction
- i. sternocostal ligament

intraaxial parenchymal brain neoplasia

intrabuccal

intrabulbar fossa

intracanalicular irradiation

intracapsular
- i. approach
- i. cataract extraction (ICCE)
- i. cataract extraction operation
- i. dissection
- i. fracture
- i. hemorrhage
- i. incision
- i. ligament
- i. metastasis
- i. osteotomy
- i. partial tonsillectomy
- i. temporomandibular joint arthroplasty

intracardiac
- i. mass
- i. pressure
- i. pressure curve
- i. shunt

intracatheter

intracavernosal
- i. injection
- i. injection treatment

intracavernous
- i. injection
- i. injection therapy
- i. plexus

intracavitary
- i. anesthesia
- i. implantation
- i. pressure-electrogram dissociation
- i. pressure gradient
- i. radiation boost therapy

intracellular
- i. fluid
- i. protein degradation
- i. volume

intracellularlike, calcium-bearing crystalloid solution, calcium-bearing crystalloid solution

intracerebral
- i. arteriovenous malformation
- i. ganglioma
- i. hematoma
- i. hemorrhage (ICH)
- i. leukostasis
- i. vascular malformation

intracerebroventricular

intracholedochal pressure

intracisternal

intracolic

intraconal lesion

intracordal silicone injection

intracorneal

intracoronal-extracoronal retention

intracoronary thrombolysis balloon valvoplasty

intracorporeal
- i. anastomosis
- i. clamp
- i. injection therapy
- i. knot
- i. knotting
- i. knotting technique
- i. laser lithotripsy (ILL)
- i. rectal transection
- i. shock wave lithotripsy
- i. suture
- i. suturing

intracostal

intracranial
- i. anatomy
- i. aneurysm
- i. arteriovenous fistula
- i. arteriovenous malformation
- i. bleeding
- i. cavity
- i. circulation
- i. dural vascular anomaly
- i. ganglion
- i. hematoma
- i. hemorrhage (ICH)
- i. hypotension
- i. mass
- i. mass lesion
- i. pathology
- i. pressure (ICP)
- i. pressure monitoring
- i. pressure value
- i. rhizotomy
- i. stimulation (ICS)
- i. tumor
- i. vascular malformation
- i. venous system

intracranial-extracranial nerve graft

intracranial-intratemporal nerve graft

intracristal space

intractable
- i. ascites
- i. diarrhea
- i. epilepsy
- i. pain
- i. vomiting

intracuff
- i. lidocaine
- i. pressure

intracutaneous segment

intracuticular stitch

intracystic
- i. hepaticojejunostomy
- i. suture ligature

intracytoplasmic sperm injection (ICSI)

intradermal, intradermic
- i. anesthetic
- i. injection
- i. mattress suture technique
- i. tattooing technique

intradermic (*var. of* intradermal)

intradiploic pseudomeningocele

intradiscal, intradiskal
- i. cleft
- i. electrothermal therapy (IDET)
- i. pressure
- i. radiofrequency thermocoagulation
- i. thermocoagulation

intradiskal (*var. of* intradiscal)

intraductal
- i. cancer
- i. carcinoma
- i. cholangioscopy
- i. component
- i. hyperplasia

intraductal (*continued*)
    i. oncocytic papillary neoplasia
    i. papillary mucinous neoplasia (IPMN)
    i. papillary mucinous tumor (IPMT)
    i. pressure
intradural
    i. abscess
    i. approach
    i. dissection
    i. dorsal spinal root rhizotomy
    i. epidermoidoma
    i. extramedullary lesion
    i. extramedullary mass
    i. tumor surgery
intraepidermal carcinoma
intraepiphysial osteotomy
intraepiploic hernia
intraepithelial
    i. excementosis
    i. nonkeratinizing carcinoma
intraesophageal
    i. peristaltic pressure
    i. variceal pressure
intrafaradization
intrafascial space
intrafollicular insemination
intragalvanization
intragastric
    i. anastomosis
    i. hydrolysis
    i. pressure
    i. prosthesis migration
    i. provocation under endoscopy
    i. resection
intraglandular fluid collection
intraglomerular pressure
intragraft expression
intrahepatic
    i. abscess
    i. anatomy
    i. arterioportal fistula
    i. AV fistula
    i. bile duct
    i. biliary cystic dilation
    i. biliary tree
    i. cholangiocarcinoma
    i. control
    i. course
    i. ductal dilation
    i. hematoma
    i. hemorrhage
    i. hepatolithiasis
    i. hypertension
    i. insulinoma
    i. lesion
    i. metastasis
    i. pathology
    i. portosystemic shunt

    i. spontaneous arterioportal fistula
    i. vascular division
intrahyoid
intrailiac hernia
intrajugular process
intralabyrinthine fistula
intralacrimal
    i. endoscopy
    i. surgery
intralesional
    i. excision
    i. injection
    i. steroid therapy
    i. therapy
intraligamentary anesthesia
intralobar sequestration
intralobular
    i. connective tissue
    i. inflammation
intraluminal
    i. cyst
    i. duodenal diverticulum
    i. esophageal pressure
    i. flow
    i. foreign body
    i. hemorrhage
    i. intubation
    i. pH-pressure relationship
    i. pouch
    i. seeding
    i. suture
    i. tonometry
    i. tumor
    i. urethral pressure
intramammary
    i. lymphatic channel
    i. sentinel node
intramedullary
    i. anesthesia
    i. arteriovenous malformation
    i. bouquet fixation
    i. canal
    i. demyelination
    i. graft
    i. lesion
    i. nail extractor
    i. nailing
    i. rod fixation
    i. tractotomy
    i. tumor
    i. tumor biopsy
intramembranous
    i. formation
    i. space
intramucosal metastasis
intramural
    i. abscess
    i. air dissection
    i. artery

i. blood perfusion
i. colonic air
i. esophageal rupture
i. extramucosal lesion
i. fistulous tract
i. hematoma
i. intestinal hemorrhage
i. involvement
i. pH
intramuscular (IM, i.m.)
    i. abscess
    i. anesthetic
    i. injection
    i. preanesthetic medication anesthetic
    technique
    i. venous malformation
intramyocardial
    i. air
    i. pressure
    i. tumor
intranasal
    i. analgesic
    i. anesthesia
    i. approach
    i. ethmoidectomy
    i. hydromorphone hydrochloride
    i. nicotine
    i. polypectomy
    i. sinus surgery
intraneural pressure
in-transit
    i.-t. disease
    i.-t. metastasis
intraoccipital joint
intraocular
    i. administration
    i. cataract extraction
    i. fistula
    i. foreign body (IOFB)
    i. hemorrhage
    i. lens (IOL)
    i. lens dislocation
    i. lens implantation
    i. pressure (IOP)
intraoperative
    i. assessment
    i. awareness
    i. bile sample
    i. biliary endoscopy
    i. biopsy
    i. bleeding
    i. blood loss
    i. bowel lavage
    i. bowel preparation
    i. cavernous nerve stimulation
    i. cell scavenging
    i. central venous pressure
    i. cholangiogram (IOC)
    i. clonidine administration

i. colonic lavage
i. complete liver devascularization
i. complication
i. computer-assisted spinal
    orientation technique
i. confirmation
i. contamination
i. core body temperature
i. core hypothermia
i. CVP
i. death
i. dilation
i. dynamic cholangiography
i. enteroscopy
i. fluid management
i. fracture
i. frozen section
i. hemorrhage
i. imaging
i. imaging method
i. inadvertent venous injury
i. intact parathyroid hormone
    assay
i. interpretation
i. iPTH assay
i. lymphatic mapping
i. monitor
i. morbidity
i. MRI
i. multiplane transesophageal
    echocardiogram
i. neurophysiologic monitoring
i. normothermia
i. oliguria
i. parathyroid hormone assay
i. parathyroid hormone monitoring
i. penile erection
i. plateletapheresis
i. procedure
i. radiation
i. radiation therapy
i. radiotherapy with electrons
i. rupture
i. stress relaxation
i. touch prep cytology
i. transcranial Doppler monitoring
i. ultrasonography (IOUS)
i. ultrasound (IOUS)
i. ultrasound finding
i. urine output
i. vascular accident
i. verification
intraoperatively donated autologous
blood
intraoral
    i. anesthesia
    i. antrostomy
    i. cone irradiation
    i. flap

intraoral (*continued*)
    i. incision
    i. pressure
    i. trauma
intraorbital
    i. anesthesia
    i. foreign body
    i. groove
    i. surgery
intraosseous
    i. abscess
    i. anesthesia
    i. bone lesion
    i. fixation
    i. injection
    i. membrane
intrapancreatic
    i. neoplasm
    i. portion
intraparavariceal procedure
intraparenchymal
    i. bleeding
    i. digital dissection
    i. hematoma
    i. hemorrhage
intraparotid plexus
intrapartum
    i. asphyxiation
    i. hemorrhage
    i. hysterectomy
intrapatellar bursa
intrapelvic hernia
intrapericardial pressure
intraperitoneal
    i. abscess
    i. adhesion
    i. air
    i. anesthesia
    i. anesthetic
    i. blood transfusion
    i. carbon dioxide insufflation
    i. cavity
    i. CO_2 insufflation
    i. dissemination
    i. drug administration
    i. endometrial metastatic disease
    i. fetal transfusion
    i. hemorrhage
    i. hyperthermic chemotherapy
    i. hyperthermic perfusion (IPHP)
    i. incision
    i. leakage
    i. method
    i. mobilization
    i. onlay mesh (IPOM)
    i. onlay mesh technique
    i. perforation
    i. position
    i. pressure

    i. procedure
    i. radiation therapy
    i. recurrence
    i. Rives-type repair
    i. seeding
    i. spillage
    i. technique
    i. viscus
    i. viscus rupture
    i. volume
intraperitoneally
intrapharyngeal space
intrapial
intraplaque hemorrhage
intrapleural
    i. approach
    i. block
    i. catheter placement
    i. pressure
    i. rupture
intraportal vein
intraprostatic
intrapulmonary
    i. metastasis (IPM)
    i. shunt ratio
intrapulpal
    i. anesthesia
    i. injection
    i. pressure
intrapyretic amputation
intrarachidian (*var. of* intrarrhachidian)
intrarenal chemolysis
intrarrhachidian, intrarachidian
intrascrotal
intrasellar
    i. extension
    i. lesion
    i. mass
intraseptal alveoloplasty
intrasheath tenotomy
intrasphincteric injection
intraspinal
    i. administration
    i. anesthesia
    i. therapy
intrasplenic
intrasynovial
intratendinous injection
intratentorial supracerebellar approach
intrathecal
    i. administration
    i. analgesic
    i. anesthesia
    i. anesthetic
    i. antinociception
    i. cannulation anesthetic technique
    i. drug delivery system
    i. hemorrhage

i. injection
i. migration
i. morphine
i. morphine anesthetic technique
i. neurolysis
i. opioid
i. opioid labor analgesia
i. therapy
intrathoracic
i. anastomosis
i. bleeding
i. disease
i. esophageal cancer
i. esophagogastric anastomosis
i. esophagogastroscopy
i. esophagogastrostomy
i. esophagoplasty
i. injury
i. leak
i. mass
i. Nissen fundoplication
i. position
i. pressure
i. stomach
intrathyroidal pathology
intrathyroid cartilage
intratracheal
i. anesthesia
i. ectopic thyroid
i. ectopic thyroid tissue
i. intubation
i. pulmonary ventilation
intratubal insemination
intratumoral
i. calcification
i. injection
intraurethral pressure
intrauterine
i. amputation
i. device (IUD)
i. foreign body
i. fracture
i. growth retardation
i. infection (IUI)
i. insemination
i. intraperitoneal fetal transfusion
i. pressure measurement
i. respiration
i. resuscitation
intravaginal
i. electrical stimulation
i. pouch
i. space
i. torsion
intravariceal
i. infusion
i. injection
i. pressure
i. sclerotherapy

intravasation
venous i.
intravascular
i. blood volume
i. coagulation
i. coagulation screen
i. endothelial proliferative lesion
i. fluid therapy
i. foreign body
i. foreign body retrieval
i. injection
i. lipolysis
i. mass
i. migration
i. pressure (IVP)
i. volume
i. volume depletion
i. volume expansion
i. volume overload
i. volume therapy
intravelar veloplasty
intravenous (I.V.)
i. administration
i. alimentation
i. analgesic
i. anesthetic
i. antibiotic therapy
i. block
i. block anesthesia
i. blood
i. cannulation
i. cannulation anesthetic technique
i. contrast
i. digital subtraction imaging
i. drip
i. fluid resuscitation
i. hydration
i. hydration therapy
i. hyperalimentation
i. hypnotic
i. injection
i. medication
i. ozone therapy
i. pyelogram (IVP)
i. regional anesthesia (IVRA)
i. regional blockade
i. regional block with guanethidine
i. regional sympathetic block
(IRSB)
i. saline
i. sedation
i. sedation anesthesia
i. sheath
i. vasopressin
intraventricular
i. aberration
i. endoscopy
i. hemorrhage
i. injection

intraventricular (*continued*)
  i. mass
  i. therapy
intravesical
  i. alum irrigation
  i. anastomosis
  i. chemotherapeutic treatment
  i. chemotherapy
  i. migration
  i. pressure
  i. ureterolysis
intravital microscopy
intravitreal injection
intrinsic
  i. brainstem lesion
  i. circuitry
  i. compression
  i. end-expiratory pressure
  i. minus deformity
  i. minus position
  i. muscle
  i. plus deformity
  i. positive end-expiratory pressure
  (PEEPi)
  i. restoration
  i. sphincter
  i. spinal cord catheter
  placement
introduction site
introflexion
introgastric
introitus
introjection
intromittent organ
introspective method
introvert
intrusive implantation
intubate
intubated ureterotomy
intubating laryngeal mask airway
  (ILMA, I-LMA)
intubation
  accidental esophageal i.
  altercursive i.
  i. anesthetic technique
  aqueductal i.
  awake i.
  awake fiberoptic i.
  blind nasotracheal i.
  bronchoscope-guided i.
  catheter-guided endoscopic i.
  double-lumen i.
  elective oral tracheal i.
  emergency tracheal i.
  emergent i.
  endobronchial i.
  endotracheal i.
  esophageal i.
  esophagogastric i.

failed i.
i. failure
fiberoptic i.
flexible lightwand-guided i.
inadvertent endobronchial i.
intraluminal i.
intratracheal i.
lighted stylet-guided oral i.
lightwand tracheal i.
Lipp maneuver for
  esophageal-tracheal i.
mainstem i.
multiple i.'s
nasal i.
nasogastric i.
nasotracheal i. (NTI)
O'Dwyer i.
oral endotracheal i.
oral lighted-stylet i.
orotracheal i.
prolonged i.
prophylactic i.
pyloric i.
rapid sequence induction i.
retrograde wire i.
RSI orotracheal i.
silicone i.
terminal ileum i.
total time to i. (TTI)
tracheal i.
translaryngeal tracheal i.
intumescence
intumescent
intumescentia
intussuscepted mass
intussuscepting
intussusception
  adult i.
  appendiceal i.
  appendicular mucosal i.
  cecal i.
  colocolic i.
  colonic i.
  enteric i.
  gastroenterostomy i.
  idiopathic adult i.
  idiopathic ileocecal i.
  ileocolic i.
  pediatric i.
  sigmoid-rectal i.
  stomal i.
inundation fever
invaded furcation
invaginate
invaginated membrane
invaginating
  i. anastomosis
  end-to-end i.
  i. suture technique

invagination
> basilar i.
> epithelial i.
> stomal i.
> stump i.
> i. technique

invasion
> advanced local i.
> blood vessel i.
> cancer i.
> capsular i.
> chest wall i.
> extrathyroid i.
> local i.
> lymphatic i.
> lymphovascular i.
> lymph vessel i.
> margin i.
> microscopic i.
> mucosal i.
> perineural i.
> serosa i.
> submucosal i.
> tumor i.
> vascular i.
> venous i.
> wall i.

invasive
> i. adenocarcinoma
> i. blood pressure
> i. breast cancer
> i. breast carcinoma
> i. ductal cancer
> i. ductal carcinoma
> i. fungal infection
> i. hemodynamic monitoring
> i. lobular carcinoma
> i. localization
> i. pressure measurement
> i. procedure
> i. recurrence
> i. signet ring cell carcinoma
> i. technique
> i. test
> i. therapy
> i. tumor

inventory
> Brief Pain I. (BPI)
> Multidimensional Pain I. (MPI)
> Neonatal Facial Pain I. (NFPI)
> Pain Appraisal I. (PAI)
> Pain Beliefs and Perception I. (PBPI)
> State-Trait Anger Expression I. (STAXI)
> State-Trait Anxiety I. (STAI)
> Westhaven-Yale Multidimensional Pain I. (WHYMPI)

inverse bevel incision

inverse-ratio ventilation
inversion appendectomy
inversion-eversion rotation
inversion-ligation appendectomy
inversus
> dextrocardia with situs i.
> situs i.

inverted
> i. bevel incision
> i. L-form osteotomy
> i. pelvis
> i. scarf osteotomy
> i. skin flap

inverted-U
> i.-U abdominal incision
> i.-U approach
> i.-U pouch

inverted-V peritoneotomy
inverted-Y
> i.-Y fracture
> i.-Y incision

inverting knot technique
invertor
Investa suture
investigation
> diagnostic i.
> direct histologic i.
> histologic i.
> preoperative i.
> soft x-ray i.

investing
> i. cartilage
> i. fascia

investment expansion
involuntary
> i. guarding
> i. sterilization

involution cyst
involved-field radiation
involvement
> bifurcation i.
> border i.
> celiac nodal i.
> diffuse breast i.
> extramedullary i.
> extraocular muscle i.
> intramural i.
> lymph node i.
> macroscopic i.
> margin resection i.
> mesocolic i.
> metastatic i.
> nervous system i.
> nodal i.
> node i.
> portal nodal i.
> pulmonary i.
> retinal i.
> segmental i.

involvement (*continued*)
  serosal i.
  trifurcation i.
inward-going rectification
inward rotation
Ioban protective skin barrier
IOC
  intraoperative cholangiogram
IOCG
  intraoperative cholangiogram
iodide
  Phospholine I.
iodide-containing medication
iodine
  i. catgut suture
  i. treatment
IOFB
  intraocular foreign body
IOL
  intraocular lens
ionization
  i. chamber pocket
  root canal i.
  specific i.
ionizing irradiation
Ionsys fentanyl iontophoretic transdermal system
IOP
  intraocular pressure
IOUS
  intraoperative ultrasonography
  intraoperative ultrasound
Iowa Satisfaction with Anesthesia Scale
IPAA
  ileal pouch-anal anastomosis
IPF
  idiopathic pulmonary fibrosis
  interstitial pulmonary fibrosis
IPHP
  intraperitoneal hyperthermic perfusion
IPM
  intrapulmonary metastasis
    macroscopic IPM
    microscopic IPM
IPMN
  intraductal papillary mucinous neoplasia
IPMT
  intraductal papillary mucinous tumor
IPN
  infected pancreatic necrosis
IPOM
  intraperitoneal onlay mesh
IPP
  intermittent positive pressure
IPPB
  intermittent positive pressure breathing
IPPS
  International Pelvic Pain Society

IPPV
  intermittent positive-pressure ventilation
IPSID
  immunoproliferative small intestine disease
ipsilateral
  i. acetabular fracture
  i. adrenalectomy
  i. femoral neck fracture
  i. femoral shaft fracture
  i. gland
  i. hemispheric symptom
  i. injection
  i. nerve root lesion
  i. pelvic fracture
  i. portal vein obstruction
  i. shoulder
  i. side
  i. thyroid lobectomy
  i. tibial fracture
iPTH
  intact parathyroid hormone
  iPTH level
I/R
  ischemia-reperfusion
  I/R injury
IRA
  ileorectal anastomosis
IRDS
  infant respiratory distress syndrome
iridectomy
  Adam i.
  argon laser i.
  basal i.
  Beer i.
  Bethke i.
  buttonhole i.
  Castroviejo i.
  central i.
  Chandler i.
  Cleasby i.
  complete i.
  Elschnig central i.
  Flajani i.
  Langenbeck i.
  laser i.
  Leveille i.
  Lusardi i.
  i. operation
  optic i.
  optic i.
  optical i.
  patent i.
  peripheral i.
  preliminary i.
  preparatory i.
  pupil-to-root i.

Quaglino i.
i. scar
sector i.
stenopeic i.
superior sector i.
therapeutic i.
Wecker i.
Weekers peripheral i.
iridencleisis
Holth i.
i. operation
irides (*pl. of* iris)
iridization
iridocapsulotomy
iridocele
iridocoloboma
iridocorneal
i. angle
i. endothelial syndrome
i. epithelial syndrome
iridocorneosclerectomy
iridocyclectomy
iridocyclochoroidectomy
Peyman i.
iridocystectomy
iridodialysis
i. operation
Scarpa i.
iridodiastasis
iridogoniocyclectomy
iridoplasty
iridosclerotomy
iridotasis operation
iridotomy, iritomy, irotomy
Abraham i.
Castroviejo radial i.
laser i.
i. operation
Physick i.
radial i.
iris, *pl.* **irides**
i. diastasis
i. ectasia
i. incarceration
i. neovascularization
i. ring
iritic
iritis
iritoectomy
iritomy (*var. of* iridotomy)
iron
i. Hudson-Stähli line
i. line
iron-stocker's line
irotomy (*var. of* iridotomy)
irradiated melanoma cell
irradiation
abdominal i.
abdominopelvic i.

adjuvant i.
breast i.
cardiac i.
i. cataract
cataract i.
cesium i.
charged-particle i.
chest wall i.
childhood thyroid i.
convergent beam i.
cranial i.
craniospinal i.
i. damage
external beam i.
extracorporeal i.
i. failure
fractionated external beam i.
gamma i.
half-body i.
heavy-ion i.
hemibody i.
hyperfractionated total body i.
i. injury
interstitial i.
intracanalicular i.
intraoral cone i.
ionizing i.
linearly polarized near-
infrared i.
local i.
low-dose i.
mantle i.
mediastinal i.
Nd:YAG laser i.
paraaortic node i.
partial-breast i.
pelvic i.
postoperative i.
prophylactic i.
selective i.
short-course i.
surface i.
therapeutic i.
total axial node i.
total body i.
total lymphoid i.
total nodal i.
ultraviolet blood i.
UV i.
whole abdomen i.
whole abdominopelvic i.
whole body i. (WBI)
whole pelvis i.
irreducible
i. fracture
i. hernia
irregular bone
irregularly widened lumen
irresectability

irresectable
    carcinoma stage i.
    i. disease
    i. finding
irrespirable
irresuscitable
irreversible
    i. coma
    i. shock
irrigating solution
irrigation
    acetohydroxamic acid i.
    i. and aspiration (I&A)
    antral i.
    i. burn
    caloric i.
    canal i.
    closed i.
    continuous bladder i.
    copious i.
    endodontic i.
    hemiacidrin i.
    heparin i.
    intravesical alum i.
    on-table i.
    oral i.
    pulsed i.
    pulse lavage i.
    rectal pulsed i.
    rectum i.
    sinus i.
    i. solution
    whole-gut i.
    wound i.
irrigation-suction
    postoperative i.-s.
irritability
    soft tissue i.
irritable lesion
irritant
    i. dermatitis
    i. patch-test reaction
    i. patch-test response
irritation
    i. callus
    i. index
    parastomal i.
    peritoneal i.
irritative lesion
irruption
irruptive
Irvine operation
Irving tubal ligation
Irwin osteotomy
ISA
    ileosigmoid anastomosis
Isaacson gastric lymphoma classification
ischemia
    acute limb i.

chronic mesenteric i.
contralateral i.
exercise i.
exercise-induced silent myocardial i.
extremity i.
hemihepatic i.
hepatic i.
inherent i.
left ventricular i.
limb i.
lower limb i.
mesenteric i.
myocardial i.
nonocclusive mesenteric i. (NOMI)
normothermic i.
pelvic i.
peripheral i.
radiation-induced i.
spinal cord i.
tourniquet i.
warm i.
ischemia-guided medical therapy
ischemia-reperfusion (I/R)
    i.-r. injury
    i.-r. phenomenon
ischemic
    i. aortic disease
    i. cardiomyopathy
    i. colitis
    i. compression
    i. encephalopathy
    i. heart disease
    i. hypoxia
    i. infected ulceration
    i. liver injury
    i. mesenteric change
    i. neuronal injury
    i. ocular inflammation
    i. optic neuritis
    i. pain stimulation
    i. preconditioning (IPC)
    i. reperfusion injury
    i. stroke
    i. ulcer
ischemic-tourniquet technique
ischia (*pl. of* ischium)
ischiadic
    i. plexus
    i. spine
ischiadicus
ischial
    i. bone
    i. bursa
    i. spine
    i. weightbearing ring
ischiatic hernia
ischioanal fossa
ischiobulbar
ischiocavernosus

ischiocavernous muscle
ischiocele
ischiococcygeal
ischiococcygeus
ischiofemoral
ischioperineal
ischiopubiotomy
> Farabeuf i.

ischiorectal
> i. abscess
> i. anorectal space
> i. fat pad
> i. fossa
> i. fossa plane

ischiovertebral
ischium, *pl.* **ischia**
ischuretic
I-shaped scalp flap
island
> endometrial i.
> i. graft
> i. nail transfer
> i. pedicle scalp flap
> i. skin flap
> i. wound dressing

island-flap procedure
islet
> i. cell
> i. cell cancer
> i. cell tumor
> i.'s of Langerhans
> pancreatic i.

ISO₂
> oxygen saturation index

isobaric spinal anesthesia
isobologram analysis
isobolographic analysis
isobolography
isocapnia
isocapnic hyperventilation
isodense subdural hematoma
isodose line
isoelectric
> i. line
> i. point

isoenzyme, isozyme
> pancreas-specific amylase i.

isoflurane
isoflurane-induced vasoconstriction
isogeneic graft
isograft
isoinertial
isokinetic collection
isolated
> i. anuloplasty
> i. arterial injury
> i. dislocation
> i. fashion
> i. hepatic perfusion (IHP)

> i. iliac artery aneurysm
> i. limb perfusion (ILP)
> i. liver injury
> i. metastatic tumor
> i. NCRLM
> i. noncolorectal liver metastasis
> i. procedure
> i. venous injury

isolation
> hepatic vascular i. (HVI)
> lung i.
> i. perfusion therapy
> i. technique
> total vascular i. (TVI)

isologous graft
isolysis
isometric
> i. cervical extension strength
> i. force dynamometry
> i. point
> i. technique
> i. tubular vacuolation
> i. venous tension

isoperistaltic
> i. anastomosis
> i. stricturoplasty

isoplastic graft
isoproterenol
isoquinoline
isorhythmic dissociation
isosulfan blue-dye mapping
isotonic
> i. crystalloid solution
> i. hyponatremia

isotope
> i. dilution-mass spectrometry
> i. injection
> i. localization

isotopic lymphoscintigraphy
isotransplantation
isotropic tissue
isovolemic hemodilution
isovolumetric
> i. relaxation
> i. relaxation time

isovolumic
> i. relaxation (IVR)
> i. relaxation time

isozyme (*var. of* isoenzyme)
ISS
> Injury Severity Score

ISSI
> interspinous segmental spinal
> instrumentation

ISTH
> International Society on Thrombosis
> and Haemostasis

isthmectomy
> thyroid i.

isthmi (*pl. of* isthmus)
isthmorrhaphy
isthmus, *pl.* **isthmi,** *pl.* **isthmuses**
    thyroid i.
isthmuses (*pl. of* isthmus)
Italian
    I. arm flap rhinoplasty method
    I. inner arm nose reconstruction
    flap
    I. rhinoplasty
ITB
    iliotibial band
itching
    burning and i.
itchy soft palate
iterative
    i. cytoreductive surgery
    i. reconstruction
Ito cells
ITP
    idiopathic thrombocytopenic
    purpura
IUD
    intrauterine device
IUD-related infection
Ivalon suture
IVC
    inferior vena cava
    intravascular coagulation
        azygos continuation of I.
        IVC ligation

IVC occlusion
IVC pressure
IVC reconstruction
retrohepatic IVC
suprahepatic IVC
thrombosis of IVC
I.V.
    intravascular
    intravenous
    I.V. contrast
    I.V. fluid therapy
IVCT
    in vitro contracture test
IVF
    in vitro fertilization
Ivor
    I. Lewis esophagectomy
    I. Lewis esophagogastrectomy
    I. Lewis esophagogastrectomy
    approach
    I. Lewis esophagus resection
    I. Lewis 2-stage subtotal
    esophagectomy
ivory membrane
IVP
    intravenous pyelogram
IVRA
    intravenous regional anesthesia
Ivy
    I. loop wiring
    I. method of bleeding time

J

J pelvic ileal pouch
J point

Jaboulay

J. amputation
J. gastroduodenostomy
J. pyloroplasty

Jaboulay-Doyen-Winkleman

J.-D.-W. hemipelvectomy
J.-D.-W. hydrocele bottleneck
technique

jackknife position

Jackson

J. and Parker classification of
Hodgkin disease
J. and Parker Hodgkin disease
classification
J. incision
J. membrane

Jackson-Babcock vein stripping

Jackson-Pratt (JP)

J.-P. drain

**Jacobaeus endoscopic thorax exploration
procedure**

Jacob membrane

Jacobs locking-hook spinal rod technique

Jacobson

J. cartilage
J. nerve

Jacoby

border tissue of J.

Jacod syndrome

Jacquart facial angle

Jacquemet recess

Jacques plexus

**Jaeger-Hamby muscle embolization of
carotid cavernous fistula procedure**

Jaesche-Arlt entropion repair

Jaesche entropion repair

Jahss

J. dorsal wedge osteotomy
procedure
J. metacarpal neck fracture
reduction maneuver

Jaime lacrimal operation

James

J. bundle
J. position

**Jameson muscle recession with scleral
reattachment operation**

jamming knot

Janecki-Nelson shoulder girdle resection

Janeway

J. gastrostomy
J. lesion

**Jannetta microvascular decompression
neurosurgical procedure**

Jansey

J. shoulder arthrodesis technique
J. toenail ablation procedure

Jansky blood type classification

Japanese

J. acupuncture
J. approach
J. cancer classification
J. Classification for Gastric
Carcinoma (JCGC)
J. standard gastrectomy

Japanese-style

J.-s. D2 lymphadenectomy
J.-s. gastrectomy
J.-s. lymphadenectomy

Japas

J. osteotomy
J. V-osteotomy

Jarjavay ligament

Jatene arterial switch procedure

jaundice

breast-milk j.
cholestatic j.
clinical j.
intensive care unit j.
nonobstructing j.
obstructive j.
preoperative j.
pruritic j.
regurgitation j.

Javid shunt

jaw

j. bone
Hapsburg j.
j. joint
j. relation
j. relation record
j. thrust maneuver
upper j.

Jaworski body

jaw-to-jaw

j.-t.-j. position
j.-t.-j. relation

JCGC

Japanese Classification for Gastric
Carcinoma

Jefferson fracture

Jeffery

J. radial fracture classification
J. technique

jejunal

j. artery
j. biopsy

jejunal (*continued*)

j. conduit
j. fasting motor activity
j. free flap
j. interposition
j. interposition of Henle loop
j. lumen
j. manometry
j. motility
j. pouch
j. puncture
j. puncture area
j. Roux-en-Y limb
j. Roux-en-Y loop
j. serosa
j. stump
j. submucosa
j. tube insertion

jejunal-ileal

j.-i. bypass (JIB)
j.-i. bypass reversal

jejunectomy
jejunization
jejunocolic fistula
jejunocolostomy
jejunoduodenal anastomosis
jejunoileal

j. anastomosis
j. bypass (JIB)
j. bypass reversal method
j. bypass reversal procedure
j. bypass reversal technique
j. bypass surgery
j. obstruction

jejunoileostomy

Roux-en-Y distal j.

jejunojejunal anastomosis
jejunojejunostomy
jejunoplasty

Hoffman j.

jejunostomy

afferent j.
decompression j.
direct percutaneous endoscopic j. (DPEJ)
j. elemental diet feeding
endoscopic j.
hepaticocutaneous j.
laparoscopic j.
loop j.
needle catheter j. (NCJ)
percutaneous endoscopic j. (PEJ)
j. tract choledochoscopy
j. tube feeding
Witzel j.

jejunotomy
jejunum

j. loop

proximal j.
upper j.

Jendrassik reflex amplification maneuver
Jensen

J. abducens palsy muscle transposition
J. muscle transposition procedure
J. trochanteric fracture classification

Jergesen incision
jerky respiration
jet

high-frequency j.
j. lesion
j. pilot position
transtracheal j.
j. ventilation
j. ventilation anesthetic technique

Jeune

J. disease
J. syndrome

Jewett

J. and Strong staging
J. and Whitmore prostate cancer classification

JIB

jejunal-ileal bypass
jejunoileal bypass
JIB reversal

J-loop

J-l. ileostomy
J-l. technique

job capacity evaluation (JCE)
Jobe-Glousman glenohumeral capsular shift procedure
Jobert

J. de Lamballe fossa
J. suture technique

Joel-Cohen abdominal wall incision
Johner-Wruhs tibial fracture classification
Johnson

J. acquired and congenital coronary artery insufficiency operation
J. chevron osteotomy
J. esophagogastroscopy
J. esophagogastrostomy
J. pelvic fracture technique
J. pronator advancement
J. root canal filling method
J. staple technique

Johnson-Spiegl hallux varus correction
Johnston

J. buttonhole arteriovenous hemodialysis fistula procedure
J. pursestring suture technique

joint

anterior intraoccipital j.
arthrodial j.
j. aspiration

J

atlantoaxial j.
atlantooccipital j.
axial rotation j.
ball-and-socket j.
biaxial j.
bicondylar j.
bilocular j.
j. branch
capitular j.
j. capsule
j. cavity
coccygeal j.
composite j.
compound j.
costochondral j.
costotransverse j.
costovertebral j.
cotyloid j.
cricoarytenoid j.
cricothyroid j.
j. deformity
dentoalveolar j.
j. depression fracture
diarthrodial j.
j. disarticulation
distal radioulnar j.
distal radius-ulnar j.
ellipsoid j.
ellipsoidal j.
enarthrodial j.
extraarticular subtalar j.
facet j.
fibrous j.
j. fusion
ginglymoid j.
glenohumeral j.
gliding j.
hinge j.
immovable j.
incudomalleolar j.
interarticular j.
intraoccipital j.
jaw j.
lateral atlantoaxial j.
j. line
j. line pain
lumbosacral j.
Luschka j.
mandibular j.
j. manipulation
manubriosternal j.
j. mobilization
j. mouse
movable j.
multiaxial j.
neurocentral j.
j. oil
peg-and-socket j.
petrooccipital j.

pivot j.
plane j.
polyaxial j.
posterior intraoccipital j.
j. protection training
j. reconstruction
j. replacement
rotary j.
rotation j.
sacrococcygeal j.
sacroiliac j.
screw j.
SI j.
simple j.
socket j.
j. space
j. space narrowing
sphenooccipital j.
spheroid j.
spiral j.
sternal j.
sternoclavicular j.
sternocostal j.
suture j.
synarthrodial j.
synchondrodial j.
syndesmodial j.
synovial j.
talocrural j.
temporomandibular j. (TMJ)
thigh j.
trochoid j.
uncovertebral j.
uniaxial j.
unilocular j.
wedge-and-groove j.
xiphisternal j.
zygapophysial j.
Jonas modification of Norwood hypoplastic left heart procedure
Jones
J. and Jones wedge technique
J. first-toe repair
J. fracture
J. position
J. resection arthroplasty
J. tube conjunctivodacryocystorhinostomy procedure
Jones-Barnes-Lloyd-Roberts classification
Jonnesco fossa
Joplin bunionectomy
Jorgensen anesthesia technique
Joseph rhinoplasty
JP
Jackson-Pratt
JP drain
J-pexy
omental J-p.

J-pouch
>colonic J-p.
>J-p. construction
>ileal J-p.
>J-p. ileoanal anastomosis

JRA
>juvenile rheumatoid arthritis

JR Moore oral and maxillofacial procedure

J-sella deformity

J-shaped
>J-s. ileal pouch
>J-s. ileal pouch-anal anastomosis
>J-s. skin incision

J-sign

J-Tip needleless injection system

J-tube insertion

J-type maneuver

Judd-Mayo overlap midline incisional hernioplasty

Judd pyloroplasty technique

Judet
>J. quadricepsplasty
>J. vascularized bone graft

Judkins selective percutaneous transfemoral coronary arteriography technique

Judkins-Sones
>J.-S. coronary arteriography technique
>J.-S. technique of cardiac catheterization

juga (*pl. of* jugum)

jugal
>j. bone
>j. point

jugomaxillary point

jugular
>j. bulb anomaly
>j. bulb catheter placement assessment
>j. bulb oximetry
>j. bulb oxyhemoglobin desaturation
>j. bulb venous oxygen saturation
>j. compression maneuver
>j. duct
>j. foramen
>j. foramen syndrome
>j. fossa
>j. ganglion
>j. lymphatic trunk
>j. nerve
>j. plexus
>j. process
>j. sinus
>j. technique
>j. tubercle
>j. vein
>j. vein dissection

>j. venous arch
>j. venous bulb
>j. venous oxygen saturation (SjVO$_2$)
>j. venous pressure (JVP)

jugularis

jugulocarotid nodule

jugulodigastric lymph node

juguloomohyoid node

jugum, *pl.* **juga**

juice
>cancer j.

jumbo biopsy

jump
>j. flap
>j. graft

jumper-knee position

junction
>anorectal j.
>atypical j.
>cavohepatic j.
>choledochoduodenal j.
>choledochopancreatic ductal j.
>costochondral j.
>cystic duct-infundibulum j.
>duodenojejunal j.
>esophagogastric j.
>gastroesophageal j. (GEJ)
>GE j.
>hard-soft palate j.
>ileocecal j.
>manubriosternal j.
>mucocutaneous j.
>neuroeffector j.
>neuromuscular j.
>rectosigmoid j.
>sacrococcygeal j.
>sclerocorneal j.
>scotoma j.
>skin-amnion j.
>squamocolumnar j.
>sternoclavicular j.
>sternomanubrial j.
>ureteropelvic j. (UPJ)
>Wirsung-choledochus j.
>xiphisternal j.

junctional
>j. dilation
>j. ectopic tachycardia
>j. epithelium

junctura, *pl.* **juncturae**

juncturae (*pl. of* junctura)

Jung muscle

Jurkat T-cell line

Juvara closing abudetory wedge for feet procedure

juvenile
>j. angiofibroma
>j. ankylosing spondylitis

j. embryonal carcinoma
j. hemangiofibroma
j. nevoxanthoendothelioma
j. pelvis
j. polyp
j. rheumatoid arthritis (JRA)
juxtaanal colostomy
juxtaarticulation
juxtaauricular fossa
juxtacardiac pleural pressure
juxtacortical
j. fracture
j. osteogenic sarcoma

juxtacrine stimulation
juxtacubital reconstruction
juxtaepiphysial
juxtaglomerular
j. body
j. complex
j. granulation index
juxtahepatic vein
juxtaposition
juxtarenal aneurysm
juxtarestiform body
JVP
jugular venous pressure

J

KACT
    kaolin-activated clotting time
Kader gastrostomy
Kader-Senn
    K.-S. gastrostomy
    K.-S. gastrotomy technique
Kadian
Kaes
    line of K.
Kajava supernumerary breast tissue
    classification
kala-azar infection
Kalamchi avascular necrosis classification
Kalicinski ureteral folding technique
    procedure
Kalish osteotomy
Kalt suture technique
Kammerer-Battle incision
kangaroo
    k. pouch
    k. tendon suture technique
kaolin-activated clotting time (KACT)
Kapandji distal radius fracture pinning
    technique
Kapel elbow dislocation technique
Kaplan
    K. oblique line
    K. open reduction
    K. osteotomy
kaposiform hemangioendothelioma
Karakousis-Vezeridis
    K.-V. hemipelvectomy procedure
    K.-V. ischiorectal fossa tumor
        resection
Karapandzic
    K. lip reconstruction flap
    K. lip reconstruction procedure
karaya powder
Karlsson ankle instability correction
    procedure
Karnofsky
    K. performance rating scale
        classification
    K. performance scale
Karydakis pilonidal sinus flap
Kasabach-Merritt syndrome
Kasai
    K. operation
    K. portoenterostomy
    K. portoenterostomy procedure
Kasai-type hepatoportoenterostomy
Kashin-Beck disease
Kashiwagi elbow arthroplasty technique
Kasser-Kennedy cineventriculographic
    ventricular volume method

Kasugai pancreatitis classification
Kates-Kessel-Kay forefoot arthroplasty
    technique
Kato thick smear technique
Katzin scleral buckle
Kaufer tendon technique
Kauffman-White Salmonella serotype
    classification
Kaufmann subpial transection
    technique
Kausch-Whipple pancreatoduodenectomy
Kavanaugh-Brower-Mann fixation
Kave knee approach
Kawamura
    K. dome osteotomy
    K. pelvic osteotomy
Kazanjian operation
Keating-Hart postexcision fulguration
    method
kebab emulsion surface graft
Keen
    K. point
    K. torticollis neurectomy
Kehr
    K. biliary drainage technique
    K. incision
    K. spleen rupture sign
Keil tumor cell classification
Keith
    K. bundle
    K. needle
Keith-Wagener-Barker (KWB)
Keith-Wagener retinal changes
    classification
Kelami penile curvature classification
Kelikian-Clayton-Loseff
    K.-C.-L. surgical syndactylia
    K.-C.-L. surgical syndactylia of toes
        technique
Kelikian lateral ankle suture anchor
    procedure
Kelikian-McFarland congenital digitus
    minimus varus correction procedure
Kelikian-Riashi-Gleason
    K.-R.-G. patellar tendon
        reconstruction technique
    K.-R.-G. patellar tendon
        repair
Kellam-Waddel tibial plafond fracture
    classification
Keller
    K. bunionectomy
    K. bunionectomy procedure
    K. resection arthroplasty
Keller-Madlener hallux valgus operation

K

415

Kelling-Madlener gastric resection procedure
Kellogg-Speed
    K.-S. fusion anterior interbody spinal fusion technique
    K.-S. lumbar spinal fusion
Kelly
    K. plication
    K. suture
    K. suture technique
    K. urethrovesical plication procedure
Kelly-Keck osteotomy
Kelly-Kennedy modification
Kelman phacoemulsification
keloid
    k. fibroblast
    k. formation
keloplasty
kelotomy
Kelsey unloading exercise therapy
Kelvin body
Kempf-Grosse-Abalo Z step osteotomy
Kendrick
    K. below-knee amputation procedure
    K. method below-knee amputation
Kendrick-Sharma-Hassler-Herndon metatarsus adductus repair technique
Kennedy
    K. area-length method
    K. ligament technique
    K. partially edentulous classification
Kennedy-Pacey urinary stress incontinence operation
Kent
    K. bundle
    K. bundle ablation
    bundle of Stanley K.
Kent-His bundle
KEP
    knee-elbow position
keratectomy
    Castroviejo k.
    excimer laser photorefractive k.
    k. operation
    photorefractive k. (PRK)
    phototherapeutic k. (PTK)
    superficial k.
keratinized tissue
keratin scale
keratitis-deafness-cornification disorder
keratitis lesion
keratoacanthoma
keratoangioma
keratocele
keratocentesis operation
keratoconjunctivitis
keratocricoid
keratodermatocele

keratoepithelioplasty
keratoglossus
keratohyal
keratoleukoma
keratolysis
    pitted k.
keratoma
keratometry
    surgical k.
keratomileusis
    Barraquer k.
    laser-assisted in situ k. (LASIK)
    laser in situ k. (LASIK)
    k. operation
keratomy
keratopathy
    band k.
    exposure k.
keratophakic keratoplasty
keratopharyngeus
keratoplasty
    allopathic k.
    Arroyo k.
    Arruga k.
    autogenous k.
    automated lamellar therapeutic k. (ALTK)
    Durr nonpenetrating k.
    Elschnig k.
    epikeratophakic k.
    Filatov k.
    Filatov penetrating k.
    Gradle k.
    heterogeneous k.
    homogenous k.
    Imre k.
    keratophakic k.
    Kraupa rotational k.
    lamellar refractive k.
    layered k.
    Magitot k.
    Morax k.
    nonpenetrating k.
    k. operation
    optic k.
    partial k.
    Paufique k.
    penetrating k.
    perforating k.
    photorefractive k. (PRK)
    punctate epithelial k.
    refractive k.
    Sourdille k.
    superficial lamellar k.
    tectonic k.
    thermal k. (TKP)
    total k.
    von Hippel k.

keratoscopy
keratostomy
keratotomy
>   arcuate transverse k.
>   astigmatic k.
>   delimiting k.
>   Gifford delimiting k.
>   laser k.
>   k. operation
>   radial k.
>   refractive k.
>   Ruiz trapezoidal k.
>   trapezoidal k.
>   Troutman radial k.

Kerckring fold
kerion formation
Kerley A, B, C lines
Kerlone
Kern lateral mass screw fixation technique
Kernohan
>   K. notch
>   K. system of glioma classification

Kerr cesarean section
KESS
>   Knowles-Eccersley-Scott Symptom
>   KESS constipation scoring system classification
>   KESS Questionnaire

Kessel-Bonney
>   K.-B. extension osteotomy
>   K.-B. hallux osteotomy procedure

Kessler
>   K. suture
>   K. suture technique
>   K. tendon repair

Kessler-Kleinert suture
Kestenbaum torticollis surgical procedure
Ketalar
ketamine gel
ketoacidosis
>   diabetic k. (DKA)

ketone body formation
ketoprofen analgesic therapy
ketorolac tromethamine
Kety-Schmidt
>   K.-S. cerebral blood flow measurement method
>   K.-S. inert gas saturation technique

Kevorkian punch biopsy
Key-Conwell pelvic fracture classification
Keyes punch biopsy
keyhole
>   k. approach
>   k. coronary bypass procedure
>   k. deformity
>   k. incision
>   k. mastopexy
>   k. method

>   k. surgery
>   k. tenodesis technique

keyhole-shaped craniectomy
key-in-lock maneuver
Key operation
keystone
>   k. anterior discectomy and fusion technique
>   k. graft
>   K. mastopexy

kg/m$_2$
>   kilogram per meter squared

KHC
>   knot holding capacity

Khodadoust line
Kidde cannula hysterosalpingogram technique
kiddie caudal
Kidner excision of accessory navicular bone procedure
kidney
>   abdominal k.
>   k. abscess
>   k. adenocarcinoma
>   k. adenoma
>   amyloid k.
>   k. anomaly
>   arciform vein of k.
>   arteriosclerotic k.
>   artificial k.
>   Ask-Upmark k.
>   atrophic k.
>   k. biopsy
>   cake k.
>   k. carbuncle
>   cicatricial k.
>   k. colic
>   contracted k.
>   cortical arch of k.
>   cystic k.
>   donor k.
>   ectopic k.
>   floating k.
>   Goldblatt k.
>   k. graft biopsy
>   granular k.
>   horseshoe k.
>   interlobular artery of k.
>   k. internal splint/stent (KISS)
>   medullary sponge k.
>   mortar k.
>   movable k.
>   pancreas after k. (PAK)
>   pelvic k.
>   k. position
>   putty k.
>   pyelonephritic k.
>   rosette k.
>   sclerotic k.

K

kidney (*continued*)
    sigmoid k.
    simultaneous pancreas and k.
     (SPK)
    k. stone
    thoracic k.
    k. transplant
    tumor-bearing k.
    unicaliceal k.
    wandering k.
    waxy k.
kidney-sparing operation
Kiehn-Earle-DesPrez plastic surgery procedure
Kiel
    K. classification
    K. heterogeneous bone graft
    K. Pediatric Tumor Registry
Kienböck dislocation
Kiernan space
Kiesselbach area
Kikuchi-MacNob-Moreau anterior cervical disectomy approach
Kilfoyle humeral medial condylar fracture classification
Kilian line
Killian
    K. bundle
    K. frontal sinusotomy
    K. frontoethmoidectomy procedure
    K. incision
Killian-Jamieson area
Killip
    K. classification of heart disease
    K. myocardial infarct classification
Killip-Kimball heart failure classification
kilogram per meter squared (kg/m^2)
kilovolt (kV)
Kimerle anomaly
Kimmelstiel-Wilson lesion
Kimura cartilage graft
kinase
    glycogen synthase k.
Kinast indirect reduction
kinesophobia
    Tampa Scale of K. (TSK)
kinesthetic
    k. method
    k. perception
kinetics
    disposition k.
kinetic venous drainage
King
    K. arytenoidopexy
    K. ASD umbrella closure
    K. biopsy method
    K. contrast venography technique
    K. curve posterior correction
    K. intraarticular hip fusion

    K. laryngeal tube
    K. open reduction
King-Richards dislocation technique
King-Steelquist
    K.-S. hindquarter amputation
    K.-S. transiliac amputation technique
kinking
    catheter k.
Kinsey
    K. atherectomy
    K. rotation atherectomy extrusion angioplasty
Kirby
    K. stapled pulmonary lobectomy
    K. superior rectus muscle blepharoptosis operation
Kirk thigh amputation technique
Kirner deformity
Kirschner
    K. pin fixation
    K. suture
    K. suture technique
    K. wire fixation
KISS
    kidney internal splint/stent
kissing
    k. balloon angioplasty
    k. balloon technique
Kitano knot
Kitaoka-Leventen medial displacement metatarsal osteotomy
Kitzinger method of childbirth
Klatskin
    K. hepatic duct bifurcation resection
    K. tumor
kleeblattschädel deformity
Kleinert
    K. flexor tendon repair
    K. modification
Klein muscle
Klippel-Feil
    K.-F. anomaly
    K.-F. deformity
    K.-F. syndrome
Klippel-Trenaunay syndrome
Klippel-Trenaunay-Weber syndrome
Knapp
    K. pterygium operation
    K. vertical transposition of horizontal recti procedure
Knapp-Wheeler-Reese operation
knee
    k. anatomy
    k. arthroplasty
    descending artery of k.
    k. dislocation
    k. extension
    k. extensor
    flail k.

k. fracture
k. fusion
lateral k.
posterior k.
k. region
k. replacement
k. replacement surgery
k. rotation
kneecap
kneecapping injury
knee-chest position (KCP)
knee-elbow position (KEP)
kneeling position
kneeling-squatting position
knife-edged finishing line
knob
aortic k.
lateral deflection control k.
Knobloch modification
knock-knee deformity
Knoll gland
knot
Aberdeen k.
Ahern k.
bow-tie k.
capstan k.
clinch k.
curved-needle surgeon's k.
enamel k.
externally releasable k.
extracorporeal jamming k.
false k.
fisherman's k.
friction k.
granny k.
half-hitch k.
1-handed k.
k. holding capacity (KHC)
ileosigmoid k.
intracorporeal k.
jamming k.
Kitano k.
laparoscopic extracorporeal k.
partial-throw surgeon's k.
primitive k.
Roeder loop k.
secure intracorporeal k.
self-tightening slip k.
slip k.
k. slippage
square k.
surgeon's k.
syncytial k.
Tim k.
Topel k.
Tripier operation throw square k.
true k.
vital k.
wire k.

knotting
catheter k.
intracorporeal k.
laparoscopic k.
Knowles-Eccersley-Scott
K.-E.-S. Symptom (KESS)
K.-E.-S. Symptom constipation
scoring system classification
Knowles pinning
knuckle of tube
Ko-Airan
K.-A. cystic artery hemostasis
maneuver
K.-A. laparoscopic cholecystectomy
bleeding control procedure
Koch
K. conduit
K. continent ileostomy
K. pouch
K. pouch cutaneous urinary
diversion
K. reservoir ileostomy
K. triangle
Kocher
K. anastomosis
K. clamp
K. curved L approach
K. fracture
K. hernia inguinalis invagination
method
K. humerus fracture classification
K. incision
K. lateral J approach
K. lateral peritoneal attachment
dissection maneuver
K. point
K. pylorectomy
K. pyloromyotomy
K. ureterosigmoidostomy procedure
Kocher-Gibson posterolateral approach
Kocher-Langenbeck
K.-L. exposure
K.-L. posterior proximal femur and
acetabulum approach
Kocher-Lorenz fracture
Kocher-McFarland hip arthroplasty
Kock pouch ileostomy procedure
Koenig coronary artery graft
Koenig-Schaefer
K.-S. incision
K.-S. medial approach
**Koerner canal wall-down mestoidectomy
flap**
Koffler operation
Köhler
K. illumination
K. line
Kohlrausch muscle
Kolobow membrane lung

K

Kondoleon operation
Kondoleon-Sistrunk elephantiasis
  procedure
Konno
    K. aortic valve anulus repair
    K. biopsy method
    K. left ventricular outflow
      enlargement procedure
Konno-Rastan aortoventriculoplasty
  operation
Korean hand acupressure
koronion
koroscopy
Korotkoff
    K. collateral circulation test
    K. sound
Kotz-Salzer rotationplasty
Koutsogiannis
    K. calcaneal displacement osteotomy
    K. sliding calcaneal osteotomy
      procedure
Koutsogiannis-Fowler-Anderson
  osteotomy
Kovalevsky canal
Krackow
    K. obese patient tourniquet
      maneuver
    K. point
    K. suture
Kramer-Craig-Noel basilar femoral neck
  osteotomy
Kraske
    K. excision of coccyx and partial
      sacrum removal operation
    K. midline posterior proctotomy
      procedure
    K. parasacral approach
    K. position
    K. transsacral proctectomy
Kraupa rotational keratoplasty
Krause
    K. bone
    K. denervation
    K. ligament
    K. muscle
    K. respiratory bundle
    transverse suture of K.
Krause-Wolfe full-thickness skin graft
Krawkow-Cohn iliac crest bone harvest
  technique
Krawkow-Thomas-Jones locking suture
  technique
Krempen-Craig-Sotelo tibial nonunion
  technique
Krempen-Silver-Sotelo infected
  pseudarthrosis operation
Kreuscher bunionectomy
Kristeller
Kroner tubal ligation

Krönig technique
Krönlein
    K. hernia
    K. lateral orbitotomy procedure
    K. orbital decompression operation
    K. orbitotomy
Krönlein-Berke orbitotomy
Kronner external fixation
Kropp
    K. cystourethroplasty
    K. onlay urethral lengthening
      operation
    K. urethral lengthening procedure
Krukenberg
    K. corneal spindle
    K. hand reconstruction
    K. reconstruction of BKA procedure
Kruskal-Wallis
Kugel
    K. anastomosis
    K. hernia patch repair technique
    K. hernia repair
    K. hernia repair approach
Kugelberg reconstruction
Kuhnt
    K. eyelid operation
    K. tarsectomy
Kuhnt-Helmbold ectropion repair
Kuhnt-Junius macular degeneration
  repair
Kuhnt-Szymanowski ectropion repair
  with lid reconstruction procedure
Kuhnt-Thorpe operation
Kulchitsky cell carcinoma
Kumar
    K. cholangiography clamp
    K.cholangiography catheter
    K. spica cast technique
Kumar-Cowell-Ramsey congenital vertical
  talus correction technique
Kümmell spondylitis
Küntscher intramedullary nailing
  technique
Kupffer cell
Kussmaul
    K. coma
    K. respiration
    K. sign
Kussmaul-Kien respiration
Küstner
    K. incision
    K. suture
    K. uterine inversion correction
Kutler
    K. digital flap
    K. double lateral advancement flap
    K. finger amputation technique
    K. V-Y flap
    K. V-Y flap graft

Kuzmak
>K. gastric banding
>K. gastroplasty

kV
>kilovolt

KWB
>Keith-Wagener-Barker

K-wire placement
Kwitko senile entropion operation
Kyle-Gustilo femoral fracture classification
Kyle-Gustilo-Premer dynamic hip screw fixation classification

Kyle internal fixation
kyphectomy
>Sharrard-type k.

kyphosis
>k. correction
>k. creation
>postlaminectomy k.
>postradiation k.

kyphos resection
kyphotic
>k. angulation
>k. deformity
>k. deformity pathomechanics

K

L
    lumbar
LA
    lateral apical
      LA segment
LABA
    laser-assisted balloon angioplasty
Labat sciatic nerve block
Labbé
    L. gastrotomy technique
    L. triangle
    L. vein
labia (*pl. of* labium)
labial
    l. cavity
    l. fusion
    l. gland
    l. hernia
    l. line
    l. pad
    l. tubercle
    l. ulceration
    l. vein
    l. vestibule
labialization
labile blood pressure
labioglossolaryngeal
labioglossomandibular approach
labioglossopharyngeal
labioincisal line angle
labiolingual
    l. plane
    l. technique
labiomandibular
    l. approach
    l. glossotomy
labiomental
labionasal
labiopalatine
labioplasty
labioscrotal fold
labium, *pl.* **labia**
    l. inferioris muscle
    l. majus
    ungual labia
labor
    l. pain
    stages of l.
laboratory (lab)
    l. monitoring
    l. parameter
labored respiration
labra (*pl. of* labrum)
labral lesion
labrum, *pl.* **labra**

L-25 absorbable surgical suture
labyrinth
    bony l.
    ethmoidal l.
    Ludwig l.
    osseous l.
    renal l.
    Santorini l.
    vestibular l.
labyrinthectomy
labyrinthine
    l. artery
    l. fistula
    l. fistula test
    l. surgery
    l. vein
labyrinthotomy
labyrinthus osseus
lacerable
lacerated foramen
laceration
    aortic l.
    birth canal l.
    bladder l.
    brain l.
    burst-type l.
    canalicular l.
    central stellate l.
    cervical l.
    chevron l.
    concurrent hepatic l.
    conjunctival l.
    corneal l.
    corneoscleral l.
    cuff l.
    diaphragm l.
    diaphragmatic l.
    eyebrow l.
    flexor tendon l.
    hallucis longus l.
    inadvertent l.
    lid margin l.
    liver l.
    longitudinal l.
    lower pole l.
    parenchymal l.
    perineal l.
    peripheral l.
    pulmonary l.
    rectal l.
    scalp l.
    splenic l.
    stellate l.
    tarsal l.
    tentorial l.

L

laceration (*continued*)
    through-and-through l.
    vaginal l.
    vascular l.
lace suture technique
Lachman knee ligament tear maneuver
lachrymal (*var. of* lacrimal)
lacmoid staining solution
lacosamide
Lacour-Gayet pediatric arterial switch operation
lacrimal, lachrymal
    l. angle duct anomaly
    l. apparatus
    l. artery
    l. bone
    l. canal
    l. canaliculus
    l. crest
    l. fascia
    l. fistula
    l. fold
    l. ganglion
    l. gland repair
    l. gland tumor
    l. irrigation test
    l. lake
    l. margin
    l. mass
    l. nerve
    l. notch
    l. papilla
    l. point
    l. punctum
    l. sac
    l. sac fossa
    l. surgery
    l. system
    l. vein
lacrimalis
    apparatus l.
lacrimation
    excessive l.
    l. reflex
lacrimoconchal suture
lacrimomaxillary suture
lacrimotomy
Lacroix
    fibroosseous ring
      of L.
    ring of L.
lactate
    blood l.
    l. clearance
    l. extraction
    l. level
    normalizing l.
    normal serum l.
lactation letdown response

lacteal
    l. fistula
    l. vessel
lactic
    l. acidosis
    l. acidosis and strokelike
      syndrome
lactiferous
    l. duct
    l. duct fistula
    l. gland
    l. sinus
lacuna, *pl.* **lacunae**
    Morgagni l.
    osteocytic l.
    urethral l.
lacunae (*pl. of* lacuna)
lacunar
    l. abscess
    l. ligament
Ladd
    L. band
    L. mobilization of intestine
      procedure
    L. operation
ladder
    WHO analgesic l.
laesa
    functio l.
Lafora body disease
lag
    l. dilation
    dilation l.
    l. phase
    l. screw fixation
    l. screw thread hole
    l. time
LAGB
    laparoscopic adjustable gastric band
Lagleyze-Trantas operation
Lagrange sclerectoiridectomy
Lahey abdominoperineal rectal cancer operation
Laimer area
Laird-McMahon anorectoplasty
laissez-faire lid operation
lake
    lacrimal l.
    lateral l.
Lallemand body
Lallemand-Trousseau body
Lallouette pyramid
LAMA
    laser-assisted microanastomosis
lambda suture line
lambdoid
    l. margin
    l. suture
Lambert canal

Lambl excrescence
Lamb-Marks-Bayne upper limb repair technique
Lambrinudi
    L. osteotomy
    L. triple arthrodesis for dropfoot technique
lamella, *pl.* **lamellae**
    corneal l.
    elastic l.
lamellae (*pl. of* lamella)
lamellar
    l. bone
    l. corneal transplant
    l. exfoliation
    l. refractive keratoplasty
lamellation
lamina, *pl.* **laminae**
    alar l.
    basal l.
    basilar l.
    cribrous l.
    deep l.
    external elastic l.
    fusca l.
    inferior epigastric l.
    pterygoid l.
    suprachoroid l.
    thyroid l.
    vascular l.
laminae (*pl. of* lamina)
laminaplasty (*var. of* laminoplasty)
laminar, laminated
    l. cortex posterior aspect
    l. flow hood
    l. fracture
laminated
    l. acellular mass
    l. clot
lamination
laminectomy
    cervical spine l.
    decompression l.
    decompressive l.
    Gill l.
    Girdlestone l.
    multilevel l.
    4-place l.
    radial l.
laminoforaminotomy
laminoplasty, laminaplasty
    expansive l.
    Tsuji l.
laminotomy
    l. and discectomy
    l. lead
lamotrigine
Lancaster scleral suture operation

Lancefield hemolytic *Streptococcus* **classification**
lanceolate deformity
lancet suture
Lanchner operation
landmark
    bony l.
    central l.
    cephalometric l.
    developmental l.
    pedicle l.
    surface l.
    thoracic spine l.
Landolt
    L. body
    L. creation of lower eyelid operation
Landzert fossa
Lane
    L. band
    L. ileorectal anastomosis
Langenbeck
    L. iridectomy
    L. operation
    L. triangle
Langendorff
    L. heart preparation
    L. perfusion
    L. perfusion of isolated heart method
Langenskiöld
    L. bone graft
    L. bony bridge resection
    L. central physeal bar excision procedure
    L. fusion
Langer
    L. arch
    L. line
Langerhans
    islets of L.
Lange tendon lengthening and repair
Langhans line
Lang suture
language
    body l.
Lannelongue ligament
LANSS
    Leeds Assessment of Neuropathic Symptoms and Signs
lanugo
Lanz
    L. incision
    L. line
    L. point
Lanza scale for drug-induced mucosal damage classification

L

LAO
    left anterior oblique
    left anterior occipital
      LAO position
lap
    laparoscopic
    laparotomy
LAP
    laparoscopy
    laparotomy
laparectomy
laparocele
laparocystidotomy
laparoenterotomy
laparogastroscopy
laparogastrostomy
laparogastrotomy
laparohepatotomy
laparohysterectomy
laparohystero-oophorectomy
laparohysteropexy
laparohysterosalpingo-oophorectomy
laparohysterotomy
laparoileotomy
laparomyomectomy
laparomyositis
laparorrhaphy
laparosalpingectomy
laparosalpingo-oophorectomy
laparosalpingotomy
laparoscopic
    l. ablative nephrectomy
    l. adjustable gastric band (LAGB)
    l. adjustable silicone gastric banding
    l. adrenalectomy
    l. antegrade transcystic sphincterotomy
    l. anterior adrenalectomy
    l. anterior partial fundoplication
    l. aortic stapler
    l. appendectomy (lap appy)
    l. artery ligation
    l. assistance
    l. autopsy
    l. bariatric surgery
    l. bilioenteric anastomosis
    l. biliopancreatic diversion
    l. bladder neck suture suspension procedure
    l. bowel resection
    l. Burch procedure
    l. bypass procedure
    l. cardiomyotomy
    l. cecopexy
    l. celiac plexus pain block
    l. cholecystectomy (lap chole, LC, LCC, LCE)
    l. cholecystotomy
    l. clip application

l. closure
l. colectomy
l. colorectal cancer surgery
l. colposuspension technique
l. common bile duct exploration
l. common bile duct exploration choledochotomy
l. common bile duct exploration transcystic approach
l. curtsy
l. cyst decortication
l. dismembered pyeloplasty
l. dissection and manipulation
l. distal pancreatectomy
l. Döderlein hysterectomy
l. donor nephrectomy (LDN)
l. donor nephrectomy technique
l. Dorr antireflux surgery
l. drift
l. duodenoileostomy ileoileostomy
l. esophageal myomectomy
l. esophagectomy
l. esophagogastric fundoplasty
l. esophagogastroplasty with Nissen fundoplication
l. esophagomyotomy
l. esophagoplasty
l. evaluation
l. examination
l. extracorporeal knot
l. feeding tube replacement
l. fenestration
l. gallbladder removal
l. gas
l. gastric banding
l. gastric bypass
l. gastroenterostomy
l. gastroplasty
l. gastrostomy
l. guidance
l. halogen light source
l. harvesting
l. Hassab gastric devascularization and splenectomy
l. Heller myotomy
l. hepatectomy
l. hepaticojejunostomy
l. hepatic resection
l. hernioplasty
l. highly selective vagotomy
l. Hill repair
l. hysterosalpingectomy
l. intracorporeal ultrasonography (LICU)
l. intragastric resection
l. intraoperative ultrasonography (LIOUS)
l. jejunostomy
l. knotting

l. laser cholecystectomy
l. left hemicolectomy
l. live donor nephrectomy
l. liver biopsy
l. liver resection
l. lymph node dissection method
l. lymph node dissection procedure
l. lymph node dissection technique
l. lymphocelectomy
l. lysis of adhesions
l. management
l. mini gastric bypass
l. needle colposuspension
l. needle driver
l. nephrectomy
l. Nissen and Toupet fundoplication
l. Nissen fundoplication (lap Nissen)
l. Nissen fundoplication method
l. Nissen fundoplication procedure
l. Nissen fundoplication technique
l. Nissen fundoplication with
  esophageal lengthening
l. no-trocar technique
l. orchiopexy
l. paraaortic lymph node sampling
l. paraaortic lymph node sampling
  method
l. paraaortic lymph node sampling
  procedure
l. paraaortic lymph node sampling
  technique
l. paraesophageal hernia repair
  (LPHR)
l. partial nephrectomy
l. pelvic lymphadenectomy
l. pelvic lymph node dissection
l. photography
l. pirouette maneuver
l. plication
l. pneumodissection
l. port site metastasis
l. posterior adrenalectomy
l. posterior hemifundoplication
l. proctectomy
l. PROST
l. prosthetic mesh repair
l. pyloromyotomy
l. radical hysterectomy
l. radical prostatectomy
l. remnant gastrectomy
l. repair of paraesophageal hernia
  (LRPH)
l. retroperitoneal lymphadenectomy
  (RPLND)
l. retropubic colposuspension
l. Roux-en-Y choledochojejunostomy
l. seromyotomy
l. sigmoidopexy
l. splenectomy

l. staging
l. stone extraction
l. stripping technique
l. surgical procedure
l. technology
l. telescope
l. total extraperitoneal herniorrhaphy
l. total gastrectomy
l. total occlusion
l. total proctocolectomy
l. Toupet antireflux surgery
l. transcystic common bile duct
  exploration (LTCBDE)
l. transcystic duct exploration
l. transcystic lithotripsy (LTCL)
l. transcystic papillotomy
l. transcystic sphincter of Oddi
  manometry
l. transhiatal esophagectomy
l. transhiatal view
l. transperitoneal adrenalectomy
l. treatment
l. trocar wound
l. tubal banding procedure
l. ultrasonography (LUS)
l. ultrasound (LUS)
l. ultrasound examination
l. ureteral reanastomosis
l. ureterolithotomy
l. uterine nerve ablation (LUNA)
l. uterolysis
l. uterosacral nerve ablation (LUNA)
l. uterosacral nerve ablation (LUNA)
l. vagotomy
l. varicocelectomy
l. varicocele repair
l. varix ligation
l. ventral hernia repair
l. vision

laparoscopically
l. assisted endorectal pullthrough
  procedure
l. assisted surgery
l. assisted vaginal hysterectomy
  (LAVH)
l. guided cryoablation
l. guided transcystic exploration

laparoscopic-assisted
l.-a. aneurysmectomy
l.-a. aortic reconstructive surgery
l.-a. colectomy
l.-a. distal gastrectomy
l.-a. esophagectomy
l.-a. gastropexy
l.-a. hemicolectomy
l.-a. hepatectomy
l.-a. living donor nephrectomy
l.-a. procedure
l.-a. small bowel resection

L

laparoscopic-assisted (*continued*)
l.-a. subtotal gastrectomy
l.-a. transverse colectomy
l.-a. vaginal hysterectomy
l.-a. vaginal hysteroscopy
laparoscopic-induced neuralgia
laparoscopist
laparoscopy (LAP)
ambulatory gynecologic l.
bedside l.
closed l.
diagnostic l.
double-puncture l.
flexible l.
full diagnostic l.
gaseous l.
gasless l.
gynecologic l.
hand-assisted l.
laser l.
mandatory l.
needle l.
open l.
pelvic l.
revision l.
robot-assisted l.
second-look l.
single-port l.
single-puncture l.
staging l.
therapeutic l.
laparoscopy-assisted sigmoidectomy
laparostomy
l. technique
l. with silo-bag technique
laparotomy (LAP)
elective l.
emergency l.
exploratory l. (ex lap)
formal l.
l. incision
negative l.
open l.
routine l.
second-look l. (SLL)
staging l.
standard midline l.
therapeutic trauma l.
xiphopubic l.
laparotrachelotomy
laparotyphlotomy
laparouterotomy
Lapides urethrocystopexy
Lapidus
L. bunionectomy
L. hammertoe technique
L. metatarsocuneiform joint
arthrodesis procedure
lappet formation

Lapra-Ty suture
LAR
low anterior resection
lardaceous liver
large
l. canal
l. cell carcinoma
l. humeral head hemiarthroplasty
l. intestine
l. intestine diverticulum
l. mask airway
l. pelvis
l. restoration
l. vestibular aqueduct syndrome
large-caliber nonabsorbable suture
large-core
l.-c. needle aspiration biopsy
l.-c. technique
large-particle biopsy
large-scale integration
Larmon
L. forefoot arthroplasty
L. forefoot procedure
LaRoque herniorrhaphy incision
**Laroyenne pelvic suppuration
drainage**
Larrey
L. cleft
L. hernia
Larsen syndrome
Larson
L. ligament reconstruction
L. posterolateral instability of knee
repair technique
laryngeal
l. aditus
l. anesthesia
l. anomaly
l. aperture
l. bursa
l. carcinoma
l. cartilage fracture
l. cavity
l. cyst
l. diaphragm
l. edema
l. electromyography
l. framework surgery
l. gland
l. hemorrhage
l. infection
l. keel operation
l. mask
l. mask airway (LMA)
l. mask insertion anesthetic
technique
l. muscle
l. nerve
l. nerve injury

l. nerve paralysis
l. oscillation
l. pharynx
l. pouch
l. prominence
l. repair
l. respiration
l. sinus
l. skeleton
l. vein
l. ventricle
l. web

laryngectomy
anterior partial l.
frontolateral l.
narrow-field l.
near-total l.
partial l.
subtotal supraglottic l.
supracricoid partial l.
supraglottic l.
total l.
vertical partial l.
wide-field total l.

larynges (*pl. of* larynx)

laryngis
corniculum l.

laryngocele

laryngofissure

laryngology

laryngopharyngeal reflux

laryngopharyngectomy
partial l.
total l.

laryngopharyngeus

laryngopharynx

laryngoplasty
sternothyroid muscle
flap l.

laryngopyocele

laryngoscope
Airtraq l.
Flexiblade l.
GlideScope Cobalt video l.
video-Macintosh l.

laryngoscopy
l. anesthetic technique
awake l.
direct l.
fiberoptic l.
indirect l.
laser l.
McCoy balloon l.
mirror-image l.
suspension l.

laryngospasm, glottidospasm
postextubation l.

laryngotomy
inferior l.

laryngotracheal
l. anesthesia (LTA)
l. resection
l. separation
l. stenosis

laryngotracheoplasty

larynx, *pl.* **larynges**
external auditory l.
folding l.
polypoid hyperplasia of l.
posterior l.
superficial anterior l.
superior l.

LASE
laser-assisted spinal endoscopy

laser
l. anterior small thoracotomy
procedure
l. arthroscopy
l. biliary lithotripsy
l. bronchoscopy
l. cavity
l. cervical conization
l. coagulation
l. coagulation vaporization procedure
(LCVP)
l. coagulation vaporization
procedure-aided resection
l. controlled area
l. dermabrasion
l. disc decompression (LDD)
l. Doppler flowmetry (LDF)
l. Doppler fluxmetry
l. hemorrhoidectomy
l. hemorrhoid excision
Ho:YAG l.
l. in situ keratomileusis (LASIK)
l. iridectomy
l. iridotomy
l. keratotomy
l. laparoscopic cholecystectomy
l. laparoscopic vagotomy
l. laparoscopy
l. laryngoscopy
l. LUNA
l. manipulation
l. method
l. partial nephrectomy
l. photoablation
l. photocoagulation
l. photovaporization
l. plume
l. recanalization
l. resection of prostate
l. surgery
l. therapy
Ti:sapphire l.
l. tissue weld
l. tissue welding

L

laser (*continued*)
    l. trabeculoplasty (LTP)
    l. uvulopalatoplasty (LUPP)
    l. vaporization
    l. welding technique
    YAG l.
laser-assisted
    l.-a. appendectomy
    l.-a. balloon angioplasty
    (LABA)
    l.-a. drug delivery
    l.-a. in situ keratomileusis
    (LASIK)
    l.-a. microanastomosis (LAMA)
    l.-a. spinal endoscopy (LASE)
    l.-a. uvulopalatoplasty (LAUP)
laser-evoked potential
laser-filtering surgery
laser-induced
    l.-i. fragmentation
    l.-i. intracorporeal shock wave
    lithotripsy
lasering
lasertripsy
Lash
    L. laparoscopic supracervical
    hysterectomy procedure
    L. operation
LASIK
    laser-assisted in situ keratomileusis
    laser in situ keratomileusis
LAST
    limited anterior small thoracotomy
    LAST coronary bypass procedure
lata, *pl.* **latae**
    fascia l.
    tensor fasciae latae
latae (*pl. of* lata)
Latarget
    L. laparoscopic highly selective
    vagotomy procedure
    L. nerve
late
    l. complication
    L. Effects of Normal
    Tissue — Subjective, Objective,
    Management, Analytic
    (LENT-SOMA)
    l. graft dysfunction
    l. graft failure
    l. infection rate
    l. transplant nephrectomy
    l. wound failure
latency
    postdrug l.
latent herpes simplex virus infection
late-onset
    l.-o. disease
    l.-o. hepatic failure

latera (*pl. of* latus)
lateral
    l. aberration
    l. adenoidectomy
    l. apex
    l. apical (LA)
    l. aspiration
    l. atlantoaxial joint
    l. band mobilization
    l. basal (LB)
    l. bending technique
    l. bicipital groove
    l. calcaneal branch
    l. canal
    l. canal entrapment
    l. canthotomy
    l. canthus
    l. cartilage flap
    l. central palmar space
    l. cerebral aperture
    l. cervical node dissection
    l. chest x-ray
    l. closing wedge osteotomy
    l. column
    l. compartment reconstruction
    l. compression
    l. compression injury
    l. condensation
    l. condylar humeral fracture
    l. condylar inclination
    l. condyle
    l. cord
    l. corticospinal tract
    l. crus
    l. decubitus position
    l. deflection control knob
    l. deltoid splitting approach
    l. edge
    l. epicondylitis
    l. excursion
    l. extensor expansion
    l. extensor release
    l. extracavitary approach
    l. fluoroscopy
    l. fusion
    l. Gatellier-Chastang ankle
    approach
    l. geniculate body
    l. ginglymus
    l. glossoepiglottic fold
    l. ground (LG)
    l. ground bundle
    l. hamstring
    l. head
    l. illumination
    l. J approach
    l. jaw projection
    l. joint line
    l. joint of ankle

l. joint space
l. knee
l. Kocher approach
l. lake
l. ligament
l. lithotomy
l. malleolus
l. mass
l. mass fracture
l. meniscectomy
l. muscle
l. nail fold
l. nasal branch
l. orbit
l. perforation
l. pole
l. portion
l. process
l. prone position
l. pterygoid
l. pterygoid muscle
l. rectus recession
l. rectus resection
l. rectus tendon
l. recumbent position
l. region
l. retraction
l. rhachotomy
l. root
l. sac
l. sector
l. sinus
l. tarsal strip procedure
l. thoracotomy
l. trap suture
l. utility incision
l. ventricle
l. wall
l. window technique
l. wound
l. x-ray view
laterality
lateralization
cortical l.
lateral-lateral pouch
lateral-sector pedicle
lateriflection (*var. of* lateriflexion)
lateriflexion, lateriflection
lateroabdominal
lateroaortic
l. lymph node dissection
l. metastasis
laterodeviation
lateroflection (*var. of* lateroflexion)
lateroflexion, lateroflection
lateropharyngeum
lateroposition
later postoperative period
late-stage disease

latex
l. allergy
l. closure
lathing procedure
latissimus
l. dorsi island flap
l. dorsi muscle flap
l. dorsi musculocutaneous flap
l. dorsi myocutaneous flap
l. dorsi procedure
l. dorsi tendon
latissimus-scapular muscle flap
latissimus-serratus muscle flap
lattice space
latus, *pl.* **latera**
Latzko
L. cesarean section
L. partial colpocleisis
L. radical abdominal hysterectomy
L. vesicovaginal fistula repair
laudable
Lauenstein ulnar head resection procedure
Lauge-Hansen ankle fracture classification
Laugier
L. fracture
L. hernia
Laumonier ganglion
LAUP
laser-assisted uvulopalatoplasty
Laurell
Lauren gastric carcinoma classification
Lauth
L. canal
L. ligament
lavage
abdominal l.
l. and suction
antral l.
bone l.
bowel l.
l. bowel preparation
bronchoalveolar l. (BAL)
colonic l.
continuous postoperative closed l.
copious peritoneal l.
diagnostic peritoneal l. (DPL)
external biliary l.
l. instillation
intraoperative bowel l.
intraoperative colonic l.
on-table l.
peritoneal l.
pulsatile pressure l.
saline l.
l. solution
unilateral l.

L

LAVH
    laparoscopically assisted vaginal hysterectomy
law
    Hilton l.
    Le Chatelier l.
    l. of association
    l. of denervation
Lawson retrograde percutaneous nephrolithotomy
layer
    aponeurotic l.
    barrier l.
    echographic l.
    fascial l.
    hidden l.
    input l.
    meningeal l.
    mesothelial cell l.
    molecular external l.
    musculoaponeurotic l.
    nerve fiber bundle l.
    nuclear external l.
    orbital l.
    output l.
    parietal l.
    plexiform external l.
    posterior l.
    pretracheal l.
    prevertebral l.
    seromuscular l.
    serous l.
    superficial l.
    suprachoroid l.
    l. technique
    visceral l.
2-layer
    2-l. anastomosis
    2-l. enteroenterostomy
    2-l. latex closure
    2-l. open technique
layered
    l. closure
    l. keratoplasty
layer-to-layer gastroplasty
laying-open fistulotomy
Lazaro da Silva technique colostomy
Lazarus-Nelson peritoneal lavage technique
lazy-C incision
lazy-H incision
lazy-S incision
lazy-Z incision
LB
    lateral basal
    LB segment
3LC
    triple-lumen catheter

LCA
    left carotid artery
    left coronary artery
LCIS
    lobular carcinoma in situ
L-curved incision
LCVP
    laser coagulation vaporization procedure
LCVP-aided
    LCVP-a. hepatectomy
    LCVP-a. hepatic resection
    LCVP-a. technique
LCVP-assisted
    LCVP-a. hepatectomy
    LCVP-a. major liver resection
LDD
    laser disc decompression
LDF
    laser Doppler flowmetry
LDN
    laparoscopic donor nephrectomy
    LDN technique
LDR
    low dose rate
    LDR intracavitary radiation therapy
Le
    L. Chatelier law
    L. Chatelier principle
    L. Dentu suture
    L. Dran suture technique
    L. Fort colpocleisis procedure
    L. Fort craniofacial dysjunction operation
    L. Fort facial fracture classification
    L. Fort fibular fracture
    L. Fort III facial advancement
    L. Fort I–III fracture
    L. Fort mandibular fracture
    L. Fort-Neugebauer uterine prolapse repair
    L. Fort osteotomy
    L. Fort partial colpocleisis
    L. Fort suture technique
    L. Fort-Wagstaffe fracture
    L. Fort-Wehrbein-Duplay hypospadias repair
LEA
    lumbar epidural anesthesia
Leach dual-imaging surgical planning technique
Leach-Igou step-cut medial osteotomy
Leach-Schepsis-Paul augmentation
lead
    l. colic
    Flexon temporary cardiac pacing l.
    laminotomy l.
    l. line

percutaneous l.
l. suture

Leadbetter
L. cystourethroplasty
L. hip manipulation
L. hip reduction maneuver
L. ureteroplasty modification
  technique
L. urethral reconstruction procedure

Leadbetter-Politano
L.-P. ureteroneocystostomy procedure
L.-P. ureterovesicoplasty

lead-pipe
l.-p. appearance
l.-p. colon
l.-p. fracture

leaf, *pl.* **leaves**
superior l.

leaflet
aortic valve l.
l. entrapment
heart valve l.
l. looping
mitral valve l.
posterior mitral valve l.
valve l.

Leahey temporary tarsorrhaphy
leak
air l.
anastomotic l.
anastomotic stump l.
bile l.
bladder l.
calyceal l.
cervical esophagogastric anastomotic
  l.
chyle l.
chylous l.
cuff l.
cystic duct stump l.
duodenal stump l.
esophageal l.
external bile l.
glue patch l.
intrathoracic l.
mask l.
pancreatic stump l.
pelvicalyceal l.
periprosthetic l.
perivalvular l.
l. point pressure
postoperative anastomotic l.
Roux limb stump l.
stump l.
l. test
transthoracic esophageal l.
trocar gas l.
uncontained l.
ureteral l.

leakage
anastomotic l.
bile l.
biliary l.
cervical l.
chylous l.
corneal l.
intestinal anastomotic l.
intraperitoneal l.
local l.
postoperative anastomotic l.
l. rate
silicone implant l.
tube l.

lean
l. body mass
l. body weight

leapfrog
L. Group for Patient Safety
l. position

leather-bottle stomach
leaves (*pl. of* leaf)
Lecompte arterial switch maneuver
ledge
eccentric l.

LeDuc
L. anastomosis
L. ureteral tunneling technique

LeDuc-Camey
L.-C. ileocolostomy
L.-C. ileocystoplasty

Lee
L. anterosuperior iliac spine graft
L. bone graft
L. ganglion
L. laryngotracheal stenosis
  management technique
L. reconstruction

leech
mechanical l.

Leeds Assessment of Neuropathic Symptoms and Signs (LANSS)
LEEP
loop electrocautery excision
  procedure
loop electrosurgical excision procedure
LEEP conization

leeway space
Lee-White clotting time
Lefèvre gastrectomy technique
left
l. anterior oblique (LAO)
l. anterior oblique position
l. anterior oblique projection
l. anterior occipital (LAO)
l. atrial isolation procedure
l. atrial pressure
l. atrium to femoral artery
  circulatory bypass

L

left (*continued*)
      l. brachiocephalic vein
      l. bundle branch block
      l. carotid artery (LCA)
      l. colectomy
      l. colic artery
      l. coronary artery (LCA)
      l. coronary valve
      l. decubitus position
      l. dominant coronary circulation
      l. frontal craniotomy
      l. gastric artery
      l. gastroomental artery
      l. gutter
      l. heart catheterization
      l. hemicolectomy
      l. hemidiaphragm
      l. hepatectomy
      l. hypochondriac region
      l. inguinal hernia
      l. internal thoracic artery
      l. lateral decubitus position
      l. lateral projection
      l. lateral region
      l. lateral sectionectomy
      l. lower extremity (LLE)
      l. lower quadrant (LLQ)
      l. pulmonary artery
      l. rotation
      l. subclavian vein
      l. thorax
      l. upper extremity
      l. upper quadrant (LUQ)
      l. upper quadrant peritonectomy
      l. ventricle
      l. ventricular assist device (LVAD)
      l. ventricular assistive device (LVAD)
      l. ventricular end-diastolic area (LVEDa)
      l. ventricular end-diastolic pressure
      l. ventricular end-systolic area (LVESa)
      l. ventricular insufficiency
      l. ventricular ischemia
      l. ventricular outflow tract (LVOT)
      l. ventricular preload
      l. ventricular pressure
      l. ventricular pressure-volume relationship (LVPVR)
      l. ventricular puncture
      l. ventricular systolic pressure
      l. ventricular volume
      l. vertebral artery
left-sided
      l.-s. colorectal obstruction
      l.-s. injury
      l.-s. nail
      l.-s. thoracotomy

left-side-down position
left-to-right subtotal pancreatectomy
leg
      bandy l.
Legat point
legged
1-legged stork test
Lehman endoscopic pancreatic sphincterotomy technique
Leibolt pantalar arthrodesis technique
leiomyoblastoma
leiomyofibroma
leiomyoma enucleation
leiomyomectomy
leiomyosarcoma
      recurrent l.
Leishman hypertensive retinopathy classification
Lejour mastopexy
Lejour-type breast reduction
Leksell stereotactic surgery technique
Lembert
      L. seromuscular stitch
      L. suture
      L. suture technique
lemniscal trigeminothalamic pathway
Lempert
      L. fenestration
      L. incision
length
      bowel l.
      l. of stay (LOS)
      optical path l.
      pedicle screw path l.
      peripheral capillary filtration slit l.
      restriction fragment l.
length-breadth index
lengthening
      distal catheter l.
      esophageal l.
      extensor l.
      laparoscopic Nissen fundoplication with esophageal l.
      surgical crown l.
      tendon l.
length-height index
length-resting tension relation
length-tension relation
lengthwise slit
Lennert
      L. lesion
      L. non-Hodgkin lymphoma classification
lens
      l. aberration
      C-loop intraocular l.
      corneal l.
      l. dislocation
      l. equator

l. exchange
intraocular l. (IOL)
l. plane
l. removal
suture of l.
l. suture technique
lensectomy
Charles l.
coal-mining l.
lentectomy
lenticular
l. loop
l. papilla
l. process
l. ring
lenticulostriate artery
lentiform bone
lentigo melanoma
LENT-SOMA
Late Effects of Normal
Tissue — Subjective, Objective,
Management, Analytic
LENT-SOMA scoring scale
LENT-SOMA system
Lepird metatarsus adductus procedure
lepirudin
L'Episcopo hip reconstruction
**L'Episcopo-Zachary brachial plexopathy
tendon transfer procedure**
leptomeningeal
l. anastomosis
l. carcinoma
l. metastasis
l. space
leptomeninges (*pl. of* leptomeninx)
leptomeninx, *pl.* **leptomeninges**
leptomyelolipoma
Leriche
L. operation
L. sympathectomy
L. syndrome
Leri-Weill disease
LES
lower esophageal sphincter
LES pressure
Lesgaft
L. hernia
L. space
LESI
lumbar epidural steroid injection
lesion
accessible l.
acetowhite l.
acneform l.
acute gastric mucosal l.
acute traumatic l.
admixture l.
aggressive l.
ampullary l.

anal squamous intraepithelial l.
(ASIL)
angiocentric immunoproliferative l.
angiocentric lymphoproliferative l.
angiodysplastic l.
angioinvasive l.
angioproliferative l.
angulated l.
anterior labrum periosteum shoulder
arthroscopic l.
anular constricting l.
aphthous-type l.
apple-core l.
l. architecture
l. arrangement
articular cartilage l.
atherosclerotic carotid artery l.
atlantoaxial l.
axial l.
axillary skin l.
Baehr-Lohlein l.
Bankart shoulder l.
barrel-shaped l.
basal ganglionic l.
benign bone l.
benign lymphoepithelial l.
benign lymphoproliferative l.
benign vascular l.
Bennett l.
biceps interval l.
bifurcation l.
bilobed polypoid l.
bird's nest l.
blanchable red l.
blastic l.
bleeding l.
blue-gray l.
Blumenthal l.
bone marrow l.
bony l.
boomerang-shaped l.
Bracht-Wachter l.
braidlike l.
brainstem l.
branch l.
bridgelike l.
brown-black l.
bubbly bone l.
bullous skin l.
bull's eye macular l.
Bywaters l.
calcified l.
cancer l.
carpet l.
cavitary lung l.
cavitary small-bowel l.
cemental l.
central l.
centrilobular l.

L

lesion (*continued*)
  cerebral l.
  cervical l.
  chest l.
  chiasmal l.
  choroidal l.
  circular cherry-red l.
  cleavage l.
  cochlear l.
  coin l.
  cold l.
  colonic vascular l.
  complete common peroneal nerve l.
  concentric l.
  congenital l.
  conjunctival melanotic l.
  constricting l.
  cornea guttate l.
  corneal punctate l.
  cortical l.
  Councilman l.
  culprit l.
  cutaneous l.
  cylindromatous l.
  cystic bone l.
  cystic lymphoepithelial
    AIDS-related l.
  demyelinating l.
  dendritic l.
  de novo l.
  depigmented l.
  depressed l.
  dermal l.
  desmoid l.
  destructive bone l.
  Dieulafoy l.
  Dieulafoy-like l.
  diffuse ulcerative l.
  dilatable l.
  disc l.
  discoid skin l.
  discrete l.
  l. distribution
  division I–IV l.
  dorsal root entry zone l.
  DREZ l.
  ductal-dependent l.
  Duret l.
  dye sham intrarenal l.
  dysarthric l.
  dysplasia-associated l.
  early cancer l.
  ectatic vascular l.
  eczematous l.
  elementary l.
  elevated l.
  enhancing brain l.
  entry zone l.
  eosinophilic fibrohistiocytic l.

  epididymis l.
  epidural extramedullary l.
  erysipelas-like skin l.
  erythrodermatous l.
  l. evolution
  excavated l.
  expansile unilocular well-demarcated
    bone l.
  extracranial mass l.
  extrahepatic l.
  extramural l.
  extratesticular l.
  extrathalamic l.
  extremity l.
  extrinsic l.
  fibrocalcific l.
  fibrohistiocytic l.
  fibromusculoelastic l.
  fibroosseous l.
  fibrous bone l.
  fibrous polypoid l.
  firm l.
  flat depressed l.
  flat elevated l.
  floor-of-mouth l.
  florid duct l.
  focal parenchymal brain l.
  focal splenic l.
  follicular l.
  Forest I, II l.
  gastrointestinal l.
  genetic l.
  genital papulosquamous l.
  Ghon primary l.
  giant cell l.
  Gill l.
  glomerular tip l.
  gross l.
  ground-glass l.
  gunpowder l.
  hamartomatous l.
  hemorrhagic l.
  hepatic mass l.
  herpetoid l.
  high-grade squamous intraepithelial
    l. (HSIL)
  high-intensity l.
  high neurological l.
  Hill-Sachs shoulder l.
  histologic l.
  honeycomb l.
  hot l.
  hyperdense brain l.
  hyperintense brain l.
  hyperkeratotic l.
  hyperpigmented l.
  hypodense brain l.
  hypoechoic l.
  l. identification

immunoproliferative l.
impaction l.
indiscriminate l.
infarctive l.
inflammatory l.
infratentorial l.
initial syphilitic l.
interpeduncular fossa l.
interradicular l.
intraabdominal l.
intraconal l.
intracranial mass l.
intradural extramedullary l.
intrahepatic l.
intramedullary l.
intramural extramucosal l.
intraosseous bone l.
intrasellar l.
intravascular endothelial
  proliferative l.
intrinsic brainstem l.
ipsilateral nerve root l.
irritable l.
irritative l.
Janeway l.
jet l.
keratitis l.
Kimmelstiel-Wilson l.
labral l.
Lennert l.
Libman-Sacks l.
lichenified l.
lipocytic l.
localized l.
Löhlein-Baehr l.
long l.
low-attenuation l.
lower motor neuron l.
low-grade squamous intraepithelial l.
  (LSIL)
lucent lung l.
lumbar spinal cord l.
lumbar spine l.
lumbosacral plexus l.
lumbosacral root l.
lymphoepithelial l.
lymphoproliferative l.
lytic bone l.
macrofollicular l.
macroscopic l.
macrovascular coronary l.
malignant pituitary l.
Mallory-Weiss l.
mammographic l.
l. margination
mass l.
melanocytic conjunctival l.
melanotic l.
mesencephalic low-density l.

mesenchymal l.
mesenteric vascular l.
metastatic l.
minute polypoid l.
mixed fat-water density l.
mixed sclerotic and lytic bone l.
molecular l.
monotypic l.
Monteggia equivalent l.
Morel-Lavallée l.
morphealike l.
l. morphology
mucocutaneous l.
mucosal l.
mucous membrane l.
mulberry l.
multifocal enhancing l.
multilocular cystic l.
napkin ring anular l.
neoplastic l.
neural l.
neurovascular l.
nickel-and-dime l.
nodular l.
nodule-in-nodule l.
nonbacterial thrombotic
  endocardial l.
nonblanchable abnormally colored l.
nonerosive gastric mucosal l.
nonmeningiomatous malignant l.
nonneoplastic tumorlike l.
nonperforative l.
nucleus ambiguus l.
nummular l.
occult talar l.
ocular adnexal l.
oil drop l.
onion scale l.
orbital l.
organic l.
Osgood-Schlatter l.
osseous l.
osteoblastic l.
osteochondral l.
osteolytic bone l.
osteopathic l.
osteosclerotic l.
ostial l.
papillary l.
papulopustular l.
papulosquamous l.
papulovesicular l.
paraorbital l.
parasagittal l.
patch l.
pathologic l.
perforative l.
periodontal l.
peripheral nerve l.

L

lesion (*continued*)

perisellar vascular l.
periventricular hyperintense l.
periventricular white matter l.
Perthes l.
photon-deficient bone l.
pigmented l.
pigment epithelial l.
plaquelike l.
plexiform l.
polypoid l.
postfracture l.
potentially resectable l.
precancerous l.
prechiasmal optic nerve l.
precipitating l.
precursor l.
preexisting l.
premalignant l.
preoperative l.
presacral cystic l.
primary l.
proliferative l.
pruritic l.
pseudocancerous l.
pseudomedial longitudinal
  fasciculus l.
pseudoverrucous l.
pulpoperiapical l.
punched-out l.
purpuric l.
pustular l.
pyodermatous skin l.
radial sclerosing l.
radiodense l.
radiofrequency l.
radiofrequency-generated thermal l.
radiolucent l.
radiopaque l.
reactive lymphoid l.
recurrent nerve l.
regurgitant l.
residual l.
restenosis l.
reticular l.
retroacetabular l.
retrochiasmal l.
retrogeniculate l.
reverse Hill-Sachs l.
right-sided l.
rim-enhancing l.
ring l.
ring-wall l.
rolled shoulder l.
rotationally induced shear-strain l.
rotator cuff l.
ruptured peliotic l.
saddle l.
satellite l.

scaling skin-colored l.
scirrhous l.
sclerosing l.
sclerotic bone l.
secondary l.
semipedunculated l.
sessile l.
shagreen l.
short-segment l.
SIL/ASCUS l.
Sinding-Larsen-Johansson l.
sinonasal l.
sinusoidal l.
l. size
skeletal l.
skin-colored l.
skip l.
SLAP l.
slope-shouldered l.
smooth skin-colored l.
soft tissue l.
space-occupying brain l.
special l.
spiculated l.
spinal l.
splenic l.
spontaneous l.
squamous intraepithelial l. (SIL)
square-shouldered l.
stellate border breast l.
Stener l.
stenotic l.
stereotactic l.
stress l.
structural l.
subtentorial l.
supranuclear l.
suprasellar low-density l.
supratentorial l.
suspicious l.
synchronous l.
systemic l.
T l.
tandem l.
target l.
thalamic l.
thoracic l.
trabeculated bone l.
transient l.
traumatic l.
trophic l.
truncal l.
tuberculous l.
tubulovillous l.
type B-1, -2 l.
typical skin l.
uncommitted metaphysial l.
undifferentiated l.
unifocal optic nerve l.

unilocular cystic l.
unresectable l.
uremic gastrointestinal l.
varicelliform l.
vasculitic l.
vegetative l.
venular l.
verrucous l.
vesicobullous l.
violaceous l.
visceral l.
vulvar pigmented l.
vulvovaginal l.
Waldeyer throat ring l.
weeping l.
well-circumscribed l.
white l.
white-spot l.
wire-loop l.
Woofry-Chandler classification of
Osgood-Schlatter l.
wraparound periapical l.
Wrisberg l.
yellow l.

lesioning
radiofrequency l.
stereotactic radiofrequency l.

Leslie-Ryan anterior axillary approach
LESR
lower esophageal sphincter relaxation

lesser
l. cul-de-sac
l. curvature
l. horn
l. omentectomy
l. omentum
l. palatine artery
l. pancreas
l. pelvis
l. peritoneal cavity
l. peritoneal sac
l. resection
l. ring
l. sac approach
l. sac hernia
l. sac technique
l. saphenous vein
l. sciatic notch
l. supraclavicular fossa
L. triangle
l. trochanter
l. trochanter fracture
l. vestibular gland

Lesshaft triangle
Lester
L. Martin modification
L. Martin modification of Duhamel
abdominoperineal pullthrough
operation

Lester-Jones
conjunctivodacryocystorhinostomy
LET
liposome-encapsulated tetracaine
lethal
l. concentration
l. osteogenesis imperfecta
Letournel-Judet
L.-J. acetabular approach
L.-J. acetabular fracture classification
letter
discharge l.
letterbox technique
leucine supplementation
leucotomy (*var. of* leukotomy)
leucovorin
leukemia
leukemic infiltration
leukochloroma
leukocyte
l. infiltration
l. recruitment
leukocytic
l. infiltration
l. margination
leukocytoclastic vasculitis
leukocytoma
leukodepletion
leukoencephalopathy
radiation-induced l.
leukolymphosarcoma
leukolysis
leukoma
adherent l.
leukoplakia
leukosarcoma
leukostasis
intracerebral l.
leukotomy, leucotomy
prefrontal l.
transorbital l.
Leung thumb loss classification
levator
l. anguli oris
l. ani syndrome
l. aponeurosis repair
Bowman transconjunctival resection
of the l.
l. glandulae thyroidea
l. hernia
l. injury
l. palati muscle
l. palpebrae
l. resection
l. scapula
l. scapulae syndrome
l. span
l. swelling
levatorplasty

L

LeVeen shunt
Leveille iridectomy
level
> anterior midpapillary l.
> antithrombin III plasma l.
> arterial lactate l.
> attenuation l.
> bilirubin l.
> CEA l.
> Clark l.
> collagenase l.
> endothelin plasma l.
> l. foundation
> heparin cofactor II plasma l.
> iPTH l.
> lactate l.
> motilin l.
> multiple shunt l.'s
> overall sound l.
> pain tolerance l.
> parathyroid hormone l.
> pentane excretion l.
> plasma l.
> plasma gelsolin l.
> plasminogen plasma l.
> postinjury l.
> pretreatment l.
> protein C, S plasma l.
> PTH l.
> sensation l.
> serum lidocaine l.
> serum total bilirubin l.
> sound pressure l.
> total bilirubin l.
> transcutaneous tissue oxygen l.
> uterine lysosome l.

level-dependent
> blood oxygenation l.-d.

leverage
Levine
> L. 1–6 cardiac murmur
> gradation
> L. dislocation operation

Levine-Harvey cardiac auscultation classification
Levin tube
levitation
levobupivacaine
levodopa dopaminergic medication
levodopa-induced dyskinesia
levosimendan
levotransposed position
Levret breech delivery maneuver
Lewis
> L. intercalary resection
> L. operation
> L. thoracotomy
> L. Y antigen

Lewis-Chekofsky femur resection

Lewis-Tanner
> L.-T. esophagectomy
> L.-T. 2-stage esophagectomy
> procedure
> L.-T. subtotal esophagectomy and
> reconstruction

Lewit stretch technique
Lewy body
Lexer eyelid ptosis operation
LFT
> liver function test

LG
> lateral ground
> LG bundle

LGD
> low-grade dysplasia

Li
> lithium

liability
> physiologic dependence l.
> psychic dependence l.

libera
> tenia l.

liberation
Libman-Sacks lesion
Lich
> L. extravesical technique
> L. ureterocystostomy procedure

lichenification
lichenified lesion
lichenoid graft-versus-host disease
Lich-Gregoir
> L.-G. anastomosis
> L.-G. kidney transplant surgery
> L.-G. ureterolysis
> L.-G. vesicoureteral reflux
> repair
> L.-G. vesicoureteral reflux repair
> technique

Lichtblau osteotomy
Lichtenstein
> L. hernia repair
> L. herniorrhaphy
> L. mesh repair
> L. tension-free hernioplasty

Lichtman staging of Kienböck disease technique
LICU
> laparoscopic intracorporeal
> ultrasonography

lid
> l. closure reaction
> l. margin laceration
> upper l.

lid-loading technique
lidocaine
> intracuff l.
> l. lollipop
> nebulized l.

Lidoderm patch
lid-splitting procedure
Lieberkühn
 L. crypt
 L. gland
Liebolt radioulnar technique
lienal artery
lienculus, lienunculus
lienectomy
lienis
lienopancreatic
lienophrenic ligament
lienorenal ligament
lienunculus
Lieutaud
 L. body
 L. triangle
 L. trigone
 L. uvula
life
 l. expectancy
 perceived quality of l. (PQOL)
 quality of l. (QOL)
 l. space
 l. table method
life-saving form of therapy
LifeSite hemodialysis access system
life-sustaining hepatic reserve
life-threatening
 l.-t. cancer
 l.-t. complication
 l.-t. illness
lift-and-cut
 l.-a.-c. biopsy
 l.-a.-c. method
lifting
 abdominal wall l.
 sternal l.
ligament
 accessory plantar l.
 accessory volar l.
 acromioclavicular l.
 alar l.
 anococcygeal l.
 anterior costotransverse l.
 anterior cruciate l. (ACL)
 anterior sternoclavicular l.
 anterior tibiotalar l.
 Arantius l.
 arcuate pubic l.
 atlantooccipital l.
 auricular l.
 Berry l.
 broad uterine l.
 Camper l.
 capsular l.
 cardinal l.
 caroticoclinoid l.
 caudal l.

ceratocricoid l.
cervical l.
cholecystoduodenal l.
chondroxiphoid l.
ciliary l.
Civinini l.
Clado l.
Cloquet l.
collateral l.
Colles l.
Cooper l.
coracoacromial l.
coracoclavicular l.
coracohumeral l.
costoclavicular l.
costocolic l.
costotransverse l.
costoxiphoid l.
cotyloid l.
Cowper l.
cricoarytenoid l.
cricothyroid l.
cricotracheal l.
cruciform l.
cystoduodenal l.
Denonvilliers l.
denticulate l.
digital retinacular l.
duodenorenal l.
epihyal l.
external l.
falciform l.
fallopian l.
Ferrein l.
fibulocalcaneal l.
fundiform l.
gastrocolic l.
gastrodiaphragmatic l.
gastrohepatic l.
gastrolienal l.
gastrophrenic l.
gastrosplenic l.
genitoinguinal l.
Gimbernat l.
l. graft
Gruber l.
Halsted l.
Hensing l.
hepatocaval l.
hepatocolic l.
hepatoduodenal l.
hepatoesophageal l.
l. hepatoesophageum
hepatogastric l.
l. hepatogastricum
hepatorenal l.
Hesselbach l.
Holl l.
Hueck l.

L

ligament (*continued*)
       hyalocapsular l.
       hyoepiglottic l.
       iliolumbar l.
       inferior glenohumeral l.
         (IGHL)
       inferior pubic l.
       inferior pulmonary l.
       inferior transverse scapular l.
       infundibuloovarian l.
       infundibulopelvic l.
       inguinal l.
       interchondral l.
       interclavicular l.
       interclinoid l.
       interfoveolar l.
       interosseous sacroiliac l.
       interphalangeal collateral l.
       interspinous l.
       intertransverse l.
       intervolar plate l.
       intraarticular sternocostal l.
       intracapsular l.
       Jarjavay l.
       Krause l.
       lacunar l.
       Lannelongue l.
       lateral l.
       Lauth l.
       lienophrenic l.
       lienorenal l.
       Lockwood l.
       longitudinal l.
       lumbocostal l.
       Luschka l.
       Mackenrodt l.
       mallear l.
       Mauchart l.
       Meckel l.
       medial puboprostatic l.
       median arcuate l.
       nuchal l.
       palpebral l.
       pancreaticosplenic l.
       pectineal l.
       peridental l.
       periodontal l.
       Petit l.
       petroclinoid l.
       petrosphenoid l.
       phrenicocolic l.
       phrenicoesophageal l.
       phrenicolienal l.
       phrenicosplenic l.
       phrenogastric l.
       phrenosplenic l.
       prostatic l.
       pterygomandibular l.
       pterygospinal l.

pterygospinous l.
pubic arcuate l.
puboprostatic l.
pubovesical l.
pulmonary l.
radiate sternocostal l.
radiocapitate l.
radiotriquetral l.
radioulnar l.
l. reconstruction
reflected inguinal l.
reflex l.
rhomboid l.
right prostatic l.
right triangular l.
round uterine l.
l. rupture
sacrococcygeal l.
sacrodural l.
sacroiliac l.
sacrospinous l.
sacrotuberous l.
serous l.
Soemmerring l.
sphenomandibular l.
spiral l.
splenocolic l.
splenorenal l.
stellate l.
sternoclavicular l.
sternopericardial l.
stylohyoid l.
stylomandibular l.
stylomaxillary l.
suprascapular l.
supraspinous l.
suspensory l.
sutural l.
synovial l.
tarsal l.
temporomandibular l.
Teutleben l.
Thompson l.
thyroepiglottic l.
thyrohyoid l.
thyrothymic l.
Treitz l.
triangular l.
urachal l.
uterosacral l.
uterovesical l.
venous l.
ventral sacrococcygeal l.
ventricular l.
vertebropelvic l.
vesicoumbilical l.
vesicouterine l.
vestibular l.
vocal l.

Whitnall l.
yellow l.
Zaglas l.
Zinn l.
ligamenta (*pl. of* ligamentum)
ligamental anesthesia
ligamentopexy
ligamentoplasty
ligamentous support tissue
ligamentum, *pl.* **ligamenta**
    l. ceratocricoideum
    l. costotransversarium
    l. hepatocolicum
    l. hyoepiglotticum
    l. teres
    l. venosum
ligand
    tissue l.
ligand-gated
    l.-g. cation channel
    l.-g. ion channel
ligated
    circumferentially l.
    doubly l.
    staple l.
    suture l.
ligate-divide-staple technique
ligation
    Abernethy external iliac artery l.
    aneurysm clip l.
    artery l.
    band l.
    Barron l.
    bidirectional l.
    bile duct l. (BDL)
    Blalock-Taussig shunt l.
    bleeding site l.
    cecal l.
    common bile duct l.
    coronary vein l.
    direct l.
    distal l.
    elastic band l.
    endoscopic band l.
    endoscopic esophagogastric
      variceal l.
    esophageal band l.
    l. hemorrhoidectomy
    high l.
    Hunter aneurysm l.
    hunterian l.
    hypogastric artery l.
    inferior vena cava l.
    interdental l.
    Irving tubal l.
    IVC l.
    Kroner tubal l.
    laparoscopic artery l.
    laparoscopic varix l.

modified Irving-type tubal l.
l. of hemorrhoid
open retroperitoneal high l.
parotid duct l.
pedicle l.
pole l.
Pomeroy tubal l.
postureteral l.
rubber-band l.
sigmoid sinus l.
sling l.
spermatic vein l.
spinal nerve l.
stump l.
subfascial l.
surgical l.
suture l.
l. suture technique
teeth l.
tracheal l.
transesophageal varix l.
transgastric l.
tubal l.
variceal band l.
varicose vein stripping and l.
varix l.
vessel l.
ligature
    intracystic suture l.
    loop l.
light
    l. coagulation
    L. criteria
    l. exposure
    l. guide bundle
    l. microscopy
    l. projection
light-around-wire technique
lighted stylet-guided oral intubation
light-reflecting wedge
lightwand tracheal intubation
light-wire torque
Likert pain scale
Lilienthal incision
Liliequist
    membrane of L.
limb
    afferent l.
    afferent jejunal l.
    alimentary l.
    antecolic Roux l.
    biliopancreatic l.
    l. deformity
    distal l.
    efferent l.
    graft l.
    l. ischemia
    l. ischemia pain
    jejunal Roux-en-Y l.

L

limb (*continued*)

l. length angulation
paretic l.
pelvic l.
phantom l.
proximal l.
l. reduction
l. reduction abnormality
l. reduction anomaly
l. replantation
Roux l.
Roux-en-Y l.
l. salvage
l. salvage index
terminal ileal l.
thoracic l.
vertebral, anal, cardiac, tracheal, esophageal, renal, l. (VACTERL)

limbal

l. approach
l. compression
l. incision
l. parallel orientation

limbal-based flap
limb-body wall complex
Limberg

L. pilonidal disease flap
L. pilonidal sinus flap repair technique

limbi (*pl. of* limbus)
limbic

l. center
l. system

limb-lengthening procedure
limb-salvage

l.-s. procedure
l.-s. surgery

limb-saving

l.-s. method
l.-s. procedure
l.-s. technique

limb-sparing

l.-s. operation
l.-s. procedure
l.-s. surgery

limbus, *pl.* **limbi**

conjunctival l.
corneal l.
l. mass
Vieussens l.

4-limb Z-plasty
lime

soda l.

limited

l. anterior small thoracotomy (LAST)
l. examination
l. fasciectomy
l. gastrectomy

l. gastric cancer lymph node dissection (D1)
l. hemorrhoidectomy
l. hepatectomy
l. obturator node dissection
l. pancreatectomy
l. resection
l. thoracotomy

limiting

adjustable pressure l. (APL)
l. membrane
l. plate erosion

limitus

hallux l.

Limoge current
LINAC

linear accelerator

LINAC-based radiosurgery
Linatrix suture
Lincoff scleral buckle
Lindell blanisotropic media classification
Lindeman laryngeal diversion procedure
Lindesmith palliative transposition of great vessels operation
Linde Walker Oxygen Program
Lindholm

L. Achilles tendon rupture repair technique
L. tendo calcaneus repair

Lindner

L. corneoscleral suture
L. sclerotomy

Lindner-Guist retinal detachment operation
Lindsay cleft lip and palate operation
Lindseth osteotomy
line

accretion l.
AC-PC l.
action l.
air-fluid l.
alveolar point-nasal point l.
alveolar point-nasion l.
alveolobasilar l.
alveolonasal l.
Amberg lateral sinus l.
anastomotic suture l.
aneuploid cell l.
l. angle
angular l.
anocutaneous l.
anorectal l.
anterior axillary l. (AAL)
anterior commissure-posterior commissure l.
antitension l.
arcuate l.
Arlt l.
arterial mean l.

atopic l.
axillary l.
azygoesophageal l.
basal l.
base l.
basinasal l.
Beau l.
bimastoid l.
bisector l.
bismuth l.
black l.
Blaschko l.
blue l.
Blumensaat l.
Bolton-nasion l.
Brödel bloodless l.
Burton l.
calcification l.
calciotraumatic l.
Camper l.
canthomeatal l.
Cantlie l.
cement l.
cemental l.
cementing l.
central venous pressure l.
cervical l.
Chaussier l.
Clapton l.
cleavage l.
clivus canal l.
colonic mucosal l.
Conradi l.
contour l.
corneal iron l.
coronoid l.
Correra l.
costoclavicular l.
costophrenic septal l.
Crampton l.
craze l.
crossarch fulcrum l.
curved radiolucent l.
CVP l.
cyma l.
D l.
Daubenton l.
delay l.
Dennie l.
Dennie-Morgan l.
dentate l.
developmental l.
digastric l.
Donders l.
Douglas l.
Ebner l.
Egger l.
Ehrlich-Türck l.
emission l.

epiphysial l.
esophageal suture l.
external oblique l.
face l.
Farre white l.
fat l.
fat-density l.
feather-edged proximal finishing l.
Feiss l.
femoral head l.
Ferry l.
fingerprint l.
Fishgold l.
Fleischner l.
l. focus principle
foramen magnum l.
fracture l.
Fränkel white l.
Frankfort horizontal light l.
Fraunhofer l.
fulcrum l.
Futcher l.
gallbladder-vena cava l.
Garrett orientation l.
gas density l.
gaussian l.
George l.
germ l.
gingival finishing l.
gluteal l.
Granger l.
gravitational l.
gravity l.
gray l.
growth arrest l.
Gubler l.
gum l.
Hampton l.
Harris growth arrest l.
Hawkins l.
Head l.
Helmholtz l.
hemostatic staple l.
high lip l.
high smile l.
Hilgenreiner horizontal Y l.
Hilgenreiner-Perkins l.
Hilton white l.
His l.
Holdaway l.
Holden l.
hot l.
Hudson l.
Hudson-Stähli l.
Hueter l.
humeral l.
Hunter l.
Hunter-Schreger l.
iliopectineal l.

L

line (*continued*)

incision l.
l. infection
infracostal l.
innominate l.
intercondylar l.
intermediate l.
internal oblique l.
interspinal l.
intertrochanteric l.
intertubercular l.
iron l.
iron Hudson-Stähli l.
iron-stocker's l.
isodose l.
isoelectric l.
l. isolation monitor
joint l.
Jurkat T-cell l.
Kaplan oblique l.
Kerley A, B, C lines
Khodadoust l.
Kilian l.
knife-edged finishing l.
Köhler l.
labial l.
lambda suture l.
Langer l.
Langhans l.
Lanz l.
lateral joint l.
lead l.
Linton l.
lip l.
load l.
long l.
lorentzian l.
lower midclavicular l.
low lip l.
lumbar gravitational l.
lymphoblastoid cell l.
M l.
Mach l.
MacNab l.
mamillary l.
mammary l.
mare's tail l.
McGregor basal l.
McKee l.
McRae foramen magnum l.
median l.
Mees l.
mercurial l.
Meyer l.
Meyerding spondylolisthesis
  classification l.
midaxillary l.
midclavicular l.
midheel l.

midhumeral l.
midmalleolar l.
midpoint to meatal l.
midscapular l.
midsternal l.
Moloney l.
Monro l.
Monro-Richter l.
Morgan l.
Morris hepatoma cell l.
mucogingival l.
mucosal l.
Muehrcke l.
myelomonocytic cell l.
mylohyoid l.
nasion-alveolar point l.
nasobasilar l.
nasolabial l.
Nélaton l.
neonatal l.
neuronal cell l.
nipple l.
nuchal l.
Obersteiner-Redlich l.
obturator l.
odontoid perpendicular l.
l. of Bekhterev
l. of direction
l. of fixation
l. of Gennari
l. of Kaes
l. of relaxation
l. of Retzius
l. of Toldt
Ohngren l.
orbital l.
orbitomeatal l.
Owen l.
oxygen supply l.
palatooccipital l.
pararectal l.
paraspinal l.
parasternal l.
paravertebral l.
Pastia l.
pectinate l.
pectineal l.
percutaneous l.
peripheral arterial l.
Perkins vertical l.
physial l.
Pickerill imbrication l.
pigmentary demarcation l.
pleural l.
pleuroesophageal l.
plumb l.
Poirier l.
Poupart l.
preaxillary l.

principal l.
properitoneal fat l.
protrusive l.
psoas l.
pubococcygeal l.
pupillary l.
radiocapitellar l.
radiolucent crescent l.
radio signal l.
recessional l.
rectal floor l.
Reid base l.
rejection l.
resonance l.
resting l.
retentive fulcrum l.
reversal l.
Rex-Cantli-Serege l.
Richter-Monro l.
right midinguinal l.
rolandic l.
Roser-Nélaton l.
sacral arcuate l.
sacral horizontal plane l.
sagittal suture l.
Salter incremental l.
Sampoelesi l.
scapular l.
Schreger l.
Schwalbe l.
sclerotic l.
scurvy l.
semicircular l.
semilunar l.
septal l.
Sergent white l.
Shenton l.
simian l.
sinus l.
Snellen l.
soleal l.
spectral l.
Spieghel l.
Spigelius l.
spinolamellar l.
spinolaminar l.
spinous interlaminar l.
spiral l.
stabilizing fulcrum l.
Stähli pigment l.
sternal l.
Stocker l.
stromal l.
subclavian l.
subcostal l.
supracondylar l.
supracrestal l.
survey l.
suture l.

Sydney l.
sylvian l.
T-cell l.
teardrop l.
temporal l.
tender l.
terminal l.
l. test
Thompson l.
tibiofibular l.
tram l.
trapezoid l.
triradiate l.
trough l.
Türk l.
Twining l.
Tycos pressure infusion l.
Ullmann l.
V l.
venous l.
Vesling l.
vibrating l.
visual l.
Voigt l.
von Ebner l.
Wackenheim clivus canal l.
water density l.
Wegner l.
white l.
l. width
Winberger l.
Z l.
Zahn l.
zero l.
Zöllner l.
Z-shaped suture l.

linea, *pl.* **lineae**
lineae (*pl. of* linea)
linear
l. accelerator (LINAC)
l. accelerator-based radiosurgery
l. calcification
l. craniectomy
l. incision
l. osteotomy
l. salpingostomy
l. skull fracture
l. tear
l. thermal expansion
l. ulceration
linearly polarized near-infrared irradiation
lined flap
linen suture
liner
streamlined pharyngeal airway l.
lingual
l. approach
l. artery

L

lingual (*continued*)
l. bone
l. branch
l. cavity
l. frenulum
l. gland
l. inclination
l. mucosa
l. nerve
l. plexus
l. split-bone technique
l. tongue flap
l. tonsil hyperplasia
l. vein
lingualplasty
lingula, *pl.* **lingulae**
lingulae pancreaticae
lingulae (*pl. of* lingula)
lingular branch
linguofacial trunk
linguoincisal line angle
linguoocclusal line angle
lining
cavity l.
linitis plastica
linnaean system of nomenclature
Linton
L. incision
L. line
L. operation
L. patch angioplasty
L. perforator interruption flap
L. varicose vein procedure
LIOUS
laparoscopic intraoperative ultrasonography
lip
acetabular l.
l. adhesion operation
anterior l.
cleft l.
l. line
l. switch flap
upper l.
lipase
apolipoprotein l.
lipectomy
abdominal l.
Malbec abdominal l.
lipid
l. infusion
l. metabolism
l. peroxidation
l. peroxidation product
lipiodol transarterial embolization treatment
lipoatrophy
postinfection l.
lipoblastoma

lipocele
lipocytic lesion
lipodermatosclerosis
lipofibroadenoma
lipofibroma
lipogranuloma
lipoid theory of narcosis
lipoleiomyoma
lipolysis
heparin-induced l.
intravascular l.
lipoma, *pl.* **lipomata**
lipomalike tissue
lipomata (*pl. of* lipoma)
lipomatous
l. infiltration
l. tissue
lipomeningocele
lipomyelocele
lipomyelocystocele
lipomyelomeningocele
lipomyxoma
liponecrosis
lipophilicity
lipophilic opioid
lipopolysaccharide
lipoprotein
liposarcoma
high-grade primary extremity l.
myxoid l.
pleomorphic l.
primary l.
round cell l.
liposomal preparation
liposome-encapsulated tetracaine (LET)
liposuction
submental l.
ultrasonic-assisted l. (UAL)
liposuctioning
Lipp maneuver for esophageal-tracheal intubation
Lipscomb-Anderson posterior cruciate ligament reconstruction procedure
Lipscomb technique
lip-splitting incision
liquefaction necrosis
liquid
l. extraction
l. nitrogen cryoablation
l. scintillation spectrometer
liquor
Scarpa l.
LIS
low intermittent suction
Lisfranc
L. amputation
L. articulation
L. disarticulation
L. dislocation

L. fracture
L. fracture-dislocation
L. tubercle
Lisofylline
Lissauer
L. bundle
L. tract
lissencephaly syndrome
lissosphincter
list
wait l.
Lister
L. antiseptic surgery method
L. flexor tendon pulley
reconstruction technique
L. tubercle
listerism
listhesis
Listing plane
lithagogue
lithectomy
lithiasis
biliary l.
pancreatic l.
renal l.
lithium (Li)
lithocystotomy
litholapaxy
Bigelow l.
litholysis
chemical l.
litholyte
litholytic
lithotomist
lithotomy
bilateral lithotomies
dorsal l.
high l.
lateral l.
marian l.
median l.
percutaneous cholangioscopic l.
percutaneous transhepatic
cholangioscopic l. (PTCSL)
perineal l.
l. position
prerectal l.
suprapubic l.
vaginal l.
vesical l.
lithotresis
ultrasonic l.
lithotripsy, lithotrity
biliary l.
blind l.
Candela l.
cystoscopic electrohydraulic l.
electrohydraulic l. (EHL)
electrohydraulic shock wave l.

endoscopic-controlled l.
endoscopic electrohydraulic l.
endoscopic pulsed dye laser l.
external shock wave l.
extracorporeal piezoelectric shock
wave l.
extracorporeal shock wave l.
(ESWL)
intracorporeal laser l. (ILL)
intracorporeal shock wave l.
laparoscopic transcystic l. (LTCL)
laser biliary l.
laser-induced intracorporeal shock
wave l.
mechanical l.
percutaneous l.
piezoelectric l.
pressure regulated electrohydraulic l.
l. retreatment
rotational contact l.
shock wave l. (SWL)
tunable dye laser l.
ultrasonic l.
lithotripsy-induced hypertension
lithotriptic
lithotriptoscopy
lithotrity (*var. of* lithotripsy)
lithuresis
litigation reaction
little
L. area
l. finger sign
Littler-Cooley opponensplasty technique
**Littler swanneck deformity repair
technique**
Littré
L. gland
L. hernia
Littré-Richter hernia
Litwak aortic bypass
Livaditis circular myotomy
live
l. donor liver transplantation without
blood products
l. donor nephrectomy
liver
l. abscess
alcoholic l.
l. allograft
l. allotransplantation
l. bed
l. biopsy
l. capsule
cirrhotic l.
l. cyst
l. cyst infection
l. damage
l. disease
l. distention

L

liver (*continued*)
l. dome stent exit site extravasation
echogenic l.
l. failure
l. flap
floating l.
frosted l.
l. function
l. function test (LFT)
l. hanging maneuver
hobnail l.
icing l.
l. injury
l. laceration
lardaceous l.
l. lobe
l. lobule
l. mass
l. metastasis
native l.
nutmeg l.
obstructed l.
l. operation
l. parenchyma
polycystic l.
l. regeneration
l. resection
split l.
stasis l.
l. steatosis
steatotic l.
sugar-icing l.
l. tissue
l. tract
l. transplant
triangular ligament of l.
l. tumor
l. volume
wandering l.
waxy l.
Livewire TC cardiac ablation
living
l. donor lobar lung transplant
l. donor nephrectomy
l. donor partial hepatectomy
l. donor renal transplant
l. lung donor
l. relative donor
l. will (LW)
living-related
l.-r. donor (LRD)
l.-r. donor transplant
l.-r. liver transplant (LRLT)
l.-r. small-bowel transplant
Livingstone therapy
Livingston peribulbar wedge
LLC
laparoscopic laser cholecystectomy
laser laparoscopic cholecystectomy

LLE
left lower extremity
Lloyd Davies modified lithotomy position
Lloyd-Roberts-Catteral-Salamon bone dysplasia classification
Lloyd-Roberts fracture technique
LLQ
left lower quadrant
LMA
laryngeal mask airway
LMWH
low-molecular weight heparin
load
fecal l.
l. line
load-bearing graft
load-deflection
l.-d. curve
l.-d. rate
load-deformation curve
load-displacement
l.-d. curve
l.-d. plot
loading
fecal l.
l. fracture
stress l.
weight l.
lobar
l. bronchus
l. collapse
l. hemorrhage
l. nephronia
l. resection
l. torsion
lobate
lobatum
hepar l.
lobe
caudate l.
inferior parietal l.
liver l.
native caudate l.
paracentral l.
renal l.
l. resection
Riedel l.
right caudate l.
Spiegel l.
spigelian l.
Spigelius l.
superior parietal l.
thyroid l.
lobectomy
caudate l.
Falconer l.
hepatic l.
ipsilateral thyroid l.
Kirby stapled pulmonary l.

pulmonary l.
sleeve l.
temporal l.
thyroid l.
total l.
unilateral l.
VATS l.
video-assisted l.
lobi (*pl. of* lobus)
lobose, lobous
lobotomy
frontal l.
prefrontal l.
radical prefrontal l.
transorbital l.
lobous (*var. of* lobose)
Lobstein ganglion
lobster-claw deformity
lobular
l. acinus
l. carcinoma
l. carcinoma in situ
l. hyperplasia
lobulate, lobulated
lobulated
l. contour
l. mass
lobule
hepatic l.
liver l.
l. of epididymis
posterior l.
posterior-lateral l.
renal cortical l.
secondary pulmonary l.
lobulet, lobulette
lobulette (*var. of* lobulet)
lobuli (*pl. of* lobulus)
lobulus, *pl.* **lobuli**
lobus, *pl.* **lobi**
local
l. abscess
l. acidosis
l. anesthesia
l. anesthetic
l. anesthetic reaction
l. anesthetic sympathetic blockade
l. bloodletting
l. epineurotomy
l. excision
l. excitatory state
l. exhaust ventilation
l. heat
l. hepatectomy
l. hypoxia
l. infection
l. ingrowth
l. injection
l. invasion

l. irradiation
l. leakage
l. lymphatic uptake
l. muscle flap
l. radical resection
l. recurrence
l. skin flap
l. standby anesthesia technique
l. surgery
l. therapy
l. tissue infiltration
l. treatment
l. tumor extension
l. twitch response (LTR)
localization
anatomic l.
bleeding site l.
bracket wire l.
estrogen receptor l.
eye tumor l.
focus l.
gamma probe l.
hooked wire l.
invasive l.
isotope l.
methylene blue dye l.
MRI-guided bracket wire l.
needle l.
l. of disease
pancreatic tumor l.
pedicle l.
percutaneous l.
placental l.
preoperative l.
radioisotope l.
sentinel lymph node l.
sentinel node l.
l. signal
SLN l.
stereotactic l.
l. study
l. technique
l. test
wire l.
localized
l. abdominal sign
l. abscess
l. inflammation
l. lesion
l. leukocyte mobilization
l. pain
l. plaque formation
l. prostate cancer
locally advanced disease
locating canal
location
extraperitoneal l.
nonaxillary l.
tumor l.

L

locator
loci (*pl. of* locus)
lock
    Howland l.
    l. stitch
locked-in syndrome
locked stitch
locking suture technique
lockout suture
lock-stitch suture technique
Lockwood ligament
locoregional
    l. adjuvant therapy
    l. management
    l. recurrence
    l. recurrence-free survival (LRRFS)
    l. relapse
    l. therapy
    l. treatment
loculation
    l. of fluid
    l. syndrome
locus, *pl.* **loci**
    l. minoris resistentiae
Loeffler-Ballard incision
Loesche periodontal disease classification
Loewenthal
    L. bundle
    L. tract
Löffler suture technique
logadectomy
logical
    l. method
    l. operation
logrolling maneuver
Löhlein-Baehr lesion
Löhlein operation
loin pain hematuria syndrome
lollipop
    lidocaine l.
    l. mastopexy
Londermann operation
lone atrial fibrillation
long
    l. axis
    l. bone
    l. bone fracture
    l. cone technique
    l. lesion
    l. line
    l. QT syndrome
    l. thoracic artery
    l. thoracic nerve
    l. thoracic vein
    l. tract sign
long- and short-lever rotational manipulation
long-chain fatty acids

longer-segment obstruction
longissimus muscle
longitudinal
    l. aberration
    l. canal
    2-chamber l. (2C-L)
    l. choledochotomy
    l. dissociation
    l. enterotomy
    l. fold
    l. fracture
    l. incision
    l. laceration
    l. ligament
    l. ligament rupture
    l. method
    l. myotomy
    l. nephrotomy of Boyce
    l. oval pelvis
    l. pancreatojejunostomy
    l. relaxation
    l. scanning
    l. section
    l. side-to-side anastomosis
    l. vertebral venous sinus
long-limb
    l.-l. gastric artery bypass
    l.-l. gastric bypass
Longmire
    L. operation
    L. valvotomy
Longmire-Gutgeman gastric reconstruction
Longo hemorrhoidectomy
long-segment spinal fusion
long-term
    l.-t. bone-instrumentation interface
    l.-t. central venous access catheter placement
    l.-t. dysphagia
    l.-t. epidural catheterization
    l.-t. followup
    l.-t. morbidity
    l.-t. opioid therapy
    l.-t. outcome
    l.-t. oxygen therapy
    l.-t. paralysis
    l.-t. restenosis
    l.-t. survival
longus
    l. capitis muscle
    l. colli muscle
    extensor carpi radialis l. (ECRL)
    extensor digitorum l. (EDL)
    extensor hallucis l. (EHL)
    extensor pollicis l. (EPL)
Look Sharpoint Ophthalmic suture

loop

air-filled l.
antiperistaltic l.
Biebl l.
bowel l.
central chemoreflex l.
cerebral-sacral l.
cervical l.
l. choledochojejunostomy
closed vascular l.
colonic l.
l. colostomy
contiguous l.
l. diathermy cervical conization
distended afferent l.
l. distribution
duodenal l.
efferent l.
elastic vascular l.
l. electrocautery excision procedure (LEEP)
l. electrosurgical excision procedure (LEEP)
l. electrosurgical excision procedure conization
l. esophagojejunostomy
expressor l.
l. fixation
flow-volume l.
l. forearm graft
foreign body l.
l. gastric bypass
l. gastric bypass method
l. gastric bypass procedure
l. gastric bypass technique
l. gastrojejunostomy
Henle l.
Hyrtl l.
ileal l.
l. ileostomy
l. ileostomy construction
intestinal l.
jejunal interposition of Henle l.
jejunal Roux-en-Y l.
l. jejunostomy
jejunum l.
lenticular l.
l. ligature
nephronic l.
N-shaped sigmoid l.
open l.
ostomy l.
l. ostomy bridge
peduncular l.
peripheral chemoreflex l.
puborectalis l.
Roux-en-Y l.
l. stoma
subclavian l.

l. transverse colostomy
vascular l.
venous l.

3-loop

3-l. ileal pouch
3-l. technique

looped cautery
loop-end ileostomy
looping

leaflet l.

2-loop J-shaped ileal pouch
loopogram
loop-on mucosa suture technique
looposcopy
loose

l. fracture
l. fragment
l. intraarticular body

loosening

screw l.

lop ear (*var. of* lop-ear)
lop-ear, lop ear
Lopez-Enriquez operation
LOR

loss of resistance

Lord

L. dilation
L. dilation of hemorrhoid
L. hemorrhoidectomy
L. operation

lordosis

l. creation
l. preservation

lorentzian line
Lorenz congenital clubfoot procedure
Loreta outlet of stomach dilatation
lorry driver's fracture
Lortat-Jacob pediatric GERD approach
LOS

length of stay

Losee

L. modification
L. modification of MacIntosh ACL repair technique
L. sling and reef ACL repair technique

loss

anticipated blood l.
articular bone l.
blood l.
bone l.
cutaneous heat l.
dermal l.
discrimination l.
excessive blood l.
excessive weight l.
extreme hearing l.
graft l.
insertion l.

L

loss (*continued*)
    intraoperative blood l.
    maximum allowable blood l.
    memory l.
    l. of airway
    l. of resistance (LOR)
    operative blood l.
    percutaneous anesthetic l.
    surgical weight l.
    third space l.
    tissue l.
    total body fluid l.
loss-of-resistance technique
loss-of-waist sign
lost wax pattern technique
Lotheissen
    L. hernia repair
    L. inguinal approach to femoral
      hernia operation
Lothrop frontoethmoidectomy procedure
lotus position
Lougheed-White coccygectomy
Louis
    L. angle
    L. mastopexy
Louis-Bar syndrome
loupe magnification
low
    l. anterior resection (LAR)
    l. back pain
    l. central venous pressure anesthesia
    l. cervical approach
    l. cervical cesarean section
    l. dose rate (LDR)
    l. dose rate radiation therapy
    l. intermittent suction (LIS)
    l. lip line
    l. lumbar spine fracture
    l. rectal cancer
    l. spinal anesthesia
    l. spousal solicitude
    l. thoracic level epidural anesthesia
    l. transverse cesarean section
    l. transverse incision
low-attenuation
    l.-a. lesion
    l.-a. mass
low-collar incision
low-current
    l.-c. electrocautery
    l.-c. monopolar coagulation
low-density mass
low-dose
    l.-d. anesthetic
    l.-d. irradiation
    l.-d. radioiodine
Lowell reduction
Löwenberg canal
low-energy fracture

lower
    l. body negative pressure
    l. cervical spine fusion
    l. cervical spine posterior
      stabilization
    l. cervical spine procedure
    l. esophageal sphincter (LES)
    l. esophageal sphincter pressure
    l. esophageal sphincter pressure
      measurement
    l. esophageal sphincter relaxation
      (LESR)
    l. extremity
    l. extremity bypass
    l. extremity edema
    l. extremity fracture
    l. extremity nerve block
    l. extremity noninvasive
    l. extremity occlusive disease
    l. extremity reconstruction
    l. extremity revascularization
    l. extremity surgery
    l. extremity vascular occlusive
      disease
    l. gastrointestinal hemorrhage
    l. gastrointestinal tract foreign body
    l. genital tract infection
    l. incisor angulation
    l. jaw bone
    l. lateral quadrant
    l. lid sling procedure
    l. limb ischemia
    l. medial quadrant
    l. midclavicular line
    l. motor neuron lesion
    l. nephron syndrome
    l. panendoscopy
    l. plexus compression
    l. pole laceration
    l. quadrant abdominal incisional
      hernia
    l. respiratory tract infection
    l. thyroid artery
    l. trapezius flap
    l. uterine segment (LUS)
    l. uterine segment incision
    l. uterine segment transverse
      (LUST)
    l. uterine segment transverse
      cesarean section
    l. uterine segment transverse
      C-section
lowest
    l. lumbar artery
    l. thyroid artery
low-field contrast-enhanced body MRA
low-flow
    l.-f. anesthetic technique
    l.-f. circuit

low-flux
low-frequency
>l.-f. jet ventilation
>l.-f. TENS

low-grade
>l.-g. dysplasia
>l.-g. glioma
>l.-g. MALT lymphoma
>l.-g. squamous intraepithelial lesion (LSIL)
>l.-g. stricture
>l.-g. suction unit

low-loop cutaneous ureterostomy
low-molecular weight heparin (LMWH)
Lown
>L. arrhythmia classification
>L. cardioverter technique

low-pressure
>l.-p. circuit leak test
>l.-p. headache
>l.-p. tamponade

low-prime circuit
low-resistance fundoplication
low-risk
>l.-r. papillary cancer
>l.-r. patient

low-segment transverse incision
Lowsley
>L. lobar anatomy
>L. ribbon gut method

low-speed rotational angioplasty
LPHR
>laparoscopic paraesophageal hernia repair

LRD
>living-related donor

LRLT
>living-related liver transplant

LRPH
>laparoscopic repair of paraesophageal hernia

LRRFS
>locoregional recurrence-free survival

LS
>lumbosacral

LSB
>lumbar sympathetic block

LSC
>laparoscopy

LSG
>lymphoscintigraphy
>preoperative LSG

L-shaped capsular incision
LSIL
>low-grade squamous intraepithelial lesion

LTA
>laryngotracheal anesthesia

LTCBDE
>laparoscopic transcystic common bile duct exploration

LTCL
>laparoscopic transcystic lithotripsy

LTH
>lingual tonsil hyperplasia

LTR
>local twitch response

lubrication
>skin l.

Lucas groove
lucent lung lesion
lucidum
>*Ganoderma l.*

lückenschädel
Ludloff
>L. bunionectomy
>L. congenital hip dislocation repair technique
>L. incision
>L. medial open reduction hip approach
>L. osteotomy

Ludwig
>L. angle
>L. ganglion
>L. labyrinth

LUE
>left upper extremity

Lukens catgut suture
Lukes and Butler Hodgkin disease classification
Lukes-Collins lymphoma classification
lumbar
>l. accessory movement technique
>l. anesthetic technique
>l. approach
>l. artery
>l. branch
>l. canal
>l. catheter
>l. cistern
>l. discectomy
>l. disc herniation
>l. discogenic pain
>l. epidural abscess
>l. epidural anesthesia (LEA)
>l. epidural catheter
>l. epidural endoscopy
>l. epidural steroid
>l. epidural steroid injection (LESI)
>l. extension
>l. extension test
>l. facet injection
>l. facet joint innervation
>l. flexure
>l. ganglion
>l. gravitational line

L

lumbar (*continued*)
   l. hemilaminectomy
   l. hernia
   l. interbody fusion
   l. lordosis preservation
   l. nephrectomy
   l. nerve (L1–L5)
   l. nerve root injection
   l. pain
   l. pedicle fixation
   l. plexus
   l. plexus block
   l. port
   l. puncture (LP)
   l. region
   l. rib
   l. rotation
   l. rotation test
   l. segment
   l. spinal cord lesion
   l. spinal fusion
   l. spine biopsy
   l. spine burst fracture
   l. spine fusion
   l. spine kyphotic deformity
   l. spine lesion
   l. spine segmental fixation
   l. spine stabilization
   l. spine transpedicular fixation
   l. spine vertebral osteosynthesis
   l. spondylodiscitis
   l. sympathectomy
   l. sympathetic block (LSB)
   l. transforaminal approach
   l. triangle
   l. triangle of Petit
   l. trunk
   l. tumor
   l. vein
   l. vertebra
   l. vertebral interbody fusion
   l. vessel
lumbarization
lumbar-peritoneal shunt
lumbi (*pl. of* lumbus)
lumboabdominal
lumbocolostomy
lumbocolotomy
lumbocostal ligament
lumbocostoabdominal triangle
lumbodorsal fascia
lumboinguinal nerve
lumboovarian
lumbosacral
   l. angle
   l. canal
   l. dislocation
   l. fusion
   l. joint

   l. junction fracture
   l. plexus
   l. plexus lesion
   l. radiculopathy
   l. root lesion
   l. trunk
lumbrical muscle flap
lumbus, *pl.* **lumbi**
lumen, *pl.* **lumina, lumens**
   bile duct l.
   gut l.
   irregularly widened l.
   jejunal l.
lumens (*pl. of* lumen)
lumina (*pl. of* lumen)
luminal
   l. contents
   l. mass
   l. side
lumpectomy
   endoscopic aspiration l.
   l. mastectomy
LUNA
   laparoscopic uterine nerve ablation
   laparoscopic uterosacral nerve ablation
   laser LUNA
lunate
   l. bone
   l. dislocation
lunchtime facelift
lung
   l. biopsy
   breathing l.
   l. cancer
   l. carcinoma
   l. cavity
   l. contusion
   l. disease
   essential brown induration of l.
   l. expansion
   fixed l.
   human l.
   inflated l.
   l. isolation
   Kolobow membrane l.
   membrane artificial l.
   nonventilated l.
   oblique fissure of l.
   pump l.
   l. rejection
   l. resection
   respirator l.
   shock l.
   stiff l.
   l. to head circumference
     ratio
   l. transplant
   trapped l.
   l. tumor

l. volume
l. volume reduction (LVR)
l. volume reduction procedure
l. volume reduction surgery
l. water
wet l.

1-lung
1-l. anesthesia
1-l. ventilation (OLV)
1-l. ventilation anesthetic technique
lung-imaging fluorescent endoscopy
lung-to-head circumference
2-lung ventilation
lunotriquetral
l. dissociation
l. fusion
lunula, *pl.* **lunulae**
azure l.
lunulae (*pl. of* lunula)
LUPP
laser uvulopalatoplasty
lupus
l. anticoagulant
l. nephritis
systemic l.
lupus-associated valve disease
LUQ
left upper quadrant
Luque
L. instrumentation concave technique
L. instrumentation convex technique
L. loop fixation
L. rod fixation
L. sublaminar wiring technique
Luque-Galveston fixation
Luria-Delbruck fluctuation test
LUS
laparoscopic ultrasonography
laparoscopic ultrasound
LUS examination
LUS scanning technique
Lusardi iridectomy
Luschka
L. cartilage
duct of L.
L. foramen
fossa of L.
L. gland
L. joint
L. ligament
L. sinus
lusitropism
LUST
lower uterine segment transverse
LUST cesarean section
LUST C-section
luster
corneal l.
lustrous central yellow point

lutea
macula l.
luteal
luteinization
luteinized thecoma
luteinoma
luteolysis
luteoma
pregnancy l.
luteum
corpus l.
luxatio erecta shoulder dislocation
luxation
habitual temporomandibular joint l.
rotatory l.
temporomandibular l.
Luys
L. body
L. body syndrome
LVAD
left ventricular assist device
left ventricular assistive device
LVEDa
left ventricular end-diastolic area
LVESa
left ventricular end-systolic area
LVOT
left ventricular outflow tract
LVPVR
left ventricular pressure-volume relationship
LVR
lung volume reduction
LVR procedure
LVRS
lung volume reduction surgery
Lyden real-time cerebral angiography technique
Lyme arthritis
lymph
l. gland
l. massage
l. nodal station
l. node basin
l. node biopsy
l. node dissection
l. node involvement
l. node metastasis
l. node sampling
l. node stage
l. node status
l. space
tissue l.
l. vessel
l. vessel invasion
lymphadenectomy
axillary l.
bilateral l.
D2 l.

L

lymphadenectomy (*continued*)
    elective l.
    endocavitary pelvic l.
    (ECPL)
    extended pelvic l.
    2-field l.
    3-field l.
    field l.
    inguinal l.
    Japanese-style l.
    Japanese-style D2 l.
    laparoscopic pelvic l.
    laparoscopic retroperitoneal l.
    (RPLND)
    mediastinal l.
    Meigs pelvic l.
    paraaortic l.
    pelvic l.
    pelvic-iliac l.
    prophylactic l.
    regional l.
    retroperitoneal l.
    selective l.
    sentinel l.
    thoracoabdominal
      retroperitoneal l.
    three-field l.
lymphadenocele
lymphadenoma
lymphadenopathy
    angioblastic l.
    angioimmunoblastic l.
    axillary l.
    cervical l.
    en bloc l.
    portal l.
lymphadenotomy
lymphangiectasia (*var. of*
  lymphangiectasis)
lymphangiectasis, lymphangiectasia
lymphangiectomy
lymphangioendothelioma
lymphangiogenesis
lymphangiography
lymphangiohemangioma
lymphangioleiomyomatosis
    pulmonary l.
lymphangioma
    cystic l.
    ileal small-bowel l.
lymphangiomyomatosis
    end-stage l.
    pulmonary l.
lymphangioplasty
    Handley l.
lymphangiosarcoma
lymphangiotomy
lymphatic
    l. canal

l. chain
l. channel
dermal l.'s
l. dissection
l. drainage
l. drainage pattern
l. duct
l. edema
extrinsic network
  of l.'s
l. invasion
l. malformation
l. mapping
l. metastasis
l. microvessel density
parenchymal l.
l. pathway
l. permeation
l. plexus
l. spread
l. system
l. tissue
l. uptake
l. valvule
l. vessel
lymphaticostomy
lymphaticovenous
    l. anastomosis
    l. bypass
lymphatolysis
lymphedema
    heart rate l.
    l. praecox
    true l.
    upper extremity l.
lymphoadenoma
**lymphoblastoid cell
line**
lymphocelectomy
    laparoscopic l.
    pelvic l.
lymphocele drainage
lymphocyte
    l. cell
    l. migration
    phenotypic l.
lymphocytic
    l. arteritis
    l. infiltration
lymphocytoma
lymphodepletion
lymphoepithelial lesion
lymphoepithelioma
lymphogenous metastasis
lymphogranuloma
lymphoid
    l. infiltration
    l. ring
    l. tissue

lymphoidectomy
lymphoma
>Ann Arbor Hodgkin l. (stage I, IE, II, IIE, IIIE, IIIS, IIISE, IV)
gastric MALT l.
gastric non-Hodgkin l.
high-grade MALT l.
low-grade MALT l.
MALT l.
mucosa-associated lymphoid tissue l.
node l.
primary gastric l. (PGL)
primary gastric non-Hodgkin l.
l. relapse
l. system

lymphomatosa
>struma l.

lymphomyeloma
lymphoplasty
lymphoproliferation
lymphoproliferative
>l. disorder
l. lesion

lymphorrhagia (*var. of* lymphorrhea)
lymphorrhea, lymphorrhagia
lymphosarcoma
lymphoscintigraphy
>internal mammary l. (IML)
isotopic l.
preoperative l.
radioactive colloid l.

lymphovascular invasion
Lynch
>L. frontoethmoidectomy procedure
L. incision

L. supravalvular stenosing ring of left atrium operation
>L. syndrome

Lynn Achilles tendon rupture repair technique
lyophilization of bone
lyophilized
>l. bone graft
l. dural patch
l. extract

Lyrica
lysate
>melanoma cell l.

lyse
Lysholm
>L. Knee Scale
L. score

lysis
>adhesion l.
direct muscle l.
endothelial l.
muscle l.
l. of adhesions

lysogenic
>l. induction
l. strain

lysosomal
>l. enzyme disorder
l. membrane
l. storage disease
l. swelling

lytic
>l. blockade
l. bone lesion
l. cocktail
l. nerve block

L

MABP
    mean arterial blood pressure
1-MAC
    1-minimum alveolar concentration
        1-MAC halothane
MAC
    minimal alveolar concentration
    minimal anesthetic concentration
    minimum alveolar concentration
    monitored anesthesia care
    monitored anesthesia control
    Mycobacterium avium complex
        MAC anesthesia
        MAC infection
        MAC ratio
        MAC stitch
MaC
    massive cuff
MacAndrew Alcoholism Scale
MacCallan trachoma classification
**MacCarthy sacral tumor excision of
    sacrum procedure**
maceration
Macewen
        M. avascular necrosis classification
        M. hernia operation
        M. herniorrhaphy
        M. triangle
Macewen-Shands osteotomy
MacFee incision
**Machek-Blaskovics eyelid entropion
    operation**
Machek-Brunswick operation
Machek-Gifford operation
Machek ptosis operation
machine
        closed-circuit anesthesia m.
        field anesthesia m.
machine-triggered breath
Mach line
MacIntosh
        M. extraarticular tenodesis
        M. laryngoscopy technique
        M. over-the-top ACL
            reconstruction
        M. over-the-top repair
MACIS
    metastasis, age, completeness of
    resection, local invasion, tumor size
        MACIS criteria
        MACIS score
Mack-Brunswick operation
Mackenrodt
        M. incision
        M. ligament

Mackenzie point
MacNab
        M. line
        M. line for facet imbrication
        M. patella operation
        M. shoulder repair
**MacNicol-Voutsinas posterior tibial tear
    classification**
macroadenoma
macrocalcification
macrochimerism
macrocirculation
macrocirculatory parameter
macrocolon
macrocyst
        multiple m.
macrocytic anemia
macroelectrode
        m. recording
        m. recording technique
macrofollicular lesion
macroglossia, megaloglossia
macronodular
macronutrient
macroorchidism
macropenis
macroperforation
macrophage
        peritoneal m.
macrophagic migration
macrophallus
macroprolactinoma
macroprosopia
macroscopic
        m. appearance
        m. evidence
        m. exploration
        m. involvement
        m. IPM
        m. lesion
        m. portal
        m. sphincter
        m. tumor removal
        m. type
macrosigmoid
macrotraumatic insult
macrovascular coronary lesion
macula, *pl.* **maculae**
        m. lutea
        retinal m.
maculae (*pl. of* macula)
macular, maculate
        m. ectopia
        m. photocoagulation
maculate (*var. of* macular)

M

macule
    hypomelanotic m.
maculopapillary bundle
maculopathy
Madden
    M. hernia repair
    M. incisional herniorrhaphy
    M. modified radical mastectomy
        technique
    M. repair of incisional hernia
Maddox
    M. rod test
    M. wing test
Madelung deformity
Madigan prostatectomy
Madlener operation
maduromycetoma
Maffucci syndrome
Magendie
    M. foramen
    M. space
Magenstrasse
    M. and Mill (M&M)
    M. and Mill antiobesity procedure
Magerl
    M. posterior cervical screw fixation
    M. translaminar facet screw fixation
        technique
maggot
    surgical m.
Magilligan femoral anteversion
 measuring technique
Magill-tip endotracheal tube
Magitot keratoplasty
magna
    cisterna m.
magnet
    m. operation
    m. therapy
magnetic
    m. control suturing
    m. extraction
    m. imaging guidance
    m. induction
    m. operation
    m. resonance (MR)
    m. resonance angiography (MRA)
    m. resonance
        cholangiopancreatography (MRCP)
    m. resonance imaging (MRI)
    m. resonance imaging
        cholangiography
    m. resonance imaging scan
    m. resonance spectroscopy
    m. seizure therapy
    m. source imaging
    m. stimulation
 magnetization precession angle
magnetoelectric stimulation

magnetoencephalography
magnification
    electronic m.
    loupe m.
    relative spectacle m.
    spot m.
magnitude matching procedure
magnum
    foramen m.
magnus
    adductor m.
Magnuson anterior dislocation of
 shoulder repair technique
Magnuson-Stack
    M.-S. shoulder arthroplasty
    M.-S. shoulder arthrotomy
    M.-S. shoulder procedure
MAGPI
    meatal advancement and glansplasty
    meatal advancement, glansplasty,
        penoscrotal junction meatotomy
    MAGPI hypospadias repair
    MAGPI operation
Ma-Griffith
    M.-G. Achilles tendon rupture repair
        technique
    M.-G. tendo calcaneus repair
Mahaim bundle
Mahan pediatric sedation
 procedure
Mahurkar catheter
MAI
    Mycobacterium avium-intracellulare
    MAI infection
Maier sinus
maim
main
    m. bundle
    m. pancreatic duct
mainstem intubation
maintainer cast space
maintenance
    m. dialysis
    m. fluid
    insufficient airway m.
Mainz
    M. I, II pouch continent urinary
        diversion
    M. neobladder
    M. pouch augmentation
    M. pouch cutaneous urinary
        diversion
Maisonneuve fibular fracture
Maissiat band
Maitland manual spinal therapy
 technique
Majestro-Ruda-Frost tendon
 technique
Majewsky operation

major

m. abdominal surgery
m. amputation
m. artery
m. calix
m. depression
m. duodenal papilla
m. fissure
m. histocompatibility complex (MHC)
m. liver resection (MLR)
m. manifestation
m. myocutaneous flap
m. nonvascular abdominal surgery
m. operation
m. sinistral branch
teres m.
teres m. (muscle)
trochanter m.
m. vascular injury
m. vascular structure

majus

labium m.

Makler insemination
malabsorptive procedure
Malacarne space
malacotomy
maladie de Graeffe operation
malar

m. fat pad
m. fold
m. foramen
m. fracture
m. node
m. periosteum-SMAS flap fixation suture

Malawer excision technique
Malbec abdominal lipectomy
Malbran retinal detachment operation
maldistribution
male

m. breast
m. castration
m. gonad
m. urethra

malformation

angel's kiss m.
angiographically occult intracranial vascular m. (AOIVM)
anorectal m.
Arnold-Chiari m.
arteriovenous m. (AVM)
atrioventricular m.
AV m.
Bing-Siebenmann m.
brain arteriovenous m.
bronchopulmonary foregut m.
capillary m.
cardiac valvular m.

cardiovascular m.
cavernous m.
central nervous system m.
cerebral arteriovenous m.
cerebral vascular m.
cerebrovascular m.
Chiari I—III m.
cloacal m.
clomiphene fetal m.
congenital brain m.
congenital cystic adenomatoid m. (CCAM)
congenital heart m.
congenital pulmonary airway m.
congenital vascular m.
craniofacial m.
cutaneous m.
cystic adenomatoid m. (CAM)
Dandy-Walker m.
DeMyer system of cerebral m.
Dieulafoy vascular m.
dural arteriovenous m.
dysraphic m.
Ebstein m.
extremity m.
faciotelencephalic m.
fetal cystic adenomatoid m.
flocculonodular arteriovenous m.
foregut m.
frontal arteriovenous m.
frontoparietal arteriovenous m.
galenic venous m.
gastric arteriovenous m.
glomus arteriovenous m.
infratentorial arteriovenous m.
intracerebral arteriovenous m.
intracerebral vascular m.
intracranial arteriovenous m.
intracranial vascular m.
intramedullary arteriovenous m.
intramuscular venous m.
lymphatic m.
mermaid m.
Michel m.
mixed venous-lymphatic m.
Mondini-Alexander m.
Mondini pulmonary arteriovenous m.
neural axis vascular m.
neural crest m.
occipital m.
occult cerebrovascular m.
occult vascular m.
orbital arteriovenous m.
pancreatobiliary m.
pulmonary arterial m.
pulmonary arteriovenous m.
radiculomeningeal spinal vascular m.
retinal arteriovenous m.
Scheibe m.

M

malformation (*continued*)
    sink-trap m.
    spinal vascular m.
    split-cord m.
    supratentorial arteriovenous m.
    telangiectatic vascular m.
    telencephalic m.
    teratogen-induced m.
    thalamocaudate arteriovenous m.
    Uhl m.
    vascular m.
    vein of Galen m.
    venous m.
malfunction
    cuff m.
    pacemaker m.
Malgaigne
    M. fossa
    M. hernia
    M. pelvic fracture
    M. triangle
malignancy
    abdominal m.
    digestive tract m.
    gastric m.
    gastrointestinal m.
    gynecologic m.
    hepatic m.
    hereditary m.
    metastatic m.
    nonhereditary m.
    pancreatic m.
    primary m.
malignant
    m. adenoma
    m. angiomyolipoma
    m. carcinoid syndrome
    m. cell
    m. degeneration
    m. etiology
    m. external otitis syndrome
    m. fasciculation
    m. glioma
    m. hyperpyrexia
    m. hypertension
    m. hyperthermia
    m. hyperthermia protocol
    m. neoplastic disease
    m. pain
    m. pancreatic disease
    m. pituitary lesion
    m. process
    m. reading
    m. renal mass
    m. synovioma
    m. transformation
    m. tumor
    m. tumor classification
malignant-appearing microcalcification

malingering questionnaire
malinterdigitation
Mallampati pharyngeal visibility classification
Mallard incision
mallear
    m. fold
    m. ligament
    m. process
    m. prominence
mallei (*pl. of* malleus)
malleoincudal
malleolar
    m. fracture
    m. osteotomy
malleoli (*pl. of* malleolus)
malleolus, *pl.* **malleoli**
    lateral m.
    medial m.
mallet
    m. finger
    m. finger deformity
    m. fracture
    m. toe
    m. toe deformity
malleus, *pl.* **mallei**
Mallory-Weiss
    M.-W. lesion
    M.-W. mucosal rupture
    M.-W. syndrome
    M.-W. tear
    M.-W. tear repair procedure
Malnutrition Universal Screening Tool
malocclusion
    Ackerman-Proffitt classification of m.
Malone
    M. ACE procedure
    M. antegrade continence enema procedure
malpighian
    m. body
    m. pyramid
    m. stigma
malposition
    catheter m.
    extension m.
    strut m.
    tube m.
malpositioning
malpresentation
    fetal m.
malrelation
malrotation
    intestinal m.
    renal m.
MALT
    mucosa-associated lymphoid tissue
    MALT lymphoma
MALToma

malunion
    humeral fracture m.
malunited
    m. calcaneus fracture
    m. forearm fracture
    m. radial fracture
mamillary (*var. of* mammillary)
    m. body
    m. duct
    m. line
    m. process
    m. tubercle
mamillothalamic tract
mamma, *pl.* **mammae**
mammae (*pl. of* mamma)
mammalian cell membrane
mammaplasty, mammoplasty, mastoplasty
    Aries-Pitanguy m.
    augmentation m.
    belly button augmentation m.
    postreduction m.
    reconstructive m.
    reduction m.
    Wise pattern m.
mammary
    m. atrophy
    m. branch
    m. duct
    m. duct ectasia
    m. fistula
    m. gland
    m. line
    m. node
    m. node biopsy
    m. plexus
    m. region
    m. tissue
mammectomy
mammilla
mammillaplasty
mammillare (*var. of* mammillary)
mammillary, mamillary, mammillare
mammogram
    abnormal m.
mammographer
mammographic
    m. abnormality
    m. appearance
    m. evaluation
    m. finding
    m. lesion
    m. malignant-appearing
      microcalcification
    m. presentation
mammography
    digital m.
    screening m.
mammoplasty (*var. of* mammaplasty)
mammotomy

management
    airway m.
    alpha-stat blood gas m.
    anesthetic m.
    anesthetic and fluid m.
    aneurysm m.
    Aneurysm Detection and M.
      (ADAM)
    emergency airway m.
    endoscopic m.
    expectant m.
    fluid m.
    foreign body m.
    interdisciplinary pain m.
    intraoperative fluid m.
    laparoscopic m.
    locoregional m.
    mechanical endoscopic m.
    medical m.
    multidisciplinary pain m.
    nonoperative m.
    nonsurgical m.
    obstetric m.
    m. of anesthesia
    operative m.
    optimal intensive medical m.
    pain m.
    perioperative m.
    postblock m.
    postoperative m.
    renal m.
    risk m.
    selective nonoperative m.
    m. strategy
    stricture m.
    surgical m.
    ventilator m.
Manchester-Fothergill uterine suspension
Manchester prolapsed uterus cervical
  amputation
mandatory
    m. celiotomy
    m. laparoscopy
Mandelbaum-Nartolozzi-Carney patellar
  tendon repair
mandible
    ramus of m.
mandibula, mandibulum, *pl.* **mandibulae**
mandibulae (*pl. of* mandibula)
mandibular
    m. articulation
    m. body fracture
    m. canal
    m. cartilage
    m. centric relation
    m. condyle
    m. condylectomy
    m. condyle fracture
    m. disc

M

mandibular (*continued*)
    m. dislocation
    m. equilibration
    m. excess
    m. fixation
    m. foramen
    m. fossa
    m. head
    m. hinge position
    m. incisor angle
    m. joint
    m. nerve
    m. nerve block
    m. node
    m. notch
    m. osteotomy advancement
    m. plane
    m. plane angle
    m. ramus fracture
    m. ramus osteotomy
    m. reconstruction
    m. rest position
    m. space
    m. surgery
    m. swing operation
    m. swing technique
    m. symphysis
    m. symphysis fracture
    m. tongue
mandibulectomy
    rim m.
    segmental m.
mandibulofacial dysotosis syndrome
mandibulomaxillary fixation (MMF)
mandibulopharyngeal
mandibulotomy
mandibulum (*var. of* mandibula)
mandrel graft
maneuver
    Adson thoracic outlet m.
    Aird pancreas exploration m.
    Allen scalenous anterior syndrome m.
    Allis hip dislocation m.
    alpha-loop m.
    Apley torn meniscus m.
    arch m.
    avoidance m.
    Barlow developmental hip dysplasia m.
    Bielschowsky vertical strabismus m.
    Bigelow posterior hip dislocation m.
    bunching m.
    BURP m.
    Buzzard patellar reflex m.
    Cairns m.
    Carlo Traverso post-trabeculectomy m.
    circumduction m.

closed manipulative m.
cold pressor testing m.
corkscrew m.
costoclavicular m.
Dandy cerebrospinal fluid leak m.
décollement m.
DeLee fetal positioning m.
Dix-Hallpike benign positional vertigo m.
doll's eye m.
doll's head m.
Ejrup collateral circulation m.
Epley benign positional vertigo m.
Finkelstein tendinitis m.
flexion-extension m.
forceps m.
Fowler-Stephens spermatic vessel ligation m.
Frenzel middle ear pressure m.
grunting m.
Halsted thoracic outlet m.
Hampton air-contrast radiograph m.
Heaney total vascular isolation m.
heel-to-ear m.
hemodynamic m.
Hillis-Müller m.
Hippocratic anterior shoulder reduction m.
Hoguet hernial sac conversion m.
Hubscher adult flatfoot m.
Hueter stomach tube introduction m.
hyperventilation m.
Jahss metacarpal neck fracture reduction m.
jaw thrust m.
Jendrassik reflex amplification m.
J-type m.
jugular compression m.
key-in-lock m.
Ko-Airan cystic artery hemostasis m.
Kocher lateral peritoneal attachment dissection m.
Krackow obese patient tourniquet m.
Lachman knee ligament tear m.
laparoscopic pirouette m.
Leadbetter hip reduction m.
Lecompte arterial switch m.
Levret breech delivery m.
liver hanging m.
logrolling m.
Martin m.
Massini m.
Mattox descending colon mobilization m.
McKenzie extension m.
McMurray circumduction m.
Mendelsohn dysphagia m.
meticulous m.

midforceps m.
modified Ritgen fetal head
delivery m.
Mueller fiberoptic nasal
endoscopy m.
Müller esophageal varices m.
Müller-Hillis 2nd stage labor m.
notch-and-roll m.
Nylen-Barany benign positional
vertigo m.
oculocephalic m.
Ortolani hip developmental
dysplasia m.
osteoclasis m.
Pajot forceps delivery m.
peroral m.
Phalen carpal tunnel m.
Pinard breech extraction m.
postural fixation back m.
Prague breech delivery m.
Prentiss cryptorchidism repair m.
Pringle liver hemorrhage m.
Proetz nasal irrigation m.
pull m.
push m.
recruiting m.
recruitment m.
reexpansion m.
relative response attributable to the
m. (RRAM)
reverse Bigelow m.
Ritgen fetal head delivery m.
rotation-compression m.
Rubin shoulder dystocia m.
Saxtorph forceps delivery m.
scalene m.
Scanzoni forceps delivery m.
Scanzoni-Smellie forceps delivery m.
scarf m.
Schatz fetal position m.
Schreiber patellar reflex m.
Sellick endotracheal intubation m.
Semont benign positional vertigo m.
shoeshine m.
Slocum knee rotatory instability m.
Spurling cervical foraminal
compression m.
squat m.
Steel m.
Stimson posterior hip dislocation
reduction m.
straightening m.
surgical m.
therapeutic m.
Thorn fetal position m.
U-turn m.
Valsalva m.
van Hoorn delivery m.
wall push m.

Wigand fetal position m.
Witzel decompression of Roux-en-Y
loop m.
Woods screw fetal position m.
Wright m.

mangled
m. extremity severity score (MESS)
m. extremity syndrome

mania

manifestation
allergic m.
articular m.
cardiopulmonary m.
central nervous system m.
clinical m.
cutaneous m.
digestive m.
hepatobiliary m.
initial m.
major m.
minor m.
mucocutaneous m.
neurologic m.
neuroophthalmic m.
ocular m.
oral m.
otolaryngologic m.
phenotypic m.
presenting clinical m.
pulmonary m.
renal m.
vascular m.

manikin
Pain Relief M.

manipulation
bile duct m.
catheter m.
cervical m.
connective tissue m.
contact m.
cranial nerve m.
digital m.
direct m.
fine m.
gamete m.
general thrust m.
gross m.
guide wire m.
Hippocrates m.
indirect m.
joint m.
laparoscopic dissection and m.
laser m.
Leadbetter hip m.
long- and short-lever rotational m.
myofascial m.
noncontact m.
opening wedge m.
optimal external laryngeal m.

M

manipulation (*continued*)
    pancreatic duct m.
    passive joint m.
    pharmacologic m.
    physical m.
    postureteroscopic m.
    shunt m.
    specific thrust m.
    spinal m. (SM)
    thrust m.
manipulation-induced PGID injury
manipulative therapy
Mankin knee resection
Manktelow transfer procedure
Mann-Bollman fistula
Mann-Coughlin-DuVries cheilectomy
Mann-Coughlin hallux valgus repair procedure
Mann-DuVries arthroplasty
Mann hallux valgus repair procedure
Mannheim peritonitis index
Mannis suture
mannitol
Mann-Williamson experimental peptic ulcer operation
manometer
    saline m.
manometric
    m. data
    m. evaluation
    m. finding
    m. recording session
    m. study
    m. technique
manometry
    anal m.
    anorectal m.
    esophageal m.
    jejunal m.
    laparoscopic transcystic sphincter of Oddi m.
    stationary m.
Mansfield Valvuloplasty Registry
Manske-McCarroll opponensplasty
Manske-McCarroll-Swanson centralization
Manske radioulnar osteoclasis technique
mantle irradiation
MANTRELS
    migration (of pain to RLQ), anorexia, nausea and vomiting, tenderness (in RLQ), rebound pain, elevated temperature, leukocytosis, shift (WBC to left)
manual
    m. endoscopic reduction
    m. extraction
    m. massage
    m. medicine

    m. method
    m. pressure
    m. push-pull technique
    m. rotation
    m. therapy
    m. ventilation
manubria (*pl. of* manubrium)
manubriosternal
    m. joint
    m. junction
    m. symphysis
manubrium, *pl.* **manubria**
MAP
    mean arterial pressure
maple leaf flap
Mapleson-type ventilating system
maplike skull
mapping
    activation-sequence m.
    advanced cardiac m.
    atrial activation m.
    body surface laplacian m.
    breast lymphatic m.
    catheter m.
    dermatomal m.
    dermatome m.
    duplex arterial m.
    endocardial m.
    intraoperative lymphatic m.
    isosulfan blue-dye m.
    lymphatic m.
    neural m.
    retrograde atrial activation m.
    sentinel lymph node m.
    SLN m.
Maquet
    M. dome osteotomy
    M. patellar realignment procedure
Maragiliano body
marantic clot
marbleization
Marcacci muscle
Marchand adrenal
march fracture
Marchi tract
Marcille triangle
Marckwald cervical os repair
Marcove-Lewis-Huvos shoulder girdle resection
Marcus Gunn phenomenon
Marcus-Balourdas-Heiple ankle fusion technique
Marcy
    M. hernia repair
    M. inguinal hernia operation
mare's tail line
Marfan syndrome

margin
    carious restoration m.
    cavity m.
    close m.
    costal m.
    dentate m.
    dissection m.
    falciform m.
    free gastric m.
    m.'s free of tumor
    frontal m.
    gastric m.
    hepatic m.
    interosseous m.
    m. invasion
    lacrimal m.
    lambdoid m.
    mastoid m.
    mesovarian m.
    negative m.
    obtuse m.
    occipital m.
    parietal m.
    positive resection m.
    positive surgical m.
    psoas m.
    pupillary m.
    resection m.
    m. resection
    m. resection involvement
    squamous m.
    superior m.
    supraorbital m.
    surgical m.
    tumor-free m.
    m.'s with tumor

marginal
    m. artery
    m. excess
    m. excision
    m. incision
    m. insertion
    m. mandibular branch
    m. myotomy
    m. resection
    m. ridge fracture
    m. sinus rupture
    m. sphincter
    m. tentorial branch
    m. tubercle
    m. ulceration

margination
    lesion m.
    leukocytic m.

margines (*pl. of* margo)
marginoplasty
margo, *pl.* **margines**
marian lithotomy
marihuana (*var. of* marijuana)

marijuana, marihuana
    medical m.
Marin Amat syndrome
Marion disease
Marion-Moschcowitz culdoplasty
mark
    ecchymotic m.
    port-wine m.
    tape m.
marked
    m. ascites
    m. tenderness
marker
    biologic m.
    blood m.
    genetic m.
    histologic m.
    immunohistochemical m.
    prognostic m.
    m. stitch
    tumor m.
    viral m.
Marks-Bayne technique for thumb duplication
Marlex
    M. band
    M. closure
    M. hernia repair
    M. mesh
    M. plug technique
    M. suture
Marquardt angulation osteotomy
Marquez-Gomez
    M.-G. conjunctival graft
    M.-G. operation
marrow
    m. ablation
    allogenic bone m.
    m. cavity
    m. graft rejection
    m. space
    spinal m.
Marseille pancreatitis classification
Marshall
    M. bladder neck test
    M. ligament repair technique
    M. oblique vein
Marshall-Marchetti urinary incontinence test
Marshall-Marchetti-Krantz
    M.-M.-K. operation
    M.-M.-K. retropubic cystourethrography suspension procedure
    M.-M.-K. urethrocystopexy
Marshall-McIntosh ACL repair technique
Marshall-Taylor vacuum extraction

M

marsupialization

    renal cyst m.
    Spence and Duckett m.
    m. technique
    transurethral m.

Martin

    M. anoplasty
    M. incision
    M. maneuver
    M. modification
    M. osteotomy
    M. patellar wiring technique
    M. reduction technique

Martin-Gruber anastomosis

Martius

    M. bulbocavernosus fat flap
    M. labial fat flap urinary fistula
      repair procedure

masculina

    vagina m.

masculine

    m. pelvis
    m. uterus

masculinization

    ovarian m.

masculinizing genitoplasty

masculinovoblastoma

mask

    ecchymotic m.
    laryngeal m.
    m. leak
    m. ventilation

masking technique

Mason

    M. incision
    M. morbid obesity vertical banded
      gastroplasty
    M. radial head fracture classification
    M. vertical banded gastroplasty

Mason-Likar limb lead modification

masquerade technique

mass

    abdominal wall m.
    abdominopelvic m.
    acellular m.
    adnexal m.
    adrenal cystic m.
    anterior mediastinal m.
    appendiceal m.
    apperceptive m.
    asymptomatic m.
    atomic m.
    benign m.
    body cell m.
    bone m.
    bony m.
    brain m.
    calcified renal m.
    carbon gelatin m.

cardiac m.
cardiophrenic angle m.
cicatricial m.
circumscribed m.
colonic m.
complex chest m.
m. concentration
congenital nasal m.
congenital renal m.
conglomerate m.
cortical m.
critical m.
cul-de-sac m.
cystic m.
m. defect
dense brain m.
discrete m.
dominant m.
doughy m.
dumbbell m.
duodenal m.
dysplasia-associated m.
echodense m.
erythrocyte m.
esophageal m.
m. excision
exophytic gut m.
expansile abdominal m.
extracardiac m.
extracellular m.
extramedullary m.
extramucosal m.
extrarenal m.
extrauterine pelvic m.
extravascular m.
extrinsic m.
fallopian tube m.
fat-free m. (FFM)
filar m.
firm m.
flank m.
fluctuant m.
fungating m.
gastric m.
groin m.
hard m.
high-attenuation m.
hilar m.
hyaline m.
ill-defined m.
m. infection
infraauricular m.
injection m.
inner cell m.
intraabdominal m.
intracardiac m.
intracranial m.
intradural extramedullary m.
intrasellar m.

intrathoracic m.
intravascular m.
intraventricular m.
intussuscepted m.
lacrimal m.
laminated acellular m.
lateral m.
lean body m.
m. lesion
limbus m.
liver mass
lobulated m.
low-attenuation m.
low-density m.
luminal m.
malignant renal m.
mediastinal high-attenuation m.
m. memory
mesenteric m.
mixed-density m.
molecular m.
mulberry-shaped m.
multiloculated renal m.
mushroom-shaped m.
mycelial m.
myocardial m.
neoplastic renal m.
noncalcified nodular m.
nonmobile m.
nonopaque intraluminal m.
ovarian m.
ovoid m.
oyster m.
palpable m.
parasellar m.
parovarian m.
pediatric m.
pelvic m.
periampullary m.
perirectal m.
perivascular m.
persistent ovarian m.
phlegmonous m.
plantar-hindfoot-midfoot bony m.
pleural m.
polypoid m.
posterior mediastinal m.
postmenopausal body m.
presacral m.
pulmonary m.
pulsatile m.
questionable m.
rectal m.
red blood cell m.
m. reflex
renal m.
retrobulbar m.
retrocardiac m.
retrosternal m.

rubbery m.
salivary m.
sclerotic cemental m.
scrotal m.
soft tissue m.
solitary pulmonary m.
m. spectrometer
m. spectrometry
stellate m.
submucosal m.
suprasellar m.
testicular m.
thymic m.
tooth m.
transformary m.
traumatic renal m.
tubular excretory m.
tumor m.
umbilical m.
uncinate process m.
unit of m.
uterine m.
vaginal m.
vascular renal m.
vertebral bone m.
well-defined m.

MASS
mitral valve prolapse, aortic anomalies, skeletal changes, skin changes
MASS syndrome

Massachusetts General Hospital (MGH)

massage
cardiac m.
connective tissue m.
deep tissue m.
external cardiac m.
hand m.
lymph m.
manual m.
nerve-point m.
prostatic m.
soft tissue m.
Swedish m.
m. therapy
trigger point m.

masse
reduction en m.

masseter
m. muscle
m. muscle flap
m. muscle rigidity
m. spasm
m. tendon

masseteric
m. artery
m. fascia
m. nerve
m. space
m. tuberosity

masseter-mandibular-pterygoid space
Massie sliding graft
Massini maneuver
massive
- m. ascites
- m. autotransfusion
- m. bowel resection
- m. bowel resection syndrome
- m. cuff (MaC)
- m. hemorrhage
- m. incisional hernioplasty
- m. lower gastrointestinal bleeding
- m. malignant infiltration
- m. pulmonary hemorrhagic edema
- m. ventral hernia

MAST
- Michigan Abuse Screening Test
- minimal access spine technology

mastadenoma
mastectomy
- areola-sparing m.
- Auchincloss modified radical m.
- axillary node dissection m.
- bilateral subcutaneous m.
- breast-sparing m.
- m. closure
- complete skin-sparing m.
- extended radical m.
- m. for gynecomastia
- Halsted radical m.
- m. incision
- lumpectomy m.
- McKissock m.
- McWhirter simple m.
- modified radical m.
- nipple-sparing m.
- partial m.
- Patey modified radical m.
- preventive m.
- prophylactic m.
- quadrantectomy m.
- radical m.
- segmental m.
- simple m.
- skin-sparing m.
- m. specimen
- 2-stage technique m.
- standard m.
- subcutaneous m.
- total m.
- transverse m.

master gland
mastication
- m. disorder
- m. muscle

masticator
- m. nerve
- m. space
- m. space infection

masticatory
- m. fat pad
- m. space

mastitis
- granulomatous m.
- periductal m.

mastoccipital
mastocytoma
mastoid
- m. antrum
- m. branch
- m. canaliculus
- m. cavity
- m. cell
- m. foramen
- m. fossa
- m. incision
- m. margin
- m. node
- m. notch
- m. obliteration operation
- m. process

mastoidea
- incisura m.

mastoidectomy
- modified radical m.
- radical m.
- simple m.
- tympanoplasty m.

mastopexy
- anchor m.
- areolar m.
- Benelli lollipop m.
- breast-lift m.
- circumareolar m.
- concentric m.
- crescent m.
- double-skin m.
- doughnut m.
- endoscopic m.
- full m.
- keyhole m.
- Keystone m.
- Lejour m.
- lollipop m.
- Louis m.
- modified m.
- periareolar m.
- pursestring m.
- reduction m.
- Regnault type B m.
- short scar technique of m.
- simple m.
- vertical m.
- Wise m.

mastoplasty
mastoscopic axillary lymph node dissection
mastotomy

Mast-Spieghel-Pappas long bone fracture classification
Matas
    M. aneurysmectomy
    M. endoaneurysmorrhaphy
Matchett-Brown hip arthroplasty
matching
    cross-modality m.
matchstick
    m. graft
    m. test
mater
    dura m.
    pia m.
material
    antithrombogenic m.
    colloid m.
    contrast m. (CM)
    m. failure break point
    hydatid m.
    nonabsorbable m.
    obstructive hydatid m.
    osteosynthetic m.
maternal
    m. abdominal pressure
    m. anesthesia
    m. birthing position
    m. deprivation syndrome
    m. fracture
    m. hydration
    m. infection
    m. rejection
    m. tissue
    m. venous
    m. venous blood
maternal-placental-fetal drug transfer
Mathews olecranon fracture classification
Mathieu
    M. hypospadias repair technique
    M. island onlay flap
Mathieu-Horton-Devine flip-flap
Mathieu-Righini hypospadias procedure
matricectomy (*var. of* matrixectomy)
matrices (*pl. of* matrix)
matrilineal
matrix, *pl.* **matrices**
    bilayered cellular m.
    bone m.
    m. calculus
    cartilage m.
    demineralized bone m. (DBM)
    distal nail m.
    extracellular m.
    germinal m.
    glomerular extracellular m.
    m. metalloprotease (MMP)
    m. metalloproteinase (MMP)
    nail m.

    proximal nail m.
    sterile m.
matrixectomy, matricectomy
    chemical m.
    partial m.
    phenol m.
    Steindler m.
    Winograd partial m.
    Zadik total m.
Matroc femoral head
Matta-Saucedo fixation
matted
    m. adhesion
    m. node
matter
    periaqueductal gray
        matter/periventricular gray m.
        (PAG/PVG)
    white m.
Matti-Russe
    M.-R. bone graft
    M.-R. scaphoid nonunion bone graft technique
Mattox descending colon mobilization maneuver
mattress
    m. stitch
    m. suture
    m. suture otoplasty
maturation
    m. division
    m. index
    m. phase
mature
    m. collagen fiber
    m. teratoma
    m. wound
maturing the stoma
Mauchart ligament
Mauck medial collateral ligament knee repair procedure
Maudsley Mentation Test
Mauksch-Maumenee-Goldberg cataract extraction
Maumenee-Goldberg cataract extraction
Maunsell-Weir coloanal anastomosis
Mau osteotomy
maxilla, *pl.* **maxillae**
maxillae (*pl. of* maxilla)
maxillary
    m. antrum
    m. antrum closure
    m. artery
    m. canal
    m. excess
    m. expansion
    m. fracture
    m. hiatus
    m. nerve

M

maxillary (*continued*)
    m. nerve block
    m. osteotomy
    m. restoration
    m. sinus carcinoma
    m. sinus cavity
    m. sinuscopy
    m. sinus mucocele
    m. surgery
    m. tubercle
maxillectomy
    Cocke m.
    partial m.
    subtotal m.
    total m.
maxillofacial
    m. anomaly
    m. fracture
    m. surgery (MFS)
maxillomandibular
    m. fixation (MMF)
    m. relation
maxillotomy
    extended m.
maximal
    m. drug concentration (Cmax)
    m. expiratory flow rate
    m. expiratory flow volume
    m. rectal diameter
    m. ventilation rate
    m. voluntary ventilation (MVV)
4-maximal breath preoxygenation technique
Maximally Discriminative Facial Coding System
maximum
    m. allowable blood loss
    m. breathing capacity (MBC)
    m. mouth opening
    m. occipital point
    m. permissible concentration
    m. stimulation test
    m. urethral closure pressure
    m. voluntary ventilation (MVV)
maximum-intensity projection
Maxon
    M. absorbable suture
    M. suture
Maxwell body
Maydl
    M. colostomy procedure
    M. hernia
    M. ureterocolostomy
Mayer trapezius transfer operation
Mayfield incision
May-Hegglin body
Maylard incision
Mayo
    M. approach

    M. carpal instability classification
    M. hysterectomy
    M. linen suture
    M. modified total elbow arthroplasty
    M. operation
    M. resection arthroplasty
    M. rheumatoid elbow classification
Mayo-Fueth inversion procedure
Mayo-Heuter bunionectomy
Mayo-Robson
    M.-R. incision
    M.-R. position
May-Thurner syndrome
maze
    m. III procedure
    m. procedure
Mazet
    M. disarticulation
    M. knee disarticulation technique
mazolysis
MBC
    maximum breathing capacity
MC
    metacarpal
MCA
    middle cerebral artery
    MCA occlusion
McArthur incision
McBride
    M. bunionectomy
    M. bunionectomy procedure
McBurney
    M. appendectomy
    M. appendectomy incision
    M. operation
    M. point
McCall
    M. culdoplasty
    M. stitch
McCall-Schumann enterocele procedure
McCannel suture
McCauley knee cartilage MRI technique
McConnell
    M. extensile knee approach
    M. median and ulnar nerve approach
    M. patellar taping technique
McCormick-Blount metatarsus adductus repair procedure
McCoy balloon laryngoscopy
McCraw gracilis myocutaneous flap
McDonald
    M. cerclage
    M. cervical encirclement suture procedure
McElfresh-Dobyns-O'Brien extension block splinting technique

McElvenny-Caldwell first metatarsocuneiform navicular joint fusion procedure
McElvenny orthopaedic technique
McFarland bone graft
McFarland-Osborne
    M.-O. hip joint lateral incision technique
    M.-O. lateral hip approach
McFarlane skin flap
McGavic bare sclera pterygium operation
McGill pain questionnaire (MPQ)
McGlamry-Downey forefoot procedure
McGoon double-switch TGA correction technique
McGregor
    M. basal line
    M. temporal z-plasty eyelid flap
McGuire prostate operation
mCi
    millicurie
McIndoe
    M. operation
    M. vaginal construction procedure
    M. vaginal creation
McIndoe-Hayes construction
McKay-Simons clubfoot operation
McKee line
McKeever
    M. and MacIntosh hemiarthroplasty
    M. medullary clavicle fixation
    M. open reduction
McKeever-Buck
    M.-B. elbow technique
    M.-B. fragment excision
McKenzie extension maneuver
McKeown esophagogastrectomy
McKissock mastectomy
McLaughlin
    M. acromioplasty
    M. approach
    M. posterior dislocated shoulder repair
    M. posterior shoulder dislocation repair procedure
McLaughlin-Ryder incision
McLean
    M. banded gastroplasty
    M. suture
McMaster
    M. bone graft
    M. Quality of Life Scale
McMurray circumduction maneuver
MCN
    mucinous cystic neoplasm
McNeer gastric carcinoma classification
MCP
    metacarpophalangeal

McRae foramen magnum line
McReynolds
    M. open reduction technique
    M. operation
MCS
    magnetic control suturing
McShane-Leinberry-Fenlin acromioplasty
McSpadden root seal method
MCTD
    mixed connective tissue disease
McVay
    M. hernia repair
    M. hernia repair procedure
    M. hernioplasty method
    M. herniorrhaphy
    M. herniorrhaphy technique
    M. incision
    M. inguinal hernial repair
    M. operation
McVay-Cooper ligament repair
McWhirter simple mastectomy
McWhorter posterior shoulder approach
MD
    muscular dystrophy
MDCT
    multidetector computed tomography
MDMQ
    Menstrual Distress Management Questionnaire
mean
    m. airway resistance
    m. arterial blood pressure (MABP)
    m. arterial pressure (MAP)
    m. circulation time
    m. diastolic left ventricular pressure
    m. foundation plane
    m. normalized systolic ejection rate
    m. pulmonary artery pressure
    m. pulmonary artery wedge pressure
    m. shunt index
    m. systolic left ventricular pressure
    m. umbilical vein to maternal vein ratio
    m. UV to MV ratio
Meares-Stamey chronic prostatitis technique
measure
    nonpharmacologic m.
    preventive m.
measurement
    acoustic reflection m.
    alveolar diffusion m.
    ankle-brachial pressure m.
    continuous intramucosal PCO_2 m.
    4-cuff technique segmental pressure m.
    diurnal intraocular pressure m.
    endpoint m.
    esophageal m.

M

measurement (*continued*)
    facial excursion m.
    Fick cardiac output m.
    hematocrit m.
    intrauterine pressure m.
    invasive pressure m.
    LES pressure m.
    lower esophageal sphincter pressure
      m.
    muscle m.
    near-infrared m.
    negative inspiratory pressure m.
    oxygen saturation m.
    pH m.
    pressure m.
    pulse-echo distance m.
    serial hematocrit m.
    skin m.
    skin temperature gradient m.
    spectral Doppler m.
    supraspinale skinfold m.
    thermographic temperature m.
    tissue pressure m.
    total exchangeable potassium m.
    transcutaneous oxygen pressure m.
    transstenotic pressure gradient m.
    tympanic membrane m.
    urethral pressure m.
    voiding urethral pressure m.
meatal
    m. advancement and glansplasty
      (MAGPI)
    m. advancement and glansplasty
      incorporated
    m. advancement, glansplasty,
      penoscrotal junction meatotomy
      (MAGPI)
    m. cartilage
meatoplasty
    V-flap m.
meatorrhaphy
meatoscopy
meatotomy
    meatal advancement, glansplasty,
      penoscrotal junction m. (MAGPI)
    ureteral m.
meatus, *pl.* **meatus**
    anterior nasal m.
    external auditory m.
    inferior m.
    middle m.
    superior m.
    ureteral m.
    m. urinarius
meaty appearance
mechanical
    m. allodynia
    m. anastomosis
    m. debridement
    m. dermabrasion
    m. endoscopic management
    m. esophagojejunostomy
    m. extrahepatic obstruction
    m. hyperalgesia
    m. leech
    m. lithotripsy
    m. low back pain
    m. obstruction
    m. occlusion
    m. paresthesia
    m. perforation
    m. pulp exposure
    m. stimulation
    m. thrombectomy
    m. ureteral dilation
    m. variceal compression
    m. ventilation
    m. ventilation anesthetic technique
    m. ventilatory support
mechanism
    antireflux flap-valve m.
    apoptotic m.
    association m.
    cardiac pump m.
    central extensor m.
    cholinergic m.
    clotting m.
    countercurrent m.
    digital extensor m.
    extensor hood m.
    extrinsic m.
    fascial shutter m.
    flap-valve m.
    hematogenous m.
    hemolytic m.
    immune m.
    inhibitory-excitatory m.
    noradrenergic m.
    obstructive m.
    pain m.
    renal m.
    screw-home m.
    sphincter m.
    surveillance m.
    thoracic pump m.
    urethral closure m.
mechanoactivation
mechanogram
mechanomyography
mechanoreflex
mèche
Meckel
    M. band
    M. cartilage
    M. cave
    M. cavity
    M. diverticulectomy
    M. diverticulum

M. ganglion
M. ligament
M. scan
M. space
M. sphenopalatine ganglionectomy

meconium

m. aspiration
m. aspiration syndrome
m. ileus
inspissated m.
m. peritonitis
m. plug syndrome
tenacious m.

Medex Hi-Flo stopcock
media (*pl. of* medius, *pl. of* medium)
medial

m. aspect
m. aspiration
m. basal segment
m. canthus
m. capsular imbrication
m. capsulorrhaphy
m. clear space
m. condyle
m. crus
m. cutaneous branch
m. direct defect
m. displacement osteotomy
m. dissection
m. extradural approach
m. flap
m. hamstring
m. malleolar network
m. malleolar subcutaneous bursa
m. malleolus
m. malleolus fixation
m. malleolus resection
m. mammary branch
m. meniscectomy
m. parapatellar capsular approach
m. parapatellar incision
m. pectoral nerve
m. process
m. pterygoid plate
m. puboprostatic ligament
m. repair
m. rotation
m. rotation procedure
m. rotator
m. sector
m. tibial stress syndrome

medialis obliquus imbrication
medialization

silicone elastomer m.

medial-sector pedicle
median

m. arcuate ligament
m. biopsy volume
m. corpectomy

m. detection threshold
m. episiotomy
m. frequency
m. glossoepiglottic fold
m. groove
m. jaw relation
m. labiomandibular glossotomy
m. line
m. lithotomy
m. longitudinal raphe
m. mandibular point
m. nerve
m. nerve compression
m. section
m. sternotomy
m. sternotomy incision
m. strumectomy
m. thoracotomy

medianum

septum m.

mediastinal

m. artery
m. branch
m. CTD
m. enlargement
m. esophagojejunostomy
m. hematoma
m. hemorrhage
m. high-attenuation mass
m. irradiation
m. lymphadenectomy
m. lymph node biopsy
m. lymph node dissection
m. pleura
m. shift
m. space
m. tumor
m. vein
m. wedge

mediastinitis
mediastinoscopic examination
mediastinoscopy

Chamberlain m.
transthoracic m.
video m.

mediastinoscopy-assisted transhiatal esophagectomy
mediastinotomy
mediastinum

anterior m.
inferior m.
middle m.
posterior m.
superior m.
upper m.

mediate transfusion
mediator

biochemical m.
inflammatory m.

M

mediator (*continued*)
    neuroinflammatory m.
    proinflammatory m.
Medicaid
medical
    m. care
    m. care evaluation
    m. chemoprevention
    m. diathermy
    m. dilation
    m. illness
    m. intervention
    m. management
    m. marijuana
    m. oncologist
    m. ophthalmoscopy
    m. problem
    m. record
    m. systemic condition
    m. therapy
    m. treatment
    m. treatment option
    m. vagotomy
Medicare
medication
    aerosolized m.
    antalgic m.
    anticholinergic m.
    antiepileptic m.
    antiinflammatory m.
    base m.
    beta-blocker m.
    m. bezoar
    concomitant m.
    dopaminergic m.
    m. efficacy
    hydrophobic topical m.
    intravenous m.
    iodide-containing m.
    levodopa dopaminergic m.
    nonsteroidal antiinfla-
      mmatory m.
    oral antibiotic m.
    over-the-counter m.
    parenteral m.
    preanesthetic m.
    pressor m.
    prophylactic m.
    psychopharmacologic m.
    psychotropic m.
    M. Quantification Scale
    systemic m.
    teratogenic m.
    vasoactive m.
medication-induced
    m.-i. injury
    m.-i. obesity
medicine
    alternative m.

    American Board of Pain M.
      (ABPM)
    American Society of Regional
      Anesthesia and Pain M. (ASRA)
    anesthesiology critical care m.
    complementary and alternative m.
    critical care m. (CCM)
    emergency m.
    evidence-based m.
    herbal m.
    manual m.
    National Center for Complementary
      and Alternative M. (NCCAM)
    nuclear m.
    palliative m.
    perioperative m.
    traditional Chinese m.
    vascular m.
medicochirurgical
medicolegal aspect
medioccipital
mediocolic sphincter
mediolateral episiotomy
medisect
Mediterranean exanthematous
  fever
medium, *pl.* **media**
    adhesive otitis media
    contrast m.
    culture m.
    otitis media (OM)
medium-chain fatty
  acids
medium-scale integration
medium-sized artery
medius
    gluteus m.
    processus clinoideus m.
    truncus m.
medulla, *pl.* **medullae**
    renal m.
    rostral ventrolateral m.
    suprarenal m.
medullae (*pl. of* medulla)
medullar
medullary
    m. adenocarcinoma
    m. bone graft
    m. canal
    m. carcinoma
    m. cavity
    m. clavicle fixation
    m. nail fixation
    m. oxygenation
    m. pyramid
    m. pyramidotomy
    m. ray
    m. space
    m. spinal artery

m. spinothalamic tractotomy
m. sponge kidney
m. substance
m. thyroid carcinoma
m. tube
medullated
medullation
medullectomy
medullization
medulloblastoma
desmoplastic m.
melanotic m.
m. metastasis
medulloepithelioma
medullomyoblastoma
medullostomy
tarsal m.
medullovasculosa
area m.
medusa, *pl.* **medusae**
caput medusae
medusae (*pl. of* medusa)
Medusa's head
Meek skin micrograft
Mees line
mefenamic acid
megabowel
megacalycosis
megacolon
toxic m.
megacystis-megaureter
m.-m. association
m.-m. syndrome
megacystis-microcolon-intestinal
hypoperistalsis syndrome
megacystis syndrome
megadolichovertebrobasilar anomaly
megaesophagus
tortuous m.
megaloblastic anemia
megaloglossia (*var. of* macroglossia)
megaloureter, megaureter
megalourethra
megarectum
megasigmoid
megaureter, megaloureter
Meibom gland
meibomian
m. gland
m. gland carcinoma
Meige disease
Meigs
M. pelvic lymphadenectomy
M. suture
M. suture technique
Meigs-Okabayashi radical hysterectomy
procedure
Meigs-Werthein hysterectomy
Meissner plexus

meizothrombin
mel
melanoma
melanization
melanoacanthoma
melanoameloblastoma
melanoblastoma
melanocarcinoma
melanocytic conjunctival lesion
melanocytoma
melanoma (mel)
acral lentiginous m. (ALM)
anorectal m.
axial m.
m. cell lysate
CTL immunity against m.
cutaneous m. (CM)
extremity m.
familial atypical mole and m.
(FAM-M)
familial atypical multiple-mole m.
(FAMMM)
lentigo m. (LM)
node-negative m.
node-positive m.
thick cutaneous m. (TCM)
m. transferrin
truncal m.
melanosarcoma
melanotic
m. carcinoma
m. lesion
m. medulloblastoma
m. oncocytic metaplasia
m. whitlow
MELAS
mitochondrial myopathy,
encephalopathy, lactacidosis, stroke
melatonin
MELD
Model for End-Stage Liver Disease
MELD Severity assessment system
Meleney
M. gangrene
M. infection
Meller lacrimal sac operation
mellitus
diabetes m.
melocervicoplasty
melolabial flap
Melone distal radius fracture
classification
melonoplasty (*var. of* meloplasty)
melon seed body
meloplasty, melonoplasty
meloschisis
melting point
Meltzer intratracheal insufflation
anesthesia method

M

memantine
membrana, *pl.* **membranae**
membranae (*pl. of* membrana)
membrane

acute inflammatory m.
acute pyogenic m.
adamantine m.
alveolocapillary m.
alveolodental m.
amniotic m.
antibasement m.
antiglomerular basement m.
antitubular basement m.
antral m.
arachnoid m.
m. artificial lung
asymmetric unit m.
atlantooccipital m.
Barkan m.
basal cell m.
basement m.
basilar m.
basolateral m.
Bichat m.
bilaminar m.
bioabsorbable m.
Bowman m.
m. bridge
Bruch m.
brush-border m.
m. catheter technique
cell m.
chorioallantoic m.
choroidal neovascular m.
cloacal m.
collodion m.
congenital pyloric m.
conjunctival m.
connective tissue m.
cricothyroid m.
cricotracheal m.
cricovocal m.
croupous m.
m. current
cuticular m.
cyclitic m.
cytoplasmic m.
Debove m.
decidual m.
Demours m.
dentinoenamel m.
Descemet m.
dialysis m.
dialyzer m.
diphtheritic m.
m. disordering
drum m.
dry mucous membranes
Duddell m.

dysmenorrheal m.
egg m.
enamel m.
endothelial cell basement m.
epipapillary m.
epiretinal m.
epithelial basement m.
erythrocyte m.
exocelomic m.
m. expansion
m. expansion theory
false m.
fenestrated m.
fetal m.
fibroproliferative m.
Fielding m.
filtration-slit m.
Fresnel m.
germinal m.
glassy m.
gliotic m.
Golgi m.
Haller m.
Henle elastic m.
Henle fenestrated m.
Heuser m.
hourglass m.
Hovius m.
hyaline basement m.
hyalitis anterior m.
hyaloid m.
hymenal m.
hyoglossal m.
idiopathic preretinal m.
inflammatory m.
inner limiting m.
m. instability
intact m.
intercostal m.
intermuscular m.
interposition m.
intraosseous m.
invaginated m.
ivory m.
Jackson m.
Jacob m.
limiting m.
lysosomal m.
mammalian cell m.
microvillous m.
moist mucous membranes
mucous m.
Nasmyth m.
neovascular m.
neuronal m.
m. of Liliequist
onion skin-like m.
otolithic m.
outer limiting m.

m. oxygenator
Payr m.
m. peeling
peridental m.
perineal m.
periodontal m.
periorbital m.
m. permeability
m. perturbation
phrenicoesophageal m.
pial-glial m.
placental m.
plasma m.
pleuroperitoneal m.
porous filter m.
postsynaptic m.
m. potential
preretinal m.
presynaptic m.
prophylactic m.
pseudoserous m.
pulpodentinal m.
pupillary m.
purpurogenous m.
pyogenic m.
quadrangular m.
Reichert m.
Reissner m.
reticular m.
retrocorneal m.
rolling m.
m. rupture
rupture of m.'s (ROM)
Ruysch m.
ruyschian m.
salpingopalatine m.
salpingopharyngeal m.
sarcolemmal m.
schneiderian respiratory m.
secondary m.
semiimpermeable m.
semipermeable m.
serous m.
Shrapnell m.
Slavianski m.
small-intestine m.
spiral m.
m. stabilizing agent
statoconic m.
stripping m.
stylomandibular m.
subepithelial m.
subimplant m.
submucous m.
subretinal neovascular m.
suprapleural m.
surface m.
synovial m.
tarsal m.

tectorial m.
Tenon m.
thickened synovial m.
thin basement m.
thyrohyoid m.
Toldt m.
Tourtual m.
trabecular m.
m. trafficking
tubular basement m.
tympanic m. (TM)
undulating m.
unit m.
urea-impermeable m.
urogenital m.
urorectal m.
urothelial basement m.
vernix m.
vestibular m.
virginal m.
vitelline m.
vitreal m.
vitreous m.
Wachendorf m.
wrinkling m.
yolk m.
Zinn m.

membrane-coating granule
membranectomy
membranocartilaginous
membranoproliferative
  glomerulonephritis
membranotomy
    transcardiac m.
membranous
    m. acute inflammation
    m. adhesion
    m. nephropathy
    m. obstruction
    m. septum
    m. urethra
Memorial Pain Assessment Card
(MPAC)
memory
    explicit m.
    m. guidance saccade test
    implicit m.
    indirect m.
    m. loss
    mass m.
    m. recall
    scratch-pad m.
    working m.
MEN
    multiple endocrine neoplasia
    MEN syndrome
Mendelsohn dysphagia maneuver
Mendelson syndrome
Ménétrier disease

M

Menghini
    M. biopsy technique
    M. technique for percutaneous liver
    biopsy
Ménière
    M. disease
    M. syndrome
meningeal
    m. branch
    m. carcinoma
    m. groove
    m. hernia
    m. layer
    m. plexus
    m. vein
meningeorrhaphy
meninges (*pl. of* meninx)
meningioma
meningioma-en-plaque
meningiomatosis
meningitic respiration
meningitides (*pl. of* meningitis)
meningitis, *pl.* **meningitides**
    postdural puncture m.
meningocele
meningoencephalitis
meningoencephalocele
meningomyelocele
meningorrhagia
meningosis
meninguria
meninx, *pl.* **meninges**
meniscal
    m. excision
    m. repair
meniscectomy
    arthroscopic m.
    lateral m.
    medial m.
    partial m.
    Patel medial m.
    subtotal lateral m.
    total m.
menisci (*pl. of* meniscus)
meniscoplasty
meniscus, *pl.* **menisci**
    Dickhaut-DeLee classification of
    discoid m.
    Watanabe classification of
    discoid m.
Mensor-Scheck hanging hip
operation
menstrual
    m. aspiration
    m. cycle induction
    M. Distress Management
    Questionnaire (MDMQ)
    m. extraction
    m. extraction abortion

menstruation
    reflux m.
mental
    m. artery
    m. block injection
    m. branch
    m. canal
    m. defeat
    m. foramen
    m. nerve
    m. nerve block
    m. point
    m. process
    m. projection
    m. region
    m. spine
    m. status evaluation
    m. status examination
    m. symphysis
    m. tubercle
mentalis muscle
mentoanterior fetal position
mentolabial
    m. furrow
    m. sulcus
mentoplasty
mentoposterior fetal position
mentotransverse fetal position
Menzies melanoma diagnosis method
MEP
    motor evoked potential
MER
    motor evoked response
meralgia paresthetica
Mercator projection
Mercedes-Benz sign for gallstones
Mercier bar
mercurial line
mercury pressure
Merendino incompetent mitral valve
  reconstruction technique
meridian
    corneal m.
    du m.
    San Jiao m.
    triple heater m.
meridional aberration
Merkel
    M. cell cancer
    M. cell carcinoma
    M. fossa
    M. muscle
mermaid malformation
Mersilene braided nonabsorbable suture
Mersilk black silk suture
Méry gland
MESA
    microsurgical epididymal sperm
    aspiration

mesangial matrix expansion
mesangiolysis
mesangium
    extraglomerular m.
mesaraic (*var. of* mesenteric)
mesareic (*var. of* mesenteric)
mesatipellic pelvis
mesencephalic
    m. cistern
    m. hemorrhage
    m. low-density lesion
    m. reticular formation
    m. tractotomy
mesencephalotomy
mesenchymal
    m. lesion
    m. tissue
mesenchymoma
mesenteric, mesaraic, mesareic
    m. angiogram
    m. angiography
    m. arterial system
    m. arteriovenous fistula
    m. artery
    m. border
    m. bypass graft
    m. circulation
    m. cyst
    m. ganglion
    m. gland
    m. hematoma
    m. hernia
    m. insufficiency
    m. ischemia
    m. lymph node
    m. mass
    m. nodal disease
    m. node
    m. plexus
    m. portion
    m. revascularization
    m. rupture
    m. tear
    m. traction syndrome
    m. vascular lesion
    m. vasodilator
    m. vasodilator infusion
    m. vein
    m. venoconstriction
    m. vessel
mesentericoparietal
    m. fossa
    m. recess
mesentericoportal axis
mesenteriopexy
mesenteriorrhaphy
mesenteriplication
mesenteritis
mesenteroaxial volvulus

mesentery
    m. abscess
    edematous m.
    sigmoid m.
    small-bowel m.
mesethmoid bone
mesh
    m. fixation
    m. herniorrhaphy
    m. implantation
    m. inguinodynia
    intraperitoneal onlay m.
    (IPOM)
    Marlex m.
    m. migration
    Parietex m.
    PGA m.
    m. plug hernioplasty
    polyester m.
    polypropylene m.
    m. removal
    m. repair
    surgical m.
    m. suture
    synthetic m.
    transabdominal onlay m.
    Vicryl m.
    Vypro m.
mesial
mesioangular position
mesiobuccal
    m. canal
    m. line angle
mesiobuccocclusal point angle
mesiodistal
    m. fracture
    m. plane
mesiolabial
    m. bilobed transposition flap
    m. line angle
mesiolabioincisal point angle
mesiolingual line angle
mesiolinguoincisal point angle
mesiolinguo-occlusal point line
  angle
mesioocclusal line angle
mesioocclusodistal (MOD)
mesoappendix
mesoatrial shunt
mesocaval
    m. anastomosis
    m. H-graft
    m. shunt
mesocecal
mesocecum
mesocolic
    m. hernia
    m. involvement
    m. tenia

M

mesocolon
- ascending m.
- descending m.
- sigmoid m.
- transverse m.

mesocolopexy
mesocoloplication
mesoderm
- extraembryonic m.
- intermediate m.

mesoduodenal
mesoduodenum
mesoenteriolum
mesoepididymis
mesoesophageal dissection
mesoesophagus
mesohepatectomy
mesoileum
mesojejunum
mesolepidoma
mesolimbic-mesocortical tract
mesometrium
mesonephric
- m. adenocarcinoma
- m. duct
- m. ridge
- m. tubule

mesonephroi (*pl. of* mesonephros)
mesonephroma
mesonephros, *pl.* **mesonephroi**
mesoneuritis
mesopexy
mesophryon
mesorchium
mesorectal excision
mesorectum
- residual m.

mesorrhaphy
mesosalpinx
mesosigmoid
mesosigmoidopexy
mesostenium
mesosternum
mesostructure
- implant m.

mesotendineum
mesotendon
mesothelial
- m. cell
- m. cell layer
- m. tissue

mesothelioma
- benign m.

mesothelium
mesovarian margin
mesovarium
MESS
- mangled extremity severity score

Messerklinger endoscopic sinus inflammation diagnostic technique
mesylate
- dolasetron m.

metabolic
- m. acidosis
- m. change
- m. coma
- m. complication
- m. disorder
- m. evaluation
- m. heat production
- m. rate
- m. response

metabolism
- aerobic m.
- lipid m.
- pyruvate m.

metabolite
metacarpal (MC)
- m. artery
- m. bone
- m. neck fracture
- m. osteotomy

metacarpophalangeal (MCP)
- m. articulation
- m. joint arthroplasty

metacarpus
metachronous
- m. emergence
- m. hernia
- m. liver metastasis

metadiaphysis
metafacial angle
metal band suture
metal-ceramic restoration
metallic
- m. cranioplasty
- m. foreign body
- m. fragment
- m. restoration
- m. rod fixation
- m. suture

metalloprotease
- matrix m. (MMP)

metalloproteinase
- matrix m. (MMP)

metalloscopy
metamorphosing respiration
metanephric
- m. cap
- m. duct

metaphyseal (*var. of* metaphysial)
metaphyses (*pl. of* metaphysis)
metaphysial, metaphyseal
- m. abscess
- m. osteotomy
- m. tibial fracture

metaphysis, *pl.* **metaphyses**

distal m.
femoral m.
fibular m.
funnelization of m.
rachitic m.
tibial m.
metaplasia
apocrine m.
Barrett m.
columnar m.
esophageal mucosa m.
melanotic oncocytic m.
squamous m.
metaplastic epithelium
metastasectomy
pulmonary m.
metastases (*pl. of* metastasis)
metastasis, *pl.* **metastases**
adnexal m.
adrenal m.
m., age, completeness of resection,
local invasion, tumor size
(MACIS)
aortic node m.
axillary node m.
bilobar liver m.
biochemical m.
biopsy-proven m.
blastic m.
blood-borne m.
bone m.
bony m.
brain m.
breast m.
calcareous m.
calcified liver m.
calcifying m.
cardiac m.
cavitating m.
celiac lymph node m.
cerebral m.
cervical m.
chiasmal m.
choroidal m.
clivus m.
colonic m.
colorectal m.
contact m.
contralateral axillary m.
cutaneous m.
cystic m.
diffuse m.
distal m.
distant m.
drop m.
duodenal m.
echopenic liver m.
extracapsular m.
extrahepatic m.

extralymphatic m.
extrathoracic m.
fallopian tube m.
gastric bed m.
gastrointestinal m.
hematogenic m.
hematogenic m.
hematopoietic m.
hemorrhagic m.
hepatic colorectal m.
hernia m.
implantation m.
incisional m.
inguinal lymph node m.
intracapsular m.
intrahepatic m.
intramucosal m.
in-transit m.
intrapulmonary m.
isolated noncolorectal liver m.
laparoscopic port site m.
lateroaortic m.
leptomeningeal m.
liver m.
lymphatic m.
lymph node m.
lymphogenous m.
medulloblastoma m.
metachronous liver m.
necrotic m.
neoplasm m.
neuroendocrine m.
nodal m.
noncolorectal liver m. (NCRLM)
nonneuroendocrine m.
occult m.
ocular m.
omental m.
orbital m.
osseous m.
osteoblastic m.
osteolytic m.
ovarian cancer m.
paracardiac m.
parasellar m.
parenchymal brain m.
peritoneal m.
placental m.
port site m.
pulmonary m.
regional m.
resectable liver m.
retrobulbar orbital m.
satellite m.
serosal m.
serosal-peritoneal m.
skeletal m.
skip m.
soft tissue m.

M

metastasis (*continued*)
    sphenoid sinus m.
    spinal m.
    stomach cancer m.
    synchronous hepatic m.
    testicular m.
    tumor, node, m. (TNM)
    unique noncolorectal liver m.
    unresectable m.
    uterine sarcoma m.
    uveal m.
    vascular m.
    Virchow m.

metastatic
    m. abscess
    m. adenocarcinoma
    m. adenopathy
    m. colorectal cancer
    m. colorectal carcinoma
    m. contamination
    m. disease
    m. implantation
    m. involvement
    m. lesion
    m. malignancy
    m. nodule
    m. prostatic carcinoma
    m. renal cell carcinoma
    m. spread
    m. tumor
    m. tumor removal

metasternum
metasynchronous bacterial urinary tract infection
metatarsal
    m. artery
    m. bone
    m. fracture
    m. head
    m. head resection
    m. pad
    m. Reverdin osteotomy
    m. V-shaped osteotomy

metatarsocuneiform articulation
metatarsophalangeal (MTP)
    m. articulation
    m. joint disarticulation
    m. joint dislocation

metatarsus primus elevatus
metathesis
meter-kilogram-second (mks)
methacholine bronchoprovocation challenge
methadone
methamphetamine exposure
methanol freezing method
metHb
    methemoglobin
methemoglobin (metHb)

methemoglobinemia
method
    Abbott scoliosis treatment m.
    acoustic m.
    analytic m.
    Anel arterial ligation m.
    antegrade m.
    Antyllus arterial ligation m.
    area-length m.
    artificial m.
    Arvidsson dimension-length m.
    Astrand 30-beat stopwatch m.
    atrial extrastimulus m.
    auditory m.
    bandage m.
    barostat m.
    Barraquer zonula ciliaris dissolution m.
    barrier m.
    Bass m.
    Bassini herniorrhaphy m.
    Beck gastric opening m.
    Belsey fundoplication m.
    Benedict-Talbot body surface area m.
    Bengston m.
    Bielschowsky ocular deviation m.
    Bier reactive hyperemia m.
    bilateral inguinal hernia repair m.
    Billroth I gastroduodenostomy m.
    bimodal m.
    bisensory m.
    Bobath therapeutic exercise m.
    Bohr isopleth m.
    Bonnaire femoral neck screw fixation m.
    Brasdor aneurysm ligation m.
    breast-conserving m.
    breathing m.
    Brisbane pediatric liver transplantation m.
    Brown and Wickham pressure profile m.
    Buck spondylolisthesis repair m.
    Budin-Chandler femoral neck anteversion measurement m.
    Buist intraabdominal pressure measurement m.
    bulkhead m.
    Burch bladder suspension m.
    Burgess m.
    bypass m.
    Callahan root canal filling m.
    Camp-Gianturco radiography m.
    Carpue rhinoplasty m.
    catheter introduction m.
    Celermajer cardiovascular profiling m.
    cellophane tape m.
    Chayes lost tooth replacement m.

chewing m.
cinefluoroscopic m.
clean-catch collection m.
closed circuit m.
Colcher-Sussman x-ray
  pelvimetry m.
cold knife m.
Collis-Nissen fundoplication m.
combined m.
composite pelvic resection m.
computer-assisted design-controlled
  alignment m.
confrontation m.
contact m.
contoured adduction
  trochanteric-controlled alignment m.
  (CAT-CAM)
contraceptive m.
conventional m.
cooled-knife m.
Crawford ptosis correction m.
cross-sectional m.
crown-contouring m.
Cuignet retinoscopy m.
cup-and-cone m.
Cüppers euthyscopy m.
Dale-Laidlaw clotting time m.
Danielson posterior annuloplasty m.
Defares rebreathing m.
definitive m.
Dieffenbach sliding flap m.
diffusion root canal filling m.
direct m.
disc diffusion m.
disc sensitivity m.
Distress Risk Assessment M.
  (DRAM)
Döderlein vaginal hysterectomy m.
Dodge area-length m.
Doppler m.
Dor fundoplication m.
double-stapled ileoanal reservoir m.
Douglas bag collection m.
downstream sampling m.
2-dye m.
dye dilution m.
dye scattering m.
dynamic traction m.
edge-detection m.
Eggleston rapid digitalization m.
Eicken hypopharyngoscopy m.
ellipsoid m.
Elmslie-Trillat patellar
  realignment m.
endorectal ileoanal pullthrough m.
endoscopic mucosal resection m.
end-to-end reconstruction m.
enucleation m.
estimated Fick m.

excisional biopsy m.
experimental m.
extension block splinting m.
extraanatomic bypass m.
extracorporeal m.
Ferguson scoliosis measuring m.
fiberoptic intubation m.
Fick oxygen extraction m.
field m.
filtration m.
floppy Nissen fundoplication m.
flow convergence m.
fluoroscopic m.
flush m.
formal m.
forward triangle m.
freehand m.
French m.
frozen section m.
Gärtner m.
gas clearance m.
gaseous laparoscopy m.
gasless laparoscopy m.
gastric valve tightening m.
Gerbert-Mellilo hallux
  Z-osteotomy m.
German m.
glass-bead retention m.
glucose oxidase m.
glycerin m.
gradient m.
gradient-reversal fat suppression m.
Granger m.
gravity m.
guidance m.
half-time m.
Hall pterygium m.
Hamilton cardiac output m.
hanging chain m.
Hanley-McNeil area under ROC
  curve m.
Harrison atrial end of
  ventriculoatrial shunt m.
Hatle pressure half-time Doppler
  echocardiography m.
head-tilt m.
helium dilution m.
hemi-double stapling m.
Hilton nerve division ulcer pain
  relief m.
Hirschberg strabismic eye
  deviation m.
hold-relax m.
hole preparation m.
Howard auditory neural prosthetic
  implant m.
hydrogen washout blood flow m.
Ilizarov limb lengthening m.
imaging m.

M

method (*continued*)

Imanaga Billroth I reconstruction m.
immersion m.
immobilization m.
impedance m.
1-inclinometer m.
2-inclinometer m.
Indian forehead flap m.
indirect restorative m.
informal m.
inhalation m.
injection m.
Insall patella alta m.
installation m.
intraoperative imaging m.
intraperitoneal m.
introspective m.
Italian arm flap rhinoplasty m.
jejunoileal bypass reversal m.
Johnson root canal filling m.
Kasser-Kennedy cineventriculographic
 ventricular volume m.
Keating-Hart postexcision
 fulguration m.
Kennedy area-length m.
Kety-Schmidt cerebral blood flow
 measurement m.
keyhole m.
kinesthetic m.
King biopsy m.
Kocher hernia inguinalis
 invagination m.
Konno biopsy m.
Langendorff perfusion of isolated
 heart m.
laparoscopic lymph node
 dissection m.
laparoscopic Nissen
 fundoplication m.
laparoscopic paraaortic lymph node
 sampling m.
laser m.
life table m.
lift-and-cut m.
limb-saving m.
Lister antiseptic surgery m.
logical m.
longitudinal m.
loop gastric bypass m.
Lowsley ribbon gut m.
manual m.
McSpadden root seal m.
McVay hernioplasty m.
Meltzer intratracheal insufflation
 anesthesia m.
Menzies melanoma diagnosis m.
methanol freezing m.
Meyerding anterior displacement of
 vertebral body m.

microinjection m.
microsurgery m.
minimal access m.
modified band lid m.
multiple cone root canal filling m.
multiple-port incision m.
Murphy intestinal anastomosis m.
nail length gauge m.
Narula sinoatrial conduction time m.
natural m.
Needles split cast m.
needle thoracentesis m.
Nissen fundoplication m.
Nissen-Rossetti fundoplication m.
noninvasive m.
nonresectional m.
nonrib-spreading thoracotomy
 incision m.
nonsurgical m.
Ollier small thin split-thickness
 graft m.
open circuit m.
optical density m.
Orsi-Grocco palpatory percussion of
 heart m.
oxygen step-up m.
Pachon cardiography m.
Papanicolaou m.
Parker-Kerr suture-closed m.
pause-squeeze m.
Payr clamp gastric surgery m.
pedicle m.
Penaz volume-clamp noninvasive
 blood pressure m.
percutaneous sampling m.
Pfeiffer-Comberg intraorbital foreign
 body localization m.
pharmacologic m.
pin-and-plaster m.
pinprick m.
plasma thrombin clot m.
polarographic tissue oxygen
 tension m.
Politzer auditory tube patency m.
Pólya gastrectomy m.
4-port m.
prick-test m.
Pringle vascular control m.
prism m.
Prochownik neonatal resuscitation m.
Purmann aneurysm sac extirpation
 m.
Puzo endoscopic cancer findings m.
pyramid m.
Rackley left ventricular mass
 determination m.
Ranawat-Dorr-Inglis atlantoaxial
 impaction m.
Ranawat triangle m.

reconstruction m.
reduction m.
reference m.
Rehfuss fractional gastric activity
  measurement m.
Reichel-Pólya partial gastrectomy m.
relaxation m.
retrofilling m.
retrograde root canal filling m.
Reverdin pinch graft m.
Risser skeletal maturity m.
Riva-Rocci blood pressure
  measurement m.
Russe-Gerhardt range of motion of
  living joints m.
Sargenti root canal m.
Scarpa aneurysm ligation m.
Schede bone defect filling m.
Schiller splint m.
Schober lumbar flexion-extension m.
Schüller oral radiography m.
scientific m.
sectional root canal filling m.
segmentation root canal
  filling m.
Seldinger catheter introduction m.
shadowing m.
Shimazaki area-length m.
silver cone root canal m.
silver point root canal filling m.
Silvester cardiopulmonary
  resuscitation m.
simultaneous m.
single cone root canal filling m.
single-stick m.
sliding scale m.
sniff m.
special reference m.
sperm washing insemination m.
sphincter-saving m.
sphincter-sparing m.
split-cast m.
Stanford biopsy m.
stapled reconstruction m.
static m.
stereotactic core biopsy m.
Stimson gravity shoulder dislocation
  reduction m.
Strauss m.
suction m. (SM)
surgical enucleation m.
swallow m.
symptothermal m.
synthetic m.
systematic m.
tetanic stimulation m.
Thal fundoplication m.
Thane central sulcus of brain
  location m.

Theden aneurysm and effusion
  treatment m.
Thiersch eyelid skin grafting m.
Thom flap laryngeal
  reconstruction m.
threshold shift m.
total fundoplication m.
Toupe pharyngocolonic
  anastomosis m.
Towako transvaginal-transmyometrial
  embryo transfer m.
traditional m.
trapezoid m.
triangulation stapling m.
trocar drainage m.
Tweed dentofacial analysis m.
twin m.
twirling scalp acupuncture m.
ultropaque rapid tissue analysis m.
uncut Collis-Nissen
  fundoplication m.
unilateral inguinal hernia repair m.
Vecchietti neovagina construction m.
vertical condensation root canal
  filling m.
vertical-cut m.
Victor Gomel microsurgical
  reconstruction m.
visual m.
volumetric m.
V-slope m.
Wardill 4-flap m.
Wardill-Kilner advancement flap m.
Wardrop aneurysm ligation m.
Waterston aorto-to-right pulmonary
  artery closure m.
Watson scapholunate treatment m.
Wheeler cicatricial ectropion
  correction m.
Wolfe full-thickness fat-free skin
  graft m.
X-line atlantooccipital dislocation
  diagnostic m.
methoxyflurane
methylation
methylene blue dye localization
methylprednisolone
methyl-*tert*-butyl ether (MTBE)
methyl-*tert*–butyl ether therapy
meticulous
  m. hemostasis
  m. maneuver
  m. surgical hemostasis
metopic point
metopion
metopoplasty
metoposcopy
metrectomy
metric ophthalmoscopy

M

metrofibroma
metroperitoneal fistula
metroplasty
    Strassman m.
metrotomy
mets
    metastasis
Meuli arthroplasty
Mexican hat incision
Meyer
    M. cartilage
    M. incision
    M. line
    M. lip carcinoma operation
Meyerding
    M. anterior displacement of
      vertebral body method
    M. orthopaedic technique
    M. spondylolisthesis classification
      line
Meyer-Overton
    M.-O. rule
    M.-O. theory of narcosis
Meyer-Schwickerath
    M.-S. light coagulation
    M.-S. retinal photocoagulation
Meyers-McKeever tibial fracture
  classification
Meyers quadratus muscle-pedicle bone
  graft
Meynert
    M. decussation
    M. retroflex bundle
Meyn reduction
MFS
    maxillofacial surgery
    monofixation syndrome
mg
    milligram
MGH
    Massachusetts General Hospital
    MGH Pain Center
MHC
    major histocompatibility complex
    MHC molecule
MI
    myocardial infarction
    occlusive MI
Miami pouch
micelle formation
Michaelson
    M. counterpressure
    M. vertebral fusion
Michal
    M. I direct anastomosis of inferior
      epigastric artery to cavernous body
    M. II direct anastomosis of inferior
      epigastric artery to dorsal penile
      artery

    M. I procedure
    M. II procedure
Michel
    M. anomaly
    M. deformity
    M. malformation
Michele vertebral aspiration
Michigan Abuse Screening Test (MAST)
Mickey Mouse sign
Micrins microsurgical suture
micro
    microscopic
    micro liquid extraction
microadenoma
    pituitary m.
microadenomectomy
microaerosol
microaldosteronoma
    contralateral m.
microamperage
    m. electrical nerve stimulation
    m. neural stimulation
microanastomosis
    laser-assisted m. (LAMA)
microaneurysm
microarchitectural deterioration
microaspiration
microatheroma
microbial
    m. contamination
    m. monitoring
microbic dissociation
microbiliary inflammation
microbubble
microcalcification
    diffuse m.
    malignant-appearing m.
    mammographic malignant-appearing m.
    suspicious m.
microcavitation
microchimerism
microchromoendoscopy
microcirculation
    native myocardial m.
    pulp m.
microcirculatory
    m. disturbance
    m. dysregulation
    m. failure
    m. flow
    m. parameter
microcoil
    computed tomography-guided
      localization using platinum
      microcoils
microcolon
microcolpohysteroscopy
microcorneal
microcurrent therapy

microcystic disease
microcytic hypochromic anemia
microdermabrasion
microdialysis
microdiffusion
microdiscectomy, microdiskectomy
    arthroscopic m. (AMD)
    uniportal arthroscopic m.
microdiskectomy (*var. of*
  microdiscectomy)
microdissection
microelectrode
    m. recording
    m. recording technique
microembolization
microfilament bundle
microfistulous communication
microflora
    endogenous m.
microfollicle
microfollicular
microgastria
microgenia
microgenitalism
microglioma
micrograft
    Meek skin m.
micrograph
microhamartoma
microincineration
microincision
microinjection method
microinvasion
microinvasive
    m. carcinoma
    m. carcinoma classification
    m. technique
microlaparoscopic
    m. cholecystectomy
    m. Nissen fundoplication
microlaparoscopy
microlaryngoscopy
    Thornell m.
microlight guide spectrophotometry
microlith
microlithiasis
microlumbar
    m. discectomy
    m. disc excision
micromanipulation
    gamete m.
    oocyte m.
    m. technique
micrometastases (*pl. of* micrometastasis)
micrometastasis, *pl.* **micrometastases**
    hematogenic m.
micrometastatic peritoneal disease
micromyelia
micron

microneurography
    sympathetic m.
microneurolysis
microneurorrhaphy
microneurovascular anastomosis
microoperative procedure
microorganism
    gram-negative m.
    gram-positive m.
micropapillary
    m. carcinoma
    m. subtype
micropenis
microperforation
microphone
micropoint suture
microprolactinoma
microproliferation
micropuncture
microscopic (micro), microscopical
    m. absence
    m. diagnosis
    m. disease
    m. epididymal sperm aspiration
    m. invasion
    m. IPM
    m. multifocal medullary carcinoma
    m. resection
    m. sphincter
microscopical (*var. of* microscopic)
microscopically controlled surgery
microscopy
    binocular m.
    cryoelectron m.
    dark-field m.
    electron m. (EM, EMC, E-MICR)
    epifluorescent m.
    fluorescence m.
    fundus m.
    immersion m.
    immune electron m. (IEM)
    immunofluorescence m.
    intravital m.
    light m. (LM)
    paraffin-section light m.
    polarization m.
    rotary shadowing electron m.
    scanning electron m. (SEM)
    scanning force m. (SFM)
    specular m.
    television m.
    transmission electron m. (TEM,
      TFM)
microshock
microspectrofluorometry
microspectroscopy
microsphere
    radioactive m.
microstomia

M

microsurgery
    m. method
    m. procedure
    m. technique
    transanal endoscopic m. (TEM)
    videoendoscopic-assisted m.
microsurgical
    m. discectomy
    m. epididymal sperm aspiration
    (MESA)
    m. epididymal sperm aspiration
    procedure
    m. free flap
    m. inguinal varicocelectomy
    m. reconstruction
    m. technique
    m. tubocornual anastomosis
microtia
microtrabecular hepatocellular carcinoma
microtransducer technique
microtraumatic insult
microtremor
    ocular m.
microtubulotomy technique
microvascular
    m. decompression (MVD)
    m. free flap
    m. free flap transfer
    m. surgical anastomosis
    m. technique
microvessel density
microvillous membrane
microwave
    m. coagulation
    m. coagulation therapy
    m. fixation
    m. radiation injury
    m. therapy
    m. thermotherapy
microwelding
micrurgical
micturition pain
midabdominal transverse incision
MIDAS
    Migraine Disability Assessment
    MIDAS questionnaire
midaxillary
    m. line
    m. line incision
midazolam-induced excitatory reaction
midbody tumor
midbrain reticular formation
MIDCAB
    minimally invasive direct coronary
    artery bypass
midcarpal
    m. arthroscopy
    m. dislocation
    m. fusion

midclavicular
    m. line
    m. port
midcoronal plane
middle
    m. cerebral artery (MCA)
    m. cerebral artery occlusion
    m. cervical fascia
    m. cervical ganglia
    m. colonic artery
    m. constrictor muscle
    m. ear infection
    m. latency auditory evoked potential
    (MLAEP)
    m. meatus
    m. mediastinum
    m. phalanx
    m. scalene muscle
midesophageal traction diverticulum
**midexpiratory to midinspiratory flow
ratio**
midface
    m. degloving technique
    m. fracture
midfoot fracture
midforceps maneuver
midfrontal
    m. plane
    m. plane coronal section
midgastric transverse sphincter
midgut volvulus
midheel line
midhumeral line
**midlatency auditory evoked potential
(MLAEP)**
midlateral approach
midline
    m. abdominal crease
    m. aponeurotic closure
    m. approach
    m. disc herniation
    m. exposure
    m. forehead flap
    m. incisional hernia
    m. incisional hernioplasty
    m. lower abdominal
    incision
    m. medial approach
    m. myelotomy
    m. nasal septum
    m. oblique incision
    m. position
    m. punctate myelotomy
    m. spinal approach
    m. upper abdominal
    incision
midmalleolar line
midoccipital
midpalatal suture opening

midpalmar
    m. abscess
    m. space
midpapillary
    anterior m. (AM)
midpapillary-longitudinal
midpapillary-transverse
midpelvis
midpoint to meatal line
midriff
midsagittal
    m. plane
    m. section
midscapular line
midsection
midshaft fracture
midsigmoid sphincter
midsternal line
midsternum
midthalamic plane
midwound healing ridge
Mielke bleeding time
MIGET
    multiple inert gas elimination
    technique
migraine
    abdominal m.
    m. abortive therapy
    basilar artery m.
    basilar-type m.
    M. Disability Assessment (MIDAS)
    familial hemiplegic m.
    hemiplegic m.
    retinal m.
    vertiginous m.
migraineur
migrainosus
    status m.
migrating abscess
migration
    m. abnormality
    calculus m.
    cell m.
    cellular m.
    clip m.
    electrode m.
    embolus m.
    epithelial m.
    fibroblast m.
    gallstone m.
    graft m.
    implant m.
    instrument m.
    intragastric prosthesis m.
    intrathecal m.
    intravascular m.
    intravesical m.
    lymphocyte m.
    macrophagic m.

mesh m.
neural crest m.
neuronal m.
neutrophil m.
m. (of pain to RLQ), anorexia,
    nausea and vomiting, tenderness
    (in RLQ), rebound pain, elevated
    temperature, leukocytosis, shift
    (WBC to left) (MANTRELS)
phagocyte m.
physiologic mesial m.
pigmentary m.
placental m.
rod m.
stage m.
subarachnoid m.
tooth m.
trochanteric m.
tube m.
m. velocity
mika operation
Mikulicz
    M. colostomy
    M. incision
    M. operation
    M. pyloroplasty
    M. sac
Milch
    M. condylar fracture classification
    M. cuff resection
    M. cuff resection of ulna
      technique
    M. elbow fracture classification
    M. elbow technique
    M. humeral fracture classification
mild
    m. acute rejection
    m. traumatic brain injury
Miles
    M. abdominoperineal resection
    M. operation
Milford mallet finger technique
miliary
    m. abscess
    m. aneurysm
    m. carcinomatosis
    m. granulomatous inflammation
military
    m. brace position
    m. tuck position
milk
    m. duct
    m. gland
    m. spot
milk-ejection reflex
milk-filled cyst
milkmaid's elbow dislocation
milkman fracture
milky ascites

Mill
  Magenstrasse and M. (M&M)
Millard
  M. advancement rotation flap
    reconstruction
  M. rotation-advancement lip repair
Millender arthroplasty
**Millen retropubic prostatectomy
  technique**
mille pattes technique
Miller
  M. cuff
  M. flatfoot operation
  M. midtarsal arthrodesis procedure
Miller-Abbott tube
Miller-Galante knee arthroplasty
Millesi
  M. interfascicular graft
  M. modified nerve graft technique
  M. nerve graft
millibar
millicurie (mCi)
Milligan-Morgan hemorrhoidectomy
milligram (mg)
milligram-hour
millimicrogram
milliosmole/kilogram (mosm/kg)
Mills valvulotome
milrinone
Milroy disease
Miltner-Wan calcaneus resection
mimetic muscle
mind-body therapy
mineral
  m. oil aspiration
  m. oil foreign body
mineralized tissue
mineralocorticoid receptor
**Ming gastric carcinoma
  classification**
minianterior thoracotomy approach
miniature
  m. end-plate potential
  m. uterine cavity
minicholecystostomy
  surgical-radiologic m.
minification
minikeratoplasty
  Castroviejo m.
minilap
  minilaparotomy
minilaparoscopic cholecystectomy
minilaparotomy (minilap)
  m. incision
  m. technique
minimal
  m. access general surgery
  m. access method
  m. access procedure

  m. access spine technology (MAST)
  m. access technique
  m. air
  m. alveolar concentration (MAC)
  m. anesthetic concentration (MAC)
  m. bactericidal concentration
  m. change nephrotic syndrome
  m. incision pubovaginal suspension
  m. incision total hip retractor
  m. leak technique
  m. lesion nephrotic syndrome
  m. sedation
  m. transurethral resection
minimal-change disease
minimally
  m. displaced fracture
  m. invasive approach
  m. invasive biopsy
  m. invasive direct coronary artery
    bypass (MIDCAB)
  m. invasive esophagectomy
  m. invasive mitral valve repair
  m. invasive nature
  m. invasive parathyroidectomy
  m. invasive plication
  m. invasive procedure (MIP)
  m. invasive robotically assisted
    mitral valve repair
  m. invasive robotic heart valve
    surgery
  M. Invasive Robotics Association
    (MIRA)
  m. invasive surgery (MIS)
  m. invasive surgical access
  m. invasive surgical technique
  m. invasive video-assisted
    parathyroidectomy (MIVAP)
minimum
  m. alveolar anesthetic
    concentration
  m. alveolar concentration (MAC)
  m. audible pressure
  m. bactericidal concentration
  m. detectable concentration
  m. effective analgesic concentration
  m. effective concentration
  m. lethal concentration (MLC)
  m. local analgesic concentration
    (MLAC)
**1-minimum alveolar concentration
  (1-MAC)**
miniplate osteosynthesis
ministernotomy
minithoracotomy
**Minkoff-Jaffe-Menendez posterior knee
  approach**
**Minkoff-Nicholas iliotibial band transfer
  knee repair procedure**
Minnesota EKG classification

minor
    m. amputation
    m. calyx
    m. duodenal papilla
    m. fissure
    m. manifestation
    m. operation
    m. splenic injury
    m. sublingual duct
    m. surgery
    teres m.
    teres m. muscle
    trochanter m.
Minsky rectal cancer operation
minute
    alveolar ventilation per m.
    physiologic dead space ventilation
      per m.
    m. polypoid lesion
    m. volume
1-minute endoscopy room test
10-minute hand scrub
MIP
    minimally invasive procedure
MIRA
    Minimally Invasive Robotics
    Association
Miralene suture
Mirizzi syndrome
mirror-image
    m.-i. breast biopsy
    m.-i. interpretation
    m.-i. laryngoscopy
    m.-i. reflection
MIS
    minimally invasive surgery
    müllerian inhibiting
    substance
misarticulation
misdirection phenomenon
mismatch
    prosthesis-patient m.
    ventilation/perfusion m.
missed fracture
missile
    m. injury
    m. track abscess
    m. trajectory
missionary position
mistranslation
Mital elbow release
  technique
Mitchell osteotomy
miter technique
mitochondrial
    m. electron transport
    m. myopathy, encephalopathy,
      lactacidosis, stroke (MELAS)
    m. permeability

mitomycin transarterial embolization
  treatment
mitoses (*pl. of* mitosis)
mitosis, *pl.* **mitoses**
mitotic activity
mitral
    m. balloon commissurotomy
    m. balloon valvotomy
    m. band anuloplasty
    m. regurgitation
    m. regurgitation murmur
    m. stenosis
    m. valve
    m. valve aneurysm
    m. valve anulus
    m. valve area
    m. valve closure index
    m. valve disorder
    m. valve gradient
    m. valve homograft graft
    m. valve insufficiency
    m. valve leaflet
    m. valve prolapse, aortic anomalies,
      skeletal changes, skin changes
      (MASS)
    m. valve prolapse syndrome
    m. valve repair
    m. valve replacement (MVR)
    m. valve-transverse
    m. valve valvotomy
    m. valvoplasty
mitralization
Mitrofanoff
    M. appendicovesicostomy
    M. appendicovesicostomy procedure
    M. conduit
    M. continent urinary diversion
      technique
    M. principle
    M. stoma
mittelschmerz
Mivacron
mivacurium
MIVAP
    minimally invasive video-assisted
      parathyroidectomy
mixed
    m. acid fermentation
    m. chancre
    m. connective tissue disease
      (MCTD)
    m. connective tissue disorder
    m. fat-water density lesion
    m. fungal/bacterial infection
    m. fungal organism
    m. hemorrhoid
    m. malignant glioma
    m. nail infection
    m. nerve

M

mixed (*continued*)
    m. nodule
    m. sclerotic and lytic bone lesion
    m. tumor
    m. venous-lymphatic malformation
    m. venous oxygen content
    m. venous oxygen saturation
      (MVO_2S)
mixed-density mass
mixture
    anesthetic gas m.
    epinephrine-anesthetic m.
    racemic m.
Mize-Bucholz-Grogen posterolateral femur approach
Mizuno double-patch ventricular septal perforation repair technique
Mizuno-Hirohata-Kashiwagi pediatric distal humeral fracture-separation repair technique
mks
    meter-kilogram-second
MLAC
    minimum local analgesic concentration
MLAEP
    middle latency auditory evoked potential
    midlatency auditory evoked potential
MLR
    major liver resection
M&M
    Magenstrasse and Mill
      M&M antiobesity procedure
MMF
    mandibulomaxillary fixation
    maxillomandibular fixation
MMK
    Marshall-Marchetti-Krantz
      MMK retropubic cystourethropexy suspension procedure
MMP
    matrix metalloprotease
    matrix metalloproteinase
Moberg
    M. advancement flap
    M. key-pinch procedure
Moberg-Gedda
    M.-G. fracture
    M.-G. open reduction
mobile
    m. arc
    m. sternum
mobility
    abdominal wall m.
    impaired m.
    muscle tissue m.
    rotation m.
    translation m.

mobilization
    circumferential m.
    colonic m.
    dorsal thyroid m.
    esophageal m.
    grade 1–5 m.
    intraperitoneal m.
    joint m.
    lateral band m.
    localized leukocyte m.
    nonthrust m.
    pericardial m.
    pretracheal space m.
    rectal m.
    soft tissue m.
    spinal joint m.
    stapes m.
    stem cell m.
    m. test
    thoracoscopic esophageal m.
    vertebral m.
    m. with impulse
Möbius anomaly
MOD
    mesioocclusodistal
    multiple organ dysfunction
modality
    adjuvant diagnostic m.
    diagnostic m.
    imaging m.
    implantable pain m.
    nonexcisional m.
    therapeutic m.
    treatment m.
mode
    Effler-Groves m.
    tumor dormancy m.
model
    corpectomy m.
    Emory Pain Estimate M. (EPEM)
    M. for End-Stage Liver Disease (MELD)
    Gail m.
    guidance-cooperation m.
    implant m.
    mortality prediction m. (MPM)
    mutual participation m.
    one-compartment pharmacokinetic m.
    Rothner headache m.
    tumor kinetic m.
    two-compartment pharmacokinetic m.
modeling-derivation
moderate
    m. hyperplasia
    m. pain
    m. rejection
    m. resuscitative hypothermia
    m. sedation
moderator band

modification

activator m.
Al-Ghorab m.
appliance m.
Astler-Coller m.
AV nodal m.
Bateman m.
beak m.
Bloom-Raney m.
Bonfiglio m.
bracket m.
Bunnell m.
Burch m.
C-D screw m.
Clark-Southwick-Odgen odontoid
  fracture m.
Counsellor-Flor m.
Deller m.
Duncan-Lovell m.
environment m.
fiber tip m.
Fielding m.
Furlow-Fisher m.
glutathione m.
Gunderson-Sosin m.
Hughes m.
interference m.
Kelly-Kennedy m.
Kleinert m.
Knobloch m.
Lester Martin m.
Losee m.
Martin m.
Mason-Likar limb lead m.
Mullins m.
Muzsnai m.
Neer m.
Pereyra-Lebhertz m.
posttranslation m.
racemic m.
Raz m.
Rosch m.
Rossetti m.
Sade m.
Sammarco-DiRaimondo m.
Schoemaker m.
Seddon m.
Sequeira-Khanuja m.
Sever m.
Smith m.
Soper m.
Stamey m.
Stauffer m.
Strickland m.
van Herick m.
Weinberg m.

modified

m. band lid method
m. Bassini herniorrhaphy
m. Belsey fundoplication
m. Belsey fundoplication procedure
m. Belsey fundoplication technique
m. Blalock-Taussig shunt
m. brachial technique
m. Cantwell technique
m. Child technique
m. coracoid approach infraclavicular
  brachial plexus block
m. dorsalis pedis myofascial flap
m. elliptical incision
m. Essed-Schroeder corporoplasty
m. flap
m. fluid gelatin
m. Frost suture
m. Gibson incision
m. Hassan open technique
m. Heller esophagomyotomy
m. Hill gastroesophageal hernia
  repair
m. Hoke-Miller flatfoot procedure
m. Irving-type tubal ligation
m. Konno procedure
m. lithotomy position
m. mastopexy
m. McVay herniorrhaphy
m. method of Pugh
m. mold and surface replacement
  arthroplasty
m. Norfolk procedure
M. Pain Disability Index (MPDI)
m. piggyback (MPB)
m. piggyback technique
m. Pomeroy technique
m. 2-portal endoscopic carpal tunnel
  release
m. radical hysterectomy
m. radical mastectomy
m. radical mastoidectomy
m. radical neck dissection
m. Raynaud phenomenon
m. Ritgen fetal head delivery
  maneuver
m. Sacks-Vine push-pull technique
m. Seldinger procedure
m. Seldinger technique
m. Shouldice hernioplasty
M. Somatic Pain Questionnaire
  (MSPQ)
M. Somatic Perception questionnaire
  (MSPQ)
m. Sturmdorf stitch
m. Sugiura procedure
m. surgical approach
m. TAPP hernioplasty
m. Toupe procedure
m. Toupe technique
m. tumescent liposuction technique
m. ultrafiltration

M

modified (*continued*)
    m. van Lint anesthesia
    m. V-Y advancement technique
    m. Weber-Fergusson procedure
    m. Whitehead hemorrhoidectomy
    m. Wies entropion procedure
    M. Yale Preoperative Anxiety Scale
    m. Young urethroplasty
    M. Zung Depression Scale
modioli (*pl. of* modiolus)
modiolus, *pl.* **modioli**
MODS
    multiorgan dysfunction syndrome
    multiple organ dysfunction syndrome
modulation
    amplitude m. (A-mode)
    antigenic m.
    autonomic m.
    biochemical m.
    brightness m. (B-mode)
    frequency m.
    immune m.
    obstruction-induced m.
    pain m.
    m. potential
    pressure amplitude m.
    sex steroid m.
    specific m.
    spinal m.
    sympathetic cutaneous m.
module
    dialysate preparation m.
    oxygen sensor m.
Moe scoliosis technique
MOF
    multiorgan failure
    multiple organ failure
mofetil
    mycophenolate m.
Mohrenheim
    M. fossa
    M. space
Mohr syndrome
Mohs
    M. fresh tissue chemosurgery
      technique
    M. micrographic surgery
    M. microsurgery technique
    M. microsurgical resection
moist
    m. gangrene
    m. mucous membranes
    m. wound environment
molar
    anchor m.
    m. teeth
    m. tooth fracture
    m. tube
mold acetabular arthroplasty

molding
    compression m.
    tissue m.
molecular
    m. biology
    m. external layer
    m. genetics
    m. lesion
    m. mass
    m. sieve
    m. technique
molecule
    adhesion m.
    amphipathic m.'s
Molesworth-Campbell elbow approach
Molesworth osteotomy
Moll gland
Moloney
    M. hernia repair
    M. line
Molteno
    M. drainage
    M. episcleral explant
moment
    activation m.
    3-point bending m.
Monakow
    M. bundle
    M. tract
Moncrieff discission
Mondini
    M. anomaly
    M. deformity
    M. pulmonary arteriovenous
      malformation
Mondini-Alexander malformation
Mondor disease
Monfort abdominal wall reconstruction
monilial infection
monitor
    acoustic m.
    AEP m.
    arterial blood pressure m.
    EEG m.
    EEG-based anesthesia m.
    entropy m.
    intraoperative m.
    line isolation m.
    muscle relaxation m.
    respiratory gas m.
monitored
    m. anesthesia care (MAC)
    m. anesthesia care anesthesia
    m. anesthesia care anesthetic
      technique
    m. anesthesia control (MAC)
monitoring
    airway gas m.
    allograft m.

ambulatory blood pressure m. (ABPM)
anesthetic m.
anticoagulant m.
anticoagulation m.
bispectral index m.
blood pressure m. ·
central venous pressure m.
close m.
depth of anesthesia m.
2-dimensional m.
ECoG m.
electrophysiologic m.
epicardial m.
esophageal pH m.
evoked external urethral sphincter potential m.
external fetal m.
fetal heart rate m.
hemodynamic m.
hospital m.
intracranial pressure m.
intraoperative neurophysiologic m.
intraoperative parathyroid hormone m.
intraoperative transcranial Doppler m.
invasive hemodynamic m.
laboratory m.
microbial m.
neuromuscular blockade m.
optoacoustic m.
outcome m.
plethysmographic pulse wave m.
posttetanic count m.
radiation m.
remote anesthetic m.
screw position perioperative m.
standard patient m.
m. technique
tissue pH m.
transcutaneous oxygen m.
vigilance m.
water vapor m.
monoamine reuptake inhibitor
monobloc
monochromatic aberration
monoclonal
m. adenoma
m. component
m. expansion
m. growth
monoclonality
Monocryl suture
monocular fixation
monodermoma
monodisperse
monofilament
m. absorbable suture

m. clear suture
m. green suture
m. nonabsorbable suture
m. nylon suture
m. polypropylene suture
m. skin suture
m. steel suture
m. suture
von Frey m.
m. wire suture
monofixation syndrome
monoinfection
monomalleolar ankle fracture
mononuclear cell infiltration
monoparesis
monophosphate
adenosine m.
monophosphoryl lipid A
monopolar
m. cautery
m. coagulation
m. diathermy
m. electrocautery
m. electrocoagulation
m. radiofrequency probe
monopulmonary ventilation
monorchid (*var. of* monorchidic)
monorchidic, monorchid
monorchidism
monorecidive chancre
Monosoft suture
monospherical total shoulder arthroplasty
monotherapy
oral m.
monotypic lesion
monoxide
carbon m. (CO)
dinitrogen m.
nitrogen m.
Monro
bursa of M.
M. foramen
M. line
Monro-Richter line
mons
m. plasty
m. pubis
Monteggia
M. dislocation
M. equivalent lesion
M. forearm fracture
Montercaux fracture
Montgomery
accessory areolar gland of M.
M. gland
M. tracheostomy
Monticelli-Spinelli distraction epiphysiolysis limb lengthening technique

M

mood
- dysphoric patient m.
- m. state

Moore
- M. fracture
- M. osteotomy-osteoclasis
- M. posterior hip approach
- M. technique
- M. tibial plateau fracture classification

Moran thoracic duct operation

Morax
- M. craniofacial reconstruction
- M. keratoplasty

morbidity
- m. and mortality
- cumulative operative m.
- m. excess
- febrile m.
- intraoperative m.
- long-term m.
- perioperative m.
- Physiological and Operative Severity Score for the Enumeration of Mortality and M. (POSSUM)
- postoperative m.

morbidly obese patient

morbid obesity

morcel

morcellation, morcellement
- m. operation
- Robinson m.
- m. technique

morcellement (*var. of* morcellation)

morcellized bone graft

Moreland-Marder-Anspach femoral stem removal

Morel-Fatio lid load operation

Morel-Lavallée lesion

Morgagni
- M. cartilage
- M. caruncle
- M. crypt
- M. foramen
- M. fossa
- M. fovea
- M. frenum
- M. hernia
- M. lacuna
- M. retinaculum
- M. ring
- M. sinus
- M. tubercle
- M. ventricle

Morgagni-Larrey type hernia

Morgan-Casscells meniscus suturing technique

Morganella morganii

morganii
- *Morganella m.*

Morgan line

moribund

Morison
- M. incision
- M. pouch

morning glory optic disc anomaly

morphallactic regeneration

morpheaform basal cell carcinoma

morphealike lesion

morphine
- m. extended-release capsule
- intrathecal m.
- m. narcotic analgesic therapy
- m. sulfate extended-release liposome injection

morphine-6-glucuronide

morphine-induced
- m.-i. lymphocyte apoptosis
- m.-i. pruritus

morphogenesis
- branching m.

morphologic
- m. change
- m. classification

morphological difference

morphology
- endometrial m.
- Gram stain m.
- lesion m.

Morquio syndrome

Morrey-Bryan total elbow arthroplasty

Morris hepatoma cell line

Morrison neurovascular free flap

Morse head

mors thymica

mortality
- cause-specific m.
- cumulative operative m.
- disease-associated m.
- hospital m.
- morbidity and m.
- operative m.
- perioperative m.
- postoperative m.
- m. prediction model (MPM)
- m. rate

mortar kidney

mortification

Morton plane

mosaicplasty
- autologous osteochondral m.

Moschcowitz culdoplasty procedure

MOSF
- multiorgan system failure
- multiple organ system failure

Mosher dacryocystorhinostomy

Mosher-Toti dacryocystorhinostomy

mosm/kg
  milliosmole/kilogram
Moss
  M. blood group
  classification
  M. Miami spinal system
  M. necrotizing enterocolitis
  operation
Motais superior rectus muscle blepharoptosis operation
moth-eaten
  m.-e. appearance
  m.-e. bone destruction
mother cyst
moth patch
motif
  binding m.
motilin
  m. effect
  m. level
motility
  contractile m.
  cyclic fasting m.
  m. disorder
  m. disturbance
  ineffective esophageal m.
  jejunal m.
  postoperative m.
  upper jejunal m.
motion
  abdominal respiratory m.
  angulation m.
  m. barrier
  helical axis of m.
  osteokinematic m.
  pattern of m.
  range of m. (ROM)
  m. segment
  translation m.
motion-preserving procedure
motivating operation
motor
  m. activity
  m. anomaly
  m. change
  m. cortex stimulation
  m. decussation
  m. disorder
  m. disturbance
  m. evoked potential (MEP)
  m. evoked response (MER)
  m. examination
  m. fusion
  m. nerve
  m. oil peritoneal fluid
  m. paraplegia
  m. pattern
  m. perseveration
  m. point

  m. point block
  m. point block anesthetic technique
  m. recording
  m. response
motor-evoked response to transcranial stimulation
Mott body
mottled appearance
Mouchet fracture
Mould arthroplasty
mounted point stone
mouse
  joint m.
mouth preparation
mouth-to-mouth
  m.-t.-m. respiration
  m.-t.-m. resuscitation
  m.-t.-m. ventilation
movable, moveable
  m. joint
  m. kidney
  m. spleen
  m. testis
moveable (*var. of* movable)
movement
  anterosuperior external ilium m.
  border tissue m.
  bowel m.
  m. disorder
  dissociation m.
  external ilium m.
  extraneous m.
  extraocular m. (EOM)
  fetal body m.
  head m.
  hepatopulmonary m.
  posteroinferior external m.
  primary rotation m.
  saccadic eye m.
  segmentation m.
  sound-stimulated fetal m.
  translational m.
  vocal cord m.
movement-related pain
moving time average
moxibustion
Moynihan
  M. colon operation
  M. position
MPAC
  Memorial Pain Assessment
  Card
MPB
  modified piggyback
  MPB technique
MPD
  main pancreatic duct
MPDI
  Modified Pain Disability Index

M

MPI
  Mannheim peritonitis index
  Multidimensional Pain Inventory
MPM
  mortality prediction model
MPQ
  McGill pain questionnaire
MPT
  multidisciplinary pain treatment
MR
  magnetic resonance
  MR spectroscopy
MRA
  magnetic resonance angiography
  low-field contrast-enhanced body
    MRA
MRCP
  magnetic resonance
    cholangiopancreatography
MRI
  magnetic resonance imaging
  MRI cholangiography
  intraoperative MRI
MRI-guided bracket wire localization
MRS
  magnetic resonance spectroscopy
MSOF
  multiple system organ failure
  multisystem organ failure
MSPQ
  Modified Somatic Pain
    Questionnaire
  Modified Somatic Perception
    questionnaire
MTBE
  methyl-*tert*-butyl ether
  MTBE therapy
MTBI
  mild traumatic brain injury
MTP
  metatarsophalangeal
  methylprednisolone
MTSS
  medial tibial stress syndrome
Mubarak-Hargens decompression technique
mucilaginous gland
mucinous
  m. adenocarcinoma
  m. ascites
  m. cystadenocarcinoma
  m. cystadenoma
  m. cystic neoplasm (MCN)
mucin-producing neoplasm
muciparous gland
mucobilia
mucobuccal
  m. fold
  m. reflection

mucocele
  appendiceal m.
  appendix m.
  breast m.
  frontal sinus m.
  frontoethmoidal m.
  maxillary sinus m.
  orbital m.
  paranasal m.
  retention m.
  sinus m.
  sphenoid m.
mucociliary
  m. clearance
  m. function
mucocutaneous
  m. hemorrhoid
  m. junction
  m. lesion
  m. lymph node syndrome
  m. manifestation
  m. muscle
  m. pigmentation of Peutz-Jeghers
    syndrome
mucoepidermal carcinoma
mucoepidermoid
  m. carcinoma
  m. tumor
mucogingival
  m. line
  m. surgery
mucoid ascites
mucoperichondrial flap
mucoperiosteal
  m. periodontal flap
  m. periodontal graft
  m. sliding flap
mucopolysaccharidoses (*pl. of*
  mucopolysaccharidosis)
mucopolysaccharidosis, *pl.*
  mucopolysaccharidoses
mucopurulent exudate
mucopyocele
Mucor **infection**
mucormycosis
mucosa, *pl.* **mucosae**
  bursa m.
  colorectal m.
  devitalize the tracheal m.
  ectopic gastric m.
  endocervical m.
  gastric m.
  gastroduodenal m.
  heterotopic gastric m.
  inlet patch m.
  lingual m.
  multifocal ectopic gastric m.
  oral m.
  pharyngeal m.

rectal m.
redundant m.
ulcerated m.
upper respiratory tract m.
mucosa-associated
    m.-a. lymphoid tissue (MALT,
      MALToma)
    m.-a. lymphoid tissue lymphoma
mucosae (*pl. of* mucosa)
mucosal
    m. ablation
    m. abnormality
    m. advancement
    m. advancement flap
    m. atrophy
    m. barrier
    m. biopsy
    m. bridge
    m. destruction
    m. esophageal ring
    m. hernia
    m. homeostasis
    m. inflammation
    m. invasion
    m. lesion
    m. line
    m. needle aspiration
    m. neuroma syndrome
    m. patch replacement
    m. periodontal flap
    m. periodontal graft
    m. proctectomy
    m. reconditioning
    m. relaxing incision technique
    m. remnant
    m. repair
    m. resection
    m. tunic
    m. ulceration
    m. vascular dilation
    m. web
    m. weight
mucosa-to-mucosa
    m.-t.-m. anastomosis
    m.-t.-m. Roux-en-Y
      hepaticojejunostomy
mucosectomy
    endoanal m.
    endoscopic m.
    rectal m.
    transabdominal m.
    transanal m.
mucositis
    radiation m.
mucous
    m. colic
    m. cystadenoma
    m. desiccation
    m. fistula

    m. gland
    m. membrane
    m. membrane graft
    m. membrane lesion
    m. membrane ulceration
    m. patch
    m. plug syndrome
    m. sheath
mucronate
mucus
    excess m.
mud bed
Muehrcke line
Mueller
    M. femoral supracondylar fracture
      classification
    M. fiberoptic nasal endoscopy
      maneuver
    M. hip arthroplasty
    M. intertrochantaric varus osteotomy
    M. operation
    M. patellar tendon graft
    M. tibial fracture classification
    M. transposition osteotomy
Mueller-type femoral head replacement
MUGA
    multiple gated acquisition
    MUGA exercise stress test
Muir-Torre syndrome
mulberry
    m. calculus
    m. lesion
mulberry-shaped mass
Mules eyelid ptosis correction
Mulholland sphincterotomy
Müller
    M. capsule
    M. duct
    M. duct body
    M. esophageal varices maneuver
Müller-Hillis 2nd stage labor maneuver
müllerian
    m. duct anomaly
    m. duct derivation syndrome
    m. duct fusion
    m. inhibiting substance (MIS)
Mullins modification
multangular
    m. bone
    m. ridge fracture
multiaxial
    m. classification
    m. joint
multicentric
    m. disease
    m. study
multicentricity
multidetector computed tomography
  (MDCT)

M

Multidimensional Pain Inventory (MPI)
multidisciplinary
    m. approach
    m. pain management
    m. pain treatment (MPT)
multidose vial
multifactorial
multifetal pregnancy reduction
multifetation
multifidus muscle
multifilament steel suture
multifocal
    m. change
    m. ectopic gastric mucosa
    m. enhancing lesion
    m. extensive DCIS
    m. extensive disease
    m. inflammation
    m. tumor
    m. variety
multigated angiogram
multigland
    m. disease
    m. hyperplasia
multiglandular
    m. disease
    m. parathyroid hyperplasia
multiinfection
multilamellar body
multilevel
    m. atherosclerotic arterial occlusive
      disease
    m. fracture
    m. laminectomy
multilocular
    m. cyst
    m. cystic lesion
multiloculated renal mass
multimerization
multimodal
    m. adjuvant therapy
    m. analgesia
    m. rehabilitation
multimodality therapy
multinodular goiter
multiorgan
    m. dysfunction syndrome (MODS)
    m. failure (MOF)
    m. hernia
    m. system dysfunction
    m. system failure (MOSF)
multiparameter sensor
multiplanar image
multiple
    m. array radiofrequency needle
      electrode
    m. calcification
    m. cone root canal filling method
    m. core biopsy

    m. diffuse intrahepatic abscesses
    m. dimension instrument
    m. endocrine neoplasia (MEN)
    m. endocrinopathy
    m. exostoses
    m. fracture
    m. gated acquisition (MUGA)
    m. gland hyperplasia
    m. hamartoma syndrome
    m. hepatic hydatidosis
    m. hepatitis virus infection
    m. hydatid disease
    m. inert gas elimination technique
      (MIGET)
    m. inert gas exchange
    m. intestinal neoplasia
    m. intubations
    m. macrocyst
    m. mucosal neuroma syndrome
    m. myeloma staging
    m. organ dysfunction (MOD)
    m. organ dysfunction syndrome
      (MODS)
    m. organ failure (MOF)
    m. organ failure syndrome
    m. organ system failure
      (MOSF)
    m. pterygium syndrome
    m. ray amputation
    m. sensitive point
    m. shunt levels
    m. site
    m. system atrophy
    m. system organ failure (MSOF)
    m. therapy
multiple-balloon valvoplasty
multiple-mechanism inhaled anesthetic
multiple-needle medial branch block
multiple-point sacral fixation
multiple-port
    m.-p. incision
    m.-p. incision method
    m.-p. incision procedure
    m.-p. incision technique
multiple-punch resection
multiple-site inhaled anesthetic
multiple-stage approach
multipolar
    m. coagulation
    m. electrocautery
    m. electrocoagulation
multiport epidural catheter
multipotential stem cell
multiray fracture
multisegmental resection
multistaged carrier flap
Multistage Maximal Effort exercise stress test
multistrand suture

multisystem
>   m. disorder
>   m. failure
>   m. organ failure (MSOF)

multivessel PTCA

multiviscera

multivisceral
>   m. graft
>   m. transplant

Mumford
>   M. distal clavicle open resection
>   procedure
>   M. distal clavicle resection

Mumford-Gurd arthroplasty

mummification
>   m. necrosis
>   pulp m.

Munro
>   M. and Parker laparoscopic
>   hysterectomy classification
>   M. point

mu receptor

murmur
>   aortic regurgitation m.
>   Austin Flint m.
>   diamond ejection m.
>   ejection m.
>   endocardial m.
>   exit block m.
>   exocardial m.
>   expiratory m.
>   extracardiac m.
>   mitral regurgitation m.
>   reduplication m.
>   systolic ejection m.

Murphy
>   M. eye of endotracheal tube
>   M. intestinal anastomosis method
>   M. sign

Murphy-tip endotracheal tube

muscarinic
>   m. agonist
>   m. receptor

muscle
>   abdominal external oblique m.
>   abdominal internal oblique m.
>   abductor hallucis m.
>   abductor longus m.
>   abductor magnus m.
>   abductor pollicis brevis m.
>   abductor pollicis longus m.
>   Aeby m.
>   airway smooth m.
>   Albinus m.
>   m. anabolism
>   anconeus m.
>   antagonistic m.
>   anterior auricular m.
>   anterior cervical intertransverse m.

anterior rectus m.
anterior scalene m.
anterior serratus m.
anterior tibial m.
antigravity m.'s
antitragicus m.
appendicular m.
arrector pili m.
aryepiglottic m.
arytenoid m.
auricular m.
axial m.
Bateman modification of Mayer
   trapezius m.
Bell m.
2-bellied m.
belt m.
m. biopsy
bipennate m.
Bovero m.
brachial m.
brachioradial m.
branchiomeric m.'s
Braune m.
m. breakdown
broadest m.
bronchoesophageal m.
buccinator m.
bulbocavernosus m.
bulbospongiosus m.
m. cachexia
Casser perforated m.
ceratocricoid m.
cervical rotator m.
cheek m.
chin m.
chondroglossus m.
circular pharyngeal m.
coccygeal m.
coccygeus m.
Coiter m.
compressor naris m.
coracobrachial m.
coracobrachialis m.
corrugator cutis m.
corrugator supercilii m.
cowl m.
cremasteric m.
cricoarytenoid m.
cricopharyngeus m.
cricothyroid m.
cruciate m.
crus m.
cutaneomucous m.
cutaneous m.
dartos m.
deepithelialized rectus abdominis m.
   (DRAM)
deltoid m.

M

muscle (*continued*)
    detrusor m.
    digastric m.
    dilator m.
    m. dissection
    m. distraction
    dorsal sacrococcygeal m.
    Duverney m.
    m. dystonia
    elevator m.
    m. energy technique
    epicranial m.
    epicranius m.
    erector spinae muscles
    extensor carpi radialis brevis m.
    extensor carpi radialis longus m.
    extensor carpi ulnaris m.
    extensor digiti minimi m.
    extensor digitorum brevis m.
    extensor digitorum longus m.
    extensor hallucis brevis m.
    extensor hallucis longus m.
    extensor indicis m.
    extensor pollicis brevis m.
    extensor pollicis longus m.
    extraocular m. (EOM)
    extrinsic m.
    facial m.
    m. fatigability
    femoral m.
    femoris rectus m.
    fibularis brevis m.
    fibularis longus m.
    fibularis tertius m.
    fixator m.
    m. flap
    flexor hallucis brevis m.
    flexor hallucis longus m.
    frontalis m.
    Gavard m.
    genioglossal m.
    geniohyoid m.
    glossopalatine m.
    gluteus maximus m.
    gluteus medius m.
    gluteus minimus m.
    greater rhomboid m.
    Guthrie m.
    hamstring m.
    m. hernia
    Horner m.
    Houston m.
    hyoglossal m.
    hyoid m.
    hypoglossus m.
    hypothenar m.
    iliac m.
    iliococcygeal m.
    iliocostal m.

iliohypogastric m.
iliopsoas m.
infrahyoid m.
m. inhibition
intercostal m.
interosseous m.
interspinal m.
intertransverse m.
intrinsic m.
ischiocavernous m.
Jung m.
Klein m.
Kohlrausch m.
Krause m.
labium inferioris m.
laryngeal m.
lateral m.
lateral pterygoid m.
levator palati m.
longissimus m.
longus capitis m.
longus colli m.
m. lysis
Marcacci m.
masseter m.
mastication m.
m. measurement
mentalis m.
Merkel m.
middle constrictor m.
middle scalene m.
mimetic m.
mucocutaneous m.
multifidus m.
mylohyoid m.
nasal m.
oblique abdominal m.
oblique arytenoid m.
oblique auricular m.
occipitofrontal m.
occipitofrontalis m.
ocular m.
omohyoid m.
orbicular m.
orbital m.
orbitalis m.
palatoglossus m.
palatopharyngeal sphincter m.
palatopharyngeus m.
palpebral m.
paraspinal m.
pectoralis m.
pectorodorsal m.
pennate m.
perineal m.
peroneal m.
peroneus brevis m.
peroneus longus m.
peroneus tertius m.

pharyngeal constrictor m.
piriform m.
plantar interosseous m.
plantar quadrate m.
platysma m.
pleuroesophageal m.
popliteal m.
posterior cricoarytenoid m.
procerus m.
pronator quadratus m.
pronator teres m.
m. proteolysis
psoas major m.
psoas minor m.
pterygoid m.
pubococcygeal m.
puboprostatic m.
puborectal m.
pubovaginal m.
pubovesical m.
pupillary m.
pyramidal auricular m.
quadrate m.
radial dilator m.
rectococcygeal m.
rectourethral m.
rectouterine m.
rectovesical m.
rectus m.
rectus abdominis m.
red m.
Reisseisen m.
m. relaxant
m. relaxation monitor
m. repositioning
m. resection
rhomboid major m.
rhomboid minor m.
ribbon m.
Riolan m.
risorius m.
rotator cuff m.
salpingopharyngeal m.
sartorius m.
scalene m.
scalenus anterior m.
scalenus medius m.
scalenus minimus m.
scalenus posterior m.
scalp m.
scapular m.
Sebileau m.
second tibial m.
semimembranosus m.
semispinal m.
semispinalis capitis m.
semispinalis cervicis m.
semitendinosus m.
serratus anterior m.

serratus posterior inferior m.
serratus posterior superior m.
shunt m.
Sibson m.
skeletal m.
m. sliding operation
smooth m.
Soemmerring m.
sphincter m.
sphincter pupillae m.
spinal m.
stapedius m.
sternal m.
sternochondroscapular m.
sternoclavicular m.
sternocleidomastoid m.
sternohyoid m.
sternomastoid m.
sternothyroid m.
strap m.
striated m. (StrAbs)
styloauricular m.
styloglossus m.
stylohyoid m.
stylopharyngeal m.
subclavian m.
subclavius m.
subcostal m.
suboccipital m.
subscapular m.
subscapularis m.
supinator m.
supraclavicular m.
suprahyoid m.
supraspinalis m.
supraspinatus m.
supraspinous m.
suspensory m.
synergistic m.
temporal m.
temporoparietal m.
tensor fasciae latae m.
Theile m.
thenar m.
thoracic interspinal m.
thoracic intertransverse m.
thoracic longissimus m.
thoracic rotator m.
thyroarytenoid m.
thyroepiglottic m.
thyrohyoid m.
thyroid m.
tibial m.
m. tissue mobility
toe extensor m.
Toynbee m.
trachealis m.
tracheloclavicular m.
tragicus m.

M

muscle (*continued*)
    transverse abdominal m.
    transverse arytenoid m.
    transverse rectus abdominis m.
      (TRAM)
    transversospinal m.
    transversus abdominis m.
    Treitz m.
    triangular m.
    true m.
    unipennate m.
    unstriated m.
    uvular m.
    Valsalva m.
    ventral sacrococcygeus m.
    vestigial m.
    visceral m.
    vocal m.
    vocalis m.
    m. wasting
    m. weakness
    white m.
    Wilson m.
    wrinkler m.
    zygomaticus major m.
    zygomaticus minor m.
muscle-balancing procedure
muscle-periosteal flap
muscle-plasty
    Speed V-Y m.-p.
muscle-sparing
    m.-s. incision
    m.-s. thoracotomy
muscle-splitting
    m.-s. incision
    m.-s. technique
muscle-tendon transplant
muscular
    m. anesthesia
    m. artery
    m. atrophy
    m. change
    m. coat
    m. contraction
    m. dystrophy (MD)
    m. esophageal ring
    m. fascia
    m. pulley
    m. substance
    m. tissue
    m. triangle
    m. tunic
muscularis
    m. propria
    tunica m.
    m. tunnel closure
musculature
musculi (*pl. of* musculus)
musculoaponeurotic layer

musculocutaneous
    m. free flap
    m. nerve
musculomembranous
musculopectineal orifice
musculophrenic
    m. artery
    m. vein
musculoplasty
    Rambo m.
musculoskeletal
    m. disorder
    m. infection
    m. system
    m. tissue
    m. tumor
musculospiral
    m. groove
    m. nerve
musculotendinous
    m. cuff
    m. flap
musculotubal canal
musculus, *pl.* **musculi**
    m. aryvocalis
    m. pleuroesophageus
mushroom
    corneal m.
    m. corneal graft
mushroom-shaped mass
mussitation
Mustard
    M. interarterial transposition of
      venous return operation
    M. interatrial transposition of
      venous return procedure
Mustardé
    M. hypospadias repair
      procedure
    M. otoplasty
    M. rotational cheek flap
mutation
    m. analysis
    breast cancer-related m.
    m. carrier
    m. carrier status
    factor V Leiden m.
    somatic m.
    true m.
mutilation
mutual participation model
Muzsnai modification
MV
    maternal venous
      MV blood
MVD
    microvascular decompression
MVO₂S
    mixed venous oxygen saturation

MVV
    maximal voluntary ventilation
    maximum voluntary ventilation
myalgia
    craniofacial m.
myasthenia gravis
myasthenic syndrome
mycelial mass
mycobacterial infection
Mycobacterium
    M. avium complex (MAC)
    M. avium complex infection
    M. avium-intracellulare (MAI)
    M. avium-intracellulare infection
mycophenolate mofetil
mycoplasma **infection**
mycotic
    m. abdominal aneurysm
    m. aneurysm
    m. club nail
    m. infection
    m. pseudoaneurysm
mydriasis
myectomy
    anorectal m.
    m. operation
    rectal m.
    septal m.
myectopia (*var. of* myectopy)
myectopy, myectopia
myelination, myelinization
    nerve fiber m.
    optic pathway m.
myelinization (*var. of* myelination)
myelinolysis
    central pontine m.
    pontine m.
myelitis
myeloablation
myeloblastoma
myelocele
myelocystocele
myelocystomeningocele
myelocytoma
myelodiastasis
myelodysplasia
myelofibrosis
myelography
myeloid tissue
myelolipoma
myelolysis
myeloma
myelomalacia
myelomeningocele
    m. operation
    m. repair
myelomonocytic cell line
myelonic
myelopathic symptom

myelopathy
    cervical spondylitic m.
    radiation m.
    spondylitic m.
myeloperoxidase determination
myelophthisic
myelophthisis
myelopoiesis
    extramedullary m.
myeloproliferative disorder
myelorrhagia
myelorrhaphy
    commissural m.
myelosarcoma
myeloschisis
myeloscopy
    flexible fiberoptic m.
myelotomy
    Bischof m.
    commissural m.
    midline m.
    midline punctate m.
    T m.
myenteric
    m. neural plexus
    m. plexus
    m. reflex
myenteron
mylohyoid
    m. artery
    m. bridge
    m. fossa
    m. groove
    m. line
    m. muscle
    m. nerve
    m. ridge
mylohyoideus
mylopharyngeus
myoablative therapy
myoarchitectonic
myoblastoma
myocardia (*pl. of* myocardium)
myocardial
    m. contractility
    m. contusion
    m. cytochrome
    m. hibernation
    m. infarction (MI)
    m. inflammation
    m. ischemia
    m. ischemic preconditioning
    m. mass
    m. necrosis
    m. oxygen demand
    m. oxygen supply
    m. perforation
    m. protection
    m. protection system

M

myocardial (*continued*)
    m. revascularization
    m. rupture
    m. stunning
    m. tissue
myocardiorrhaphy
myocarditis
myocardium, *pl.* **myocardia**
    postischemic stunned m.
    m. retrograde
    stunned m.
myocele
myoclonus
myocutaneous
    m. flap
    m. graft
myocytolysis
    coagulative m.
myocytoma
myodegeneration
myodermal flap
myodesis
myodiastasis
myoepithelioma
myofascial
    m. dehiscence
    m. dysfunction
    m. flap
    m. manipulation
    m. pain
    m. pain syndrome (MPS)
    m. release
    m. trigger point
myofeedback
myofibril
myofibroblastoma
myofibroma
myofilament disintegration
myofunctional therapy
myogenic
    m. headache
    m. motor-evoked potential (MEP)
myogenous temporomandibular disorder
myoglobin tubular obstruction
myoid cyst
myolipoma
myolysis
    cardiotoxic m.
myoma
    uterine m.
myomatectomy (*var. of* myomectomy)
myomectomy, myomatectomy
    abdominal m.
    laparoscopic esophageal m.
    vaginal m.
myomedulloblastoma
myometrial
myometrium

myomotomy
myonecrosis
    clostridial m.
myoneural blockade
myoneurectomy
myoneuroma
myoneurotization
myopathy
    acute quadriplegic m. (AQM)
    critical illness polyneuropathy and m. (CIPNM)
    familial visceral m.
    hollow visceral m.
    hollow viscus m.
myopectineal
    m. diaphragm
    m. orifice
myopia
    space m.
myoplastic muscle stabilization
myoplasty
myorrhaphy
myorrhexis
myosalpinx
myosarcoma
myositis
myosteoma
myotenontoplasty
myotenotomy
myotomy
    circular m.
    cricoid m.
    cricopharyngeal m.
    diverticulectomy with m.
    esophageal m.
    extended m.
    Heller m.
    laparoscopic Heller m.
    Livaditis circular m.
    longitudinal m.
    marginal m.
    m. operation
    pyloric m.
    septal m.
    Z m.
myotomy-myectomy-septal resection
myotonia fluctuans
myotonic
    m. dystrophy
    m. syndrome
myotoxicity
myovascular sphincter
myovenous sphincter
myringitis
    chronic granular m.
myringoplasty
myringostapediopexy
myringotomy with aspiration
myrinx

myxadenoma
myxedema
    m. ascites
    m. coma
myxochondrofibrosarcoma
myxochondroma
myxofibroma
myxofibrosarcoma

myxoid liposarcoma
myxolipoma
myxoliposarcoma
myxoma sarcomatosum
myxomatosis
myxoneuroma
myxopapilloma
myxosarcoma

M

N
newton
N pelvic ileal pouch
Na
sodium
nabothian cyst
Naclerio
V-sign of N.
NACS
Neurologic and Adaptive Capacity Score
nadir pressure
naevoid (*var. of* nevoid)
Naffziger exophthalmos operation
Nagamatsu incision
nail
anteroposterior n.
beak n.
n. bed
boat n.
brittle n.
cannulated n.
n. change
closed n.
clubbed n.
n. clubbing
condylocephalic n.
convex n.
digital n.
n. disorder
dystrophic n.
eggshell n.
n. fold
n. fold capillaroscopy
n. fold removal
n. groove
half-and-half n.
hooked intramedullary n.
n. horn
ingrown n.
left-sided n.
n. length gauge method
n. matrix
mycotic club n.
nested n.
onychocryptosis n.
open-section n.
parrot-beak n.
pincer n.
n. pit
pitted n.
n. pitting
n. plate fixation
n. plate removal

racket n.
ram horn n.
reamed n.
reedy n.
n. root
shell n.
sliding n.
telescoping n.
thickened n.
titanium flexible humeral n.
n. wall
yellow n.
Zickel n.
nailing
antegrade n.
femoral n.
intramedullary n.
reamed femoral n.
retrograde n.
tibiocalcaneal medullary n.
unreamed n.
nail-patella-elbow syndrome
nail-patella syndrome
nail-to-nail bed angle
NAIS
neoaortoiliac system
naive recipient
Nakajima cheiloplasty fan flap
Nakayama anastomosis
nalbuphine
Nalebuff-Millender swan-neck deformity lateral band mobilization technique
Nalebuff swan-neck deformity classification
naloxone
naltrexone
Nance leeway space
nanogram (ng)
napkin-ring
n.-r. carcinoma
n.-r. compression
n.-r. defect
napkin ring anular lesion
naprapathic therapy
naprapathy
naproxen
narcosis
adsorption theory of n.
carbon dioxide n.
colloid theory of n.
lipoid theory of n.
Meyer-Overton theory of n.
nitrogen n.
oxygen deprivation theory of n.
permeability theory of n.

N

narcosis (*continued*)
  surface tension theory of n.
  thermodynamic theory of n.
narcotic
  n. analgesic
  n. reversal
narcotism
nares (*pl. of* naris)
naris, *pl.* **nares**
Naropin
narrow-complex supraventricular
 tachycardia resuscitation algorithm
narrowed pulse pressure
narrow-field laryngectomy
narrowing
  disc space n.
  eccentric n.
  joint space n.
narrow internal ring
narrow-slit illumination
Narula sinoatrial conduction time
 method
nasal
  n. airway
  n. alar necrosis
  n. antrostomy
  n. border
  n. canal
  n. cavity
  n. cavity cancer
  n. concha
  n. crest
  n. deformity
  n. dissection
  n. endoscopic surgery
  n. endoscopy
  n. foramen
  n. fracture
  n. granuloma gravidarum
  n. height
  n. hemorrhage
  n. index
  n. intubation
  n. mucosal identification
  n. mucosal ulceration
  n. muscle
  n. oxygen
  n. packing
  n. pharynx
  n. placode
  n. port
  n. provocation test
  n. pyramid
  n. reconstruction
  n. respiration
  n. septal perforation
  n. septum
  n. tip
  n. tract

  n. trumpet
  n. vestibule
  n. wall
nasioiniac
nasion-alveolar point line
nasion soft tissue
Nasmyth membrane
nasobasilar line
nasobregmatic arc
nasociliary
  n. ganglion
  n. nerve
nasoendoscopy
nasoenteric feeding tube
nasofrontal
  n. duct
  n. suture
  n. vein
nasofrontalis
nasogastric (NG, N-G)
  n. decompression
  n. intubation
  n. suction
  n. tonometry
  n. tube (NGT)
nasoileal
nasojejunal
  n. nutrition
  n. tube
nasojugal fold
nasolabial
  n. groove
  n. line
  n. rotation flap
nasolacrimal
  n. canal
  n. sac
nasomandibular fixation
nasomaxillary suture
nasooccipital arc
nasooral
nasoorbital fracture
nasopalatine injection
nasopharyngeal
  n. airway (NPA)
  n. biopsy
  n. carcinoma (NPC)
  n. groove
  n. hematoma
  n. hemorrhage
  n. passage
  n. suction
nasopharyngoscopy
nasopharynx (NP, NPhx)
nasorostral
nasotracheal
  n. intubation (NTI)
  n. intubation anesthetic technique
  n. suction

n. suctioning
n. tube fixation using infant feeding tube
nasovesicular catheter technique
NASPE
North American Society of Pacing and Electrophysiology
NASS
North American Spine Society
natal cleft
natatorium
nates
Nathanson retractors
Nathan-Trung modification of Krukenberg hand reconstruction
national
N. Blood Resource Education Committee
N. Cancer Data Base (NCDB)
N. Cancer Institute (NCI)
N. Center for Complementary and Alternative Medicine (NCCAM)
N. Football Head and Neck Injury Registry
N. Marrow Donor Program (NMDP)
N. Nosocomial Infections Surveillance System (NNIS)
N. Pediatric Trauma Registry (NPTR)
N. Surgical Adjuvant Breast and Bowel Project (NSABP)
N. Surgical Quality Improvement Program (NSQIP)
N. Survey on Drug Use and Health (NSDUH)
N. Trauma Data Bank (NTDB)
native
n. caudate lobe
n. coronary anatomy
n. esophagus
n. liver
n. myocardial microcirculation
n. portal vein
n. renal biopsy
natriuresis
pressure n.
natural
n. method
n. suture
nature
benign n.
dense n.
minimally invasive n.
pathologic n.
n. root canal filling
secretomotor n.
nausea
postprandial n.

navel
navicular
n. abdomen
n. bone
n. fracture
naviculocapitate
n. fracture
n. fracture syndrome
naviculocuneiform fusion
navigated
n. brain tumor surgery
n. neurosurgery
n. surgical resection
navigation
image-guided n.
surgical microscope n.
n. system
navigational surgery
NCCAM
National Center for Complementary and Alternative Medicine
NCCPC
Non-Communicating Children's Pain Checklist
NCDB
National Cancer Data Base
NCI
National Cancer Institute
NCJ
needle catheter jejunostomy
NCPB
neurolytic celiac plexus block
NCRLM
noncolorectal liver metastasis
isolated NCRLM
unique NCRLM
Nd
neodymium
NDSA
nondermatomal sensory abnormality
NDT
noise detection threshold
Nd:YAG
neodymium:yttrium-aluminum-garnet
Nd:YAG cyclophotocoagulation
Nd:YAG laser ablation
Nd:YAG laser irradiation
Nd:YAG laser therapy
Nealon provisional dental restoration technique
near
n. fixation
n. infrared(NIR)
n. visual point
near-anatomic position
near-and-far suture technique
near-infrared
n.-i. measurement

N

near-infrared (*continued*)
    n.-i. spectrophotometry
    n.-i. spectroscopy (NIRS, NIS)
near-point relative
near-total
    n.-t. esophagectomy
    n.-t. gastrectomy
    n.-t. laryngectomy
    n.-t. pancreatectomy
    n.-t. splenectomy
    n.-t. thyroidectomy
NEB
    New England Baptist
    NEB hip arthroplasty
nebula, *pl.* **nebulae**
    corneal n.
nebulae (*pl. of* nebula)
nebulization
nebulized lidocaine
nebulizer
    spinning disc n.
    ultrasonic n.
NEC
    necrotizing enterocolitis
neck
    anterolateral n.
    aortic n.
    deep anterior n.
    N. Disability Index
    n. dissection
    n. exploration
    n. extension position
    n. flap
    n. flexion
    n. fracture
    gallbladder n.
    implant n.
    implant superstructure n.
    innervation of head and n.
    pancreatic n.
    residual n.
    superficial n.
    surgical n.
    virgin n.
necrectomy
necrolysis
    epidermal n.
    toxic epidermal n.
necrolytic migratory erythema
necropsy, necroscopy
necroscopy (*var. of* necropsy)
necrosectomy
    initial n.
    operative n.
    reoperative n.
necroses (*pl. of* necrosis)
necrosis, *pl.* **necroses**
    acute tubular n. (ATN)
    aminoglycoside tubular n.

    avascular n. (AVN)
    bloodless zone of n.
    bony n.
    caseation n.
    centrilobular n.
    cerebral radiation n.
    cheesy n.
    coagulation n.
    coumarin n.
    CT-proven n.
    cystic medial n.
    diffuse n.
    electrocoagulation n.
    Erdheim cystic medial n.
    ethanol-induced tumor n.
    fat n.
    flap n.
    frank n.
    hepatic n.
    hepatocytic n.
    infected n.
    infected pancreatic n.
    liquefaction n.
    mummification n.
    myocardial n.
    nasal alar n.
    pancreatic n.
    periodontal membrane n.
    peripancreatic n.
    pressure n.
    radiation n.
    skin flap n.
    soft tissue n.
    splenic n.
    strangulation n.
    subcutaneous n.
    thermal n.
    tissue n.
    tumor n.
necrotic
    n. abscess
    n. flap
    n. focus
    n. hemorrhoid
    n. hyalinized tissue
    n. inflammation
    n. metastasis
    n. remains
    n. ulceration
necrotic/fibrotic tissue
necrotizing
    n. angiitis
    n. enterocolitis (NEC)
    n. fasciitis
    n. granulomatous inflammation
    n. infection
    n. pancreatitis
necrotomy
    osteoplastic n.

needle
    n. ablation
    access n.
    n. arthroscopy
    n. aspiration
    n. aspiration cytology
    n. catheter jejunostomy (NCJ)
    Chang n.
    n. core biopsy
    Crawford epidural n.
    n. electrode examination
    Espocan epidural n.
    Greene spinal n.
    n. holder
    Huber n.
    Hustead epidural n.
    n. insertion
    insulated epidural n.
    Keith n.
    n. laparoscopy
    n. localization
    noninsulated n.
    n. prick
    Quick Stitch n.
    Quincke spinal n.
    n. reaction
    sham n.
    Sprotte spinal n.
    n. suspension procedure
    n. thoracentesis
    n. thoracentesis method
    n. thoracentesis procedure
    n. thoracentesis technique
    n. tracheoesophageal puncture
    n. tract
    n. tract implantation
    n. tract tumor seeding
    Veress n.
    warming n.
    Weiss epidural n.
    Whitacre spinal n.
needle-free system
needle-knife
    n.-k. papillotomy
    n.-k. sphincterotomy
    n.-k. technique
needleless
    n. intravenous administration
        system
    n. suturing
needle-localized
    n.-l. excisional biopsy
    n.-l. open biopsy (NLOB)
needlepoint electrocautery
needlescopic
    n. appendectomy
    n. laparoscopic
        cholecystectomy
needlescopy

Needles split cast method
Needless Wound suture
needlestick injury
2-needle technique
needle-through-needle single interspace
    technique
needling
    dry n.
Neer
    N. acromioplasty
    N. capsular shift procedure
    N. femur fracture classification
    N. hemiarthroplasty
    N. modification
    N. open reduction
    N. posterior shoulder reconstruction
    N. shoulder fracture classification
    N. unconstrained shoulder
        arthroplasty
nefopam
negative
    n. abdominal pressure
    n. appendectomy
    n. aspiration
    axillary node n.
    n. breast biopsy
    n. celiotomy
    n. correlation
    n. cytology
    n. effect
    n. end-expiratory pressure
    false n.
    n. inotropy
    n. inspiratory breathing
    n. inspiratory pressure measurement
    n. laparotomy
    n. margin
    n. peritoneal cytology
    n. predictive value (NPV)
    n. pressure
    n. pressure closure technique
    n. pressure operating theater
    n. pressure pulmonary edema
    n. pressure therapy
    n. pressure ventilation (NPV)
    n. tropism
    true n.
    tumor receptor protein n.
negative-pressure
neglected rupture
neglectlike phenomena
Neher acute pancreatitis operation
Nehra esophageal operation
Neill-Mooser body
neisserial infection
Nélaton
    N. ankle dislocation
    N. fiber
    N. fold

N

Nélaton (*continued*)
    N. line
    N. sphincter
nematode infection
neoadjuvant
    n. chemoradiation
    n. therapy
    n. total androgen ablation
    n. treatment
neoaortoiliac system (NAIS)
neoatrial cuff
neobladder
    Hartmann n.
    Mainz n.
    Studer n.
    T-pouch ileal n.
neocartilage formation
neocystostomy
neodymium (Nd)
neodymium:yttrium-aluminum-garnet (Nd:YAG)
neoesophagus
neoformation
neoglottic reconstruction
neointima formation
neointimal hyperplasia
neonatal
    n. anesthesia
    N. Facial Coding System (NFCS)
    N. Facial Pain Inventory (NFPI)
    N. Infant Pain Scale (NIPS)
    n. infection
    n. intracranial hemorrhage
    n. intraventricular hemorrhage
    n. line
    n. pulmonary transplant
    n. resuscitation
    n. ring
    n. severe hyperparathyroidism (NSHPT)
    n. testicular torsion
    n. thymectomy
neonate
    n. examination
    surgical n.
    n. ventilation
neoplasia
    colonic n.
    cystic n.
    hepatic n.
    intraaxial parenchymal brain n.
    intraductal oncocytic papillary n.
    intraductal papillary mucinous n. (IPMN)
    multiple endocrine n. (MEN)
    multiple intestinal n.
    pancreatic n.

    pancreatic endocrine n.
    parenchymal brain n.
    pediatric n.
    thymic n.
    thyroid n.
    vascular n.
neoplasm
    asymptomatic n.
    brain n.
    colon n.
    cystic n.
    follicular n.
    hepatic n.
    histoid n.
    intrapancreatic n.
    n. metastasis
    mucinous cystic n. (MCN)
    mucin-producing n.
    pancreatic n.
    pediatric n.
    second malignant n. (SMN)
    thymic n.
    thyroid n.
neoplastic
    n. dissemination
    n. fracture
    n. lesion
    n. pathology
    n. port site implant
    n. renal mass
    n. tissue
    n. transformation
neorectal function
neosalpingostomy
    terminal n.
neosaxitoxin
neosphincter
    gracilis n.
neostigmine toxicity
neostomy
neotrigeminothalamic tract
neoumbilicus
neovagina
    skin graft n.
neovascular
    n. bundle
    n. membrane
    n. network
neovascularization
    choroidal n.
    corneal n.
    disc n.
    disseminated asymptomatic unilateral n.
    interstitial n.
    iris n.
    pathologic n.
    preretinal n.
    retinal quadrant n.

stromal n.
subretinal n.
vitreous n.
neovasculature
tumor n.
nephradenoma
nephralgia
nephralgic
nephratonia
nephrectomy
abdominal n.
adjuvant n.
anterior n.
apical polar n.
Balkan n.
extracorporeal partial n.
extraperitoneal laparoscopic n.
hand-assisted laparoscopic
live-donor n.
laparoscopic n.
laparoscopic ablative n.
laparoscopic-assisted living
donor n.
laparoscopic donor n. (LDN)
laparoscopic live donor n.
laparoscopic partial n.
laser partial n.
late transplant n.
live donor n.
living donor n.
lumbar n.
open partial n.
paraperitoneal n.
partial n.
perifascial n.
posterior n.
radical n.
retroperitoneoscopic n.
transperitoneal laparoscopic n.
transplant n.
unilateral n.
nephredema
nephrelcosis
nephric
nephritic
n. calculus
n. colic
n. syndrome
nephritides (*pl. of* nephritis)
nephritis, *pl.* **nephritides**
interstitial n.
lupus n.
nephritogenic
nephroblastoma
nephroblastomatosis
nephrocalcinosis
nephrocapsectomy
nephrocardiac
nephrocele

nephrogenetic, nephrogenic
n. cord
n. tissue
nephrogenic (*var. of* nephrogenetic)
nephrogenous
nephrohydrosis
nephroid
nephrolith
nephrolithiasis
nephrolithotomy
anatrophic n.
Lawson retrograde percutaneous n.
percutaneous n. (PCN, PCNL,
PNL)
simultaneous bilateral percutaneous
n.'s (SBPN)
nephrolithotripsy
percutaneous n. (PCNL)
nephrology
nephrolysis
nephrolytic
nephroma
nephron
nephronia
lobar n.
nephronic loop
nephronophthisis (*var. of* nephrophthisis)
nephron-sparing surgery (NSS)
nephropathia (*var. of* nephropathy)
nephropathic
nephropathy, nephropathia
contrast n.
contrast-induced n.
diabetic peripheral n.
end-stage reflux n.
membranous n.
nephropexy
nephrophthisis, nephronophthisis
nephroptosia (*var. of* nephroptosis)
nephroptosis, nephroptosia
nephropyeloplasty
nephropyosis
nephrorrhaphy
nephros
nephrosclerosis
nephroscopic fulguration
nephroscopy
anatrophic n.
flexible n.
percutaneous n.
nephrosis
nephrospasia
nephrostolithotomy
calyceal n.
percutaneous n. (PCNL)
nephrostomy
circle wire n.
n. drainage
open n.

N

nephrostomy (*continued*)
    percutaneous n. (PCN)
    n. puncture
    U-loop n.
nephrotic
    n. edema
    n. syndrome
nephrotomic cavity
nephrotomy
    anatrophic n.
nephrotoxic
nephrotoxicity
    acute n.
    fluoride-induced n.
nephrotoxin
nephrotrophic, nephrotropic
nephrotropic (*var. of* nephrotrophic)
nephrotuberculosis
nephroureterectomy
    bilateral nephroureterectomies
    radical n.
    retroperitoneoscopic n.
    transperitoneal laparoscopic n.
nephroureterocystectomy
nephroureteroscopy
nerve
    abdominopelvic splanchnic n.
    abducent n. [CN VI]
    accelerator n.
    accessory n.
    acoustic n.
    n. allografting
    alveolar n.
    n. anastomosis
    Andersch n.
    ansa cervicalis n.
    anterior auricular n.
    anterior cutaneous n.
    anterior ethmoidal n.
    anterior labial n.
    anterior scrotal n.
    anterior supraclavicular n.
    Arnold n.
    articular recurrent n.
    auditory tube n.
    augmentor n.
    auricular n.
    auriculotemporal n.
    autonomic n.
    axillary n.
    baroreceptor n.
    Bell respiratory n.
    n. biopsy
    n. block
    n. block anesthesia
    n. block infusion
    Bock n.
    brachial plexus n.
    buccal n.

buccinator n.
cardiac n.
caroticotympanic n.
cavernous n.
centrifugal n.
centripetal n.
cervical splanchnic n.
chorda tympani n.
ciliary n.
circumflex n.
n. coaptation
coccygeal n.
cochlear n.
common peroneal n.
communicating n.
n. compression anesthesia
n. compression-degeneration
    syndrome
n. conduction velocity examination
corneal n.
cranial n. (CN1–CN12)
n. cross section
cutaneous cervical n.
n. decompression
deep peroneal n.
deep petrosal n.
deep temporal n.
dental n.
descending n.
dorsal interosseous n.
dorsal rami n.
dorsal scapular n.
eighth cranial n.
eleventh cranial n.
entrapped n.
esodic n.
ethmoidal n.
n. excitability test
excitor n.
excitoreflex n.
exodic n.
external branch of superior
    laryngeal n.
external nasal n.
external saphenous n.
external spermatic n.
extrinsic n.
facial n.
femoral n.
n. fiber bundle
n. fiber bundle layer
n. fiber myelination
fifth cranial n.
first cranial n.
fold of laryngeal n.
fourth cranial n.
fourth lumbar n.
furcal n.
Galen n.

gangliated n.
genitocrural n.
genitofemoral n.
glossopharyngeal n.
n. graft
great auricular n.
greater occipital n. (GON)
n. growth factor receptor
gustatory n.
hemorrhoidal n.
Hering n.
hypogastric n.
hypoglossal n.
iliohypogastric n.
ilioinguinal n.
n. implantation
inferior alveolar n.
inferior hemorrhoidal n.
inferior laryngeal n.
inferior palpebral n.
inferior rectal n.
inferior vesical n.
infraorbital n.
infratrochlear n.
inhibitory n.
n. injury
intercarotid n.
intercostal n.
intercostobrachial n.
intercostohumeral n.
intermediary n.
internal rectal n.
interosseous n.
Jacobson n.
jugular n.
lacrimal n.
laryngeal n.
Latarget n.
lingual n.
long thoracic n.
lumbar n. (L1–L5)
lumboinguinal n.
mandibular n.
masseteric n.
masticator n.
maxillary n.
medial pectoral n.
median n.
mental n.
mixed n.
motor n.
musculocutaneous n.
musculospiral n.
mylohyoid n.
nasociliary n.
ninth cranial n.
obturator n.
occipital n.
oculomotor n.

olfactory n.
olivocochlear n.
Oort n.
ophthalmic n.
optic n.
palatine n.
palpebral n.
n. paralysis
parasympathetic n.
pericardiophrenic n.
perineal n.
peripheral n.
peritonsillar n.
peroneal communicating n.
petrosal n.
phrenic n. (PN)
plantar digital n.
pneumogastric n.
popliteal communicating n.
posterior auricular n.
presacral n.
pterygoid n.
pterygopalatine n.
pudendal n.
pudic n.
rectal n.
recurrent laryngeal n. (RLN)
recurrent meningeal n.
n. regeneration
right common iliac n.
n. root
n. root compression
n. rootlet ablation
n. root sleeve injection
sacral splanchnic n.
second cranial n.
secretory n.
sensory n.
seventh cranial n.
sinocarotid n.
sinuvertebral n.
sixth cranial n.
somatic n.
sphenopalatine n.
spinal accessory n.
splanchnic n.
statoacoustic n.
n. stimulator anesthetic technique
subclavian n.
subcostal n.
suboccipital n.
subscapular n.
supraclavicular n.
supraorbital n.
suprascapular n.
supratrochlear n.
sural n.
n. suture
n. suture technique

N

nerve (*continued*)
    sympathetic n.
    temporal n.
    temporomandibular n.
    tenth cranial n.
    tentorial n.
    third cranial n.
    third occipital n.
    thoracic cardiac n.
    thoracic spinal n.
    thoracoabdominal n.
    thoracodorsal n.
    Tiedemann n.
    n. tract
    transverse cervical n.
    trifacial n.
    trigeminal n.
    trochlear n.
    n. trunk
    twelfth cranial n.
    upper subscapular n.
    vaginal n.
    vagus n.
    vascular n.
    vasomotor n.
    vesical n.
    vestibular n.
    vestibulocochlear n.
    vidian n.
    visceral n.
    vomeronasal n.
    Wrisberg n.
    zygomatic n.
nerve-containing plate
nerve-point massage
nerve-preserving parotidectomy
nerve-sparing
    n.-s. dissection
    n.-s. radical retropubic prostatectomy
nervi (*pl. of* nervus)
nervosa
    foramina n.
nervous
    n. damage
    n. exhaustion
    n. respiration
    n. system (NS)
    n. system involvement
nervus, *pl.* **nervi**
    nervi erigentes
    n. furcalis
    n. hypogastricus
    n. infratrochlearis
Nesbit
    N. congenital curvature of penis
      operation
    N. corporeal plication
    N. tuck penis straightening
      procedure

nesidiectomy
nesidioblastoma
nest
    Brunn n.
    choristoma n.
nested nail
net
    vascular n.
network
    acromial arterial n.
    articular vascular n.
    calcaneal arterial n.
    Cancer Genetics N.
    cytokine n.
    medial malleolar n.
    neovascular n.
    neural n
    Organ Procurement and
      Transplantation N. (OPTN)
    patellar n.
    peritarsal n.
    plantar venous n.
    Purkinje n.
    somatotrophic n.
    trabecular n.
Neubauer artery
Neugebauer-Le Fort colpocleisis
  procedure
neural
    n. arch
    n. arch resection technique
    n. axis vascular malformation
    n. canal
    n. crest malformation
    n. crest migration
    n. lesion
    n. mapping
    n. network
    n. plasticity
    n. spine
    n. stimulator
    n. tissue
    n. tube
    n. tube defect
neuralgia
    acute and postherpetic n.
    acute herpetic n.
    geniculate n.
    glossopharyngeal n.
    inguinal n.
    intercostal n.
    laparoscopic-induced n.
    occipital n.
    petrosal n.
    postherpetic n. (PHN)
    postsympathectomy n.
    posttraumatic gustatory n.
    secondary n.
    Sluder n.

trigeminal n.
vagoglossopharyngeal n.
vidian n.
neuralgic
neurapophysis
neurasthenia, neurosthenia
experimental n.
neuraxial
n. analgesia
n. anesthesia
n. blockade
n. medication trial
n. neurolytic block
n. opioid
neurectasia (*var. of* neurectasis)
neurectasis, neurectasia, neurectasy
neurectasy (*var. of* neurectasis)
neurectomy, neuroectomy
cochleovestibular n.
Cotte presacral n.
Eggers n.
genitofemoral n.
Green and McDermott gastrocnemius
lengthening at origin with/
without n.
iliohypogastric n.
ilioinguinal n.
inguinal n.
Keen torticollis n.
obturator n.
occipital n.
opticociliary n.
peripheral n.
pharyngeal plexus n.
Phelps n.
presacral n.
retrogasserian n.
retrolabyrinthine-retrosigmoid
vestibular n.
retrolabyrinthine vestibular n.
Sonnenberg n.
transcochlear cochleovestibular n.
transcochlear vestibular n.
transtympanic n.
tympanic n.
ulnar motor n.
vestibular n.
neurenteric canal
neurepithelium (*var. of*
neuroepithelium)
neurilemmoma (*var. of* neurilemoma)
neurilemmosarcoma
neurilemoma, neurilemmoma,
neurolemmoma
neurinoma
neuritic plaque
neuritis
ischemic optic n.
vibration n.

neuroablation
cryogenic n.
neuroablative technique
neuroadenolysis
pituitary n.
neuroanastomosis
neuroanatomic acupuncture
neuroanatomy
neuroanesthesia
neuroastrocytoma
neuroaugmentation
neuroaxial opioid
neuroblastoma
neuroborreliosis
neurocele
neurocentral
n. joint
n. suture
neurochemical stimulation
neurocirculation
neurocladism
neurocognitive change
neurocranium
neurocutaneous island flap
neurocytolysis
neurocytoma
neurodiagnostic evaluation
neuroectomy (*var. of* neurectomy)
neuroeffector junction
neuroelectric
n. event
n. source imaging
neuroendocrine
n. cancer
n. exhaustion
n. metastasis
n. skin carcinoma
n. stress response
n. system
n. tumor
neuroepithelioma
neuroepithelium, neurepithelium
neurofibroma
plexiform n.
neurofibromatosis
neurofibrosarcoma
neuroganglion
neurogastric
neurogenetic (*var. of* neurogenic)
neurogenic, neurogenetic, neurogenous
n. bladder
n. bladder dysfunction
n. blockade
n. dysregulation
n. fracture
n. hypertension
n. incontinence
n. intermittent claudication
n. PGID

N

neurogenic (*continued*)
    n. pulmonary edema (NPE)
    n. shock
    n. theory
neurogenous (*var. of* neurogenic)
neurogliomatosis
neuroglycopenia
neurohypophysial
neurohypophysis
neuroimaging
neuroinflammatory mediator
neurolemmoma (*var. of* neurilemoma)
neuroleptanalgesia (NLA)
    n. anesthesia
    n. anesthetic technique
neuroleptanesthesia (NLA)
neuroleptic
    n. agent
    n. malignant syndrome (NMS)
neurologic, neurological
    N. and Adaptive Capacity Score (NACS)
    n. complication
    n. deficit
    n. disease
    n. disorder
    n. examination
    n. failure
    n. function
    n. injury
    n. manifestation
    n. recovery
    n. surgery
    n. symptom
neurological (*var. of* neurologic)
    n. evaluation
    n. surgery
neurology
    surgical n.
neurolysis
    distal n.
    internal n.
    intrathecal n.
    sympathetic n.
neurolytic
    n. agent
    n. blockade
    n. celiac plexus block (NCPB)
neuroma, neurinoma, *pl.* **neuromata, neuromas**
    acoustic n.
    n. relocation surgery
neuromagnetic source imaging
neuroma-in-continuity
neuromas (*pl. of* neuroma)
neuromata (*pl. of* neuroma)
neuromatosis
neuromediator
    excitatory n.

neuromodulation technique
neuromodulator
    inhibitory n.
neuromotor dysfunction
neuromuscular
    n. block
    n. blockade (NMB)
    n. blockade monitoring
    n. blocking agent (NMBA)
    n. blocking drug (NMBD)
    n. electrical stimulation
    n. facilitation
    n. junction
    n. pedicle graft
    n. proprioception exercise
    n. relaxant
    n. system electric induction
    n. transmission
neuron, neurone
    inspiratory bulbospinal n.
    nondopaminergic n.
neuronal
    n. cell line
    n. excitability
    n. membrane
    n. migration
    n. nicotinic acetylcholine receptor
    n. nicotinic receptor activation
    n. plasticity
    n. regeneration
    n. windup
neuronavigation
neuronavigational system
neurone (*var. of* neuron)
neuronephric
neuronoma
Neurontin
neuroophthalmic manifestation
neuroophthalmologic examination
neuropathic
    n. bladder
    n. central pain
    n. fracture
    n. pain
    n. pain diagnostic questionnaire (DN4)
    n. pain from amputation
    n. ulcer
neuropathicum
    papilloma n.
neuropathologist
neuropathology
neuropathophysiology
    normalization of n.
neuropathy
    acquired immunodeficiency virus-associated distal sensory n. (AADSN)
    antiretroviral toxic n. (ATN)

autoimmune n.
diabetic n.
focal n.
hereditary sensory and autonomic n. (HSAN)
inherited n.
optic n.
stretch-induced n.
traumatic optic n.
neurophysiologic examination
neuroplasticity
neuroplasty
epidural n.
neuropsychological deficit
neuropsychologic test
neuroradiologic evaluation
neuroradiology
interventional n.
neurorrhaphy
epineurial n.
perineurial n.
neurosarcocleisis
neurosarcoma
neuroschwannoma
neurosthenia (*var. of* neurasthenia)
neurostimulating procedure
neurostimulation trial
neurosurgeon
pediatric n.
neurosurgery
decompressive n.
functional stereotactic n.
image-guided interactive n.
navigated n.
stereotactic n.
neurosurgical
n. anesthesia
n. approach
n. intensive care unit (NSICU)
n. intervention
n. procedure
n. suture
neurosuture
neurotendinous
neurothekeoma
neurotic excoriation
neuroticism
neurotization
neurotize
neurotologic examination
neurotomy
Dandy retroganglial n.
opticociliary n.
percutaneous radiofrequency n.
radiofrequency cervical zygapophysial joint n.
retrogasserian n.
neurotoxicity
chloroprocaine-related n.

neurotoxicology
neurotransmission
glutamatergic n.
neurotransmitter system
neurotrauma
neurotripsy
neurotrophic factor
neurotrosis
neuroureterectomy
neurourology
neurovaricosis, neurovaricosity
neurovaricosity (*var. of* neurovaricosis)
neurovascular
n. anatomy
n. bundle
n. complication
n. compression syndrome
n. crosscompression
n. free flap
n. island graft
n. island pedicle flap
n. lesion
n. pain
n. sheath
neuroxanthoendothelioma
neutral
n. hip position
n. point
n. rotation
n. spine position
neutralization
n. plate fixation
serum n.
n. test
neutron
n. activation analysis
n. beam therapy
n. capture therapy
neutropenia-related bacterial infection
neutrophil, neutrophile
n. activation
n. migration
polymorphonuclear n. (PMN)
neutrophil-dependent tissue destruction
neutrophile (*var. of* neutrophil)
neutrophilic
n. infiltration
n. inflammation
nevi (*pl. of* nevus)
Neviaser
N. acromioclavicular technique
N. old shoulder dislocation operation
Neviaser-Wilson-Gardner first dorsal interosseus replacement technique
nevocarcinoma
nevoid, naevoid
n. anomaly
n. basal cell carcinoma syndrome

N

nevoxanthoendothelioma
 juvenile n.
nevus, *pl.* **nevi**
 bathing trunk n.
 spider n.
new
 N. England Baptist (NEB)
 N. England Baptist hip arthroplasty
 N. York Heart Association heart
  disease classification
 N. York State Trauma Registry
  (NYSTR)
newborn
 n. anesthesia
 n. examination
 n. resuscitation
**Newman radial neck and head fracture
 classification**
newton (N)
newtonian
 n. aberration
 n. body
NFCS
 Neonatal Facial Coding System
NFPI
 Neonatal Facial Pain Inventory
NG
 nasogastric
 NG suction
 NG tube
NHBD
 nonheart-beating donor
NIBP
 noninvasive blood pressure
nicardipine hydrochloride
NICH
 noninvoluting congenital hemangioma
Nicholas
 N. coracoclavicular congenital knee
  dislocation ligament technique
 N. 5-in-1 knee reconstruction
  technique
Nichols
 N. bowel prep
 N. sacrospinous fixation
nick
 skin n.
nickel-and-dime lesion
**Nicks aortic anulus enlargement
 procedure**
Nicola
 N. incision
 N. shoulder tenodesis procedure
Nicoll
 N. cancellous bone graft
 N. cancellous insert graft
 N. fracture reconstruction
 N. fracture repair procedure
 N. spinal fracture classification

**nicotinamide adenine dinucleotide
 phosphate oxidase**
nicotine
 intranasal n.
nicotinic
 n. excitation
 n. receptor
nictation (*var. of* nictitation)
nictitation, nictation
nidi (*pl. of* nidus)
nidus, *pl.* **nidi**
 cellular n.
**Niebauer-King congenital knee
 dislocation open reduction technique**
**Niebauer trapeziometacarpal
 arthroplasty**
Niemeier
 N. gallbladder perforation
 N. gallbladder perforation
  classification
nightstick fracture
nigroid body
Nigro protocol
nigrostriatal tract
**Nikaidoh-Bex TGA with VSD repair
 technique**
nil disease
ninth cranial nerve
nipple
 accessory n.
 aortic n.
 n. aspiration cytology
 n. line
 n. reconstruction
 n. retraction
 n. stimulation test
nipple-areola reconstruction
nippled stoma
nipple-flat duct resection
nipple-sparing mastectomy
NIPS
 Neonatal Infant Pain Scale
 noninvasive programmed electrical
  stimulation
NIR
 near infrared
NIRS
 near-infrared spectroscopy
Nirschl
 N. lateral epicondylitis mini-open
  technique
 N. tennis elbow release
Nissen
 N. antireflux operation
 N. fundoplasty
 N. fundoplication
 N. fundoplication method
 N. fundoplication of stomach
  procedure

N. fundoplication technique
N. fundoplication wrap
N. fundus repair
Nissen-Rossetti
N.-R. fundoplication
N.-R. fundoplication method
N.-R. fundoplication procedure
N.-R. fundoplication technique
nitrate-induced venodilation
nitric
n. oxide (NO)
n. oxide bioavailability
n. oxide blocked sphincter relaxation
n. oxide signaling
nitrogen
blood urea n. (BUN)
n. concentration
expiratory n.
n. monoxide
n. narcosis
n. partial pressure
nitroglycerine
nitroprusside-induced cyanide production
nitrous
n. oxide (N_2O)
n. oxide-opioid-barbiturate anesthetic technique
n. oxide-oxygen (N_2O-O_2)
n. oxide-oxygen-opioid anesthetic technique
nitrovasodilator
Nizetic corneal transplant
NLOB
needle-localized open biopsy
NMB
neuromuscular blockade
NMBA
neuromuscular blocking agent
NMBD
neuromuscular blocking drug
NMDP
National Marrow Donor Program
N-methyl-D aspartate receptor
NMR
nuclear magnetic resonance
NMR spectroscopy
NMS
neuroleptic malignant syndrome
NMT
neuromuscular transmission
NNIS
National Nosocomial Infections Surveillance
NNIS system
NO
nitric oxide
no
n. infection-no rejection

n. rejection
n. residual disease (R0)
N_2O
nitrous oxide
Noble
N. bowel plication
N. position
N. surgical plication of bowel
Noble-Mengert perineal repair
nocebo
nociception
nociceptive
n. pain
n. stimulation
nociceptor afferent peripheral terminal
nocturia, nycturia
nocturnal
n. enuresis
n. painful tonic spasm (NPTS)
nodal
n. disease
n. extirpation
n. involvement
n. metastasis
n. plane
n. point
n. recurrence
n. step-sectioning
n. tissue
n. yield
node (N)
aberrant n.
atrioventricular n.
AV n.
n. biopsy
buccinator n.
Cloquet n.
companion lymph n.
coronary n.
cystic n.
delphian n.
diaphragmatic n.
n. dissection
foraminal n.
free n.
gastroomental n.
hot sentinel n.
inferior mesenteric lymph n.
infraclavicular n.
intercostal lymph n.
internal mammary n.
intramammary sentinel n.
n. involvement
jugulodigastric lymph n.
juguloomohyoid n.
n. lymphoma
malar n.
mammary n.
mandibular n.

N

node (*continued*)
    mastoid n.
    matted n.
    mesenteric n.
    mesenteric lymph n.
    nonsentinel n.
    occipital n.
    parasternal lymph n.
    paratracheal n.
    parietal n.
    parotid n.
    perigastric n.
    prelaryngeal n.
    pretracheal n.
    radiolabeled sentinel n.
    Ranvier n.
    regional n.
    retroauricular n.
    retroperitoneal n.
    retropharyngeal n.
    retropyloric n.
    Rosenmüller n.
    SA n.
    sentinel n.
    sentinel lymph n. (SLN)
    sinuatrial n.
    n. station
    sternal lymph n.
    subdigastric n.
    submandibular n.
    submental n.
    subpyloric n.
    superior mesenteric lymph n.
    supraclavicular n.
    suprapyloric n.
    Tawara n.
    tracheal n.
    tracheobronchial n.
    visceral n.
node-negative
    n.-n. disease
    n.-n. melanoma
node-positive
    n.-p. breast cancer
    n.-p. disease
    n.-p. melanoma
nodi (*pl. of* nodus)
nodose ganglion
nodoventricular tract
nodular
    n. chondrodermatitis
    n. hidradenoma
    n. lesion
nodulation
nodule
    cold n.
    hot n.
    hyperfunctioning n.
    jugulocarotid n.

    metastatic n.
    mixed n.
    posterior n.
    subependymal brain n.
    thyroid n.
nodulectomy
nodule-in-nodule lesion
nodulus cutaneus
nodus, *pl.* **nodi**
    nodi lymphoidei parauterini
    n. lymphoideus foraminalis
noise
    n. detection threshold
    n. exposure
no-leak technique
nomenclature
    Anglo-Saxon n.
    Couinaud n.
    linnaean system of n.
NOMI
    nonocclusive mesenteric ischemia
nomogram
    prognostic n.
    Radford n.
nonabsorbable
    n. material
    n. surgical suture
nonadherent
nonalcoholic
    n. cirrhosis
    n. fatty liver disease
    n. steatohepatitis
nonamide analogue
nonanatomic
    n. renal bypass
    n. wedge resection
nonanesthetic gas
nonaneurysmal perimesencephalic subarachnoid hemorrhage
nonappendiceal carcinoid
nonarticular distal radial fracture
nonawakening
    persistent n.
nonaxillary location
nonbacterial thrombotic endocardial lesion
nonbench surgery
nonbiologic liver support
nonblanchable abnormally colored lesion
nonbulbar polio
nonbullous emphysema
noncalcified nodular mass
noncancer death
noncardiac surgery
noncausal association
noncemented total hip arthroplasty
noncircumferential antireflux procedure
noncirrhotic metabolic liver disease
nonclassic nodal basin

noncolorectal
    n. liver metastasis (NCRLM)
    n. primary
Non-Communicating Children's Pain Checklist (NCCPC)
Noncommunicative Patient's Pain Assessment Instrument (NOPPAIN)
noncontact manipulation
noncontiguous fracture
nondepolarizer
nondepolarizing
    n. block
    n. blockade
    n. muscle relaxant
    n. relaxant
nondermatomal sensory abnormality (NDSA)
nondermatophyte fungal infection
nondiabetic
nondiagnostic FNA
nondismembered anastomosis
nondisplaced fracture
nondistended abdomen
nondominant gland
nondopaminergic neuron
nondysgerminoma
nonencapsulated
nonerosive gastric mucosal lesion
nonexcisional modality
nonfamilial
    n. malignant endocrine tumor
    n. multiglandular disease
    n. untreated HPT
nonfatal
    n. complication
    n. stroke
nonfenestrated Fontan procedure
nonfunction
    primary graft n.
nonfunctional malignant tumor
nonfunctioning
    n. islet cell tumor
    n. tumor of pancreas
nonheart-beating donor (NHBD)
nonhemolytic febrile reaction
nonhereditary malignancy
nonideal solution
nonimmunologic complication
noninfective extraabdominal complication
noninhalation
noninsulated needle
noninvasive
    n. assessment
    n. blood pressure (NIBP)
    n. diagnosis
    n. evaluation
    n. imaging
    n. infestation

    n. localization study
    lower extremity n.
    n. method
    n. positive-pressure ventilation (NPPV)
    n. procedure
    n. programmed electrical stimulation
    n. recurrence
    n. technique
    n. venous study
noninvoluting congenital hemangioma (NICH)
nonisometric graft
nonkeratinization
nonlaparoscopic
    n. series
    n. technique
nonmalignant
    chronic n.
    n. disease
    n. pain
nonmeningiomatous malignant lesion
nonmobile mass
nonmucosal hemorrhoidectomy
nonnecrotizing granulomatous inflammation
nonneoplastic tumorlike lesion
nonneuroendocrine metastasis
nonobstructing jaundice
nonocclusive
    n. mesenteric ischemia (NOMI)
    n. mesenteric ischemia syndrome
nonopaque intraluminal mass
nonoperative
    n. approach
    n. closure
    n. diagnosis
    n. management
    n. reduction
    n. staging
nonoperatively
nonophthalmologic surgical specialty
nonopioid analgesic
nonopportunistic infection
nonoptimal technique
nonorganic stridor
nonpain symptom control
nonpalpable
    n. invasive breast cancer
    n. mammographic abnormality
nonparametric test
nonparasitic liver cyst
nonpathologic scar
nonpenetrating
    n. keratoplasty
    n. rupture
    n. wound
nonperforative lesion

N

nonpharmacologic
n. measure
n. pain
nonphysial fracture
nonphysiologic position
nonplicated appendicocystostomy
nonpolypoid tumor
nonprogressive dilational technique
nonprosthetic closure
nonpulmonary route of elimination
nonpulsatile flow
nonrebreathing anesthesia
nonresectional method
nonrib-spreading
n.-s. thoracotomy incision
n.-s. thoracotomy incision method
n.-s. thoracotomy incision procedure
n.-s. thoracotomy incision technique
nonrigid registration algorithm
nonrotation
nonrotational burst fracture
nonsecretory sigmoid cystoplasty
nonselective opioid receptor antagonist
nonseminomatous
n. component
n. testicular tumor
nonsentinel node
nonseptate cavity
nonsevered injury
nonshivering thermogenesis
nonspecific
n. symptom
n. therapy
nonstereospecific action
nonsteroidal
n. antiinflammatory drug (NSAID)
n. antiinflammatory medication
nonsurgical
n. clinician
n. management
n. method
n. therapy
n. treatment
nonsurvivor
nonsympathetically mediated pain
nontherapeutic
nonthoracotomy
nonthrust mobilization
nontraumatic hernia
nontuberculous mycobacterial infection
nontumoral gastric wall
nonunion fracture
nonunited fracture
nonvariceal gastrointestinal bleeding
nonvascular abdominal surgery
nonventilated lung
nonviable tissue
nonvisualization
nonvital tissue
N_2O-O2
nitrous oxide-oxygen
noose
Dormia n.
n. suture technique
NOPPAIN
Noncommunicative Patient's Pain Assessment Instrument
no-punch technique
noradrenergic
n. mechanism
n. system
norepinephrine
Norfolk
N. phalloplasty procedure
N. phalloplasty technique
norma
normal
n. anatomic alignment
n. anatomic position
n. base deficit
n. body temperature
n. CI
n. colon
n. intravascular pressure
n. ovariotomy
n. planar MR anatomy
n. saline
n. saline solution
n. serum lactate
n. tissue
n. transformation zone
normalization
assay n.
n. of neuropathophysiology
normalizing lactate
normal-pressure hydrocephalus
Norman Miller vaginopexy
normocalcemia
normocalcemic
normocapnia
normocephalic
normosensitivity
pain n.
normotensive
normothermia
intraoperative n.
normothermic
n. ischemia
n. temperature
normoventilation
normovolemic hemodilution
North
N. American Bassini inguinal hernia repair
N. American Society of Pacing and Electrophysiology (NASPE)
N. American Spine Society (NASS)

N. American Spine Society Lumbar Spine Outcome Assessment Instrument

Northwick Park Neck Pain Questionnaire (NPQ)

Norton operation

Norwood
N. neonatal univentricular heart with subaortic stenosis repair
N. univentricular heart procedure

no-scalpel vasectomy

nose
n. anesthesia
artificial n.
cleft n.
electronic n.
external n.

nosocomial
n. fire
n. fungal infection
n. gangrene
n. infection
n. pneumonia

nostril

notal

notancephalia

notch
acetabular n.
anacrotic n.
angular n.
auricular n.
costal n.
craniofacial n.
ethmoidal n.
frontal n.
greater sciatic n.
inferior thyroid n.
inferior vertebral n.
infraorbital n.
interarytenoid n.
interclavicular n.
intercondylar n.
intervertebral n.
Kernohan n.
lacrimal n.
lesser sciatic n.
mandibular n.
mastoid n.
n. of acetabulum
pancreatic n.
parietal n.
parotid n.
preoccipital n.
presternal n.
pterygoid n.
scapular n.
sciatic n.
sternal n.
superior thyroid n.

superior vertebral n.
supraorbital n.
suprascapular n.
suprasternal n.
tentorial n.
thyroid n.
tympanic n.
umbilical n.
vertebral n.

notch-and-roll maneuver

notching
rib n.

notchplasty procedure

notencephalocele

notochord

no-touch technique

Novafil suture

noxious
n. event
n. stimulus

Noyes flexion rotation drawer test

NPA
nasopharyngeal airway

NPC
nasopharyngeal carcinoma

NPE
neurogenic pulmonary edema

NPQ
Northwick Park Neck Pain Questionnaire

NPTR
National Pediatric Trauma Registry

NPTS
nocturnal painful tonic spasm

NPV
negative predictive value
negative pressure ventilation

NSABP
National Surgical Adjuvant Breast and Bowel Project

NSAID
nonsteroidal antiinflammatory drug
NSAID analgesic

NSDUH
National Survey on Drug Use and Health

N-shaped sigmoid loop

NSICU
neurosurgical intensive care unit

NSQIP
National Surgical Quality Improvement Program

NSS
nephron-sparing surgery

NTDB
National Trauma Data Bank

NTI
nasotracheal intubation

N

N-type voltage-sensitive calcium channel

Nu

nucleus

nub

fibrotic n.

nucha

nuchal

n. fascia

n. ligament

n. line

n. plane

n. region

Nuck canal

nuclear

n. atypia

n. external layer

n. grade

n. magnetic resonance (NMR)

n. magnetic resonance spectroscopy (NMRS)

n. matrix protein

n. medicine

n. tissue

nuclear-annular boundary

nucleation time

nuclei (*pl. of* nucleus)

nucleic acid testing

nucleolysis

percutaneous laser n.

nucleus, *pl.* **nuclei**

n. ambiguus lesion

centrolateral n.

Edinger-Westphal n.

external cuneate n.

extrapyramidal n.

ossifying n.

prosthetic disc n. (PDN)

n. pulposus herniation

n. rotator

Nuhn gland

nulliparity

null point

numbness

numerary renal anomaly

numeric rating scale

nummular lesion

nummulation

Nurolon suture

nurse

n. anesthetist

visiting n.

Nuss pectus excavatum procedure

nutcracker

n. esophagus

n. fracture

nutmeg

n. appearance

n. liver

nutricius

nutrient

n. absorption

n. artery

n. canal

n. flap

n. foramen

hepatotrophic n.

n. vessel

nutrition

enteral n.

home parenteral n.

nasojejunal n.

parenteral n.

peripheral parenteral n.

tissue n.

total parenteral n.

nutritional

n. assessment

n. status

Nuttall incisional hernia repair

nycturia

Nyhus inguinal hernia classification

Nylen-Barany benign positional vertigo maneuver

nylon

n. monofilament suture

n. retention suture

n. 66 suture

nympha, *pl.* **nymphae**

nymphae (*pl. of* nympha)

nymphal

nymphectomy

nymphocaruncularis

nymphocaruncular sulcus

nymphohymenal sulcus

nymphotomy

nystagmogram

nystagmoidlike oscillation

nystagmus (nyst)

NYSTR

New York State Trauma Registry

nyxis

O, O2
  oxygen
OAA/S
  Observer's Assessment of Alertness
    and Sedation
  Observer's Assessment of Alertness
    and Sedation scale
    OAA/S scale
oat cell carcinoma
OAV
  oculoauriculovertebral
    OAV syndrome
OAVD
  oculoauriculovertebral dysplasia
O'Beirne sphincter
Ober
  O. incision
  O. tendon transfer for footdrop
    technique
Ober-Barr
  O.-B. procedure for brachioradialis
    transfer
  O.-B. tendon transfer for footdrop
    technique
Obersteiner-Redlich line
obese patient
obesity
  androgenic o.
  central o.
  clinically severe o. (CSO)
  o. hypoventilation syndrome (OHS)
  medication-induced o.
  morbid o.
obex
object
  O. Classification Test
  fixation o.
  o. program
  o. space
objective
  O. Pain Scale
  surgical treatment o.
object-space focus
oblique
  o. abdominal muscle
  o. aberration
  o. arytenoid muscle
  o. auricular muscle
  o. base wedge osteotomy
  o. cord
  o. coronal plane
  o. displacement osteotomy
  external o.
  o. facial cleft
  o. fissure of lung

  o. flap
  o. fracture
  o. head
  o. hernia
  o. illumination
  left anterior o. (LAO)
  o. pericardial sinus
  o. projection
  right anterior o. (RAO)
  o. section
obliterans
  arteriosclerosis o. (ASO)
  bronchiolitis o. (BO)
  thromboangiitis o. (TAO)
obliterate
obliterated abdomen
obliteration
  balloon-occluded retrograde
    transvenous o.
  cicatricial o.
  dead space o.
  fibrous o.
  percutaneous transhepatic o.
  radiographic o.
  subdeltoid fat plane o.
  total ear o.
obliterative
  o. bronchiolitis
  o. inflammation
  o. peritonitis
  o. scarring
oblongata
  rostral ventrolateral medulla o.
O'Brien
  O. akinesia ocular anesthesia
    technique
  O. anesthesia
  O. capsular shift procedure
  O. pelvic halo operation
obscuration
  transient visual o.
observation
  o. period
  o. ward
observer-dependent criteria
observer's
  O. Assessment of Alertness and
    Sedation (OAA/S)
  O. Assessment of Alertness and
    Sedation scale (OAA/S)
obstetric, obstetrical
  o. anesthesia
  o. complication
  o. hysterectomy
  o. management

O

obstetric (*continued*)
    o. operation
    o. pain
    o. position
    o. traction injury
obstetrical (*var. of* obstetric)
obstetrics
    International Federation of
      Gynecology and O. (FIGO)
obstipation
obstructed
    o. bowel
    o. liver
    o. tube
obstructing
    o. colorectal cancer
    o. pathology
obstruction
    acute intestinal o.
    adherence o.
    adhesive small bowel o.
    airway o.
    anorectal outlet o.
    ball-valve o.
    biliary tract o.
    bowel o.
    cannula o.
    catheter o.
    chronic upper airways o.
    closed loop intestinal o.
    clot-induced urinary tract o.
    colon o.
    colonic o.
    common duct o.
    complete o.
    complex left ventricular outflow
      tract o.
    ductal o.
    esophageal o.
    extrahepatic bile duct o.
    extrahepatic biliary o.
    extrahepatic portal vein o.
    extramural upper airway o.
    gastric outlet o. (GOO)
    hepatic venous outflow o.
    inguinal vasal o.
    intermittent subclavian vein o.
    intestinal o.
    ipsilateral portal vein o.
    jejunoileal o.
    left-sided colorectal o.
    longer-segment o.
    mechanical o.
    mechanical extrahepatic o.
    membranous o.
    myoglobin tubular o.
    outflow tract o.
    pancreatic duct o.
    paralytic gastrointestinal o.

    partial mechanical o.
    portal vein o.
    postoperative airway o.
    shunt o.
    site of o.
    small-bowel o.
    stop-valve airway o.
    superior venal caval o.
    upper airway o.
    ureteral o.
    ureteropelvic o.
    ureterovesical o.
    urinary tract o.
    vein o.
    ventricular inflow tract o.
    ventricular outflow tract o.
obstruction-induced modulation
obstructive
    o. apnea
    o. azoospermia
    o. esophagogastric cancer
    o. hydatid material
    o. hydrocephalus
    o. jaundice
    o. lung disease (OLD)
    o. mechanism
    o. pulmonary dysfunction
    o. uropathy
obstruent
obtundation
obtunded gag reflex
obturation
    canal o.
    retrograde o.
    root canal filling technique o.
obturator
    o. artery
    o. avulsion fracture
    o. bypass
    o. canal
    o. crest
    o. fascia
    o. foramen
    o. groove
    o. hernia
    o. line
    o. lymphatic chain
    o. lymph node packet
    o. nerve
    o. nerve block
    o. nerve damage
    o. nerve injury
    o. neurectomy
    o. shelf cystourethropexy
    o. sign
    o. test
    o. tubercle
obtuse margin
obviate

occipital

o. angle
o. artery
o. belly
o. bone
o. border
o. branch
o. cephalocele
o. cerebral vein
o. condyle
o. condyle fracture
o. condyle syndrome
o. emissary vein
o. fontanelle
o. groove
o. headache
left anterior o. (LAO)
o. malformation
o. margin
o. nerve
o. nerve block
o. nerve blockade
o. neuralgia
o. neurectomy
o. node
o. plane
o. plexus
o. point
right anterior o. (RAO)
o. sinus
o. suture
o. triangle

occipitalization
occipitoanterior fetal position
occipitoatlantal dislocation
occipitoatlantoaxial anomaly
occipitoatloid
occipitoaxial, occipitoaxoid
occipitoaxoid (*var. of* occipitoaxial)
occipitobregmatic
occipitocervical

o. approach
o. fixation
o. fusion
o. stabilization

occipitocollicular tract
occipitofacial
occipitofrontalis muscle
occipitofrontal muscle
occipitomastoid suture
occipitomental projection
occipitoparietal suture
occipitopontine tract
occipitoposterior fetal position
occipitosphenoid suture
occipitotectal tract
occipitotemporal
occipitothalamic radiation
occipitotransverse fetal position

occiput
occluded segment
occluding

o. centric relation record
o. relation

occlusal

o. cavity
o. correction
distal o.
o. equilibration
o. plane
o. plane angle
o. position
o. pressure
o. projection
o. relation
o. therapy

occlusion

acute embolic arterial o.
angioplasty-related vessel o.
aortic o.
arterial o.
artery o.
carotid artery o.
centric relation o.
clip o.
contralateral carotid artery o.
eccentric o.
endovascular balloon o.
graft o.
hemihepatic vascular o.
inferior vena cava o.
inferior vena cava balloon o.
inflow o.
intermittent inflow o.
IVC o.
laparoscopic total o.
MCA o.
mechanical o.
middle cerebral artery o.
2-plane o.
plastic stent o.
o. pressure
rapid o.
subclavian artery o.
temporary balloon o.
o. therapy
tourniquet o.
vascular o.
vein o.
venous o.

occlusive

o. carotid artery disease
o. coronary artery disease
o. ileus
o. MI
o. patch test
o. surgical glue dressing
o. therapy

O

535

occult
- o. bleeding
- o. blood
- o. cerebrovascular malformation
- o. diaphragmatic injury
- o. enterotomy
- o. extrahepatic disease
- o. fracture
- o. hepatic disease
- o. irresectable disease
- o. metastasis
- o. spinal dysraphism
- o. systemic disease
- o. talar lesion
- o. vascular malformation

occupational
- o. therapy
- o. toxin exposure

Occup Rx

OCD
- osteochondral defect

Ochsenbein gingivectomy

Ockerblad-Boari ureteral flap

O'Connor operation

O'Connor-Peter operation

OCR
- oculocardiac reflex

octanol/water coefficient

octogenarian

octreotide

ocular
- o. adnexa
- o. adnexal lesion
- o. barrier
- o. cul-de-sac
- o. inflammation
- o. manifestation
- o. metastasis
- o. microtremor
- o. microtremor during general anesthesia
- o. motility disorder
- o. muscle
- o. oscillation
- o. pain
- o. radiation therapy
- o. tumor

ocular-mucous membrane syndrome

oculi (*pl. of* oculus)

oculoauriculovertebral (OAV)
- o. dysplasia (OAVD)
- o. syndrome

oculobuccogenital syndrome

oculocardiac reflex (OCR)

oculocephalic
- o. maneuver
- o. vascular anomaly

oculofacial

oculogyration

oculomandibulofacial syndrome

oculomotor
- o. decussation
- o. foramen
- o. ganglion
- o. nerve

oculopharyngeal muscular dystrophy

oculoplastic
- o. surgeon
- o. surgery

oculovertebral syndrome

oculozygomatic

Oddi sphincter

ODI
- Oswestry Disability Index

O'Donnell operation

O'Donoghue
- O. ACL reconstruction
- O. facetectomy
- O. triad knee repair procedure

odontectomy

odontoameloblastoma

odontoblastoma

odontocele

odontoclastoma

odontogenic
- o. infection
- o. pain

odontoid
- o. condyle fracture
- o. fracture internal fixation
- o. fracture stabilization
- o. neck fracture
- o. perpendicular line
- o. process osteosynthesis
- o. screw fixation
- o. screw placement

odontoidectomy

odontolysis

odontoplasty

odontoscopy

odontosteophyte

odontotomy
- prophylactic o.

odoriferous gland

ODQ
- Oswestry Disability Questionnaire

O'Dwyer intubation

OFD
- oral-facial-digital
- orofaciodigital
- OFD syndrome

off-center isoperistaltic technique

office
- Surgeon General's O. (SGO)

off-label use

off-loading

off-pump
- o.-p. coronary artery bypass (OPCAB)
- o.-p. coronary bypass grafting

off-set V-osteotomy

Ogata

Ogden
- O. epiphysial fracture classification
- O. knee dislocation classification

Ogilvie
- O. herniorrhaphy
- O. syndrome

Ogston-Luc frontal sinus operation

Ogura orbital decompression

Ohngren line

OHS
- obesity hypoventilation syndrome
- open heart surgery

OHT
- orthotopic heart transplant

OI
- oxygenation index

oil
- o. drop lesion
- o. gland
- joint o.

oil-aspiration pneumonia

oiled silk suture

oil-gas partition coefficient

Okamura ACL repair technique

Okuda transhepatic obliteration of varix

OLBPQ
- Oswestry Low Back Pain Questionnaire

OLD
- obstructive lung disease

O'Leary stitch

olecranization

olecranon
- o. bursa
- o. fracture
- o. process

oleogranuloma

oleoma

olfactoria

olfactory
- o. anesthesia
- o. bulb
- o. bundle
- o. nerve
- o. tract

oligoanalgesia

oligoastrocytoma
- recurrent vermian o.

oligoclonal growth

oligodendroblastoma

oligodendroglioma

oligomerization

oligosegmental correction

oligospermatism (*var. of* oligospermia)

oligospermia, oligospermatism

oligozoospermatism

oliguresia

oliguresis (*var. of* oliguria)

oliguria, oliguresis, oliguresia
- intraoperative o.

olisthesis

olivary body

olivocerebellar tract

olivocochlear
- o. bundle
- o. nerve

olivospinal tract

Ollier
- O. arthrodesis approach
- O. incision
- O. lateral hip approach
- O. small thin split-thickness graft method
- O. thick split free graft
- O. transtrochanteric hip technique

Ollier-Thiersch split-thickness skin graft

Olshausen
- O. uterine ligaments suspension
- O. uterine suspension procedure

OLT
- orthotopic liver transplant
- OLT recipient

OLV
- 1-lung ventilation

Olympus gastrostomy

Ombrédanne transscrotal orchiopexy

omega-conopeptide toxin

omega jejunoduodenal anastomosis

omega-shaped incision

omenta (*pl. of* omentum)

omental
- o. appendage
- o. arcade
- o. branch
- o. bursa
- o. cyst
- o. enterocleisis
- o. flap
- o. hammock
- o. hernia
- o. J-pexy
- o. metastasis
- o. nodal disease
- o. patch
- o. patch closure
- o. pedicle
- o. pedicle wrapping
- o. pouch
- o. recess
- o. reinforcement
- o. sac
- o. spread

O

omental (*continued*)
 o. tenia
 o. tuber
omentectomy
 greater o.
 lesser o.
omentitis
omentofixation
 Drummond-Morison o.
omentopexy
omentoplasty
 pedicled o.
omentorrhaphy
omentosplenopexy
omentotomy
omentovolvulus
omentulum
omentum, *pl.* **omenta**
 colic o.
 gastrocolic o.
 gastrohepatic o.
 gastrosplenic o.
 greater o.
 lesser o.
 o. majus flap procedure
 pancreaticosplenic o.
 permanent mesh o.
 splenogastric o.
 vascularized o.
omentumectomy
omentum-to-brain transposition
Omer-Capen
 O.-C. carpectomy
 O.-C. proximal row carpectomy
  technique
omniplane scan
omocervical flap
omoclavicular
 o. fossa
 o. triangle
omohyoideus
omohyoid muscle
omothyroid
omotracheal triangle
omphalectomy
omphalic
omphalocele
 o. hernia
 infraumbilical o.
omphalomesenteric
omphalos (*var. of* omphalus)
omphalospinous
omphalotomy
omphalotripsy
omphalovesical
omphalus, omphalos
OMS
 oral and maxillofacial surgery
onchoosteodysplasia

oncocytoma
oncogene
 tumor suppressor o.
oncologic, oncological
 o. clearance
 o. consideration
oncological (*var. of* oncologic)
oncologist
 medical o.
 radiation o.
 surgical o.
oncology
 GI o.
 surgical o.
 urologic o.
oncolysate
 polyvalent melanoma o.
 vaccinia melanoma o.
  (VMO)
oncoma
oncometric
oncoplastic surgery
oncotic pressure
oncotomy
ondansetron
Ondine curse
one-compartment pharmacokinetic model
oneirogmus
oneiroscopy
ONH
 optic nerve head
onion
 o. bulb
 o. bulb changes
 o. bulb changes on biopsy
 o. peel appearance
 o. scale lesion
 o. skin-like membrane
onlay
 o. island flap
 o. island flap urethroplasty
 o. patch anastomosis
 o. technique
onlay-tube-onlay urethroplasty technique
on-line data
on-off weaning
onset of blockade
on-site first aid
on-table
 o.-t. angiography
 o.-t. irrigation
 o.-t. lavage
onychectomy
onychocryptosis nail
onychogryposis
onycholysis
onychoma

onychomycosis
onychoosteodysplasia
onychoplasty
onychotomy
onyx
oocyte
    o. extrusion
    o. micromanipulation
oophorectomy
    prophylactic o.
oophorocystectomy
oophorohysterectomy
oophoroma
oophoropeliopexy
oophoropexy
oophoroplasty
oophororrhaphy
oophorosalpingectomy
oophorostomy
oophorotomy
Oort nerve
OP
    operative procedure
OPA
    oral pharyngeal airway
    oropharyngeal airway
opacification
opacity
Opana ER
opaque wire suture
OPCAB
    off-pump coronary artery bypass
open
    o. adjustable silicone gastric banding
    o. adrenalectomy
    o. amputation
    o. anesthesia system
    o. anterior adrenalectomy
    o. antireflux surgery
    o. appendectomy
    o. application test
    o. bone graft epiphysiodesis
    o. brain biopsy
    o. cavity
    o. cholecystectomy
    o. circuit method
    o. colectomy
    o. common bile duct exploration
    o. disc surgery
    o. diverticulectomy
    o. drainage
    o. drop anesthesia
    o. drop technique
    o. endarterectomy
    o. esophagectomy
    o. esophagomyotomy
    o. eye-full stomach

    o. flap
    o. flap technique
    o. fundoplication
    o. gastric bypass
    o. Hasson technique
    o. head injury
    o. heart surgery (OHS)
    o. hemorrhoidectomy
    o. hernia operation
    o. herniorrhaphy
    o. intraoperative ultrasonography
    o. laparoscopic approach
    o. laparoscopic technique
    o. laparoscopy
    o. laparotomy
    o. liver biopsy
    o. loop
    o. lung approach
    o. lung biopsy
    o. neck surgery
    o. nephrostomy
    o. Nissen fundoplication
    o. Nissen operation
    o. osteotomy
    o. palm technique
    o. partial nephrectomy
    o. patch test
    o. pinning
    o. pneumothorax
    o. pyelolithotomy
    o. pyelotomy
    o. pyloromyotomy
    o. reconstruction
    o. reconstructive procedure
    o. reduction
    o. reduction and internal fixation (ORIF)
    o. repair
    o. retroperitoneal high ligation
    o. skull fracture
    o. sphincteroplasty
    o. splenectomy
    o. stereotactic craniotomy
    o. surgical biopsy
    o. surgical cordotomy
    o. surgical therapy
    o. surgical treatment
    o. thoracoabdominal adrenalectomy
    o. thoracotomy
    o. type I, II, III, IIIA, IIIB, IIIC fracture
    o. venous channel
    o. vertical banded gastroplasty
    o. wedge
    o. wound
open-book fracture
open-break fracture
open-end ostomy pouch
open-gloving technique

O

opening

> appendiceal o.
> o. flap
> ileocecal o.
> maximum mouth o.
> midpalatal suture o.
> o. pressure
> saphenous o.
> tendinous o.
> urethral o.
> vaginal o.
> o. wedge manipulation

open-section nail

open-sky

> o.-s. cryoextraction operation
> o.-s. technique
> o.-s. trephination
> o.-s. vitrectomy

operable

opera-glass deformity

operant conditioning

operating

> o. room (OR)
> o. theater
> o. time

operation

> Abbott-Lucas shoulder o.
> ab externo filtering o.
> ab interno filtering o.
> Adams hip o.
> Adler o.
> Agnew lacrimal sac o.
> Agrikola o.
> Allport o.
> Alvis cataract o.
> Amsler o.
> Amussat transverse abdominal
>   incision o.
> Anagnostakis entropion o.
> anastomotic o.
> Anel aneurysm o.
> Anel lacrimal fistula o.
> Angelucci cataract o.
> Anson-McVay inguinal
>   hernia o.
> antiperistaltic o.
> antireflux o.
> anular corneal graft o.
> Appolito intestinal o.
> Arion o.
> Arlt o.
> Armistead ulnar lengthening o.
> Arrowhead o.
> Arruga-Berens ophthalmologic o.
> Arruga retinal reattachment o.
> arterial switch o. (ASO)
> Ashford retracted nipple o.
> atrial baffle o.
> Badal cicatricial entropion o.

Badal conical cornea o.
Baer cataract o.
Baker-Hill posterior tibial tendon
  translocation o.
Baker translocation o.
Baldy uteropexy o.
Baldy-Webster o.
Ball-Hoffman o.
Band-Aid o.
Bangerter pterygium o.
Bankart-Putti-Platt shoulder o.
bariatric o.
Barkan-Cordes linear cataract o.
Barkan goniotomy o.
Barr tendon transfer o.
Bassini o.
Battle appendix o.
Bauer-Tondra-Trusler o.
Baynton leg ulcer o.
Belsey Mark IV antireflux o.
Benedict orbit o.
Berens pterygium transplant o.
Berens-Smith cataract o.
Berger interscapulothoracic
  amputation o.
Berke o.
Bielschowsky o.
biliary-enteric anastomosis o.
Billroth I, II o.
Birch-Hirschfeld entropion o.
Blair cleft lip o.
Blalock-Hanlon o.
Blalock-Taussig o.
Blasius lid flap o.
Blaskovics lid o.
bloodless o.
Bonaccolto-Flieringa vitreous o.
Bonnet enucleation o.
Bonzel artificial pupil o.
Bora o.
Bose hip resurfacing o.
Bowman o.
Boyd o.
Bricker ileal conduit o.
Bridge o.
bridge pedicle flap o.
Briggs strabismus o.
Bristow o.
Bromley foreign body o.
Buschke-Löwenstein tumor o.
Butler fifth toe o.
buttonhole o.
Buzzi artificial pupil o.
bypass o.
Byron Smith ectropion o.
Cairns o.
Caldwell-Luc o.
Calhoun-Hagler lens extraction o.
Callahan cataract o.

Callahan silicone tube
  blepharoplasty o.
Callahan silicone tube
  blepharoplasty o.
Camey I, II detubalarized
  neobladder o.
Campodonico pterygium o.
capital o.
Carrel experimental coronary artery
  bypass o.
Carter o.
Casanellas lacrimal o.
Casey o.
Castroviejo corneal transplantation o.
Castroviejo-Scheie cyclodiathermy o.
cataract extraction o.
Cattell o.
cautery o.
Celsus-Hotz entropion o.
Celsus spasmodic entropion o.
cerclage o.
cesarean o.
Chandler-Verhoeff vitreous o.
Chandler vitreous o.
Chaput anal o.
Chaput tibial o.
Charles o.
Cheyne antiseptic o.
Child o.
Cibis retinal detachment o.
cinching o.
Clagett o.
clean o.
clean-contaminated o.
Cloward cervical spine fusion o.
cluster o.
Collis antireflux o.
colorectal o.
Comberg foreign body o.
comparison o.
complete wrap Nissen o.
Conn o.
Conrad orbital blowout fracture o.
conventional o.
Cooper inguinal hernia o.
corneal graft o.
Cotte presacral neurotomy for
  dysmenorrhea o.
Cotting toenail o.
Counsellor-Davis artificial vagina o.
crescent o.
Crespo o.
Critchett corneal staphyloma o.
Crock anterior cervical spine
  encircling o.
cryoextraction o.
cryotherapy o.
curative-intent o.
curative sphincter-saving o.

Cushing pituitary o.
Cusick blepharoptosis o.
Cusick-Sarrail ptosis o.
Cutler ophthalmic o.
cyclodiathermy o.
Czermak pterygium o.
dacryoadenectomy o.
dacryocystectomy o.
dacryocystorhinotomy o.
dacryocystostomy o.
Dallas o.
Damus-Kaye-Stansel pulmonary
  artery to ascending aorta
  anastomotic o.
Dana o.
Danforth fetal o.
day-case o.
debulking o.
de Grandmont o.
Deiter o.
Denker sinus o.
Derby fascia lata eyelid sling o.
Desmarres o.
DeWecker glaucoma o.
Diamond-Gould syndactyly o.
diathermy o.
Dickey rectus muscle
  blepharoptosis o.
Dickson-Wright fascial transplant o.
Dieffenbach o.
DKS pulmonary artery to ascending
  aorta anastomotic o.
D'ombrain o.
Doyle o.
Duhamel colon o.
Duke-Elder strabismus o.
Durham flatfoot o.
Durr o.
Duverger-Velter o.
Dwyer clawfoot o.
Eagleton o.
Eaton-Malerich fracture-dislocation o.
Edlan-Mejchar mucogingival
  subperiosteal vestibule extension o.
effector o.
Elschnig canthorrhaphy o.
Ely protruding ear corrective o.
emergency o.
emergent o.
Emmet o.
equilibrating o.
Escapini cataract o.
Esmarch-Rizzoli ankylosed
  temporomaxillary articulation o.
Esser inlay skin graft o.
Estlander o.
Eversbusch eyelid ptosis o.
eversion o.
evisceration o.

O

operation (*continued*)
Ewing sarcoma o.
exploratory o.
extraabdominal o.
extracapsular cataract extraction o.
Faden esotropia repair o.
Falk-Shukuris o.
Fanta cataract o.
Farmer in utero myelomeningocele
  repair o.
Fasanella o.
Fasanella-Servat ptosis o.
fenestrated Fontan o.
fenestration o.
Filatov-Marzinkowsky o.
filtering o.
Finney o.
Flajani o.
flap o.
floating forehead o.
Foerster o.
Foley o.
Fontan o.
Fothergill-Donald o.
Fothergill prolapsed uterus
  suspension o.
Fox o.
Franceschetti deviation o.
Franceschetti keratoplasty o.
Franceschetti pupil deviation o.
Franke tabes o.
Frazier-Spiller o.
French supracondylar fracture o.
Friedenwald eyelid ptosis o.
Friedenwald-Guyton blepharoptosis o.
Frost-Lang implantation of metal
  ball in Tenon capsule o.
Furlow-Fisher modification of Virag
  1 erectile failure microsurgical o.
Galeazzi patellar o.
Gardner o.
Gauderer-Ponsky percutaneous
  endoscopic o.
Gilliam o.
Gilliam-Doleris o.
Giordano suburethral sling o.
Girard keratoprosthesis o.
Goldmann-Larson foreign body o.
Goldsmith o.
gold weight and wire spring facial
  paralysis reanimation o.
Gomez-Marquez lacrimal o.
goniotomy o.
Gonzalez-Ulloa body lift o.
Gonzalez-Ulloa facelifting o.
Grant-Ward head and neck o.
Graves epiphora o.
Grimsdale eye o.
Grossmann retinal detachment o.

Gussenbauer pancreatic cyst external
  drainage o.
Guyton ptosis o.
Halsted o.
Hampton o.
Handley carcinoma of
  breast o.
hanging hip o.
hanging toe o.
Hartmann o.
Hasner injured eye o.
Hassab gastric variceal o.
Haultain inverted uterus o.
Heaney vaginal hysterectomy o.
Heine o.
Heller-Belsey esophageal o.
Heller-Dor esophageal o.
hemi-Fontan o.
Henry incarcerated and strangulated
  femoral hernia o.
Herbert scleral flap o.
Hess eyelid o.
Hess ptosis o.
Hiff o.
Hill antireflux o.
Hinsberg labyrinth o.
Hippel o.
Hirst cystocele o.
Hofmeister o.
Hogan o.
Hoguet inguinal hernia o.
Holth scleral punch o.
Hopkins tetralogy of Fallot o.
Horay cataract o.
Hotz entropion o.
Hughes colorectal o.
Hummelsheim transposition of
  vertical recti o.
Hunt cerebral aneurysm o.
Hunt-Transley lid ptosis o.
I-beam hip o.
indentation o.
initial o.
interval o.
intracapsular cataract extraction o.
iridectomy o.
iridencleisis o.
iridodialysis o.
iridotasis o.
iridotomy o.
Irvine o.
Jaime lacrimal o.
Jameson muscle recession with
  scleral reattachment o.
Johnson acquired and congenital
  coronary artery insufficiency o.
Kasai o.
Kazanjian o.
Keller-Madlener hallux valgus o.

Kennedy-Pacey urinary stress
  incontinence o.
keratectomy o.
keratocentesis o.
keratomileusis o.
keratoplasty o.
keratotomy o.
Key o.
kidney-sparing o.
Kirby superior rectus muscle
  blepharoptosis o.
Knapp pterygium o.
Knapp-Wheeler-Reese o.
Koffler o.
Kondoleon o.
Konno-Rastan aortoventriculoplasty o.
Kraske excision of coccyx and
  partial sacrum removal o.
Krempen-Silver-Sotelo infected
  pseudarthrosis o.
Krönlein orbital decompression o.
Kropp onlay urethral lengthening o.
Kuhnt eyelid o.
Kuhnt-Thorpe o.
Kwitko senile entropion o.
Lacour-Gayet pediatric arterial
  switch o.
Ladd o.
Lagleyze-Trantas o.
Lahey abdominoperineal rectal
  cancer o.
laissez-faire lid o.
Lancaster scleral suture o.
Lanchner o.
Landolt creation of lower eyelid o.
Langenbeck o.
laryngeal keel o.
Lash o.
Le Fort craniofacial dysjunction o.
Leriche o.
Lester Martin modification of
  Duhamel abdominoperineal
  pullthrough o.
Levine dislocation o.
Lewis o.
Lexer eyelid ptosis o.
limb-sparing o.
Lindesmith palliative transposition of
  great vessels o.
Lindner-Guist retinal detachment o.
Lindsay cleft lip and palate o.
Linton o.
lip adhesion o.
liver o.
logical o.
Löhlein o.
Londermann o.
Longmire o.
Lopez-Enriquez o.

Lord o.
Lotheissen inguinal approach to
  femoral hernia o.
Lynch supravalvular stenosing ring
  of left atrium o.
Macewen hernia o.
Machek-Blaskovics eyelid
  entropion o.
Machek-Brunswick o.
Machek-Gifford o.
Machek ptosis o.
Mack-Brunswick o.
MacNab patella o.
Madlener o.
magnet o.
magnetic o.
MAGPI o.
Majewsky o.
major o.
maladie de Graeffe o.
Malbran retinal detachment o.
mandibular swing o.
Mann-Williamson experimental peptic
  ulcer o.
Marcy inguinal hernia o.
Marquez-Gomez o.
Marshall-Marchetti-Krantz o.
mastoid obliteration o.
Mayer trapezius transfer o.
Mayo o.
McBurney o.
McGavic bare sclera pterygium o.
McGuire prostate o.
McIndoe o.
McKay-Simons clubfoot o.
McReynolds o.
McVay o.
Meller lacrimal sac o.
Mensor-Scheck hanging hip o.
Meyer lip carcinoma o.
mika o.
Mikulicz o.
Miles o.
Miller flatfoot o.
minor o.
Minsky rectal cancer o.
Moran thoracic duct o.
morcellation o.
Morel-Fatio lid load o.
Moss necrotizing enterocolitis o.
Motais superior rectus muscle
  blepharoptosis o.
motivating o.
Moynihan colon o.
Mueller o.
muscle sliding o.
Mustard interarterial transposition of
  venous return o.
myectomy o.

o

operation (*continued*)
>myelomeningocele o.
>myotomy o.
>Naffziger exophthalmos o.
>Neher acute pancreatitis o.
>Nehra esophageal o.
>Nesbit congenital curvature of penis o.
>Neviaser old shoulder dislocation o.
>Nissen antireflux o.
>Norton o.
>O'Brien pelvic halo o.
>obstetric o.
>O'Connor o.
>O'Connor-Peter o.
>O'Donnell o.
>Ogston-Luc frontal sinus o.
>open hernia o.
>open Nissen o.
>open-sky cryoextraction o.
>orbital implant o.
>orthotopic hemi-Koch o.
>outpatient thyroid o.
>Owen o.
>palliative o.
>Panas lid ptosis o.
>pancreatic o.
>parallel o.
>parathyroid o.
>Partsch o.
>pattern cut corneal graft o.
>pedicle flap o.
>Peet o.
>Pemberton o.
>Peter o.
>Peters exstrophy of bladder o.
>Pico o.
>Pirogoff o.
>plastic o.
>plombage o.
>pocket o.
>Pollock o.
>Pólya o.
>Pomeroy o.
>Porro o.
>portacaval shunt o.
>Potts pulmonary stenosis o.
>Power o.
>Preziosi hemorrhagic glaucoma o.
>probing lacrimonasal duct o.
>protective antireflux o.
>pubovaginal o.
>pull-through o.
>pulsed-mode o.
>Ramstedt o.
>Ransohoff aneurysm wiring o.
>Rashkind o.
>Rastan o.
>Rastelli transposition of great arteries o.
>Raverdino retinal detachment photocoagulation o.
>Ray-Brunswick-Mack o.
>Ray-McLean o.
>Récamier o.
>reconstructive o.
>Reese-Cleasby cataract o.
>Reese-Jones-Cooper cataract o.
>Reese ptosis o.
>repeat o.
>resectional phase of o.
>resurfacing o.
>Richet ectropion o.
>Ripstein rectal prolapse o.
>Rosenburg o.
>Roux-en-Y o.
>Roux-Goldthwait dislocation o.
>Rovsing polycystic kidney o.
>Rowbotham neurological o.
>Rowinski kidney transplant o.
>Rubbrecht malocclusion o.
>Ruedemann enucleation o.
>Rutkow and Robbins direct or indirect inguinal hernia o.
>Rycroft empty eye socket o.
>Saemisch corneal transfixion o.
>Saenger cesarean o.
>Sanders thoracic outlet decompression o.
>Sato radial keratotomy o.
>Savin cryorectal o.
>Sawyer afferent loop o.
>Sayoc orbicularis levator fixation o.
>Scarpa o.
>Schepens retinal detachment o.
>Schimek blepharoptosis o.
>Schirmer lacrimal sac o.
>Schmalz lacrimal o.
>Schönbein o.
>Schroeder o.
>Schuchardt o.
>scleral shortening o.
>Scott o.
>scrotal pouch o.
>Scudder tuberculous parotid gland o.
>second-look o. (SLO)
>sector iridectomy o.
>Selinger o.
>semielective o.
>Senning o.
>Senn ventriculosubgaleal shunt o.
>sensor o.
>serial o.
>seton o.
>sex change o.
>Shaffer glaucoma o.
>Shirodkar o.

Shouldice indirect inguinal hernia o.
Shugrue orbital o.
Sichi o.
single-stage o.
slant muscle o.
Smith-Boyce renal calculus o.
Smith eyelid o.
Smith-Indian o.
Smith Indian intracapsular
  cataract o.
Snellen ptosis o.
1-snip punctum o.
3-snip punctum o.
Soria o.
Soriano o.
Sourdille ptosis o.
Spaeth cystic bleb o.
Spaeth ptosis o.
Spencer-Watson Z-plasty
  entropion o.
sphincter-saving o.
Spinelli o.
splitting lacrimal papilla o.
stage o.
staging o.
Stallard flap o.
Stallard-Liegard o.
Stallard tarsectomy for ptosis
  secondary to trachoma o.
Stamey antiincontinence o.
step graft o.
stereotactic o.
Stock o.
Stocker o.
Straith eyelid o.
Strampelli-Valvo o.
Streatfield-Fox eyelid o.
Streatfield lid ptosis o.
Streatfield-Snellen o.
Stretta GERD radiofrequency o.
Sturmdorf o.
subcutaneous o.
Sugiura esophageal varices o.
Summerskill o.
suspensory sling o.
switch o.
symmetry o.
synchrocyclotron o.
Szymanowski o.
tagliacotian rhinoplasty o.
talc o.
Tanner stomach devascularization o.
Tansini osteomyocutaneous intercostal
  transposition flap o.
Tansley lid ptosis o.
Taussig o.
Taussig-Morton modified
  Blalock-Taussig o.
Teale-Knapp symblepharon o.

tenotomy o.
Terson ectropion o.
Tessier craniofacial o.
Thal fundic patch o.
Thiersch anal incontinence o.
Thiersch graft o.
Thomson o.
thyroid o.
Tillett blepharoptosis o.
tongue-in-groove o.
Torek esophagus o.
total excisional o.
Toti o.
Toti-Mosher o.
trabeculectomy o.
Trainor o.
transsphenoidal o.
Trantas o.
Trendelenburg II great saphenous
  vein ligation o.
Trendelenburg I pulmonary
  embolism o.
Treves appendicitis o.
Treves lumbar and last dorsal
  vertebrae o.
Treves psoas abscess o.
Truc o.
Tudor-Thomas o.
tumbling technique o.
Turnbull blowhole o.
Turnbull ostomy o.
unattended laboratory o.
Urban o.
urologic o.
Uyemura o.
Valvo full-thickness lid o.
van Buren artificial anus o.
Vecchietti neovagina o.
Verhoeff-Chandler o.
Vermale o.
Verneuil o.
Verwey eyelid o.
Virag o.
Vogt cyclodiathermy o.
von Ammon epichanthus o.
von Blaskovics-Doyen vesicouterine
  fistula o.
von Giordano suburethral sling o.
von Graefe o.
Waldhauer entropion o.
Walter Reed o.
Warren splenorenal shunt o.
Waterston o.
Watson o.
Waugh abdominoanal pullthrough o.
Webster o.
Wendell Hughes cataract o.
Werb o.
Wertheim o.

O

operation (*continued*)
 Wertheim-Schauta o.
 West o.
 Weve o.
 Wharton Jones o.
 Wheeler o.
 Whipple o.
 Whitehead o.
 Whitnall sling o.
 Wicherkiewicz eyelid o.
 Wies lower lid entropion o.
 Williams copulating pouch o.
 Winiwarter o.
 Wise o.
 Witzel o.
 Wolfe ptosis o.
 Woodward o.
 Worst o.
 Worth ptosis o.
 Wright caries of spine o.
 Zickel subtrochanteric fracture o.
 Ziegler o.
 Zylik o.
operational homeostasis
operationoperation
operative
 o. approach
 o. arthroscopy
 o. arthrotomy
 o. biliary bypass
 o. blood loss
 o. cholangiography
 o. choledochoscopy
 o. correction
 o. débridement
 o. diagnosis
 o. drainage
 o. excision
 o. exposure
 o. field
 o. finding
 o. intervention
 o. management
 o. mortality
 o. mortality rate
 o. necrosectomy
 o. perforation
 o. procedure (OP)
 o. reconstruction
 o. reexploration
 o. result
 o. site complication
 o. specimen
 o. stabilization
 o. stress
 o. technique
 o. therapy
 o. time
 o. treatment

operatively stabilized
operator exposure
operculectomy
operculum
O'Phelan technique
ophryon
ophryospinal angle
ophthalmectomy
ophthalmic
 o. activating solution
 o. anesthesia
 o. artery
 o. cul-de-sac
 o. examination
 o. nerve
 o. vein
ophthalmocarcinoma
ophthalmocele
ophthalmologic anesthesia
ophthalmomyotomy
ophthalmopathy
ophthalmophlebotomy
ophthalmoplasty
ophthalmoplegia
ophthalmoscopy
 binocular indirect o.
 direct o.
 indirect o.
 medical o.
 metric o.
 slit-lamp o.
ophthalmospectroscopy
ophthalmostasis
ophthalmotomy
opiate-induced
 o.-i. endocrinopathy
 o.-i. hypogonadism
opiate receptor antagonist
opioid
 o. agonist
 o. analgesia
 o. analgesic
 o. anesthesia
 o. anesthetic
 o. antagonist
 o. antinociceptive activity
 endogenous o.
 epidural o.
 o. escalation
 esterase-metabolized o.
 intrathecal o.
 lipophilic o.
 neuraxial o.
 neuroaxial o.
 o. prescreening
 o. receptor
 o. rescue
 o. rotation
 single-shot intrathecal o.

o. system
o. therapy
o. therapy addiction
opioid-based technique
opioid-induced hyperalgesia
opioid-insensitive pain
opisthion
opisthionasial
opisthotonos, opisthotonus
o. position
opisthotonus (*var. of* opisthotonos)
OPO
organ procurement organization
opponensplasty
abductor digiti minimi o.
abductor digiti quinti o.
Bunnell o.
Huber adductor digiti quinti o.
Manske-McCarroll o.
opportunistic
o. complication
o. organism
o. systemic fungal infection
opposition respiration
opposure
opsonization
optic, optical
o. aberration
o. biopsy
o. canal
o. chiasm compression
o. correction
o. cul-de-sac
o. cup
o. cup to disc ratio
o. decussation
o. disc
o. evagination
o. foramen
o. ganglion (OG)
o. iridectomy
o. iridectomy
o. keratoplasty
o. keratoplasty
o. nerve (ON)
o. nerve atrophy
o. nerve head (ONH)
o. nerve tumor
o. neuropathy (ON)
o. nodal point
o. papilla (p, P)
o. papilla cavity
o. pathway myelination
o. radiation (OR)
o. rotation
o. sheath
o. system
o. tracking
o. tract (OT)

o. tract compression
o. tract syndrome
o. vesicle
optical (*var. of* optic)
o. density method
o. iridectomy
o. path length
o. scanner
opticociliary
o. neurectomy
o. neurotomy
optimal
o. cytoreduction
o. external laryngeal manipulation
o. intensive medical management
O. Observation Score
o. technique
o. therapy
opting
o. in
o. out
option
interventional o.
medical treatment o.
surgical treatment o.
therapeutic o.
treatment o.
OPTN
Organ Procurement and Transplantation Network
optoacoustic monitoring
optometrist
OR
operating room
orthopedic
OR technician
ora, *pl.* **orae**
orad
orae (*pl. of* ora)
O'Rahilly limb deficiency classification
oral
o. administration
o. analgesic
o. and maxillofacial surgery (OMS)
o. anesthetic
o. anesthetic technique
o. anomaly
o. antibiotic medication
o. anticoagulant
o. anticoagulation
o. antimotility agent
o. aphthous ulcer
o. cavity
o. cavity abnormality
o. cavity cytology
o. cavity tumor
o. cephalocele
o. competence
o. complication

O

oral (*continued*)
    o. condyloma planus
    o. endotracheal intubation
    o. feeding
    o. fissure
    o. immediate-release oxymorphone
    o. infection
    o. irrigation
    o. lighted-stylet intubation
    o. manifestation
    o. monotherapy
    o. mucosa
    o. peripheral examination
    o. pharyngeal airway (OPA)
    o. pharynx
    o. reconstruction
    o. region
    o. respiration
    o. tissue
    o. transmucosal fentanyl citrate
    o. ulceration
oral-facial-digital (OFD)
    o.-f.-d. syndrome
Orandi vascularized flap technique
OraVescent fentanyl
orbicular
    o. muscle
    o. zone
orbit
    deep o.
    lateral o.
    superficial o.
    superior o.
orbita
orbital
    o. adipose tissue
    o. anesthesia
    o. angioma
    o. apex syndrome
    o. arteriovenous malformation
    o. blow-out fracture
    o. branch
    o. canal
    o. cavity
    o. cellulitis
    o. decompression
    o. eminence
    o. exenteration
    o. exenteration gastroscopic access
      technique
    o. extension
    o. fascia
    o. fat pad
    o. fissure
    o. floor fracture
    o. height
    o. hematoma
    o. hernia
    o. implant operation

    o. index
    o. layer
    o. lesion
    o. line
    o. metastasis
    o. mucocele
    o. muscle
    o. pain
    o. phlebogram
    o. plane
    o. pyramid
    o. region
    o. rim fracture
    o. rim reconstruction
    o. section
    o. septum
    o. surface
    o. surgery
    o. tumor
    o. vein
    o. wall
    o. wall fracture
orbitalis muscle
orbitofrontal artery
orbitomaxillectomy
orbitomeatal line
orbitonasal
    o. index
    o. tissue
orbitosphenoid
orbitotomy
    Berke-Krönlein o.
    Krönlein o.
    Krönlein-Berke o.
orbitozygomatic
    o. mandibular osteotomy
    o. temporopolar approach
orchalgia (*var. of* orchialgia)
orchectomy
orchialgia, orchalgia, orchioneuralgia, ,
  orchidalgia, testalgia
orchichorea
orchidalgia (*var. of* orchialgia)
orchidectomy
    partial o.
    radical o.
orchidic
orchiditis
orchidoblastoma
orchidopexy (*var. of* orchiopexy)
    Torek cryptorchidism o.
orchidoptosis
orchidorraphy
orchidorrhaphy (*var. of* orchiorrhaphy,
  orchiopexy)
orchidotomy (*var. of* orchiotomy)
orchiectomy, orchidectomy, orchectomy,
  testectomy
    Huggins o.

prophylactic o.
radical inguinal o.
orchiepididymitis
orchioblastoma
orchiocele
orchiodynia
orchioneuralgia
orchiopathy
orchiopexy, orchidopexy,
 orchidorrhaphy
 Bevan o.
 Cabot-Nesbit o.
 eversion o.
 Fowler-Stephens o.
 laparoscopic o.
 Ombrédanne transscrotal o.
 Prentiss o.
 scrotal pouch o.
 staged o.
 2-step o.
 Torek o.
 transseptal o.
orchioplasty
orchiorrhaphy, orchidorrhaphy
orchiotherapy
orchiotomy, orchotomy, orchidotomy
orchis, *pl.* **orchises**
orchises (*pl. of* orchis)
orchitic
orchitis, orchiditis, testitis
orchotomy
ordinal classification
orexigenic
organ
 o. ablation
 o. allograft
 o. compromise
 Corti o.
 o. donation
 o. donor
 o. dysfunction
 effector o.
 external female genital o.
 external male genital o.
 o. failure criteria
 floating o.
 genital o.
 o. harvest
 internal female genital o.
 internal male genital o.
 intraabdominal o.
 intromittent o.
 o. of Zuckerkandl
 o. perfusion
 O. Procurement and Transplantation
  Network (OPTN)
 o. procurement organization (OPO)
 O. Procurement Program
 ptotic o.

secondary retroperitoneal o.
size-matched o.
solid o.
o. space
o. space infection
supernumerary o.
o. system
o. transplant
urinary o.
wandering o.
Weber o.
organic
 o. articulation disorder
 o. lesion
 o. short bowel syndrome
organ-induced intolerance
organism
 aerobic gram-negative o.
 Campylobacter-like o. (CLO)
 colonizing o.
 commensal o.
 enteric o.
 fungal o.
 gram-negative aerobic o.
 gut-derived gram-negative aerobic o.
 mixed fungal o.
 opportunistic o.
 pure fungal o.
organization
 organ procurement o. (OPO)
 World Health O. (WHO)
organized
 o. clot
 o. hematoma
organizing inflammation
organoaxial
 o. rotation
 o. volvulus
organogenesis
organology
organopexia (*var. of* organopexy)
organopexy, organopexia
organoscopy
organ-specific
 o.-s. pattern
 o.-s. pattern of injury
organum
Oriental
 O. cholangiohepatitis
 O. V-Y flap
orientation
 angle of o.
 limbal parallel o.
 phalangeal articular o.
 temporal o.
 visual o.
ORIF
 open reduction and internal
 fixation

O

orifice
anal o.
appendiceal o.
esophagogastric o.
eustachian tube o.
exocranial o.
external urethral o.
gastroduodenal o.
golf-hole ureteral o.
ileocecal o.
internal urethral o.
musculopectineal o.
myopectineal o.
pharyngeal o.
pulmonary o.
pyloric o.
renal artery o.
root canal o.
vaginal o.
vein o.
orificia (*pl. of* orificium)
orificium, *pl.* **orificia**
o. ureteris
origin
aberrant bronchial o.
biliodigestive o.
ectal o.
flexor-pronator o.
pancreatic head o.
pectoralis major muscle o.
primary o.
sternocleidomastoid muscle o.
tumor o.
oris
levator anguli o.
Ormond disease
oroantral fistula
orocutaneous fistula
oroendotracheal
orofacial
o. carcinoma
o. fistula
o. pain
orofaciodigital (OFD)
o. syndrome
orogastric
o. pathway
o. suction
oromandibular
o. defect
o. reconstruction
oronasal fistula
oropharyngeal
o. airway (OPA)
o. anesthesia
o. approach
o. carcinoma
o. hemorrhage
o. passage

o. reconstruction
o. wall
oropharynx
ororespiratory tract
orostoma
orotracheal intubation
Orr
O. incision
O. rectal prolapse repair
Orr-Loygue transabdominal proctopexy
Orsi-Grocco palpatory percussion of heart method
orthodifluorobenzene
orthodontia
surgical o.
orthodontic
o. procedure
o. therapy
orthodontics
surgical o.
orthodox procedure
orthognathic surgery
orthogonal
o. plane
o. polarization spectral imaging
o. projection
orthokeratinization
orthopaedic (*var. of* orthopedic)
O. Trauma Association classification
orthopedic, orthopaedic
o. anesthesia
o. anomaly
o. problem
o. surgical procedure
o. traumatologist
orthoptic transplant
orthoradioscopy
orthoscopy
orthoses (*pl. of* orthosis)
orthosis, *pl.* **orthoses**
cervicothoracic o. (CTO)
o. drop-lock ring
orthostatic hypotension
orthotopic
o. appendicocystostomy
o. bladder
o. graft
o. heart transplant (OHT)
o. hemi-Koch operation
o. liver transplant (OLT)
o. liver transplant recipient
o. ureterocele
o. urinary diversion
Orticochea
O. scalping technique
O. sphincter pharyngoplasty procedure
Ortner syndrome
Ortolani hip developmental dysplasia maneuver

os
>o. calcis osteotomy
>cervical o.
>external o.
>o. planum

Osborne-Cotterill
>O.-C. elbow technique
>O.-C. procedure

Osborne posterior hip approach
oscheal
oscheoplasty
oscillation
>grade I, II o.
>high-frequency o.
>laryngeal o.
>nystagmoidlike o.
>ocular o.

oscillatory ventilation
oscillometric
>o. blood pressure cuff
>o. calibration

oscillometry
>automated o.

Osgood
>O. modified technique
>O. rotational osteotomy

Osgood-Schlatter lesion
osmication, osmification
osmification (*var. of* osmication)
Osmond-Clarke staged congenital vertical talus repair technique
osmotic pressure
osseointegration
osseoligamentous ring
osseous, osteal
>o. anomaly
>o. fixation
>o. flap
>o. labyrinth
>o. lesion
>o. metastasis
>o. surgery
>o. tissue

osseus
>labyrinthus o.

ossicle
ossicular
>o. chain reconstruction
>o. prosthesis

ossiculectomy
ossiculoplasty
>tympanoplasty o.

ossiculum
ossification
ossificationis
>centrum o.

ossifying
>o. epiphysis
>o. fibroma

>o. inflammation
>o. nucleus

osteal (*var. of* osseous)
ostectomy, osteoectomy
>buccal o.
>fibular o.
>partial o.
>periodontal o.

osteitis
>bone flap o.

osteoaneurysm
osteoarthritis disease
osteoarthropathy
osteoarticular
>o. allograft
>o. allograft transplant
>o. defect
>o. graft

osteoblast
osteoblastic
>o. bone regeneration
>o. lesion
>o. metastasis

osteoblastoma
osteobunionectomy
osteocachexia
osteocarcinoma
osteocartilaginous
>o. graft
>o. loose body

osteocementum
osteochondral
>o. allograft
>o. defect
>o. fragment
>o. graft
>o. injury
>o. lesion
>o. loose body
>o. prominence
>o. ridge

osteochondritis
osteochondrodesmodysplasia
osteochondrodysplasia
osteochondrodystrophy
>familial o.

osteochondrofibroma
osteochondrolysis
osteochondroma
osteochondromatosis
osteochondropathy
osteochondrophyte
osteochondrosarcoma
osteochondrosis
osteochrondral slice fracture
osteoclasia (*var. of* osteoclasis)
osteoclasis, osteoclasia
>Blount technique for o.
>o. maneuver

O

osteoclast
osteoclastic
osteoclastoma
osteoconduction
osteocranium
osteocutaneous flap
osteocystoma
osteocyte
osteocytic lacuna
osteocytoma
osteodentin
osteodentinoma
osteodermatopoikilosis
osteodermatous
osteodermia
osteodiastasis
osteodysplasty
osteodystrophia (var. of osteodystrophy)
osteodystrophy, osteodystrophia
    renal o.
osteoectasia
osteoectomy (var. of ostectomy)
osteoenchondroma
osteoepiphysis
osteofibrochondrosarcoma
osteofibroma
osteofibromatosis
osteofibrosis
osteogenesis
    distraction o.
    o. imperfecta
    o. imperfecta congenita syndrome
osteogenetic fiber
osteogenic sarcoma
osteohalisteresis
osteohypertrophy
osteoid osteoma
osteoinduction
osteointegration phenomenon
osteokinematic motion
osteokinematics
osteolathyrism
osteolipochondroma
osteolipoma
osteologia (var. of osteology)
osteologist
osteology, osteologia
osteolysis
osteolytic
    o. bone lesion
    o. metastasis
osteoma
    extraspinal osteoid o.
    osteoid o.
osteomalacia
osteomalacic pelvis
osteomatoid
osteomatosis
osteomere

osteomesopyknosis
osteometry
osteomized
osteomuscular flap
osteomusculocutaneous flap
osteomyelitic sinus
osteomyelitis
osteomyelodysplasia
osteomyelofibrosis
osteomyelofibrotic syndrome
osteomyelosclerosis
osteomyocutaneous flap
osteon, osteone
osteonal
    o. bone union
    o. lamellar bone
osteoncus
osteone (var. of osteon)
osteonecrosis
osteonectin
osteoneogenesis
osteoneuralgia
osteopathia striata syndrome
osteopathic lesion
osteopathy
osteopedion
osteopenia
osteoperiosteal
    o. bone graft
    o. flap
osteoperiostitis
osteopetrosis
    cranial o.
osteopetrotic scar
osteophlebitis
osteophyma
osteophyte formation
osteophytosis
osteoplastic
    o. bone flap
    o. craniotomy
    o. flap
    o. flap approach
    o. frontal sinus procedure
    o. necrotomy
    o. reconstruction
osteoplasty
osteopoikilosis
osteopontin
osteoporosis pseudoglioma syndrome
osteoporotic
    o. bone
    o. fracture
    o. spine
osteopsathyrosis
osteopulmonary arthropathy
osteoradionecrosis
osteosarcoma
osteosarcomatosis

osteosclerotic lesion
osteosis
osteospongioma
osteosteatoma
osteosynovitis
Osteosynthesefragen
    Arbeitsgemeinschaft für O. (AO)
osteosynthesis
    anterior column o.
    cranial o.
    facial o.
    lumbar spine vertebral o.
    miniplate o.
    odontoid process o.
    plate-screw o.
    posterior column o.
    thoracic spine vertebral o.
    thoracolumbar spine vertebral o.
    vertebral o.
    wire o.
osteosynthetic material
osteotelangiectasia
osteothrombophlebitis
osteothrombosis
osteotomize
osteotomy
    Abbott-Gill o.
    abduction o.
    abductor o.
    abductory wedge o.
    adduction o.
    Agliette supracondylar o.
    Akin proximal phalangeal o.
    Amspacher-Messenbaugh closing
      wedge o.
    Amstutz-Wilson o.
    Anderson-Fowler calcaneal
      displacement o.
    angular o.
    angulation o.
    anterior calcaneal o.
    anterior innominate o.
    Austin o.
    Axer lateral opening wedge o.
    Axer varus derotational o.
    Bailey-Dubow o.
    Baker-Hill o.
    Balacescu closing wedge o.
    ball-and-socket trochanteric o.
    base-of-neck o.
    base wedge o.
    basilar o.
    Bellemore-Barrett closing wedge o.
    Berman-Gartland metatarsal o.
    Bernese periacetabular o.
    bifurcation o.
    biplane trochanteric o.
    blind o.
    block o.

Blount displacement o.
Brackett o.
Brett-Campbell tibial o.
calcaneal L o.
Campbell o.
Canale o.
canal innominate o.
Carstan reverse wedge o.
Cartam-Treander reverse wedge o.
cervical o.
C-form o.
Chambers o.
chevron o.
chevron-type transmalleolar o.
Chiari innominate o.
Chiari-Salter-Steel pelvic o.
closed intramedullary o.
closed wedge o.
closing abductory wedge o.
  (CAWO)
closing base wedge o.
Cole o.
compensatory basilar o.
controlled rotational o.
countersinking o.
Coventry distal femoral o.
Coventry vagal o.
craniofacial o.
Crego femoral o.
crescentic o.
crescentic calcaneal o.
C sliding o.
cuneiform o.
cup-and-ball o.
cylindrical o.
Dega pelvic o.
delayed femoral o.
derotational o.
dial pelvic o.
dial periacetabular o.
diaphysial o.
Dickinson-Coutts-Woodward-
  Handler o.
Dickson geometric o.
Dillwyn-Evans o.
Dimon-Hughston intertrochanteric o.
displacement o.
dome o.
dome-shaped o.
dorsal closing wedge o.
dorsal proximal metatarsal o.
dorsal V o.
dorsiflexory wedge o.
double o.
Dunn o.
Dunn-Hess trochanteric o.
Dwyer o.
Elizabethtown o.
Emmon o.

O

osteotomy (*continued*)

endoscopic vertical ramus o.
epiphysial-metaphysial o.
Eppright dial o.
Estersohn o.
ethmoidal o.
Evans anterior calcaneal o.
eversion o.
extension o.
failed femoral o.
femoral o.
Fernandez o.
flexion o.
French lateral closing wedge o.
frontonasomaxillary o.
frontoorbital o.
geometric supracondylar extension o.
Gerbert o.
Giannestras oblique metatarsal o.
Gibson-Piggott o.
glabellar exposure o.
Gleich o.
glenoid o.
Golden closing wedge o.
Grant-Small-Lehman supracondylar
  extension o.
Greenfield o.
Green-Reverdin o.
greenstick dorsal proximal
  metatarsal o.
Green-Watermann o.
Gudas scarf Z-plasty o.
Haber-Kraft o.
Haddad metatarsal o.
Herman-Gartland o.
high tibial o.
hinge o.
Hirayma o.
horizontal o.
iliac o.
Ingram-Canle-Beaty
  epiphysial-metaphysial o.
innominate o.
intertrochanteric varus o.
intraarticular o.
intracapsular o.
intraepiphysial o.
inverted L-form o.
inverted scarf o.
Irwin o.
Japas o.
Johnson chevron o.
Kalish o.
Kaplan o.
Kawamura dome o.
Kawamura pelvic o.
Kelly-Keck o.
Kempf-Grosse-Abalo Z step o.
Kessel-Bonney extension o.

Kitaoka-Leventen medial
  displacement metatarsal o.
Koutsogiannis calcaneal
  displacement o.
Koutsogiannis-Fowler-Anderson o.
Kramer-Craig-Noel basilar femoral
  neck o.
Lambrinudi o.
lateral closing wedge o.
Leach-Igou step-cut medial o.
Le Fort o.
Lichtblau o.
Lindseth o.
linear o.
Ludloff o.
Macewen-Shands o.
malleolar o.
mandibular ramus o.
Maquet dome o.
Marquardt angulation o.
Martin o.
Mau o.
maxillary o.
medial displacement o.
metacarpal o.
metaphysial o.
metatarsal Reverdin o.
metatarsal V-shaped o.
Mitchell o.
Molesworth o.
Mueller intertrochantaric varus o.
Mueller transposition o.
oblique base wedge o.
oblique displacement o.
open o.
orbitozygomatic mandibular o.
os calcis o.
Osgood rotational o.
Pauwels proximal o.
Pauwels valgus o.
pedicle subtraction o.
peg-in-hole o.
Peimer reduction o.
pelvic o.
Pemberton pericapsular o.
perforation o.
pericapsular o.
phalangeal o.
Platou o.
posterior iliac o.
posterior spinal wedge o.
Pott eversion o.
radial wedge o.
Ranawat-DeFiore-Straub o.
Rappaport o.
reduction o.
Reverdin o.
Reverdin-Laird o.
reverse Dillwyn-Evans calcaneal o.

reverse wedge o.
Root-Siegal varus derotational o.
rotational o.
sagittal-split mandibular o.
Sakoff o.
Salter innominate o.
Salter pelvic o.
Samilson crescentic calcaneal o.
Sarmiento intertrochanteric o.
scarf o.
Schanz angulation o.
Schanz femoral o.
Schwartz dorsiflexory o.
segmental alveolar o.
Siffert intraepiphysial o.
Siffert-Storen intraepiphysial o.
Silver-Hildreth o.
Simmonds-Menelaus metatarsal o.
Simmonds-Menelaus proximal
  phalangeal o.
Simmons o.
o. site
sliding oblique o.
Smith-Petersen o.
Smith-Robinson mandible open o.
Sofield o.
Southwick biplane trochanteric o.
Speas o.
spinal o.
Sponsel oblique o.
Stamm metatarsal o.
Steel triple innominate o.
step o.
step-cut o.
stepdown o.
Stren intraepiphysial o.
subcapital o.
subcondylar oblique o.
subtrochanteric o.
Sugioka transtrochanteric
  rotational o.
supracondylar varus o.
supramalleolar varus derotation o.
Sutherland-Greenfield o.
tarsal wedge o.
Tessier o.
Thompson telescoping V o.
through-and-through V-shaped
  horizontal o.
tibial tuberosity o.
transtrochanteric rotational o.
trapezoidal o.
Trethowan metatarsal o.
triplane o.
triple innominate o.
trochanteric o.
tubercle o.
unplanned valgus o.
valgus wedge o.

valgus Y-shaped o.
varus rotation shortening o.
vertical o.
V-shaped o.
Waterman o.
Weber humeral o.
Weber subcapital o.
wedge o.
wedge-shaped o.
Whitman o.
Wilson oblique displacement o.
Wiltse ankle o.
Wiltse varus supramalleolar o.
Yancey o.
Yu o.

osteotomy-bunionectomy
  scarf o.-b.
osteotomy-osteoclasis
  Moore o.-o.
osteotripsy
osteotrite
osteotympanic bone conduction
ostia (*pl. of* ostium)
ostial
  o. lesion
  o. sphincter
ostiomeatal complex
ostium, *pl.* **ostia**
  abdominal o.
  o. cardiacum
  celiac o.
  ileocecal o.
  o. primum
  o. secundum
ostomate
ostomy
  o. loop
  o. skin
Ostrum-Furst syndrome
Ostrup
  O. bone graft harvesting technique
  O. vascularized rib graft
Oswestry
  O. Disability Index (ODI)
  O. Disability Questionnaire (ODQ)
  O. Low Back Pain Questionnaire
    (OLBPQ)
Osypka rotational angioplasty
otic
  o. ganglion
  o. periotic shunt procedure
  o. vesicle
otitis
  o. externa
  o. media
otoconia
  degenerating o.
otolaryngologic manifestation
otolaryngologist

O

otolaryngology
    pediatric o.
otolith
otolithic membrane
otomandibular syndrome
otomicrosurgical transtemporal
  approach
otoplasty
    mattress suture o.
    Mustardé o.
otorhinolaryngology
otorrhea
    clear o.
otosclerosis
otoscopy
    pneumatic o.
OTR
    Ovarian Tumor Registry
Otto pelvis dislocation
ouabain
Oudard shoulder bone block procedure
out
    opting o.
outcome
    adverse o.
    clinical o.
    cosmetic o.
    final o.
    functional o.
    long-term o.
    o. monitoring
    perioperative o.
    short-term o.
    surgical o.
Outerbridge chondral knee lesion
  classification
outer limiting membrane
outermost
outflow
    cerebrospinal fluid o.
    o. control
    craniosacral o.
    thoracolumbar o.
    o. tract
    o. tract obstruction
    venous o.
out-in-out technique
outlet strut fracture
out-of-phase endometrial biopsy
outpatient
    o. anesthesia
    o. biopsy
    o. dialysis
    o. dialysis clinic
    o. endoscopy
    o. physical therapy
    o. surgical setting
    o. thyroidectomy
    o. thyroid operation

output
    cardiac o. ($\mathring{Q}$)
    chest tube o. (CTO)
    intraoperative urine o.
    o. layer
    pacemaker o.
    radiation o.
    saturation o.
    thermodilution cardiac o. (TDCO)
outside-to-outside arthroscopy technique
outward rotation
ova (*pl. of* ovum)
ovale
    patent foramen o. (PFO)
oval window
ovarian
    o. ablation
    o. artery
    o. branch
    o. bursa
    o. cancer
    o. cancer metastasis
    o. carcinoma
    o. carcinoma debulking
    o. clear cell adenocarcinoma
    o. cortex
    o. cystectomy
    o. dermoid cyst
    o. fimbria
    o. follicle exhaustion
    o. hernia
    o. hyperstimulation syndrome
    o. incision
    o. masculinization
    o. mass
    o. overstimulation syndrome
    o. plexus
    o. stimulation
    o. surface
    o. thecoma
    o. tumor
    O. Tumor Registry (OTR)
    o. vein
    o. vein syndrome
    o. wedge resection
ovariectomy
ovariocele
ovariohysterectomy
ovariosalpingectomy
ovariostomy
ovariotomy
    Beatson o.
    normal o.
ovary
    celomic epithelium carcinoma of o.
    premenopausal o.
    right o.
overall sound level
over-and-over suture technique

overangulation
overbite
overcirculation
    pulmonary o.
overcompensation
overcorrected position
overcorrection
overdetermination
overdilation
overfilled canal
overflow incontinence
overgrafting
overgrowth
    bacterial o.
    cartilage o.
    fungal o.
overhang
overhanging restoration
Overholt colonoscopy procedure
overinflation
overinstrumentation
overlap
    o. midline incisional hernioplasty
    suture o.
overlapping
    o. incision
    o. suture technique
overlay restoration
overload
    circulatory o.
    compression o.
    intravascular volume o.
    pressure o.
overpressurization
overprojecting nasal tip
override
    sternal o.
overrotation
oversedation
oversewing
    early o.
oversewn
overshoot
    calibration o.
    o. phenomenon
overstimulation
over-the-counter medication
over-the-head CPR
over-the-top position
over-the-wire technique
Overton dowel graft
overventilation
overwhelming
    o. postsplenectomy infection
    o. postsplenectomy sepsis
oviduct
oviductal
ovoid mass
ovotestes (*pl. of* ovotestis)

ovotestis, *pl.* **ovotestes**
ovulation
    estimated time of o.
    o. induction
    o. rate
    o. stimulation
ovum, *pl.* **ova**
Owen
    interglobular space of O.
    O. line
    O. operation
owl's
    o. eye
    o. eye inclusion body
oxalate calculus
Oxford cleft palate repair technique
oxidase
    nicotinamide adenine dinucleotide
      phosphate o.
oxidation
    o. of solution
    o. state
oxidation-reducing potential
oxide
    ethylene o. (ETO)
    inhaled nitrous o. (INO)
    nitric o. (NO)
    nitrous o. (N_2O)
oxide-oxygen
    nitrous o.-o. (N_2O-O_2)
oximetry
    cerebral o.
    exercise o.
    forehead reflectance o.
    jugular bulb o.
    pulse o. (pulse ox)
    spinal o.
    transesophageal
      echocardiograph-guided left
      ventricular o.
    transesophageal
      echocardiograph-guided right
      ventricular o.
oxycarbonate
oxycardiorespirogram
oxycephalia
oxycephalic, oxycephalous
oxycephalous (*var. of* oxycephalic)
oxycephaly, oxycephalia
oxycodone HCl and ibuprofen
OxyContin
oxygen (O_2, oxy)
    o. administration
    o. analyzer
    o. analyzer calibration
    o. concentration
    o. concentration in pulmonary
      capillary blood
    o. consumption (VO_2)

O

oxygen (*continued*)
o. cylinder A–E
o. debt
o. deprivation theory of narcosis
o. desaturation
o. dissociation curve
o. effect
o. extraction rate
flow-dependent o.
hyperbaric o. (HBO)
o. in air
nasal o.
partial pressure of o. (PO_2)
partial pressure of alveolar o.
partial pressure of arterial o. (PaO_2)
o. poisoning
rapid recompression-high pressure o.
o. reduction product
o. saturation (O_2 sat.)
o. saturation index
o. saturation measurement
o. saturation of hemoglobin of
  arterial blood
o. sensor module
o. step-up method
supplementary o.
o. supply line
o. tension
o. therapy
o. toxicity
transcutaneous partial pressure of o.
o. under high pressure
o. utilization)
o. washout technique

oxygenation
apneic o.
brain tissue o.
bubble o.
cell o.
disc o.
extracorporeal membrane o. (ECMO)
fetal scalp o.
film o.
hyperbaric o. (HBO)
inadequate postoperative o.
o. index (OI)
medullary o.
pump o.
rotating disc o.
screen o.
splanchnic o.
tissue o.
tumor o.

oxygenator
membrane o.

oxygen-carrying resuscitative fluid
oxygen-enriched atmosphere
oxygen-hemoglobin dissociation curve
oxygen-ratio monitoring controller
oxygen-related response
Oxyglobin
oxyhemoglobin dissociation curve
oxymorphone
o. HCl
oral immediate-release o.
oyster mass
ozonization
ozonolysis

PA
    posteroanterior
    pulmonary artery
      PA filling pressure
      PA projection
pacchionian granulation
pacemaker
    p. adaptive rate
    p. artifact
    p. burst pacing
    p. capture
    p. escape interval
    p. failure
    p. impedance
    p. lead fracture
    p. malfunction
    p. output
    p. pocket
    p. potential
    p. syndrome
    p. threshold
    p. undersensing
pacemaker-mediated tachycardia
Pacey anterior colporrhaphy technique
Pachon
    P. cardiography method
    P. collateral circulation test
pachydermatocele
pachymeningitis
pachyperitonitis
pachyvaginalitis
pacing
    external transcutaneous p.
    implantable
      cardioverter-defibrillator/atrial
      tachycardia p.
    pacemaker burst p.
    transesophageal atrial p. (TAP)
    transesophageal echocardiography
      with p. (TEEP)
    transesophageal ventricular p.
      (TEVP)
packed red blood cells (PRBC)
Pack-Ehrlich deep iliac dissection
packet
    obturator lymph node p.
packing
    nasal p.
    perihepatic p.
PaCO2
    arterial partial pressure of CO_2
    partial pressure of arterial carbon
      dioxide
Pacquin ureterolysis

PACU
    postanesthesia care unit
PAD
    percutaneous abscess drainage
pad
    abdominal fat p.
    adenoid p.
    adenoidal p.
    antimesenteric fat p.
    artificial fat p.
    axillary fat p.
    Bichat fat p.
    branch p.
    buccal fat p.
    bulbocavernosus fat p.
    buttocks p.
    digital p.
    epicardial fat p.
    esophagogastric fat p.
    fat p.
    heel fat p.
    herniated presacral fat p.
    Hoffa fat p. (HFP)
    ileocecal fat p.
    ischiorectal fat p.
    labial p.
    malar fat p.
    masticatory fat p.
    metatarsal p.
    orbital fat p.
    patellar fat p.
    pericardial fat p.
    pubic p.
    retrodiscal p.
    retromolar p.
    retropatellar fat p.
PADE
    Pain Assessment for the Dementing
    Elderly
paediatric (*var. of* pediatric)
PAF
    paroxysmal atrial fibrillation
    platelet activating factor
    pulmonary arteriovenous fistula
Pagenstecher
    P. circle
    P. intracapsular cataract
      extraction
    P. linen nonabsorbable suture
      technique
Paget
    P. carcinoma
    P. extramammary disease
Paget-Eccleston stain
Paget-von Schrötter syndrome

P

PAG/PVG
periaqueductal gray
matter/periventricular gray matter
PAG/PVG region
PAH
pulmonary artery hypertension
PAI
Pain Appraisal Inventory
pain
acute p.
allodynic p.
anorectal p.
p. anxiety symptoms scale
P. Appraisal Inventory (PAI)
p. assessment
P. Assessment for the Dementing
Elderly (PADE)
P. Assessment in Advanced
Dementia (PAINAD)
P. Assessment in Noncommunicative
Elderly Persons (PAINE)
back p.
p. behavior
P. Beliefs and Perception Inventory
(PBPI)
benign p.
bone p.
breakthrough p. (BTP)
burn p.
burning p.
cancer p.
cancer-related p.
p. catastrophizing scale (PCS)
cementum p.
central p.
central neuropathic p.
central poststroke p. (CPSP)
chronic nonmalignant p. (CNMP)
chronic nonterminal p.
chronic postsurgical p. (CPSP)
chronic widespread p.
Cognitive Risk Profile for P.
(CRPP)
colicky p.
colorectal distention p.
committee for classification of
chronic p.
concordant p.
consultation for low back p.
P. Coping Questionnaire (PCQ)
craniofacial p.
cyclic p.
deafferentation p.
p. deception
dentin p.
p. diary
diffuse abdominal p.
discogenic p.
p. drawing

dysesthetic p.
dystonic p.
Edmonton Staging System for
Cancer P.
epicritic p.
epigastric p.
episodic p.
exacerbation of p.
experimental p.
p. expression
expulsive p.
exquisite p.
facet p.
facial p.
gynecologic p.
head and neck cancer p.
herpes zoster p.
HIV-related abdominal p.
p. hypersensitivity
p. hyposensitivity
IASP classification of chronic p.
idiopathic neck p.
incident p.
incisional p.
p. induction
inflammatory p.
p. intensity score
p. interference
International Association for the
Study of P. (IASP)
intractable p.
joint line p.
labor p.
limb ischemia p.
localized p.
P. Locus of Control Questionnaire
(PLCQ)
low back p.
lumbar p.
lumbar discogenic p.
malignant p.
p. management
mechanical low back p.
p. mechanism
micturition p.
moderate p.
p. modulation
movement-related p.
myofascial p.
neuropathic p.
neuropathic central p.
neurovascular p.
nociceptive p.
nonmalignant p.
nonpharmacologic p.
nonsympathetically mediated p.
p. normosensitivity
obstetric p.
ocular p.

odontogenic p.
opioid-insensitive p.
orbital p.
orofacial p.
palliation of p.
pancreatic cancer p.
pediatric p.
perceived intensity of p.
p. perception profile
periauricular p.
periocular p.
phantom foot p.
phantom limb p.
phantom tooth p.
p. phenomenology
pillar p.
postherniorrhaphy p.
postmastectomy p.
postoperative cesarean section p.
poststroke p.
postsurgical p.
postsurgical truncal p.
postthoracotomy p.
posttraumatic p.
procedural p.
p. projection
protopathic p.
psychogenic p.
radicular p.
recurrent radicular p.
referred p.
referred trigger point p.
P. Relief Manikin
P. Relief Scoring System
residual limb p.
scleratomal distribution of p.
P. Self-Efficacy Questionnaire
  (PSEQ)
p. sensitivity range (PSR)
shortcut sciatic p.
sickle cell p.
p. signaling
somatic p.
spinal cord injury p.
spontaneous p.
stump p.
sympathetically independent p. (SIP)
sympathetically maintained p.
  (SMP)
p. syndrome
temporal summation p.
temporomandibular p.
thalamic p.
p. threshold reduction
p. tolerance level
tourniquet p.
tourniquet-induced p.
tourniquet ischemic p.
venous cannulation p.

visceral p.
zygapophysial joint p.
PAINAD
  Pain Assessment in Advanced
  Dementia
pain-coping strategies
PAINE
  Pain Assessment in Noncommunicative
  Elderly Persons
painful
  p. anesthesia
  p. point
painless rectal bleeding
pain-related fear
painter's colic
paired
  p. arytenoid
  p. electrical stimulation
  p. vasomotor response
Pais fracture
PAJB
  primary antecubital jump bypass
Pajot forceps delivery maneuver
PAK
  pancreas after kidney
  PAK transplant
palatal
  p. approach
  p. expansion
  p. flap
  p. implant
  p. index
  p. lengthening procedure
  p. vein
palate
  Byzantine arch p.
  cleft p.
  hard p.
  itchy soft p.
  p. reconstruction
  soft p.
palatine
  p. bone
  p. canal
  p. flap
  p. foramen
  p. gland
  p. nerve
  p. suture
  p. tonsil
palatoethmoidal suture
palatoglossal
  p. arch
  p. fold
palatoglossus muscle
palatomaxillary
  p. canal
  p. index
  p. suture

P

palatooccipital line
palatopharyngeal
    p. closure
    p. fold
    p. ring
    p. sphincter
    p. sphincter muscle
palatopharyngeus muscle
palatopharyngoplasty
palatopharyngorrhaphy
palatoplasty
palatorrhaphy
palatosalpingeus
palatostaphylinus
palatovaginal
    p. canal
    p. groove
paleotrigeminothalamic tract
Paley fibular hemimelia classification
Palfyn sinus
palladium (Pd)
palladium-103
    transperineal p.-1. (^{103}Pd)
palliation of pain
palliative
    p. bypass
    p. care
    p. cerebrospinal shunt procedure
    p. esophagostomy
    p. exeresis
    p. gastrostomy
    p. hepaticojejunostomy
    p. intent
    p. medicine
    p. operation
    p. resection
    p. sedation
    p. splenectomy
    p. surgery
    p. surgical procedure
    p. technique
    p. therapy
    p. total gastrectomy
    p. treatment
pallidectomy
pallidoamygdalotomy
pallidoansotomy
pallidotomy
    posteroventral p.
    stereotactic p.
    unilateral p.
    VPL p.
pallor
Palma crossover saphenous vein graft
palmar
    p. advancement flap
    p. angulation
    p. approach
    p. branch

    p. crease
    p. cross-finger flap
    p. hyperhidrosis
    p. incision
    p. interosseous artery
    p. synovectomy
palmate fold
Palmaz stent
Palmer
    P. all-inside TFCC repair technique
    P. transscaphoid perilunar dislocation
Palmer-Dobyns-Linscheid ligament repair
Palmer-Widen shoulder technique
palmoscopy
palm space
Palomo
    P. varicocelectomy
    P. varicocelectomy procedure
    P. varicocele ligation technique
palpable
    p. mass
    p. rib diastasis
palpation
    bimanual p.
    point p.
    p. testing
palpatory examination
palpebra, *pl.* **palpebrae**
    levator palpebrae
palpebrae (*pl. of* palpebra)
palpebral
    p. artery
    p. branch
    p. fascia
    p. fissure
    p. ligament
    p. muscle
    p. nerve
    p. rim
palpebration
palpebronasal fold
palpitation
    paroxysmal p.
    premonitory p.
PALS
    pediatric advanced life support
    PALS pulseless arrest algorithm
palsy
    Bell p.
    temporary p.
    vocal cord p.
pamidronate
pampiniform
    p. body
    p. venous plexus
pampinocele
Panacryl suture
Panalok absorbable suture
Panas lid ptosis operation

panclavicular dislocation
Pancoast
    P. suture
    P. suture technique
    P. tumor
pancolectomy
pancolonoscopy
pancreas
    aberrant p.
    accessory p.
    p. after kidney (PAK)
    anular p.
    artificial endocrine p.
    Aselli p.
    p. cancer
    denervation of p.
    distal p.
    ectopic p.
    endocrine p.
    esophageal heterotopic p.
    exocrine p.
    p. graft perfusion
    lesser p.
    nonfunctioning tumor of p.
    retroperitoneal p.
    small p.
    splanchnic denervation of p.
    p. transplant
    p. transplant alone (PTA)
    uncinate p.
    whole organ p. (WOP)
    Willis p.
    Winslow p.
pancreas-kidney transplant
pancreas-specific amylase isoenzyme
pancreatectomy, pancreectomy
    Child radical p.
    complete laparoscopic distal p.
    conventional distal p.
    distal p.
    distal laparoscopic p.
    donor p.
    en bloc distal p.
    laparoscopic distal p.
    left-to-right subtotal p.
    limited p.
    near-total p.
    partial p.
    proximal subtotal p.
    spleen-preserving distal p.
    subtotal distal p.
    total p.
    transduodenal p.
pancreatemphraxis
pancreatic
    p. abscess
    p. adenocarcinoma
    p. anastomosis
    p. artery

p. ascites
p. autotransplantation
p. bacterial infection
p. biopsy
p. body
p. branch
p. bypass
p. calculus
p. cancer pain
p. capsule
p. carcinoma
p. colic
p. complication
p. cyst
p. cystogastrostomy
p. cystoduodenostomy
p. cystoenterostomy
p. disease
p. duct
p. ductal disruption
p. duct dilation
p. duct manipulation
p. duct obstruction
p. duct pressure
p. duct sphincterotomy
p. ductule
p. dysfunction
p. endocrine neoplasia
p. endocrine tumor
p. endoscopy
p. enzyme
p. enzyme secretion
p. extract
p. fascia
p. fistula
p. fistula formation
p. fluid
p. fluid collection
p. fungal detection
p. fungus
p. head
p. head cancer
p. head origin
p. imaging
p. incidentaloma
p. insulinoma
p. intraluminal radiation therapy
p. islet
p. lithiasis
p. malignancy
p. neck
p. necrosis
p. necrosis prognostic score
p. neoplasia
p. neoplasm
p. neuroendocrine tumor
p. notch
p. operation
p. parenchyma

P

pancreatic (*continued*)
    p. plexus
    p. pseudocyst
    p. pseudocystogastrostomy
    p. resection
    p. rest
    p. sphincter
    p. sphincteroplasty
    p. stump
    p. stump closure
    p. stump leak
    p. surgeon
    p. surgery
    p. tail
    p. tail resection
    p. tissue
    p. transplant
    p. transplantation alone (PTA)
    p. trauma
    p. tumor localization
    p. vein
pancreaticae
    insulae p.
    lingulae p.
    venae p.
pancreatic-cutaneous fistula
pancreatici
    rami p.
pancreaticobiliary, panreatobiliary,
    p. canal
    p. endoscopy
    p. tract
pancreaticoblastoma
pancreaticocystostomy
pancreaticoduodenal, pancreatoduodenal
    p. allograft
    p. arcade vessel
    p. arterial arcade
    p. artery
    p. resection
    p. transplantation
    p. vein
pancreaticoduodenectomy (*var. of*
  pancreatoduodenectomy)
    pylorus-sparing p.
pancreaticoduodenostomy (*var. of*
  pancreatoduodenostomy)
    Whipple p.
pancreaticoenterostomy,
  pancreatoenterostomy
pancreaticogastrostomy (*var. of*
  pancreatogastrostomy)
    p. reconstruction
pancreaticojejunal
    p. anastomosis
    p. diversion
pancreaticojejunostomy (*var. of*
  pancreatojejunostomy)
    Cattell-Warren p.

distal p.
duct-to-mucosa p.
Duval p.
end-to-end intussuscepted p.
end-to-end inverting p.
Frey p.
Partington-Rochelle p.
retrocolic end-to-end p.
pancreaticopleural fistula
pancreaticosplenectomy
pancreaticosplenic
    p. ligament
    p. omentum
pancreatic-preserving total
  gastrectomy
pancreatic-renal
    simultaneous p.-r. (SPR)
pancreatitis
    acute p.
    biliary p.
    centrilobular p.
    chronic p.
    clinical acute p.
    diffuse hemorrhagic p.
    gallstone p.
    hemosuccus p.
    necrotizing p.
    recurrent p.
    severe acute p. (SAP)
pancreatitis-related hemorrhage
pancreatobiliary malformation
pancreatoblastoma
pancreatocholecystostomy
pancreatoduodenal (*var. of*
  pancreaticoduodenal)
pancreatoduodenectomy,
  pancreaticoduodenectomy
    Billroth II p.
    Brunschwig p.
    conventional p.
    extended p.
    Kausch-Whipple p.
    partial p.
    pylorus-preserving p. (PPPD)
    radical p.
    2-step p.
    subtotal p.
    Whipple p.
pancreatoduodenostomy,
  pancreaticoduodenostomy
    Child p.
    Dennis-Varco p.
    Waugh-Clagett p.
    Whipple p.
pancreatoenterostomy (*var. of*
  pancreaticoenterostomy)
pancreatogastric anastomosis
pancreatogastrointestinal
  anastomosis

pancreatogastrostomy,
pancreaticogastrostomy
    p. anastomosis (PGA)
pancreatography
pancreatojejunostomy,
pancreaticojejunostomy
    p. afferent
    p. anastomosis (PJA)
    caudal p.
    longitudinal p.
    Puestow p.
    Puestow-Gillesby p.
    Roux-en-Y p.
pancreatolith, pancreolith
pancreatolithectomy (*var. of*
  pancreatolithotomy)
pancreatolithiasis
pancreatolithotomy, pancreatolithectomy,
  pancreolithotomy
pancreatologist
pancreatolysis, pancreolysis
pancreatolytic, pancreolytic
pancreatomy (*var. of* pancreatotomy)
pancreatoscopy, pancreoscopy
    infragastric p.
    peroral p.
pancreatosplenectomy
    radical antegrade modular p.
    (RAMPS)
pancreatotomy, pancreatomy
pancreectomy
pancreolith (*var. of* pancreatolith)
pancreolithotomy (*var. of*
  pancreatolithotomy)
pancreolysis (*var. of* pancreatolysis)
pancreolytic (*var. of* pancreatolytic)
pancreoscopy
pandiculation
panel
    bleeding time coagulation p.
    clot retraction coagulation p.
    clotting time coagulation p.
    partial thromboplastin time
      coagulation p.
    plasma assay coagulation p.
    prediluted antibody p.
    prothrombin time coagulation p.
panendoscopy
    fiberoptic p.
    lower p.
    primary p.
    upper gastrointestinal p.
panenteric inflammatory ileus
panhysterectomy
panmetatarsal head resection
panmucosal inflammatory cell infiltration
panni (*pl. of* pannus)
pannicular hernia
panniculectomy

panniculi (*pl. of* panniculus)
panniculitis
    xanthogranulomatous p.
panniculus, *pl.* **panniculi**
    abdominal p.
    p. retraction
pannus, *pl.* **panni**
    p. formation
panoramic surface projection
PANP
    pelvic autonomic nerve preservation
panphotocoagulation
panproctocolectomy
panreatobiliary (*var. of* pancreaticobiliary)
panretinal
    p. ablation
    p. argon laser photocoagulation
pantalar fusion
pantaloon
    p. hernia
    p. patch
pants-over-vest
    p.-o.-v. capsulorrhaphy
    p.-o.-v. hernial repair
    p.-o.-v. herniorrhaphy
    p.-o.-v. technique
Panum fusion area
PaO₂
    partial pressure of arterial oxygen
PAOD
    popliteal artery occlusive disease
PAP
    positive airway pressure
    pulmonary artery pressure
Pap
    Papanicolaou
    Pap smear classification
Papanicolaou (Pap)
    P. method
Papavasiliou olecranon fracture
  classification
paper point
papilla, *pl.* **papillae**
    bile p.
    circumvallate p.
    duodenal p.
    foliate p.
    inferior lacrimal p.
    interdental p.
    lacrimal p.
    lenticular p.
    major duodenal p.
    minor duodenal p.
    optic p.
    renal p.
    retrocuspid p.
    retromolar p.
    sublingual p.
    superior lacrimal p.

P

papilla (*continued*)
    urethral p.
    vallate p.
    Vater p.
papillae (*pl. of* papilla)
papillary, papillate
    p. adenoma
    p. cancer
    p. cystadenocarcinoma
    p. duct
    p. ectasia
    p. foramen
    p. gastric carcinoma
    p. hidradenoma
    p. hyperplasia
    p. lesion
    p. muscle rupture
    p. muscle tip
    p. pedicle graft
    p. process
    p. projection
    p. reconstruction
    p. subtype
    p. thyroid carcinoma
papillate (*var. of* papillary)
papillectomy
papillitis
papilloadenocystoma
papillocarcinoma
papillogram
papilloma
    choroid plexus p.
    p. neuropathicum
papillomacular nerve fiber bundle
papillomatosis
    diffuse p.
papillomavirus
    human p. (HPV)
    p. infection
Papillon-Léage and Psaume syndrome
papillotome
papillotomy
    accessory p.
    endoscopic p.
    laparoscopic transcystic p.
    needle-knife p.
    precut p.
Papineau
    P. bone graft
    P. open bone grafting technique
Pappenheimer body
papulopustular lesion
papulosis
papulosquamous lesion
papulovesicular lesion
papyracea
Paquin ureterocystoneostomy technique
paraaortic
    p. hematoma

    p. lymphadenectomy
    p. lymph node dissection
    p. node irradiation
    p. region
paraaortica
paraappendicitis
parabiosis
parabiotic flap
paracancerous tissue
paracanthoma
paracardiac metastasis
paracentesis
    abdominal p.
paracentetic
paracentral
    p. lobe
    p. nerve fiber bundle
paracervical
    p. block (PCB)
    p. block anesthesia
    p. injection
paracervix
parachroma, parachromatosis
parachromatosis (*var. of* parachroma)
parachute
    p. deformity
    p. jumper's dislocation
    p. mitral valve
paraclavicular thoracic outlet decompression
paracoagulation
paracolic
    p. gutter
    p. recess
    p. sulcus
paracollicular biopsy
paracolpium
paracystic pouch
paracystitis
paracystium
paradidymal
paradidymis
paradoxic (*var. of* paradoxical)
paradoxical, paradoxic
    p. embolism
    p. embolus
    p. extensor reflex
    p. incontinence
    p. reaction
    p. respiration
    p. technique
paraduodenal
    p. fossa
    p. hernia
    p. recess
paraesophageal
    p. diaphragmatic hernia
    p. hiatal hernia

paraesophagogastric devascularization
paraesthesia (*var. of* paresthesia)
paraexstrophy skin flap
paraffin
    p. film application
    p. gauze dressing
    p. graft
paraffin-film treatment
paraffinoma
paraffin-section light microscopy
parafunctional habit
paraganglioma
paragenital tubule
paraglenoid groove
paraglottic
    p. area
    p. space
paragranuloma
parahepatic abscess
parahiatal hernia
parahypophysis
paraileostomal hernia
parainfluenza virus infection
parainguinal incision
parajejunal fossa
parakeratinization
parakeratosis
paralaryngeal space
parallel
    p. operation
    p. robot
    p. technique
paralleling
    p. cone position
    p. technique
parallelism
paralyses (*pl. of* paralysis)
paralysis, *pl.* **paralyses**
    compression p.
    cord p.
    hernia p.
    hysteric p.
    laryngeal nerve p.
    long-term p.
    nerve p.
    permanent p.
    pharmacologic p.
    pharmacologically induced p.
    polio p.
    postoperative residual p.
    pressure p.
    recurrent nerve p.
    soft palate p.
    thoracic motor p.
    tourniquet p.
    transient p.
    unilateral laryngeal p.
    unilateral vocal cord p.
    vocal cord p. (VCP)

paralytic
    p. gastrointestinal obstruction
    p. ileus
    p. strabismus
paramagnetic contrast injection
paramedial incision
paramedian
    p. approach
    p. incision
    p. pontine reticular
      formation
    p. sagittal plane
    p. sheath
paramedical personnel
paramesonephric duct
paramesonephricus
parameter
    canonical univariate p.
    clinical p.
    clotting p.
    conventional p.
    effect p.
    laboratory p.
    macrocirculatory p.
    microcirculatory p.
    postprandial motor p.
parametrectomy
    radical p.
parametrial
parametric test
parametritis
    posterior p.
parametrium
paranalgesia
paranasal
    p. cell
    p. mucocele
    p. sinus
    p. sinus drainage
paraneoplastic
    p. ectopic ACTH
      production
    p. syndrome
paranephric
    p. abscess
    p. body
paranephros
paranesthesia
paraneural infiltration
paraomphalic
paraoperative
paraoral tissue
paraorbital lesion
paraovarian
parapancreatic
paraparesis
parapatellar
    p. arthrotomy
    p. incision

P

paraperitoneal
    p. hernia
    p. nephrectomy
parapharyngeal
    p. space
    p. space abscess
paraphasia
    extended jargon p.
paraphimosis
paraphysis
parapineal
paraplegia
    complete motor p.
    p. in extension
    motor p.
    postoperative p.
parapneumonic empyema
paraproctium
paraprostatitis
parapubic hernia
pararectal
    p. fistula
    p. fossa
    p. line
    p. pouch
pararectus
    p. approach
    p. incision
pararenal
    p. aortic aneurysm
    p. space
parasaccular hernia
parasacral approach
parasagittal
    p. incision
    p. lesion
    p. plane
    p. section
parascapular
    p. flap
    p. incision
parasellar
    p. mass
    p. metastasis
    p. syndrome
parasinoidal
parasite
    bile duct p.
parasitic
    p. castration
    p. cyst
    p. flap
    p. infection
paraspinal
    p. approach
    p. line
    p. muscle
    p. rod application
paraspinous aspect

parasternal
    p. block
    p. defect
    p. examination
    p. line
    p. lymph node
parastomal
    p. hernia
    p. infection
    p. irritation
parasympathectomy
    sinuatrial nodal p.
parasympathetic
    p. fiber
    p. ganglion
    p. innervation
    p. nerve
    p. projection
paraterminal body
parathyroid
    p. adenoma
    p. artery
    p. autograft
    p. biopsy
    p. carcinoma
    p. extract
    p. gland
    p. hormone (PTH)
    p. hormone level
    p. hyperplasia
    p. operation
    p. remnant
    superior p.
    p. surgeon
    p. surgery
    p. tissue
    p. tumor
    p. tumor ablation
    p. vascularity
parathyroidectomy
    endoscopic p.
    incidental p.
    minimally invasive p.
    minimally invasive video-assisted p.
      (MIVAP)
    radioguided p.
    reoperative p.
    subtotal p.
    total p.
    unilateral p.
paratonsillar vein
paratracheal
    p. node
    p. tissue stripe
paratrachoma
paratrigeminal syndrome
paratrooper's fracture
paraumbilical
    p. hernia

p. incision
p. vein
paraurethral
p. duct
p. gland
parauterini
nodi lymphoidei p.
paravaccinia virus infection
paravaginal
p. defect repair
p. hysterectomy
p. incision
p. soft tissue
paravalvular regurgitation
paravariceal
p. injection
p. sclerotherapy
paravertebral
p. anesthesia
p. ganglion
p. gutter
p. line
p. lumbar sympathetic block
p. somatic nerve blockade
paravesical
p. fossa
p. pouch
Paré
P. reduction
P. suture technique
parectasis
parencephalia
parencephalocele
parenchyma
breast p.
cirrhotic liver p.
damaged p.
functional p.
hepatic p.
liver p.
pancreatic p.
pulmonary p.
parenchymal
p. brain metastasis
p. brain neoplasia
p. cell
p. change
p. destruction
p. dissection
p. laceration
p. lymphatic
p. route of injection
p. sparing surgery
p. transection
parenchymatous
p. hematoma
p. intracerebral hemorrhage
p. tissue
parental pain perception

parenteral
p. administration
p. alimentation
p. analgesia
p. analgesic
p. anesthesia
p. hyperalimentation
p. medication
p. nutrition
p. nutritional support
p. therapy
parent vessel
parepicele
parepididymis
paresis
elevation p.
paresthesia pressure p.
paresthesia, paraesthesia
p. anesthetic technique
mechanical p.
p. pressure paresis
paresthetica
meralgia p.
postlaparoscopy meralgia p.
paretic limb
paries, *pl.* **parietes**
parietal
p. angle
p. artery
p. bone
p. border
p. branch
p. cell vagotomy
p. defect
p. eminence
p. emissary vein
p. fistula
p. foramen
p. hernia
p. layer
p. margin
p. node
p. notch
p. pelvic fascia
p. pericardiectomy
p. pericardium
p. peritoneal closure
p. peritoneum
p. pleura
p. region
p. suture
p. tuber
p. wall
parietes (*pl. of* paries)
Parietex mesh
parietofrontal
parietography
parietomastoidea
parietomastoid suture

P

parietooccipital
    p. approach
    p. artery
parietooccipitalis
parietopontine tract
parietosphenoid
parietosplanchnic
parietosquamosal
parietotemporal
parietovisceral
Paris endoscopic superficial neoplastic lesion classification
park-bench position
Parker incision
Parker-Kerr
    P.-K. suture-closed method
    P.-K. suture technique
Parkinson disease
parkinsonian tremor
Parks
    P. hemorrhoidectomy
    P. ileoanal anastomosis
    P. method of anal fistulotomy
    P. partial sphincterotomy
    P. staged fistulotomy
Parks-Bielschowsky 3-step, head-tilt test
paroccipital process
Parodi flow reversal technique
parolivary
paromphalocele
Parona space
paronychial infection
parorchidium
parorchis
parosteal
parotic
parotid
    p. bed
    p. branch
    p. carcinoma
    p. dissection
    p. duct
    p. duct ligation
    p. fascia
    p. gland
    p. node
    p. notch
    p. plexus
    p. recess
    p. region
    p. resection
    p. sheath
    p. space
    p. vein
parotidectomy
    facial nerve-preserving p.
    nerve-preserving p.
    radical p.
    superficial p.

    supraneural p.
    total p.
parotideomasseteric fascia
parotidoauricularis
parovarian mass
parovariotomy
parovarium
paroxysmal
    p. atrial fibrillation (PAF)
    p. hemicrania
    p. nocturnal hemoglobinuria (PNH)
    p. palpitation
Parrish-Mann hammertoe technique
Parrish microvascular decompression procedure
parrot-beak nail
Parry-Jones vulvectomy
pars, *pl.* **partes**
    p. flaccida
    p. flaccida cholesteatoma
Parsonage-Turner syndrome
Parsonnet cardiac surgery risk score
partes (*pl. of* pars)
1-part fracture
2-part fracture
3-part fracture
4-part fracture
partial
    p. alveolectomy
    p. atrioventricular canal
    p. breech extraction
    p. cardiopulmonary bypass
    p. central hypophysectomy
    p. colectomy
    p. cricotracheal resection
    p. cystectomy
    p. discectomy
    p. dislocation
    p. duplication
    p. encircling endocardial ventriculotomy
    p. ethmoidectomy
    p. facetectomy
    p. fasciectomy
    p. fibulectomy
    p. gastrectomy
    p. gastric resection
    p. glossectomy
    p. hemilaminectomy
    p. hepatectomy
    p. hepatic vascular exclusion (PHVE)
    p. ileal bypass
    p. inferior retrocolic end-to-side gastrojejunostomy
    p. internal hemipelvectomy
    p. keratoplasty
    p. lamellar sclerouvectomy

p. laparoscopic decapsulation
p. laryngectomy
p. laryngopharyngectomy
p. lateral internal sphincterotomy
p. left ventriculectomy
p. liquid ventilation
p. mastectomy
p. matrixectomy
p. maxillectomy
p. mechanical obstruction
p. meniscectomy
p. mesh excision
p. nephrectomy
p. orchidectomy
p. ostectomy
p. pancreatectomy
p. pancreatoduodenectomy
p. patellectomy
p. pericystectomy
p. pressure
p. pressure of alveolar oxygen
p. pressure of arterial carbon dioxide ($PaCO_2$)
p. pressure of arterial oxygen (PaO_2)
p. pressure of carbon dioxide (PCO_2)
p. pressure of intramuscular carbon dioxide
p. pressure of mesenteric venous carbon dioxide
p. pressure of oxygen (PO_2)
p. pressure of water vapor
p. proctectomy
p. pulpectomy
p. pulpotomy
p. saturation
p. superior retrocolic end-to-side gastrojejunostomy
p. thromboplastin time coagulation panel
p. wrist fusion
p. zonal dissection
partial-breast irradiation
partial-thickness
p.-t. burn
p.-t. craniectomy
p.-t. flap
partial-throw surgeon's knot
particle
p. beam radiation therapy
free-floating p.
particulate
p. cancellous bone graft
p. embolization
Partington-Rochelle pancreaticojejunostomy
Partipilo gastrostomy
partition

Partsch operation
parturient canal
parturient-controlled epidural analgesia (PCEA)
parumbilical
paruresis
Parvin
P. gravity technique
P. reduction
PAS
peripheral access system
PAS port
passage
antegrade p.
duodenal p.
false p.
nasopharyngeal p.
oropharyngeal p.
p. pressure
transforaminal p.
transperineurial p.
wire p.
Passavant
P. bar
P. fold
P. ridge
passé
coma dé p.
passer
suture p.
passive
p. clot
p. gliding technique
p. incontinence
p. joint manipulation
p. pain coping
p. reciprocation
p. safety intravenous catheter
p. tissue cooling
Pastia line
PAT
percutaneous aspiration thromboembolectomy
prism adaptation test
patch
achromic p.
p. amnesia
aortic p.
p. aortoplasty
ash-leaf p.
autologous pericardial p.
Bard modified Kugel p.
blood p.
butterfly p.
cardiac p.
Carrel p.
p. clamp electrophysiology
colic p.
colonic p.

P

patch (*continued*)
    cotton-wool p.
    eczematous p.
    electrodispersive skin p.
    epidural blood p. (EBP)
    p. esophagoplasty
    fundic p.
    glue p.
    gray p.
    herald p.
    Hutchinson p.
    p. lesion
    Lidoderm p.
    lyophilized dural p.
    moth p.
    mucous p.
    omental p.
    pantaloon p.
    pedicle pericardial p.
    pericardial p.
    peritoneal p.
    Peyer patches
    pigskin p.
    prophylactic epidural blood p.
    prosthetic p.
    pruritic erythematous p.
    sandwich p.
    S-Caine topical anesthetic p.
    sclerotic calvarial p.
    scopolamine antiemetic p.
    shagreen p.
    soldier's p.
    p. stage
    Synera topical anesthetic p.
    p. technique
    p. testing
    p. test scarring
    Thal fundic p.
    Transderm Scop antiemetic p.
    vein p.
    venous sheath p.
    Ventralex p.
    white p.
patch-graft angioplasty
patchplasty
2-patch technique
patchy
    p. colonic ulceration
    p. infiltration
patefaction
patella, *pl.* **patellae**
    chondromalacia patellae (CMP, CP)
    p. turndown approach
patellae (*pl. of* patella)
patellapexy
patellar
    p. fat pad
    p. intraarticular dislocation
    p. network

    p. retinaculum
    p. sleeve fracture
    p. tendon graft donor site (PTGDS)
    p. tendon repair
patellectomy
    partial p.
    total p.
    West and Soto-Hall p.
patelliform
patellofemoral
    p. articulation
    p. pain syndrome
Patel medial meniscectomy
patency
    biliary stent p.
    catheter p.
    graft p.
    shunt p.
    stent p.
    valve p.
patent
    p. ductus arteriosus (PDA)
    p. foramen ovale (PFO)
    p. iridectomy
    p. portal vein
Paterson
Patey modified radical mastectomy
path
    p. of insertion
    p. of removal
pathogen
    fungal p.
    initial primary p.
    primary p.
pathogenesis
pathologic, pathological
    p. amputation
    p. barrier
    p. breast discharge
    p. cause
    p. characteristic
    p. diagnosis
    p. dislocation
    p. entity
    p. examination
    p. lesion
    p. nature
    p. neovascularization
    p. perforation
    p. response
    p. retraction ring
    p. specimen
    p. sphincter
pathological (*var. of* pathologic)
    p. anatomy
    p. fracture
pathology
    adrenal p.
    airway p.

anatomic p.
clinical p.
colorectal p.
p. examination
experimental p.
inciting p.
intracranial p.
intrahepatic p.
intrathyroidal p.
neoplastic p.
obstructing p.
p. scarring
surgical p.
synchronous p.
thyroid p.
venous p.

pathomechanics
kyphotic deformity p.
spinal fusion p.
pathophysiologic factor
pathophysiology
pathostimulation
pathway
ascending p.
ascending nociceptive p.
beta oxidation p.
coagulation p.
descending pain p.
effector p.
extrapyramidal p.
extrinsic p.
lemniscal trigeminothalamic p.
lymphatic p.
orogastric p.
P. pain and sensory evaluation
system
proteolytic p.
receptor-mediated endocytosis p.
sensory p.
shunt p.
somatosensory p.
spinothalamic p.
taste p.
visual p.

PATI
penetrating abdominal trauma
index
patient
adult p.
ambulatory p.
asymptomatic p.
bariatric p.
brain-dead p.
debilitated p.
diabetic p.
dialysis-dependent p.
disease-free p.
endoscopically normal p.
head-injured p.

hemodialysis-dependent p.
high-risk p.
immunosuppressed p.
inoperable p.
intermediate-risk p.
low-risk p.
morbidly obese p.
obese p.
pediatric p.
poor-risk p.
p. population
sentinel node-positive p.
septic p.
p. state analyzer
p. state index (PSI)
super-obese p.
surgical p.
surgically treated p.
symptomatic p.
toxic-traumatized p.
trauma p.
tube-fed p.
vascular access p.

**patient-activated transdermal system
(PATS)**
patient-controlled
p.-c. analgesia (PCA)
p.-c. analgesia anesthetic technique
p.-c. anesthesia (PCA)
p.-c. epidural analgesia (PCEA)
p.-c. epidural with intravenous
analgesia
p.-c. intranasal analgesia (PCINA)
p.-c. regional analgesia (PCRA)
patient-dependent factor
patient-triggered breath
Patrick sacroiliitis test
patrilineal
PATS
patient-activated transdermal system
pattern
abdominal wall venous p.
airway p.
p. arborization
architectural p.
butterfly p.
p. cut corneal graft operation
distribution p.
drainage p.
flow p.
histologic p.
lymphatic drainage p.
motor p.
p. of breathing
p. of distribution
p. of drainage
p. of motion
p. of staining
organ-specific p.

P

pattern (*continued*)
  p. recognition
  sinusoidal p.
  strain p.
  upper jejunal motor p.
pattern-cut corneal graft
patulous
Pauchet gastrectomy procedure
paucity
Paufique
  P. keratoplasty
  P. synechiotomy
Paul-Mikulicz
  P.-M. sigmoid colectomy
  P.-M. staged bowel resection
Paulos ligament technique
Pauly point
pause-squeeze method
Pauwels
  P. femoral neck fracture
    classification
  P. fracture
  P. osteotomy technique
  P. proximal osteotomy
  P. valgus osteotomy
  P. Y-osteotomy
PAV
  proportional assist ventilation
  proportional assist ventilator
PAVF
  pulmonary arteriovenous fistula
PAW
  pulmonary artery wedge
Payne-DeWind jejunoileal bypass
**Payne morbid obesity jejunoileal
  bypass**
Payr
  P. clamp gastric surgery method
  P. membrane
Pb
  lead
PBAV
  percutaneous balloon aortic
    valvoplasty
PBPI
  Pain Beliefs and Perception Inventory
  penile-brachial pressure index
PCA
  patient-controlled analgesia
  patient-controlled anesthesia
  posterior cerebral artery
  prostate cancer
    PCA by proxy
PCB
  paracervical block
PCC
  percutaneous catheter cecostomy
PCEA
  patient-controlled epidural analgesia

PCINA
  patient-controlled intranasal analgesia
PCIRV
  pressure control inverse ratio
    ventilation
  pressure controlled inverse ratio
    ventilation
PCN
  percutaneous nephrolithotomy
  percutaneous nephrostomy
PCNA
  proliferating cell nuclear antigen
PCNL
  percutaneous nephrolithotomy
  percutaneous nephrolithotripsy
  percutaneous nephrostolithotomy
PCO$_2$
  partial pressure of carbon dioxide
PCoA
  posterior communicating artery
PCom
  posterior communicating artery
PComA
  posterior communicating artery
PCPS
  peroral cholangiopancreatoscopy
PCQ
  Pain Coping Questionnaire
PCRA
  patient-controlled regional analgesia
  percutaneous coronary rotational
    atherectomy
PCS
  pain catastrophizing scale
  peroral cholangioscopy
PCT
  percutaneous transhepatic
    cholangiography
PCV
  pressure controlled ventilation
  pressure-control ventilation
PCWP
  pulmonary capillary wedge pressure
Pd
  palladium
^{103}Pd
  transperineal palladium-103
PDA
  patent ductus arteriosus
PDGF
  platelet-derived growth factor
PDN
  prosthetic disc nucleus
PDPH
  postdural puncture headache
PDS
  polydioxanone suture
    PDS II suture
    PDS suture

PDT
    percutaneous dilational tracheostomy
    photodynamic therapy
PE
    pulmonary embolism
      submassive PE
PEA
    pulseless electrical activity
Peabody-Mitchell bunionectomy
Peacock neurovascular island pedicle
  flap technique
peak
    p. exercise oxygen consumption
    p. expiratory flow
    p. expiratory flow rate (PEFR)
    p. inspiratory ventilator pressure
    p. pressure analysis
    p. systolic aortic pressure
    p. systolic gradient
    p. systolic gradient pressure
    p. transaortic valve gradient
Péan incision
pearl
    cholesteatoma p.
    perineal p.
PEBB
    percutaneous excisional breast biopsy
Pecquet
    P. cistern
    P. duct
pecten
    anal p.
    p. band
pectinata
    zona p.
pectinate
    p. body
    p. line
    p. zone
pectineal
    p. fascia
    p. hernia
    p. ligament
    p. line
pectiniforme
    septum p.
pectiniform septum, septum pectiniforme
pectora (*pl. of* pectus)
pectoral
    p. branch
    p. fascia
    p. groove
pectoralis
    p. fascia
    p. major muscle flap
    p. major muscle origin
    p. major myocutaneous flap
      (PMMF)
    p. minor syndrome

    p. muscle
    p. myocutaneous esophagoplasty
    p. myocutaneous flap
    p. myofascial flap
pectoriloquy
    whispered p.
pectoris (*pl. of* pectus)
pectorodorsal muscle
pectus, *pl.* **pectoris,** *pl.* **pectora**
    p. carinatum
    p. carinatum deformity
    p. excavatum
    p. excavatum deformity
    p. excavatum repair
    p. index
PED
    percutaneous external drainage
pediatric, paediatric
    p. advanced life support (PALS)
    p. airway
    p. analgesic
    p. anesthesia system
    p. anesthetic
    p. cardiovascular surgery
    p. circle
    p. colonoscopy
    p. endoscopy
    p. end-stage liver disease (PELD)
    p. esophagogastroduodenoscopy
    p. esophagoplasty
    p. hepaticojejunostomy
    p. hernia
    p. hypothermia
    p. injury
    p. intussusception
    p. laparoscopic surgical procedure
    p. mass
    p. neoplasia
    p. neoplasm
    p. neurosurgeon
    p. ophthalmic surgery
    p. otolaryngology
    p. pain
    p. patient
    p. population
    p. portal hypertension
    p. radiotherapy anesthesia
    p. surgeon
    P. Surgery Board
    p. tracheotomy
    p. trauma scale (PTS)
    p. urologist
    p. urology
    p. vaginoscopy
pedicellation
pedicle
    p. anatomy
    p. cannulation
    p. entrance point

P

pedicle (*continued*)
    p. evaluation
    p. fat graft
    Filatov-Gillies tubed p.
    p. flap operation
    p. flap urethroplasty
    p. fracture
    glissonian p.
    p. groin flap
    hepatic p.
    intercostal muscle p.
    p. landmark
    lateral-sector p.
    p. ligation
    p. localization
    medial-sector p.
    p. method
    omental p.
    p. pericardial patch
    portal p.
    posterior p.
    p. screw construct
    p. screw hardware prominence
    p. screw path length
    p. screw plating
    p. screw-rod fixation
    sectoral p.
    p. subtraction osteotomy
    vascular p.
    vasculobiliary p.
    p. wrapping
pedicled
    p. jejunal reconstruction
    p. myocutaneous flap
    p. omentoplasty
pedicolaminar fracture-dislocation
pedicular fixation
pediculation
pediculus
pediphalanx
pedodontic endodontics
peduncle
peduncular loop
pedunculated
    p. loose body
    p. polyp
pedunculation
pedunculotomy
peel
    chemical p.
    fibrin p.
peeling
    membrane p.
PEEP
    positive end-expiratory pressure
PEEP/CPAP
    positive end-expiratory
    pressure/continuous positive airway
    pressure

PEEPi
    intrinsic positive end-expiratory
      pressure
PEER
    pronation eversion external rotation
peer review
Peet
    P. operation
    P. splanchnic resection
    P. Z-plasty
PEFR
    peak expiratory flow rate
PEG
    percutaneous endoscopic gastrostomy
    polyethylene glycol
peg
    p. bone graft
    p. flap
    P. tube insertion
peg-and-socket
    p.-a.-s. articulation
    p.-a.-s. joint
    p.-a.-s. technique
peg-in-hole osteotomy
PEG-J
    percutaneous endoscopic
      gastrojejunostomy
      PEG-J tube
PEI
    percutaneous ethanol injection
Peimer reduction osteotomy
PEJ
    percutaneous endoscopic jejunostomy
PELD
    pediatric end-stage liver disease
pelidnoma (*var. of* pelioma)
pelioma, pelidnoma
peliosis hepatitis
Pell-Gregory tooth position classification
pellucida
    zona p.
pellucidum
    cavum septum p.
    septum p.
pelma
pelmatic
peltation
pelves (*pl. of* pelvis)
pelvic
    p. abscess
    p. adhesive disease
    p. appendix
    p. aspiration biopsy
    p. autonomic nerve preservation (PANP)
    p. autonomic plexus
    p. avulsion fracture
    p. axis
    p. brim
    p. canal

p. cavity
p. collection
p. colonic surgery
p. diaphragm
p. direction
p. examination
p. exenteration
p. fascia
p. fixation
p. floor dysfunction
p. floor physical therapy
p. floor procedure
p. ganglion
p. girdle
p. hematocele
p. hemorrhage volume
p. ileal reservoir construction
p. inclination
p. infection
p. inflammation
p. inflammatory disease (PID)
p. irradiation
p. ischemia
p. kidney
p. laparoscopy
p. limb
p. lymphadenectomy
p. lymph node dissection (PLND)
p. lymphocelectomy
p. mass
p. node dissection
p. organ dysfunction syndrome
p. osteotomy
P. Pain Assessment form
p. peritonectomy
p. plane
p. pouch
p. pouchoscopy
p. pouch procedure
p. promontory
p. relaxation
p. ring
p. ring fracture
p. rotation
p. sidewall
p. skeleton
p. stimulation
p. straddle fracture
p. type A, B, C fracture
p. type I, II AP compression
   fracture
p. type I, II lateral compression
   fracture
pelvicaliceal (*var. of* pelvicalyceal)
pelvicalyceal, pelvicaliceal
   p. leak
pelvic-floor procedure
pelvic-iliac lymphadenectomy
pelvifixation

pelvilithotomy (*var. of* pyelolithotomy)
pelviolithotomy (*var. of* pyelolithotomy)
pelvioplasty (*var. of* pyeloplasty)
pelvioscopy, pelvoscopy, pelviscopy
pelviotomy, pelvitomy
pelvirectal sphincter
pelvis, *pl.* **pelves**
   android p.
   anthropoid p.
   assimilation p.
   brachypellic p.
   contracted p.
   cordate p.
   Deventer p.
   dolichopellic p.
   dwarf p.
   extrarenal renal p.
   false p.
   flat p.
   funnel-shaped p.
   greater p.
   gynecoid p.
   heart-shaped p.
   inclinatio p.
   inverted p.
   juvenile p.
   large p.
   lesser p.
   longitudinal oval p.
   masculine p.
   mesatipellic p.
   osteomalacic p.
   platypellic p.
   pseudoosteomalacic p.
   renal p.
   reniform p.
   Robert p.
   round p.
   small p.
   spider p.
   transverse oval p.
   true p.
   ureteric p.
pelvisacral
pelviscopic
   p. clip ligation technique
   p. intrafascial hysterectomy
pelviscopy (*var. of* pelvioscopy)
pelvitomy (*var. of* pelviotomy)
pelvivertebral angle
pelvoscopy (*var. of* pelvioscopy)
Pemberton
   P. acetabuloplasty
   P. operation
   P. pericapsular osteotomy
PEMF
   pulsed electromagnetic field
   PEMF therapy
pemphigoid

P

pemphigus
**Pena anorectal malformation corrective
  procedure**
penalization
**Penaz volume-clamp noninvasive blood
  pressure method**
pencil-in-cup deformity
pendulous abdomen
pendulum
penectomy
penes (*pl. of* penis)
penetrance
penetrating
    p. abdominal trauma index
      (PATI)
    p. corneal transplant
    p. fracture
    p. keratoplasty
    p. liver injury
    p. rupture
    p. thoracoabdominal injury
    p. trauma
    p. ulcer
    p. wound
penetration
    peritoneal p.
    serosal p.
    p. test
penial
penicillary
penicillate
penicilli (*pl. of* penicillus)
penicillus, *pl.* penicilli
penile, penial
    p. amputation
    p. block
    p. blockade
    p. cancer
    p. carcinoma
    p. deformity
    p. erection
    p. extensibility
    p. fracture
    p. incarceration
    p. injection testing
    p. injection therapy
    p. island flap
    p. raphe
    p. revascularization
    p. rupture
    p. trauma
    p. urethra
    p. vein occlusion therapy
    p. venous ligation surgery
**penile-brachial pressure index
  (PBPI)**
penile-preserving surgery
penis, *pl.* penes, penises
    bifid p.

    buried p.
    clubbed p.
    concealed p.
    deep p.
    dorsal p.
    glans p.
    webbed p.
penischisis
peniscopy
penises (*pl. of* penis)
penitis
**Pennal pelvic fracture
  classification**
pennate muscle
penoplasty
penoscrotal transposition
penotomy
PENS
    percutaneous electrical nerve
      stimulation
pentad
    Reynolds p.
pentadactyl, pentadactyle
pentadactyle (*var. of* pentadactyl)
pentagonal block excision
pentalogy
    Cantrell p.
pentane excretion level
pentoxifylline
    preincisional intravenous p.
penumbral region
PEP
    positive expiratory pressure
pepsic (*var. of* peptic)
peptic, pepsic
    p. aspiration pneumonitis
    p. gland
    p. stricture
    p. ulcer
    p. ulcer disease (PUD)
peptide
    atrial natriuretic p. (ANP)
    brain natriuretic p. (BNP)
    connective tissue activating p.
    endogenous opioid p.
    fusion p.
    gastric inhibitory p.
    glucagonlike p. 1
    vasoactive intestinal p. (VIP)
per
    p. anum
    p. contiguum
    p. continuum
peraxillary
perceived
    p. exertion
    p. intensity of pain
    p. quality of life (PQOL)
percentage of ideal body weight

perception
    augmented pain p.
    cutaneous p.
    kinesthetic p.
    parental pain p.
perceptual expansion
perched facet
percolation
percussion
    hard p.
    p. therapy
percutaneous
    p. abscess drainage (PAD)
    p. access
    p. alcohol injection
    p. anesthetic loss
    p. angioplasty
    p. anterior gastropexy
    p. appendectomy
    p. arterial cannulation
    p. aspirate
    p. aspiration thromboembolectomy (PAT)
    p. balloon angioplasty
    p. balloon aortic valvoplasty (PBAV)
    p. balloon aspiration
    p. balloon compression
    p. balloon dilation
    p. balloon mitral valvoplasty
    p. balloon pericardiotomy
    p. balloon pulmonic valvoplasty
    p. bone marrow infection
    p. catheter cecostomy (PCC)
    p. catheter drainage
    p. catheter insertion
    p. cholangioscopic lithotomy
    p. cholecystectomy
    p. cholecystolithotomy
    p. cholecystostomy
    p. compression device-toe deformity
    p. cordotomy
    p. coronary rotational atherectomy (PCRA)
    p. corticotomy
    p. CT-guided aspiration
    p. dilational tracheostomy (PDT)
    p. disc decompression
    p. electrical nerve stimulation (PENS)
    p. embolization therapy
    p. endofluoroscopy
    p. endopyeloureterotomy
    p. endoscopic approach
    p. endoscopic gastrojejunostomy (PEG-J)
    p. endoscopic gastrojejunostomy tube
    p. endoscopic gastrostomy (PEG)
    p. endoscopic gastrostomy tube insertion

    p. endoscopic jejunostomy (PEJ)
    p. endoscopic removal
    p. endoscopic tube insertion
    p. endoscopy
    p. endovascular treatment
    p. enterostomy
    p. epididymal sperm aspiration (PESA)
    p. ethanol ablation
    p. ethanol injection (PEI)
    p. ethanol injection therapy
    p. excisional breast biopsy (PEBB)
    p. external drainage
    p. fetal cystoscopy
    p. fetal tissue sampling
    p. fine-needle aspiration (PFNA)
    p. fine-needle aspiration biopsy
    p. fine-needle pancreatic biopsy
    p. fixation
    p. FNA
    p. gastroenterostomy (PGE)
    p. glycerol rhizolysis (PGR)
    p. injury
    p. insertion technique
    p. interventional technique
    p. intraaortic balloon counterpulsation
    p. laser nucleolysis
    p. lead
    p. line
    p. lithotripsy
    p. local ablative therapy
    p. localization
    p. low-stress angioplasty
    p. lumbar discectomy
    p. mechanical thrombectomy (PMT)
    p. microwave coagulation therapy
    p. mitral balloon commissurotomy
    p. mitral balloon valvotomy
    p. native renal biopsy
    p. needle liver biopsy
    p. needle puncture
    p. nephrolithotomy (PCN, PCNL, PNL)
    p. nephrolithotripsy (PCNL)
    p. nephroscopy
    p. nephrostolithotomy (PCNL)
    p. nephrostomy (PCN)
    p. nephrostomy tube placement
    p. neurolytic intercostal block
    p. pancreas biopsy
    p. patent ductus arteriosus closure
    p. pin insertion
    p. pinning
    p. plantar fasciotomy
    p. portocaval anastomosis
    p. pressure ureteral perfusion test
    p. radical cryosurgical ablation
    p. radiofrequency catheter ablation

P

percutaneous (*continued*)
- p. radiofrequency dorsal rhizotomy
- p. radiofrequency gangliolysis
- p. radiofrequency neurotomy
- p. radiofrequency rhizolysis
- p. radiofrequency thermoablation
- p. reduction
- p. renal puncture
- p. retrogasserian glycerol chemoneurolysis
- p. retrogasserian glycerol rhizolysis
- p. rotational thrombectomy
- p. sampling method
- p. stimulation
- p. stone removal
- p. stricture dilation (PSD)
- p. tenotomy
- p. thrombectomy
- p. tracheotomy
- p. transatrial mitral commissurotomy
- p. transcatheter therapy
- p. transhepatic approach
- p. transhepatic balloon dilatation (PTBD)
- p. transhepatic biliary drainage (PTBD)
- p. transhepatic biliary procedure
- p. transhepatic cardiac catheterization
- p. transhepatic catheter
- p. transhepatic cholangiography (PTC)
- p. transhepatic cholangioscopic lithotomy (PTCSL)
- p. transhepatic cholangioscopy
- p. transhepatic cholecystoscopy
- p. transhepatic direct portography
- p. transhepatic obliteration
- p. transhepatic obliteration of esophageal varix
- p. transhepatic placement
- p. transluminal angioplasty (PTA, PTAB)
- p. transluminal angioscopy (PTAS)
- p. transluminal balloon valvoplasty
- p. transluminal coronary angioplasty (PTCA)
- p. transluminal renal angioplasty
- p. transtracheal jet ventilation (PTJV)
- p. transtracheal ventilation (PTV)
- p. transvenous mitral commissurotomy

- p. tumor ablation
- p. venoablation
- p. vertebroplasty

Pereyra
- P. bladder neck suspension
- P. bladder neck suspension procedure
- P. needle suspension

Pereyra-Lebhertz modification

Pereyra-Raz cystourethropexy

perflation

perfluorocarbon emulsion

perforans

perforantes

perforated
- p. appendix
- p. cancer
- p. cholecystitis
- p. cyst
- p. peptic ulcer
- p. space

perforating
- p. abscess
- p. branch
- p. canal
- p. keratoplasty
- p. wound

perforation
- advanced tumor p.
- amebic p.
- appendiceal p.
- barogenic esophageal p.
- bladder p.
- bowel p.
- cardiac p.
- colon p.
- colonic p.
- corneal p.
- cortical p.
- diaphragm p.
- ductal system p.
- duodenal p.
- esophageal p.
- frank p.
- gallbladder p.
- gastric p.
- guide wire p.
- iatrogenic colonic p.
- ileal p.
- inflammatory p.
- instrumental p.
- intestinal p.
- intraperitoneal p.
- lateral p.
- mechanical p.
- myocardial p.
- nasal septal p.
- Niemeier gallbladder p.
- operative p.

p. osteotomy
pathologic p.
peritoneal p.
p. peritonitis
prepyloric p.
retroduodenal p.
retroperitoneal p.
p. risk
root p.
sealing p.
septal p.
spontaneous p.
spontaneous intestinal p. (SIP)
strip p.
sublabial p.
tooth p.
traumatic p.
ureteral p.
uterine p.
vascular p.
ventricular p.
visceral p.
perforative lesion
perforator
Cockett p.
p. flap
incompetent p.
subfascial p.
superior gluteal artery p.
p. vein
performance
psychomotor p.
p. status
perfrigeration
perfusate
perfusion
aortic p.
blood p.
cerebral p.
continuous hyperthermic peritoneal p. (CHPP)
continuous sanguineous p.
distal aortic p.
distal visceral p.
extracorporeal liver p. (ECLP)
ex vivo p.
p. flow rate
hepatic p.
hyperthermic isolated limb p. (HILP)
p. hypothermia technique
hypothermic hepatic p.
in-line p.
in situ hypothermic p.
intramural blood p.
intraperitoneal hyperthermic p. (IPHP)
isolated hepatic p. (IHP)
isolated limb p. (ILP)

Langendorff p.
p. measurement technique
organ p.
pancreas graft p.
portal p.
p. pressure
renal p.
sanguineous p.
selective antegrade cerebral p. (SACP)
splanchnic p.
superficial renal cortical p. (SRCP)
p. system
systemic p.
p. therapy
tissue p.
visceral p.
perfusion-limited clearance
perfusion/ventilation
periadventitial
p. dissection
p. tissue
periampullary
p. cancer
p. carcinoma
p. duodenal diverticulum
p. incidentaloma
p. mass
p. tumor
perianal
p. abscess
p. anorectal space
p. condyloma
p. Crohn disease
p. dermatitis
p. fistula
p. fistula abscess
p. hematoma
p. incision
p. infection
perianesthetic thermoregulation
perianeurysmal hemorrhage
periangiocholitis
periaortic mediastinal hematoma
periaortitis
periapical
p. curettage
p. infection
p. pressure
p. surgery
p. tissue
p. tooth repair
periappendiceal abscess
periappendicitis
periappendicular
periaqueductal
p. gray area
p. gray matter/periventricular gray matter (PAG/PVG)

P

periaqueductal (*continued*)
    p. gray matter-periventricular gray matter region
    p. gray matter stimulation
periaqueductal-periventricular stimulation
periareolar
    p. incision
    p. mastopexy
periarterial
    p. plexus
    p. sympathectomy
periarticular
    p. fluid collection
    p. fracture
    p. tissue
periauricular pain
periaxial
periaxillary
peribronchial
peribronchiolar lymphocyte infiltration
peribuccal
peribulbar
    p. anesthesia
    p. anesthetic technique
    p. block
    p. injection
peribursal
pericallosal artery
pericanalicular connective tissue
pericapsular
    p. fat infiltration
    p. osteotomy
pericardectomy
pericardiacae
    venae p.
pericardiacophrenic
    p. artery
    p. vein
pericardial
    p. biopsy
    p. branch
    p. cavity evacuation
    p. decompression
    p. effusion
    p. eventration
    p. fat pad
    p. flap
    p. fluid examination
    p. hematoma
    p. hood aortic flap technique
    p. mobilization
    p. patch
    p. pressure
    p. puncture
    p. reflection
    p. reflex
    p. reinforcement

    p. ring
    p. sac
    p. sinus
    p. tamponade
    p. vein
    p. window
pericardicentesis (*var. of* pericardiocentesis)
pericardiectomy
    parietal p.
    thoracoscopic p.
    visceral p.
pericardiocentesis, pericardicentesis
pericardiophrenic nerve
pericardioplasty in pectus excavatum repair
pericardiorrhaphy
pericardioscopy
pericardiostomy
pericardiotomy, pericardotomy
    percutaneous balloon p.
    subxiphoid limited p.
    p. syndrome
pericarditis
    constrictive p.
pericardium
    parietal p.
    visceral p.
pericardotomy (*var. of* pericardiotomy)
pericecal fossa
pericholecystic
    p. edema
    p. fluid collection
pericholecystitis
perichondral, perichondrial
    p. circulation
    p. ring
    p. sheath
perichondrial (*var. of* perichondral)
perichondrium
perichoroidal space
pericolic membrane syndrome
pericolonitis
pericolostomy
    p. area
    p. hernia
pericorneal plexus
pericoronal flap
pericostal suture technique
pericranial temporalis flap
pericranium
pericystectomy
    closed p.
    partial p.
    sterile p.
    total p.
pericystic resection
pericystitis
pericystium

peridectomy
peridental
    p. ligament
    p. membrane
    p. space
peridentinoblastic space
peridentium (*var. of* periodontium)
peridesmic
peridesmium
peridiaphragmatic hematoma
perididymis
perididymitis
peridiverticular abscess
periductal
    p. fibrosis
    p. mastitis
peridural anesthesia
perienteric
periependymal
periesophageal
    p. abscess
    p. blood vessel
    p. fat
    p. fibrosis
    p. lymph node dissection
    p. structure
    p. tissue
perifascial nephrectomy
periganglionic
perigastric
    p. node
    p. node station
perigenicular vascular injury
perigraft
    p. hematoma
    p. seroma
perihepatic
    p. abscess
    p. lymph nodal station
    p. packing
    p. space
perihepatitis
    gonococcal p.
perihernial
perihilar cholangiocarcinoma
periimplant
    p. space
    p. tissue
periimplantation
perikaryon
perilaryngeal airway (PLA)
perilenticular space
periligamentous
perilimbal
    p. incision
    p. suction
perilobular connective tissue
perilunar transscaphoid dislocation
perilunate

    p. carpal dislocation
    p. fracture-dislocation
perilymphatic
    p. cavity
    p. duct
    p. fistula
    p. fluid
    p. space
perilymph fistula
perimesencephalic cistern
perimeter
    p. corneal reflex test
    Goldmann p.
    p. projection
perimetric
perimetrium
perimyelis
perimylolysis
perimysium
perinatal
    p. biliary atresia
    p. infection
    p. torsion
perinea (*pl. of* perineum)
perineal
    p. abscess
    p. analgesia
    p. anesthesia
    p. artery
    p. body
    p. defect
    p. flap
    p. flexure
    p. hernia
    p. hernia ring
    p. impact trauma
    p. incision
    p. infection
    p. laceration
    p. lithotomy
    p. membrane
    p. muscle
    p. nerve
    p. nerve terminal motor latency test
    p. pearl
    p. polyp
    p. proctectomy
    p. prostatectomy
    p. raphe
    p. region
    p. repair
    p. scar
    p. section
    p. sinus
    p. sinus tract
    p. space
    p. urethrostomy
    p. urethrotomy
    p. urinary fistula

P

perineocele
perineoplasty
perineorrhaphy
    vaginal p.
perineoscrotal
perineostomy
perineosynthesis
perineotomy
perineovaginal fistula
perinephria (*pl. of* perinephrium)
perinephrial
perinephric
    p. abscess
    p. fluid collection
    p. hematoma
    p. space hemorrhage
    p. tissue
perinephritis
perinephrium, *pl.* **perinephria**
perineum, *pl.* **perinea**
perineural
    p. anesthesia
    p. catheter
    p. infiltration
    p. invasion
    p. tissue
perineuria (*pl. of* perineurium)
perineurial neurorrhaphy
perineurium, *pl.* **perineuria**
perinodal tissue
perinuclear
    p. cisterna
    p. space
periocular
    p. injection
    p. pain
period
    early postoperative p.
    immediate postoperative p.
    interdigestive p.
    later postoperative p.
    observation p.
    postimplantation p.
    postoperative p.
    postprandial p.
    postresuscitation p.
    preinduction p.
    preoperative p.
    resuscitation p.
periodic respiration
periodontal
    p. disease
    p. flap
    p. inflammation
    p. lesion
    p. ligament
    p. ligament anesthesia
    p. membrane
    p. membrane necrosis

    p. ostectomy
    p. therapy
periodontia (*pl. of* periodontium)
periodontium, peridentium, *pl.*
  periodontia
periodontolysis
periomphalic
perioperative
    p. adjunct
    p. analgesia
    p. antibiotic
    p. antibiotic prophylaxis
    p. antibiotic therapy
    p. aspiration risk
    p. bacteremia
    p. blood conservation
    p. complication
    p. corneal abrasion
    p. death
    p. echocardiography
    p. management
    p. medicine
    p. morbidity
    p. mortality
    p. outcome
    p. reduction
    p. risk factor
    p. shock
    p. standardized protocol
    p. stroke
    p. transfusion
    p. wound infection
perioptic subarachnoid space
periorbital
    p. infection
    p. membrane
periostea (*pl. of* periosteum)
periosteal
    p. elevation
    p. flap
    p. implantation
    p. new bone formation
    p. tissue
periosteoma
periosteophyte
periosteotomy
periosteous
periosteum, *pl.* **periostea**
    posterior p.
periostoma
periotic
    p. bone
    p. duct
    p. space
peripancreatic
    p. abdominal
      drainage
    p. fat plane
    p. infection

p. necrosis
p. necrotic tissue
p. tissue
peripartum endoscopy
peripenial
peripharyngeal space
peripheral
p. access system (PAS)
p. aneurysm
p. antinociceptive action
p. arterial aneurysmal disease
p. arterial line
p. artery control
p. atheroembolism
p. balloon angioplasty
p. bruit
p. capillary filtration slit length
p. cavity wall
p. chemoreflex loop
p. circulation
p. examination
p. extremity edema
p. fusion
p. hepaticojejunostomy
p. hyperalimentation
p. hyperinsulinemia
p. insulin resistance
p. intravenous alimentation
p. iridectomy
p. ischemia
p. laceration
p. laser angioplasty
p. lymphoid tissue
p. nerve
p. nerve allografting
p. nerve block
p. nerve block anesthesia
p. nerve block anesthetic
    technique
p. nerve injury
p. nerve lesion
p. nerve regeneration
p. nerve stimulation
p. nervous system (PNS)
p. neurectomy
p. panretinal ablation
p. parenteral nutrition (PPN)
p. pressure
p. pulse
p. sensitization
p. thrombus
p. vascular disease (PVD)
p. vascular surgery
p. vasoconstriction
p. vein
p. venous cannulation
peripherally inserted central catheter
  (PICC)
periportal sinusoidal dilation

periproctic
periprostatic tissue
periprostatitis
periprosthetic
p. fracture
p. leak
peripylephlebitis
peripylic
peripyloric
perirectal
p. abscess
p. inflammation
p. mass
p. pelvic dissection
perirenal
p. fascia
p. hematoma
p. insufflation
p. space
perisalpinx
periscapular incision
periscleral space
perisellar vascular lesion
perisinusoidal space
perisplanchnic
perisplenic
perispondylic
peristalsis
absent p.
dropped p.
peristaltic
peristasis
peristomal, peristomatous
p. fistula
p. hernia
p. infection
p. varix
peristomatous (*var. of* peristomal)
peritarsal network
peritectomy
peritendineum
perithelioma
perithoracic
peritomist
peritomy
peritonea (*pl. of* peritoneum)
peritoneal
p. access
p. adenocarcinoma
p. adhesion
p. anatomy
p. aspiration
p. band
p. biopsy
p. cancer
p. carcinomatosis
p. cavity
p. cavity abscess
p. cavity fluid

P

peritoneal (*continued*)
    p. cytological assessment
    p. cytology
    p. cytology sample
    p. defect
    p. dialysis
    p. disease
    p. dissemination
    p. drainage
    p. encapsulation
    p. envelope
    p. equilibration test
    p. exchange volume
    p. fluid examination
    p. friction rub
    p. fungal infection
    p. hernia
    p. incision
    p. insufflation
    p. irritation
    p. lavage
    p. macrophage
    p. membrane permeability
    p. metastasis
    p. patch
    p. penetration
    p. perforation
    p. pocket
    p. reconstruction
    p. recurrence
    p. reflection
    p. reinforcement
    p. sac
    p. seeding
    p. sepsis
    p. soilage
    p. space
    p. spill
    p. spread
    p. studding
    p. surface
    p. tap
    p. toilet
    p. transfusion
    p. tuberculosis
    p. vein
    ventricular p.
    p. villus
    p. violation
    p. washing
    p. washout
    p. window
peritonectomy
    left upper quadrant p.
    pelvic p.
    right upper quadrant p.
peritoneocentesis
peritoneoclysis
peritoneopericardial diaphragmatic hernia

peritoneopexy
peritoneoplasty
peritoneoscopy
peritoneotomy
    inverted-V p.
peritoneovenous shunt patency scan
peritoneum, *pl.* **peritonea**
    abdominal p.
    parietal p.
    visceral p.
peritonitis
    adhesive p.
    amebic p.
    aseptic p.
    barium p.
    chemical p.
    diffuse p.
    focal p.
    gastric perforation p.
    generalized p.
    infectious p.
    meconium p.
    obliterative p.
    perforation p.
    primary bacterial p.
    purulent p.
    P. Severity Score (PSS)
    talc p.
peritonization
peritonize
peritonsillar
    p. nerve
    p. space
peritracheal
peritrochanteric fracture
peritubal syndrome
peritumoral site
perityphlic
periumbilical
    p. abscess
    p. hernia
    p. incision
    p. port
periureteral abscess
periureteric venous ring
periurethral abscess
periurethritis
periuterine
perivalvular leak
perivascular
    p. canal
    p. mass
    p. space
perivaterian therapeutic endoscopic procedure
periventricular
    p. hyperintense lesion
    p. white matter lesion

periventricular-intraventricular hemorrhage
perivertebral
perivesical
perivisceral
perivitelline space
periwound erythema
Perkins vertical line
Perlon suture
Permahand braided silk suture
permanent
    p. anticoagulant therapy
    p. bipolar magnet placement
    p. end colostomy
    p. hypoparathyroidism
    p. loop ileostomy
    p. mesh omentum
    p. pacemaker placement
    p. paralysis
    p. pedicle flap
    p. proctectomy
    p. restoration
    p. section
    p. stoma
Perma Sharp suture
permeability
    capillary p.
    intestinal p.
    membrane p.
    mitochondrial p.
    peritoneal membrane p.
    sarcoplasmic reticulum p.
    p. theory of narcosis
    p. transition pore
    tubal p.
permeation
    analgesia p.
    lymphatic p.
permissive hypercapnia (PHC)
permutation
perone
peronea
peroneae
    venae p.
peroneal
    p. artery
    p. brevis tendon
    p. communicating nerve
    p. compartment syndrome
    p. dislocation
    p. groove
    p. island flap
    p. longus tendon
    p. muscle
    p. muscle atrophy
    p. nerve entrapment
    p. nerve injury
    p. phenomenon
    p. pulley

    p. retinaculum
    p. somatosensory evoked potential
    p. spastic flatfoot
    p. tendon sheath injection
    p. vein
peroneus
    p. brevis muscle
    p. longus muscle
    p. tertius muscle
peroral
    p. approach
    p. cholangiopancreatoscopy (PCPS)
    p. cholangioscopy (PCS)
    p. endoscopy
    p. esophageal dilation
    p. intestinal biopsy
    p. maneuver
    p. pancreatoscopy
peroxidation
    lipid p.
perpendicular
    p. fashion
    p. of ethmoid plate
    p. plane
Perry extensile anterior distal humerus approach
Perry-Nickel halo traction technique
Perry-O'Brien-Hodgson orthopaedic technique
Perry-Robinson cervical technique
perseveration
    infantile p.
    motor p.
persistent
    p. anovulation
    p. breast abnormality
    p. common atrioventricular canal
    p. fetal circulation
    p. hypercalcemia
    p. hyperinsulinemia and hyperglycemia of infancy
    p. ileus
    p. müllerian duct syndrome
    p. nonawakening
    p. occiput posterior fetal position
    p. ovarian mass
    p. sciatic artery (PSA)
    p. tolerant infection
person
    Pain Assessment in Noncommunicative Elderly P.'s (PAINE)
personnel
    paramedical p.
perspective
    surgical p.
    p. volume rendering (PVR)
perspiratory gland

P

Perthes
P. deep femoral vein patency test
P. incision
P. lesion
perturbation
hemodynamic p.
membrane p.
pes
dorsalis pedis
p. planus
p. planus deformity
PESA
percutaneous epididymal sperm
aspiration
PET
positron emission tomography
PETCO₂
end-tidal carbon dioxide pressure
petechiae (*pl. of* petechia)
petechial hemorrhage
Peter operation
Peters
P. anomaly
P. exstrophy of bladder
operation
Peterson hernia
PET-guided biopsy
Petit
P. aponeurosis
P. canal
P. hernia
P. herniotomy
P. ligament
P. lumbar triangle
lumbar triangle of P.
P. suture technique
petrobasilar suture
petroccipital
petroclinoid ligament
petromastoid
petrooccipital
p. fissure
p. joint
petropharyngeus
petrosa, *pl.* **petrosae**
petrosae (*pl. of* petrosa)
petrosal
p. approach
p. artery
p. bone
p. branch
p. foramen
p. fossa
p. fossula
p. ganglion
p. nerve
p. neuralgia
p. vein
p. venous sinus

petrosectomy
total p.
petrositis
petrosomastoid
petrosphenoid ligament
petrospheno-occipital suture
petrosquamosal, petrosquamous
petrosquamous (*var. of*
petrosquamosal)
p. fissure
p. suture
p. venous sinus
petrostaphylinus
petrotympanic
p. fissure
p. suture
p. tissue
petrous
p. apex cell
p. ganglion
p. pyramid
p. pyramid air cell exploration
p. pyramid exenteration
p. pyramid fracture
p. ridge
p. to supraclinoid bypass
Peutz-Jeghers syndrome
Peyer
P. gland
P. patches
Peyman
P. full-thickness eye wall resection
P. iridocyclochoroidectomy
Peyronie disease
Peyrot thorax
Pfannenstiel
P. incision
P. transverse approach
**Pfeiffer-Comberg intraorbital foreign
body localization method**
PFNA
percutaneous fine-needle aspiration
PFO
patent foramen ovale
PFRIA
proximal femoral resection-interposition
arthroplasty
PGA
pancreatogastrostomy anastomosis
polyglycolic acid
PGA mesh
PGA synthetic absorbable suture
PGE
percutaneous gastroenterostomy
PGID
postoperative gastrointestinal tract
dysfunction
analgesia-induced PGID
anesthesia-induced PGID

hypoperfusion-induced PGID
neurogenic PGID
surgery-induced PGID
PGL
primary gastric lymphoma
PGR
percutaneous glycerol rhizolysis
pH
hydrogen ion concentration
power of hydrogen
pH electrode placement
esophageal pH
gastric mucosal pH
intramural pH
pH measurement
phaco
phacoemulsification
phacoanaphylactic endophthalmitis
phacocele
phacocystectomy
phacoemulsification (phaco), phakoemulsification
Kelman p.
phacofragmentation
phacoglaucoma
phacolysis
phacoma, phakoma
retinal p.
phacomatosis, phakomatosis
phacoscopy
phagocyte migration
phagocytosis
phagolysis
phakoemulsification (*var. of* phacoemulsification)
phakoma (*var. of* phacoma)
phakomatosis (*var. of* phacomatosis)
phalangeal
p. articular orientation
p. diaphysial fracture
p. dislocation
p. fracture fixation
p. malunion correction
p. osteotomy
phalangectomy
intermediate p.
phalanges (*pl. of* phalanx)
phalangization
phalanx, *pl.* **phalanges**
distal p.
middle p.
proximal p.
Phalen
P. carpal tunnel maneuver
P. position
P. sign
phalalgia
phallectomy
phalli (*pl. of* phallus)

phallic
phalliform
phallitis
phallocampsis
phallocrypsis
phallodynia
phalloid
phalloncus
phalloplasty
phallotomy
phallus, *pl.* **phalli**
Phaneuf-Graves enterocele repair
phantasmoscopy
phantom
p. aneurysm
p. foot pain
p. limb
p. limb pain
p. sensation
p. tooth pain
pharaonic circumcision
pharmacodynamics
pharmacologic, pharmacological
p. immunosuppression
p. manipulation
p. method
p. paralysis
pharmacological (*var. of* pharmacologic)
p. sleeve
pharmacologically
p. induced erection
p. induced paralysis
pharyngeal
p. airway
p. anesthesia
p. branch
p. bursa
p. canal
p. cell
p. constrictor muscle
p. exudate
p. flap
p. fornix
p. gland
p. gonococcal infection
p. mucosa
p. orifice
p. plexus
p. plexus neurectomy
p. pouch
p. pouch syndrome
p. raphe
p. recess
p. region
p. residue
p. ridge
p. space
p. tissue
p. tubercle

P

pharyngeal (*continued*)
   p. vein
   p. wall carcinoma
pharyngealis
   tonsilla p.
pharyngectomy
pharyngei
   rami p.
pharynges (*pl. of* pharynx)
pharyngis (*pl. of* pharynx)
pharyngobasilar fascia
pharyngocutaneous fistula
pharyngoepiglottic fold
pharyngoesophageal
   p. diverticulectomy
   p. diverticulum
   p. reconstruction
pharyngoesophagogastroduodenoscopy
pharyngoesophagoplasty
pharyngoglossal
pharyngoglossus
pharyngolaryngeal
pharyngolaryngectomy
pharyngomaxillary space
pharyngometer
pharyngometry
   acoustic p.
pharyngonasal cavity
pharyngooral
pharyngopalatine
pharyngoplasty
   Hynes p.
   sphincter p.
   Wardill p.
pharyngoscleroma
pharyngoscopy
pharyngostoma
pharyngotomy
   transhyoid p.
pharyngotympanic groove
pharynx, *pl.* **pharynges**
   laryngeal p.
   nasal p.
   oral p.
   posterior p.
phase
   anhepatic p.
   eclipse p.
   ejection p.
   end-expiratory p.
   excitement p.
   exponential p.
   extradural p.
   granulation p.
   p. I, II block
   implantation p.
   lag p.
   maturation p.

   posthepatic resection p.
   prehepatic resection p.
   preinduction p.
   presensitization p.
   prolonged expiratory p.
   resectional p.
   reservoir p.
   transverse magnetization p.
   vector p.
phase-encoding direction
1-phase subperiosteal implant technique
phasic pressure wave
PHC
   permissive hypercapnia
PHCA
   profoundly hypothermic circulatory arrest
Phelps
   P. neurectomy
   P. partial resection
   P. scapulectomy
Phemister
   P. acromioclavicular pin fixation
   P. incision
   P. medial epiphysiodesis approach
   P. onlay bone graft
   P. onlay bone graft technique
Phemister-Bonfiglio femoral neck bone grafting technique
phenol
   p. cauterization
   p. matrixectomy
phenolization
   angular p.
phenol-preserved extract
phenomena (*pl. of* phenomenon)
phenomenology
   pain p.
phenomenon, *pl.* **phenomena**
   all-or-nothing p.
   anoxic preconditioning p.
   Ascher glass-rod p.
   common cavity p.
   declamping p.
   doll's head p.
   entry p.
   extinction p.
   extravasation p.
   gelling p.
   glass-rod negative p.
   glass-rod positive p.
   Goldblatt p.
   hesitation p.
   identification p.
   ischemia-reperfusion p.
   Marcus Gunn p.
   misdirection p.
   modified Raynaud p.
   neglectlike phenomena

osteointegration p.
overshoot p.
peroneal p.
preconditioning p.
Raynaud p.
referred trigger point p.
relaxation p.
specificity p.
staircase p.
steal p.
temporary cavity p.
truncation p.

phenotypic
p. lymphocyte
p. manifestation

phenozygous
phentolamine infusion
phenylethylbarbituric acid
pheochrome cell
pheochromoblastoma
pheochromocytoma
adrenal p.
p. crisis

pheresis (*var. of* apheresis)
philtra (*pl. of* philtrum)
philtrum, *pl.* **philtra**
phimoses (*pl. of* phimosis)
phimosis, *pl.* **phimoses**
phimotic
phlebectomy
greater saphenous p.
rotablator p.
stab p.
transilluminated power p.

phlebitis
phlebogram
orbital p.

phlebography
saphenous p.

phlebolite
phlebolith
phlebophlebostomy
phlebophthalmotomy
phleboplasty
phleborrhagia
phleborrhaphy
phleborrhexis
phlebostasis
phlebostrepsis
phlebotomy
bloodless p.
therapeutic p.

phlegmasia
p. alba dolens
p. cerulea dolens

phlegmon
phlegmonous
p. abscess
p. gastritis

p. inflammation
p. mass

PHN
postherpetic neuralgia

Phocas syndrome
phonation
phonomyography
phonophoresis
phonoscopy
phosphatase
serum alkaline p.

phosphatase-antiphosphatase
alkaline p.-a.

phosphate
p. buffered saline (PBS)
p. excretion index
primary sodium p.

phosphodiesterase III inhibitor
Phospholine Iodide
phospholipid
photic stimulation
photoablation
laser p.

photoactivation
photoaged skin
photocoagulation
argon laser p. (ALP)
infrared p.
in situ p.
laser p. (LPC)
macular p.
Meyer-Schwickerath retinal p.
panretinal argon laser p.
retinal scatter p.
scatter p.
transendoscopic laser p.
p. treatment
xenon arc p.

photodisintegration
photodissociation
photodocumentation
photodynamic therapy (PDT)
photoelectric plethysmography
photoepilation
photoexcitation
photography
cross-polarization p.
endoscopic p.
laparoscopic p.

photoinactivation
photoirradiation
photolysis
flash p.

photomicrograph
photomicroscopy
photon-deficient bone lesion
photoonycholysis
photoplethysmographic waveform
photoplethysmography

P

photopolymerize
photopsia, photopsy
photopsy (*var. of* photopsia)
photoradiation therapy
photorefractive
    p. keratectomy (PRK)
    p. keratoplasty (PRK)
photorejuvenation
photoresection
photoscopy
photoselective laser vaporization of
  prostate
photosensitive cell
phototherapeutic keratectomy (PTK)
photothermal laser ablation
photothermolysis
    selective p. (SPTL)
photovaporization
    laser p.
phrenectomy (*var. of* phrenicectomy)
phrenemphraxis
phrenic
    p. ganglion
    p. nerve
    p. nerve block
    p. nerve block anesthetic
      technique
    p. pleura
    p. plexus
    p. stimulation
    p. vein
phrenicectomy, phrenectomy,
  phrenicoexeresis, phreniconeurectomy
phreniclasia, phreniclasis, phrenicotripsy
phreniclasis (*var. of* phreniclasia)
phrenicoabdominal branch
phrenicocolic, phrenocolic
    p. ligament
phrenicocostal sinus
phrenicoesophageal, phrenoesophageal
    p. ligament
    p. ligament
    p. membrane
phrenicoexeresis (*var. of* phrenicectomy)
phrenicogastric, phrenogastric
phrenicoglottic
phrenicohepatic, phrenohepatic
phrenicolienal ligament
phrenicomediastinalis
    recessus p.
phrenicomediastinal recess
phreniconeurectomy (*var. of*
  phrenicectomy)
phrenicopleural fascia
phrenicosplenic ligament
phrenicotomy
phrenicotripsy
phrenicus
phrenocolic (*var. of* phrenicocolic)

phrenocolopexy
phrenoesophageal (*var. of*
  phrenicoesophageal)
phrenogastric (*var. of* phrenicogastric)
    p. ligament
phrenohepatic (*var. of* phrenicohepatic)
phrenosplenic ligament
phrictopathic
phrygian
    p. cap
    p. cap deformity
PHTC
    pulmonary hypertensive crisis
PHVE
    partial hepatic vascular exclusion
phyllodes
    cystosarcoma p.
    p. tumor
physeal (*var. of* physial)
physial, physeal
    p. fracture
    p. line
physical
    p. barrier
    p. capacity evaluation
    p. examination
    p. finding
    p. manipulation
    p. problem
    p. restoration
    p. therapy (PT)
    p. therapy index
Physick iridotomy
physiologic, physiological
    p. aspect
    p. barrier
    p. breast discharge
    p. change
    p. dead space
    p. dead space ventilation per
      minute
    p. dependence liability
    p. dose
    p. excavation
    p. mesial migration
    p. pattern release
    p. rest position
    p. retraction ring
    p. saline solution
    p. salt solution
    p. sphincter
physiological (*var. of* physiologic)
    P. and Operative Severity Score for
      the Enumeration of Mortality and
      Morbidity (POSSUM)
physiology
    colorectal p.
    exercise p.
    flap p.

physiolysis
    central p.
physis
physocele
physostigmine
phytobezoar
piagetian theory
pial-glial membrane
pia mater
piano-wire adhesion
PIC
    plasmin inhibitor
      complex
PICA
    posterior inferior cerebellar artery
PICC
    peripherally inserted central
      catheter
Pichlmayer
    P. orthotopic liver transplantation
      procedure
    P. split liver transplantation
      technique
Pick bundle
Pickerill
    P. imbrication line
    imbrication line of P.
pickling solution
pickup spatula suture
Pico operation
Picot incision
picrotoxin
picture
    clinical p.
    p. frame vertebra
PID
    pelvic inflammatory disease
piece
    Y p.
1-piece ostomy pouch
2-piece
    2-p. dental implant
    2-p. ostomy pouch
pie-crusting skin graft
Piedmont fracture
Pierre Robin anomalad
**Pierrot and Murphy transplantation of
insertion of tendo Achillis**
Pierrot-Murphy
    P.-M. advancement insertion
    P.-M. tendon technique
Piersol point
piezoelectric lithotripsy
pigeon-breast deformity
piggyback
    p. approach
    p. liver transplant
    modified p. (MPB)
piggybacking

pigment
    p. cell transplant
    p. epithelial lesion
pigmentary
    p. demarcation line
    p. migration
pigmented lesion
pigskin
    p. graft
    p. patch
pile
    sentinel p.
pileus
pilimiction
pillar
    p. pain
    p. rib
pill-induced esophagitis
pillion fracture
pillow fracture
pill-rolling tremor
piloerection
pilojection
piloleiomyoma
pilomatrixoma
pilon ankle fracture
pilonidal
    p. abscess
    p. cyst
    p. cystectomy
    p. fistula
    p. sinus
pilorum
pilot application
pin
    cranial p.
    p. fixation
    p. retention
    p. site
    p. suture
    p. suture technique
    p. track
    p. tract infection
pin-and-plaster
    p.-a.-p. fixation
    p.-a.-p. method
Pinard breech extraction maneuver
pin-bone interface
pincer nail
pinch
    p. biopsy
    p. restoration
    p. skin graft
pinch-grasp injection technique
pincushion distortion
pineal
    p. body
    p. eye
    p. gland

P

pineal (*continued*)
    p. recess
    p. region
    p. teratocarcinoma
pinealectomy
pinealoma
pineoblastoma
pineocytoma
ping-pong
    p.-p. ball
    p.-p. ball deformity
    p.-p. fracture
piniform
pin-index safety system
pink
    p. frothy sputum
    p. twisted cotton suture
pinning
    closed p.
    hip p.
    in situ p.
    Knowles p.
    open p.
    percutaneous p.
    Sherk-Probst percutaneous p.
    Sofield p.
    Wagner closed p.
pinpoint
    p. electrocoagulation
    p. gastric mucosal defect
    p. gastric mucosal defect
      bleeding
pinprick
    p. analgesia
    p. method
pins-and-needles
pin-supported restoration
Pioneer catheter
PIP
    positive inspiratory pressure
pipe bone
pipeline supply source
Pipelle biopsy
Pipkin
    P. femoral fracture classification
    P. posterior hip dislocation
      classification
    P. subclassification of
      Epstein-Thomas classification
PIPP
    Premature Infant Pain Profile
Pippi Salle urethral lengthening
  procedure
Pirie bone
piriform, pyriform
    p. fossa
    p. muscle
    p. recess
    p. sinus

piriformis, pyriformis
    p. syndrome
Pirogoff
    P. amputation
    P. angle
    P. operation
    P. triangle
pisiform
    p. bone
    p. fracture
pisotriquetral arthritis
pit
    p. and fissure cavity
    p. cell
    commissural lip p.
    costal p.
    gastric p.
    granular p.
    herniation p.
    inferior articular p.
    inferior costal p.
    nail p.
    p. of atlas for dens
    pterygoid p.
    sublingual p.
    superior costal p.
    suprameatal p.
pitted
    p. erythrocyte count
    p. keratolysis
    p. nail
pitting
    nail p.
pituicytoma
pituitary
    p. ablation
    p. adenoma
    p. body
    p. endocrine disorder
    p. fossa
    p. gland
    p. gland transplant
    p. microadenoma
    p. neuroadenolysis
    p. stalk section
    p. tumor
    p. tumor cell
pituitectomy
pituitous
pivot
    p. joint
    p. point
PJA
    pancreatojejunostomy
    anastomosis
      PJA afferent
      PJA efferent
PKD
    polycystic kidney disease

PLA
    perilaryngeal airway
place of articulation
placebo
    p. therapy
    p. treatment
4-place laminectomy
placement
    aortic graft p.
    band p.
    biliary sphincterotomy and
      stent p.
    bone graft p.
    bur hole p.
    catheter tip p.
    clip p.
    dilator p.
    electrode p.
    endoscopic biliary stent p.
    endotracheal tube p.
    epidural catheter p.
    feeding tube p.
    filter p.
    fluoroscopic p.
    graft p.
    implant p.
    infrarenal endograft p.
    intrapleural catheter p.
    intrinsic spinal cord catheter p.
    K-wire p.
    long-term central venous access
      catheter p.
    odontoid screw p.
    percutaneous nephrostomy
      tube p.
    percutaneous transhepatic p.
    permanent bipolar magnet p.
    permanent pacemaker p.
    pH electrode p.
    plate p.
    4-port diamond p.
    5-port fan p.
    posterolateral bone graft p.
    radiologic biliary stent p.
    rod p.
    sacral screw p.
    screw p.
    shunt p.
    stent p.
    suprarenal filter p.
    surgical p.
    temporary pacemaker p.
    trocar p.
    T-tube p.
    tube p.
    ultrasound-guided caudal epidural
      needle p.
    ureteral stent p.
    variable screw p. (VSP)

    ventriculoperitoneal shunt p.
    wire-guided p.
placenta
    endotheliochorial p.
    endothelio-endothelial p.
    extrachorial p.
    p. fetalis
    premature separation of p.
    p. uterina
placentae
    ablatio p.
    abruptio p. (AP)
placental
    p. barrier
    p. circulation
    p. extrusion
    p. fragment
    p. hemangioma syndrome
    p. hematoma
    p. hemorrhage
    p. implantation
    p. localization
    p. membrane
    p. metastasis
    p. migration
    p. respiration
    p. tissue
    p. tissue transplant
    p. transfer
    p. uptake
placentation bleeding
placentoma
Placido ring
placode
    nasal p.
pladaroma, pladarosis
pladarosis (*var. of* pladaroma)
plafond fracture
plagiocephaly
plain
    p. abdominal film
    p. abdominal radiography (PAR)
    p. catgut suture
    p. collagen suture
    p. gut suture
plana (*pl. of* planum)
plane
    Aeby p.
    alveolar point-meatus p.
    anatomic p.
    auriculoinfraorbital p.
    axial p.
    axiobuccolingual p.
    axiolabiolingual p.
    axiomesiodistal p.
    base p.
    bite p.
    Broca visual p.
    buccolingual p.

P

plane (*continued*)
Camper p.
cleavage p.
coronal p.
cove p.
cusp p.
Daubenton p.
diffuse p.
equatorial p.
equivalent refracting p.
eye-ear p.
facet p.
facial p.
fascial p.
fat p.
first parallel pelvic p.
flexion-extension p.
focal p.
fourth parallel pelvic p.
Frankfort horizontal p.
French p.
frontal p.
guide p.
guiding p.
Hensen p.
His p.
Hodge p.
horizontal p.
internervous p.
interspinal p.
intertubercular p.
ischiorectal fossa p.
p. joint
labiolingual p.
lens p.
Listing p.
mandibular p.
mean foundation p.
mesiodistal p.
midcoronal p.
midfrontal p.
midsagittal p.
midthalamic p.
Morton p.
nodal p.
nuchal p.
oblique coronal p.
occipital p.
occlusal p.
p. of dissection
orbital p.
orthogonal p.
paramedian sagittal p.
parasagittal p.
pelvic p.
peripancreatic fat p.
perpendicular p.
preglenoid p.
primary movement p.

principal p.
sagittal p.
scan p.
second parallel pelvic p.
sensitive p.
short-axis p.
slant of occlusal p.
spectacle p.
spinous p.
sternal p.
sternoxiphoid p.
subcostal p.
subcutaneous p.
subpectoral p.
supracrestal p.
supracristal p.
suprasternal p.
symmetry p.
temporal p.
terminal p.
thalamic p.
third parallel pelvic p.
thoracic p.
tooth p.
transaxial scan p.
transection p.
transpyloric p.
transtubercular p.
transverse p.
umbilical p.
varus-valgus p.
vertical p.
visual p.
wide p.

1-plane
1-p. deformity
1-p. instability
1-p. view
2-plane
2-p. deformity
2-p. fluoroscopy
2-p. occlusion
3-plane deformity
planimetry
planithorax
planned
p. awakening
p. extracapsular cataract extraction
p. reoperation
planning
image-integrated surgery treatment p.
planta, *pl.* **plantae**
plantae (*pl. of* planta)
plantar
p. angulation
p. approach
p. artery bypass
p. aspect
p. compartmental anatomy

p. condylectomy
p. digital nerve
p. fascial release
p. fasciitis
p. fasciotomy
p. flexion-inversion
p. flexion-inversion deformity
p. interosseous muscle
p. longitudinal incision
p. plate release
p. pressure
p. quadrate muscle
p. space
p. tendon sheath
p. venous network

plantar-hindfoot-midfoot bony mass
plantaris tendon
planum, *pl.* **plana**
os p.
planuria
planus
condyloma p.
oral condyloma p.
pes p.
plaque
atheromatous p.
atherosclerotic p.
augmentation p.
carotid p.
echogenic p.
echolucent p.
eczematoid pruritic p.
p. formation
p. fracture
p. incision
neuritic p.
Randall p.
p. rupture
senile p.
p. technique
p. ulceration
plaquelike
p. hamartoma
p. lesion
plaquing
plasm (*var. of* plasma)
plasma, plasm
p. assay coagulation panel
p. atrial natriuretic protein
p. cell portal infiltration
p. clotting time
p. colloid osmotic pressure
p. endotoxin concentration
p. exchange
p. exchange therapy
expanded p.
extracellular p.
fresh frozen p. (FFP)
p. gastrin concentration

p. gelsolin level
p. half-life
p. iron concentration
p. level
p. membrane
p. norepinephrine concentration
p. oncotic pressure
p. product concentrate
p. renin concentration
p. separation rate
p. substitute
target p.
p. thrombin clot method
p. urea concentration
p. volume expansion

plasmacytoma
plasma-mediated ablation
plasmapheresis
plasmatic coagulation factor
plasmin
p. coagulation
p. inhibitor complex (PIC)
plasminogen plasma level
plasmolysis
plaster
capsicum p.
p. cast application burn
plastic
p. and reconstructive surgery
p. bowing fracture
p. clot
p. induration
p. matrix technique
p. operation
p. reconstruction
p. repair
p. section
p. stent occlusion
p. surgeon
p. suture
p. suture technique
plastica
linitis p.
plasticity
connective tissue p.
neural p.
neuronal p.
plasticizer
plastron
plasty
Coleman p.
Durham p.
endoventricular circular patch p.
Foley Y-V p.
mons p.
posterior bladder flap p.
rotation p.
skin p.
sliding p.

P

plasty (*continued*)
    sliding leaflet p.
    V-Y p.
    Y-V p.
plate
    cribriform p.
    dorsal p.
    ethmoidal p.
    p. fixation
    gallbladder p.
    hilar p.
    medial pterygoid p.
    nerve-containing p.
    p. of Arantius
    perpendicular of ethmoid p.
    p. placement
    pterygoid p.
    tarsal p.
    umbilical p.
    vessel-containing p.
    volar p.
plateau
    alveolar p.
    p. pressure
plate-guided
    p.-g. distraction device
    p.-g. distractor
platelet
    p. activating factor
    p. aggregation
    p. concentrate
    p. function analyzer
    p. function assay
    p. gene polymorphism
    p. nucleotide content
plateletapheresis, plateletpheresis
    intraoperative p.
platelet-derived growth factor (PDGF)
platelet-inhibiting drug
plateletpheresis (*var. of* plateletapheresis)
plate-screw
    p.-s. fixation
    p.-s. osteosynthesis
platform
    dual-delivery p.
    p. posturography
plating
    compression p.
    pedicle screw p.
    posterior cervical lateral p.
Platou osteotomy
platybasia
platycephaly
platycrania
platyhieric
platymeric
platyopia

platyopic
platypellic, platypelloid
    p. pelvis
platypelloid (*var. of* platypellic)
platyrrhine
platyrrhiny
platysma
    p. muscle
    p. myocutaneous flap
platyspondylia, platyspondylisis
platyspondylisis (*var. of* platyspondylia)
platystencephaly
Plavix
PLCQ
    Pain Locus of Control Questionnaire
Pleatman sac
pledgeted
    p. Ethibond suture
    p. mattress suture
pledget suture
pleiotropic endocrine response
pleomorphic
    p. adenoma
    p. liposarcoma
pleoptics
    Bangerter method of p.
    Cüppers method of p.
plethysmographic
    p. pulse wave amplitude
    p. pulse wave monitoring
plethysmography
    air p.
    forearm p.
    impedance p.
    photoelectric p.
    venous-occlusion volume p.
    volume p.
pleura, *pl.* **pleurae**
    cervical p.
    costal p.
    diaphragmatic p.
    mediastinal p.
    parietal p.
    phrenic p.
    pulmonary p.
    visceral p.
pleuracentesis
pleuracotomy
pleurae (*pl. of* pleura)
pleural
    p. biopsy
    p. calculus
    p. cavity
    p. cupula
    p. effusion
    p. empyema
    p. fluid
    p. fluid aspiration
    p. fluid collection

p. fluid examination
p. line
p. mass
p. patch reinforcement
p. recess
p. reflection
p. sac
p. sinus
p. space
p. stoma
p. symphysis
p. villus
p. violation
pleurapophysis
pleurectomy
thorascopic apical p.
pleurisy
pleuritis
biliary p.
pleurobiliary fistula
pleurocele
pleurocentesis, pleuracentesis
pleurocentrum
pleuroclysis
pleurodesis
talc p.
pleuroesophageal
p. fistula
p. line
p. muscle
pleuroesophageus
musculus p.
pleurolith
pleuroparietopexy
pleuropericardial
pleuropericarditis
pleuroperitoneal
p. canal
p. fold
p. foramen
p. hernia
p. hiatus
p. membrane
p. shunt
p. space
pleuropneumonectomy
pleuropulmonary
pleuroscopy
pleurotomy
pleurovisceral
plexectomy
plexiform
p. external layer
p. lesion
p. neurofibroma
plexopathy
brachial p.
idiopathic brachial p.
postradiation p.

plexus, *pl.* **plexus, plexuses**
abdominal aortic p.
abdominal aortic sympathic p.
ascending pharyngeal p.
Auerbach p.
axillary p.
basilar venous p.
Batson p.
brachial p.
cardiac p.
carotid venous p.
cavernous p.
celiac nervous p.
cervical p.
choroid p.
coccygeal p.
colic p.
colonic mesenteric p.
common carotid p.
coronary p.
Cruveilhier p.
deep cardiac p.
deferential p.
dorsal venous p.
enteric p.
esophageal p.
Exner p.
external carotid p.
external iliac p.
external maxillary p.
extrapancreatic nerve p.
facial p.
femoral p.
gastroesophageal variceal p.
Heller p.
hemorrhoidal p.
hepatic p.
hypogastric p.
hypoglossal canal venous p.
iliac p.
inferior hemorrhoidal p.
inferior hypogastric p.
inferior mesenteric p.
inferior rectal p.
inferior thyroid p.
inferior vesical p.
infraclavicular part of brachial p.
inguinal p.
intermesenteric p.
internal carotid venous p.
internal mammary p.
internal maxillary p.
internal thoracic lymphatic p.
intracavernous p.
intraparotid p.
ischiadic p.
Jacques p.
jugular p.
lingual p.

P

plexus (*continued*)
  lumbar p.
  lumbosacral p.
  lymphatic p.
  mammary p.
  Meissner p.
  meningeal p.
  mesenteric p.
  myenteric p.
  myenteric neural p.
  p. (nervosus) entericus
  occipital p.
  ovarian p.
  pampiniform venous p.
  pancreatic p.
  parotid p.
  pelvic autonomic p.
  periarterial p.
  pericorneal p.
  pharyngeal p.
  phrenic p.
  popliteal p.
  posterior auricular p.
  posterior coronary p.
  prostaticovesical p.
  prostatic venous p.
  pterygoid p.
  pulmonary p.
  Quénu hemorrhoidal p.
  rectal venous p.
  Remak p.
  renal p.
  sacral venous p.
  Santorini p.
  Sappey p.
  sciatic p.
  solar p.
  spermatic p.
  splenic p.
  subclavian periarterial p.
  submucosal p.
  suboccipital venous p.
  superficial cardiac p.
  superficial cervical p.
  superficial temporal p.
  superior hemorrhoidal p.
  superior hypogastric p.
  superior mesenteric p.
  superior rectal p.
  superior thyroid p.
  suprarenal p.
  testicular p.
  thoracic aortic p.
  thyroid p.
  tympanic p.
  ureteral p.
  uterine venous p.
  uterovaginal p.
  vaginal venous p.

  vascular p.
  venous p.
  vertebral venous p.
  vesical p.
  vesicular venous p.
  Walther p.
plexuses (*pl. of* plexus)
plica, *pl.* **plicae**
  plicae tubariae tubae uterinae
  p. urachi
plicae (*pl. of* plica)
plicated appendicocystostomy
plicating suture technique
plication
  bowel p.
  buccinator p.
  Childs-Phillips bowel p.
  disc p.
  fundal p.
  Graham p.
  Kelly p.
  laparoscopic p.
  minimally invasive p.
  Nesbit corporeal p.
  Noble bowel p.
  Rehne-Delorme p.
  retractor p.
  soft tissue p.
  surgical p.
  suture p.
  tongue p.
  transgastric p.
  transmesenteric p.
plicectomy
plicotomy
PLIF
  posterior lumbar interbody fusion
  posterolateral interbody fusion
  PLIF procedure
PLND
  pelvic lymph node dissection
ploidy
  tumor p.
plombage operation
plop
  cardiac tumor p.
  tumor p.
plot
  load-displacement p.
  pressure-flow p.
plug
  bioabsorbable hernia p.
  p. flow
  p. prosthetic mesh repair
plumb line
plume
  laser p.
Plummer disease
plyometric exercise

PMI
    point of maximum impulse
PMMF
    pectoralis major myocutaneous flap
PMN
    polymorphonuclear neutrophil
PMR
    progressive muscle relaxation
PMT
    percutaneous mechanical thrombectomy
pneumatic
    p. bag esophageal dilation
    p. balloon catheter dilation
    p. bone
    p. compression
    p. dilation
    p. otoscopy
    p. reduction
    p. retinopexy
    p. space
pneumatinuria (*var. of* pneumaturia)
pneumatization
pneumatocele
pneumatorrhachis
pneumatosis
    intestinal p.
pneumaturia, pneumatinuria
pneumectomy
pneumobulbar
pneumocardial
pneumocele
pneumocentesis
pneumocephalus
pneumococcal infection
pneumococcolysis
pneumoconioses (*pl. of* pneumoconiosis)
pneumoconiosis, pneumokoniosis, *pl.*
  pneumoconioses
pneumoconstriction
pneumocystography
pneumocystosis
pneumodissection
    laparoscopic p.
pneumogastric nerve
pneumography
    impedance p.
    retroperitoneal p.
pneumohydroperitoneum
pneumokoniosis (*var. of* pneumoconiosis)
pneumolysis
pneumomediastinum
pneumonectomy
    p. chest
    sleeve p.
    p. stump
pneumonia
    aspiration p.
    bacterial p.
    congenital aspiration p.

endogenous lipid p.
    extensive bilateral p.
    gram-negative p.
    inhalation p.
    nosocomial p.
    oil-aspiration p.
    postoperative p.
    ventilator-associated p. (VAP)
pneumonic
pneumonitis
    acute radiation p.
    aspiration p. (AP)
    chemical p.
    peptic aspiration p.
    radiation p.
pneumonocele
pneumonocentesis
pneumonopexy
pneumonoresection
pneumonorrhaphy
pneumonotomy, pneumotomy
pneumoorbitography
pneumopericardium
    tension p.
    ventilator-induced p.
pneumoperitoneum
    ambulatory p.
    CO_2 p.
    hospital p.
    positive-pressure p.
    preoperative p.
    stent-induced p.
pneumopexy
pneumopleuroparietopexy
pneumopreperitoneum
pneumopyelography
pneumoresection
pneumoretroperitoneum
    unilateral p.
pneumostatic dilation
pneumotachogram
pneumotachograph
pneumothoraces (*pl. of* pneumothorax)
pneumothorax, *pl.* **pneumothoraces**
    delayed p.
    extrapleural p.
    iatrogenic tension p.
    induced tension p.
    open p.
    posttraumatic persistent p. (PPP)
    pressure p.
    spontaneous p.
    tension p.
    underwater seal for p.
    ventilator-induced p.
pneumotomy (*var. of* pneumonotomy)
pneupreperitoneum-induced hypercapnia
PNL
    percutaneous nephrolithotomy

PNPB
> positive-negative pressure breathing

PNS
> peripheral nervous system

PO₂
> partial pressure of oxygen

POA
> power of attorney

POCD
> postoperative cognitive dysfunction

pocket
> circulating air p.
> elimination p.
> ionization chamber p.
> p. operation
> pacemaker p.
> peritoneal p.
> subpectoral p.

pocketed calculus

POD
> postoperative day

podalic extraction

PODVT
> postoperative deep venous
> thrombosis

pogonion

Pogrund lateral meniscectomy approach

point
> p. A
> abrasive p.
> absorbent p.
> Addison p.
> alveolar p.
> anchoring p.
> p. angle
> anterior focal p.
> apophysial p.
> associated myofascial trigger p.
> auricular p.
> axial p.
> p. B
> B p.
> bleeding p.
> blur p.
> Boas p.
> Bolton craniometric p. (Bo)
> bounce p.
> Boyd p.
> break p.
> Brinell hardness indenter p.
> Broadbent registration p.
> Cannon p.
> Capuron p.
> cardinal p.
> Castellani p.
> central bearing p.
> central yellow p.
> p. centric

> change p.
> Chauffard p.
> choroid p.
> Clado p.
> condenser p.
> conjugate p.
> contact area p.
> convenience p.
> convergence p.
> copular p.
> corresponding p.
> craniometric p.
> Crowe pilot p.
> cut p.
> D p.
> de Mussy p.
> Desjardins p.
> disparate p.
> dorsal p.
> E p.
> electrodesiccated bleeding p.
> end p.
> entry p.
> equivalence p.
> Erb p.
> ethmoid registration p.
> exit p.
> eye p.
> far p.
> faulty contact p.
> fibromyalgia trigger p.
> fixation p.
> fixed p.
> focal bleeding p.
> focal image p.
> freezing p.
> fusing p.
> gingival p.
> glenoid p.
> growing p.
> Guéneau de Mussy p.
> Halle p.
> Hartmann p.
> hinge-axis p.
> ice p.
> identical p.
> ignition p.
> image p.
> p. imaging
> impaction p.
> incident p.
> incisal p.
> incisor p.
> insertion p.
> isoelectric p.
> isometric p.
> J p.
> jugal p.
> jugomaxillary p.

Keen p.
Kocher p.
Krackow p.
lacrimal p.
Lanz p.
Legat p.
lustrous central yellow p.
Mackenzie p.
material failure break p.
maximum occipital p.
McBurney p.
median mandibular p.
melting p.
mental p.
metopic p.
motor p.
multiple sensitive p.
Munro p.
myofascial trigger p.
near visual p.
neutral p.
nodal p.
null p.
occipital p.
p. of abscess
p. of Arrhigi
p. of inflection
p. of maximum impulse (PMI)
optic nodal p.
painful p.
p. palpation
paper p.
Pauly p.
pedicle entrance p.
Piersol p.
pivot p.
posterior focal p.
power p.
preauricular p.
pressure inversion p.
primary myofascial trigger p.
principal p.
purchase p.
Ramond p.
referred p.
respiratory inversion p.
restoration p.
retention p.
retrograde insertion p.
retromandibular p.
Robson p.
root canal p.
rotary mounted p.
sacral brim target p.
satellite myofascial trigger p.
p. scanning
secondary focal p.
secondary myofascial trigger p.
sensitive p.

separation p.
set p.
p. source
spinal p.
stereo-identical p.
Sudeck critical p.
supraauricular p.
supraorbital p.
sylvian p.
taper p.
tender p.
thermal death p.
trial p.
trigger p.
triple p.
Trousseau p.
Valleix p.
virtual p.
visual p.
Weber p.
white p.
Z p.
zygomaxillary p.
2-point
    2-p. discrimination test
    2-p. nerve block
3-point
    3-p. bending moment
    3-p. touch
4-point
    4-p. biopsy
    4-p. fixation
point-counting image
pointed condyloma
point-in-space stereotactic biopsy
Poirier
    P. gland
    P. line
    space of P.
Poiseuille space
poisoning
    oxygen p.
    radiation p.
Poland
    P. anomaly
    P. epiphysial fracture
      classification
    P. physical injury classification
polarimetry
    scanning laser p.
polariscopy
polarization microscopy
**polarographic tissue oxygen tension
  method**
pole (P)
    inferior p.
    lateral p.
    p. ligation
    superior p.

P

poli (*pl. of* polus)
polio
    poliomyelitis
        bulbar polio
        nonbulbar polio
        polio paralysis
poliomyelitis (PM, polio)
Politano-Leadbetter
        P.-L. anastomosis
        P.-L. reimplantation
        P.-L. tunnel creation
        P.-L. ureterolysis
        P.-L. ureteroneocystostomy
Politzer auditory tube patency method
pollakiuria
pollex
        adductor pollicis (AP)
pollicization
        Buck-Gramcko p.
        index p.
        Riordan p.
pollination
Pollock operation
polus, *pl.* **poli**
Pólya
        P. anastomosis
        P. gastrectomy
        P. gastrectomy method
        P. gastrectomy procedure
        P. gastroduodenal anastomosis
          technique
        P. gastroenterostomy
        P. operation
polyadenous
polyadenylation
polyagglutination
Polyak endonasal dacryocystorhinostomy
polyamide suture
polyaxial joint
polybutester suture
polycentric rotation
polychondritis
        relapsing p.
polyclonal
        p. growth
        p. hyperplasia
polycystic
        p. kidney disease (PKD)
        p. liver
polycythemia vera
polydactylous
polydactyly
Polydek suture
polydioxanone
        p. surgical suture
        p. suture (PDS)
polydysplasia
polyembryoma

polyester
        p. fiber suture
        p. mesh
polyethylene
        p. glycol
        p. suture
polyfilament suture
polygalactic acid suture
polyganglionic
polyglactin 910 suture
polyglandular
polyglecaprone 25 suture
polyglycolate suture
polyglycolic
        p. acid (PGA)
        p. acid suture
polyglyconate suture
polyhydramnios
polymer anesthetic
polymerization
        fibrin p.
polymethylmethacrylate injection
polymicrobial infection
polymorphism
        platelet gene p.
polymorphonuclear neutrophil (PMN)
polymyalgia rheumatica
polymyositis
polyneuropathy
        critical illness p. (CIPN)
polyorchidism (*var. of* polyorchism)
polyorchism, polyorchidism
polyp
        adenomatous p.
        cellular p.
        colon p.
        colorectal p.
        cystic p.
        dental p.
        endocervical p.
        endometrial p.
        hyperplastic p.
        juvenile p.
        pedunculated p.
        perineal p.
        rectal p.
polypapilloma
polypectomy
        colonoscopic p.
        duodenal endoscopic p.
        electrosurgical snare p.
        endoscopic sessile p.
        gastric p.
        incomplete p.
        intranasal p.
polypiform (*var. of* polypoid)
polypoid, polypiform
        p. hyperplasia
        p. hyperplasia of larynx

p. lesion
p. mass
p. superficial gastric carcinoma
p. tissue
p. tumor
polyposis
carpetlike p.
diffuse GI p.
diffuse mucosal p.
familial adenomatous p. (FAP)
familial juvenile p. (FJP)
polypropylene
p. button suture
p. mesh
p. mesh herniorrhaphy
polyradiculoneuropathy
chronic inflammatory demyelinating
p. (CIDP)
polyradiculopathy
polysinusectomy
Polysorb suture
polyspermia, polyspermism, polyspermy
polyspermism (*var. of* polyspermia)
polyspermy (*var. of* polyspermia)
polysyndactyly
PolySyn Ophthalmic suture
polytetrafluoroethylene
p. graft
p. suture
polythelia
polytrauma
polyuria
polyvalent
p. melanoma oncolysate
p. VMO
Pomeroy
P. operation
P. tubal ligation
Poncet perineal urethrostomy
pond fracture
Ponka
P. herniorrhaphy
P. technique for local anesthesia
pons
**Ponsky pull PEG tube insertion
  technique**
Pontén fasciocutaneous flap
pontile, pontine
pontine (*var. of* pontile)
p. artery
p. cistern
p. hemorrhage
p. myelinolysis
p. paramedian reticular formation
p. spinothalamic tractotomy
PONV
postoperative nausea and vomiting
pool
abdominal p.

donor p.
p. therapy
poor exercise tolerance
poorly compliant bladder
poor-risk patient
popliteal
p. artery
p. artery entrapment
p. artery occlusive disease
  (PAOD)
p. artery trifurcation
p. catheter
p. communicating nerve
p. fascia
p. fossa
p. groove
p. incision
p. muscle
p. plexus
p. region
p. space
p. vein
p. web syndrome
**popliteus fossa muscle
  tendon**
pop-off
p.-o. suture
p.-o. valve
population
adult p.
patient p.
pediatric p.
p. sample
porcelain
p. cervical ditching technique
p. condensation
p. fracture
p. gallbladder
p. jacket restoration
porcelain-bonded restoration
porcelain-fused-to-metal restoration
pore
permeability transition p.
pori (*pl. of* porus)
porocarcinoma
poroid hidradenoma
poroma
porotomy
porous
p. filter membrane
p. ingrowth fixation
p. polyethylene implant
p. tantalum implant
porphyria
acute intermittent p.
intermittent acute p.
Porro
P. cesarean section
P. operation

P

Porstmann patent ductus arteriovenosus closure technique
port
    camera p.
    chest p.
    p. displacement
    Hasson p.
    implantable infusion p.
    p. incision
    infusion p.
    inlet p.
    lumbar p.
    midclavicular p.
    nasal p.
    PAS p.
    periumbilical p.
    side p.
    p. site
    p. site hernia
    p. site metastasis
    p. site sinus
    p. stopper
    subcostal p.
    subcutaneous implanted injection p.
    subxiphoid p.
    suprapubic p.
    umbilical p.
    velopharyngeal p.
    p. vitrectomy
    working p.
4-port
    4-p. diamond placement
    4-p. method
    4-p. procedure
    4-p. technique
5-port fan placement
portable
    p. C-arm image intensifier fluoroscopy
    p. infusion pump
portacaval, portocaval
    p. anastomosis
    p. H graft
    p. shunt
    p. shunt operation
port-access technique for coronary bypass surgery
porta hepatis
portal
    arthroscopic entry p.
    aspiration p.
    p. azygos disconnection
    p. bifurcation
    p. canal
    p. collateral
    p. decompression
    p. decompression surgery
    p. delta
    p. drainage

    p. eosinophilic inflammation
    p. fissure
    p. hypertension
    p. hypertensive bleeding
    p. inflow
    p. infusion
    p. lymphadenopathy
    p. lymph node basin
    macroscopic p.
    p. mesenteric shunt
    p. nodal involvement
    p. pedicle
    p. perfusion
    p. scissura
    p. shunt index
    p. space
    p. steal
    p. thrombosis
    p. tract
    p. tract inflammation
    p. triad
    p. triad clamping
    p. tumor thrombus
    p. vein
    p. vein approach
    p. vein catheterization
    p. vein embolization
    p. vein obstruction
    p. vein reconstruction
    p. vein resection
    p. vein tumor thrombus (PVTT)
    p. venous pressure
    p. venous system
    p. vessel
portal-collateral circulation
portal-hypophysial circulation
6-portal synovectomy
portal-systemic
    p.-s. anastomosis
    p.-s. collateral
    p.-s. collateral vein
    p.-s. encephalopathy (PSE)
    p.-s. encephalopathy index
    p.-s. shunt
    p.-s. shunt surgery
2-portal technique
3-portal technique
Porter fascia
Porter-Richardson-Vainio
    P.-R.-V. arthroscopic synovectomy technique
    P.-R.-V. synovectomy
portio, *pl.* **portiones**
portion
    distal p.
    intrapancreatic p.
    lateral p.
    mesenteric p.

proximal p.
subcutaneous p.
portiones (*pl. of* portio)
portiplexus
Portmann posterior crus of stapes interposition
portobilioarterial
portocaval (*var. of* portacaval)
portoenterostomy
Kasai p.
portography
computed tomography arterial p. (CTAP)
CT p.
indirect p.
percutaneous transhepatic direct p.
portojejunostomy
hepatic p.
portoportal anastomosis
portopulmonary venous anastomosis
portosystemic, portal-systemic
p. anastomosis
p. collateral circulation
p. shunt
port-site wound recurrence
port-wine
p.-w. hemangioma
p.-w. mark
p.-w. stain
porus, *pl.* **pori**
Posada fracture
position
abdominal brace p.
Adams p.
airplane p.
p. ametropia
angular p.
anomalous p.
antecolic p.
anterior oblique p.
antiembolic p.
anti-Trendelenburg p.
arch-and-slouch p.
arm p.
arm-extension p.
asynclitic p.
back-up p.
backward p.
barber chair p.
batrachian p.
bayonet fracture p.
beach chair p.
Bertel p.
birthing p.
bisecting angle cone p.
body p.
Bonner p.
Boyce p.
Bozeman p.

Brickner p.
brow p.
brow-anterior p.
brow-down p.
brow-posterior p.
brow-up p.
Buie p.
calcaneal stance p.
cardiac p.
cardinal p.
Casselberry p.
catheter p.
centric p.
cervical p.
chin p.
Concorde p.
condylar hinge p.
consonant p.
convergence p.
corrected sternal p.
cotton-loader p.
curved flank p.
cuspid-molar p.
decubitus p.
deep extubation in tonsil p.
dissociated p.
distoangular p.
dorsal decubitus p.
dorsal elevated p.
dorsal inertia p.
dorsal lithotomy p.
dorsal recumbent p.
dorsal rigid p.
dorsal supine p.
dorsosacral p.
Duncan p.
eccentric jaw p.
Edebohls p.
electrical heart p.
Elliot p.
emprosthotonos p.
en face p.
English p.
equinus p.
exaggerated sniffing p.
extraabdominal p.
extrathoracic p.
face-down p.
face-to-pubes fetal p.
Feist-Mankin p.
fetal head p.
Fick p.
figure-of-4 p.
flank p.
flexed p.
forehead-nose p.
French p.
frogleg p.
frontoanterior fetal p.

P

position (*continued*)
    frontoposterior fetal p.
    frontotransverse fetal p.
    Fuchs p.
    fusion-free p.
    Gaynor-Hart p.
    genucubital p.
    genufacial p.
    genupectoral p.
    gingival p.
    greater curve p.
    head dependent p.
    head elevated p.
    head-up tilt p.
    heart p.
    heterophoric p.
    hinge p.
    hook-lying p.
    horizontal p.
    hornpipe p.
    infraumbilical p.
    initial consonant p.
    p. in space
    intercuspal p.
    intraperitoneal p.
    intrathoracic p.
    intrinsic minus p.
    jackknife p.
    James p.
    jaw-to-jaw p.
    jet pilot p.
    Jones p.
    jumper-knee p.
    kidney p.
    knee-chest p.
    knee-elbow p.
    kneeling p.
    kneeling-squatting p.
    Kraske p.
    LAO p.
    lateral decubitus p.
    lateral prone p.
    lateral recumbent p.
    leapfrog p.
    left anterior oblique p.
    left decubitus p.
    left lateral decubitus p.
    left-side-down p.
    levotransposed p.
    lithotomy p.
    Lloyd Davies modified lithotomy p.
    lotus p.
    mandibular hinge p.
    mandibular rest p.
    maternal birthing p.
    Mayo-Robson p.
    mentoanterior fetal p.
    mentoposterior fetal p.
    mentotransverse fetal p.

mentum anterior fetal p.
mentum posterior fetal p.
mentum transverse fetal p.
mesioangular p.
midline p.
military brace p.
military tuck p.
missionary p.
modified lithotomy p.
Moynihan p.
near-anatomic p.
neck extension p.
neutral hip p.
neutral spine p.
Noble p.
nonphysiologic p.
normal anatomic p.
obstetric p.
occipitoanterior fetal p.
occipitoposterior fetal p.
occipitotransverse fetal p.
occlusal p.
opisthotonos p.
overcorrected p.
over-the-top p.
paralleling cone p.
park-bench p.
persistent occiput posterior fetal p.
Phalen p.
physiologic rest p.
posterior border p.
postural resting p.
prayer p.
premuscular p.
primary p.
Proetz p.
prone split-leg p.
protrusive occlusal p.
proximal bow p.
pterygoid p.
pulmonary p.
quasistatic stressed p.
RAO p.
ready-ready p.
reclining p.
rectus p.
recumbent p.
rest p.
retrocolic p.
retromuscular p.
retruded p.
reverse Trendelenburg p.
Rhese p.
right acromiodorsoposterior fetal p.
right anterior oblique p.
right-side-down p.
Robson p.
Rose p.
sacroanterior fetal p.

sacroposterior fetal p.
sacrotransverse fetal p.
Samuel p.
scapuloanterior fetal p.
scapuloposterior fetal p.
Schüller p.
scissor-leg p.
Scultetus p.
sea lion p.
semi-Fowler p.
semilateral p.
semioblique p.
semiprone p.
semireclining p.
semirecumbent p.
semiupright p.
shock p.
shoe-and-stocking p.
Simon p.
Sims p.
sitting p.
ski p.
smiley face up p.
sniffing p.
sphinx p.
spinal fusion p.
split-leg p.
static p.
steep lateral decubitus p.
steep Trendelenburg p.
sternal p.
subcostal p.
sulcus fixated p.
supine p.
terminal hinge p.
tooth p.
tooth-to-tooth p.
translational p.
Trendelenburg p.
tricuspid p.
tuck p.
upright p.
Valentine p.
ventral decubitus p.
vertex p.
vertical divergence p.
W p.
Walcher p.
W-sitting p.
positional
p. release therapy
p. vertigo
positioner
hip p.
positioning
Automated Endoscopic System for
Optimal P. (AESOP)
prone p.
surgical p.

positive
p. airway pressure (PAP)
p. correlation
p. cytology
p. end-expiratory pressure (PEEP)
p. end-expiratory pressure/continuous
positive airway pressure
(PEEP/CPAP)
p. expiratory pressure
false p.
p. inspiratory pressure
p. peritoneal cytology
p. predictive value (PPV)
p. resection margin
resection margin macroscopic p.
(R2)
resection margin microscopic p.
(R1)
p. spousal reinforcement
p. surgical margin
p. tropism
true p.
**positive-negative pressure breathing
(PNPB)**
positive-pressure
p.-p. pneumoperitoneum
p.-p. ventilation (PPV)
positron
p. emission tomography (PET)
p. emission tomography-guided
biopsy
possible operative arthrotomy
POSSUM
Physiological and Operative Severity
Score for the Enumeration of
Mortality and Morbidity
post
p. herniorrhaphy inguinodynia
P. total shoulder arthroplasty
postactivation
p. exhaustion
p. facilitation
postadrenalectomy syndrome
postage stamp skin graft
postanal repair
postanesthesia
p. care unit (PACU)
p. emergence reaction
postanesthetic
p. central nervous system
dysfunction
p. shivering
postangioplasty
p. intimal flap
p. restenosis
postaugmentation
postauricular incision
postaxial
postballoon angioplasty restenosis

P

postbiopsy
 p. renal AV fistula
 p. vascular complication
postblock management
postbrachial
postbulbar ulceration
postburn
 p. bone marrow failure
 p. hypermetabolic response
postcardiotomy
 p. shock
 p. syndrome
postcatheterization
postcaval ureter
postcementation
postcentral
 p. gyrectomy
 p. sulcal artery
postcesarean anesthesia
postcholecystectomy
 p. flatulent dyspepsia
 p. syndrome
postclavicular
postcoiling
postcoital
 p. bleeding
 p. test
postcolonoscopy distention syndrome
postcommissurotomy syndrome
postcondensation
postconditioning
 anesthetic-induced p.
postcordial
postcore restoration
postcoronary angioplasty
postcostal
postcricoid web
postdiagnosis
postdischarge nausea and vomiting
postdrug latency
postductal coarctation
postdural
 p. puncture headache
 p. puncture meningitis
postembolization syndrome
postendoscopy
posterior
 p. alveolar artery
 p. antebrachial region
 anterior and p. (A&P)
 p. anterior jugular vein
 p. arch
 p. arch fracture
 p. arm
 p. aspect
 p. auricular artery
 p. auricular groove
 p. auricular nerve

p. auricular plexus
p. auricular vein
p. basal branch
p. basal segment
p. belly
p. bladder flap plasty
p. border jaw relation
p. border position
p. brachial region
p. capsular zonular barrier
p. capsulorrhaphy
p. capsulotomy
p. cartilage graft
p. cecal artery
p. cerebral artery (PCA)
p. cervical fixation
p. cervical fusion
p. cervical lateral plating
p. cervical space
p. choroidal artery
p. circulation aneurysm
p. circumflex humeral artery
p. clinoid process
p. colporrhaphy
p. column
p. column cordotomy
p. column fracture
p. column osteosynthesis
p. communicating artery (PCoA)
p. condyloid foramen
p. coronary plexus
p. costotransversectomy approach
p. cranial fossa
p. cricoarytenoid muscle
p. cyst
p. diaphragmatic gastropexy
p. element fracture
p. explant
p. extraperitoneal approach
p. facial vein
p. flap
p. flap technique
p. flap vaginoplasty
p. focal point
p. fontanelle
p. fornix of vagina
p. fossa circulation
p. fossa decompression
p. fracture-dislocation
p. fundoplasty
p. glenoplasty
p. great vessel
p. hemicircular incision
p. hip dislocation
p. humeral circumflex artery
p. iliac osteotomy
p. inferior cerebellar artery (PICA)
p. inferior iliac spine
p. inferior pancreaticoduodenal artery

p. innominate rotation
p. interbody lumbar spinal fusion
p. intercostal artery
p. intercostal vein
p. intermuscular septum
p. interosseous artery
p. interosseous nerve compression
  syndrome
p. interosseous vein
p. intraoccipital joint
p. inverted-U approach
p. knee
p. knee region
p. labial artery
p. labial commissure
p. labial vein
p. laparoscopic approach
p. larynx
p. layer
p. limiting ring
p. lobule
p. longitudinal bundle
p. lower cervical spine surgery
p. lumbar approach
p. lumbar interbody fusion (PLIF)
p. lumbar spine and sacrum
  surgery
p. mediastinal artery
p. mediastinal esophagoplasty
p. mediastinal mass
p. mediastinum
p. meningeal artery
p. midline approach
p. mitral valve leaflet
p. neck region
p. nephrectomy
p. nodule
p. occipitocervical approach
p. oropharyngeal wall
p. pancreaticoduodenal artery
p. parametritis
p. parietal artery
p. parotid vein
p. pedicle
p. pelvic exenteration
p. periosteum
p. pharynx
p. Pólya gastrectomy procedure
p. primary division
processus clinoideus p.
p. proctotomy
p. radial approach
p. radicular artery
p. rectopexy
p. rectus sheath
p. rectus sheath wall
p. repair
p. reversible encephalopathy
  syndrome

p. rhizotomy
p. ring fracture
p. root
p. sagittal anorectoplasty (PSARP)
p. sagittal anorectoplasty procedure
p. sclerotomy
p. screw fixation
p. scrotal vein
p. segmental fixation
p. shoulder approach
p. shoulder dislocation
p. side
p. spinal artery (PSA)
p. spinal fusion
p. spinal wedge osteotomy
p. spinocerebellar tract
p. stomach
p. superior alveolar artery
p. superior iliac spine
superior labrum anterior and p.
  (SLAP)
p. superior pancreaticoduodenal
  artery
p. surface
p. synechia formation
p. temporal artery
p. thalamic syndrome
p. thermal sclerostomy
p. thigh
p. tibialis tendon
p. tibial nerve block
p. tibial recurrent artery
p. tibiotalar
p. translation
p. transolecranon approach
p. transthoracic incision
p. triangle
p. truncal vagotomy
p. ulnar recurrent artery
p. upper cervical spine surgery
p. urethra
p. uveitis
p. vaginal fornix
p. vaginal hernia
p. vaginal trunk
p. vertical canal
p. vitrectomy
p. wall fracture
posterior-anterior pressure
posterioris
posterior-lateral
  p.-l. lobule
  p.-l. lumbar spinal fusion
posterior-superior oblique projection
posteroanterior (PA)
  p. projection
posteroinferior
  p. external
  p. external movement

posterolateral
- p. approach
- p. aspect
- p. bone graft placement
- p. bundle
- p. central artery
- p. costotransversectomy incision
- p. costotransversectomy technique
- p. herniation
- p. interbody fusion (PLIF)
- p. lumbosacral fusion

posteromedial
- p. approach
- p. central artery
- p. dislocation

posterosuperior segment
posteroventral pallidotomy
postesophageal
postevacuation
postexcision cavity
postextraction hemorrhage
postextubation
- p. apnea
- p. croup
- p. laryngospasm
- p. stridor

postfixation radiography
postfracture lesion
postfundoplication syndrome
postganglionic
- p. parasympathetic fiber
- p. sympathetic fiber

postgastrectomy
- p. bleeding
- p. cancer
- p. dysfunction
- p. hemorrhage
- p. syndrome

posthemorrhagic
posthepatic resection phase
postherniorrhaphy pain
postherpetic neuralgia (PHN)
posthetomy
posthioplasty
posthitis
postholith
posthyoid
posthypercapnic state
posthyperventilation apnea
posticus
postimplantation period
postinfarction ventricular septal defect
postinfection lipoatrophy
postinflammatory hypopigmentation
postinjury
- p. immunologic defect
- p. level

postinsufflation

postintervention
postintubation croup
postirradiation
- p. fracture
- p. study
- p. syndrome

postischemic
- p. administration
- p. stunned myocardium

postischial
postkeratoplasty
postlaminectomy
- p. kyphosis
- p. syndrome

postlaparoscopic subcutaneous emphysema
postlaparoscopy meralgia paresthetica
post-living donor liver transplant
postlumpectomy skin thickening
postlymphangiography abdomen
postmastectomy pain
postmastoid
postmedian
postmediastinal
postmediastinum
postmembrane
- p. pressure
- p. rupture

postmenopausal
- p. bleeding
- p. body mass

postmortem
- p. clot
- p. examination
- p. hypostasis
- p. suggillation

postnatal
- p. therapy
- p. torsion

postobstructive pulmonary edema
postocular
postop
- postoperative

postoperative (postop)
- p. abscess
- p. airway obstruction
- p. analgesia
- p. analgesic
- p. analgesic technique
- p. anastomotic leak
- p. anastomotic leakage
- p. anesthesia
- p. anisocoria
- p. antibiotic
- p. anticoagulation therapy
- p. apnea
- p. bleeding
- p. cesarean section pain
- p. choledochoscopy

p. cognitive dysfunction (POCD)
p. course
p. CT scan
p. day (POD)
p. death
p. deconditioning
p. deep venous thrombosis (PODVT)
p. delirium
p. diagnosis
p. dialysis
p. ductal dilation
p. dysphagia
p. ERCP
p. extubation
p. fatigue
p. followup evaluation
p. fracture
p. gastrointestinal tract dysfunction (PGID)
p. hemorrhage
p. hepatic failure
p. hernia
p. hour
p. hydrocele
p. hypocalcemia
p. ileus
p. immobilization
p. infection
p. irradiation
p. irrigation-suction
p. irrigation-suction drainage
p. liver failure
p. management
p. morbidity
p. mortality
p. motility
p. nausea and vomiting (PONV)
p. paraplegia
p. pelvic radiation
p. period
p. pleurobiliary fistula
p. pneumonia
p. recovery
p. regimen for oral early feeding (PROEF)
p. renal dysfunction
p. repair
p. residual paralysis
p. respiratory complication
p. result
p. shivering
p. supplementation
p. survival
p. survival probability (PSP)
p. symptom
p. systemic chemotherapy
p. tetany
p. ventilation

postpartum
　　p. hemorrhage
　　p. infection
postpericardiotomy syndrome
postpharyngeal space
postphlebitic syndrome
postpneumonectomy tuberculous empyema
postpolypectomy
　　p. bleeding
　　p. coagulation syndrome
　　p. hemorrhage
postprandial
　　p. AUC
　　p. distention
　　p. flushing
　　p. hour
　　p. hyperglycemia
　　p. motor activity
　　p. motor parameter
　　p. motor result
　　p. nausea
　　p. period
　　p. value
postprostatectomy incontinence
postpyloric
　　p. feeding
　　p. sphincter
postradiation
　　p. change
　　p. fistula
　　p. kyphosis
　　p. plexopathy
　　p. therapy
postradical neck dissection
postreduction mammaplasty
postresection
　　p. defect
　　p. filling
　　p. filling technique
postresuscitation period
postreversal
postsacral
postscapular
postsclerotherapy ulcer
postsensation
postshunt
postsphenoid bone
postsphincterotomy ERCP cannulation
postsplenectomy
　　p. complication
　　p. infection
　　p. sepsis
postsplenic
poststenotic dilation
poststroke pain
postsubarachnoid hemorrhage hydrocephalus
postsulcal

P

postsurgical
- p. abdomen
- p. disturbance
- p. endoscopy
- p. gastroparesis
- p. motor anomaly
- p. motor change
- p. nervous damage
- p. pain
- p. truncal pain

postsympathectomy neuralgia

postsynaptic membrane

posttecta

posttetanic
- p. count
- p. count monitoring
- p. facilitation

postthoracotomy
- p. change
- p. pain

posttranslation modification

posttransplant
- p. day
- p. diabetes
- p. immunosuppression therapy
- p. lymphoproliferative disease (PTLD)
- p. lymphoproliferative disorder (PTLD)

posttransverse

posttraumatic
- p. autotransplantation
- p. cervical dystonia
- p. chondrolysis
- p. diaphragmatic hernia
- p. gustatory neuralgia
- p. hemorrhage
- p. intradiploic pseudomeningocele
- p. pain
- p. pancreatic-cutaneous fistula
- p. persistent pneumothorax (PPP)
- p. renal failure
- p. seizure
- p. spinal deformity
- p. stress disorder (PTSD)
- p. subcapsular hepatic fluid collection

posttreatment hemorrhage

posttubal ligation syndrome

postural
- p. deformity
- p. drainage
- p. fixation back maneuver
- p. headache
- p. orthostatic tachycardia syndrome (POTS)
- p. reduction
- p. resting position
- p. therapy

posture
- compensatory head p.
- forward head p.
- head p.

postureteral ligation

postureteroscopic manipulation

posturography
- platform p.

postuterine

postvagotomy
- p. dysphagia
- p. gastroparesis
- p. syndrome

postvalvar, postvalvular

postvalvular (*var. of* postvalvar)

postvasectomy

postvitrectomy fibrin

postzygomatic space

potassium space

potato tumor

potency
- anesthetic p.
- sphincteric p.

potential
- auditory evoked p. (AEP)
- p. complications of postoperative ileus
- compound muscle action p. (CMAP)
- curative p.
- demarcation p.
- denervation p.
- electrode p.
- endogenous event-related p.
- excitatory junction p.
- excitatory postsynaptic p.
- extreme somatosensory evoked p.
- fasciculation p.
- fibrillation p.
- laser-evoked p.
- membrane p.
- middle latency auditory evoked p. (MLAEP)
- midlatency auditory evoked p. (MLAEP)
- miniature end-plate p.
- modulation p.
- motor evoked p. (MEP)
- myogenic motor-evoked p.
- oxidation-reducing p.
- pacemaker p.
- peroneal somatosensory evoked p.
- reduction p.
- regeneration motor unit p.
- resting membrane p.
- somatosensory evoked p. (SEP)
- standard electrode p.
- standard reduction p.

potentially
    p. curative procedure
    p. lethal x-ray damage repair
    p. resectable lesion
potentiation
potent inhaled anesthetic
potentiometric titration
POTS
    postural orthostatic tachycardia
    syndrome
Pott
    P. aneurysm
    P. ankle fracture
    P. eversion osteotomy
    P. fracture
    P. gangrene
Potter
    P. facies
    P. polycystic kidney classification
Potts
    P. anastomosis
    P. pulmonary stenosis operation
Potts-Smith
    P.-S. anastomosis
    P.-S. descending aorta to left
      pulmonary artery anastomosis
      procedure
pouch
    anal p.
    antibiotic bead p.
    arachnoid retrocerebellar p.
    bead p.
    p. biopsy
    bladder replacement urinary p.
    blind rectal p.
    blind upper esophageal p.
    Broca p.
    colonic p.
    coloplasty p.
    continent ileal p.
    continent urinary p.
    copulating p.
    deep perineal p.
    dermal p.
    p. development
    p. dilation
    double-loop p.
    Douglas p.
    drainable ostomy p.
    endorectal ileal p.
    p. failure
    gastric p.
    Hartmann p.
    haustral p.
    hepatorenal p.
    hernia p.
    Hunt-Lawrence jejunal p.
    ileal neobladder urinary p.
    p. ileitis

    ileoanal p.
    ileocecal p.
    ileocolic p.
    Indiana urinary diversion p.
    inflamed synovial p.
    intraluminal p.
    intravaginal p.
    inverted-U p.
    jejunal p.
    J pelvic ileal p.
    J-shaped ileal p.
    kangaroo p.
    Koch p.
    laryngeal p.
    lateral-lateral p.
    3-loop ileal p.
    2-loop J-shaped ileal p.
    Miami p.
    Morison p.
    N pelvic ileal p.
    omental p.
    open-end ostomy p.
    paracystic p.
    pararectal p.
    paravesical p.
    pelvic p.
    pharyngeal p.
    1-piece ostomy p.
    2-piece ostomy p.
    Prussak p.
    p. reconstruction
    rectal blind p.
    rectouterine p.
    rectovaginal p.
    rectovaginouterine p.
    rectovesical p.
    renal p.
    self-seal p.
    sigmoid rectum p.
    S pelvic ileal p.
    superficial perineal p.
    supradiaphragmatic p.
    suprapatellar p.
    terminal ileal p.
    triple loop p.
    U p.
    U-shaped jejunal p.
    uterovesical p.
    VBG p.
    vertical banded gastroplasty p.
    vesicouterine p.
    visceral p.
    W p.
    wallaby p.
    Willis p.
    W pelvic p.
    Zenker p.
pouched ileostomy
pouchitis

P

pouchoscopy
pelvic p.
pouch-vaginal fistula
Poupart line
1-pour technique
2-pour technique
powder
karaya p.
powdered bone graft
power
p. Doppler imaging
p. of attorney (POA)
p. of hydrogen (pH)
P. operation
p. point
PPG
pylorus-preserving gastrectomy
PPH
primary pulmonary hypertension
PPI
proton pump inhibitor
PPM
prosthesis-patient mismatch
PPN
peripheral parenteral nutrition
PPP
posttraumatic persistent
pneumothorax
PPPD
pylorus-preserving
pancreatoduodenectomy
PPS
presurgical psychological
screening
PPT
pressure pain threshold
PPV
positive predictive value
positive-pressure ventilation
PQOL
perceived quality of life
practice
value-based anesthesia p.
practitioner
praecox
lymphedema p.
Prague breech delivery maneuver
Pratt open reduction
prayer position
PRBC
packed red blood cells
preadaptation
preanal
preanesthetic
p. medication
p. skin-surface warming
preantiseptic
preaortic
preaseptic

preauricular
p. cyst
p. fistula
p. fossa
p. groove
p. incision
p. point
p. sulcus
preauricularis
preaxial
preaxillary line
prebiotic
precancerous lesion
precapillary anastomosis
precatheterization
precaution
full-stomach p.'s
radiation p.'s
Precedex
precentral
p. cortical stimulation
p. gyrectomy
p. gyrus
p. sulcal artery
prechiasmal
p. compression
p. optic nerve lesion
precipitate in solution
precipitating
p. lesion
p. noxious event
precise dissection
preclotted graft
precommissural bundle
preconditioning
anesthetic p.
cerebral p.
ischemic p.
myocardial ischemic p.
p. phenomenon
precordial
p. Doppler
p. thump
p. wound
precordium
precorneal
precostal
precuneal artery
precursor lesion
precut
p. incision
p. papillotomy
p. sphincterotomy
predental space
predialysis plasma phosphate
concentration
prediction
breast cancer risk p.
Gail model of breast cancer risk p.

predictive value
prediluted antibody panel
predisposing
> p. condition
> p. factor

predisposition
> hereditary p.

predorsal bundle
preeclamptic liver disease
preemergence
preemptive
> p. analgesia
> p. anesthesia

preendoscopy
preepiglottic
> p. soft tissue
> p. space

preexcitation
> p. syndrome
> ventricular p.

preexisting lesion
prefabrication
prefrontal
> p. leukotomy
> p. lobotomy

pregabalin
preganglionic
> p. cardiac sympathetic blockade
> p. parasympathetic fiber
> p. sympathectomy
> p. sympathetic block
> p. sympathetic denervation
> p. sympathetic fiber

preglenoid plane
pregnancy
> abdominal p.
> p. complication
> ectopic p.
> p. luteoma

prehepatic resection phase
prehospital resuscitation
prehyoid gland
preincision
preincisional intravenous pentoxifylline
preincubation
preinduction
> p. period
> p. phase

preinsufflation
preinterparietal bone
preintervention
preischemic administration
Preiser disease
prelabor membrane rupture
prelaryngeal node
prelimbic
preliminary iridectomy
preload
> decreased p.

> p. dependency
> left ventricular p.
> p. recruitable stroke work
> p. reduction

premalignant
> p. condition
> p. lesion

premasseteric
> p. space
> p. space abscess

premature
> p. airway closure
> p. amnion rupture
> p. ductus arteriosus closure
> P. Infant Pain Profile (PIPP)
> p. membrane rupture
> p. separation
> p. separation of placenta

premaxilla
premed
> premedication

premedicate
premedication (premed)
premembrane
> p. pressure
> p. rupture

premenopausal ovary
PremiCron nonabsorbable suture
premicturition pressure
premolar teeth
premonitory palpitation
premorbid performance status
premuscular
> p. mesh technique
> p. position
> p. prosthetic repair

prenatal
> p. diethylstilbestrol exposure
> p. dislocation
> p. therapy
> p. torsion

Prentiss
> P. cryptorchidism repair maneuver
> P. orchiopexy

preoccipital notch
preoperative
> p. analgesia
> p. anesthetic
> p. biopsy
> p. chemoradiotherapy
> p. diagnosis
> p. dose
> p. ERCP
> p. evolution time
> p. factor
> p. fasting
> p. feature
> p. FNA specimen
> p. imaging

P

preoperative (*continued*)
    p. induction chemotherapy
    p. investigation
    p. jaundice
    p. lesion
    p. liver function
    p. localization
    p. localization signal
    p. LSG
    p. lymphoscintigraphy
    p. percutaneous aspiration
    p. period
    p. pneumoperitoneum
    p. preparation
    p. retrograde cholangiogram
    p. scoring
    p. scoring system
    p. skin-surface warming
    p. staging
    p. staging evaluation
    p. study
    p. systemic chemotherapy
    p. therapy
    p. ultrasound
preoperatively donated autologous blood
preoxygenation
    head-up p.
prep
    preparation
    Nichols bowel prep
    shave prep
prepancreatic arch
prepapillary sphincter
preparation (prep)
    access p.
    p. and draping
    bevel p.
    biomechanical p.
    bone-patellar tendon-bone p.
    bowel p.
    Brown dietary method for colon p.
    cavity p.
    chamfer p.
    ChloraPrep skin p.
    chlorhexidine gluconate skin p.
    colon p.
    corrosion p.
    crush p.
    facet joint p.
    facial butt joint p.
    figure-of-8 p.
    fortified topical p.
    full shoulder p.
    galenic p.
    graft p.
    heart-lung p.
    impression p.
    incisal p.
    initial p.

insulin p.
intraoperative bowel p.
Langendorff heart p.
lavage bowel p.
liposomal p.
mouth p.
preoperative p.
rod contour p.
shoulder with bevel p.
skin p.
slice p.
slot p.
slot-type p.
step p.
surgical p.
unfiltered p.
vertical versus horizontal p.
wire contour p.
preparatory iridectomy
prepared
    p. cavity
    p. cavity impression
    p. large bowel
prepatellar
    p. bursa
    p. bursa inflammation
preperitoneal
    p. anesthesia
    p. approach
    p. fat
    p. space
    transabdominal p. (TAPP)
PREPIC
    Prévention du Risque d'Embolie
    Pulmonaire par Interruption Cave
    PREPIC study group
preplacental hemorrhage
prepontine
    p. cistern
    p. white epidermoidoma
prepped and draped
preprostate urethral sphincter
preprosthetic surgery
prepubic fascia
prepuce
preputial
    p. calculus
    p. continent vesicostomy
    p. gland
    p. sac
preputiotomy
prepyloric
    p. perforation
    p. sphincter
    p. vein
prepyramidal tract
prerecruitment
prerectal lithotomy
prerenal

preretinal
- p. hemorrhage
- p. membrane
- p. neovascularization

prerolandic artery

presacral
- p. anesthesia
- p. anomaly
- p. cystic lesion
- p. fascia
- p. insufflation
- p. mass
- p. nerve
- p. neurectomy
- p. rectopexy
- p. resection
- p. space
- p. sympathectomy

presaturation technique

presbyopia

presbyopic vision

prescreening
- opioid p.

presence
- arteriographic p.

presensitization phase

presentation
- acute p.
- chronic p.
- clinical p.
- mammographic p.
- p. of cord

presenting
- p. clinical manifestation
- p. symptom

Present Pain Index

preseptal space

preservation
- autonomic nerve p.
- breast p.
- cadaver renal p.
- carotid p.
- extracorporeal renal p.
- extremity p.
- lordosis p.
- lumbar lordosis p.
- pelvic autonomic nerve p. (PANP)
- renal p.
- simple cold storage p.
- sphincter p.
- spleen p.
- splenic p.
- p. technique
- p. time
- tissue p.
- visual p.

preservative solution

presigmoid-transtransversarium intradural approach

presphenoid bone

prespinal

presplenic fold

pressoreceptor

pressor medication

pressure
- abdominal p.
- acoustic p.
- airway p. (AWP)
- p. alopecia
- alveolar carbon dioxide p.
- alveolar partial p.
- p. amaurosis
- p. amplitude modulation
- anal resting p.
- anal sphincter squeeze p.
- p. anesthesia
- aortic blood p.
- aortic dicrotic notch p.
- aortic pullback p.
- applanation p.
- p. area
- arterial blood p.
- arterial carbon dioxide p.
- arterial dicrotic notch p.
- arterial partial p.
- ascending aortic p.
- atmospheres of p.
- atrial filling p.
- p. atrophy
- average mean p.
- backward, upward, rightward p. (BURP)
- barometric p.
- basal anal canal p.
- basal anal sphincter p.
- bile duct p.
- bilevel positive airway p. (BiPAP)
- biliary tract p.
- biting p.
- bladder p.
- bleeding controlled with direct p.
- p. blister
- blood p. (BP)
- bone marrow p.
- capillary wedge p.
- carbon dioxide p.
- cardiovascular p.
- carotid artery stump p.
- central posterior-anterior p.
- central venous p. (CVP)
- cerebral perfusion p.
- cerebrospinal fluid p.
- choledochal basal p.
- closing p.
- closure p.
- coaxial p.
- colloidal osmotic p.
- colloid osmotic p.

P

pressure (*continued*)

compartmental p.
compliance, rate, oxygenation, p.
  (CROP)
p. condensation
continuous distending airway p.
continuous negative p.
continuous negative airway p.
  (CNAP)
continuous positive airway p.
  (CPAP)
p. control inverse ratio ventilation
  (PCIRV)
p. controlled inverse ratio ventilation
  (PCIRV)
p. controlled ventilation (PCV)
p. conversion
coronary perfusion p.
coronary venous p.
cricoid p.
critical closing p.
CSF p.
detrusor p.
diastolic blood p.
diastolic filling p.
differential blood p.
digital p.
direct p.
disc p.
downstream venous p.
dynamic closure p.
dynamic negative airway p. (DNAP)
elastic recoil p.
end-diastolic left ventricular p.
end-expiratory intragastric p.
end-systolic left ventricular p.
end-tidal carbon dioxide p.
  ($PETCO_2$)
p. epiphysis
esophageal p.
esophageal peristaltic p.
esophageal sphincter p.
expiratory positive airway p.
external direct p.
free hepatic venous p.
p. gangrene
gastric p.
glomerular capillary p.
p. gradient
p. half-time technique
high blood p.
high-frequency positive p.
high intraluminal p.
hydrostatic p.
hyperbaric p.
increased p.
p. increment rate
inferior vena cava p. (IVCP)
inspiratory occlusion p.

inspiratory positive airway p. (IPAP)
insufflation p.
intermittent positive p. (IPP)
interstitial p.
intraabdominal p. (IAP)
intraanal p.
intracardiac p.
intracholedochal p.
intracranial p. (ICP)
intracuff p.
intradiscal p.
intraductal p.
intraesophageal peristaltic p.
intraesophageal variceal p.
intragastric p.
intraglomerular p.
intraluminal esophageal p.
intraluminal urethral p.
intramyocardial p.
intraneural p.
intraocular p.
intraoperative central venous p.
intraoral p.
intrapericardial p.
intraperitoneal p.
intrapleural p.
intrapulpal p.
intrathoracic p.
intraurethral p.
intravariceal p.
intravascular p.
intravesical p.
intrinsic end-expiratory p.
intrinsic positive end-expiratory p.
  (PEEPi)
invasive blood p.
p. inversion point
IVC p.
jugular venous p. (JVP)
juxtacardiac pleural p.
labile blood p.
leak point p.
left atrial p.
left ventricular p.
left ventricular end-diastolic p.
left ventricular systolic p.
LES p.
lower body negative p.
lower esophageal sphincter p.
manual p.
maternal abdominal p.
maximum urethral closure p.
mean arterial p. (MAP)
mean arterial blood p. (MABP)
mean diastolic left ventricular p.
mean pulmonary artery p.
mean pulmonary artery wedge p.
mean systolic left ventricular p.
p. measurement

mercury p.
minimum audible p.
nadir p.
narrowed pulse p.
p. natriuresis
p. necrosis
negative p.
negative abdominal p.
negative end-expiratory p.
nitrogen partial p.
noninvasive blood p. (NIBP)
normal intravascular p.
occlusal p.
occlusion p.
oncotic p.
opening p.
osmotic p.
p. overload
oxygen under high p.
PA filling p.
p. pain threshold (PPT)
pancreatic duct p.
p. paralysis
partial p.
passage p.
peak inspiratory ventilator p.
peak systolic aortic p.
peak systolic gradient p.
perfusion p.
periapical p.
pericardial p.
peripheral p.
plantar p.
plasma colloid osmotic p.
plasma oncotic p.
plateau p.
p. pneumothorax
portal venous p.
positive airway p. (PAP)
positive end-expiratory p. (PEEP)
positive end-expiratory
  pressure/continuous positive airway
  p. (PEEP/CPAP)
positive expiratory p. (PEP)
positive inspiratory p. (PIP)
posterior-anterior p.
postmembrane p.
premembrane p.
premicturition p.
proximal p.
pullback p.
pulmonary artery p. (PAP)
pulmonary artery diastolic p.
pulmonary artery occlusion p.
pulmonary artery occlusive wedge p.
pulmonary artery systolic p.
pulmonary capillary wedge p.
  (PCWP)
pulmonary hypertension p.

pulmonary vascular p.
pulp p.
pulse p.
p. rate quotient
p. receptor
p. recovery
rectal resting p.
p. regulated electrohydraulic
  lithotripsy
p. relief valve
resting anal sphincter p.
p. reversal
right atrial p.
right ventricular end-diastolic p.
right ventricular systolic p.
p. ring
p. rise
screen filtration p.
selection p.
shock wave p.
sinusoidal capillary p.
p. sore
sphincter of Oddi p.
spinal cord perfusion p. (SCPP)
splanchnic capillary p.
squeeze p.
static closure p.
p. study
stump p.
subambient p.
subatmospheric epidural p.
subglottic p.
systolic arterial p. (SAP)
systolic blood p.
systolic left ventricular p.
p. technique filling
tentorial p.
time p.
tissue p.
p. tolerance
tongue p.
tourniquet p.
transglomerular hydrostatic
  filtration p.
transmembrane hydraulic p.
p. transmission
p. transmission ratio
transmural p.
transmyocardial perfusion p.
p. ulcer
ureteral p.
urethral p.
p. value
vapor p.
variable positive airway p. (VPAP)
variceal p.
vascular p.
venous p.
venous dialysis p.

P

pressure (*continued*)
    ventilation peak p.
    ventricular diastolic p.
    ventricular filling p.
    p. wave
    p. waveform
    wedge p.
    wedged hepatic vein p. (WHVP)
    wedged hepatic venous p.
    (WHVP)
    p. welding
    white without p.
    zero end-expiratory p. (ZEEP)
    zero end-inspiratory p.
    Z-point p.
pressure-control ventilation (PCV)
pressure-flow
    p.-f. electromyography study
    p.-f. plot
    p.-f. relation
    p.-f. relationship
pressure-limited ventilation
pressure-natriuresis curve
pressure-point tension ring
pressure-regulated volume control ventilation
pressure-sensitive
    p.-s. area
    p.-s. tissue
pressure-support ventilation (PSV)
pressure-tolerant tissue
pressure-volume
    p.-v. analysis
    p.-v. curve
    p.-v. index
    p.-v. relation
pressurized reservoir
prestenotic dilatation
presternal
    p. notch
    p. region
    p. space
presternum
presulcal
presumptive diagnosis
presurgical
    p. medical evaluation
    p. psychological screening (PPS)
    p. state
presynaptic
    p. and postsynaptic nicotinic
    activation
    p. membrane
presystolic pressure and volume
pretarsal space
pretecta
pretemporal space
prethyroid, prethyroideal, prethyroidean
prethyroideal (*var. of* prethyroid)

prethyroidean (*var. of* prethyroid)
pretracheal
    p. fascia
    p. layer
    p. node
    p. space
    p. space mobilization
pretransplant
    p. evaluation
    p. lymphoid depletion
pretreatment
    p. evaluation
    p. level
pretympanic
prevention
    DVT p.
    extension for p.
    heterotopic ossification p.
    infection p.
    injury p.
    rod rotation p.
Prévention
    P. du Risque d'Embolie Pulmonaire
    par Interruption Cave (PREPIC)
    P. du Risque d'Embolie Pulmonaire
    par Interruption Cave study group
preventive
    p. intravesical therapy
    p. mastectomy
    p. measure
prevertebral
    p. fascia
    p. ganglion
    p. layer
    p. soft tissue
    p. space
    p. space abscess
prevesical fascia
prewarming
Preziosi hemorrhagic glaucoma operation
prezonular space
priapus
prick
    needle p.
    p. puncture test
prickle cell carcinoma
prick-test
    p.-t. concentration
    p.-t. method
Pridie incision
Pridie-Koutsogiannis calcaneous displacement osteotomy procedure
Primacor
primarily
    p. healing wound
    p. vascularized organ transplant
primarium
    centrum ossificationis p.

primary
p. adenocarcinoma
p. adhesion
p. afferent depolarization
p. amputation
p. anesthetic
p. antecubital jump bypass (PAJB)
p. arteriovenous fistula
p. bacterial peritonitis
p. bile duct carcinoma
p. biliary cirrhosis
p. cancer
p. cesarean section
p. closure
colorectal p.
p. cough headache
p. diagnostic endoscopy
p. endpoint
p. end-to-end anastomosis
p. exertional headache
p. extremity synovial sarcoma
p. fibrinolysis
p. fungal infection
p. gangrene
p. gastric lymphoma
p. gastric lymphoma staging
p. gastric non-Hodgkin lymphoma
  (PGL)
p. graft nonfunction
p. headache
p. healing
p. hemorrhage
p. hepatic
p. herpes simplex infection
p. hyperparathyroidism
p. indirect inguinal hernia
p. inguinal herniorrhaphy
p. intervention
p. intraosseous carcinoma
p. lesion
p. liposarcoma
p. malignancy
p. movement plane
p. myofascial trigger point
noncolorectal p.
p. origin
p. panendoscopy
p. parathyroid hyperplastic tumor
p. pathogen
p. perineal hypospadias surgery
p. position
p. procedure
p. proctocolectomy
p. prophylaxis
p. pulmonary hypertension (PPH)
p. radiation
p. rejection
p. renal calculus
p. repair

p. resection
p. rhabdomyosarcoma
p. rotation movement
p. sclerosing cholangitis (PSC)
p. shock
p. sodium phosphate
p. stabbing headache
p. stenting
p. surgeon
p. suture technique
p. thyrotracheal anastomosis
p. tumor site
p. union
p. untreated HPT
p. vascular incompetence
p. wound closure
p. yolk sac
primer
Bowen cavity p.
cavity p.
priming
autologous p.
p. dose
primitive
p. dislocation
p. knot
p. yolk sac
primordial cyst
primum
ostium p.
primus
princeps
p. cervicis artery
p. pollicis artery
Princeteau tubercle
principal
p. fiber bundle
p. line
p. plane
p. point
p. visual direction
principle
anatomic fracture reduction p.
axial compression p.
clinical p.
closure p.
Fick p.
Goodwin cup-patch p.
Hennemans size p.
image formation p.
Le Chatelier p.
line focus p.
Mitrofanoff p.
Venturi p.
Pringle
P. hepatectomy vascular control
  procedure
P. liver hemorrhage maneuver
P. vascular control

P

Pringle (*continued*)
P. vascular control method
P. vascular control technique
prior drug exposure
priority
ICU care p.
prism
p. adaptation test
p. method
PRK
photorefractive keratectomy
photorefractive keratoplasty
proactive hemostasis
probability
bone cyst fracture p.
postoperative survival p. (PSP)
survival p.
proband
probe
cryoablation p.
3D ultrasound p.
monopolar radiofrequency p.
probing
p. lacrimonasal duct operation
robotic p.
probiotic bacteria
problem
biliary p.
clinical p.
colon p.
comorbid medical p.
Coping with Health, Injuries, and
P.'s (CHIP)
cosmetic p.
dermatologic p.
functional p.
gastrointestinal p.
inflammatory p.
innervation p.
medical p.
orthopedic p.
physical p.
psychological p.
rectal p.
surgical p.
wound p.
procallus formation
procedural pain
procedure
Abbe-McIndoe total endoscopic
vaginal reconstruction p.
Abbe-McIndoe-Williams
vaginoplasty p.
Abbe-Wharton-McIndoe vaginal
reconstruction p.
abdominal p.
ablative p.
Adams hallux valgus interphalangeus
correction p.

advancement p.
aesthetic p.
Akin p.
Akiyama p.
Aldridge urethral sling p.
Al-Ghorab p.
Allison antireflux p.
Altemeier perineal rectal
pullthrough p.
anchovy tendon interposition p.
Anderson abnormal mixed head
position correction p.
Anderson-Fowler laparascopic colon
resection p.
anecdotal p.
antegrade continence enema p.
antenna p.
anterior Pólya gastrectomy p.
anterior stabilization p.
antiincontinence p.
antireflux p.
AO p.
arterial limb salvage p.
arterial reconstructive p.
arterial switch p.
articulatory p.
Axer-Clark muscle-tendon transfer
for elbow paralysis p.
Badgley combination cervical
discectomy and fusion p.
Baldy-Webster uterine displacement
repair p.
balloon fenestration p.
Bandi knee p.
Bankart shoulder p.
Barsky cleft hand repair p.
Bassini inguinal hernia p.
Batista experimental open heart p.
Baxter-D'Astous proximal femoral
resection-interposition
arthroplasty p.
Bell-Tawse radial head p.
Belsey fundoplication p.
Bentall aortic graft p.
Berman-Gartland adduction of
forepart of foot p.
Bernard lip reconstruction p.
BH Moore p.
Bickel-Moe osteoid osteoma p.
bilateral inguinal hernia repair p.
Bilhaut-Cloquet polydactyly p.
Billroth I, II gastric p.
Bing-Taussig heart p.
Björk method of Fontan tricuspid
atresia repair p.
bladder chimney p.
Blair-Brown p.
Blalock-Hanlon transposition of great
vessels repair p.

Blalock-Taussig subclavian to pulmonary artery shunt p.
Blatt-Ashworth trapezium excision p.
Blatt capsulodesis p.
blocking p.
Boari bladder flap p.
bone block p.
bony p.
Bose hip resurfacing p.
bowel refashioning p.
Boyce-Vest bladder exstrophy p.
Boyd-Bosworth tennis elbow p.
Boyd-McLeod tennis elbow p.
Boytchev shoulder p.
Brantigan lung volume reduction p.
Brantigan-Voshell posterior cruciate ligament p.
Braun gastric p.
breast-conserving p.
Bricker ileoureterostomy p.
Bridle foot drop p.
Bristow-Helfet glenohumeral joint p.
Bristow-May glenohumeral joint p.
Brock pulmonary valvotomy and infundibular resection p.
bronchial sleeve p.
bronchoplastic p.
Broström-Gould ankle instability repair p.
Broström lateral ankle instability p.
Bunnell-Williams p.
Burch bladder suspension p.
burnout p.
Butler congenital varus correction p.
bypass p.
Calandriello orthopedic p.
Caldwell-Luc sinus window p.
Camey total gastrectomy p.
Campbell-Akbarnia bone graft of radius p.
Campbell-Goldthwait distal realignment osteotomy of patella p.
canalith repositioning p.
Cantwell-Ransley hypospadias repair p.
capsular shift p.
Carolinas Laparoscopic Advanced Surgery Program minimal accessory surgery p.
carotid ablative p.
Castaneda tetralogy of Fallot repair p.
Castle femoral resection p.
cataract p.
catheter-directed interventional p.
Cawthorne-Day labyrinthectomy p.
cecal imbrication p.
Cecil hypospadias repair p.

Celestin tube carcinoma palliation p.
central ablative p.
cervical spine stabilization p.
Chamberlain mediastinoscopy p.
Charles lymphedema debulking p.
Chassar Moir pubovaginal sling p.
Chassar Moir-Sims urinary fistula repair p.
Chester-Winter urinary stress incontinence repair p.
Chrisman-Snook lateral ankle reconstruction p.
Cibis liquid silicone retinal detachment p.
ciliary p.
circulatory arrest p.
Clancy peroneal tenodesis p.
CLASP minimal access surgery p.
Clayton first metatarsophalangeal joint fusion p.
Cleveland p.
Cloward cervical spine fusion p.
Cockett varicose vein p.
Cohen antireflux p.
Cole intubation p.
Collis gastroplasty p.
Collis-Nissen esophageal lengthening p.
Collis-Nissen fundoplication p.
colon p.
coloplasty p.
Commando radical glossectomy p.
compartment p.
composite pelvic resection p.
concentration p.
Connolly p.
conventional p.
core drilling p.
coronary artery revascularization p.
coronary bypass p.
corporeal rotation p.
corridor p.
Cox maze III for atrial fibrillation p.
Cracchiolo hallux limitus implant arthroplasty p.
curative p.
curative-intent p.
Custodis nondraining p.
cyclodestructive p.
cyclops p.
Damian graft p.
Damus-Kaye-Stansel pulmonary artery to ascending aorta anastomosis p.
Darrach extensor carpi ulnaris tendesis p.
dartos pouch p.

P

625

procedure (*continued*)

Das Gupta transbronchial needle aspiration p.
Davis-Kitlowski otoplasty p.
Davydov vaginoplasty p.
DAWG p.
deairing p.
debubbling p.
debulking p.
degloving p.
Delorme rectal prolapse repair p.
dental prosthetic laboratory p.
Desmarres pterygium p.
Dewar posterior cervical fixation p.
diagnostic p.
Dickson-Diveley total joint replacement p.
DKS pulmonary artery to ascending aorta anastomosis p.
Dohlman pharyngeal pouch repair p.
domino p.
Dor fundoplication p.
Dorrance push-back cleft palate p.
dorsal root entry zone lesioning p.
double-stapled ileoanal reservoir p.
DREZ ankle joint arthroscopy p.
DREZ lesioning p.
Duckett tubularized neourethra p.
Duhamel abdominoperineal pullthrough p.
Dukes p.
duodenal diverticularization p.
Duval pancreaticojejunostomy p.
Dwyer orthopaedic p.
Ebbehoj penile straightening-reinforcing p.
Eden-Hybbinette anterior glenoid bone block p.
Eden-Lange trapezius p.
Edwards transposing atrial septum p.
Effler-Groves mode of Allison antireflux p.
elective p.
elective surgical p.
elimination p.
Elmslie-Trillat patellar p.
emergency p.
endolacrimal p.
endorectal ileoanal pullthrough p.
endoscopic mucosal resection p.
endoscopy p.
end-to-end reconstruction p.
enucleation p.
epidural p.
esophageal sling p.
Estes ovarian transfer p.
esthetic p.
evacuation p.
Evans ankle instability p.
Everard Williams retropubic cystourethropexy suspension p.
excisional biopsy p.
EXIT p.
ex situ-in vivo p.
extended Ross p.
extraanatomic bypass p.
extraarticular p.
extracorporeal p.
ex utero intrapartum treatment p.
Faden esotropia repair p.
failed p.
Fairbanks-Sever brachial plexus repair p.
Fasanella-Servat blepharoptosis repair p.
fascial sling p.
fiberoptic intubation p.
Ficat hip p.
filling p.
filtering p.
flip-flap p.
floppy Nissen fundoplication p.
Fontan-Baudet tricuspid atresia repair p.
Fontan-Kreutzer atriopulmonary anastomosis p.
Fontan modification of Norwood heart p.
forage p.
Fowler-Stephens spermatic vessel division p.
Fox-Blazina pes anserinus transfer p.
Fredet-Ramstedt extramucosal longitudinal myotomy p.
Frey pancreatic head resection and lateral pancreaticojejunostomy p.
Froimson tendon interposition thumb p.
frontalis sling p.
Frost ingrown nail p.
Fulford subtalar arthrodesis p.
Furlow palatal lengthening p.
Gallie ankle arthrodesis p.
Gartland forefoot reconstruction p.
gaseous laparoscopy p.
gasless laparoscopy p.
gastric bypass p. (GBP)
gastric drainage p.
gastric emptying p. (GEP)
gastric partitioning p.
gastric pullthrough p.
gastric pullup p.
gastric valve tightening p.
general laparoscopic surgical p.
Gilchrist urinary diversion p.

Gill-Jonas modification of Norwood hypoplastic left heart p.
Gill laminectomy p.
Gillquist p.
Gil-Vernet ileocecocystoplasty p.
Girdlestone orthopedic p.
Girdlestone-Taylor muscle transfer clawtoe repair p.
Gittes endoscopic bladder neck suspension p.
Gittes-Loughlin needle bladder suspension p.
Glenn superior vena cava to right pulmonary artery anastomosis p.
Goebel-Stoeckel-Frangenheim urethrovesical suspension p.
Goldner-Hayes clubfoot release p.
Goldthwait-Hauser orthopedic p.
Gould ankle p.
gracilis p.
Gregoir-Lich ureteroneocystostomy p.
Gurd distal clavicle open resection p.
Halban culdoplasty p.
hallux valgus p.
hamular p.
Hanley rectal bladder p.
Harada-Ito excyclotorsion correction p.
Hartmann resection of intestine p.
Hass p.
Haultain uterine inversion repair p.
Hauser patellar tendon p.
Hawkins shoulder p.
Heifetz nail matrix excision p.
hemi-Fontan p.
hemi-Koch p.
heparinization p.
Hepp-Couinaud biliary tract p.
hex p.
Heyman-Herndon clubfoot p.
Hibbs lumbar fusion p.
Hill antireflux p.
Hinman stress incontinence p.
Hoffmann-Clayton panmetatarsal excision p.
Hofmeister gastrectomy p.
Hohmann hallux osteotomy p.
Hoke foot arthrodesis p.
Hoke-Miller pes planus p.
Horton-Devine hypospadias flip-flap p.
Howorth hip p.
Hughston-Hauser patellar dislocation repair p.
Hughston lateral knee instability p.
Hui-Linscheid ulnotriquetral augmentation tenodesis p.

Hummelsheim transposition of vertical recti p.
Huntington uterine inversion repair p.
hypoglossal facial transfer p.
ileoanal pouch p.
ileoanal pullthrough p.
iliac buttressing p.
4-incision p.
5-incision p.
infrarenal template p.
Ingelman-Sundberg gracilis muscle vesicovaginal fistula repair p.
initial screening p.
inner ear tack p.
Insall patellar instability repair p.
in situ p.
instillation p.
intercalary allograft p.
interventional p.
intestinal bypass p.
intraarticular p.
intraoperative p.
intraparavariceal p.
intraperitoneal p.
invasive p.
island-flap p.
isolated p.
Jacobaeus endoscopic thorax exploration p.
Jaeger-Hamby muscle embolization of carotid cavernous fistula p.
Jahss dorsal wedge osteotomy p.
Jannetta microvascular decompression neurosurgical p.
Jansey toenail ablation p.
Jatene arterial switch p.
jejunoileal bypass reversal p.
Jensen muscle transposition p.
Jobe-Glousman glenohumeral capsular shift p.
Johnston buttonhole arteriovenous hemodialysis fistula p.
Jonas modification of Norwood hypoplastic left heart p.
Jones tube conjunctivodacryocystorhinostomy p.
JR Moore oral and maxillofacial p.
Juvara closing abudetory wedge for feet p.
Kalicinski ureteral folding technique p.
Karakousis-Vezeridis hemipelvectomy p.
Karapandzic lip reconstruction p.
Karlsson ankle instability correction p.
Kasai portoenterostomy p.

procedure (*continued*)

Kelikian lateral ankle suture anchor p.

Kelikian-McFarland congenital digitus minimus varus correction p.

Keller bunionectomy p.

Kelling-Madlener gastric resection p.

Kelly urethrovesical plication p.

Kendrick below-knee amputation p.

Kessel-Bonney hallux osteotomy p.

Kestenbaum torticollis surgical p.

keyhole coronary bypass p.

Kidner excision of accessory navicular bone p.

Kiehn-Earle-DesPrez plastic surgery p.

Killian frontoethmoidectomy p.

Knapp vertical transposition of horizontal recti p.

Ko-Airan laparoscopic cholecystectomy bleeding control p.

Kocher ureterosigmoidostomy p.

Kock pouch ileostomy p.

Kondoleon-Sistrunk elephantiasis p.

Konno left ventricular outflow enlargement p.

Koutsogiannis sliding calcaneal osteotomy p.

Kraske midline posterior proctotomy p.

Krönlein lateral orbitotomy p.

Kropp urethral lengthening p.

Krukenberg reconstruction of BKA p.

Kuhnt-Szymanowski ectropion repair with lid reconstruction p.

Ladd mobilization of intestine p.

Langenskiöld central physeal bar excision p.

laparoscopically assisted endorectal pullthrough p.

laparoscopic-assisted p.

laparoscopic bladder neck suture suspension p.

laparoscopic Burch p.

laparoscopic bypass p.

laparoscopic lymph node dissection p.

laparoscopic Nissen fundoplication p.

laparoscopic paraaortic lymph node sampling p.

laparoscopic surgical p.

laparoscopic tubal banding p.

Lapidus metatarsocuneiform joint arthrodesis p.

Larmon forefoot p.

laser anterior small thoracotomy p.

laser coagulation vaporization p. (LCVP)

Lash laparoscopic supracervical hysterectomy p.

LAST coronary bypass p.

Latarget laparoscopic highly selective vagotomy p.

lateral tarsal strip p.

lathing p.

latissimus dorsi p.

Lauenstein ulnar head resection p.

Leadbetter-Politano ureteroneocystostomy p.

Leadbetter urethral reconstruction p.

Le Fort colpocleisis p.

left atrial isolation p.

Lepird metatarsus adductus p.

L'Episcopo-Zachary brachial plexopathy tendon transfer p.

Lewis-Tanner 2-stage esophagectomy p.

Lich ureterocystostomy p.

lid-splitting p.

limb-lengthening p.

limb-salvage p.

limb-saving p.

limb-sparing p.

Lindeman laryngeal diversion p.

Linton varicose vein p.

Lipscomb-Anderson posterior cruciate ligament reconstruction p.

loop electrocautery excision p. (LEEP)

loop electrosurgical excision p. (LEEP)

loop gastric bypass p.

Lorenz congenital clubfoot p.

Lothrop frontoethmoidectomy p.

lower cervical spine p.

lower lid sling p.

lung volume reduction p.

LVR p.

Lynch frontoethmoidectomy p.

MacCarthy sacral tumor excision of sacrum p.

Magenstrasse and Mill antiobesity p.

magnitude matching p.

Magnuson-Stack shoulder p.

Mahan pediatric sedation p.

malabsorptive p.

Mallory-Weiss tear repair p.

Malone ACE p.

Malone antegrade continence enema p.

Manktelow transfer p.

Mann-Coughlin hallux valgus repair p.

Mann hallux valgus repair p.

Maquet patellar realignment p.

Marshall-Marchetti-Krantz retropubic cystourethrography suspension p.

Martius labial fat flap urinary fistula repair p.
Mathieu-Righini hypospadias p.
Mauck medial collateral ligament knee repair p.
Maydl colostomy p.
Mayo-Fueth inversion p.
Maze p.
Maze III p.
McBride bunionectomy p.
McCall-Schumann enterocele p.
McCormick-Blount metatarsus adductus repair p.
McDonald cervical encirclement suture p.
McElvenny-Caldwell first metatarsocuneiform navicular joint fusion p.
McGlamry-Downey forefoot p.
McIndoe vaginal construction p.
McLaughlin posterior shoulder dislocation repair p.
McVay hernia repair p.
medial rotation p.
Meigs-Okabayashi radical hysterectomy p.
Michal I p.
Michal II p.
microoperative p.
microsurgery p.
microsurgical epididymal sperm aspiration p.
Miller midtarsal arthrodesis p.
minimal access p.
minimally invasive p. (MIP)
Minkoff-Nicholas iliotibial band transfer knee repair p.
Mitrofanoff appendicovesicostomy p.
M&M antiobesity p.
MMK retropubic cystourethropexy suspension p.
Moberg key-pinch p.
modified Belsey fundoplication p.
modified Hoke-Miller flatfoot p.
modified Konno p.
modified Norfolk p.
modified Seldinger p.
modified Sugiura p.
modified Toupe p.
modified Weber-Fergusson p.
modified Wies entropion p.
Moschcowitz culdoplasty p.
motion-preserving p.
multiple-port incision p.
Mumford distal clavicle open resection p.
muscle-balancing p.
Mustardé hypospadias repair p.

Mustard interatrial transposition of venous return p.
needle suspension p.
needle thoracentesis p.
Neer capsular shift p.
Nesbit tuck penis straightening p.
Neugebauer-Le Fort colpocleisis p.
neurostimulating p.
neurosurgical p.
Nicks aortic anulus enlargement p.
Nicola shoulder tenodesis p.
Nicoll fracture repair p.
Nissen fundoplication of stomach p.
Nissen-Rossetti fundoplication p.
noncircumferential antireflux p.
nonfenestrated Fontan p.
noninvasive p.
nonrib-spreading thoracotomy incision p.
Norfolk phalloplasty p.
Norwood univentricular heart p.
notchplasty p.
Nuss pectus excavatum p.
O'Brien capsular shift p.
O'Donoghue triad knee repair p.
Olshausen uterine suspension p.
omentum majus flap p.
open reconstructive p.
operative p. (OP)
orthodontic p.
orthodox p.
orthopedic surgical p.
Orticochea sphincter pharyngoplasty p.
Osborne-Cotterill p.
osteoplastic frontal sinus p.
otic periotic shunt p.
Oudard shoulder bone block p.
Overholt colonoscopy p.
palatal lengthening p.
palliative cerebrospinal shunt p.
palliative surgical p.
Palomo varicocelectomy p.
Parrish microvascular decompression p.
Pauchet gastrectomy p.
pediatric laparoscopic surgical p.
pelvic floor p.
pelvic pouch p.
Pena anorectal malformation corrective p.
percutaneous transhepatic biliary p.
Pereyra bladder neck suspension p.
perivateran therapeutic endoscopic p.
Pichlmayer orthotopic liver transplantation p.
Pippi Salle urethral lengthening p.
PLIF p.

P

procedure (*continued*)

Pólya gastrectomy p.

4-port p.

posterior Pólya gastrectomy p.

posterior sagittal anorectoplasty p.

potentially curative p.

Potts-Smith descending aorta to left pulmonary artery anastomosis p.

Pridie-Koutsogiannis calcaneous displacement osteotomy p.

primary p.

Pringle hepatectomy vascular control p.

PSARP p.

psoas hitch p.

pull-through p.

push-back cleft palate repair p.

Putti-Platt shoulder p.

Quaegebeur infant heart surgery p.

QUART p.

Quickert nonincisional entropion repair p.

Ramstedt pyloromyotomy with wedge resection p.

Rastan-Konno anterior aortoventriculoplasty p.

Rastelli right ventricle and pulmonary artery conduit p.

Ravitch pectus excavatum repair p.

Raz bladder neck suspension p.

realignment p.

Récamier uterine curettage p.

reconstruction p.

reconstructive surgical p.

reefing p.

Rehbein colonic pullthrough p.

Reichel-Pólya subtotal gastrectomy p.

Reichenheim-King biceps tendon transplantation p.

repeat p.

restorative p.

resurfacing p.

retrogasserian p.

revascularization p.

reverse filling p.

reverse Mauck p.

reverse Putti-Platt p.

revision p.

Richter and Albrich vaginal sacrospinous suspension p.

Riedel frontoethmoidectomy p.

Ripstein prolapsed rectum repair p.

Rockwood acromioclavicular joint dislocation repair p.

Rockwood-Matsen capsular shift shoulder repair p.

Ross aortic valve replacement p.

Roux-en-Y gastrointestinal system p.

Roux-Goldthwait repair of recurrent patellar dislocation p.

Ruiz astigmatic keratotomy p.

Ruiz-Mora proximal phalangectomy for hammertoe p.

Ryerson triple arthrodesis of foot p.

sacroiliac buttressing p.

Sade modification of Norwood p.

salvage p.

Samilson sliding osteotomy of calcaneus p.

sartorial slide p.

Sato radial keratotomy p.

Sauve-Kapandji distal radioulnar joint repair p.

Sayoc upper lid fold creation p.

Schauta-Aumreich radical vaginal hysterectomy p.

Schenk-Eichelter vena cava plastic filter p.

Schoemaker transscrotal orchiopexy p.

Schrock scapula elevation repair p.

scleral buckling p.

Scopinaro biliopancreatic bypass p.

screening p.

Scuderi urethral reconstruction p.

secondary p.

second-look p.

segment-oriented p.

Selakovich sustenaculum tali p.

Seldinger vascular access p.

semitendinosus p.

Senning transposition of great arteries p.

septation p.

Shirodkar cervix encirclement suture p.

short lever specific contact p.

Silfverskiöld gastrocnemius soleus recession p.

Silver bunionectomy p.

simultaneous pancreas and kidney transplant p.

single-stage p.

Sistrunk excision of thyroglossal cyst p.

sling p.

Smith-Robinson open osteotomy of mandible p.

Soave transanal pullthrough p.

Sondergaard epicardial incision p.

spatial localization p.

Spence urethral diverticulum p.

sphincter-saving p.

sphincter-sparing p.

spinal-locking p.

Spira scapulothoracic arthrodesis p.

Spittler ankle disarticulation p.

SPLATT p.
split anterior tibial tendon p.
split anterior tibial tendon
 transfer p.
Stack shoulder p.
2-stage p.
3-stage p.
Staheli hip osteotomy shelf p.
Stamey-Martius antiincontinence p.
Stamey modification of Pereyra
 bladder neck suspension p.
Stamm temporary gastrostomy p.
standard gastric resection
 Whipple p.
standard stripping p.
standard surgical p.
Stanley Way radical vulvectomy p.
stapled reconstruction p.
Steindler elbow flexion
 restoration p.
2-step p.
STEP p.
stereotactic needle core biopsy p.
Stone anoplasty p.
Stoppa bilateral inguinal hernia
 repair p.
Strayer gastrocnemius recession p.
Stretta radiofrequency for GERD p.
strip p.
Studer pouch ileal neobladder p.
suburethral rectus fascial sling p.
Sugiura esophageal varices repair p.
supplementary sling p.
suprainguinal vascular p.
supramesocolic surgical p.
surgical enucleation p.
Swenson colonic pullthrough p.
switch p.
Syme ankle amputation p.
Syme external urethrotomy p.
Tachdjian external fixation for cavus
 fixation p.
takedown p.
tarsal strip p.
terminal Syme toe-tip amputation p.
Thal fundoplication p.
Thal-Woodward antireflux p.
thermal-assisted capsular shift p.
Thiersch anus p.
Thiersch-Duplay proximal tube
 urethroplasty p.
Thiersch hand p.
Thiersch skin graft p.
Thompson cleft lip repair p.
Thompson correction of
 lymphedema p.
Thompson quadricepsplasty p.
Thompson thumb apposition with
 bone graft p.

Tikhoff-Linberg proximal humerus
 resection p.
p. time
TIPS p.
total fundoplication p.
Toti dacryocystorhinostomy p.
touch-up p.
Toupe fundoplication p.
Toupet antireflux p.
TRAM flap p.
transendoscopic p.
transhepatic antegrade biliary
 drainage p.
transjugular intrahepatic
 portosystemic shunt p.
transthoracic antireflux p.
transvaginal Burch p.
transverse rectus abdominis muscle
 flap p.
Trillat shoulder bone block p.
triple-wire p.
Tsai-Stillwell distal radioulnar joint
 repair p.
tuck p.
tumbling p.
Turco release of joint capsule in
 clubfoot p.
uncut Collis-Nissen fundoplication p.
unilateral inguinal hernia
 repair p.
untethering p.
up-and-down staircases p.
UPLIFT p.
upper cervical spine p.
ureteral patch p.
urethral vesicle suspension p.
urologic laparoscopic surgical p.
uterine positioning via ligament
 investment fixation and
 truncation p.
vaginal needle suspension p.
vaginal wall sling p.
valvotomy p.
van Ness lower limb amputation
 with foot reversal p.
vascular p.
VATS p.
venous bypass p.
ventriculoperitoneal shunting p.
video-assisted thoracic surgical p.
Vineberg internal mammary artery
 implantation p.
Vulpius lengthening of
 gastrocnemius muscle p.
Vulpius-Stoffel gastrocnemius
 intramuscular aponeurotic
 recession p.
V-Y p.
W p.

P

procedure (*continued*)
  Waldhausen subclavian flap angioplasty p.
  Wardill-Kilner palatoplasty p.
  Waterhouse transpubic urethroplasty p.
  Waterston-Cooley aorto-to-right pulmonary artery anastomosis p.
  Watson Cheyne-Burghard segmental matrix toenail excision p.
  Watson-Jones shoulder p.
  Weaver-Dunn acromioclavicular joint stabilization p.
  Weber-Fergusson maxillofacial skeleton exposure p.
  Weir appendicostomy p.
  Weir correction of nostrils p.
  Wheeler entropion repair p.
  Whipple radical pancreatoduodenectomy p.
  White slide lengthening of tendo Achillis p.
  Whitman talectomy p.
  Wies transconjunctival lower eyelid involutional entropion repair p.
  Williams vaginal construction p.
  Wilson angulation osteotomy for hallux valgus p.
  Winograd ingrown nail p.
  Winter priapism repair p.
  Womack portal systemic shunting p.
  Woodward release of high-riding scapula p.
  yoke transposition p.
  York-Mason repair of postoperative rectoprostatic-urethral fistula p.
  Young-Dees bladder neck repair p.
  Young epispadias repair p.
  Yount gluteal-iliotibial fasciotomy p.
  Z p.
  Zancolli biceps tendon transfer p.
  Zarins-Rowe semitendinosus and iliotibial band knee repair p.
  Zoellner-Clancy sliding fibular graft repair of peroneal tendon p.
  Z-plasty p.
procephalic
procerus muscle
process
  accessory p.
  acromial p.
  alveolar p.
  anterior clinoid p.
  articular p.
  basilar p.
  benign p.
  calcaneal p.
  caudate p.
  ciliary p.

  Civinini p.
  clinoid p.
  cochleariform p.
  condylar p.
  condyloid p.
  conoid p.
  coracoid p.
  corniculate p.
  coronoid p.
  costal p.
  ensiform p.
  epileptogenic p.
  exocrinopathic p.
  falciform p.
  frontosphenoidal p.
  funicular p.
  healing p.
  hypersecretory p.
  inferior articular p.
  intrajugular p.
  jugular p.
  lateral p.
  lenticular p.
  malignant p.
  mallear p.
  mammillary p.
  mastoid p.
  medial p.
  mental p.
  olecranon p.
  papillary p.
  paroccipital p.
  posterior clinoid p.
  pterygoid p.
  pterygospinous p.
  resuscitation p.
  space-occupying p.
  sphenoid p.
  spinous p.
  Stieda p.
  superior articular p.
  supracondylar p.
  supraepicondylar p.
  temporal p.
  thrombotic p.
  transverse p.
  trochlear p.
  uncinate p.
  vaginal p.
  vermiform p.
  vertebral spine infectious p.
  vocal p.
  xiphoid p.
processus, *pl.* **processus**
  p. clinoideus anterior
  p. clinoideus medius
  p. clinoideus posterior
  p. coronoideus
  p. vermiformis

procheilon, prochilon
prochilon (*var. of* procheilon)
prochordal
Prochownik neonatal resuscitation method
procidentia
procoagulant
procreate
procreation
   assisted medical p. (AMP)
procreative
proctalgia fugax
proctectasia
proctectomy
   abdominoperineal p.
   intersphincteric p.
   Kraske transsacral p.
   laparoscopic p.
   mucosal p.
   partial p.
   perineal p.
   permanent p.
   proctomucosal p.
   radical p.
   restorative p.
   sphincter-preserving p.
   stapled ileal pouch-anal anastomosis
     without proctomucosal p.
   subtotal p.
   total p.
   transsacral p.
procteurynter
procteurysis
proctitis
   radiation p.
   radiation-induced p.
proctocele
proctoclysis
proctococcypexy
proctocolectomy
   abdominal p.
   laparoscopic total p.
   primary p.
   restorative p.
   secondary stage p.
   single-stage total p.
   subtotal p.
   total p.
   totally stapled restorative p.
proctocolitis
   radiation p.
proctocolonoscopy
proctocolpoplasty
proctocystocele
proctocystoplasty
proctocystotomy
proctodynia
proctoelytroplasty
proctography

proctologic
proctologist
proctology
proctomucosal proctectomy
proctoperineoplasty
proctoperineorrhaphy
proctopexy
   Orr-Loygue transabdominal p.
   transabdominal p.
proctoplasty
proctoptosia, proctoptosis
proctoptosis (*var. of* proctoptosia)
proctorrhagia
proctorrhaphy
proctorrhea
proctoscopic examination
proctoscopy
   rigid p.
proctosigmoidectomy
proctosigmoidoscopy
   rigid p.
proctospasm
proctostasis
proctostat
proctostenosis
proctostomy
proctotomy
   posterior p.
proctotresia
proctovalvotomy
procumbent
procurement
   in situ split liver p.
procurvation
prodrug design
product
   altered gene p.
   blood p.
   contact activation p.
   degradation p.
   fibrin degradation p.
   lipid peroxidation p.
   live donor liver transplantation
     without blood p.'s
   oxygen reduction p.
   pyrolysis p.
   rate pressure p.
   tumor-cell p.
   vector p.
production
   biofilm p.
   collagen p.
   cytokine p.
   ectopic parathormone p.
   excessive heat p.
   metabolic heat p.
   nitroprusside-induced cyanide p.
   paraneoplastic ectopic ACTH p.
   sputum p.

P

productive inflammation
PROEF
postoperative regimen for oral early feeding
Proetz
P. displacement sinus irrigation technique
P. nasal irrigation maneuver
P. position
profile
aortic valve velocity p.
coagulation p.
extraoral radiographic examination p.
facial p.
pain perception p.
Premature Infant Pain P. (PIPP)
projection p.
resting urethral pressure p.
sickness impact p. (SIP)
stress urethral pressure p.
thrombogenic p.
urethral closure pressure p.
vector p.
profound hypothermia
profoundly hypothermic circulatory arrest (PHCA)
profunda
p. brachii artery
p. cervicalis artery
colitis cystica p.
progenitalis
progestational
p. protection
p. therapy
prognosis
prognostic
p. block
p. determinant
p. factor
p. finding
p. indicator
p. information
p. marker
p. nomogram
p. value
prognosticator
progonoma
prograde technique
program
aquatic stabilization p.
back-propagation neural network p.
Cancer Surveillance P.
Carolinas Laparoscopic Advanced Surgery P. (CLASP)
conditioning p.
diagnostic p.
electronic prescription-monitoring p. (ePMP)
independent exercise p.

Linde Walker Oxygen P.
National Marrow Donor P. (NMDP)
National Surgical Quality Improvement P. (NSQIP)
object p.
Organ Procurement P.
Rothman Institute total hip p.
safety p.
SEER P.
Solid Tumor Autologous Marrow Transplant P. (STAMP)
source p.
standard bone algorithm p.
4-star exercise p.
Starkey matrix p.
stripping p.
Surgical Education and Self-Assessment P. (SESAP)
surveillance p.
survey p.
walking p.
work hardening p.
programmed
p. electrical stimulation
p. therapy
progression
tumor p.
progressive
p. abdominal distention
P. Ambulation Scale
p. ascites
p. bacterial synergistic gangrene
p. compression
p. dilation
p. dilational technique
p. disease
p. encephalopathy
p. extraction
p. fibroplasia
p. liver failure
p. muscle relaxation
p. parenchymal destruction
p. respiratory failure
p. spin saturation
proinflammatory
p. mediator
p. mediator synthesis
project
Alabama Breast Cancer P.
Breast Cancer Detection Demonstration P. (BCDDP)
National Surgical Adjuvant Breast and Bowel P. (NSABP)
projection
afferent p.
anterior oblique p.
anteroposterior p.
A&P p.
apical lordotic p.

ascending pathway of pain p.
axial calcaneal p.
axial sesamoid p.
back p.
base p.
bony p.
bregma-mentum p.
bursal p.
Caldwell p.
convergence p.
coronal oblique p.
cross-sectional p.
crosstable lateral p.
Didiee p.
divergent ray p.
dorsoplantar p.
enamel p.
erroneous p.
extradental p.
false p.
fan beam p.
p. fiber
p. fiber damage
filtered-back p.
Fischer p.
frogleg lateral p.
frontal p.
Granger p.
half-axial p.
Harris-Beath p.
Hermodsson tangential p.
horizontal p.
lateral jaw p.
left anterior oblique p.
left lateral p.
light p.
maximum-intensity p.
mental p.
Mercator p.
oblique p.
occipitomental p.
occlusal p.
orthogonal p.
PA p.
pain p.
panoramic surface p.
papillary p.
parasympathetic p.
perimeter p.
posterior-superior oblique p.
posteroanterior p.
p. profile
reverse topographic p.
Rhese p.
Rungstrom p.
sagittal p.
Schüller p.
spider p.
Stenvers p.

stress dorsiflexion p.
submental vertex p.
submentovertical p.
surface p.
sympathetic p.
tangential p.
topographic p.
Towne p.
p. tract imaging
transmandibular p.
transorbital p.
transverse p.
visual p.
Waters p.

projection-reconstruction
p.-r. imaging
p.-r. technique

projective technique
prolabial
prolabium
prolactin inducible protein
prolapse
Altemeier repair of rectal p.
anorectal mucosal p.
rectal p.
stomal p.
uterine p.
vaginal vault p.

prolapsed
p. hemorrhoid
p. mitral valve syndrome
p. stoma

Prolene suture
proliferating cell nuclear antigen (PCNA)
proliferation
p. area
cellular p.
ductal p.
fibroblast p.
follicular p.
p. zone

proliferative, proliferous
p. factor
p. inflammation
p. lesion

proliferous (*var. of* proliferative)
prolongation
expiratory p.
P2 p.
pulse repetition time p.

prolonged
p. expiratory phase
p. hospital stay
p. intubation
p. neural blockage
p. postoperative ventilation
p. prothrombin time
p. rupture

P

prominence
    hypothenar p.
    laryngeal p.
    mallear p.
    osteochondral p.
    pedicle screw hardware p.
    styloid p.
    thenar p.
    thyroid p.
prominens
prominentia
prominent indentation
promontoria (*pl. of* promontorium)
promontorium, *pl.* **promontoria**
promontory, promontorium
    pelvic p.
    sacral p.
    p. stimulation test
promoter
    tumor p.
pronate
pronation
    p. control
    p. eversion external rotation (PEER)
    p. injury
pronation-abduction
    p.-a. fracture
    p.-a. injury
pronation-eversion
    p.-e. fracture
    p.-e. injury
pronation-eversion-external rotation injury
pronation-supination
pronator
    p. quadratus muscle
    p. reflex
    p. teres muscle
    p. teres release
    p. teres syndrome
    p. teres tendon
prone
    p. extension test
    p. positioning
    p. reduction
    p. split-leg position
pronephric duct
pronephroi (*pl. of* pronephros)
pronephros, *pl.* **pronephroi**
pronglike excementosis
pronograde
Pronova suture
pronuclear stage transfer (PROST)
prootic
prop
    rubber mouth p.
propacetamol
propagate

propagating clustered contraction
propagation
    clot p.
propagative
proper
    p. hepatic artery (PHA)
    p. palmar digital artery
    p. plantar digital artery
properitoneal
    p. fat
    p. fat line
    p. flank stripe
    p. inguinal hernia
    p. space
property
    chemotactic p.
    vasodilatory p.
prophylactic
    p. angiographic intervention
    p. antibiotic
    p. antibiotic therapy
    p. anticoagulation
    p. antiemetic
    p. antifungal treatment
    p. bone graft
    p. cholecystectomy
    p. colectomy
    p. epidural blood patch
    p. fasciotomy
    p. gastroenterostomy
    p. gastrojejunostomy
    p. hemofiltration
    p. hysterectomy
    p. inspiratory muscle training
    p. intravenous antibiotic
    p. intubation
    p. irradiation
    p. lymphadenectomy
    p. mastectomy
    p. medication
    p. membrane
    p. odontotomy
    p. oophorectomy
    p. operative stabilization
    p. orchiectomy
    p. resection
    p. skeletal fixation
    p. surgery
    p. therapy
    p. thyroidectomy
prophylaxes (*pl. of* prophylaxis)
prophylaxis, *pl.* **prophylaxes**
    acustimulation antiemetic p.
    antibiotic p.
    antiemetic p.
    antifungal p.
    antithromboembolic p.
    antiviral p.

aspiration p.
CMV p.
cytomegalovirus p.
deep venous thrombosis p.
DVT p.
perioperative antibiotic p.
primary p.
stricture p.
thromboembolic p.
venous thromboembolism p.
propofol
    p. infusion
    p. rescue
proportional
    p. assist ventilation
    p. assist ventilator (PAV)
propria, *pl.* **propriae**
    muscularis p.
propriae (*pl. of* propria)
proprioceptive
    p. head-turning reflex
    p. neuromuscular facilitation
    p. neuromuscular facilitation
      approach
proptosis
prosection
prosector tubercle
prosopalgia
prospective study
prospermia
PROST
    pronuclear stage transfer
    laparoscopic PROST
prostacyclin
prostanoid
prostata
prostatalgia
prostate
    p. cancer
    contact laser ablation of p.
      (CLAP)
    female p.
    p. gland
    laser resection of p.
    photoselective laser vaporization of
      p.
    radical cryosurgical ablation of p.
      (RCSA)
    transurethral electrovaporization of p.
      (TEVAP, TUEP, TUEVP, TUVP,
      TVP)
    transurethral resection of p.
      (TURP)
    transurethral vaporization of p.
      (TUVP)
    visual laser ablation of p. (VLAP)
prostatectomy
    Alexander perineal p.
    Alexander suprapubic p.

anatomic radical retropubic p.
cavernous nerve-sparing p.
laparoscopic radical p.
Madigan p.
nerve-sparing radical retropubic p.
perineal p.
Puntenney radical p.
radical perineal p.
radical retropubic p.
radical transcoccygeal p.
salvage p.
Stanford radical retropubic p.
suprapubic p.
total perineal p.
transurethral ablative p.
transurethral ultrasound-guided
  laser-induced p. (TULIP)
visual laser-assisted p. (VLAP)
Walsh radical retropubic p.
Young perineal p.
prostatic
    p. adenocarcinoma
    p. adenoma
    p. calculus
    p. carcinoma
    p. duct
    p. ductule
    p. fluid
    p. ligament
    p. massage
    p. sheath
    p. sinus
    p. urethra
    p. urethroplasty
    p. utricle
    p. venous plexus
prostaticovesicalis
prostaticovesical plexus
prostatism
prostatitis
prostatocystitis
prostatocystotomy
prostatodynia
prostatolith
prostatolithotomy
prostatomegaly
prostatomy (*var. of* prostatotomy)
prostatorrhea
prostatoseminal vesiculectomy
prostatotomy, prostatomy
prostatovesiculectomy
prostatovesiculitis
prostheses (*pl. of* prosthesis)
prosthesis, *pl.* **prostheses**
    femoral p.
    p. interface
    ossicular p.
    scrotal p.
prosthesis-cement interface

P

prosthesis-patient mismatch (PPM)
prosthetic
 p. arterial graft
 p. arthroplasty
 p. disc nucleus (PDN)
 p. hemiarthroplasty
 p. implant
 p. incisional hernioplasty
 p. mesh repair
 p. patch
 p. restoration
 p. ring anuloplasty
 totally extraperitoneal p.
 p. valve endocarditis (PVE)
prosthetist
prosthokeratoplasty
protamine
 p. correction
 p. sulfate
protection
 airway p.
 automated boundary p.
 barrier p.
 Baxter venous/arterial
  management p.
 cerebral p.
 digital artery p.
 endogenous p.
 gastroduodenal mucosal p.
 myocardial p.
 progestational p.
 radiation p.
 spinal cord p.
 p. test
 venous/arterial management p.
  (VAMP)
protective
 p. airway reflex
 p. antireflux operation
 p. ventilatory strategy
protein
 bone morphogenetic p.
  (BMP)
 p. C deficiency
 p. content
 p. C, S plasma level
 p. degradation
 p. electrophoresis
 heparin-binding p.
 nuclear matrix p.
 plasma atrial natriuretic p.
 prolactin inducible p.
 p. shock therapy
 p. truncation
 p. truncation test
proteinaceous aqueous exudation
proteinase
proteinuria
 steroid-resistant p.

proteolysis
 burn-induced muscle p.
 muscle p.
 sepsis-induced muscle p.
proteolytic pathway
proteome
 human p.
protheses (*pl. of* prothesis)
prothesis, *pl.* **protheses**
prothrombin
 p. time (protime, pro-time,
  PTT)
 p. time coagulation panel
prothrombogenic agent
protime, pro-time
 prothrombin time
protocol
 anticoagulation p.
 antiplatelet p.
 chemotherapy p.
 evaluation p.
 exsanguination p.
 flashback p.
 fractionation p.
 malignant hyperthermia p.
 Nigro p.
 perioperative standardized p.
 reinjection p.
 resuscitation p.
 standardized p.
protoduodenum
proton
 p. beam therapy
 p. pump inhibition therapy
 p. pump inhibitor (PPI)
protopathic pain
protopianoma
protoplasmolysis
protozoal infection
protracted venous infusion
protrude
protruded disc
protrusio
 p. acetabuli
 p. deformity
 p. ring
protrusion
 corneal p.
protrusive
 p. excursion
 p. jaw relation
 p. line
 p. occlusal position
protuberance
protuberant abdomen
protuberantia
proud graft
Proust space
provesicalis

provisional
 p. fixation
 p. restoration
 p. stabilization
provocation test
provocative
 p. chelation test
 p. discography
 p. food thyroidectomy
Prowazek-Greeff body
proximad
proximal
 p. aorta
 p. bowel distention
 p. bowel tenderness
 p. bow position
 p. cavity
 p. centriole
 p. clot
 p. diverting stoma
 p. end
 p. endoleak
 p. esophagus
 p. femoral epiphysiolysis
 p. femoral fracture
 p. femoral resection
 p. femoral resection-interposition
  arthroplasty (PFRIA)
 p. gastrectomy
 p. gastric cancer
 p. gastric resection
 p. gastric vagotomy
 p. humeral fracture
 p. incision
 p. interphalangeal joint
  approach
 p. jejunum
 p. limb
 p. loop syndrome
 p. myofascial dysfunction
 p. nail matrix
 p. phalanx (PP)
 p. portion
 p. pressure
 p. radioulnar articulation
 p. reflux
 p. saphenous vein
 p. space
 p. subclavian injury
 p. subtotal pancreatectomy
 p. tendon rupture
 p. tibial metaphysial fracture
 p. tibiofibular joint dislocation
 p. tumor
 p. urethral sphincter
 p. vascular control
 p. vein
proximal-row carpectomy
proximal-to-distal ring

proximate space
proximity
 close p.
Proxi-Strip suture
proxy
 PCA by p.
prune-belly
 p.-b. abdomen
 p.-b. syndrome
prune-juice
 p.-j. expectoration
 p.-j. peritoneal fluid
pruritic
 p. erythematous patch
 p. jaundice
 p. lesion
pruritus
 morphine-induced p.
Prussak
 P. pouch
 P. space
PS
 postcardiotomy shock
PSA
 persistent sciatic artery
 posterior spinal artery
psammocarcinoma
psammoma body
psammomatoid ossifying fibroma
psammomatous
psammosarcoma
PSARP
 posterior sagittal anorectoplasty
  PSARP procedure
psauoscopy
PSC
 primary sclerosing cholangitis
PSD
 percutaneous stricture dilation
PSE
 portal-systemic encephalopathy
  PSE index
PSEQ
 Pain Self-Efficacy Questionnaire
pseudarthrosis repair
pseudesthesia, pseudoesthesia
pseudoaddiction
pseudoagglutination
pseudoaneurysm
 p. formation
 hepatic artery p.
 mycotic p.
 ruptured p.
pseudoaneurysmectomy
pseudoangiosarcoma
pseudoankylosis
pseudoarthritis
pseudoarthrosis repair
pseudoarticulation

P

pseudobiopsy technique
pseudo-blind loop syndrome
pseudoboutonnière deformity
pseudocalcification
pseudocancerous lesion
pseudocarcinoma
pseudocavitation
pseudocele
pseudocephalocele
pseudocholesteatoma
pseudocholinesterase deficiency
pseudochylous ascites
pseudoclaudication
pseudocoarctation of aorta
pseudocoloboma
pseudocoma
pseudocryptorchism
pseudocyst
    p. drainage
    pancreatic p.
pseudocystobiliary fistula
pseudocystogastrostomy
    pancreatic p.
pseudodefecation
pseudodislocation
pseudoepiphysis
pseudoepithelioma
pseudoesthesia (*var. of*
  pseudesthesia)
pseudoexfoliation syndrome
pseudofacilitation
pseudoganglion
    Cloquet p.
pseudogestational sac
pseudoglioma
pseudohernia
pseudohydrocephaly
pseudoinfection
pseudointimal hyperplasia
pseudolipoma
pseudolymphoma syndrome
pseudomasturbation
pseudomedial longitudinal fasciculus
  lesion
pseudomelanoma
pseudomembranous
    p. acute inflammation
    p. colitis
pseudomeningocele
    intradiploic p.
    posttraumatic intradiploic p.
    traumatic p.
pseudomigration
Pseudomonas **infection**
pseudomucinous cystadenocarcinoma
pseudomyxoma
pseudoneurogenic bladder
pseudoneuroma
pseudoobstruction

    acute colonic p.
    colonic p.
    p. syndrome
pseudoomphalocele
pseudoosteomalacia
pseudoosteomalacic pelvis
pseudoprolactinoma
pseudoretinoblastoma
pseudosacculation
pseudosarcoma
pseudoserous membrane
pseudostoma
pseudostratified
    p. ciliated epithelium
    p. epithelium
pseudosubluxation
pseudotabes
    diabetic p.
pseudotrachoma
pseudotumor
    p. cerebri
    p. formation
    inflammatory p.
pseudounipolar
pseudoureterocele
pseudoverrucous lesion
pseudoxanthoma elasticum
  syndrome
PSI
    patient state index
    portal shunt index
    posterior superior iliac spine
psoas
    p. fascia
    p. hernia
    p. hitch procedure
    p. line
    p. major muscle
    p. margin
    p. minor muscle
    p. minor tendon
    p. sheath block
    p. sign
psoriatic arthritis
PSP
    postoperative survival probability
PSR
    pain sensitivity range
PSS
    Peritonitis Severity Score
PSV
    pressure-support ventilation
psychic dependence liability
psychoactive
psychogenetic (*var. of* psychogenic)
psychogenic, psychogenetic
    p. colic
    p. pain
    p. symptom

psychologic
    p. consequence
    p. implication
    p. therapy
psychological
    p. problem
    p. screening
psychometric test
psychomotor
    p. performance
    p. retardation
psychopharmacologic medication
psychoprophylaxis
psychorelaxation
psychosedation
    dental p.
psychoses (*pl. of* psychosis)
psychosis, *pl.* **psychoses**
    intensive care unit p.
psychostimulant
psychosurgery
psychotherapy
psychotropic medication
psychrophore
PT
    physical therapy
    prothrombin time
PTA
    pancreas transplant alone
    pancreatic transplantation alone
    percutaneous transluminal angioplasty
PTBD
    percutaneous transhepatic balloon
      dilatation
    percutaneous transhepatic biliary
      drainage
PTC
    percutaneous transhepatic
      cholangiography
PTCA
    percutaneous transluminal coronary
      angioplasty
      multivessel PTCA
PTCSL
    percutaneous transhepatic
      cholangioscopic lithotomy
PTE
    pulmonary thromboendarterectomy
pterion
pterional
    p. approach
    p. craniotomy
pterygoid
    p. artery
    p. branch
    p. canal
    p. fissure
    p. fossa
    p. fovea

    p. hamulus
    p. lamina
    lateral p.
    p. muscle
    p. nerve
    p. notch
    p. pit
    p. plate
    p. plexus
    p. position
    p. process
    p. tubercle
    p. tuberosity
    p. venous complex
pterygomandibular
    p. ligament
    p. raphe
    p. space
    p. space abscess
pterygomaxillary
    p. fissure
    p. fossa
    p. space
pterygopalatine
    p. canal
    p. fossa
    p. fossa syndrome
    p. ganglion
    p. groove
    p. nerve
    p. space
pterygopharyngeal space
pterygospinal ligament
pterygospinous
    p. ligament
    p. process
PTGDS
    patellar tendon graft donor site
PTH
    parathyroid hormone
      PTH level
PTI
    persistent tolerant infection
PTJV
    percutaneous transtracheal jet
      ventilation
PTK
    phototherapeutic keratectomy
PTLD
    posttransplant lymphoproliferative
      disease
    posttransplant lymphoproliferative
      disorder
ptosed
ptoses (*pl. of* ptosis)
ptosis, *pl.* **ptoses**
ptotic organ
PTS
    pediatric trauma scale

P

PTSD
>posttraumatic stress disorder

PTX
>pancreas transplant

ptyalocele

pubalgia
>athletic p.

pubes, *pl.* **pubes**

pubic
>p. angle
>p. arch
>p. arcuate ligament
>p. artery
>p. body
>p. bone
>p. branch
>p. crest
>p. diastasis
>p. fixation
>p. hairline
>p. pad
>p. region
>p. spine
>p. symphysis
>p. tubercle

pubiotomy

pubis
>mons p.

pubocapsular

pubococcygeal
>p. line
>p. muscle

pubofemoral

puboprostatic
>p. ligament
>p. muscle

puboprostaticus

puborectalis
>p. division
>p. fasciocutaneous flap
>p. loop

puborectal muscle

pubourethral triangle

pubovaginal
>p. muscle
>p. operation

pubovaginalis

pubovesical
>p. ligament
>p. muscle

PUD
>peptic ulcer disease

Puddu tendon technique

pudenda (*pl. of* pudendum)

pudendal
>p. anesthesia
>p. canal
>p. cleft
>p. hematocele

>p. hernia
>p. nerve
>p. sac
>p. slit
>p. vein

pudendum, *pl.* **pudenda**

pudic nerve

puerile respiration

puerperal
>p. hematoma
>p. infection

Puestow-Gillesby pancreatojejunostomy

Puestow pancreatojejunostomy

Pugh
>P. liver disease classification
>modified method of P.

Pugh-Child bleeding esophageal varices grading scale classification

Pulec and Freedman congenital ear abnormality classification

pullback
>p. pressure
>p. pressure gradient

pulled-down colon

pull-enteroscopy

pulley
>muscular p.
>peroneal p.
>p. reconstruction
>p. suture technique

pulling
>suture p.

pull maneuver

pull-out wire suture technique

pull-through, pullthrough
>abdominal p.-t.
>Duhamel laparoscopic p.-t.
>ileoanal endorectal p.-t.
>p.-t. operation
>p.-t. procedure
>rapid p.-t. (RPT)
>sacroabdominoperineal p.-t.
>slow p.-t. (SPT)
>Soave endorectal p.-t.
>station p.-t. (SPT)
>Swenson endorectal p.-t.
>p.-t. technique

pullthrough (*var. of* pull-through)
>Babcock rectal p.
>endorectal ileal p.
>endorectal ileoanal p.

pull-up, pullup
>gastric p.-u.
>total gastric p.-u.

pullup (*var. of* pull-up)

pulmo, *pl.* **pulmones**

pulmoaortic canal

pulmonale
>cor p. (CP)

pulmonary
    p. acid aspiration syndrome
    p. angioma
    p. apoptosis
    p. arborization
    p. arterial malformation
    p. arterial web
    p. arteriovenous fistula (PAVF)
    p. arteriovenous malformation
    p. artery
    p. artery catheter
    p. artery catheterization
    p. artery catheterization anesthetic
      technique
    p. artery diastolic pressure
    p. artery hypertension (PAH)
    p. artery occlusion pressure
    p. artery occlusive wedge
      pressure
    p. artery pressure (PAP)
    p. artery systolic pressure
    p. artery wedge (PAW)
    p. aspiration
    p. atresia
    p. autograft
    p. bacterial infection
    p. blastoma
    p. capillary blood
    p. capillary wedge pressure
      (PCWP)
    p. carbon dioxide elimination
      (VECO$_2$)
    p. cavitation
    p. cavity
    p. circulation
    p. circulation tear
    p. collateral
    p. compliance
    p. complication
    p. contusion
    p. dysfunction
    p. edema
    p. effect
    p. embolectomy
    p. embolism (PE)
    p. embolization
    p. epithelial cell
    p. fibrosis
    p. function
    p. fungal infection
    p. gas exchange
    p. glomangiosis
    p. homograft
    p. hypertension pressure
    p. hypertensive crisis (PHTC)
    p. hypoplasia
    p. hypostasis
    p. intralobar sequestration
    p. involvement

    p. laceration
    p. ligament
    p. lobectomy
    p. lymphangioleiomyomatosis
    p. lymphangiomyomatosis
    p. manifestation
    p. mass
    p. metastasectomy
    p. metastasis
    p. orifice
    p. outflow tract
    p. overcirculation
    p. parenchyma
    p. parenchymal infection
    p. pleura
    p. plexus
    p. position
    p. resection
    p. sinus
    p. stenosis repair
    p. sulcus
    p. sulcus syndrome
    p. support
    p. suppuration
    p. sympathetic blockade
    p. thromboendarterectomy (PTE)
    p. tissue
    p. toilet
    p. transplant
    p. trunk
    p. tuberous sclerosis
    p. tumor
    p. valve anomaly
    p. valve area
    p. valve disease
    p. valve gradient
    p. valve insufficiency
    p. valve replacement
    p. valve restenosis
    p. valve stenosis
    p. valvoplasty
    p. vascular abnormality
    p. vascular pressure
    p. vascular resistance (PVR)
    p. vascular resistance index (PVRI)
    p. vein
    p. venous connection anomaly
    p. venous return
    p. venous return anomaly
    p. ventilation
    p. ventilation scan
pulmonectomy
pulmones (*pl. of* pulmo)
pulmonic valve stenosis (PVS)
pulmonis
pulp
    p. amputation
    p. approach
    p. canal

P

pulp (*continued*)
    p. canal therapy
    p. cavity
    p. devitalization
    digital p.
    exposed p.
    p. extirpation
    p. flap
    p. microcirculation
    p. mummification
    p. pressure
    red p.
    splenic p.
    white p.
pulpa
pulpal wall
pulpation
pulpectomy
    complete p.
    partial p.
pulpifaction
pulpiform
pulpify
pulpitis
pulpodentinal membrane
pulpoma
pulpoperiapical lesion
pulposus
pulpotomy
    complete p.
    formocresol p.
    partial p.
    total p.
pulsatile
    p. flow
    p. hematoma
    p. mass
    p. pressure lavage
pulsation
pulse
    abdominal p.
    p. contour analysis
    p. dye laser therapy
    p. lavage irrigation
    p. oximetry (pulse ox)
    peripheral p.
    p. pressure
    p. repetition time prolongation
    p. trisection
    p. value recording (PVR)
    p. width
pulsed
    p. electromagnetic field (PEMF)
    p. electromagnetic field technique
    p. electromagnetic field therapy
    p. irrigation
    p. laser ablation
    p. radiofrequency
pulsed-mode operation

pulse-echo distance measurement
pulseless electrical activity (PEA)
pulsion
    p. diverticulum
    p. hernia
pultaceous
pulverization
Pulvertaft
    P. fishmouth incision
    P. weave suture
    P. weave tendon graft technique
pump
    p. case
    centrifugal p.
    elastomeric p.
    extracorporeal bypass p.
     (ECBP)
    p. failure
    implantable intrathecal p.
    intraaortic balloon p. (IABP)
    p. lung
    p. oxygenation
    portable infusion p.
    syringe p.
    syringe infusion p.
punch
    p. biopsy
    p. graft
    p. resection
punched-out lesion
puncta (*pl. of* punctum)
punctate
    p. epithelial keratoplasty
    p. hemorrhage
    p. stimulation
punctation
punctoplasty
    Viers p.
punctum, *pl.* **puncta**
    inferior lacrimal p.
    lacrimal p.
    renal p.
    scleral p.
    superior lacrimal p.
puncture
    antegrade p.
    anterior p.
    apical left ventricular p.
    Bernard p.
    bone marrow p.
    brain p.
    calyx p.
    cecal ligation and p.
    cisternal p.
    cystic p.
    dental p.
    diabetic p.
    diathermy p.
    direct cardiac p.

direct cautery p.
direct needle p.
dural p.
endoscopic fine-needle p.
exploratory p.
femoral p.
p. incision
jejunal p.
left ventricular p.
lumbar p. (LP)
needle tracheoesophageal p.
nephrostomy p.
percutaneous needle p.
percutaneous renal p.
pericardial p.
Quincke p.
retrograde nephrostomy p.
self-sealing scleral p.
p. site
skin p.
spinal p.
splenic p.
stereotactic p.
sternal p.
subdural p.
suprapubic p.
tracheoesophageal p. (TEP)
transseptal p.
ultrasound-guided nephrostomy p.
venous p.
ventricular p.
p. wound
Ziegler p.

Puntenney radical prostatectomy
pupil
Beer artificial p.
p. dilation
exit p.
Himly artificial p.
pupilla
pupillary
p. dilation
p. line
p. margin
p. membrane
p. membrane remnant
p. muscle
p. zone
pupillodilator fiber
pupilloscopy
pupil-to-root iridectomy
puppet technique
purchase point
pure
p. cutting cautery
p. fungal infection
p. fungal organism
p. insular carcinoma
p. refractive surgery

p. rotation
p. translation
purgation
purging
immunologic method of p.
tumor cell p.
puriform aspect
Purkinje network
**Purmann aneurysm sac extirpation
method**
purpose-made tube holder
purpura
idiopathic thrombocytopenic p.
(ITP)
thrombotic thrombocytopenic p.
(TTP)
purpuric lesion
purpurogenous membrane
pursestring
p. atriotomy
p. mastopexy
p. suture technique
purulence, purulency
purulency (var. of purulence)
purulent
p. exudate
p. exudation
p. inflammation
p. peritonitis
p. rhinorrhea
pus
p. collection
p. culture
frank p.
push
p. enteroscopy
hemodynamic p.
p. maneuver
p. plus refraction technique
push-back
p.-b. cleft palate repair procedure
p.-b. technique
push-pull T technique
push-type enteroscopy
pustular
p. inflammation
p. lesion
p. patch-test reaction
pustulation
pustule
Putti-Platt
P.-P. arthroplasty
P.-P. shoulder capsulorrhaphy
P.-P. shoulder procedure
Putti posterior knee approach
putty kidney
Puzo endoscopic cancer findings method
PVD
peripheral vascular disease

P

PVE
prosthetic valve endocarditis
PVR
pulmonary vascular resistance
pulse value recording
PVTT
portal vein tumor thrombus
pyelectasia (*var. of* pyelectasis)
pyelectasis, pyelectasia
pyelitic
pyelitis
pyelocaliceal, pyelocalyceal
pyelocaliectasis (*var. of* caliectasis)
pyelocalyceal (*var. of* pyelocaliceal)
pyelocalycotomy
pyelocystitis
pyelogram
intravenous p. (IVP)
pyeloileocutaneous anastomosis
pyelolithotomy, pelvilithotomy,
pelviolithotomy
coagulum p.
open p.
pyelolymphatic
pyelolysis
pyelonephritic kidney
pyelonephritis
xanthogranulomatous p. (XGP)
pyelonephrosis
pyeloplasty, pelvioplasty
Anderson-Hynes p.
capsular flap p.
Culp spiral flap p.
disjoined p.
dismembered p.
Foley Y-plasty p.
laparoscopic dismembered p.
robotic-assisted p.
Scardino vertical flap p.
Thompson capsule flap p.
pyeloplication
pyeloscopy
pyelostomy
pyelotomy
extended p.
open p.
pyeloureterectasis
pyeloureterography
pyeloureterostomy
pyelovenous backflow
pyelovesicostomy
pyencephalus
pyesis
pygal
pyknic
pyknotic body
pylemphraxis
pylephlebectasis
pylethrombosis

pylorectomy
Kocher p.
pylori (*pl. of* pylorus)
pyloric
p. antrum
p. artery
p. autotransplantation
p. canal
p. constriction
p. dilation
p. gland
p. intubation
p. myotomy
p. orifice
p. part of stomach
p. ring
p. sphincter
p. stenosis
p. vein
pyloricum
pyloricus
pyloristenosis, pylorostenosis
pylorodiosis
pylorogastrectomy
pyloromyotomy
circumumbilical p.
extramucosal p.
Fredet-Ramstedt p.
Kocher p.
laparoscopic p.
open p.
Ramstedt p.
Ramstedt-Fredet p.
pyloroplasty
double p.
Finney p.
Heineke p.
Heineke-Mikulicz p.
Jaboulay p.
Mikulicz p.
Ramstedt p.
reconstructive p.
transhiatal p.
truncal vagotomy and p.
vagotomy and p. (V&P)
Weinberg modification of p.
Yu p.
pyloroptosia (*var. of* pyloroptosis)
pyloroptosis, pyloroptosia
pylorostenosis (*var. of* pyloristenosis)
pylorostomy
pylorotomy
pylorus, *pl.* **pylori**
pylorus-preserving
p.-p. gastrectomy
p.-p. pancreatoduodenectomy (PPPD)
p.-p. surgery
p.-p. total duodenectomy
pylorus-sparing pancreaticoduodenectomy

pyocele
pyocelia
pyocephalus
pyocolpocele
pyocystis
pyoderma gangrenosum
pyodermatous
    p. infection
    p. skin lesion
pyogen
pyogenesis
pyogenetic (*var. of* pyogenic)
pyogenic, pyogenetic, pyogenous
    p. abscess
    p. arthritis
    p. granuloma
    p. hepatic abscess
    p. membrane
    p. spinal infection
pyogenicum
pyogenous (*var. of* pyogenic)
pyomyoma
pyonephritis
pyonephrolithiasis
pyonephrosis, nephropyosis
pyoperitoneum
pyoperitonitis
pyopneumothorax
pyopoiesis
pyopyelectasis
pyorrhea
pyosemia, pyospermia
pyosis
pyospermia (*var. of* pyosemia)
pyothorax
pyoureter ectopic ureterocele
pyramid
      Ferrein p.
      Lallouette p.
      malpighian p.

      medullary p.
    p. method
    nasal p.
    orbital p.
    petrous p.
    renal p.
pyramidal
    p. auricular muscle
    p. bone
    p. decussation
    p. eminence
    p. epithelium
    p. fracture
    p. process of thyroid
    p. radiation
    p. tip
    p. tract
    p. tractotomy
pyramidale
pyramidalis
pyramidal-shaped cartilage
pyramides (*pl. of* pyramis)
pyramidotomy
      medullary p.
      spinal p.
pyramis, *pl.* **pyramides**
pyretic therapy
pyridostigmine
pyriform
pyriformis (*var. of* piriformis)
pyrogen
      endogenous p.
pyrolysis product
pyropoikilocytosis
pyrosequencing
pyruvate
    p. dehydrogenase inhibition
    p. kinase deficiency
    p. metabolism
pyuria

P

Q̊
    cardiac output
QALY
    quality adjusted life year
QOL
    quality of life
QST
    Quantitative Sensory
    Testing
Q-tip test
quadrangular
    q. cartilage
    q. membrane
    q. space
    q. therapy
quadrant
    circumareolar q.
    left lower q. (LLQ)
    left upper q. (LUQ)
    lower lateral q.
    lower medial q.
    right lower q. (RLQ)
    right upper q. (RUQ)
    q. sampling technique
    upper lateral q.
    upper medial q.
quadrantectomy
    quadrantectomy, axillary dissection,
    radiation therapy (QUART)
    q. mastectomy
2-quadrant hemorrhoidectomy
3-quadrant hemorrhoidectomy
4-quadrant hemorrhoidectomy
quadrate
    q. femoral tubercle
    q. muscle
quadratus
quadriceps femoris tendon
quadricepsplasty
    Judet q.
    Thomas q.
    Thompson q.
    V-Y q.
quadrigeminal cistern
quadrilateral
    q. space
    q. space syndrome
quadripedal extensor reflex
quadripolar
quadruple
    q. amputation
    q. therapy
Quaegebeur infant heart surgery
  procedure

Quaglino iridectomy
quality
    q. adjusted life year (QALY)
    q. of life (QOL)
    Q. of Well-Being Scale
    Self-Administered (QWB-SA)
    Q. of Well-Being Scale
    Self-Administered form
quantification
    acoustic q.
    shunt q.
quantitative
    q. evaluation
    Q. Sensory Testing (QST)
    q. stool collection
    Q. Sudomotor Axon Reflex
    Test
quantity
    sound q.
    vector q.
QUART
    quadrantectomy, axillary dissection,
    radiation therapy
    QUART procedure
    QUART procedure for breast
    cancer
Quartey pedicled penile flap
  urethroplasty technique
quasistatic stressed position
Quatrefages angle
quenching
    thermal q.
Quénu
    Q. hemorrhoidal plexus
    Q. nail plate removal technique
Quénu-Küss tarsometatarsal injury
  classification
questionable mass
questionnaire
    Acute Low Back Pain Screening Q.
    (ALBPSQ)
    Barriers Pain Q.
    CAGE alcohol addiction q.
    Cognitive Errors Q.
    Coping Strategies Q. (CSQ)
    Fear Avoidance Beliefs Q.
    KESS Q.
    malingering q.
    McGill pain q. (MPQ)
    Menstrual Distress Management Q.
    (MDMQ, MDQ)
    MIDAS q.
    Modified Somatic Pain Q.
    (MSPQ)

questionnaire (*continued*)
  Modified Somatic Perception q.
    (MSPQ)
  neuropathic pain diagnostic q.
    (DN4)
  Northwick Park Neck Pain Q.
    (NPQ)
  Oswestry Disability Q. (ODQ)
  Oswestry Low Back Pain Q.
    (OLBPQ)
  Pain Coping Q. (PCQ)
  Pain Locus of Control Q.
    (PLCQ)
  Pain Self-Efficacy Q. (PSEQ)
  Roland-Morris disability q.
  SF36 q.
  short-form-36 q.
  short form McGill Pain Q.
Quetelet body mass index
quick
  q. angulation technique
  Q. Stitch needle

Quickert
  Q. nonincisional entropion repair
    procedure
  Q. suture
  Q. 3-suture ectropion and entropion
    technique
quilt suture technique
Quinby pelvic fracture classification
Quincke
  Q. puncture
  Q. spinal needle
quinsy tonsil
quinti
Quinton dialysis catheter
quotient
  pressure rate q.
  respiratory q.
  ventilation/perfusion q.
QWB-SA
  Quality of Well-Being Scale
    Self-Administered
  QWB-SA form

R0

no residual disease

resection margin free of tumor

R1

resection margin microscopic positive

residual disease

R2

gross residual disease

resection margin macroscopic positive

RA

rheumatoid arthritis

racemic

r. mixture

r. modification

racemization

rachial

rachidial

rachidian

rachiotomy, rachitomy

rachis

rachitic metaphysis

rachitomy (*var. of* rachiotomy)

racket (*var. of* racquet)

r. incision

r. nail

racket-shaped

r.-s. flap

r.-s. incision

Rackley left ventricular mass determination method

racquet, racket

r. incision

racquet-shaped incision

radectomy

Radford nomogram

radiad

radial

r. artery

r. bursa

r. club hand

r. collateral artery

r. dilator muscle

r. forearm flap

r. fracture reduction

r. head

r. head dislocation

r. head fracture

r. index artery

r. iridotomy

r. keratotomy (RK)

r. laminectomy

r. neck fracture

r. recurrent artery

r. scar

r. sclerosing lesion

r. skin incision

r. styloid fracture

r. suture track

r. tear

r. wedge osteotomy

r. wrist extensor

radial-based flap

radiate sternocostal ligament

radiation

r. angiopathy

braking r.

r. burn

r. cataract

characteristic r.

r. chimera

r. damage

diagnostic r.

r. enteritis

r. enteropathy

r. exposure

general r.

geniculocalcarine r.

Gratiolet r.

r. hepatitis

r. hepatopathy

high dose r. (HDR)

homogenous r.

r. injury

intraoperative r.

involved-field r.

r. lung disease

r. monitoring

r. mucositis

r. myelopathy

r. necrosis

occipitothalamic r.

r. oncologist

optic r.

r. output

r. pneumonitis

r. poisoning

postoperative pelvic r.

r. precautions

primary r.

r. proctitis

r. proctocolitis

r. protection

pyramidal r.

rectosigmoid r.

r. response

r. risk

single fraction r.

superficial r.

r. survey

temporal lobe r.

R

radiation (*continued*)
  r. therapy
  r. treatment
  Wernicke r.
  whole abdominal r.
  whole-body r.
radiation-associated stricture
radiation-induced
  r.-i. carcinoma
  r.-i. colitis
  r.-i. disease
  r.-i. ischemia
  r.-i. leukoencephalopathy
  r.-i. proctitis
  r.-i. pulmonary toxicity
  r.-i. ulceration
radiatum
radical
  r. abdominal hysterectomy
  r. antegrade modular
    pancreatosplenectomy (RAMPS)
  r. axillary dissection
  r. compartmental excision
  r. cryosurgical ablation of prostate
    (RCSA)
  r. curative surgery
  r. cystectomy
  r. en bloc removal
  r. gastric resection
  r. glossectomy
  r. hemorrhoidectomy
  r. hysterectomy
  r. inguinal orchiectomy
  r. lymph node dissection
  r. mastectomy
  r. mastoidectomy
  r. mediastinal dissection
  r. neck dissection (RND)
  r. nephrectomy
  r. nephroureterectomy
  r. orchidectomy
  r. palmar fasciectomy
  r. pancreatoduodenectomy
  r. parametrectomy
  r. parotidectomy
  r. pericystic resection
  r. perineal prostatectomy
  r. prefrontal lobotomy
  r. proctectomy
  r. retropubic prostatectomy
  r. subtotal resection
  r. therapy
  r. total gastrectomy
  r. transcoccygeal prostatectomy
  r. vaginal hysterectomy
  r. vulvectomy
radices (*pl. of* radix)
radicle
radicotomy

radicular
  r. artery
  r. canal
  r. pain
  r. pain syndrome
radiculectomy
radiculomedullary fistula
**radiculomeningeal spinal vascular
  malformation**
radiculopathy
  lumbosacral r.
  thoracic r.
radiectomy
radii (*pl. of* radius)
radioactive
  r. colloid lymphoscintigraphy
  r. concentration
  r. iodine uptake
  r. microsphere
  r. scan
  r. seed implantation
radioactivity
radiobicipital
radiocapitate ligament
radiocapitellar
  r. articulation
  r. line
radiocarpal
  r. arthroscopy
  r. articulation
  r. dislocation
radiocolloid
radiodense lesion
radiodigital
radiofluoroscopy
  televised r.
radiofrequency (RF)
  r. ablation (RFA)
  r. catheter ablation (RFCA)
  r. cervical zygapophysial joint
    neurotomy
  r. denervation
  r. electrocoagulation
  r. electrophrenic respiration
  r. identification (RFID)
  r. lesion
  r. lesioning
  pulsed r.
  r. rhizotomy
  temperature-controlled r. (TCRF)
  r. thermal ablation (RFTA)
  r. tissue ablation (RFTA)
radiofrequency-generated thermal lesion
radiograph
  sequential r.'s
  serial r.'s
  specimen r.
radiographic
  r. evaluation

r. examination
r. image
r. obliteration
r. technique
r. tooth repair
radiography
radioguided
r. parathyroidectomy
r. technique
radiohumeral
radioimmunoglobulin therapy
radioimmunoguided surgery (RIGS)
radioimmunoscintimetry
radioiodination
radioiodine
r. ablation
r. ablation therapy
low-dose r.
r. treatment
radioisotope
filtered r.
r. localization
unfiltered r.
r. uptake
radiolabeled
r. sentinel node
r. serum albumin
radioligand binding assay
radiolocalization
gamma-probe r.
SLN r.
radiologic, radiological
r. biliary stent placement
r. evaluation
r. evidence
r. examination
r. percutaneous gastrostomy
(RPG)
r. sphincter
r. study
r. technique
radiological (*var. of* radiologic)
radiologist
interventional r.
vascular r.
radiology
interventional r.
radiolucent
r. crescent line
r. lesion
r. operating room table extension
radiolunate fusion
radiolus
radiolysis
radiomuscular
radiomutation
radionecrosis
radionuclide
radiopalmar

radiopaque
r. foreign body
r. lesion
radiopharmaceutical therapy
radiopotentiation
radioprotector
radioscaphoid fusion
radiosensitization
radio signal line
radiosurgery
LINAC-based r.
linear accelerator-based r.
stereotactic r. (SRS)
radiotherapy
adjuvant r.
radiotriquetral ligament
radioulnar
r. articulation
r. dissociation
r. ligament
radisectomy
radius, *pl.* **radii**
r. of angulation
scaphoid r.
radix, *pl.* **radices**
**Radley-Liebig-Brown pubic bone
chondrosarcoma resection**
radon seed implantation
Raeder syndrome
RAFF
rectus abdominis free flap
Rai leukemia classification
raise
single heel r.
raising
straight-leg r. (SLR)
rale
**Ralston-Thompson pseudoarthrosis
technique**
RAM
rectus abdominis muscle
Raman spectroscopy
Rambo musculoplasty
RAMCF
rectus abdominis myocutaneous
flap
ram horn nail
rami (*pl. of* ramus)
ramicotomy
ramification
apical r.
ramisection
Ramond point
ramotomy
superior pubic r.
RAMPS
radical antegrade modular
pancreatosplenectomy
Ramsay Hunt syndrome

Ramstedt
  R. operation
  R. pyloromyotomy
  R. pyloromyotomy with wedge
  resection procedure
  R. pyloroplasty
Ramstedt-Fredet pyloromyotomy
ramus, *pl.* **rami**
  cephalic arterial r.
  rami communicans
  r. communicans block
  interganglionic rami
  r. of mandible
  rami pancreatici
  r. perforans
  rami pharyngei
Ranawat
  R. pneumatoid spondylitis
  classification
  R. triangle method
Ranawat-DeFiore-Straub
  R.-D.-S. correction of Madelung
  deformity technique
  R.-D.-S. osteotomy
**Ranawat-Dorr-Inglis atlantoaxial
  impaction method**
Randall plaque
random
  r. bladder biopsy
  r. controlled trial
  r. cutaneous flap
  r. pattern flap
randomization
range
  r. of excursion
  r. of motion (ROM)
  pain sensitivity r. (PSR)
Ransley-Cantwell epispadias repair
**Ransohoff aneurysm wiring
  operation**
Ranson
  R. acute pancreatitis classification
  R. pancreatitis criteria
  R. prognostic scoring index
Ranvier node
RAO
  right anterior oblique
  right anterior occipital
  RAO angulation
  RAO position
rapacuronium
Rapamune
rapamycin
raphe, rhaphe
  anogenital r.
  median longitudinal r.
  penile r.
  perineal r.
  pharyngeal r.

  pterygomandibular r.
  scrotal r.
rapid
  r. bedside imaging
  r. intraoperative parathormone
  assay
  r. intraoperative parathormone
  immunoradiometric assay
  r. maxillary expansion
  r. occlusion
  r. opiate detoxification
  r. pull-through (RPT)
  r. pullthrough esophageal manometry
  technique
  r. pullthrough technique
  r. recompression-high pressure
  oxygen
  r. scan fluoroscopy
  r. scan technique
  r. sequence induction (RSI)
  r. sequence induction intubation
  r. shallow breathing index
  r. tumor lysis syndrome
  r. volume resuscitation
Rapide suture
rapid-flush technique
**rapidly involuting congenital hemangioma
  (RICH)**
rapid-sequence
  r.-s. induction anesthetic technique
  r.-s. induction of anesthesia
rapid-volume approach
Rapoport renal function technique
Rappaport
  R. lymphoma classification
  R. osteotomy
RAPS
  recurrent abdominal pain syndrome
Rapunzel syndrome
rare system reaction
RAS
  robot-assisted surgery
rasceta
rash
  acneform r.
Rashkind
  R. balloon technique
  R. operation
raspberrylike density
**Rastan-Konno anterior
  aortoventriculoplasty procedure**
Rastan operation
Rastelli
  R. classification (A–C) of
  atrioventricular septal defect
  R. conduit
  R. pericardial roll graft
  R. right ventricle and pulmonary
  artery conduit procedure

R. transposition of great arteries operation
R. transposition of great arteries repair
R. ventricular septal defect classification

rate
anastomotic complication r.
anastomotic stricture r.
average flow r.
beat-to-beat variation of fetal heart r.
blood flow r.
cerebral metabolic r.
circulation r.
complication r.
disease recurrence r.
disintegration r.
early infection r.
ejection r.
expiratory flow r.
fecundity r.
fetal heart r.
flotation r.
fusion nonunion r.
gallbladder ejection r.
glomerular filtration r.
heart r.
high dose r. (HDR)
ideal flow r.
implant survival r.
infection r.
infusion r.
in-hospital mortality r.
late infection r.
leakage r.
load-deflection r.
low dose r. (LDR)
maximal expiratory flow r.
maximal ventilation r.
mean normalized systolic ejection r.
metabolic r.
mortality r.
r. of fluid filtration
operative mortality r.
ovulation r.
oxygen extraction r.
pacemaker adaptive r.
peak expiratory flow r. (PEFR)
perfusion flow r.
plasma separation r.
pressure increment r.
r. pressure product
recurrence r.
relapse r.
relaxation r.
resectability r.
stricture r.
stroke ejection r.

success r.
systolic ejection r.
transverse relaxation r.
T2 relaxation r.
ventilatory flow r.
vertebral osteosynthesis fusion r.
voiding flow r.
rated perceived exertion
Rathke
R. bundle
R. pouch cyst
rating of perceived exertion
ratio (R)
acceleromyographic train-of-four r.
adenoma hyperplastic polyp r.
adenoma to nonadenoma r.
ankle brachial blood pressure r.
body hematocrit to venous hematocrit r. (BH:VH)
common mode rejection r. (CMRR)
cough pressure transmission r.
cup to disc r. (C:D)
dead space to tidal volume r.
external to internal rotation r.
fetal head to abdominal circumference r.
hand r.
head circumference to abdominal circumference r.
head to body r.
inspiratory to expiratory r.
international normalized r. (INR)
intrapulmonary shunt r. (Qs/Qt)
lung to head circumference r.
MAC r.
mean umbilical vein to maternal vein r.
mean UV to MV r.
midexpiratory to midinspiratory flow r.
optic cup to disc r.
pressure transmission r. (PTR)
respiratory rate to tidal volume r. (f/VT)
sentinel node to background r. (SNBR)
shunt r.
stereoselectivity r.
TOF r.
train-of-four r.
tumor to cerebellum r.
umbilical vein to maternal vein r. (UV:MV)
UV to MV r. (UV:MV)
ventilation/perfusion r.
rationalization
rat-tail deformity
Rauwolfia **extract**

655

rave
> fracture en r.

RAVECAB
> robotically assisted vision-enhanced coronary artery bypass

Raverdino retinal detachment photocoagulation operation

Ravitch pectus excavatum repair procedure

raw hepatic surface

ray
> r. amputation
> medullary r.
> r. resection

Ray-Brunswick-Mack operation

Ray-Clancy-Lemon semitendinosus tendon transfer technique

Rayhack ulnar shortening osteotomy technique

Ray-McLean operation

Raynaud
> R. phenomenon
> R. syndrome

Raz
> R. bladder neck suspension
> R. bladder neck suspension procedure
> R. modification
> R. needle suspension
> R. 4-quadrant suspension
> R. urethral suspension

RCA
> right carotid artery

rCABG
> reoperative coronary artery bypass graft

rCBF
> regional cerebral blood flow

RCSA
> radical cryosurgical ablation of prostate

RDS
> respiratory distress syndrome

REA
> rollerball endometrial ablation

reabsorb

reabsorbable suture

reaction
> acute hemolytic transfusion r.
> anaphylactoid r.
> anaphylactoid-type r.
> anesthetic r.
> compensation r.
> cutaneous graft-versus-host r.
> delayed hemolytic r.
> dextran r.
> eczematous r.
> elimination r.
> exergonic r.

> extrapyramidal r.
> fibrotic r.
> foreign body r.
> r. formation
> general adaptation r.
> graft-versus-host disease r.
> hemolytic r.
> homograft r.
> immediate asthmatic r. (IAR)
> implant r.
> inflammation r.
> influence r.
> irritant patch-test r.
> lid closure r.
> litigation r.
> local anesthetic r.
> midazolam-induced excitatory r.
> needle r.
> nonhemolytic febrile r.
> paradoxical r.
> postanesthesia emergence r.
> pustular patch-test r.
> rare system r.
> scar tissue r.
> transfusion r.
> whitegraft r.

reactivation
> incremental r.
> r. tuberculosis

reactive
> r. arthritis
> r. dilation
> r. hyperemia
> r. lymphoid lesion

reactivity
> airway r.

reading
> benign r.
> malignant r.

ready-ready position

real
> r. adaptive relaxation
> r. reconstruction

realignment procedure

realimentation

reality
> virtual r.

real-time
> r.-t. colonoscopy
> r.-t. 3D biplanar transperineal prostate implantation
> r.-t. echo-planar image
> r.-t. endoscopic ultrasound-guided fine-needle aspiration
> r.-t. multiplanar image
> r.-t. sector scanning

reamed
> r. femoral nailing
> r. nail

reamputation
reanastomosed
reanastomosis
 laparoscopic ureteral r.
reanimation
 facial r.
reapproximation
reassignment
reattachment
 Harris 4-wire trochanter r.
 4-wire trochanter r.
reattribution technique
rebound
 r. headache
 r. tenderness
rebreathing
 r. anesthesia
 intentional r.
 r. technique
Rebuck skin window technique
recalcification time
recall
 memory r.
Récamier
 R. operation
 R. uterine curettage procedure
recanalization
 balloon occlusive intravascular lysis
  enhanced r.
 excimer vascular r.
 laser r.
 TCD r.
 r. technique
 tibial r.
 transcranial Doppler r.
 umbilical vein r.
 r. versus recannulization
recannulization
 recanalization versus r.
receiver saturation
recent dislocation
recently healed surgical incision
receptacula (*pl. of* receptaculum)
receptaculum, *pl.* **receptacula**
receptoma
receptor
 acetylcholine r.
 alpha-adrenergic r.
 alpha-2 adrenergic r.
 r. antagonist
 beta-2 adrenergic r.
 beta-adrenergic r.
 calcium-sensing r.
 cannabinoid r.
 dopamine r.
 endogenous opiate r.
 endometrial r.
 endothelin A, B r.
 gamma-amino butyric acid r.

 glucocorticoid r.
 glycine r.
 high-affinity progestin r.
 high threshold r.
 intensity-encoded r.
 mineralocorticoid r.
 mu r.
 muscarinic r.
 nerve growth factor r.
 neuronal nicotinic acetylcholine r.
 nicotinic r.
 N-methyl-D aspartate r.
 opioid r.
 pressure r.
 silent r.
 vanilloid r.
receptor-mediated endocytosis
 pathway
recess
 azygoesophageal r.
 cecal r.
 costodiaphragmatic r.
 costomediastinal r.
 duodenal r.
 duodenojejunal r.
 elliptical r.
 epitympanic r.
 frontal r.
 hepatorenal r.
 ileocecal r.
 inferior duodenal r.
 inferior ileocecal r.
 inferior omental r.
 intersigmoid r.
 Jacquemet r.
 mesentericoparietal r.
 omental r.
 paracolic r.
 paraduodenal r.
 parotid r.
 pharyngeal r.
 phrenicomediastinal r.
 pineal r.
 piriform r.
 pleural r.
 retrocecal r.
 retroduodenal r.
 Rosenmüller r.
 sacciform r.
 sphenoethmoidal r.
 spherical r.
 splenic r.
 subhepatic r.
 subphrenic r.
 subpopliteal r.
 superior duodenal r.
 superior ileocecal r.
 superior omental r.
 suprabullar r.

recess (*continued*)
    suprapineal r.
    supratonsillar r.
recession
    clitoral r.
    Dunnington lateral rectus r.
    Fink inferior oblique r.
    lateral rectus r.
recessional line
recession-resection
recessive
    autosomal r.
recessus phrenicomediastinalis
recidivation
recidivism
    trauma r.
recipient
    adult r.
    r. hepatectomy
    high-risk r.
    naive r.
    OLT r.
    orthotopic liver transplant r.
    Scientific Registry of Transplant R.'s
      (SRTR)
    transplant r. (TR)
reciprocal relaxation
reciprocation
    active r.
    passive r.
recirculation
    instrument r.
Recklinghausen type I disease
reclamping
reclination
reclining position
Reclus I syndrome
recoarctation of aorta
recognition
    pattern r.
    within-list r. (WLR)
recoil
    elastic r.
recombinant
    r. activated coagulation factor VII
    r. activated factor VII
    r. factor VIIa
recommendation
    FDA Anesthesia Apparatus Checkout
      R.'s
    screening r.
reconciliation
reconditioning
    mucosal r.
reconstruction
    Abbe-McIndoe vaginal r.
    ACL r.
    aesthetic r.
    alar r.

    anal sphincter r.
    analytic r.
    Andrews iliotibial band r.
    anterior capsulolabral r. (ACLR)
    anterior cruciate ligament r.
    aortic root r.
    aortorenal r.
    artery r.
    arthroscopic anterior cruciate
      ligament r. (AACLR)
    Bankart anterior capsolabral r.
    Beard-Cutler eyelid r.
    Bernard lip r.
    biliary r.
    Billroth I, II gastrointestinal r.
    bladder outlet r.
    breast r.
    Brown knee joint r.
    chest wall r.
    Cho anterior cruciate ligament r.
    Chrisman-Snook ankle
      ligament r.
    circumferential esophageal r.
    Clancy cruciate ligament r.
    columellar r.
    commissure r.
    constrained r.
    coronal r.
    corporeal r.
    craniofacial r.
    cruciate ligament r.
    Dalgleish eyelid r.
    d'Aubigné femoral r.
    d'Aubigné resection r.
    3D computer r.
    dermal pouch r.
    Dibbell cleft lip-nasal r.
    distal vertebral artery r.
    dural patch r.
    Eaton-Littler ligament r.
    Ellison lateral knee r.
    endoscopic anterior cruciate
      ligament r.
    endoscopic condylectomy and
      costochondral graft r.
    end-to-end r.
    epiglottic r.
    Evans ankle tenodesis r.
    exogenous r.
    extraarticular r.
    gastrojejunal r.
    genital r.
    Gilles soft palate r.
    Goldner thumb r.
    hand r.
    Harmon hip r.
    hemimandible r.
    House upper limb r.
    Hughston-Degenhardt ACL r.

Hughston-Jacobson lateral
   compartment r.
immediate breast r. (IBR)
index metacarpophalangeal joint r.
inferior vena cava r.
infrarenal aortic r.
innominate artery r.
Insall anterior cruciate ligament r.
in situ r.
intraarticular r.
iterative r.
IVC r.
joint r.
juxtacubital r.
Krukenberg hand r.
Kugelberg r.
Larson ligament r.
lateral compartment r.
Lee r.
L'Episcopo hip r.
Lewis-Tanner subtotal esophagectomy
   and r.
ligament r.
Longmire-Gutgeman gastric r.
lower extremity r.
MacIntosh over-the-top ACL r.
mandibular r.
r. method
microsurgical r.
Millard advancement rotation flap r.
Monfort abdominal wall r.
Morax craniofacial r.
nasal r.
Nathan-Trung modification of
   Krukenberg hand r.
Neer posterior shoulder r.
neoglottic r.
Nicoll fracture r.
nipple r.
nipple-areola r.
r. occlusal surface (RecOS)
O'Donoghue ACL r.
open r.
operative r.
oral r.
orbital rim r.
oromandibular r.
oropharyngeal r.
ossicular chain r.
osteoplastic r.
palate r.
pancreaticogastrostomy r.
papillary r.
pedicled jejunal r.
peritoneal r.
pharyngoesophageal r.
plastic r.
portal vein r.
pouch r.

r. procedure
pulley r.
real r.
renal artery r.
Rosenberg endoscopic anterior
   cruciate ligament r.
Roux-en-Y r.
Roux gastric r.
sagittal r.
secondary r.
septal r.
Sheen airway r.
Smith-Kuhnt-Szymanowski ectropion
   repair with eyelid r.
socket r.
soft tissue r.
sphincter r.
S-pouch r.
staged r.
2-stage tendon graft r.
stapled r.
sternoclavicular joint r.
Swanson midfacial defect r.
synchronous bladder r.
Szymanowski-Kuhnt ectropion repair
   with lid r.
Tanagho bladder neck r.
r. technique
tenoplastic r.
thumb r.
Torg knee r.
tracheal r.
tubular r.
tubularized bladder neck r.
urinary tract r.
vascular r.
Verdan osteoplastic thumb r.
vertebral artery r.
Watson-Jones ankle r.
Whitman femoral neck r.
Wookey laryngopharyngeal r.
Young-Dees bladder neck r.
Young-Dees-Leadbetter bladder
   neck r.
Zancolli upper limb r.

reconstructive
r. mammaplasty
r. operation
r. preprosthetic surgery
r. pyloroplasty
r. surgical procedure
r. technique

record
anesthesia r.
anesthetic r.
automated anesthesia r. (AAR)
centric occluding relation r.
eccentric interocclusal r.
eccentric maxillomandibular r.

record (*continued*)
    jaw relation r.
    medical r.
    occluding centric relation r.
    terminal jaw relation r.
recording
    continuous on-line r.
    duodenojejunal motor r.
    fasting r.
    macroelectrode r.
    microelectrode r.
    motor r.
    pulse value r. (PVR)
    segmental limb pressure r.
    r. session
    venous outflow r.
    whole-cell patch clamp r.
RecOS
    reconstruction occlusal surface
recovery
    r. and reorganization
    anesthetic immediate r.
    r. index
    neurologic r.
    postoperative r.
    pressure r.
    r. room
    r. room time
    saturation r.
    selective saturation r.
    r. time
    time to r.
recruiting maneuver
recruitment
    alveolar r.
    leukocyte r.
    r. maneuver
recta (*pl. of* rectum)
rectal
    r. alimentation
    r. ampulla
    r. anesthesia
    r. anesthetic
    r. anesthetic technique
    r. blind pouch
    r. cancer
    r. carcinoma
    r. column
    r. diameter
    r. dilation
    r. distention
    r. evacuation
    r. examination
    r. excision
    r. fascia
    r. fissure
    r. fistula
    r. flap
    r. floor

    r. floor line
    r. fold
    r. foreign body
    r. hernia
    r. laceration
    r. mass
    r. mobilization
    r. mucosa
    r. mucosectomy
    r. muscle cuff
    r. myectomy
    r. nerve
    r. polyp
    r. probe electroejaculation
    r. problem
    r. prolapse
    r. prolapse repair
    r. pulsed irrigation
    r. resection
    r. resting pressure
    r. shelf
    r. sinus
    r. sphincter
    r. stricture
    r. stump
    r. suction biopsy
    r. surgery
    r. tip
    r. ulceration
    r. valvotomy
    r. vault
    r. venous plexus
rectalgia
rectalis
rectangular amputation
rectectomy
rectification
    anomalous r.
    inward-going r.
rectify
recto
    hernia in r.
rectoanal
    r. angulation
    r. inhibitory reflex
rectocele repair
rectoclysis
rectococcygeal muscle
rectococcygeus
rectococcypexy
rectolabial fistula
rectoperineal
rectoperineorrhaphy
rectopexy
    abdominal r.
    anterior r.
    Ekehorn r.
    posterior r.
    presacral r.

Ripstein anterior sling r.
Wells posterior r.
rectoplasty
 vertical reduction r.
rectorrhaphy
rectoscopic endometrial ablation
rectoscopy
rectoscrotal fistula
rectosigmoid
 r. anastomosis
 r. carcinoma
 r. colon
 r. junction
 r. radiation
 r. rupture
 r. sphincter
 r. stump
 r. vein
rectosigmoidectomy
rectosigmoidoscopy
rectosphincteric reflex
rectostenosis
rectostomy
rectotomy
rectourethral
 r. fistula
 r. muscle
rectourinary fistula
rectouterine
 r. cul-de-sac
 r. fold
 r. muscle
 r. pouch
rectovaginal
 r. examination
 r. fistula
 r. pouch
 r. septum
 r. surgery
 r. surgical treatment
rectovaginouterine pouch
rectovesical
 r. fascia
 r. fistula
 r. fold
 r. muscle
 r. pouch
 r. septum
rectovestibular fistula
rectovulvar fistula
rectum, *pl.* **rectums, recta**
 aganglionic r.
 r. cancer
 colonoscopy per r.
 r. irrigation
rectums (*pl. of* rectum)
rectus
 r. abdominis free flap (RAFF)
 r. abdominis muscle (RAM)

 r. abdominis muscle flap
 r. abdominis musculocutaneous flap
 r. abdominis myocutaneous flap
 (RAMCF)
 r. diastasis
 r. fascial wrap
 femoris r.
 r. femoris fasciocutaneous flap
 r. femoris flap
 r. femoris (muscle)
 r. femoris musculocutaneous flap
 r. femoris tendon
 r. muscle
 r. muscle-splitting incision
 r. position
 r. sheath
 r. sheath hematoma (RSH)
 r. sheath incision
 r. sheath wall
recumbent
 r. hypertension
 r. incision
 r. position
recurarization
recurrence
 distant r.
 goiter r.
 intraperitoneal r.
 invasive r.
 local r.
 locoregional r.
 nodal r.
 noninvasive r.
 peritoneal r.
 port-site wound r.
 r. rate
 resectable extrahepatic r.
 suprapubic midline r.
 tumor r.
 wound r.
recurrence-free survival
recurrent
 r. abdominal pain syndrome (RAPS)
 r. arthralgia
 r. ascites
 r. aspiration
 r. attack
 r. corneal erosion
 r. dysphagia
 r. enterocolitis
 r. exophthalmos
 r. hypercalcemia
 r. incisional hernia
 r. inflammation
 r. interosseous artery
 r. laryngeal nerve (RLN)
 r. leiomyosarcoma
 r. meningeal branch
 r. meningeal nerve

recurrent (*continued*)
  r. nerve injury
  r. nerve lesion
  r. nerve lymphatic chain
  r. nerve paralysis
  r. pancreatitis
  r. patellar dislocation
  r. pyogenic cholangiohepatitis (RPC)
  r. radial artery
  r. radicular pain
  r. sarcoma
  r. thromboembolic complication
  r. thromboembolic disease
  r. thromboembolism
  r. thrombophlebitis
  r. thrombosis
  r. tumor
  r. ulnar artery
  r. upper respiratory tract infection
  r. vermian oligoastrocytoma
recurvatum angulation deformity
red
  r. blood cell mass
  r. blood cell substitute
  r. desaturation
  r. ear syndrome
  r. granulation
  r. hepatization
  r. induration
  r. man syndrome
  r. muscle
  r. pulp
redébridement
red-eyed shunt syndrome
red-filter therapy
redilation
redintegration
redistribution hypothermia
Redman approach
Redmond Smith ab externo trabeculectomy
redo
  r. CABG
  r. fundoplication
redox indicator
redressement forcé
REDTCAB
  robot-enhanced Dresden technique coronary artery bypass
reduced liver transplant (RLT)
reduced-size
  r.-s. graft
  r.-s. transplant
reducible hernia
reduction
  afterload r.
  Agee force-couple splint r.
  alar base r.
  Allen lung volume r.

r. anuloplasty
Aries-Pitanguy breast r.
axillary endoscopic r.
Barsky macrodactyly r.
Becton open r.
r. before resection
Bircher stomach r.
Boitzy open r.
breast r.
Brenner lung volume r.
calcaneal fracture r.
Carmody-Batson zygoma and zygomatic arch fracture r.
central cone technique r.
closed r.
cluster r.
concentric r.
Cooper lung volume r.
Cotton lung volume r.
Crosby lung volume r.
Cubbins open r.
delayed open r.
Dias-Giegerich open r.
r. division
Eaton closed r.
Eaton-Malerich r.
embryo r.
r. en masse
Essex-Lopresti open r.
femoral neck fracture r.
fetal r.
Flynn femoral neck fracture r.
force-couple splint r.
Fowles open r.
fracture r.
fracture-dislocation r.
funic r.
Hankin lung volume r.
Hastings open r.
hip r.
Houghton-Akroyd open r.
incomplete r.
indirect r.
internal fixation, closed r.
interproximal r.
Kaplan open r.
Kinast indirect r.
King open r.
Lejour-type breast r.
limb r.
Lowell r.
lung volume r. (LVR)
r. mammaplasty
manual endoscopic r.
r. mastopexy
McKeever open r.
r. method
Meyn r.
Moberg-Gedda open r.

multifetal pregnancy r.
Neer open r.
nonoperative r.
open r. (OR)
r. osteotomy
pain threshold r.
Paré r.
Parvin r.
percutaneous r.
perioperative r.
pneumatic r.
postural r.
r. potential
Pratt open r.
preload r.
prone r.
radial fracture r.
r. ring
risk r.
short scar technique breast r.
shoulder r.
side posture r.
sigmoid loop r.
Speed-Boyd open r.
Speed open r.
spondylolisthesis r.
stable r.
staged r.
stapled lung r.
sternoclavicular joint r.
stress r.
surgical r.
swan-neck deformity r.
r. syndactylia
r. technique
tongue base r.
trial r.
r. tuberosity
tuberosity r.
tumescent technique breast r.
r. ventriculoplasty
vertical pedicle technique
  breast r.
volvulus r.
Wayne County General Hospital r.
Weber-Brunner-Freuler open r.
weight r.
wet technique with liposuction
  breast r.
reduction-stabilization
redundant
r. mucosa
r. sac tissue
r. triangular-shaped skin
reduplication
r. cataract
r. murmur
redux
chancre r.

REE
resting energy expenditure
reedy nail
reefing
r. procedure
stomach r.
reendothelialization
reentry
bundle branch r.
reepithelialization
Reese-Cleasby cataract operation
Reese-Jones-Cooper cataract operation
Reese ptosis operation
reexcision
reexpansion
r. maneuver
r. pulmonary edema (REPE)
reexploration
operative r.
reexplore
refashioning
refeeding syndrome
reference method
referred
r. pain
r. point
r. trigger point pain
r. trigger point phenomenon
refixation
reflectance
endoscopic r.
r. spectroscopy
reflected inguinal ligament
reflection
angle of r.
Campbell triceps r.
corneal r.
diaphragmatic r.
diffuse r.
r. filter
guide wire r.
hepatoduodenal r.
hepatoduodenal-peritoneal r.
internal r.
mirror-image r.
mucobuccal r.
pericardial r.
peritoneal r.
pleural r.
shiny cellophane r.
specular r.
total internal r.
reflectometry
acoustic r.
reflex
abdominal cardiac r.
absent gag r.
accommodation r.
airway r.

R

reflex (*continued*)
    antebrachial r.
    r. arc
    Bezold-Jarisch r.
    body righting r.
    Breuer-Hering inflation r.
    cardiopressor r.
    celiac plexus r.
    copper-wire r.
    corneal light r.
    cremasteric r.
    crossed extension r.
    crossed extensor r.
    Cushing r.
    r. erection
    erector-spinal r.
    r. examination
    extensor thrust r.
    external oblique r.
    eyeball compression r.
    eye-closure r.
    eyelash r.
    eyelid-closure r.
    fixation r.
    flexion-extension r.
    fusion r.
    gastropancreatic vagovagal r.
    grasp r.
    Head paradoxical r.
    head-turning r.
    Hering-Breuer r.
    r. incontinence
    inflation r.
    inhibitory r.
    lacrimation r.
    r. ligament
    mass r.
    milk-ejection r.
    myenteric r.
    r. neurogenic bladder
    obtunded gag r.
    oculocardiac r. (OCR)
    paradoxical extensor r.
    pericardial r.
    pronator r.
    proprioceptive head-turning r.
    protective airway r.
    quadripedal extensor r.
    rectoanal inhibitory r.
    rectosphincteric r.
    renal r.
    silver-wire r.
    supination r.
    supinator longus r.
    r. sympathetic dystrophy (RSD)
    sympathoexcitation r.
    r. therapy
    vagovagal r.
    r. venoconstriction
    vertical suspension r.
    visceral traction r.

reflexive saccade
reflexogenic erection
Refludan
reflux
    abdominal r.
    abdominojugular r.
    acid r.
    alkaline r.
    r. disease
    r. esophagitis
    gastric r.
    gastrocolic r.
    gastroesophageal r.
    laryngopharyngeal r.
    r. menstruation
    proximal r.
    saphenofemoral r.
    r. stricture
    upright r.
    venous r.
    vesicoureteral r.
reformation
    fornix r.
    inferior fornix r.
reformulation
refractile body
refractive
    r. keratoplasty
    r. keratotomy
    r. operative technique
    r. surgery
refractory
    r. ascites
    r. atrial fibrillation
    r. encephalopathy
    r. headache
    r. stricture
    r. variceal hemorrhage
reframing
refrigeration anesthesia
regainer space
regenerate
regenerated esophageal
  epithelium
regeneration
    aberrant r.
    r. aberration
    atypical r.
    axonal r.
    bone r.
    compensatory r.
    epimorphic r.
    hepatic r.
    incomplete r.
    liver r.
    morphallactic r.
    r. motor unit potential

R

nerve r.
neuronal r.
osteoblastic bone r.
peripheral nerve r.
squamous r.
tibial bone defect r.
tissue r.
tubular r.

regimen
adjuvant r.
antifungal r.
antiplatelet r.
treatment r.

regio, *pl.* **regiones**
r. hypochondriaca

region
abdominal r.
anal r.
ankle r.
antebrachial r.
anterior antebrachial r.
anterior brachial r.
anterior knee r.
argyrophilic nucleolar organizer r.
(AgNOR)
axillary r.
brachial r.
brain r.
calcaneal r.
carpal r.
choledochal r.
epigastric r.
femoral r.
gastric pacemaker r.
gluteal r.
hilar r.
hypochondriac r.
hypogastric r.
ileocecal r.
iliac r.
inframammary r.
infraorbital r.
infrascapular r.
inguinal r.
knee r.
lateral r.
left hypochondriac r.
left lateral r.
lumbar r.
mammary r.
mental r.
nuchal r.
oral r.
orbital r.
PAG/PVG r.
paraaortic r.
parietal r.
parotid r.
penumbral r.

periaqueductal gray
matter-periventricular gray matter r.
perineal r.
pharyngeal r.
pineal r.
popliteal r.
posterior antebrachial r.
posterior brachial r.
posterior knee r.
posterior neck r.
presternal r.
pubic r.
retroperitoneal r.
right hypochondriac r.
right iliac r.
right lateral r.
sacral r.
scapular r.
sternocleidomastoid r.
suboccipital r.
subphrenic r.
supraomental r.
suprapubic r.
sural r.
thoracoabdominal r.
umbilical r.
urogenital r.
vertebral r.
zygomatic r.

regional
r. anesthesia
r. anesthetic
r. anesthetic technique
r. block
r. blockade
r. cerebral blood flow (rCBF)
r. enteritis
r. flap
r. hepatectomy
r. hypoperfusion
r. hypothermia
r. lymphadenectomy
r. lymph node basin
r. metastasis
r. node
r. saturation
r. ventilation
r. wall motion abnormality (RWMA)

regiones (*pl. of* regio)

Registered Nurse, First Assist (RNFA)

registration
r. algorithm
image r.
robot-assisted r.

registry
Acoustic Neuroma R.
Autologous Bone and Marrow
Transplant R. (ABMTR)
Balloon Valvuloplasty R.

registry (*continued*)
    Brain Tumor R.
    Kiel Pediatric Tumor R.
    Mansfield Valvuloplasty R.
    National Football Head and Neck
      Injury R.
    National Pediatric Trauma R.
      (NPTR)
    New York State Trauma R.
      (NYSTR)
    Ovarian Tumor R. (OTR)
    Renal Allograft Disease R.
    St. Mark polyposis r.
    tumor r.
    United Kingdom Heart Valve R.
Regnault type B mastopexy
regression
    clot r.
    disease r.
    r. of thrombus
    tumor r.
regular
    r. body acupuncture
    r. diet
regurgitant lesion
regurgitation
    r. jaundice
    mitral r.
    paravalvular r.
    r. test
    tricuspid r.
rehabilitation
    exercise-based r.
    multimodal r.
    r. stage
    vocational r.
rehalation
Rehbein colonic pullthrough procedure
rehepatectomy
**Rehfuss fractional gastric activity
measurement method**
Rehne-Delorme plication
rehydrating solution
rehydration therapy
Reichel-Pólya
    R.-P. gastric resection technique
    R.-P. partial gastrectomy method
    R.-P. stomach resection
    R.-P. subtotal gastrectomy procedure
**Reichenheim elbow surgical stabilization
technique**
**Reichenheim-King biceps tendon
transplantation procedure**
Reichert
    R. cartilage
    R. membrane
Reid base line
Reifenstein syndrome
Reilly body

reimplantation
    aortorenal r.
    Cohen crosstrigonal r.
    end-to-side r.
    intentional tooth r.
    Politano-Leadbetter r.
    ureteral r.
**Reinert acetabular extensile
approach**
reinfection tuberculosis
reinforce
    giant prosthetic r.
reinforcement
    omental r.
    pericardial r.
    peritoneal r.
    pleural patch r.
    positive spousal r.
    Stoppa giant prosthetic r.
reinjection protocol
Reinke
    R. crystalloid
    R. space
reinnervation
reinoculation
reinsemination
reintegrate
reintegration
reintubation
reinversion
reirrigation
Reisseisen muscle
Reissner membrane
**Reis-Wertheim vaginal
hysterectomy**
Reiter
    R. disease
    R. syndrome
rejection
    accelerated transplant r.
    acute r.
    acute allograft r.
    acute cellular r.
    acute lung r.
    acute vascular r.
    allograft corneal r.
    r. cardiomyopathy transplant
    cellular xenograft r.
    chronic allograft r.
    chronic transplant r.
    corneal r.
    delayed hyperacute transplant r.
    ductopenic r.
    fetal r.
    fierce cellular r.
    first-set graft r.
    graft r.
    homograft r.
    hyperacute r.

interstitial r.
r. line
lung r.
marrow graft r.
maternal r.
mild acute r.
moderate r.
no r.
no infection-no r.
primary r.
renal allograft r.
second-set graft r.
severe r.
total graft area r.
transplant r.
treatment-resistant r.
vascular r.

rejuvenation

relapse

axillary r.
locoregional r.
lymphoma r.
r. rate

relapsing polychondritis

relation

acentric r.
acquired centric r.
acquired eccentric jaw r.
buccolingual r.
centric jaw r.
centric occluding r.
concentration-effect r.
convenience jaw r.
cusp-fossa r.
diastolic pressure-volume r.
dynamic r.
eccentric jaw r.
end-systolic pressure-volume r.
end-systolic stress-dimension r.
equivalence r.
force-frequency r.
force-length r.
force-velocity r.
force-velocity-length r.
force-velocity-volume r.
Frank-Starling r.
intermaxillary r.
interval-strength r.
jaw r.
jaw-to-jaw r.
length-resting tension r.
length-tension r.
mandibular centric r.
maxillomandibular r.
median jaw r.
occluding r.
occlusal r.
posterior border jaw r.
pressure-flow r.

pressure-volume r.
protrusive jaw r.
resting length-tension r.
rest jaw r.
retruded jaw r.
ridge r.
static r.
tension-length r.
unstrained jaw r.
ventilation/perfusion r.
ventricular end-systolic
  pressure-volume r.
vertical r.
working bite r.

relationship

cause-effect r.
endoscope-body position r.
end-systolic pressure-length r.
  (ESPLR)
intraluminal pH-pressure r.
left ventricular pressure-volume r.
  (LVPVR)
pressure-flow r.
tissue-base r.
tumor cell-host bone r.
ventilation/perfusion r.

relative

r. curative resection
r. humidity
near-point r.
r. noncurative resection
r. response attributable to the
  maneuver
r. spectacle magnification

relaxant

depolarizing r.
muscle r.
neuromuscular r.
nondepolarizing r.
nondepolarizing muscle r.
r. reversal
skeletal muscle r.
smooth muscle r.

relaxation

adaptive r.
breathing-focused r.
cardioesophageal r.
complete sphincter r.
diastolic r.
differential r.
dynamic r.
endothelial-dependent r.
endothelium-mediated r.
esophageal sphincter r.
incomplete r.
intraoperative stress r.
isovolumetric r.
isovolumic r. (IVR)
line of r.

relaxation (*continued*)
    longitudinal r.
    lower esophageal sphincter r.
    (LESR)
    r. method
    nitric oxide blocked sphincter r.
    pelvic r.
    r. phenomenon
    progressive muscle r. (PMR)
    r. rate
    real adaptive r.
    reciprocal r.
    r. response
    sinusoidal r.
    smooth muscle r.
    sphincter r.
    stress r.
    r. technique
    r. time
    r. time index
    transverse r.
    upper esophageal sphincter r.
    (UESR)
    uterine r.
    ventricular r.
relaxing
    r. incision
    r. solution
release
    de Quervain stenosing
    tenosynovitis r.
    endoscopic carpal tunnel r.
    (ECTR)
    endoscopic gastrocnemius r.
    extended r. (ER, XR)
    flexor-pronator origin r.
    glutamatergic r.
    hilar r.
    lateral extensor r.
    modified 2-portal endoscopic carpal
    tunnel r.
    myofascial r.
    Nirschl tennis elbow r.
    physiologic pattern r.
    plantar fascial r.
    plantar plate r.
    pronator teres r.
    soft tissue r.
    suprahyoid laryngeal r.
    sustained r.
reliability
    interrater r.
relief
    r. incision
    r. space
    symptomatic r.
relieving incision
remain
    necrotic r.'s

Remak
    R. ganglion
    R. plexus
remargination
remedial
    r. inguinal exploration
    r. parathyroid surgery
    r. surgery
remifentanil
remission induction
remnant
    cirrhotic liver r.
    Cloquet canal r.
    devascularized parathyroid r.
    distal r.
    esophageal r.
    gastric r.
    r. gland
    r. liver volume
    mucosal r.
    parathyroid r.
    pupillary membrane r.
remobilization
remodeling
    extracellular matrix r.
    r. of wound
    tissue r.
remote
    r. anesthetic monitoring
    r. pedicle flap
    r. tier
removable maintainer space
removal
    Baudelocque extrauterine
    pregnancy r.
    Bronson foreign body r.
    Cameron femoral component r.
    cast r.
    cement r.
    chordee r.
    Collis-Dubrul femoral stem r.
    colonoscopic r.
    en bloc r.
    endoscopic r.
    excisional r.
    extracorporeal carbon dioxide r.
    ($ECCO_2R$)
    femoral stem r.
    forceps r.
    foreign body r.
    Fukala lens r.
    gallbladder r.
    gastric coin r.
    gland r.
    Harris femoral component r.
    hump r.
    implant r.
    laparoscopic gallbladder r.
    lens r.

macroscopic tumor r.
mesh r.
metastatic tumor r.
Moreland-Marder-Anspach femoral
  stem r.
nail fold r.
nail plate r.
r. of foreign body
path of r.
percutaneous endoscopic r.
percutaneous stone r.
radical en bloc r.
rib r.
1-session r.
small polyp r.
stem r.
stone r.
Sugarbaker pseudomyxoma peritonei
  complete tumor r.
through-the-scope balloon r.
total surgical r.
transsphenoidal r.
tube r.
tumor r.
ureteral stoma r.
Winograd nail plate r.
remyelination, remyelinization
remyelinization (*var. of* remyelination)
renal
r. abnormality
r. adenocarcinoma
r. adenoma
r. allograft
R. Allograft Disease Registry
r. allograft rejection
r. allograft rupture
r. angiomyolipoma
r. angioplasty
r. anomaly
r. arterial embolization
r. artery
r. artery occlusive disease
r. artery orifice
r. artery reconstruction
r. artery response
r. artery rupture
r. artery stenosis
r. artery stenotic disease
r. artery stenting
r. artery thrombosis
r. autotransplantation
r. biopsy
r. branch
r. calculus
r. capsule
r. capsulotomy
r. cell carcinoma
r. colic
r. collecting system

r. column
r. complication
r. compromise
r. cortex
r. cortical lobule
r. crush syndrome
r. cyst
r. cyst ablation
r. cyst decortication
r. cyst hemorrhage
r. cyst infection
r. cyst marsupialization
r. duplication
r. dysfunction
r. ectopia
r. failure
r. fascia
r. fistula
r. function
r. fungal infection
r. ganglion
r. hematoma
r. hyperfiltration
r. hypertension
r. impression
r. infarction
r. infusion therapy
r. injury repair
r. insufficiency
r. labyrinth
r. lithiasis
r. lobe
r. malrotation
r. management
r. manifestation
r. mass
r. mechanism
r. medulla
r. osteodystrophy
r. papilla
r. pelvis
r. pelvis carcinoma
r. perfusion
r. plexus
r. pouch
r. preservation
r. punctum
r. pyramid
r. reflex
r. replacement therapy
r. resistive index
r. revascularization
r. scintography
r. segment
r. sinus
r. sonography
r. stone
r. surface
r. thromboendarterectomy

R

renal (*continued*)
    r. transplantation
    r. trauma
    r. tubular acidosis
    r. tumor
    r. vascular disease
    r. vein
    r. vein renin concentration
    vertebral, anus, tracheoesophageal, radial, r. (VATER)
    r. vessel
renal-sparing surgery
renal-splanchnic steal
renaturation
rendering
    interactive volume r.
    perspective volume r.
renewal
    tissue r.
renicapsule
renicardiac
reniculi (*pl. of* reniculus)
reniculus, *pl.* **reniculi**
reniform pelvis
renin-angiotensin inhibitor
reninoma
renipelvic end-to-side shunt
reniportal
renocutaneous
renogastric fistula
renointestinal
renomegaly
renopathy
renoprival
renopulmonary
renorrhaphy
renovascular hypertension (RVH)
rent
    dural r.
Rentrop cardiac collateral circulation classification
renunculus
reopening
    chest r.
reoperation
    planned r.
reoperative
    r. aesthetic surgery
    r. bariatric surgery
    r. blepharoplasty
    r. carotid surgery
    r. coronary artery bypass graft (rCABG)
    r. laparoscopic technique
    r. necrosectomy
    r. parathyroidectomy
    r. pelvic surgery
    r. thoracotomy technique
    r. ureteroneocystostomy

reorganization
    recovery and r.
reoxygenation
repair
    Abraham-Pankovich tendo calcaneus r.
    ACL r.
    acromioclavicular joint r.
    all-inside r.
    Allison gastroesophageal reflux r.
    Allison hiatal hernia r.
    anal sphincter r.
    anatomic r.
    aneurysm r.
    Anson-McVay hernia r.
    anterior and posterior r.
    aortic valve r.
    A&P r.
    Arlt epicanthus r.
    Arlt eyelid r.
    Bankart dislocated shoulder capsular r.
    Bankart shoulder r.
    Bassini inguinal hernia r.
    Bassini-Stetten hernia r.
    Belsey Mark IV r.
    Belt-Fuqua hypospadias r.
    Bethke sacrococcygeal chordoma r.
    bilateral inguinal hernia r.
    bilayer patch hernia r.
    Black r.
    Blair epicanthus r.
    blepharochalasis r.
    blepharoptosis r.
    Boari ureteral flap r.
    Boerema hernia r.
    bone graft r.
    Bosworth tendo calcaneus r.
    Boyd-Anderson biceps tendon r.
    brachial plexus r.
    Brom supravalvular aortic stenosis r.
    Bryant vascular r.
    Bunnell tendon r.
    Cantwell-Ransley epispadias r.
    cartilage r.
    Caspari transglenoid r.
    cemental r.
    coarctation r.
    Collis thoracoabdominal r.
    columellar r.
    complex syndactyly r.
    crosstrigonal r.
    crural r.
    Csapody orbital r.
    Cutler-Beard eyelid r.
    cystocele r.
    DeBakey-Creech aneurysm r.
    delayed primary r.
    Delorme rectal prolapse r.

density-dependent r.
Devine hypospadias r.
diaphragmatic crural r.
dog-ear r.
dural r.
DuVries hammertoe r.
dynamic r.
early thoracoscopic r.
Ecker-Lotke-Glazer patellar tendon r.
Effler hiatal hernia r.
Ekehorn rectal prolapse r.
elective hernia r.
endoluminal r.
endoscopic mitral valve r.
endovascular r.
endovascular aneurysm r.
end-to-end r.
end-to-end ductal r.
end-to-end tendon r.
end-to-side r.
epineural r.
episiotomy r.
epispadias r.
Eriksson-Drez intraarticular ACL r.
extensor tendon r.
exteriorized uterine r.
extracorporeal r.
extraperitoneal endoscopic hernia r.
fascicular r.
fibrous r.
first stage r.
flexor tendon r.
Fontan r.
Fothergill-Hunter uterine prolapse r.
fracture r.
Froimson-Oh upper limb tendon
  interposition r.
functional r.
Gardner meningocele r.
glenohumeral dislocation r.
Goodall-Power uterine prolapse r.
group fascicular r.
Halsted-Bassini hernia r.
Harrington-Allison hiatal hernia r.
Hatafuku fundus onlay patch
  esophageal r.
Heaton hernia r.
hernia r.
Hill hiatus hernia r.
Hill median arcuate r.
Hoguet pantaloon hernia r.
hypoplastic left heart r.
in situ uterine r.
intraperitoneal Rives-type r.
Jaesche-Arlt entropion r.
Jaesche entropion r.
Jones first-toe r.
Kelikian-Riashi-Gleason patellar
  tendon r.

Kessler tendon r.
Kleinert flexor tendon r.
Konno aortic valve anulus r.
Kugel hernia r.
Kuhnt-Helmbold ectropion r.
Kuhnt-Junius macular degeneration r.
lacrimal gland r.
Lange tendon lengthening and r.
laparoscopic Hill r.
laparoscopic paraesophageal hernia r.
  (LPHR)
laparoscopic prosthetic mesh r.
laparoscopic varicocele r.
laparoscopic ventral hernia r.
laryngeal r.
Latzko vesicovaginal fistula r.
Le Fort-Neugebauer uterine
  prolapse r.
Le Fort-Wehrbein-Duplay
  hypospadias r.
levator aponeurosis r.
Lich-Gregoir vesicoureteral
  reflux r.
Lichtenstein hernia r.
Lichtenstein mesh r.
Lindholm tendo calcaneus r.
Lotheissen hernia r.
MacIntosh over-the-top r.
MacNab shoulder r.
Madden hernia r.
MAGPI hypospadias r.
Ma-Griffith tendo calcaneus r.
Mandelbaum-Nartolozzi-Carney
  patellar tendon r.
Marckwald cervical os r.
Marcy hernia r.
Marlex hernia r.
McLaughlin posterior dislocated
  shoulder r.
McVay-Cooper ligament r.
McVay hernia r.
McVay inguinal hernial r.
medial r.
meniscal r.
mesh r.
Millard rotation-advancement lip r.
minimally invasive mitral valve r.
minimally invasive robotically
  assisted mitral valve r.
mitral valve r.
modified Hill gastroesophageal
  hernia r.
Moloney hernia r.
mucosal r.
myelomeningocele r.
Nissen fundus r.
Noble-Mengert perineal r.
North American Bassini inguinal
  hernia r.

repair (*continued*)

Norwood neonatal univentricular heart with subaortic stenosis r.
Nuttall incisional hernia r.
open r.
Orr rectal prolapse r.
Palmer-Dobyns-Linscheid ligament r.
pants-over-vest hernial r.
paravaginal defect r.
patellar tendon r.
pectus excavatum r.
periapical tooth r.
pericardioplasty in pectus excavatum r.
perineal r.
Phaneuf-Graves enterocele r.
plastic r.
plug prosthetic mesh r.
postanal r.
posterior r.
postoperative r.
potentially lethal x-ray damage r.
premuscular prosthetic r.
primary r.
prosthetic mesh r.
pseudarthrosis r.
pseudoarthrosis r.
pulmonary stenosis r.
radiographic tooth r.
Ransley-Cantwell epispadias r.
Rastelli transposition of great arteries r.
rectal prolapse r.
rectocele r.
renal injury r.
reverse sigma penoscrotal transposition r.
Rives-Stoppa-Wantz retrorectus r.
rod fracture r.
Rodney Smith biliary stricture r.
rotator cuff r.
Scuderi hypospadias r.
secondary r.
Senning transposition of great arteries r.
Sever-L'Episcopo tendon r.
shoulder r.
Shouldice-Bassini hernia r.
Shouldice hernia r.
simple syndactyly r.
slipped Nissen r.
Soave congenital megacolon r.
spatulated r.
Speed sternoclavicular r.
sphincter r.
2-stage r.
staged abdominal r. (STAR)
1-stage hypospadias r.
Staples-Black-Broström ligament r.
Staples ligament r.
Stoppa hernia r.
Stoppa-type laparoscopic r.
Strickland tendon r.
sublethal x-ray damage r.
surgical r.
suture r.
Talesnick scapholunate r.
tendon r.
Tennison-Randall lip r.
tension-free mesh r.
tension-free prosthetic mesh r.
TEP r.
Teuffer tendo calcaneus r.
Thal esophageal stricture r.
Theirsch-Duplay hypospadias r.
thoracic aortic aneurysm r.
thoracoabdominal aortic aneurysm r.
thoracoscopic r.
tight Nissen r.
tissue r.
totally extraperitoneal r.
tracheal r.
tracheoesophageal puncture r.
transabdominal preperitoneal r.
transthoracic r.
triad knee r.
trichiasis r.
tricuspid valve r.
triple ligamentous r.
Turco-Spinella tendo calcaneus r.
ultrasound-guided compression r. (UGCR)
unilateral inguinal hernia r.
vaginal-psoas suspension r.
vaginal wall r.
vascular laceration r.
Veirs canaliculus r.
vesicovaginal r.
vest-over-pants hernia r.
videoscopic r.
volar plate r.
Watson-Jones fracture r.
Wheeler halving r.
Y mesh hernia r.
York-Mason rectourinary fistula r.
Young-Dees bladder neck r.
Young type epispadias r.
Zancolli clawhand deformity r.

repairable parietal defect
reparative cardiac surgery
REPE

reexpansion pulmonary edema

repeat

r. balloon mitral valvotomy
r. cesarean section
r. operation
r. procedure
r. revascularization

repeated
    r. exposure
    r. respiratory infection
    r. tissue expansion
reperfusion
    controlled r.
    r. injury
    thoracic aortic ischemia r.
reperfusion-induced hemorrhage
reperitonealization
repetitive
    r. cluster
    r. magnetic stimulation
    r. motion injury
    r. nerve stimulation
    r. transcranial magnetic stimulation
rephasing
    even-echo r.
replacement
    anatomic porous r. (APR)
    aortic root r.
    aortic valve r. (AVR)
    Cosgrove mitral valve r.
    fluid r.
    heart valve r.
    hip r.
    homograft aortic valve r.
    joint r.
    knee r.
    laparoscopic feeding tube r.
    mitral valve r. (MVR)
    mucosal patch r.
    Mueller-type femoral head r.
    pulmonary valve r.
    supraannular mitral valve r. (SMVR)
    tile plate facet r.
    total hip r. (THR)
    total joint r.
    total knee r.
    tube r.
    valve r.
    valve-sparing aortic root r.
replant
replantation
    intentional r.
    limb r.
replication
    viral r.
repolarization
reposit
reposition
repositioning
    muscle r.
repreparation
reproductive
    r. tract
    r. tract abnormality
requirement
    anticoagulation monitoring r.

reresected
reresecting
reresection
rerouting insertion
rerupture
rescue
    r. analgesia
    r. angioplasty
    r. antiemetic
    r. breathing
    failure to r.
    opioid r.
    propofol r.
    r. surgery
    r. technique
    r. therapy
research
    U.S. Army Institute of Surgical R. (USAISR)
resect
resectability
    r. rate
    surgical r.
    tumor r.
resectable
    r. carcinoma
    r. extrahepatic recurrence
    r. hepatic disease
    r. liver metastasis
    r. periampullary cancer
    r. tumor
resection
    abdominal-perineal r. (APR)
    abdominoperineal r. (APR)
    abdominosacral r.
    absolute curative r.
    absolute noncurative r.
    activation map-guided surgical r.
    anatomic r.
    anterior r.
    r. arthroplasty
    atrial septal r.
    Badgley iliac wing r.
    bar r.
    bilateral r.
    bilobar r.
    bleb r.
    Bloch-Paul-Mikulicz extraperitoneal colon r.
    Böhm spine and limb bony metastasis r.
    bone r.
    bony bridge r.
    bowel r.
    breast r.
    bronchial sleeve r.
    calcaneonavicular bar r.
    carinal r.
    Carrell distal fibula r.

R

resection (*continued*)

caudal lamina r.
central duct r.
cesarean r.
classical subtotal r.
Clayton procedure with panmetatarsal head r.
cold-cup r.
coloanal r.
colon r.
colonic r.
colorectal cancer r.
colosigmoid r.
combined gastrointestinal r.
combined organ r.
complete r.
composite pelvic r.
condyle r.
conservative r.
craniofacial en bloc r.
CRC r.
cricotracheal r.
cryoassisted r.
cuff r.
curative r.
Darrach distal ulna r.
definitive r.
r. dermodesis
diathermic r.
Dillwyn-Evans relapsed club foot r.
duodenopancreatic r.
duodenum-preserving r.
elective sigmoid r.
electrocautery r.
en bloc celiac axis r.
en bloc vein r.
endocardial r.
endometrial r.
endoscopic mucosal r. (EMR)
endoscopic snare r.
end-to-end ileoanal anastomosis without mucosal r.
epidermoid r.
epiphysial bar r.
esophageal r.
esophagogastric r.
ex situ-in situ liver r.
extended r.
extraarticular r.
ex vivo r.
femoral r.
formal hepatic r.
Freund thorax r.
Friede full-thickness eye wall r.
gastric leiomyoma r.
gastrointestinal r.
Girdlestone arthroplasty of hip r.
Guller sigmoid r.

gum r.
Gurd distal clavicle r.
Hartmann perforated sigmoid diverticulitis r.
Henry femoral neck r.
hepatic r.
Hoffmann panmetatarsal head r.
hyoid bone r.
ileal r.
ileocolic r.
ileocolonic r.
iliac crest r.
iliac wing r.
incomplete tumor r.
infundibular wedge r.
Ingram bony bridge r.
initial r.
innominate bone r.
intercalary r.
interdental r.
intestinal r.
intragastric r.
Ivor Lewis esophagus r.
Janecki-Nelson shoulder girdle r.
Karakousis-Vezeridis ischiorectal fossa tumor r.
Klatskin hepatic duct bifurcation r.
kyphos r.
Langenskiöld bony bridge r.
laparoscopic-assisted small bowel r.
laparoscopic bowel r.
laparoscopic hepatic r.
laparoscopic intragastric r.
laparoscopic liver r.
laryngotracheal r.
laser coagulation vaporization procedure-aided r.
lateral rectus r.
LCVP-aided hepatic r.
LCVP-assisted major liver r.
lesser r.
levator r.
Lewis-Chekofsky femur r.
Lewis intercalary r.
limited r.
liver r.
lobar r.
lobe r.
local radical r.
low anterior r. (LAR)
lung r.
major liver r. (MLR)
Mankin knee r.
Marcove-Lewis-Huvos shoulder girdle r.
r. margin
margin r.
marginal r.
r. margin free of tumor (R0)

r. margin macroscopic positive (R2)
r. margin microscopic positive (R1)
massive bowel r.
medial malleolus r.
metatarsal head r.
microscopic r.
Milch cuff r.
Miles abdominoperineal r.
Miltner-Wan calcaneus r.
minimal transurethral r.
Mohs microsurgical r.
mucosal r.
multiple-punch r.
multisegmental r.
Mumford distal clavicle r.
muscle r.
myotomy-myectomy-septal r.
navigated surgical r.
nipple-flat duct r.
nonanatomic wedge r.
ovarian wedge r.
palliative r.
pancreatic r.
pancreaticoduodenal r.
pancreatic tail r.
panmetatarsal head r.
parotid r.
partial cricotracheal r.
partial gastric r.
Paul-Mikulicz staged bowel r.
Peet splanchnic r.
pericystic r.
Peyman full-thickness eye wall r.
Phelps partial r.
portal vein r.
presacral r.
primary r.
prophylactic r.
proximal femoral r.
proximal gastric r.
pulmonary r.
punch r.
R0 r.
R1 r.
R2 r.
radical gastric r.
radical pericystic r.
radical subtotal r.
Radley-Liebig-Brown pubic bone
  chondrosarcoma r.
ray r.
rectal r.
reduction before r.
Reichel-Pólya stomach r.
relative curative r.
relative noncurative r.
rim r.
Rockwood sternoclavicular joint r.
root end r.

scleral r.
sectoral r.
sectorial r.
segmental colonic r.
segmental lung r.
segmental pulmonary r.
segment-oriented hepatic r.
segment-oriented liver r.
septal r.
shoulder girdle r.
sleeve r.
sphincter-saving r.
sphincter-sparing r.
spleen-preserving pancreatic r.
standard gastric r.
stapled transanal rectal r.
  (STARR)
Stener-Gunterberg abdominal sacral
  rectal cancer r.
stomach r.
strip r.
subcomplete r.
submucous r.
subperiosteal r.
subtotal gastric r.
subtotal parenchymal r.
surgical r.
synchronous r.
terminal ileal r.
Thompson r.
thyroid r.
Tikhoff-Linberg shoulder girdle r.
Torek thoracic esophagus cancer r.
Torpin cul-de-sac r.
tracheal r.
transanal endoscopic microsurgical r.
transcervical r.
transgastric laparoscopic r.
transoral odontoid r.
transsphenoidal microsurgical r.
transsphenoidal pituitary r.
transthoracic vertebral body r.
transurethral r.
transverse r.
tumor r.
ultralow anterior r.
unilateral r.
VATS wedge r.
vertebral r.
video-assisted thoracoscopic wedge r.
Weaver-Dunn distal clavicle r.
wedge r.
Whipple pancreatic r.

resectional
r. phase
r. phase of operation
r. technique
resection-arthrodesis
resection-realignment

resective
    r. colostomy
    r. surgery
resectoscopy
resedation
reserve
    hepatic function r.
    life-sustaining hepatic r.
reservoir
    r. host
    hydrogel r.
    r. mucosal absorption
    r. of infection
    r. phase
    pressurized r.
residual
    r. abscess
    r. body
    r. cleft
    r. cyst
    r. cystic cavity
    r. DCIS
    r. disease (R1)
    r. ductal carcinoma
    r. ductal carcinoma in situ
    r. ductal tissue
    r. focus
    r. fragment
    r. lesion
    r. limb pain
    r. mesorectum
    r. neck
    r. neuromuscular blockade
residue
    pharyngeal r.
resin
    r. condensation
    r. restoration
resiniferatoxin
resistance
    activated protein C r.
    alkylation r.
    aortic valve r.
    cerebrovascular r.
    drug r.
    extreme drug r. (EDR)
    increased systemic vascular r.
    insulin r.
    loss of r. (LOR)
    mean airway r.
    peripheral insulin r.
    pulmonary vascular r. (PVR)
    respiratory system r.
    systemic vascular r. (SVR)
    tissue r.
resistentiae
    locus minoris r.
resolution
    spontaneous r.

resolvent
resonance
    r. line
    magnetic r. (MR)
    nuclear magnetic r. (NMR)
resonant abdomen
resorption
respirable aerosol
respiration
    abdominal r.
    absent r.
    accelerated r.
    aerobic r.
    agonal r.
    amphoric r.
    anaerobic r.
    apneustic r.
    artificial r.
    assisted r.
    asthmoid r.
    Austin Flint r.
    Biot r.
    Bouchut r.
    bronchial r.
    bronchocavernous r.
    bronchovesicular r.
    cavernous r.
    central r.
    cerebral r.
    Cheyne-Stokes r.
    cogwheel r.
    collateral r.
    controlled diaphragmatic r.
    Corrigan r.
    cortical r.
    costal r.
    cyclic r.
    decreased r.
    diaphragmatic r.
    diaphragmatic-abdominal r.
    diffusion r.
    direct r.
    divided r.
    electrophrenic r.
    external r.
    forced r.
    granular r.
    grunting r.
    harsh r.
    internal r.
    interrupted r.
    intrauterine r.
    jerky r.
    Kussmaul r.
    Kussmaul-Kien r.
    labored r.
    laryngeal r.
    meningitic r.
    metamorphosing r.

mouth-to-mouth r.
nasal r.
nervous r.
opposition r.
oral r.
paradoxical r.
periodic r.
placental r.
puerile r.
radiofrequency electrophrenic r.
rude r.
Seitz metamorphosing r.
shallow r.
sighing r.
slow r.
sonorous r.
stertorous r.
stridulous r.
supplementary r.
suppressed r.
temperature, pulse, r. (TPR)
thoracic r.
tissue r.
transitional r.
tubular r.
ventilator-assisted r.
vesiculocavernous r.
vicarious r.
wavy r.

respirator
r. brain
r. lung

respiratory
r. ataxia
r. bronchiole
r. bundle
r. burst
r. care
r. complication
r. compromise
r. decompensation
r. depression
r. diaphragm
r. distress syndrome (RDS)
r. drive
r. exchange
r. excursion
r. failure
r. frequency
r. gas monitor
r. insufficiency
r. inversion point
r. kinetic therapy
r. minute volume
r. quotient
r. rate to tidal volume ratio
r. status
r. support
r. syncytial virus conduit

r. syncytial virus infection
r. system resistance
r. tract
r. tract fluid
r. tract infection

respiratory-esophageal fistula
response
anabolic r.
baroreflex r.
biobehavioral r.
brainstem evoked r. (BSER)
callus r.
canal resonance r.
carbon dioxide r.
central carbon dioxide ventilatory r.
clinical r.
Cushing pressure r.
deconditioned exercise r.
detector r.
discography-provoked pain r.
efferent sympathetic r.
r. entropy
foreign body r.
foreign-body fibroblastic r.
hemodynamic r.
hepatic arterial buffer r.
hypercapnic ventilatory r. (HCVR)
hypercontractile external sphincter r.
hypermetabolic r.
hypnotic r.
hypoxic ventilatory r.
immune r.
implantation r.
inflammatory r.
irritant patch-test r.
lactation letdown r.
local twitch r. (LTR)
metabolic r.
motor r.
motor evoked r. (MER)
neuroendocrine stress r.
oxygen-related r.
paired vasomotor r.
pathologic r.
pleiotropic endocrine r.
postburn hypermetabolic r.
radiation r.
relaxation r.
renal artery r.
sensitization r.
severe systemic inflammatory r.
skin potential r.
snout r.
steady-state ventilatory r.
stress r.
stress hormone r.
sympathetic flow r.
sympathetic sweat r.
sympathoadrenal r.

R

response (*continued*)
    sympathoexcitatory r.
    transient hyperemic r.
    twitch r.
    ventilatory r.
    white line r.
responsiveness
    airway r.
    baroreflex r.
rest
    bowel r.
    r. jaw relation
    pancreatic r.
    r. position
    thyroid r.
    thyrothymic thyroid r.
restenosis
    aortic valve r.
    in-stent r.
    r. lesion
    long-term r.
    postangioplasty r.
    postballoon angioplasty r.
    pulmonary valve r.
restiform body
resting
    r. anal sphincter pressure
    r. energy expenditure
    r. length-tension relation
    r. line
    r. membrane potential
    r. urethral pressure profile
restless legs syndrome
restoration
    acid-etched r.
    adhesive resin-bonded cast r.
    alloy r.
    amalgam r.
    Berens-Smith cul-de-sac r.
    bonded cast r.
    buccal r.
    ceramic r.
    ceramometal r.
    combination r.
    composite resin r.
    compound r.
    r. contour
    contour r.
    crown r.
    cul-de-sac r.
    cusp r.
    dental r.
    direct acrylic r.
    direct composite resin r.
    direct gold r.
    distal extension r.
    esthetic r.
    facial r.
    facilitating r.

    faulty r.
    foreskin r.
    full cast r.
    implant r.
    inlay r.
    intermediate r.
    intrinsic r.
    large r.
    maxillary r.
    metal-ceramic r.
    metallic r.
    overhanging r.
    overlay r.
    permanent r.
    physical r.
    pinch r.
    pin-supported r.
    r. point
    porcelain-bonded r.
    porcelain-fused-to-metal r.
    porcelain jacket r.
    postcore r.
    prosthetic r.
    provisional r.
    resin r.
    root canal r.
    silicate r.
    surgical ventricular r.
     (SVR)
    temporary r.
    ventricular r.
    voice r.
restorative
    r. colectomy
    r. fixation
    r. procedure
    r. proctectomy
    r. proctocolectomy
    r. proctocolectomy technique
restriction
    extension r.
    r. fragment length
    soft tissue r.
result
    angiographic r.
    cosmetic r.
    cytologic r.
    false-negative r.
    false-positive r.
    histologic r.
    indocyanine green clearance r.
    operative r.
    postoperative r.
    postprandial motor r.
    short-term r.
    Surveillance, Epidemiology, End R.
     (SEER)
    true-negative r.
    true-positive r.

resurfacing
    facial laser r.
    r. operation
    r. procedure
resurgence
resuscitate
resuscitated by volume
resuscitation
    blood substitute r.
    cardiac r.
    cardiopulmonary r. (CPR)
    delayed r.
    emergency department r.
    r. endpoint
    fluid r.
    heart-lung r.
    hypertonic-hyperoncotic fluid r.
    hypertonic saline r.
    hypotensive r.
    inotrope r.
    intrauterine r.
    intravenous fluid r.
    mouth-to-mouth r.
    neonatal r.
    newborn r.
    r. period
    prehospital r.
    r. process
    r. protocol
    rapid volume r.
    Safar cardiopulmonary r.
    simultaneous compression-ventilation
      cardiopulmonary r. (SCV-CPR)
    supranormal r.
    supraphysiologic r.
resuscitation-induced pulmonary apoptosis
resuscitative
    r. endpoint
    r. fluid
    r. thoracotomy
resuscitator
    self-inflating manual r.
retained
    r. foreign body
    r. gastric antrum syndrome
    r. papilla technique
    r. placental fragment
    r. valvular tissue
retainer closure
retard
    expiratory r.
retardation
    developmental r.
    fetal growth r.
    growth r.
    healing r.
    intrauterine growth r.
    psychomotor r.
retching, vomiturition

rete, *pl.* **retia**
    r. cord
    Haller r.
retention
    r. cyst
    extracoronal r.
    intracoronal-extracoronal r.
    r. mucocele
    pin r.
    r. point
    surgical r.
    r. suture bridge
    r. suture technique
    throat pack r.
    urinary r.
    viscera r.
retentive fulcrum line
Rethi incision
retia (*pl. of* rete)
retial
reticula (*pl. of* reticulum)
reticular, reticulated
    r. endothelial system
    r. formation
    r. lesion
    r. membrane
    r. vein
reticulated (*var. of* reticular)
reticulate pigmented anomaly
reticulation
reticuloendothelial system
reticuloendothelioma
reticulogranuloma
reticulohistiocytoma
reticulospinal tract
reticulotomy
reticulum, *pl.* **reticula**
    Ebner r.
    endoplasmic r.
    extraconal fat r.
retina
retinacula (*pl. of* retinaculum)
retinaculum, *pl.* **retinacula**
    antebrachial flexor r.
    caudal r.
    extensor r.
    Morgagni r.
    patellar r.
    peroneal r.
    superior peroneal r.
retinae
    ablatio r.
retinal
    r. arteriovenous malformation
    r. circulation
    r. examination
    r. excavation
    r. exudate
    r. flap

R

retinal (*continued*)
    r. fold
    r. hemorrhage
    r. imbrication
    r. involvement
    r. macula
    r. migraine
    r. phacoma
    r. pigment epithelial cell
    r. quadrant neovascularization
    r. scatter photocoagulation
    r. surgeon
    r. surgery
    r. treatment
retinectomy
retinitis
retinoblastoma
retinoblastoma-mental retardation syndrome
retinochoroidectomy
retinocytoma
retinoic acid
retinopathy
    diabetic r.
    r. hemorrhage
retinopexy
    pneumatic r.
    Rosengren r.
retinophotoscopy
retinoscopy
    Copeland r.
    cylinder r.
    fogging r.
    streak r.
retinotomy
retothelioma
retract
retracted stoma
retractile testis
retraction
    anterior r.
    clot r.
    downward r.
    lateral r.
    nipple r.
    r. of clot
    panniculus r.
    scar r.
    soft palate r.
    r. space
    stomal r.
    wound r.
retractor
    acetabular r.
    Bookwalter r.
    fan-type r.
    minimal incision total hip r.
    Nathanson r.'s
    r. plication

    sciatic nerve r.
    Thompson-Farley r.
retraining
    computerized diaphragmatic breathing r. (CDBR)
retransplantation
    cardiac r.
retreat
    stabilization on r.
retreatment
    lithotripsy r.
retrenchment
retrieval
    foreign body r.
    intravascular foreign body r.
    stent r.
    transvaginal oocyte r. (TVOR)
    transvaginal ultrasonically guided oocyte r.
retroacetabular lesion
retroadductor space
retroanastomotic hernia
retroarytenoidal edema
retroauricular
    r. free flap
    r. incision
    r. node
retrobulbar
    r. anesthesia
    r. anesthetic technique
    r. hemorrhage
    r. injection
    r. mass
    r. nerve block
    r. orbital metastasis
    r. space
retrocalcaneal bursa
retrocardiac
    r. mass
    r. space
retrocaval ureter
retrocecal
    r. abscess
    r. hernia
    r. recess
retrocervical
retrochiasmal
    r. lesion
    r. optic tract
retroclavicular injury
retroclination
retroclival structure
retroclusion
retrocolic
    r. approach
    r. end-to-end pancreaticojejunostomy
    r. end-to-side choledochojejunostomy
    r. end-to-side gastrojejunostomy

r. hernia
r. position
retrocorneal membrane
retrocrural
r. approach
r. celiac plexus block
r. space
retrocuspid papilla
retrodeviation
retrodiscal, retrodiskal
r. pad
r. temporomandibular joint pad inflammation
retrodiskal (*var. of* retrodiscal)
retrodisplacement
retroduodenal
r. artery
r. fossa
r. perforation
r. recess
retroesophageal
r. artery
r. space
retrofilling method
retroflected (*var. of* retroflexed)
retroflection (*var. of* retroflexion)
retroflexed, retroflected
retroflexion, retroflection
endoscopic r.
retrogasserian
r. glycerol injection
r. neurectomy
r. neurotomy
r. procedure
retrogastric
r. dissection
r. space
retrogeniculate lesion
retrograde
r. atrial activation mapping
r. balloon rupture
r. cannulation
r. catheter insertion
r. catheterization
r. cholangiogram
r. cholecystectomy
r. collateral endoleak
r. direction
r. duodenogastroscopy
r. ejaculation
r. endoscopic approach
r. femoral approach
r. hernia
r. incarceration
r. insertion point
r. intrarenal surgery (RIRS)
myocardium r.
r. nailing
r. nephrostomy puncture

r. obturation
r. percutaneous gastrostomy tube
r. root canal filling method
r. sphincterotomy
r. tracheal intubation anesthetic technique
r. transurethral prostatic urethroplasty
r. valvulotome
r. vascularization of superior mesenteric artery
r. wire intubation
retrohepatic
r. inferior vena cava
r. IVC
r. vein
retrohyoid bursa
retroiliac ureter
retroillumination
retroinguinal space
retrojection
retrojector
retrolabyrinthine
r. presigmoid approach
r. vestibular neurectomy
retrolabyrinthine-retrosigmoid vestibular neurectomy
retrolental space
retrolenticular syndrome
retrolingual
retrolisthesis positional dyskinesia
retromammary
r. bursa
r. space
retromandibular
r. fossa
r. point
r. vein
retromastoid suboccipital craniectomy
retromolar
r. fossa
r. pad
r. papilla
r. triangle
r. trigone
retromuscular
r. position
r. prosthetic technique
r. space
retromylohyoid space
retroocular space
retropancreatic lymph node basin
retropatellar fat pad
retroperitoneal
r. abscess
r. adenopathy
r. approach (RPA)
r. bleeding
r. cavity
r. cutaneous ureterostomy

retroperitoneal (*continued*)
  r. decompression
  r. fibrosis
  r. fistula
  r. gas insufflation
  r. hematoma
  r. hemorrhage
  r. hernia
  r. iliopsoas abscess
  r. incision
  r. infection
  r. lymphadenectomy
  r. lymph node dissection
    (RPLND)
  r. node
  r. pancreas
  r. pelvic lymph node
    dissection
  r. perforation
  r. pneumography
  r. primary rhabdomyosarcoma
  r. region
  r. sarcoma
  r. soft tissue
  r. space
  r. structure
  r. tumor
  r. viscus
retroperitoneoscopic
  r. nephrectomy
  r. nephroureterectomy
retroperitoneoscopy
retroperitoneum
retroperitonitis
retropharyngeal
  r. approach
  r. hematoma
  r. hemorrhage
  r. node
  r. soft tissue
  r. space
retropharynx
retroplacental hematoma
retroposed
retroposition
retropubic
  r. anatomy
  r. colpourethrocystopexy
  r. hernia
  r. Lapides-Ball bladder neck
    suspension
  r. space
  r. urethrocystopexy
  r. urethrolysis
  r. urethroscopy
  r. vesiculoprostatectomy
retropulsed bone excision
retropulsion
retropyloric node

retrorectal
  r. abscess
  r. tumor
retrosacral fascia
retrosellar structure
retrosigmoid approach
retrospection
retrospective analysis
retrosphenoidal syndrome
retrosternal
  r. air space
  r. approach
  r. dislocation
  r. gland
  r. hernia
  r. mass
  r. route
retrotracheal space
retrouterine
retroversioflexion
retroversion
retroverted
retrovesical
  r. hernia
  r. space
retrovirus infection
retrovisceral
  r. fascia
  r. space
retrozygomatic space
retruded
  r. jaw relation
  r. position
retrusive excursion
return
  pulmonary venous r.
  total anomalous pulmonary venous
    r. (TAPVR)
  venous r.
Retzius
  R. cavity
  line of R.
  R. space
  R. vein
reunient
reuptake-inhibitor
revaccination
revascularization
  arrested-heart r.
  arterial r.
  brain r.
  cerebral r.
  coronary r.
  heart laser r.
  hybrid myocardial r.
  infrapopliteal r.
  lower extremity r.
  mesenteric r.
  myocardial r.

penile r.
r. procedure
renal r.
repeat r.
STA-MCA r.
superficial temporal artery to middle
  cerebral artery r.
transmyocardial carbon dioxide
  laser r.
transmyocardial laser r. (TMLR,
  TMR)
revascularized tissue
reverberation room
Reverdin
  R. bunionectomy
  R. epidermal free graft
  R. osteotomy
  R. pinch graft method
Reverdin-Laird
  R.-L. bunionectomy
  R.-L. osteotomy
Reverdin-McBride bunionectomy
reversal
  ileostomy r.
  jejunal-ileal bypass r.
  JIB r.
  r. line
  narcotic r.
  r. of jejunoileal bypass
    surgery
  r. pedicle flap
  pressure r.
  relaxant r.
  sex r.
  unfractionated heparin r.
  vasectomy r.
reverse
  r. augmentation
  r. Barton fracture
  r. bevel incision
  r. Bigelow maneuver
  r. Colles fracture
  r. cross-finger flap
  r. Dillwyn-Evans calcaneal
    osteotomy
  r. Eck fistula
  r. filling procedure
  r. forearm island flap
  r. gastric tube esophagoplasty
  r. Hill-Sachs lesion
  r. Mauck procedure
  r. Monteggia fracture
  r. Putti-Platt procedure
  r. sigma penoscrotal transposition
    repair
  r. steal effect
  r. topographic projection
  r. Trendelenburg position
  r. vein bypass technique

r. wedge osteotomy
r. wedge technique
reversed
  r. left saphenous vein bypass
    graft
  r. reimplanted appendicocystostomy
reverse-Y incision
reversible
  r. decortication
  r. ischemic neurologic deficit
    (RIND)
  r. shock
review
  peer r.
revision
  Fontan r.
  r. hip arthroplasty
  r. laparoscopy
  r. procedure
  scar r.
  shunt r.
  surgical scar r.
revivification
revulsion
rewarming
Rex-Cantli-Serege line
Reynolds pentad
RF
  radiofrequency
RFA
  radiofrequency ablation
  right femoral artery
RFCA
  radiofrequency catheter ablation
RFID
  radiofrequency identification
RFTA
  radiofrequency thermal
    ablation
  radiofrequency tissue ablation
rhabdomyolysis
  acute recurrent r.
  exertional r.
  familial paroxysmal r.
  hypoxia-induced r.
  idiopathic paroxysmal r.
rhabdomyoma
  cardiac r.
  clinically silent r.
rhabdomyosarcoma, rhabdosarcoma
  abdominal wall r.
  advanced retroperitoneal r.
  alveolar r.
  primary r.
  retroperitoneal primary r.
  vaginal r.
rhabdosarcoma (*var. of*
  rhabdomyosarcoma)
rhabdosphincter

rhachotomy
Capener lateral r.
decompression r.
lateral r.
rhaphe (*var. of* raphe)
rhegma
rhegmatogenous
rheologic therapy
rheolytic catheter thrombectomy
Rhese
R. position
R. projection
rheumatica
polymyalgia r.
rheumatoid arthritis (RA)
rheumatoid-related ulceration
rhexis
hemorrhage per r.
rhinitis
rhinocanthectomy
rhinocerebral infection
rhinocheiloplasty (*var. of*
rhinochiloplasty)
rhinochiloplasty, rhinocheiloplasty
rhinocleisis
rhinodymia
rhinokyphectomy
rhinology
rhinometry
acoustic r.
rhinopharyngeal
rhinopharynx
rhinoplasty
aesthetic r.
English r.
esthetic r.
Indian r.
Italian r.
Joseph r.
rhinorrhea
purulent r.
rhinoscleroma
rhinoscopy
rhinoseptal approach
rhinotomy
rhizolysis
chemical r.
percutaneous glycerol r. (PGR)
percutaneous radiofrequency r.
percutaneous retrogasserian glycerol
r.
Rhizopus **infection**
rhizotomy
anterior r.
bilateral ventral r.
cranial nerve r.
Dana posterior r.
Dandy trigeminal r.
dorsal r.

facet r.
Frazier-Spiller r.
glycerol r.
intracranial r.
intradural dorsal spinal root r.
percutaneous radiofrequency dorsal r.
posterior r.
radiofrequency r.
selective posterior r. (SPR)
selective sacral r.
thermal r.
trigeminal r.
rhombic
rhomboatloideus
rhombocele
rhomboid, rhomboidal
r. ligament
r. major muscle
r. minor muscle
r. transposition flap
rhomboidal (*var. of* rhomboid)
r. sinus
rhomboidalis
sinus r.
Rhoton suction
rhythm
ectopic r.
fibrillation r.
sinus r.
rhythmic, rhythmical
r. initiation technique
r. stabilization
rhythmical (*var. of* rhythmic)
rhytide
rhytidectomy
rhytidoplasty
rib
bicipital r.
bifid r.
cervical r.
r. diastasis
double-exposed r.
false r.
floating r.
r. fracture
lumbar r.
r. notching
pillar r.
r. removal
slipping r.
r. tip syndrome
true r.
vertebral r.
vertebrochondral r.
vertebrosternal r.
ribbon
r. arch technique
r. muscle
rib-cage volume

Ribes ganglion
rice body
RICH
    rapidly involuting congenital
    hemangioma
Richard fringe
Richardson suture technique
Riche-Cannieu anastomosis
Richet ectropion operation
Richmond bolt
Richter
        R. and Albrich vaginal sacrospinous
          suspension procedure
        R. hernia
        R. suture technique
Richter-Monro line
rickets
        celiac r.
Ricketts-Abrams 2-catheter coronary
  arteriography technique
rickettsial infection
Rideau hip contracture release
  technique
ridge
        bicipital r.
        epidermal r.
        r. extension
        external oblique r.
        healing r.
        mesonephric r.
        midwound healing r.
        mylohyoid r.
        osteochondral r.
        Passavant r.
        petrous r.
        pharyngeal r.
        r. relation
        sphenoidal r.
        supraorbital r.
        temporal r.
        trapezoid r.
        urogenital r.
Ridley sinus
Riedel
        R. frontoethmoidectomy procedure
        R. lobe
        R. thyroiditis
Rieger syndrome
Rieux hernia
right
        r. acromiodorsoposterior fetal
          position
        r. anterior oblique (RAO)
        r. anterior oblique angulation
        r. anterior oblique position
        r. anterior occipital (RAO)
        r. anterior pararenal space
        r. atrial pressure
        r. branch

r. bundle branch block
r. carotid artery (RCA)
r. caudate lobe
r. colic artery
r. colic flexure
r. common iliac nerve
r. coronary artery (RCA)
r. coronary valve
r. crural area
deviation to r.
r. femoral artery (RFA)
r. fibrous trigone
r. gastric vein
r. gastroepiploic vein
r. gastroomental vein
r. heart catheterization
r. hemicolectomy
r. hemidiaphragm
r. hepatectomy
r. hepatic vein
r. hypochondriac region
r. iliac region
r. inguinal hernia (RIH)
r. internal thoracic artery (RITA)
r. lateral region
r. lobe hepatectomy
r. lower extremity (RLE)
r. lower quadrant (RLQ)
r. lymphatic duct
r. main bronchus
r. middle suprarenal artery
r. midinguinal line
r. obturator artery
r. ovary
r. prostatic ligament
r. replaced hepatic artery
r. rotation
r. sagittal fissure
r. septal valve
r. sigmoid sinus
r. subclavian artery
r. subclavian vessel
r. temporoparietal craniotomy
r. testicular artery
r. thorax
r. triangular ligament
r. umbilical fold
r. upper extremity (RUE)
r. upper quadrant (RUQ)
r. upper quadrant peritonectomy
r. ventricle
r. ventricle-pulmonary artery conduit
  surgery
r. ventricular assistive device
  (RVAD)
r. ventricular ejection fraction
  (RVEF)
r. ventricular end-diastolic pressure
r. ventricular outflow tract (RVOT)

R

right (*continued*)
    r. ventricular outflow tract
      tachycardia
    r. ventricular stroke work index
      (RVSWI)
    r. ventricular systolic pressure
    r. vertebral artery
right-angled end-to-side anastomosis
right-angle technique
right-sided
    r.-s. injury
    r.-s. lesion
    r.-s. submandibular transverse
      incision
    r.-s. thoracotomy
right-side-down position
rightward pressure
rigid
    r. body
    r. bronchoscopy
    r. cervical immobilization
    r. endofluoroscopy
    r. endoscopic surgery
    r. graft
    r. internal fixation
    r. plate fixation
    r. proctoscopy
    r. proctosigmoidoscopy
    r. ureteroscopy
rigidity
    abdominal r.
    boardlike r.
    chest wall r.
    masseter muscle r.
    spinal fixation r.
rigidus
    hallux r.
rigors
    frank r.
RIGS
    radioimmunoguided surgery
RIH
    right inguinal hernia
Riley-Day syndrome
Riley-Smith syndrome
rim
    r. incision
    r. mandibulectomy
    palpebral r.
    r. resection
    surgical occlusion r.
rima, *pl.* **rimae**
    r. glottidis
    r. vestibuli
rimae (*pl. of* rima)
rim-enhancing lesion
RIND
    reversible ischemic neurologic
    deficit

ring
    abdominal r.
    r. abscess
    abscess r.
    acetabular reinforcement r.
    amnion r.
    anorectal r.
    anterior limiting r.
    aortic r.
    r. apophysis
    arterial r.
    atrial r.
    atrioventricular r.
    B r.
    r. block
    r. block digital anesthetic
    Bochdalek r.
    cardiac lymphatic r.
    cataract mask r.
    choroidal r.
    ciliary r.
    Coats white r.
    collagenous trabecular r.
    common annular r.
    common tendinous r.
    congenital r.
    conjunctival r.
    constriction r.
    contractile r.
    coronary r.
    cricoid r.
    crural r.
    r. D chromosome syndrome
    deep inguinal r.
    distal esophageal r.
    double r.
    doughnut r.
    drop-lock r.
    dural r.
    enhancing r.
    epiphysial r.
    r. epiphysis
    esophageal A, B r.
    esophageal contractile r.
    esophageal contraction r.
    esophageal mucosal r.
    esophageal muscular r.
    external inguinal r.
    extracapsular arterial r.
    femoral r.
    fibrous r.
    r. finger
    r. fracture
    glaucomatous r.
    glial r.
    gold r.
    greater r.
    head r.
    hernial r.

R

hymenal r.
ilioinguinal r.
iliopsoas r.
inguinal r.
internal abdominal r.
internal inguinal r.
iris r.
ischial weightbearing r.
lenticular r.
r. lesion
lesser r.
lymphoid r.
Morgagni r.
mucosal esophageal r.
muscular esophageal r.
narrow internal r.
neonatal r.
r. of Lacroix
orthosis drop-lock r.
osseoligamentous r.
palatopharyngeal r.
pathologic retraction r.
pelvic r.
pericardial r.
perichondral r.
perineal hernia r.
periureteric venous r.
physiologic retraction r.
Placido r.
posterior limiting r.
pressure r.
pressure-point tension r.
protrusio r.
proximal-to-distal r.
pyloric r.
reduction r.
rust r.
Schatzki esophageal r.
Schwalbe anterior
  border r.
scotoma r.
Soemmerring r.
r. structure
subcutaneous r.
suture r.
symblepharon r.
tentorial r.
tracheal r.
trigonal r.
T-shaped constriction r.
tympanic r.
r. ulcer
umbilical r.
vascular r.
Vieussens r.
Waldeyer r.
white r.
wide internal inguinal r.
ring-disrupting fracture

Ringer arthroscopy
ring-form congenital cataract
ring-shaped cataract
ring-wall lesion
ringworm
Rinkel serial endpoint
  titration
Riolan
    R. anastomosis
    R. arc
    R. arcade
    R. bone
    R. muscle
Riordan
    R. pollicization
    R. tendon transfer technique
rip-cord suture
Ripstein
    R. anterior sling rectopexy
    R. prolapsed rectum repair
      procedure
    R. rectal prolapse operation
RIRS
    retrograde intrarenal surgery
Risdon submandibular approach
rise
    pressure r.
Riseborough-Radin intercondylar fracture
  classification
risk
    anesthetic r.
    bleeding r.
    breast cancer r.
    r. classification
    r. factor
    Goldman classification operative r.
    r. index
    inherent r.
    r. management
    r. management of anesthesia
    perforation r.
    perioperative aspiration r.
    radiation r.
    r. reduction
    surgical r.
risorius muscle
Risser
    R. cast technique
    R. skeletal maturity method
RITA
    right internal thoracic artery
Ritgen fetal head delivery maneuver
Riva-Rocci blood pressure measurement
  method
Rives splenectomy
Rives-Stoppa incisional hernia repair
  technique
Rives-Stoppa-Wantz retrorectus
  repair

Rivinus
  R. canal
  R. duct
  R. gland
Rizzoli arthroplasty
RK
  radial keratotomy
RLE
  right lower extremity
RLN
  recurrent laryngeal nerve
RLND
  retroperitoneal lymph node
  dissection
RLQ
  right lower quadrant
RLT
  reduced liver transplant
RND
  radical neck dissection
RNFA
  Registered Nurse, First Assist
Roaf syndrome
Robert pelvis
Roberts
  R. approach
  R. fat grafting technique
  R. syndrome
robertsonian fusion
Robertson incision
Robinson
  R. anterior cervical discectomy
  R. cervical spine fusion
  R. morcellation
  R. nephrostomy tube
Robinson-Southwick cervical spine fusion
  technique
robot
  da Vinci r.
  parallel r.
robot-assisted
  r.-a. laparoscopy
  r.-a. registration
  r.-a. surgery (RAS)
robot-enhanced Dresden technique
  coronary artery bypass (REDTCAB)
robotic
  r. approach
  r. probing
  r. surgery
robotically assisted vision-enhanced
  coronary artery bypass (RAVECAB)
robotic-assisted
  r.-a. laparoscopic bariatric surgery
  r.-a. pyeloplasty
Robson
  R. point
  R. position
Rockey-Davis incision

Rockwood
  R. acromioclavicular injury
  classification
  R. acromioclavicular joint dislocation
  repair procedure
  R. clavicular fracture classification
  R. posterior capsulorrhaphy
  R. sternoclavicular joint resection
Rockwood-Green orthopaedic casting
  technique
Rockwood-Matsen capsular shift shoulder
  repair procedure
rocuronium bromide
rocuronium-desflurane
rod
  r. cell
  r. contour preparation
  r. fiber
  r. fracture repair
  r. granule
  r. migration
  r. placement
  r. rotation prevention
  r. sleeve fixation
  r. spherule
rodless end-loop stoma
Rodman incision
Rodney Smith biliary stricture repair
Roeder loop knot
roentgenographic evaluation
rofecoxib
Rogers cervical fusion technique
Röhrer index
Rokitansky hernia
rolandic
  r. artery
  r. line
  r. vein
Roland-Morris disability questionnaire
Rolando
  R. fissure
  R. fracture
  R. vein
role
  r. fixation
  inhibitory r.
roll
  iliac r.
  scleral r.
  r. stitch
rolled shoulder lesion
rollerball
  r. endometrial ablation (REA)
  r. technique
Rollet incision
rolling
  r. hiatal hernia
  r. membrane
roll-tube technique

ROM
 range of motion
 rupture of membranes
rongeur
rongeured
Rood neuromuscular facilitation technique
roof fracture
roof-patch graft
room
 emergency r. (ER)
 operating r. (OR)
 recovery r.
 reverberation r.
 surgical dressing r.
 trauma r.
Roos transaxillary 1st rib resection approach
root
 accessory nerve r.
 r. amputation
 anatomical r.
 r. anomaly
 ansa cervicalis r.
 anterior r.
 bifurcation of r.
 r. canal
 r. canal access
 r. canal débridement
 r. canal disinfection
 r. canal electrosterilization
 r. canal filling
 r. canal filling technique obturation
 r. canal ionization
 r. canal orifice
 r. canal point
 r. canal restoration
 r. canal shaping
 r. canal sterilization
 r. canal therapy
 r. canal treatment
 ciliary ganglion r.
 r. compression
 dorsal r.
 dural nerve r.
 r. end resection
 facial r.
 facial nerve r.
 r. formation
 r. fracture
 r. furcation
 r. fusion
 glossopharyngeal nerve r.
 r. infiltration
 r. injection
 lateral r.
 nail r.
 nerve r.
 r. perforation

 posterior r.
 spinal r.
 trigeminal nerve r.
 vagus nerve r.
 ventral r.
rootlet
 cranial nerve r.
Root-Siegal varus derotational osteotomy
rope flap
ropivacaine
Rorabeck fasciotomy
Rosch modification
rosebud stoma
Rosenberg endoscopic anterior cruciate ligament reconstruction
Rosenburg operation
Rosengren retinopexy
Rosen incision
Rosenmüller
 R. body
 R. fossa
 R. gland
 R. node
 R. recess
 valve of R.
Rosenthal
 basal vein of R.
 R. fiber
 R. nail injury classification
 R. vein
Rose position
Roser-Nélaton line
rosette kidney
Ross
 R. aortic valve replacement procedure
 R. body
 R. mitral valve replacement technique
Rossetti
 R. modification
 R. modification of Nissen fundoplication
Rossetti-Hell modification of Nissen fundoplication
rostrad
rostral
 r. anterior cingulate cortex
 r. cingulotomy
 r. transtentorial herniation
 r. ventrolateral medulla
 r. ventrolateral medulla oblongata
rostralis
rostrate
rostriform
rostrocaudal extent signal abnormality
rostrum
rotablator phlebectomy

R

rotary
r. joint
r. mounted point
r. shadowing electron microscopy
r. subluxation

rotated
externally r.

rotating
r. aspiration thromboembolectomy (RAT)
r. disc oxygenation
r. frame imaging
r. frame zeugmatography

rotating-frame zeugmatography

rotation
abduction-external r. (AER)
adduction-internal r.
anisotropic r.
anterior innominate r.
axial r.
axis of r.
Borggreve limb r.
caudal-cranial r.
cervical general r.
clockwise r.
counterclockwise r.
r. drawer test
eversion-external r.
external r.
external/internal r.
eye r.
r. flap
flexion, abduction, external r. (faber)
flexion in abduction and external r. (faber)
flexion in adduction and internal r. (fadir)
flexion-internal r.
foot r.
forceps r.
r. fracture
gantry r.
hip r.
horizontal external r.
intentional r.
internal r.
internal-external r.
intersegmental r.
intestinal r.
inversion-eversion r.
inward r.
r. joint
knee r.
left r.
lumbar r.
manual r.
medial r.
r. mobility

neutral r.
opioid r.
optic r.
organoaxial r.
outward r.
pelvic r.
r. plasty
polycentric r.
posterior innominate r.
pronation eversion external r. (PEER)
pure r.
r. recurvatum test
right r.
sagittal r.
shoulder r.
specific r.
spine r.
sternal r.
supination-external r. (SER)
synchronous scapuloclavicular r.
r. testing
r. therapy
timed intermittent r.
twin bracket tooth r.
vertebral r.
visceral r.
wheel r.

rotational
r. ablation
r. angioplasty
r. blood flow
r. burst fracture
r. contact lithotripsy
r. coronary atherectomy
r. correction
r. deformity
r. dislocation
r. flap
r. osteotomy
r. thrombectomy

rotationally induced shear-strain lesion
rotation-compression maneuver
rotation-plasty
Borggreve r.-p.

rotationplasty
Kotz-Salzer r.
van Ness r.
Winkelmann r.

rotator
r. cuff
r. cuff advancer
r. cuff arthropathy
r. cuff lesion
r. cuff muscle
r. cuff repair
r. cuff tear
r. cuff tear arthroplasty
external r.

R

r. flap
internal r.
medial r.
nucleus r.

rotatory
r. fixation
r. luxation

rotavirus infection
Rothman Institute total hip program
Rothner headache model
Rotterdam Symptom Checklist
rotunda
Rouget bulb
rough tissue handling
rouleaux formation
round
r. back deformity
r. body
r. cell liposarcoma
r. foramen
r. hemorrhage
r. pelvis
r. shoulder deformity
r. spermatid
r. uterine ligament

rounded contour
round-robin classification
route
endoscopic r.
external r.
r. of administration
r. of injection
r. of insertion
retrosternal r.
subcutaneous r.
transthoracic r.

routine
r. bilateral neck exploration
r. laparotomy
r. unilateral exploration

Roux
R. gastric reconstruction
R. gastroenterostomy
R. limb
R. limb stump
R. limb stump dehiscence
R. limb stump leak
R. stasis syndrome

Roux-duToit staple capsulorrhaphy
Roux-en-Y
R.-e.-Y biliary bypass
R.-e.-Y biliary bypass with antrectomy
R.-e.-Y choledochojejunostomy
R.-e.-Y cystojejunostomy
R.-e.-Y distal jejunoileostomy
R.-e.-Y esophagojejunostomy
R.-e.-Y gastric bypass
R.-e.-Y gastroenterostomy

R.-e.-Y gastrointestinal system procedure
R.-e.-Y gastrojejunostomy
R.-e.-Y hepaticojejunal anastomosis
R.-e.-Y hepaticojejunostomy
R.-e.-Y jejunal loop incision
R.-e.-Y limb
R.-e.-Y limb enteroscopy
R.-e.-Y loop
R.-e.-Y operation
R.-e.-Y pancreatojejunostomy
R.-e.-Y procedure with vagotomy
R.-e.-Y reconstruction

Roux-Goldthwait
R.-G. dislocation operation
R.-G. repair of recurrent patellar dislocation procedure

Roveda epicanthus and blepharophimosis correction
Rovsing
R. polycystic kidney operation
R. sign

Rowbotham
R. neurological operation
R. orbital decompression

Rowe
R. calcaneal fracture classification
R. posterior shoulder approach

Rowe-Lowell
R.-L. hip dislocation classification
R.-L. system for fracture-dislocation classification

Rowe-Zarins shoulder immobilization
Rowinski
R. dacryostomy
R. kidney transplant operation

Royle posterior hemivertebra approach
Royle-Thompson tendon transfer technique
RPC
recurrent pyogenic cholangiohepatitis

RPG
radiologic percutaneous gastrostomy
RPG tube

RPH
retroperitoneal hemorrhage

RPLND
retroperitoneal lymph node dissection

RPT
rapid pull-through
RPT technique

RSD
reflex sympathetic dystrophy

RSI
rapid sequence induction
RSI orotracheal intubation

rub
peritoneal friction r.
textured fabric r.

rubber
>   r. mouth prop
>   r. suture
>   r. tissue

rubber-band
>   r.-b. extraction
>   r.-b. hemorrhoidectomy
>   r.-b. ligation
>   r.-b. ligation of hemorrhoid

rubbery
>   r. mass
>   r. texture

rubbing
>   desensitization with towel r.

Rubbrecht
>   R. extirpation
>   R. malocclusion operation

Rubens breast flap

Rubin
>   R. shoulder dystocia maneuver
>   R. tubal insufflation

rubrobulbar tract

rubroreticular tract

rubrospinal
>   r. decussation
>   r. tract

Rucker body

Ruddy incision

rude respiration

RUE
>   right upper extremity

Ruedemann enucleation operation

Ruedi-Allgower pilon fracture classification

ruffed canal

ruga, *pl.* **rugae**

rugae (*pl. of* ruga)

rugal column

rugine

rugose, rugous

rugosity

rugous (*var. of* rugose)

Ruiz
>   R. astigmatic keratotomy procedure
>   R. trapezoidal keratotomy

Ruiz-Mora
>   R.-M. correction
>   R.-M. proximal phalangectomy for hammertoe procedure

rule
>   Goodsall anal fistula r.
>   Meyer-Overton r.

rumination

Rungstrom projection

running
>   r. continuous suture technique
>   r. locked stitch
>   r. stitch

>   r. vascular technique
>   r. vascular technique without tension

runoff

Runyon nontuberculous mycobacteria classification

rupture
>   Achilles tendon r.
>   acute hepatic r.
>   adductor longus muscle r.
>   amnion r.
>   aneurysmal r.
>   anterior talofibular ligament r.
>   aortic r.
>   balloon r.
>   cardiac r.
>   chamber r.
>   chordae tendineae r.
>   chordal r.
>   choroidal r.
>   collateral ligament r.
>   complete r.
>   contained r.
>   crescentic r.
>   diaphragmatic r.
>   distal biceps brachii tendon r.
>   ERCP-induced splenic r.
>   esophageal r.
>   flexor tendon r.
>   frank intrabiliary r.
>   free r.
>   gastric r.
>   hemidiaphragm r.
>   hepatic r.
>   hernia r.
>   hydatid cyst intrahepatic r.
>   incidental r.
>   inflammatory r.
>   infrapatellar tendon r.
>   interventricular septal r.
>   intramural esophageal r.
>   intraoperative r.
>   intraperitoneal viscus r.
>   intrapleural r.
>   ligament r.
>   longitudinal ligament r.
>   Mallory-Weiss mucosal r.
>   marginal sinus r.
>   membrane r.
>   mesenteric r.
>   myocardial r.
>   neglected r.
>   nonpenetrating r.
>   r. of membranes (ROM)
>   papillary muscle r.
>   penetrating r.
>   penile r.
>   plaque r.
>   postmembrane r.
>   prelabor membrane r.

premature amnion r.
premature membrane r.
premembrane r.
prolonged r.
proximal tendon r.
rectosigmoid r.
renal allograft r.
renal artery r.
retrograde balloon r.
scar r.
scleral r.
splenic r.
spontaneous r.
spontaneous esophageal r.
stress r.
tendon r.
testicular r.
total perineal r.
transverse ligament r.
traumatic aortic r.
traumatic choroidal r.
tubal r.
ulnar collateral ligament r.
umbilical hernia r.
urinary bladder r.
uterine r.
valve r.
ventricular septal r.
ruptured
r. abdominal aortic aneurysm
r. appendicitis
r. disc
r. disc excision
r. episiotomy
r. peliotic lesion
r. pseudoaneurysm
rupture-delivery interval
RUQ
right upper quadrant
Russe
R. classification

R. scaphoid fracture technique
R. scaphoid nonunion bone grafting
technique
**Russe-Gerhardt range of motion of
living joints method**
Russell
R. fibular head autograft
hooked bundle of R.
R. percutaneous endoscopic
gastrostomy
uncinate bundle of R.
Russell-Taylor hip fracture classification
rust ring
Rüter classification
**Rutkow and Robbins direct or indirect
inguinal hernia operation**
**Rutkow-Robbins-Gilbert inguinal hernia
classification**
**Rutledge extended hysterectomy
classification**
ruyschian membrane
Ruysch membrane
RVAD
right ventricular assistive device
RVEF
right ventricular ejection fraction
RVH
renovascular hypertension
RVOT
right ventricular outflow tract
RVSWI
right ventricular stroke work index
RWMA
regional wall motion abnormality
ryanodine test
Rycroft empty eye socket operation
Rye Hodgkin disease classification
Ryerson
R. bone graft
R. triple arthrodesis of foot
procedure

R

S

S incision
S pelvic ileal
  pouch

SA

septal apical
sinuatrial
spinal anesthesia
splenic artery
  SA node
  SA segment

S-A

sinuatrial

SAA

splenic artery aneurysm

SAB

subarachnoid block

saber-cut

s.-c. approach
s.-c. incision

saber-sheath trachea
sabre-shin deformity
sac

abdominal s.
air s.
allantoic s.
alveolar s.
amniotic s.
aneurysmal s.
aortic s.
bursal s.
caudal s.
chorionic s.
common dural s.
conjunctival s.
cupular blind s.
dental s.
double decidual s.
embryonic s.
empty gestational s.
enamel s.
endolymphatic s.
enterocele s.
s. extirpation
fluid-filled s.
s. formation
gestational s.
giant prosthetic reinforcement of
  visceral s. (GPRVS)
greater peritoneal s.
heart s.
hernia s.
hydrocele s.
indirect hernial s.
lacrimal s.

lateral s.
lesser peritoneal s.
Mikulicz s.
nasolacrimal s.
omental s.
pericardial s.
peritoneal s.
Pleatman s.
pleural s.
preputial s.
primary yolk s.
primitive yolk s.
pseudogestational s.
pudendal s.
secondary yolk s.
serous s.
Stoppa giant prosthetic reinforcement
  of visceral s.
tear s.
thecal s.
tooth s.
vestibular blind s.
vitelline s.
wide-mouth s.
yolk s.

saccade

intentional s.
reflexive s.
volitional s.

saccadic

s. eccentric target
s. eye movement

saccate
sacciform recess
saccular

s. aneurysm
s. collection
s. spot

sacculated
sacculation
saccule
sacculi (*pl. of* sacculus)
sacculotomy
sacculus, *pl.* **sacculi**
saccus
sack

entrapment s.

saclike cavity
SACP

selective antegrade cerebral perfusion

sacrad
sacral

s. ala
s. anesthesia
s. arcuate line

sacral (*continued*)
    s. bar technique
    s. bone tumor
    s. brim target point
    s. canal
    s. crest
    s. foramen
    s. fracture
    s. ganglion
    s. hiatus
    s. horizontal plane line
    s. horn
    s. index
    s. pedicle screw fixation
    s. promontory
    s. region
    s. screw placement
    s. spine fixation
    s. spine fusion
    s. spine stabilization
    s. splanchnic nerve
    s. triangle
    s. venous plexus
    s. vertebra
sacral-foraminal approach
sacralization
sacrectomy
sacred bone
sacroabdominoperineal pull-through
sacroanterior fetal position
sacrococcygeal
    s. cyst
    s. disc
    s. joint
    s. junction
    s. ligament
    s. tumor
sacrococcygeus
sacrocolpopexy
    abdominal s.
sacrodural ligament
sacrofixation
sacrogenital fold
sacroiliac (SI)
    s. approach
    s. articulation
    s. buttressing procedure
    s. disarticulation
    s. dislocation
    s. extension fixation
    s. flexion fixation
    s. fracture
    s. joint
    s. joint dysfunction
    s. ligament
sacrolisthesis
sacrolumbar
sacropelvic
sacroperineal approach

sacropexy
    abdominal s.
sacroposterior fetal position
sacrosciatic
sacrospinal
sacrospinous
    s. ligament
    s. ligament suspension
    s. ligament vaginal fixation
sacrotomy
sacrotransverse fetal position
sacrotuberous ligament
sacrouterine fold
sacrovaginal fold
sacrovertebral
sacrovesical fold
sacrum
    assimilation s.
    s. fracture
    s. fusion screw fixation
saddle
    s. block
    s. block anesthesia
    s. connector base
    s. lesion
    syringe s.
    Turkish s.
saddle-nose deformity
Sade
    S. modification
    S. modification of Norwood
        procedure
SAE
    serious adverse event
Saeed esophageal banding technique
Saemisch
    S. corneal transfixion operation
    S. section
Saenger
    S. cesarean operation
    S. suture technique
Safar cardiopulmonary resuscitation
safety
    Leapfrog Group for Patient S.
    s. program
Safil synthetic absorbable surgical suture
Sage-Clark cheilectomy
SAGES
    Society of American Gastrointestinal
    Endoscopic Surgeons
Sage-Salvatore acromioclavicular joint injury classification
sagittal
    s. deformity
    s. fissure
    s. plane
    s. plane imaging
    s. plane instability

s. projection
s. reconstruction
s. rotation
s. section
s. slice fracture
s. spin-echo image
s. suture line
s. venous sinus
sagittal-split mandibular osteotomy
Saha
S. shoulder muscle classification
S. trapezius muscle transfer
technique
Sakati-Nyhan syndrome
Sakellarides calcaneal fracture classification
Sakellarides-DeWeese ulnar collateral ligament reconstuction technique
Sakoff osteotomy
saline
hypertonic lactated s.
ice-cold s.
s. injection
s. injection therapy
intravenous s.
s. lavage
s. manometer
normal s.
phosphate buffered s.
s. solution
s. technique
saline-epinephrine
Salinem infection
saliva
salivary
s. duct
s. duct carcinoma
s. EGF
s. epithelium
s. fistula
s. gland
s. gland carcinoma
s. gland infection
s. gland tumor
s. mass
salivation
Salmon backcut incision
salmon-patch
s.-p. hemorrhage
s.-p. hue
salmon-pink epithelium
salpingectomy
salpinges (*pl. of* salpinx)
salpingian
salpingioma
salpingitis
salpingocele
salpingolysis
salpingoneostomy

salpingo-oophorectomy
abdominal s.-o.
bilateral s.-o. (BSO)
total abdominal hysterectomy and
bilateral s.-o. (TAHBSO)
unilateral s.-o.
salpingo-oophorocele
salpingoovariectomy
salpingo-ovariolysis
salpingopalatine
s. fold
s. membrane
salpingopexy
salpingopharyngeal
s. fascia
s. fold
s. membrane
s. muscle
salpingoplasty
salpingorrhaphy
salpingoscopy
salpingostomatomy
salpingostomy
linear s.
salpingotomy
abdominal s.
salpinx, *pl.* **salpinges**
Salter
S. epiphysial fracture classification
S. incremental line
S. innominate osteotomy
S. innominate osteotomy technique
S. I–VI fracture
S. pelvic osteotomy
Salter-Harris
S.-H. epiphysial fracture
classification
S.-H. fracture
saltwater solution
salvage
s. balloon angioplasty
s. cystectomy
s. cytology
limb s.
s. procedure
s. prostatectomy
splenic s.
s. surgery
s. therapy
SAMBA
simultaneous areolar mastopexy and
breast augmentation
same-day
s.-d. admit
s.-d. discharge
Samilson
S. crescentic calcaneal osteotomy
S. sliding osteotomy of calcaneus
procedure

S

Sammarco-DiRaimondo
    S.-D. modification
    S.-D. modification of Elmslie lateral
    ankle reconstruction technique
sample
    bile s.
    biopsy s.
    cytology s.
    FNA s.
    intraoperative bile s.
    peritoneal cytology s.
    population s.
    wire-guided biopsy s.
sampling
    adrenal vein s.
    endocervical s.
    endometrial s.
    fetal tissue s.
    incremental blood s.
    laparoscopic paraaortic lymph
    node s.
    lymph node s.
    percutaneous fetal tissue s.
    selective venous s.
    tissue s.
    venous s.
Sampoelesi line
Sampson cyst
Samuel position
sand
    s. body
    urinary s.
Sanders
    S. incision
    S. pediatric bronchoscopy
    technique
    S. thoracic outlet decompression
    operation
Sandimmune
Sandström body
sandwich
    s. patch
    s. staghorn calculus therapy
sandwiched iliac bone graft
Sanger incision
sanguification
sanguineous
    s. exudate
    s. infiltration
    s. inflammation
    s. perfusion
sanitation
sanitization
San Jiao meridian
Santiani-Stone pancreas head gunshot
  classification
Santorini
    S. canal
    S. cartilage

    S. duct
    S. fissure
    S. labyrinth
    S. major caruncle
    S. minor caruncle
    S. plexus
    S. vein
SaO$_2$
    arterial oxygen saturation
SAP
    severe acute pancreatitis
    systolic arterial pressure
saphena
saphenectomy
saphenofemoral
    s. incompetence
    s. reflux
saphenous
    s. branch
    s. flap
    s. hiatus
    s. ICA bypass
    s. nerve block
    s. opening
    s. phlebography
    s. vein
    s. vein bypass (SVB)
    s. vein bypass graft
    s. vein patch graft
    s. vein stripping
Sappey
    S. fiber
    S. plexus
saprophyte
SAPS
    simplified acute physiology
    score
sarcocele
sarcoid
sarcoidosis
sarcolemmal membrane
sarcology
sarcoma
    Abernethy s.
    embryonal s.
    high-grade s.
    juxtacortical osteogenic s.
    osteogenic s.
    primary extremity synovial s.
    recurrent s.
    retroperitoneal s.
    soft tissue s. (STS)
    spindle cell s.
    s. surgery
    undifferentiated embryonal s.
sarcomatosis
sarcomatosum
    glioma s.
    myxoma s.

sarcomere
sarcoplasmic reticulum permeability
sarcotripsy
Sargenti root canal method
Sarmiento
    S. intertrochanteric osteotomy
    S. trochanteric fracture technique
sartorial slide procedure
sartorius muscle
Sassouni skeletal facial classification
satellite
    s. abscess
    s. lesion
    s. metastasis
    s. myofascial trigger point
satellitosis
Satinsky clamp
Sato
    S. radial keratotomy operation
    S. radial keratotomy procedure
saturated solution
saturation
    s. analysis
    arterial oxygen s. (SaO_2)
    arterial oxyhemoglobin s.
    color s.
    s. current
    hepatovenous oxygen s.
    s. index
    jugular bulb venous oxygen s.
    jugular venous oxygen s. ($SjVO_2$)
    mixed venous oxygen s. (MVO_2S)
    s. output
    oxygen s. (O_2 sat.)
    partial s.
    progressive spin s.
    receiver s.
    s. recovery
    regional s.
    secondary s.
    selective s.
    sensorial s.
    step-up in oxygen s.
    s. time
    s. transfer
    venous s.
saturnine colic
saucerization
saucerized biopsy
sausage-shaped appearance
Sauve-Kapandji distal radioulnar joint repair procedure
Savage perineal body
Savary-Miller endoscopic reflux esophagitis classification
Savin cryorectal operation
Sawyer afferent loop operation
Saxtorph forceps delivery maneuver

Sayoc
    S. orbicularis levator fixation operation
    S. upper lid fold creation procedure
S-B
    Sengstaken-Blakemore
    S-B tube
SB
    septal basal
    SB segment
SBP
    systolic blood pressure
SBR
    Scarff-Bloom-Richardson
    SBR breast cancer classification
    SBR breast cancer grade
    SBR staging
SC
    supraclavicular
    supracondylar
    SC suspension
scaffold
    biodegradable polymer s.
Scaglietti
    S. closed reduction technique
    S. procedure scale
S-Caine topical anesthetic patch
scala
scalar classification
scale
    abbreviated injury s. (AIS)
    Aches and Pains S.
    addiction acknowledgment s.
    addiction potential s.
    alcohol dependence s.
    Attitudes to Back Pain S. (ABPS)
    Barratt Impulsivity S.
    behavioral pain s.
    Borg treadmill exertion s.
    Bromage motor block s.
    Charrière catheter size s.
    children's coma s.
    Children's Hospital of Eastern Ontario Pain S. (CHEOPS)
    Children's Revised Impact of Event S. (CRIES)
    CHIP s.
    Cleveland Clinic weighted s.
    clinical grading s. (CGS)
    Colored Visual Analogue S. (CVAS)
    coma s.
    Coping with Health Injuries and Problems S.
    dissociation, analgesia, immobility, and tension s.
    ECoG performance status s.
    Edinburgh 2 Coma S. (E2CS)
    Faces Pain S.
    French s. (F, Fr)

scale (*continued*)
    Glasgow coma s. (GCS)
    Glasgow Outcome S. (GOS)
    Graphic Rating S. (GRS)
    Hospital Anxiety and Depression S.
    Iowa Satisfaction with Anesthesia S.
    Karnofsky performance s.
    keratin s.
    LENT-SOMA scoring s.
    Likert pain s.
    Lysholm Knee S.
    MacAndrew Alcoholism S.
    McMaster Quality of Life S.
    Medication Quantification S.
    Modified Yale Preoperative
      Anxiety S.
    Modified Zung Depression S.
    Neonatal Infant Pain S. (NIPS)
    numeric rating s.
    OAA/S s.
    Objective Pain S.
    Observer's Assessment of Alertness
      and Sedation s. (OAA/S)
    pain anxiety symptoms s.
    pain catastrophizing s. (PCS)
    pediatric trauma s. (PTS)
    Progressive Ambulation S.
    Scaglietti procedure s.
    Sessing pressure ulcer assessment s.
    Shea pressure ulcer assessment s.
    sound pressure level s.
    Symptom Distress S. (SDS)
    University of Michigan Sedation S.
      (UMSS)
    verbal descriptor s.
    verbal-rank s.
    visual analog s. (VAS)
    Volpicelli functional ambulation s.
    Zung Depression S.
scalene
    s. fascia
    s. fat pad biopsy
    s. hiatus
    s. lymph node biopsy
    s. maneuver
    s. muscle
    s. node biopsy
    s. triangle
    s. tubercle
scalenectomy
scalenotomy
    Adson-Coffey s.
scalenus
    s. anterior muscle
    s. anticus syndrome
    s. medius muscle
    s. minimus muscle
    s. posterior muscle
scaling skin-colored lesion

scalloped closure
scalp
    s. closure
    s. incision
    s. infection
    s. laceration
    s. muscle
    s. nerve block
    s. sickle flap
    subcutaneous s.
scalpel
    s. cricothyrotomy
    Harmonic S.
scalping
    s. flap
    s. flap of Converse
scan
    biplane s.
    bone s.
    computed tomography s.
    contrast-enhanced CT s.
    crossvector A s.
    CT s.
    EMI s.
    HIDA s.
    high-dose s.
    magnetic resonance imaging s.
    Meckel s.
    omniplane s.
    peritoneovenous shunt patency s.
    s. plane
    postoperative CT s.
    pulmonary ventilation s.
    radioactive s.
    scintillation s.
    sector s.
    serial transverse s.
    stimulation s.
    time position s.
    transesophageal echocardiography s.
    transverse s.
    ventilation lung s.
    ventilation/perfusion lung s.
scan-directed biopsy
Scanlon early neonatal neurobehavioral
  score
scanner
    optical s.
scanning
    body s.
    contrast-enhanced CT s.
    CT s.
    s. electron microscopy
    external s.
    s. force microscopy
    functional activation PET s.
    s. laser Doppler flowmetry
    s. laser polarimetry
    longitudinal s.

point s.
real-time sector s.
scintillation s.
sector s.
s. technique
thallium-technetium s.
total body s.
transverse s.
whole-body s.
Scanzoni forceps delivery maneuver
Scanzoni-Smellie forceps delivery
  maneuver
scaphocapitate fusion
scaphocephaly
scaphohydrocephalus, scaphohydrocephaly
scaphohydrocephaly (*var. of*
  scaphohydrocephalus)
scaphoid
s. abdomen
s. bone
s. fossa
s. fracture
s. radius
scapholunate
s. dislocation
s. dissociation
scaphotrapezial trapezoid arthritis
scaphotrapeziotrapezoidal fusion
scapi (*pl. of* scapus)
scapula, *pl.* **scapulae**
s. entrapment
levator s.
scapulae (*pl. of* scapula)
scapular
s. approximation test
s. elevation
s. flap
s. line
s. muscle
s. notch
s. peroneal atrophy
s. region
scapulectomy
Das Gupta s.
Phelps s.
scapuloanterior fetal position
scapuloclavicular articulation
scapulocostal syndrome
scapulohumeral
scapuloperoneal syndrome
scapulopexy
scapuloposterior fetal position
scapulothoracic
s. disarticulation
s. dissociation
s. fusion
scapus, *pl.* **scapi**
scar
s. carcinoma

s. dehiscence
dermal s.
episiotomy s.
facetted corneal s.
fibrous s.
s. force
s. formation
gray-white corneal s.
hypertrophic s.
incisional s.
iridectomy s.
nonpathologic s.
osteopetrotic s.
perineal s.
radial s.
s. retraction
s. revision
s. rupture
sternotomy s.
thoracotomy s.
s. tissue
s. tissue reaction
Scardino
S. vertical flap pyeloplasty
S. vertical pyeloplasty flap
scarf
s. maneuver
s. osteotomy
s. osteotomy-bunionectomy
s. Z-osteotomy
s. Z-osteotomy-bunionectomy
s. Z-plasty
Scarff-Bloom-Richardson (SBR)
S.-B.-R. breast cancer classification
S.-B.-R. breast cancer grade
S.-B.-R. staging
scarification test
scarify
scarless endoscopic thyroidectomy
Scarpa
S. aneurysm ligation method
S. fascia
S. ganglion
S. hiatus
S. iridodialysis
S. liquor
S. operation
S. sheath
S. triangle
scarred skin
scarring
corneal s.
duodenal s.
gastrostomy s.
hypertrophic s.
obliterative s.
patch test s.
pathology s.
scatoma

S

scatoscopy
scatter
    s. correction
    s. photocoagulation
scavenger
    free radical s.
    superoxide s.
scavenging
    intraoperative cell s.
    s. system
SCFE
    slipped capital femoral epiphysis
Schaberg-Harper-Allen arthroscopic iliopsoas release technique
Schacher ganglion
Schanz
    S. angulation osteotomy
    S. femoral osteotomy
Schatz fetal position maneuver
Schatzker tibial plateau fracture classification
Schatzki esophageal ring
Schaumann body
Schauta-Aumreich radical vaginal hysterectomy procedure
Schauta radical vaginal hysterectomy
Schauwecker patellar wiring technique
Schede
    S. bone defect filling method
    S. clot
    S. thoracoplasty
schedule
    Edmonton Symptom Assessment S.
    Support Team Assessment S. (STAS)
Scheibe malformation
Scheie
    S. cataract scleral flap technique
    S. hypertensive retinopathy classification
    S. scleral cauterization
    S. syndrome
    S. thermal sclerostomy
schema, scheme, *pl.* **schemata**
    body s.
schemata (*pl. of* schema)
schematic
scheme
    chemotherapeutic s.
Schenk-Eichelter vena cava plastic filter procedure
Schepens
    S. retinal detachment operation
    S. transvitreal probe testing technique
Schepsis-Leach hamstring reconstruction technique
Scher nail biopsy

Schiller-Duvall body
Schiller splint method
Schimek blepharoptosis operation
schindylesis
Schiotz tonometry
Schirmer lacrimal sac operation
schistocystis
schistorrhachis
schistosomal
    s. bladder carcinoma
    s. cystitis
schistosomiasis
    ectopic cutaneous s.
schistothorax
Schlatter
    S. gastrectomy technique
    S. total gastrectomy with side-to-side esophagojejunostomy
Schlein elbow arthroplasty
Schlemm canal
Schmalz lacrimal operation
Schmidel anastomosis
Schneider fixation
schneiderian
    s. carcinoma
    s. respiratory membrane
Schnute wedge resection technique
Schober
    S. lumbar flexion-extension method
    S. lumbar spine mobility measuring technique
Schobinger incision
Schoemaker
    S. anastomosis
    S. gastroenterostomy
    S. modification
    S. transscrotal orchiopexy procedure
Schonander imaging technique
Schönbein operation
Schoonmaker-King single-catheter technique
Schreger line
Schreiber patellar reflex maneuver
Schrock scapula elevation repair procedure
Schroeder operation
Schuchardt
    S. operation
    S. relaxing incision
Schuknecht age-related hearing loss classification
Schüller
    S. duct
    S. oral radiography method
    S. position
    S. projection
Schütz
    S. bundle
    tract of S.

Schwalbe
    S. anterior border ring
    S. line
    S. space
Schwann cell
schwannoma
Schwartz
    S. dorsiflexory osteotomy
    S. tractotomy
SCI
    spinal cord injury
sciatic
    s. hernia
    s. nerve block
    s. nerve palsy hematoma
    s. nerve retractor
    s. notch
    s. plexus
    s. spine
sciatic-femoral nerve block
scientific
    s. method
    S. Registry of Transplant Recipients (SRTR)
scimitar syndrome
scintigraphy
    hepatic s.
    somatostatin receptor s.
    splenic s.
scintillation
    s. scan
    s. scanning
    s. vial
scintography
    renal s.
scirrhous lesion
scissor-leg position
scissors
    s. dissection
    suture wire-cutting s.
scissors-excision hemorrhoidectomy
scissura
    portal s.
SCL90
    Symptom Checklist 90
SCLC
    small-cell lung carcinoma
sclera, *pl.* **sclerae**
sclerae (*pl. of* sclera)
scleral
    s. buckle
    s. buckling
    s. buckling procedure
    s. canal
    s. ectasia
    s. exoplant
    s. fistula
    s. fistulectomy
    s. flap

    s. hemorrhage
    s. punctum
    s. resection
    s. roll
    s. rupture
    s. search coil technique
    s. shortening operation
    s. sulcus
scleratomal distribution of pain
sclerectoiridectomy
    Lagrange s.
sclerectomy
    Berens s.
    Holth s.
    thermal s.
scleriritomy
scleroatrophic cholecystitis
sclerocorneal
    s. junction
    s. sulcus
scleroderma
sclerodermoid graft-versus-host disease
sclerokeratectomy
scleroma
scleroplasty
sclerosant
sclerosing
    s. adenosis
    s. inflammation
    s. lesion
    s. osteomyelitis of Garré
    s. solution
    s. therapy
sclerosis
    pulmonary tuberous s.
    systemic s.
    tuberous s.
sclerostomy
    posterior thermal s.
    Scheie thermal s.
sclerotherapy
    s. complication
    emergent endoscopic s.
    endoscopic injection s. (EIS)
    endoscopic retrograde s.
    endoscopic variceal s. (EVS)
    esophageal variceal s. (EVS)
    ethanol s.
    s. failure
    fiberoptic injection s. (FIS)
    injection s.
    intravariceal s.
    paravariceal s.
    variceal s.
sclerotic
    s. bone lesion
    s. calvarial patch
    s. cemental mass
    s. kidney

S

sclerotic (*continued*)
    s. line
    s. stomach
scleroticectomy
scleroticotomy
sclerotomy
    anterior s.
    Dianoux s.
    foreign body s.
    Lindner s.
    posterior s.
    s. with drainage
    s. with exploration
sclerouvectomy
    partial lamellar s.
SCM
    sternocleidomastoid
scolicidal fluid
scoliosis
    s. correction
    s. surgery
scoliotic
    s. curve fixation
    s. deformity
scope
    arthroscopy
Scopinaro
    S. biliopancreatic bypass
      procedure
    S. pancreaticobiliary bypass
scopolamine
    s. antiemetic patch
    transdermal s.
score
    Abbreviated Injury S. (AIS)
    airway s.
    Aldrete s.
    alertness/sedation s.
    Alvarado iliac fossa pain s.
    American Society of
      Anesthesiology s.
    Apgar s.
    BI-RADS s.
    Child-Pugh chronic liver disease s.
    cosmetic s.
    cumulative s.
    cumulative pain s. (CPS)
    defecation s.
    discrimination s.
    Dripps-American Surgical
      Association s.
    evacuation s.
    French cardiac surgery risk s.
    GIQLI s.
    Glasgow coma s. (GCS)
    Glasgow Outcome S. (GOS)
    Gleason s.
    Higgins cardiac surgery
      risk s.

    Injury Severity S. (ISS)
    International Classification of
      Diseases-9 Version of Injury
      Severity S. (ICISS)
    Lysholm s.
    MACIS s.
    mangled extremity severity s.
      (MESS)
    Neurologic and Adaptive Capacity
      S. (NACS)
    Optimal Observation S.
    pain intensity s.
    pancreatic necrosis prognostic s.
    Parsonnet cardiac surgery risk s.
    Peritonitis Severity S. (PSS)
    Scanlon early neonatal
      neurobehavioral s.
    simplified acute physiology s.
      (SAPS)
    Steward Recovery S.
    surgical Apgar s. (SAS)
    symptom s.
    Total Pain Rating S.
    Total Tenderness S.
    Trauma Score and Injury Severity
      S. (TRISS)
    Tu cardiac surgery risk s.
    VASPI s.
    verbal pain s.
    verbal stress s.
    visual analog pain s. (VAPS)
    visual analog scale of pain
      intensity s.
    Yale Optimal Observation S.
scoring
    s. incision
    preoperative s.
    severity of illness s.
    s. system
scotoma, *pl.* **scotomata**
    s. junction
    s. ring
scotomata (*pl. of* scotoma)
scotomization
scotoscopy
Scott
    S. glenoplasty technique
    S. jejunoileal bypass
    S. operation
    S. posterior glenoplasty
scotty
    s. dog fracture
    s. dog graft
    s. dog sign
SCPP
    spinal cord perfusion
      pressure
scratch-pad memory
scratch-type incision

screen
    coagulation s.
    s. filtration pressure
    intravascular coagulation s.
    s. oxygenation
    throat s.
screening
    colonoscopy s.
    endocrine s.
    s. mammography
    presurgical psychological s. (PPS)
    s. procedure
    psychological s.
    s. recommendation
    s. test
screw
    s. angulation
    s. epiphysiodesis
    s. fixation
    headless bone s.
    s. implantation
    s. insertion
    s. insertion technique
    s. joint
    s. loosening
    s. placement
    s. position perioperative
      monitoring
    s. stabilization
    s. stripout
screw-and-plate fixation
screw-and-wire fixation
screw-home mechanism
screw-in
screw-plate approach
screw-type abutment
scrota (*pl. of* scrotum)
scrotal
    s. artery
    s. hematocele
    s. hematoma
    s. hernia
    s. mass
    s. pouch operation
    s. pouch orchiopexy
    s. prosthesis
    s. raphe
    s. septum
    s. skin
    s. skin ulcer
    s. swelling
    s. vein
scrotectomy
    total s.
scrotiform
scrotitis
scrotocele
scrotoplasty
scrotoscopy

scrotum, *pl.* **scrota,** *pl.* **scrotums**
scrotums (*pl. of* scrotum)
scrub
    10-minute hand s.
scrubbing technique
SCS
    spinal canal stenosis
    spinal cord stimulation
Scudder
    S. energy-based healing technique
    S. tuberculous parotid gland
      operation
Scuderi
    S. hypospadias repair
    S. ruptured quadriceps repair
      technique
    S. urethral reconstruction
      procedure
Scultetus position
scurvy line
SCV-CPR
    simultaneous compression-ventilation
      cardiopulmonary resuscitation
scybala
scyphiform
scyphoid
SDS
    Symptom Distress Scale
SEA
    spinal epidural abscess
seal
    cavity s.
sealant
    Crosseal human fibrin s.
    fibrin s.
sealed envelope technique
sealer
    dissecting s.
    s. extrusion
sealing
    s. perforation
    wound s.
sea lion position
seamless graft
seatbelt
    s. fracture
    s. sign
Seattle graft-versus-host disease
  classification
sebaceous
    s. adenocarcinoma
    s. cyst
    s. gland
sebaceum
    adenoma s.
Sebileau
    S. hollow
    S. muscle
seborrhea

S

second
  s. cranial nerve
  s. cuneiform bone
  forced expiratory volume in 1 s. (FEV_1)
  s. gas effect
  s. intention
  s. lumbar artery
  s. malignant neoplasm (SMN)
  s. pain windup
  s. parallel pelvic plane
  s. tibial muscle
secondary
  s. adhesion
  s. amputation
  s. anesthetic
  s. arrest (SA)
  s. arrest of dilation
  s. articulation
  s. closure
  s. diagnostic biopsy
  s. expansion
  s. fixation
  s. focal point
  s. fracture
  s. fungal infection
  s. gangrene
  s. headache
  s. hemorrhage
  s. hernia
  s. HPT
  s. hyperalgesia
  s. hypersplenism
  s. intention
  s. lesion
  s. membrane
  s. myofascial trigger point
  s. neuralgia
  s. procedure
  s. ptosis correction
  s. pulmonary lobule
  s. reconstruction
  s. renal calculus
  s. repair
  s. retroperitoneal organ
  s. saturation
  s. stage proctocolectomy
  s. surgery
  s. suture technique
  s. union
  s. wound healing
  s. yolk sac
second-degree
  s.-d. burn
  s.-d. hemorrhoid
  s.-d. radiation injury
second-echo image
second-generation
second-grade fusion

second-line
  s.-l. chemotherapy
  s.-l. drug
second-look
  s.-l. laparoscopy
  s.-l. laparotomy (SLL)
  s.-l. operation (SLO)
  s.-l. procedure
  s.-l. surgery
second-set graft rejection
secretin stimulation
secretion
  biliary s.
  cholecystokinin s.
  gastrin s.
  insulin s.
  pancreatic enzyme s.
  tracheal s.
secretomotor
  s. nature
  s. parasympathetic fiber
secretory
  s. adenocarcinoma
  s. diarrhea
  s. duct
  s. nerve
sectile
sectio, *pl.* **sectiones**
section
  abdominal s.
  attached cranial s.
  axial s.
  bar s.
  cesarean s. (C-section)
  classical cesarean s.
  coronal s.
  cranial s.
  cross s.
  cryostat s.
  cryostat tissue s.
  s. cutting
  detached cranial s.
  diagonal s.
  distal shave s.
  extraperitoneal cesarean s.
  s. freeze substitution technique
  frontal s.
  frozen s.
  Giemsa-stained s.
  Gigli lateral os pubis s.
  horizontal s.
  intraoperative frozen s.
  Kerr cesarean s.
  Latzko cesarean s.
  longitudinal s.
  low cervical cesarean s.
  lower uterine segment transverse cesarean s.
  low transverse cesarean s.

LUST cesarean s.
median s.
midfrontal plane coronal s.
midsagittal s.
nerve cross s.
oblique s.
orbital s.
parasagittal s.
perineal s.
permanent s.
pituitary stalk s.
plastic s.
Porro cesarean s.
primary cesarean s.
repeat cesarean s.
Saemisch s.
sagittal s.
tangential s.
thin s.
transperitoneal cesarean s.
transverse s.
vertical s.
vestibular nerve s.
Waters extraperitoneal cesarean s.

sectional
s. root canal filling method
s. technique

sectionectomy
left lateral s.

sectiones (*pl. of* sectio)

sectioning
surgical s.

sector
s. cut
end-viewing s.
s. iridectomy
s. iridectomy operation
lateral s.
medial s.
s. scan
s. scanning

sectoral
s. pedicle
s. resection

sectorial
s. branch
s. resection

secundarium
centrum ossificationis s.

secundum
centrum ossificationis s.
ostium s.

secure intracorporeal knot

sedation
adjunctive s.
chemical s.
conscious s.
ICU s.
intravenous s.

IV s.
minimal s.
moderate s.
Observer's Assessment of Alertness
and S. (OAA/S)
palliative s.
terminal s.

sedation-induced hypoventilation
sedative
s. effect
s. therapy

Seddon
S. dorsal spine costotransversectomy
S. modification
S. nerve graft
S. nerve injury classification

sedimentation
s. equilibrium
s. index

seeding
instrument-tract s.
intraluminal s.
intraperitoneal s.
needle tract tumor s.
peritoneal s.
surgical s.
tumor s.

SEER
Surveillance, Epidemiology, End Result
SEER Program

segment
AA s.
AB s.
AM s.
anterior apical s.
anterior basal s.
anterior inferior s.
anterior midpapillary s.
anterior superior s.
apical s.
apicoposterior s.
bronchopulmonary s.
cardiac s.
cervical s.
colorectal s.
demucosalized augmentation with
gastric s. (DAWG)
extramedullary s.
gastric s.
hepatic s.
IA s.
IB s.
inferior apical s.
inferior basal s.
inferior lingular s.
intracutaneous s.
LA s.
LB s.
lower uterine s. (LUS)

S

segment (*continued*)
    lumbar s.
    medial basal s.
    motion s.
    occluded s.
    posterior basal s.
    posterosuperior s.
    renal s.
    SA s.
    SB s.
    septal apical s.
    septal basal s.
    subapical s.
    subsuperior s.
    superior lingular s.
    venous s.
segmenta (*pl. of* segmentum)
segmental
    s. alveolar osteotomy
    s. blocking technique
    s. bronchus
    s. colectomy
    s. colonic resection
    s. compression construct
    s. dilation
    s. duct
    s. epidural anesthesia
    s. explant
    s. fixation
    s. fracture
    s. gastrectomy
    s. hepatectomy
    s. involvement
    s. limb pressure recording
    s. lung resection
    s. mandibulectomy
    s. mastectomy
    s. neural blockade
    s. peridural spinal anesthesia
    s. pressure index
    s. pulmonary resection
    s. sphincter
    s. spinal instrumentation (SSI)
    s. surgery
    s. tendon graft
    s. vessel
    s. wall motion abnormality
    (SWMA)
segmentalis
segmentation
    s. anomaly
    s. movement
    s. root canal filling method
    s. sphere
    volume s.
segmentectomy
segmented flap
segment-oriented
    s.-o. hepatic resection

s.-o. liver resection
s.-o. procedure
s.-o. technique
segmentum, *pl.* **segmenta**
    s. cardiacum
Segond fracture
segregation
Seidelin body
Seiler cartilage
Seinsheimer femoral fracture
    classification
Seitz metamorphosing respiration
seizure
    posttraumatic s.
    self-limiting grand mal s.
Selakovich sustenaculum tali procedure
Seldinger
    S. catheter introduction method
    S. cystic duct catheterization
    S. introducer sheath
    S. percutaneous technique
    S. retrograde wire intubation
    technique
    S. vascular access procedure
selection pressure
selective
    s. anesthesia
    s. angiography
    s. antegrade cerebral perfusion
    (SACP)
    s. arterial embolization
    s. arterial stimulation
    s. blockade
    s. bowel decontamination
    s. bronchial catheterization anesthetic
    technique
    s. catheterization
    s. ductal cannulation
    s. inguinal node dissection
    s. injection
    s. intracoronary thrombolysis (SICT)
    s. irradiation
    s. lectin-triggered apoptosis
    s. lymphadenectomy
    s. nonoperative management
    s. obturator nerve block
    s. photothermolysis
    s. portal decompression
    s. posterior rhizotomy (SPR)
    s. proximal vagotomy (SPV)
    s. relaxant binding agent
    s. sacral rhizotomy
    s. saturation
    s. saturation recovery
    s. serotonin reuptake inhibitor
    (SSRI)
    s. shunt
    s. spinal analgesic
    s. thoracic spine fusion

s. vascular clamping
s. venous sampling
selenoid body
self-administered
Quality of Well-Being Scale S.-A. (QWB-SA)
self-breast examination
self-catheterization
clean intermittent s.-c.
self-expandable
self-expanding metallic stent
self-help
self-infection
self-inflating manual resuscitator
self-limiting grand mal seizure
self-mutilation
self-obturation
intermittent s.-o.
self-reduction
self-sealing scleral puncture
self-seal pouch
self-tightening slip knot
Selinger operation
sella
empty s.
s. structure
sellar tumor
Sell-Frank-Johnson extensor shift technique
Sellheim incision
Sellick endotracheal intubation maneuver
Selye
adaptation syndrome of S.
Semb
S. apicolysis
S. nephrectomy technique
semenuria, seminuria, spermaturia
SEMI
subendocardial myocardial infarction
semicanal
semicanalis
semicartilaginous
semicircular
s. canal
s. duct
s. line
semicircularis
semiclosed
s. anesthesia
s. circle
semicoma
semiconductor
extrinsic s.
semiconstrained total elbow arthroplasty
semielective
s. operation
s. status
semiflexed incision

semi-Fowler position
semiimpermeable membrane
semilateral
s. approach
s. position
semilinear canonical correlation
semilunar
s. bone
s. cartilage
s. fibrocartilage
s. flap
s. ganglion
s. hiatus
s. incision
s. line
s. valvular septum
semilunate cut
semimembranosus
s. muscle
s. tendon
semimembranous
seminal
s. colliculus
s. duct
s. fluid
s. gland
s. granule
s. hillock
s. tract
s. tract washout
s. vesicle
s. vesicle aspiration
semination
seminiferous
seminoma
seminomatous
seminuria (*var. of* semenuria)
semioblique position
semiopen
s. anesthesia
s. hemorrhoidectomy
s. sliding tenotomy
semipedunculated lesion
semipermeable membrane
semipronation
semiprone position
semireclining position
semirecumbent position
semispinalis
s. capitis muscle
s. cervicis
s. cervicis muscle
semispinal muscle
semisulcus
semisupination
semisupine
semitendinosus
s. muscle
s. procedure

semitendinosus (*continued*)
    s. technique
    s. tendon
semitendinous
semiupright position
Semm Z-stab laparoscope insertion technique
Semont benign positional vertigo maneuver
Sengstaken-Blakemore (S-B)
    S.-B. tube
SENIC
    Study of the Efficacy of Nosocomial Infection Control
senile
    s. ectasia
    s. plaque
Senning
    S. operation
    S. transposition of great arteries procedure
    S. transposition of great arteries repair
Senn ventriculosubgaleal shunt operation
sensate
sensation
    du qi s.
    globus s.
    s. level
    phantom s.
    s. time
sense of defecation
sensitive
    s. plane
    s. point
    s. visceral postsurgical disturbance
sensitivity
sensitization
    central s.
    peripheral s.
    s. response
sensitizing injection
sensor
    calcium s.
    multiparameter s.
    s. operation
    wireless biomedical s.
sensorial saturation
sensorimotor stimulation approach
sensorineural acuity level technique
sensorium
sensory
    s. abnormality
    s. block
    s. blockade
    s. dermatome
    s. dysregulation
    s. examination
    s. extinction

    s. fusion
    s. innervation
    s. nerve
    s. nerve fiber bundle
    s. pathway
    s. stimulation
    s. testing
    s. tract
sentinel
    s. blood clot
    s. event
    s. lymphadenectomy
    s. lymph node (SLN)
    s. lymph node biopsy (SLNB)
    s. lymph node detection (SLND)
    s. lymph node localization
    s. lymph node mapping
    s. node
    s. node biopsy (SNB)
    s. node excision
    s. node localization
    s. node-positive patient
    s. node staging
    s. node to background ratio (SNBR)
    s. pile
    s. spinous process fracture
SEP
    somatosensory evoked potential
separation
    cotton-wool s.
    dermal wound s.
    laryngotracheal s.
    s. point
    premature s.
Seprafilm adhesion barrier
SEPS
    subfascial endoscopic perforator surgery
sepses (*pl. of* sepsis)
sepsis, *pl.* **sepses**
    anorectal s.
    catheter s.
    graft s.
    gram-negative s.
    gram-positive s.
    hypermetabolic s.
    intraabdominal s.
    overwhelming postsplenectomy s.
    peritoneal s.
    postsplenectomy s.
    severe human s.
    systemic s.
sepsis-induced
    s.-i. disseminated intravascular coagulation
    s.-i. metabolic change
    s.-i. muscle breakdown
    s.-i. muscle proteolysis

septa (*pl. of* septum)
septal
    s. apical (SA)
    s. apical segment
    s. basal (SB)
    s. basal segment
    s. defect
    s. hematoma
    s. line
    s. myectomy
    s. myotomy
    s. perforation
    s. reconstruction
    s. resection
    s. space
septate
septation procedure
septectomy
    atrial s.
    balloon s.
    Blalock-Hanlon atrial s.
    Edwards s.
    transampullary s.
septic
    s. arthritis
    s. complication
    s. focus
    s. patient
    s. shock
septicemia
septodermoplasty
septomarginal tract
septoplasty
    frontal sinus s.
septorhinoplasty
    esthetic s.
septostomy
    atrial balloon s.
    balloon atrial s.
    blade atrial s.
septula (*pl. of* septulum)
septulum, *pl.* **septula**
septum, *pl.* **septa**
    anorectal s.
    anterior intermuscular s.
    Bigelow s.
    bridgelike s.
    cartilaginous s.
    Cloquet s.
    colorectal s.
    comblike s.
    crural s.
    deviated s.
    s. endovenosum
    endovenous s.
    femoral s.
    interatrial s.
    intercavernosus s.
    intermuscular s.

    interpulmonary s.
    interradicular s.
    interventricular s.
    s. medianum
    membranous s.
    midline nasal s.
    nasal s.
    orbital s.
    pectiniform s.
    s. pectiniforme
    s. pellucidum
    posterior intermuscular s.
    rectovaginal s.
    rectovesical s.
    scrotal s.
    semilunar valvular s.
    transverse s.
    urogenital s.
    urorectal s.
    valvular s.
    ventricular s.
Sequeira-Khanuja modification
sequela, *pl.* **sequelae**
    thromboembolic s.
sequelae (*pl. of* sequela)
sequence
    caudal dysplasia s.
    turbo spin-echo s.
sequencing
    treatment s.
sequential
    s. administration
    s. organ failure assessment (SOFA)
    s. radiographs
sequestration
    s. bronchopneumonia
    extralobar s.
    intralobar s.
    pulmonary intralobar s.
sequestrectomy
sequestrotomy
SER
    supination-external rotation
        SER stage I–IV
        SER type I–IV fracture
sera (*pl. of* serum)
Serafini hernia
Sergent white line
serial
    s. blood gas
    s. dilation
    s. extraction
    s. hematocrit measurement
    s. imaging
    s. operation
    s. percutaneous liver biopsy
    s. radiographic evaluation
    s. radiographs
    s. sonography

S

serial (*continued*)
    s. transverse enteroplasty (STEP)
    s. transverse scan
series
    diagnostic small-bowel s.
    nonlaparoscopic s.
serioscopy
serious adverse event (SAE)
seriscission
serofibrinous inflammation
serofibrous
serologic
    s. adhesion
    s. examination
serological test
seroma
    s. cavity
    perigraft s.
seromembranous
seromucosa
seromucous gland
seromuscular
    s. coat
    s. colocystoplasty
    s. enterocystoplasty
    s. layer
    s. stitch
    s. suture technique
seromyectomy
    duodenal s.
seromyotomy
    anterior s.
    laparoscopic s.
seroprotection
serosa
    cecal s.
    gastric s.
    intact gastric s.
    s. invasion
    jejunal s.
serosal
    s. breach
    s. fluid
    s. involvement
    s. metastasis
    s. penetration
    s. tear
serosal-peritoneal metastasis
serosanguineous fluid
seroserous suture technique
serotonergic
    s. activity
    s. system
    s. tract
serotonin syndrome
serous
    s. acute inflammation
    s. adenocarcinoma
    s. cystadenocarcinoma

    s. exudate
    s. gland
    s. layer
    s. ligament
    s. membrane
    s. sac
serovaccination
serpentine
    s. aneurysm
    s. incision
serpent infection
serpiginosum
    angioma s.
serpiginous ulceration
Serralnyl suture
Serralsilk suture
serrated suture
serration
serratus
    s. anterior muscle
    s. anterior muscle flap
    s. posterior inferior muscle
    s. posterior superior muscle
Serres angle
Sertoli-cell-only syndrome
serum, *pl.* **serums,** *pl.* **sera**
    s. alkaline phosphatase
    s. ALT
    s. bactericidal concentration
    s. bilirubin
    s. bilirubin concentration
    s. calcium concentration
    s. carcinoembryonic antigen
    s. CEA
    s. EGF
    s. lidocaine level
    s. lithium concentration
    s. neutralization
    s. total bilirubin level
serums (*pl. of* serum)
service
    acute pain s.
    trauma s.
sesamoid
    s. bone
    s. cartilage
sesamoidectomy
    fibular s.
SESAP
    Surgical Education and Self-Assessment
    Program
sessile
    s. adenoma
    s. lesion
Sessing pressure ulcer assessment scale
session
    manometric recording s.
    recording s.
1-session removal

sestamibi-directed parathyroid surgery
sestamibi systemic imaging
set
> insufflation test s.
> s. point

SET
> signal extraction technology

seton
> anal s.
> s. operation
> s. suture
> s. wound

setpoint
setting
> s. expansion
> outpatient surgical s.

setup
> ambulatory s.

seventh cranial nerve
severe
> s. acute pancreatitis (SAP)
> s. deforming osteogenesis imperfecta
> s. human sepsis
> s. hypoxemia
> s. rejection
> s. systemic inflammatory response
> s. traumatic brain injury

Severin radiographic residual hip
dysplasia classification
severity of illness scoring
Sever-L'Episcopo
> S.-L. repair of shoulder
> S.-L. tendon repair

Sever modification
sevoflurane
Sewall-Boyden frontal sinus surgery
technique
sewing machine technique
sex
> s. change operation
> s. reversal
> s. steroid modulation

sextant technique
sexual
> s. aberration
> s. evaluation
> s. gland

sexualization
SFA
> superficial femoral artery

S-flap incision
SF36 questionnaire
SG
> surgical gastrostomy
> Swan-Ganz
>> SG catheter
>> SG tube

SGA
> supraglottic airway

SGB
> stellate ganglion block

SGO
> Surgeon General's Office

SGPA
> supragenicular popliteal artery

shadowing
> acoustic s.
> s. method

Shaffer glaucoma operation
Shaffer-Weiss central retinal vein
occlusion classification
shaft
> femoral s.
> s. fracture

shagreen
> s. lesion
> s. patch

Shaher-Puddu coronary arterial anatomy
classification
shallow
> s. inspiration
> s. respiration

sham
> s. injection
> s. needle
> s. surgery
> s. treatment

Shambaugh incision
shank bone
shape
> airway s.

shaping
> root canal s.

sharing
> United Network for Organ S.
> (UNOS)

sharp
> s. and blunt dissection
> s. angle
> s. dilaceration
> s. dissection
> s. dissection technique

Sharpey fiber
Sharpoint ophthalmic microsurgical
suture
Sharrard iliopsoas transfer technique
Sharrard-type kyphectomy
shave
> s. biopsy
> s. excision technique
> s. prep

Shea pressure ulcer assessment scale
shear
> s. fracture
> vascular s.

sheath
> anterior s.
> anterior rectus s.

S

sheath (*continued*)
    axillary s.
    carotid s.
    cervicoaxillary s.
    common flexor s.
    contralateral s.
    crural s.
    femoral s.
    fenestrated s.
    fibrous tendon s.
    flexor s.
    glissonian s.
    infundibuliform s.
    intertubercular s.
    intravenous s.
    mucous s.
    neurovascular s.
    optic s.
    paramedian s.
    parotid s.
    perichondral s.
    plantar tendon s.
    posterior rectus s.
    prostatic s.
    rectus s.
    Scarpa s.
    Seldinger introducer s.
    synovial tendon s.
    vascular s.
    Waldeyer s.
sheathed artery
shedding
    endometrial s.
Sheehan syndrome
Sheen
    S. airway reconstruction
    S. tip graft
sheet mesh excision
shelf, *pl.* **shelves**
    s. acetabuloplasty
    Blumer s.
    rectal s.
    vocal s.
shell
    s. nail
    total hip arthroplasty with internal
      eccentric s.'s (THARIES)
Shelton femoral fracture classification
shelves (*pl. of* shelf)
shelving
    s. edge
    s. incision
Shenton line
Shepherd fracture
shepherd's crook deformity
Sherk-Probst
    S.-P. pediatric humeral epiphysis
      fracture technique
    S.-P. percutaneous pinning

shift
    fluid s.
    mediastinal s.
    migration (of pain to RLQ),
      anorexia, nausea and vomiting,
      tenderness (in RLQ), rebound
      pain, elevated temperature,
      leukocytosis, s. (WBC to left)
      (MANTRELS)
***Shigella* infection**
Shimazaki area-length method
shin bone
shingles
shiny cellophane reflection
ship
    Fabricius s.
Shirodkar
    S. cervical cerclage
    S. cervix encirclement suture
      procedure
    S. operation
    S. suture
    S. suture technique
shish
    s. kebab graft
    s. kebab technique
shivering
    postanesthetic s.
    postoperative s.
Shoch suture
shock
    allergic s.
    anesthetic s.
    burn s.
    cardiogenic s.
    declamping s.
    deferred s.
    defibrillation s.
    defibrillatory s.
    early unequivocal s.
    endotoxic s.
    endotoxin s.
    heat s.
    hemorrhagic s.
    hyperdynamic s.
    hypovolemic s.
    irreversible s.
    s. lung
    neurogenic s.
    perioperative s.
    s. position
    postcardiotomy s.
    primary s.
    reversible s.
    septic s.
    spinal s.
    s. wave lithotripsy (SWL)
    s. wave pressure
shoe-and-stocking position

shoelace
    s. fasciotomy closure
    s. stitch
shoeshine maneuver
Shone anomaly
short
    s. bone
    s. bowel
    s. bowel syndrome
    s. central artery
    s. esophagus type hiatal hernia
    s. form McGill Pain Questionnaire
    s. gastric artery
    s. gastric vein
    s. gastric vessel
    s. head
    s. hepatic vein
    s. incubation hepatitis
    s. lever accessory movement
        technique
    s. lever specific contact procedure
    s. limb Roux-en-Y gastroenterostomy
    s. oblique fracture
    s. saphenous vein
    s. scar technique breast reduction
    s. scar technique of mastopexy
    s. stricture
    s. wave diathermy
short-axis plane
short-cone technique
short-course irradiation
shortcut sciatic pain
shortening
    chordal s.
    esophageal s.
short-form-36 (SF36)
short-lasting
    s.-l. unilateral neuralgiaform
        headache with conjunctival
        injection and tearing (SUNCT)
    s.-l. unilateral neuralgiaform
        headache with conjunctival
        injection and tearing syndrome
short-limb gastric bypass
short-segment
    s.-s. disease
    s.-s. lesion
    s.-s. spinal fusion
    s.-s. tracheal stenosis
short-term
    s.-t. convalescence
    s.-t. immunosuppression
    s.-t. outcome
    s.-t. result
    s.-t. total continence
shotgun wound
shotted suture
shoulder
    s. amputation

    s. arthroplasty
    s. blade
    s. deformity
    s. disarticulation
    s. dislocation
    s. dislocation bone bank
    s. flap
    s. girdle
    s. girdle resection
    ipsilateral s.
    S. Pain and Disability Index
    s. reduction
    s. repair
    s. rotation
    Sever-L'Episcopo repair of s.
    s. strap incision
    s. with bevel preparation
Shouldice
    S. hernia repair
    S. hernia repair technique
    S. hernioplasty
    S. herniorrhaphy
    S. indirect inguinal hernia operation
Shouldice-Bassini hernia repair
SH pop-off suture
Shrapnell membrane
shrinkage
    thermal-assisted capsular s.
    tumor s.
Shugrue orbital operation
shunt
    airway s.
    atriocaval s.
    Beck II aorta to coronary sinus s.
    bidirectional Glenn s.
    Blalock-Taussig s.
    s. blockage
    cavoatrial s.
    central renosplenic s. (CRSS)
    central systemic-to-pulmonary s.
    s. cyanosis
    distal splenoadrenal s.
    distal splenorenal s. (DSRS)
    end-to-side portocaval s.
    end-to-side splenorenal s.
    Glenn s.
    s. index
    s. infection
    interposition mesocaval s.
    intracardiac s.
    intrahepatic portosystemic s.
    Javid s.
    LeVeen s.
    lumbar-peritoneal s.
    s. manipulation
    mesoatrial s.
    mesocaval s.
    modified Blalock-Taussig s.
    s. muscle

S

shunt (*continued*)
    s. obstruction
    s. patency
    s. pathway
    s. placement
    pleuroperitoneal s.
    portacaval s.
    portal mesenteric s.
    portal-systemic s.
    portosystemic s.
    s. quantification
    s. ratio
    renipelvic end-to-end s.
    s. revision
    selective s.
    side-to-side portacaval s. (SSPCS)
    splenoadrenal s.
    splenocaval s.
    splenorenal s. (SRS)
    s. surgery
    surgical portosystemic s.
    s. tap
    transjugular intrahepatic
      portosystemic s. (TIPS)
    ventricular peritoneal s.
    ventriculoperitoneal s.
    Warren-Zeppa s.

SI
    sacroiliac
    SI joint

SIA
    stimulation-induced analgesia

SIADH
    syndrome of inappropriate secretion of
    antidiuretic hormone

sialadenitis, sialoadenitis
sialoadenectomy
sialoadenitis (*var. of* sialadenitis)
sialoadenotomy
sialocarcinoma
sialocele
sialolithotomy
sibilant rhonchus
Sibson
    S. fascia
    S. groove
    S. muscle
Sichi operation
sick
    s. building syndrome
    s. sinus syndrome
sickle
    s. cell disease
    s. cell pain
    s. flap
sickle-shaped canal
sickness impact profile (SIP)
SICT
    selective intracoronary thrombolysis

side
    antimesenteric s.
    contralateral s.
    depressed s.
    ipsilateral s.
    luminal s.
    s. port
    posterior s.
    s. posture reduction
side-bending barrier
side-entry access
side-lying iliac compression test
sideration
sideswipe elbow fracture
side-to-side
    s.-t.-s. anastomosis
    s.-t.-s. gastroenterostomy
    s.-t.-s. hepaticojejunostomy
    s.-t.-s. portacaval shunt (SSPCS,
      SSPS)
sidewall
    pelvic s.
    s. structure
SIDS
    sudden infant death syndrome
sieve
    s. bone
    s. graft
    molecular s.
Siewert type I–III tumor
Siffert intraepiphysial osteotomy
Siffert-Storen intraepiphysial
    osteotomy
sighing respiration
sigma receptor agonist
sigmoid
    s. artery
    s. colon
    s. colon carcinoma
    s. cutaneous fistula
    s. cystoplasty
    s. end colostomy
    s. enterocystoplasty
    s. flexure
    s. fold
    s. fossa
    s. kidney
    s. loop reduction
    s. loop rod colostomy
    s. mesentery
    s. mesocolon
    s. rectum pouch
    s. sinus ligation
    s. sulcus
    s. venous sinus
    s. volvulus
sigmoidectomy
    laparoscopy-assisted s.
sigmoidocystoplasty

sigmoidopexy
    band s.
    endoscopic s.
    laparoscopic s.
sigmoidoproctostomy
sigmoidorectostomy
sigmoidoscopy
    fiberoptic s.
    flexible s.
sigmoidostomy
sigmoidotomy
sigmoidovesical fistula
sigmoid-rectal intussusception
sign
    Aaron s.
    absent bow tie s.
    accordion s.
    adverse prognostic s.
    alien hand s.
    Allis s.
    Apley s.
    Aufrecht s.
    Babinski s.
    banana s.
    Battle s.
    bent inner tube s.
    bite s.
    blue dot s.
    Blumberg s.
    Boas s.
    bone bruise s.
    bow-tie s.
    brim s.
    Brudzinski s.
    Chadwick s.
    chain-of-lakes s.
    chandelier s.
    coiled spring s.
    Cole s.
    comb s.
    cortical ring s.
    cotton-wool s.
    Courvoisier s.
    crowded carpal s.
    Cullen s.
    dagger s.
    Dalrymple s.
    Dance s.
    David Letterman s.
    double bubble s.
    double-density s.
    double halo s.
    drawer s.
    echo s.
    extrapyramidal s.
    fabere s.
    fat pad s.
    fish-eye s.
    Grey Turner s.

    halo s.
    Hannington-Kiff s.
    Homans s.
    Howship-Romberg s.
    impingement s.
    Kehr s.
    Kehr spleen rupture s.
    Kussmaul s.
    Leeds Assessment of Neuropathic Symptoms and S.'s (LANSS)
    little finger s.
    localized abdominal s.
    long tract s.
    loss-of-waist s.
    Mickey Mouse s.
    Murphy s.
    obturator s.
    Phalen s.
    psoas s.
    Rovsing s.
    scotty dog s.
    seatbelt s.
    stacked coin s.
    T s.
    target s.
    Thomas s.
    Tillaux s.
    Tinel s.
    Trousseau s.
    Waddell nonorganic s.
signal
    abnormal preoperative localization s.
    s. attenuation
    Doppler s.
    electromagnetic s.
    s. extraction technology (SET)
    s. hemorrhage
    localization s.
    preoperative localization s.
signaling
    afferent spinal s.
    downstream s.
    excitatory synaptic s.
    nitric oxide s.
    pain s.
signature
    surgical s.
signet-ring
    s.-r. adenocarcinoma
    s.-r. appearance
    s.-r. cell carcinoma
significance
    atypical squamous cells of undetermined s. (ASCUS)
    squamous intraepithelial lesion/atypical squamous cell of undetermined s. (SIL/ASCUS)
significant organ dysfunction

SIH
    stress-induced hyperthermia
SIL
    squamous intraepithelial lesion
SIL/ASCUS
    squamous intraepithelial lesion/atypical
    squamous cell of undetermined
    significance
    SIL/ASCUS lesion
silastic
    s. collar-reinforced stoma
    S. lunate arthroplasty
    S. ring vertical-banded gastric
    bypass (SRVGB)
Silber testicular autotransplantation
  technique
silence
    EEG s.
    electrocerebral s. (ECS)
silencing
    gene s.
silent
    s. aspiration
    s. autonephrectomy
    s. gallstone
    s. receptor
Silfverskiöld
    S. Achilles tendon lengthening
    technique
    S. gastrocnemius soleus recession
    procedure
    S. transplantation of heads of origin
    of gastrocnemius
silhouette sign of Felson
silicate restoration
silicone
    s. elastomer medialization
    s. elastomer ring vertical
    gastroplasty (SRVG)
    s. implant arthroplasty
    s. implant leakage
    s. intubation
    s. rubber arthroplasty
    s. wrist arthroplasty
silicone-treated surgical silk suture
silk
    s. braided suture
    s. nonabsorbable suture
    s. pop-off suture
    s. stay suture
    s. traction suture
silkworm gut suture
Sillence type I-IV osteogenesis
  imperfecta
Silva Costa combined
  trabeculotomy-trabeculectomy
silver (Ag)
    S. and Simon modification of
    Silfverskiöld procedure with

    selective neurectomy of
    gastrocnemius
    S. bunionectomy
    S. bunionectomy procedure
    s. cone root canal method
    s. dollar technique
    s. point root canal filling method
    s. suture
silver-fork deformity
Silver-Hildreth osteotomy
silver-wire
    s.-w. arteriole
    s.-w. reflex
Silvester cardiopulmonary resuscitation
  method
simian line
Simmonds-Menelaus
    S.-M. metatarsal osteotomy
    S.-M. proximal phalangeal osteotomy
Simmons
    S. cervical spine fusion
    S. osteotomy
Simon
    S. expansion arch
    S. incision
    S. position
    S. suture technique
Simonart band
Simonton biofeedback technique
simple
    s. bypass
    s. cold storage preservation
    s. cyst
    s. diversion
    s. external drainage
    s. hepaticojejunostomy
    s. interrupted stitch
    s. joint
    s. liver cyst
    s. mastectomy
    s. mastoidectomy
    s. mastopexy
    s. periodontal flap
    s. shoulder test
    s. skull fracture
    s. suture technique
    s. syndactyly repair
    s. tetralogy of Fallot
    s. transfusion
    s. vulvectomy
simplification
simplified acute physiology score (SAPS)
Simpson atherectomy
Sims
    S. position
    S. suture
    S. suture technique
simulation
    surgical s.

Simulect
simultaneous
    s. areolar mastopexy and breast augmentation (SAMBA)
    s. bilateral percutaneous nephrolithotomies
    s. compression-ventilation cardiopulmonary resuscitation (SCV-CPR)
    s. kidney-pancreas transplant (SKPT)
    s. method
    s. pancreas and kidney (SPK)
    s. pancreas and kidney transplant procedure
    s. pancreas-kidney transplant
    s. pancreatic-renal (SPR)
    s. segmental hepatectomy
SIMV
    spontaneous intermittent mandatory ventilation
    synchronized intermittent mandatory ventilation
sincipital
sinciput
Sinding-Larsen-Johansson lesion
sinew
Singer-Blom endoscopic tracheoesophageal puncture technique
Singh
    S. osteoporosis classification
    S. osteoporosis index
single
    s. adenoma
    s. biopsy
    s. cone root canal filling method
    s. denture construction
    s. fraction radiation
    s. fracture
    s. GSW
    s. heel raise
    s. hydatid disease
    s. injection ultrasound-assisted femoral nerve block
    s. lung ventilation
    s. midline extraperitoneal incision
    s. pedicle TRAM flap
    s. proximal portal technique
    s. site
    s. space technique
single-armed
    s.-a. suture
    s.-a. suture technique
single-balloon
    s.-b. valvoplasty
    s.-b. valvotomy
single-breath
    s.-b. diffusing capacity
    s.-b. induction
    s.-b. induction of anesthesia

single-incision fasciotomy
single-layer continuous closure
single-level spinal fusion
single-lung transplant (SLT)
single-mechanism inhaled anesthetic
single-needle
    s.-n. medial branch block
    s.-n. technique
single-port
    s.-p. epidural catheter
    s.-p. laparoscopy
    s.-p. technique
single-pour dental material technique
single-puncture laparoscopy
single-shot
    s.-s. caudal block
    s.-s. conduction block
    s.-s. intrathecal opioid
    s.-s. spinal
    s.-s. spinal anesthesia
    s.-s. subarachnoid block
single-site inhaled anesthetic
single-stage
    s.-s. operation
    s.-s. procedure
    s.-s. tissue transfer
    s.-s. total proctocolectomy
single-step esophagoplasty
single-stick method
Singleton incision
Singleton-Merten syndrome
single-trocar access thoracoscopy
sinister
sinistra
sinistrogyration
sinistrorotation
sinistrorse
sinistrotorsion
sinistrum
sink-trap malformation
sinoaortic denervation
sinoatrial (*var. of* sinuatrial)
sinocarotid nerve
sinonasal
    s. carcinoma
    s. cavity
    s. disease
    s. lesion
    s. tumor
sinoscopy
sinuatrial (SA), sinoatrial
    s. exit block
    s. nodal branch
    s. nodal function
    s. nodal parasympathectomy
    s. node
sinus
    air s.
    anal s.

S

sinus (*continued*)

basilar venous s.
branchial s.
carotid s.
cavernous venous s.
s. cavity
cerebral s.
cervical s.
circular venous s.
s. closure
coronary s.
costomediastinal s.
cranial venous s.
dural venous s.
endodermal s.
s. endoscopy
Englisch s.
epigastric s.
s. exit block
frontal s.
Guérin s.
Huguier s.
inferior longitudinal s.
inferior petrosal s.
inferior sagittal s.
intercavernous venous s.
s. irrigation
jugular s.
lactiferous s.
laryngeal s.
lateral s.
s. line
longitudinal vertebral
  venous s.
Luschka s.
Maier s.
Morgagni s.
s. mucocele
oblique pericardial s.
occipital s.
osteomyelitic s.
Palfyn s.
paranasal s.
pericardial s.
perineal s.
petrosal venous s.
petrosquamous venous s.
s. petrosus superior
phrenicocostal s.
pilonidal s.
piriform s.
pleural s.
port site s.
prostatic s.
pulmonary s.
rectal s.
renal s.
rhomboidal s.
s. rhomboidalis

s. rhythm
Ridley s.
right sigmoid s.
sagittal venous s.
sigmoid venous s.
sphenoidal s.
sphenoparietal venous s.
splenic s.
straight s.
s. surgery
s. tarsi syndrome
tentorial s.
s. tract
transverse pericardial s.
transverse venous s.
tympanic s.
urogenital s.
s. venosus
venous s.

sinuscopy

maxillary s.

sinusitis

allergic fungal s.
chronic s.
fungal s.

sinusoid

hepatic s.

sinusoidal

s. capillary pressure
s. congestion
s. endothelium
s. endothelium cornucopia
s. lesion
s. pattern
s. relaxation

sinusotomy

Killian frontal s.

sinuvertebral nerve

SIP

sickness impact profile
spontaneous intestinal perforation
sympathetically independent pain

siphon

carotid s.

siphonage

sirolimus

SIRS

systemic inflammatory response
  syndrome

SIS

small-intestine submucosa
Surgical Infection Society

Sistrunk excision of thyroglossal cyst procedure

site

alternative introduction s.
anesthetic binding s.
arterial bleeding s.
arterial entry s.

biopsy s.
bleeding s.
carcinoma of uncertain
  primary s.
catheter s.
coaptation s.
contralateral s.
endoscopic biopsy s.
entry s.
excisional biopsy s.
exit s.
extraabdominal s.
extraction s.
extrahepatic tumor s.
extranodal s.
extrapulmonary s.
fracture s.
graft s.
implantation s.
injection s.
introduction s.
multiple s.
s. of obstruction
osteotomy s.
patellar tendon graft donor s.
  (PTGDS)
peritumoral s.
pin s.
port s.
primary tumor s.
puncture s.
single s.
stoma s.
suprapubic extraction s.
tumor s.
wound s.

site-specific
s.-s. analgesia
s.-s. surgery

sitting
s. position
W s.

1-sitting endodontics
situ
carcinoma in s. (CIS)
ductal carcinoma in s. (DCIS)
ex s.
fusion in s.
in s.
lobular carcinoma in s. (LCIS)
residual ductal carcinoma in s.
tumor in s.

situation
anatomic s.

situs, *pl.* **situs**
s. inversus
s. inversus viscerum

sitz bath
Siurala gastritis classification

sixth
s. cranial nerve
s. venereal disease

size
aerodynamic s.
age, metastases, extent, s. (AMES)
breast s.
clot s.
crosslink plate s.
gland s.
heterogeneous gland s.
in-between s.
lesion s.
metastasis, age, completeness of
  resection, local invasion, tumor s.
  (MACIS)
true s.
tumor s.

size-matched organ
Sjöqvist intramedullary tractotomy
SjVO₂
jugular venous oxygen saturation

skate flaps
skeletal
s. abnormality
s. biopsy
s. correction
s. deformity
s. fixation
s. lesion
s. metastasis
s. muscle
s. muscle atrophy
s. muscle hypotonia
s. muscle relaxant
s. tissue

skeletal-extraskeletal angiomatosis
skeletology
skeleton
appendicular s.
axial s.
cardiac fibrous s.
fibrous s.
laryngeal s.
pelvic s.
spine s.

skeletonization
Skene
external genitalia, Bartholin, urethral,
  S. (EG/BUS)
S. gland

skewer technique
skew flap
skier's fracture
Skillern fracture
skin
alligator s.
s. approximation
atrophic s.

skin (*continued*)
  s. barrier
  s. biopsy
  s. cancer
  s. closure
  combination s.
  s. conductance
  s. crease
  s. crease incision
  s. deficit wound
  s. erosion
  s. expansion technique
  s. flap
  s. flap necrosis
  s. flora
  s. folding
  s. graft
  s. graft neovagina
  s. groove
  hidden nail s.
  s. infection
  s. knife incision
  s. lubrication
  s. lubrication therapy
  s. measurement
  s. nick
  ostomy s.
  photoaged s.
  s. plasty
  s. potential response
  s. preparation
  s. puncture
  s. puncture test
  redundant triangular-shaped s.
  scarred s.
  scrotal s.
  s. surfacing technique
  surplus s.
  s. temperature
  s. temperature gradient measurement
  thin glossy s.
  triangular-shaped s.
  s. ulcer
  s. window technique
skin-amnion junction
skin-colored lesion
skin-epidural distance
skinfold
  supraspinale s.
  s. thickness
skinned muscle fiber
Skinner partially edentulous classification
skinning
  s. colpectomy
  s. vulvectomy
skinny-needle biopsy
skin-sparing
  s.-s. mastectomy
  s.-s. mastectomy approach

skin-to-tumor distance
skip
  s. area
  s. graft
  s. lesion
  s. metastasis
ski position
skived incision
Skoog
  S. fasciotomy
  S. female genitalia construction
    technique
SKPT
  simultaneous kidney-pancreas transplant
skull
  s. base approach
  s. base tumor
  s. block
  cloverleaf s.
  s. deformity
  s. fracture
  maplike s.
  steeple s.
  tower s.
skullcap
slack
  tissue s.
slant
  s. muscle operation
  s. of occlusal plane
SLAP
  superior labrum anterior and posterior
  SLAP lesion
Slavianski membrane
sleep
  s. apnea-hypoventilation syndrome
  s. dissociation
  twilight s.
sleeve
  s. fracture
  s. gastrectomy
  s. graft
  s. lobectomy
  pharmacological s.
  s. pneumonectomy
  s. resection
  s. technique
2-sleeve technique
slice
  s. fracture
  s. preparation
slide tracheoplasty
sliding
  s. abdominal hernia
  s. esophageal hiatal hernia
  s. flap
  s. hiatal hernia
  s. inlay bone graft
  s. leaflet plasty

s. nail
s. oblique osteotomy
s. plasty
s. scale method
s. tenotomy
s. valvoplasty

sling
s. and blanket technique
s. and reef technique
Crawford eyelid tarsofrontalis s.
s. immobilization
s. ligation
s. procedure
s. suture technique

sling-ring complex
sling/wrapping technique
slip knot
slippage
band s.
knot s.
stomach s.

slipped
s. capital femoral epiphysis (SCFE)
s. hernia
s. Nissen fundoplication
s. Nissen repair
s. rib cartilage syndrome
s. vertebral apophysis

slipping
s. rib
s. rib syndrome

slit
s. catheter technique
Cheatle s.
s. hemorrhage
s. illumination
lengthwise s.
pudendal s.
s. valve
s. ventricle syndrome
vulvar s.

slit-lamp ophthalmoscopy
slitlike defect
SLL
second-look laparotomy

SLN
sentinel lymph node
SLN biopsy
SLN localization
SLN mapping
SLN radiolocalization

SLNB
sentinel lymph node biopsy

SLND
sentinel lymph node detection

SLO
second-look operation

Sloan incision
Sloan-Kettering thyroid cancer staging

Slocum
S. amputation technique
S. knee rotatory instability maneuver
S. spinal fusion technique

slope-shouldered lesion
slot
s. fracture
s. preparation

slotted acetabular augmentation
slot-type preparation
slow
s. exchange soft tissue
s. maxillary expansion
s. pull-through (SPT)
s. pullthrough technique
s. respiration

slowly absorbable continuous suture
slow-pathway radiofrequency ablation
SLR
straight-leg raising
SLR with external rotation test

SLS
Society of Laparoendoscopic Surgeons

SLT
single-lung transplant
split-liver transplant

Sluder
S. guillotine tonsillectomy
S. neuralgia

sludge
biliary s.

sludging of circulation
slush
ice s.

SMA
superior mesenteric artery

small
s. capillary syndrome
s. fenestra stapedotomy
s. intestinal endoscopy
s. intestine
s. intestine adenoma
s. nerve fiber dysfunction
s. pancreas
s. pelvis
s. polyp removal
s. round cell carcinoma
s. trochanter

small-bowel
s.-b. evisceration
s.-b. infarction
s.-b. mesentery
s.-b. obstruction

small-cell lung carcinoma (SCLC)
small-intestine
s.-i. membrane
s.-i. submucosa (SIS)

S

SMART
   sperm microaspiration retrieval
   technique
SMAS
   superficial musculoaponeurotic system
Smead-Jones closure
smear
   buccal s.
smegma
smegmalith
smile
   endogenous s.
   exogenous s.
smiley-face knotting technique
smiley-face-up position
smiling incision
Smith
   S. dislocation
   S. eyelid operation
   S. flexor pollicis longus
   abductorplasty
   S. fracture
   S. Indian intracapsular cataract
   operation
   S. Indian intracapsular cataract
   removal technique
   S. modification
   S. physical capacity evaluation
   S. trabeculectomy
Smith-Boyce renal calculus operation
Smith-Gibson tetralogy of Fallot
correction
Smith-Indian operation, Smith
operation
Smith-Kuhnt-Szymanowski ectropion
repair with eyelid reconstruction
Smith-Lemli-Opitz syndrome
Smith-Petersen
   S.-P. anterior hip approach
   S.-P. anterior hip joint incision
   S.-P. cup arthroplasty
   S.-P. hemiarthroplasty
   S.-P. osteotomy
   S.-P. sacroiliac joint fusion
   S.-P. synovectomy
Smith-Petersen-Cave-Van Gorder
anterolateral hip approach
Smith-Robinson
   S.-R. anterior cervical discectomy
   S.-R. anterior cervical discectomy
   and fusion technique
   S.-R. anterior fusion
   S.-R. cervical disc approach
   S.-R. cervical fusion
   S.-R. interbody fusion
   S.-R. mandible open osteotomy
   S.-R. open osteotomy of mandible
   procedure
Smithwick sympathectomy

SMN
   second malignant neoplasm
   surgical microscope navigation
smoldering appendix
smooth
   s. muscle (SM)
   s. muscle relaxant
   s. muscle relaxation
   s. muscular sphincter
   s. skin-colored lesion
   s. surface cavity
   s. wrap
smooth-brain syndrome
SMP
   sympathetically maintained pain
SMV
   superior mesenteric vein
SMVR
   supraannular mitral valve replacement
snap-frozen biopsy
snapping
   s. hip syndrome
   s. iliopsoas tendon
snare
   s. cautery
   s. electrocoagulation
   s. excision biopsy
   s. loop biopsy
   s. technique
SNB
   sentinel node biopsy
SNBR
   sentinel node to background ratio
SNCB
   stereotactic needle core biopsy
Snellen
   S. line
   S. ptosis operation
   S. suture
   S. suture technique
sniffing position
sniff method
snip
1-snip punctum operation
3-snip punctum operation
snout response
snuffbox
   anatomic s.
Snuggle Warm blanket
Snyder SLAP lesion classification
soaking solution
soak therapy
Soave
   S. congenital megacolon repair
   S. endorectal pull-through
   S. transanal pullthrough procedure
social
   s. consequence
   s. interaction therapy

society
>American Pain S. (APS)
>American Thoracic S. (ATS)
>Canadian Infectious Disease S.
>Heart Rhythm S. (HRS)
>International Pelvic Pain S. (IPPS)
>North American Spine S. (NASS)
>S. of American Gastrointestinal Endoscopic Surgeons (SAGES)
>S. of Laparoendoscopic Surgeons (SLS)
>Surgical Infection S. (SIS)

socket
>hard s.
>s. joint
>s. reconstruction
>suspension-type s.

soda lime

sodium (Na)
>s. channel blocker

Soemmerring
>S. ganglion
>S. ligament
>S. muscle
>S. ring
>S. ring cataract
>S. spot

SOFA
>sequential organ failure assessment

Sofield
>S. femoral deficiency leg-lengthening technique
>S. osteotomy
>S. pinning

SOFS
>superior orbital fissure syndrome

Sofsilk
>S. coated braided silk suture
>S. nonabsorbable silk suture

soft
>s. abdomen
>s. callus stage
>s. cataract
>s. chancre
>s. corn
>s. event
>s. exudate
>s. palate
>s. palate cancer
>s. palate cleft
>s. palate paralysis
>s. palate retraction
>s. pigment stone
>s. sore
>s. stool
>s. tissue
>s. tissue abnormality
>s. tissue abscess
>s. tissue damage
>s. tissue dissection
>s. tissue extremity injury
>s. tissue flap
>s. tissue healing
>s. tissue hinge
>s. tissue integrity
>s. tissue interface
>s. tissue interposition
>s. tissue irritability
>s. tissue lesion
>s. tissue mass
>s. tissue massage
>s. tissue metastasis
>s. tissue mobilization (STM)
>s. tissue necrosis
>s. tissue plication
>s. tissue reconstruction
>s. tissue release
>s. tissue restriction
>s. tissue sarcoma (STS)
>s. tissue stranding
>s. tissue stretching
>s. tissue structure
>s. tissue swelling
>s. tissue thickness
>s. tissue undercut
>s. tissue window
>s. tissue xerography
>s. tubercle
>s. wall
>s. x-ray examination
>s. x-ray investigation

soft-tissue
>s.-t. curettage
>s.-t. envelope

SOHND
>supraomohyoid neck dissection

soilage
>peritoneal s.

soiling
>colostomy s.
>fecal s.

solar
>s. ganglion
>s. plexus

Solcia gastric dysplasia classification

soldier's patch

soleal line

sole laser therapy

soleus
>Baumann and Koch intramuscular lengthening of gastrocnemius and/or s.

solicitude
>low spousal s.

solid
>s. hidradenoma
>s. hyperplasia
>s. organ

solid (*continued*)
    s. organ injury
    s. subtype
    s. tumor
    S. Tumor Autologous Marrow
      Transplant Program (STAMP)
    s. visceral hematoma
solitaire
    cholesterol s.
solitary
    s. bundle
    s. foramen
    s. gland
    s. pulmonary arteriovenous fistula
    s. pulmonary mass
    s. rectal ulcer
    s. rectal ulcer syndrome
    s. testicle
    s. tract
solubility
    anesthetic s.
solubilization
soluble gas technique
solute
    total body s.
solution
    activating s.
    aqueous s.
    azeotropic s.
    cardioplegic s.
    cleaning s.
    cold soak s.
    cold vein graft s.
    colloid s.
    colonic lavage s.
    crystalloid cardioplegic s.
    disclosing s.
    disinfecting s.
    electrolyte flush s.
    electrolytic s.
    extracellularlike calcium-free s.
    extravasation irrigation s.
    eye irrigating s.
    hardening s.
    Hartman s. (dentin desensitizer)
    Hartmann s. (lactated Ringer)
    hydrolysis of s.
    hypotonic s.
    ideal s.
    intracellularlike, calcium-bearing
      crystalloid s.
    irrigating s.
    irrigation s.
    isotonic crystalloid s.
    lacmoid staining s.
    lavage s.
    nonideal s.
    normal saline s.
    s. of contiguity

    s. of continuity
    ophthalmic activating s.
    oxidation of s.
    physiologic saline s.
    physiologic salt s.
    pickling s.
    precipitate in s.
    preservative s.
    rehydrating s.
    relaxing s.
    saline s.
    saltwater s.
    saturated s.
    sclerosing s.
    soaking s.
    solvent s.
    standard s.
    sterility of s.
    surgical marking s.
    volumetric s.
    wetting s.
    whole-gut lavage activating s.
solvation
solvent
    s. extraction
    s. solution
solvolysis
soma
somatectomy
    subtotal s.
somatic
    s. gene-transfer approach
    s. hypoalgesia
    s. mutation
    s. nerve
    s. pain
    s. therapy
somaticosplanchnic
somaticovisceral
somatization disorder
somatoprosthetics
somatosensory
    s. cortex
    s. evoked potential (SEP)
    s. pathway
    s. testing
somatostatin
    s. analogue
    s. receptor scintigraphy
somatostatinoma syndrome
somatotrophic network
somatotropinoma
somatovisceral
Somerville anterior hip approach
SOMI
    sternal-occipital-mandibular
      immobilization
somite formation
somnolence, somnolency

somnolency (*var. of* somnolence)
Sondergaard epicardial incision procedure
Sondermann canal
Sones coronary arteriography technique
sonication technique
sonic thrombolysis
sonification
Sonnenberg
    S. classification
    S. neurectomy
sonographic evidence
sonography
    abdominal s.
    focused abdominal s.
    renal s.
    serial s.
sonography-guided aspiration
sonoguided biopsy
sonohysterography
sonolucent tissue
sonomicrometry
sonomicroscopy
SonoPrep therapeutic ultrasound device
sonorous respiration
Soper modification
Sorbie calcaneal fracture classification
sore
    fungating s.
    hard s.
    pressure s.
    soft s.
    venereal s.
Soren ankle fusion
soreness
    delayed onset muscle s. (DOMS)
Soriano operation
Soria operation
Sorondo-Ferré hindquarter amputation
Sorrin periodontal abscess flap
sorter
Soto-Hall bone graft
sound
    absent bowel s.'s
    s. analysis
    bowel s.'s
    hypoactive bowel s.'s
    Korotkoff s.
    s. pressure level (SPL)
    s. pressure level scale
    s. quantity
sound-stimulated fetal movement
source
    cold light s.
    discrete bleeding s.
    endoscopic light s.
    laparoscopic halogen light s.
    pipeline supply s.

    point s.
    s. program
Sourdille
    S. keratoplasty
    S. ptosis operation
Southwick biplane trochanteric osteotomy
Southwick-Robinson anterior cervical approach
space
    abdominal s.
    acromioclavicular s.
    air s.
    alveolar dead s.
    anatomic dead s.
    anorectal s.
    antecubital s.
    anterior clear s.
    apical s.
    arachnoid s.
    axillary s.
    Berger s.
    Bogros s.
    Böttcher s.
    Bowman s.
    buccal s.
    buccinator s.
    buccopharyngeal s.
    Burns s.
    capsular s.
    carotid s.
    central palmar s.
    cervical s.
    Chassaignac s.
    circumlental s.
    Colles s.
    coracoclavicular s.
    costoclavicular s.
    Cotunnius s.
    cranial epidural s.
    craniospinal s.
    danger s.
    dead s.
    deep perineal s.
    deep postanal anorectal s.
    Denonvilliers s.
    denture s.
    digastric s.
    disc s.
    Disse s.
    edentulous s.
    embrasure s.
    endolymphatic s.
    epidural s.
    episcleral s.
    extracellular s.
    extraction s.
    extradural s.
    extraperitoneal s.
    extrapleural s.

S

space (*continued*)
    extravascular s.
    fascial s.
    fat cell s.
    first web s.
    fixed maintainer s.
    Fontana s.
    freeway s.
    geniohyoid s.
    gingival s.
    H s.
    Henke s.
    His perivascular s.
    Holzknecht s.
    incisural s.
    increased lateral joint s.
    infraglottic s.
    inframesocolic s.
    infraorbital s.
    infratemporal s.
    interalveolar s.
    intercellular s.
    intercondylar s.
    intercostal s.
    intercristal s.
    interdental s.
    interfascial s.
    interlamellar s.
    interocclusal rest s.
    interprismatic s.
    interproximal s.
    interradicular s.
    intersheath s.
    intersphincteric anorectal s.
    interstitial s.
    intervaginal s.
    intracristal s.
    intrafascial s.
    intramembranous s.
    intrapharyngeal s.
    intravaginal s.
    ischiorectal anorectal s.
    joint s.
    Kiernan s.
    lateral central palmar s.
    lateral joint s.
    lattice s.
    leeway s.
    leptomeningeal s.
    Lesgaft s.
    life s.
    lymph s.
    Magendie s.
    maintainer cast s.
    Malacarne s.
    mandibular s.
    marrow s.
    masseteric s.
    masseter-mandibular-pterygoid s.

    masticator s.
    masticatory s.
    Meckel s.
    medial clear s.
    mediastinal s.
    medullary s.
    midpalmar s.
    Mohrenheim s.
    s. myopia
    Nance leeway s.
    object s.
    s. of Donders
    s. of Fontana
    s. of Poirier
    s. of Retzius abscess
    organ s.
    palm s.
    paraglottic s.
    paralaryngeal s.
    parapharyngeal s.
    pararenal s.
    Parona s.
    parotid s.
    perforated s.
    perianal anorectal s.
    perichoroidal s.
    peridental s.
    peridentinoblastic s.
    perihepatic s.
    periimplant s.
    perilenticular s.
    perilymphatic s.
    perineal s.
    perinuclear s.
    perioptic subarachnoid s.
    periotic s.
    peripharyngeal s.
    perirenal s.
    periscleral s.
    perisinusoidal s.
    peritoneal s.
    peritonsillar s.
    perivascular s.
    perivitelline s.
    pharyngeal s.
    pharyngomaxillary s.
    physiologic dead s.
    plantar s.
    pleural s.
    pleuroperitoneal s.
    pneumatic s.
    Poiseuille s.
    popliteal s.
    portal s.
    position in s.
    posterior cervical s.
    postpharyngeal s.
    postzygomatic s.
    potassium s.

predental s.
preepiglottic s.
premasseteric s.
preperitoneal s.
presacral s.
preseptal s.
presternal s.
pretarsal s.
pretemporal s.
pretracheal s.
prevertebral s.
prezonular s.
properitoneal s.
Proust s.
proximal s.
proximate s.
Prussak s.
pterygomandibular s.
pterygomaxillary s.
pterygopalatine s.
pterygopharyngeal s.
quadrangular s.
quadrilateral s.
regainer s.
Reinke s.
relief s.
removable maintainer s.
retraction s.
retroadductor s.
retrobulbar s.
retrocardiac s.
retrocrural s.
retroesophageal s.
retrogastric s.
retroinguinal s.
retrolental s.
retromammary s.
retromuscular s.
retromylohyoid s.
retroocular s.
retroperitoneal s.
retropharyngeal s.
retropubic s.
retrosternal air s.
retrotracheal s.
retrovesical s.
retrovisceral s.
retrozygomatic s.
Retzius s.
right anterior pararenal s.
Schwalbe s.
septal s.
sphenomaxillary s.
sphenopalatine s.
subacromial s.
subaponeurotic s.
subarachnoid s.
subchorial s.
subcoracoid s.

subdiaphragmatic s.
subdural s.
subgingival s.
subhepatic s.
sublingual s.
submandibular s.
submasseteric s.
submaxillary s.
submental s.
submucosal s.
subperitoneal s.
subphrenic s.
subpulmonic pleural s.
subretinal s.
subumbilical s.
superficial perineal s.
superior joint s.
supracolic s.
suprahepatic s.
suprahyoid s.
supralevator anorectal s.
supraomental s.
suprasternal s.
supratentorial s.
Tarin s.
temporal s.
Tenon s.
thenar s.
tibiofibular clear s.
tissue s.
Traube semilunar s.
Trautmann triangular s.
triangular s.
vascular s.
vertebral epidural s.
vesicocervical s.
Virchow-Robin s.
visceral s.
Waldeyer s.
web s.
Westberg s.
widened retrogastric s.
yolk s.
Zang s.
zonular s.
zygomaticotemporal s.

space-occupying
s.-o. brain lesion
s.-o. disease
s.-o. process
s.-o. tumor

spacer
disc s.
suture s.

spacing
excessive s.

Spaeth
S. cystic bleb operation
S. ptosis operation

spall
span
    levator s.
Spanish silk suture
sparganoma
sparing therapy
spasm
    diffuse esophageal s.
    esophageal s.
    masseter s.
    nocturnal painful tonic s. (NPTS)
    tonic s.
    trismus s.
spasmodic colic
spasmolysis
spastic
    s. colon
    s. diplegia
    s. thumb-in-palm
    s. thumb-in-palm deformity
spasticity
spatia (*pl. of* spatium)
spatial
    s. contiguity
    s. facilitation
    s. localization procedure
    S. Orientation Memory Test
    (SOMT)
spatium, *pl.* spatia
spatula
    suture pickup s.
spatulate
spatulated repair
spatulation
    s. condensation
    graft s.
    ureteral s.
Spaulding sterilization of medical devices
  classification
Speas osteotomy
special
    s. lesion
    s. reference method
specialized intralobular connective
  tissue
specialty
    nonophthalmologic surgical s.
    surgical s.
species
    fungal s.
specific
    s. adjuvant exercise
    s. ionization
    s. modulation
    s. rotation
    s. survival
    s. thrust manipulation
    tumor s.
specificity phenomenon

specimen
    biopsy s.
    catheter s.
    colorectal s.
    cytologic s.
    cytology s.
    excised s.
    FNA s.
    gastrectomy s.
    mastectomy s.
    operative s.
    pathologic s.
    preoperative FNA s.
    s. radiograph
    trichrome-stained s.
    s. volume
speckled appearance
spectacle
    s. correction
    s. plane
spectacular shrinking deficit syndrome
spectral
    s. Doppler measurement
    s. edge frequency capnography
    s. entropy
    s. line
spectrometer
    liquid scintillation s.
    mass s.
spectrometry
    gas chromatography-mass s.
    (GC-MS)
    isotope dilution-mass s.
    mass s.
spectrophotometry
    endoscopic reflectance s.
    fluorescence s.
    microlight guide s.
    near-infrared s.
spectroscopic
spectroscopy
    bioelectrical impedance s. (BIS)
    clinical s.
    image-selected in vivo s.
    infrared s.
    in vivo optical s.
    magnetic resonance s.
    MR s.
    near-infrared s.
    NMR s.
    nuclear magnetic resonance s.
    (NMRS)
    Raman s.
    reflectance s.
specular
    s. echo
    s. microscopy
    s. reflection
speculum examination

speech
    s. correction
    s. detection threshold
Speed
    S. arthroplasty
    S. open reduction
    S. osteotomy graft
    S. radial head fracture classification
    S. sternoclavicular repair
    S. V-Y muscle-plasty
Speed-Boyd
    S.-B. open reduction
    S.-B. radial-ulnar fracture treatment
    technique
Spence
    S. and Duckett marsupialization
    axillary tail of S.
    S. urethral diverticulum procedure
Spencer plication of vena cava
Spencer-Watson
    S.-W. Z-plasty
    S.-W. Z-plasty entropion operation
sperm, spermatozoon
    s. aspiration
    epididymal s.
    s. immobilization test
    s. microaspiration retrieval technique
    (SMART)
    s. washing insemination method
spermagglutination
spermatic
    s. cord
    s. cord dissection
    s. duct
    s. fistula
    s. plexus
    s. vein
    s. vein ligation
spermatid
    round s.
spermatocele, spermatocyst
spermatocelectomy
spermatocyst (*var. of* spermatocele)
spermatogram
spermatolysis, spermolysis
spermatorrhea
spermatozoa
spermatozoon (*var. of* sperm)
spermaturia (*var. of* semenuria)
spermiduct
spermolith
spermolysis
Spetzler anterior transoral approach
Spetzler-Martin arteriovenous
  malformation classification
sphacelation
sphenethmoid
sphenion
sphenobasilar

sphenoccipital
sphenocephaly
sphenoethmoid
sphenoethmoidal recess
sphenoethmoidectomy
sphenofrontal suture
sphenoid
    s. bone
    s. emissary foramen
    s. emissary vein
    s. mucocele
    s. process
    s. sinus metastasis
sphenoidal, sphenoid
    s. angle
    s. concha
    s. fissure
    s. herniation
    s. ridge
    s. sinus
    s. spine
    s. turbinated bone
sphenoidectomy
sphenoidostomy
sphenoidotomy
sphenomalar
sphenomandibular ligament
sphenomaxillary
    s. fissure
    s. fossa
    s. space
    s. suture
sphenooccipital
    s. joint
    s. suture
sphenoorbital suture
sphenopalantine ganglion blockade
sphenopalatine
    s. artery
    s. canal
    s. foramen
    s. ganglion
    s. ganglionectomy
    s. nerve
    s. space
sphenoparietal
    s. suture
    s. venous sinus
sphenopetrosa
sphenopetrosal fissure
sphenorbital
sphenosalpingostaphylinus
sphenosquamosal
sphenosquamous suture
sphenotemporal
sphenotic foramen
sphenoturbinal
sphenovomerine suture
sphenozygomatic suture

S

sphere
    segmentation s.
spherica
spherical
    s. lens aberration
    s. recess
spherocytosis
    hereditary s.
spheroid, spheroidal
    s. articulation
    s. joint
spheroidal (*var. of* spheroid)
spherule
    rod s.
sphincter
    anatomic s.
    anorectal s.
    antral s.
    anular s.
    artificial s.
    basal s.
    bicanalicular s.
    Boyden s.
    canalicular s.
    choledochal s.
    colic s.
    s. constrictor cardiae
    deep anal s.
    duodenal s.
    duodenojejunal s.
    esophageal s.
    external rectal s.
    external urethral s.
    extrinsic s.
    functional s.
    Glisson s.
    hepatopancreatic s.
    hypertensive lower esophageal s.
    Hyrtl s.
    ileal s.
    ileocecocolic s.
    iliopelvic s.
    incompetent s.
    s. injury
    internal anal s. (IAS)
    internal urethral s.
    intrinsic s.
    lower esophageal s. (LES)
    macroscopic s.
    marginal s.
    s. mechanism
    mediocolic s.
    microscopic s.
    midgastric transverse s.
    midsigmoid s.
    s. muscle
    myovascular s.
    myovenous s.
    Nélaton s.

    O'Beirne s.
    Oddi s.
    s. of Oddi dysfunction
    s. of Oddi pressure
    ostial s.
    palatopharyngeal s.
    pancreatic s.
    pathologic s.
    pelvirectal s.
    s. pharyngoplasty
    physiologic s.
    postpyloric s.
    prepapillary s.
    preprostate urethral s.
    prepyloric s.
    s. preservation
    proximal urethral s.
    s. pupillae muscle
    pyloric s.
    radiologic s.
    s. reconstruction
    rectal s.
    rectosigmoid s.
    s. relaxation
    s. repair
    segmental s.
    smooth muscular s.
    striated muscular s.
    superior esophageal s.
    unicanalicular s.
    urethral s.
    Varolius s.
    velopharyngeal s.
sphincteral
sphincteralgia
sphincterectomy
    endoscopic s.
sphincterial, sphincteric
sphincteric
    s. construction
    s. continence
    s. potency
sphincterismus
sphincteroid tract
sphincterolysis
sphincteroplasty
    open s.
    pancreatic s.
    transduodenal s.
sphincteroscopy
sphincterotomy
    antegrade transcystic s.
    biliary s.
    Doublet s.
    endoscopic s.
    endoscopic pancreatic duct s.
    Erlangen pull-type s.
    external s.
    Geenen s.

internal s.
laparoscopic antegrade transcystic s.
Mulholland s.
needle-knife s.
pancreatic duct s.
Parks partial s.
partial lateral internal s.
precut s.
retrograde s.
transduodenal s.
transendoscopic s.
transurethral s.
urethral s.
zipper s.

sphincter-preserving proctectomy
sphincter-saving
    s.-s. method
    s.-s. operation
    s.-s. procedure
    s.-s. resection
    s.-s. surgery
    s.-s. technique
sphincter-sparing
    s.-s. method
    s.-s. procedure
    s.-s. resection
    s.-s. technique
sphinx position
sphygmopalpation
sphygmoscopy
SPI
    structured pain interview
spica cast immobilization
spiculated lesion
spider
    s. angioma
    s. nevus
    s. pelvis
    s. projection
    vascular s.
    s. veins
spider-web clot
Spiegel lobe
Spieghel line
spigelian
    s. hernia
    s. lobe
    s. vein
Spigelius
    S. hernia
    S. line
    S. lobe
spike-burst on electromyogram of colon
spiking temperature
spill
    endobronchial s.
    peritoneal s.
spillage
    intraabdominal s.

intraperitoneal s.
tumor s.
**Spiller-Frazier intracranial trigeminal
  neurotomy technique**
spina, *pl.* **spinae**
    s. bifida
    s. bifida aperta
spinae (*pl. of* spina)
spinal
    s. accessory nerve
    s. accessory nerve-facial nerve
    anastomosis
    afferent s.
    s. analgesia
    s. analgesic
    s. anesthesia (SA)
    s. anesthetic
    s. anesthetic technique
    s. angioma
    s. artery
    s. block
    s. canal
    s. canal stenosis
    s. column
    s. column stabilization
    s. compression fracture
    s. cord
    s. cord circulation
    s. cord compression
    s. cord concussion
    s. cord injury (SCI)
    s. cord injury pain
    s. cord ischemia
    s. cord perfusion pressure (SCPP)
    s. cord protection
    s. cord shock syndrome
    s. cord stimulation (SCS)
    s. cord tumor
    s. coronal plane deformity
    s. deafferentation
    s. decompression
    s. deformity-instability
    s. delivery
    s. dermal sinus tract
    s. dural arteriovenous fistula
    S. Dynamics Corporation
    s. dysraphism
    s. epidural abscess (SEA)
    failed s.
    s. fixation
    s. fixation rigidity
    s. flexibility test
    s. fluid drainage
    s. fusion
    s. fusion pathomechanics
    s. fusion position
    s. fusion technique
    s. ganglion
    s. gate

S

spinal (*continued*)
- s. headache
- s. hematoma
- s. infection
- s. infection biopsy
- s. inflammation
- s. injury operative stabilization
- s. instability
- s. joint mobilization
- s. lesion
- s. manipulation
- s. marrow
- s. metastasis
- s. mobilization technique
- s. modulation
- s. muscle
- s. nerve ligation
- s. osteotomy
- s. osteotomy stabilization
- s. oximetry
- s. point
- s. puncture
- s. pyramidotomy
- s. root
- s. shock
- single-shot s.
- s. surgery
- s. tractotomy
- s. trauma
- s. vascular malformation
- s. vein

spinal-epidural
- combined s.-e. (CSE)

spinal/epidural

spinal-locking procedure

spinally administered

spinaloscopy

spinate

spindle
- s. cell carcinoma
- s. cell sarcoma
- s. cell thymoma
- Krukenberg corneal s.

spindle-shaped incision

spine
- alar s.
- angular s.
- anterior inferior iliac s. (AIIS)
- anterior superior iliac s. (ASIS)
- bamboo s.
- Chance fracture thoracolumbar s.
- s. deformity
- dorsal s.
- s. fracture
- hemal s.
- iliac s.
- inferior iliac s.
- ischiadic s.

- ischial s.
- mental s.
- neural s.
- osteoporotic s.
- posterior inferior iliac s.
- posterior superior iliac s.
- pubic s.
- s. rotation
- sciatic s.
- s. skeleton
- sphenoidal s.
- thoracic s. (T-spine)

spin-echo image

Spinelli operation

spinning disc nebulizer

spinning-top deformity

spinocerebellar tract

spinogalvanization

spinoglenoid

spinolamellar line

spinolaminar line

spinomuscular

spinoneural

spinoolivary tract

spinotectal tract

spinothalamic
- s. cordotomy
- s. pathway
- s. tract (STT)
- s. tractotomy

spinous
- s. aspect
- s. interlaminar line
- s. plane
- s. process
- s. process fracture

spiradenoma

spiral
- s. CT technique
- s. dissection
- s. fold
- s. foraminous tract
- s. ganglion
- s. groove
- s. incision
- s. joint
- s. ligament
- s. line
- s. membrane
- s. oblique fracture
- s. of Tillaux
- s. suture technique
- Tillaux s.
- s. vein graft

Spira scapulothoracic arthrodesis procedure

spirochetal infection

spirochete infection

spirochetolysis

spirogram
    forced expiratory s.
spirometer
    incentive s.
spirometry
    continuous intraoperative s.
spiroscopy
Spittler ankle disarticulation procedure
Spitzka marginal tract
Spivack
    S. gastrostomy
    S. gastrotomy technique
SPK
    simultaneous pancreas and kidney
    SPK transplant
    SPK transplantation
splanchnapophyseal (*var. of*
  splanchnapophysial)
splanchnapophysial, splanchnapophyseal
splanchnapophysis
splanchnectopia
splanchnemphraxis
splanchnic
    s. anesthesia
    s. artery aneurysm
    s. AV fistula
    s. capillary pressure
    s. circulation
    s. congestion
    s. denervation of pancreas
    s. ganglion
    s. hypoperfusion
    s. nerve
    s. oxygenation
    s. oxygen consumption
    s. oxygen extraction
    s. oxygen transport
    s. perfusion
    s. venous stasis
    s. vessel
    s. wall
splanchnicectomy
    chemical s.
    thoracoscopic s.
splanchnicotomy
splanchnocele
splanchnocranium
splanchnodiastasis
splanchnolith
splanchnologia
splanchnology
splanchnomicria
splanchnoptosia (*var. of* splanchnoptosis)
splanchnoptosis, splanchnoptosia
splanchnorenal bypass
splanchnoscopy
splanchnoskeletal
splanchnoskeleton
splanchnosomatic

splanchnotomy
splanchnotribe
S-plasty
SPLATT
    split anterior tibial tendon
    SPLATT procedure
    SPLATT transfer
SPLATTT
    split anterior tibial tendon transfer
splayed carina
splayfoot deformity
spleen
    accessory s.
    adult wandering s.
    ectopic s.
    enlarged s.
    floating s.
    movable s.
    s. preservation
    supernumerary s.
    s. tip
    wandering s.
spleen-preserving
    s.-p. distal pancreatectomy
    s.-p. pancreatic resection
splenectomy
    abdominal s.
    Henry s.
    incidental s.
    laparoscopic s.
    laparoscopic Hassab gastric
      devascularization and s.
    near-total s.
    open s.
    palliative s.
    Rives s.
    subcapsular s.
splenectopia, splenectopy
splenectopy (*var. of* splenectopia)
splenetic
splenial
splenic
    s. abscess
    s. artery (SA)
    s. artery aneurysm (SAA)
    s. AV fistula
    s. branch
    s. conservation
    s. cord
    s. cord of Billroth
    s. cyst
    s. flexure
    s. flexure carcinoma
    s. flexure colonoscopy
    s. fossa
    s. hilum
    s. injury
    s. laceration
    s. lesion

S

splenic (*continued*)
    s. necrosis
    s. plexus
    s. preservation
    s. pulp
    s. puncture
    s. recess
    s. rupture
    s. salvage
    s. scintigraphy
    s. sequestration syndrome
    s. sinus
    s. tissue
    s. tuberculosis
    s. vein
    s. vein deformity
    s. vein stump
spleniform
spleniserrate
splenium
splenius capitis
splenoadrenal
    s. anastomosis
    s. shunt
splenobronchial fistula
splenocaval shunt
splenocele
splenocleisis
splenocolic ligament
splenogastric omentum
splenogonadal fusion
splenoid
splenolymphatic
splenoma
splenomegalia (*var. of* splenomegaly)
splenomegaly, splenomegalia
    congenital s.
splenonephric
splenopancreatic
splenopexia (*var. of* splenopexy)
splenopexy, splenopexia
splenophrenic
splenoptosia (*var. of* splenoptosis)
splenoptosis, splenoptosia
splenorenal
    s. angle
    s. bypass
    s. ligament
    s. shunt (SRS)
    s. venous anastomosis
splenorenale
splenorrhagia
splenorrhaphy
    Dexon mesh s.
splenosis
splenotomy
splenule
splenulus
splenunculus

splintered fracture
splinter hemorrhage
splinting
    closed reduction/chemical s.
    extracoronal s.
    s. of abdomen
    Strong dorsal extension block s.
splint/stent
    kidney internal s. (KISS)
split
    s. anterior tibial tendon (SPLATT)
    s. anterior tibial tendon procedure
    s. anterior tibial tendon transfer
        (SPLATTT)
    s. anterior tibial tendon transfer
        procedure
    s. fixation
    s. fracture
    s. ileostomy
    s. incision
    s. liver
    s. renal function test
    upper sternal s.
split-and-roll technique
split-bone technique
split-cast method
split-cord malformation
split-course technique
split-cuff nipple technique
split-hand deformity
split-heel
    s.-h. approach
    s.-h. fracture
    s.-h. incision
split-leg position
split-liver transplant (SLT)
split-lung ventilation
split-nail deformity
split-patellar approach
split-sternum esophagectomy
split-thickness
    s.-t. periodontal flap
    s.-t. skin graft (STSG)
splitting
    s. fracture
    s. lacrimal papilla operation
spoke-wheel appearance
spondylectomy
spondylitic
    s. deformity
    s. myelopathy
spondylitis
    ankylosing s.
    juvenile ankylosing s.
    Kümmell s.
spondylodesis
spondylodiscitis, spondylodiskitis
    lumbar s.
spondylodiskitis (*var. of* spondylodiscitis)

spondylolisthesis reduction
spondylolysis
spondylophyte
spondylosis
    symptomatic s.
spondylothoracic
spondylotomy
spondylous
sponge
    s. biopsy
    s. dissection
    s. explant
spongioblastoma
spongioplasty
spongiositis
spongy
    s. body
    s. urethra
Sponsel oblique osteotomy
spontaneous
    s. adenocarcinoma
    s. aliquorrhea
    s. amputation
    s. ascites filtration
    s. breathing
    s. breech extraction
    s. coronary artery dissection
    s. dialytic ultrafiltration
    s. esophageal rupture
    s. fistula closure
    s. fracture
    s. hyperemic dislocation
    s. intermittent mandatory ventilation (SIMV)
    s. intestinal perforation (SIP)
    s. lateral ventricle hernia
    s. lesion
    s. nipple discharge
    s. pain
    s. perforation
    s. pneumothorax
    s. renal hemorrhage
    s. resolution
    s. rupture
    s. ventilation
    s. ventilation anesthetic technique
    s. ventrolateral hernia
sporadic
    s. CRC
    s. islet cell tumor
    s. multigland disease
    s. multigland hyperplasia
    s. multiple gland parathyroid hyperplasia
    s. pituitary adenoma
    s. primary HPT
    s. primary hyperparathyroidism
    s. renal cell carcinoma

sports hernia
spot
    ash-leaf s.
    cold s.
    s. compression
    corneal s.
    hottest s.
    s. magnification
    milk s.
    saccular s.
    Soemmerring s.
    utricular s.
S-pouch reconstruction
spout
    ileostomy s.
SPR
    selective posterior rhizotomy
    simultaneous pancreatic-renal
Sprague orthopaedic arthroscopic technique
sprain fracture
spray-wipe-spray disinfection
spread
    block s.
    extrathyroid s.
    lymphatic s.
    metastatic s.
    omental s.
    peritoneal s.
spreader graft
spreading
    s. fistulation
    s. hypoperfusion
Sprengel
    S. anomaly
    S. deformity
spring fixation
sprinter's fracture
Sprotte spinal needle
sprouting
    ephaptic s.
    sympathetic s.
sprue
    collagenous s.
SPT
    slow pull-through
    station pull-through
    SPT technique
spur formation
spurious hyponatremia
spurium
Spurling cervical foraminal compression maneuver
spurring
sputa (*pl. of* sputum)
sputum, *pl.* **sputa**
    carbonaceous s.
    s. culture

S

sputum (*continued*)
   s. induction
   pink frothy s.
   s. production
SPV
   selective proximal vagotomy
squama, *pl.* **squamae**
   frontal s.
   temporal s.
squamae (*pl. of* squama)
squamatization
squame
squamocolumnar junction
squamofrontal
squamomastoid suture
squamooccipital
squamoparietal
squamopetrosal
squamosal suture
squamosomastoidea
squamotemporal
squamotympanic fissure
squamous
   s. border
   s. cell carcinoma (SCC)
   s. epithelium
   s. hyperplasia
   s. intraepithelial lesion (SIL)
   s. intraepithelial lesion/atypical
   squamous cell of undetermined
   significance (SIL/ASCUS)
   s. margin
   s. metaplasia
   s. regeneration
   s. suture
squamozygomatic
squared
   kilogram per meter s.
   (kg/m^2)
3-square flap
square knot
square-shouldered lesion
squat maneuver
squeak
   bronchopleural leak s.
squeeze pressure
SR
   sustained release
SRCP
   superficial renal cortical perfusion
SRS
   splenorenal shunt
   stereotactic radiosurgery
SRTR
   Scientific Registry of Transplant
   Recipients
SRVG
   silicone elastomer ring vertical
   gastroplasty

SRVGB
   Silastic ring vertical-banded gastric
   bypass
SS
   stainless steel
   SS suture
Ssabanejew-Frank gastrostomy
SSEP
   somatosensory evoked potential
S-shaped
   S-s. body
   S-s. deformity
   S-s. ileal pouch-anal anastomosis
   S-s. incision
SSI
   segmental spinal instrumentation
   surgical site infection
   anterior-posterior fusion with SSI
SSL
   subtotal supraglottic laryngectomy
SSNB
   suprascapular nerve block
SSPCS
   side-to-side portacaval shunt
   direct SSPCS
   emergency SSPCS
SSRI
   selective serotonin reuptake inhibitor
   SSRI discontinuation syndrome
SSS
   subclavian steal syndrome
ST segment elevation
STA
   superficial temporal artery
stab
   s. avulsion microphlebotomy
   technique
   s. phlebectomy
   s. skin incision
   s. wound
   s. wound incision
stability
   cardiovascular s.
   detrusor s.
   hemodynamic s.
stabilization
   anterior internal s.
   anterior short-segment s.
   s. approach
   atlantoaxial s.
   atlantooccipital s.
   cervical spine s.
   cervicothoracic junction s.
   chest wall s.
   coronoradicular s.
   definitive s.
   distal radioulnar joint s.
   dynamic lumbar s.
   flexion compression spine injury s.

fracture s.
Gruca s.
iliac crest bone graft s.
lower cervical spine posterior s.
lumbar spine s.
myoplastic muscle s.
occipitocervical s.
odontoid fracture s.
s. on retreat
operative s.
prophylactic operative s.
provisional s.
rhythmic s.
sacral spine s.
screw s.
spinal column s.
spinal injury operative s.
spinal osteotomy s.
subluxation s.
Texas Scottish Rite Hospital
  crosslink s.
thoracolumbar spine s.
s. training
TSRH crosslink s.
wire s.

stabilized
operatively s.
stabilizing fulcrum line
stable
s. burst fracture
s. cavitation
hemodynamically s.
s. reduction
stacked coin sign
stacking
breath s.
Stack shoulder procedure
Stafne idiopathic bone cavity
stage
s. B, C carcinoma
disease s.
Dukes s.
hard callus s.
implant s.
s.'s of labor
lymph node s.
s. migration
s. operation
patch s.
rehabilitation s.
soft callus s.
symptom experience s.
tumor s.
1-stage
1-s. amputation
1-s. hypospadias repair
1-s. left colectomy
2-stage
2-s. hip fusion

2-s. procedure
2-s. repair
2-s. Syme amputation
2-s. technique mastectomy
2-s. tendon grafting technique
2-s. tendon graft reconstruction
staged
s. abdominal repair (STAR)
s. approach
s. bilateral stereotactic
  thalamotomy
s. orchiopexy
s. pullthrough technique
s. reconstruction
s. reduction
s. repair of extensive aortic
  aneurysm
s. tympanoplasty
3-stage procedure
staghorn calculus
staging
Ann Arbor classification of Hodgkin
  disease s.
Astwood-Coller s.
Boden-Gibb tumor s.
s. celiotomy
s. evaluation
FAB s.
FIGO classification s.
French-American-British s.
International Federation of
  Gynecology and Obstetrics s.
Jewett and Strong s.
laparoscopic s.
s. laparoscopy
s. laparotomy
multiple myeloma s.
nonoperative s.
s. operation
preoperative s.
primary gastric
  lymphoma s.
SBR s.
Scarff-Bloom-Richardson s.
sentinel node s.
Sloan-Kettering thyroid
  cancer s.
surgical s.
surgical-pathologic s.
TNM system for tumor s.
tumor s.
tumor, node, metastasis s.
Whitmore-Jewett classification
  prostate cancer s.
stagnant
s. anoxia
s. hypoxemia
s. hypoxia
s. loop syndrome

S

stagnation

Staheli
    S. congenital hip dislocation containment technique
    S. hip osteotomy shelf procedure

Stähli pigment line

STAI
    State-Trait Anxiety Inventory

stain
    Alcian blue s.
    endocardial s.
    immunohistochemical s.
    Paget-Eccleston s.
    port-wine s.

staining
    anal canal s.
    argyrophilic nucleolar organizer region s.
    blue s.
    corneal blood s.
    extrinsic environmental s.
    immunohistochemical s.
    pattern of s.

stainless
    s. steel (SS)
    s. steel suture
    s. steel wire suture

staircase phenomenon

stairstep fracture

stalk
    body s.

Stallard
    S. flap operation
    S. tarsectomy for ptosis secondary to trachoma operation

Stallard-Liegard operation

staltic

STA-MCA
    superficial temporal artery to middle cerebral artery
    STA-MCA anastomosis
    STA-MCA bypass
    STA-MCA bypass surgery
    STA-MCA revascularization

Stamey
    S. antiincontinence operation
    S. modification
    S. modification of Pereyra bladder neck suspension procedure
    S. needle suspension
    S. urethrocystopexy

Stamey-Martius antiincontinence procedure

Stamm
    S. enterostomy
    S. gastroplasty
    S. gastrostomy
    S. metatarsal osteotomy
    S. procedure for intraarticular hip fusion
    S. temporary gastrostomy procedure

Stamm-Kader gastrotomy technique

STAMP
    Solid Tumor Autologous Marrow Transplant Program

standard
    s. biopsy technique
    s. bone algorithm program
    s. clavicular incision
    s. D1 gastrectomy
    s. electrode potential
    s. fashion
    s. formalin fixation
    s. gastric bypass
    s. gastric resection
    s. gastric resection Whipple procedure
    s. Kocher incision
    s. mastectomy
    s. midline laparotomy
    s. neck exploration
    s. open approach
    s. organ failure criteria
    s. patient monitoring
    s. reduction potential
    s. retroperitoneal flank incision
    s. right hemicolectomy
    s. solution
    s. stripping procedure
    s. surgical procedure
    s. technique
    s. thoracotomy

standardization

standardized
    s. curative radical total gastrectomy
    s. hepatectomy
    s. protocol
    s. surveillance criteria
    s. uptake value

stand-off weapon

Stanford
    S. biopsy method
    S. radical retropubic prostatectomy
    S. (type A, B) aortic dissection

Stanisavljevic knee reconstruction technique

Stanley Way radical vulvectomy procedure

Stanmore shoulder arthroplasty

stapedectomy
    House s.

stapedius
    s. muscle
    s. tendon

stapedotomy
    small fenestra s.

stapes mobilization
staphylectomy
staphylococcal
    s. infection
    s. scalded skin syndrome
Staphylococcus epidermidis
staphylopharyngorrhaphy
staphyloplasty
staphylorrhaphy
    Brophy s.
staphylotomy
staple
    s. capsulorraphy bone bank
    s. capsulorrhaphy
    s. fixation
    s. ligated
    s. line dehiscence
stapled
    s. blind end
    s. coloanal anastomosis
    s. esophagojejunostomy
    s. hemorrhoidectomy
    s. ileal pouch-anal anastomosis
    s. ileal pouch-anal anastomosis
      without proctomucosal
      proctectomy
    s. ileoanal anastomosis
    s. lung reduction
    s. reconstruction
    s. reconstruction method
    s. reconstruction procedure
    s. reconstruction technique
    s. stricturoplasty
    s. transanal rectal resection
      (STARR)
    s. vascular anastomosis
staple-line
    s.-l. bleeding
    s.-l. reinforcement device
stapler
    EEA s.
    laparoscopic aortic s.
Staples-Black-Broström ligament
repair
Staples ligament repair
stapling
    s. diverticulotomy
    gastric s.
    hemidouble s.
    surgical s.
    s. technique
star
    s. formation
    S. technique
STAR
    staged abdominal repair
starch
    hydroxyethyl s.
4-star exercise program

Stark
    S. cleft lip/palate classification
    S. iliac bone to mandibular body
      graft
Starkey matrix program
Stark-Moore-Ashworth-Boyes first
metacarpotrapezial joint fusion
technique
STARR
    stapled transanal rectal resection
startle technique
Starzl intraluminal venous anastomosis
technique
STAS
    Support Team Assessment Schedule
stases (*pl. of* stasis)
stasis, *pl.* **stases**
    s. edema
    s. gallbladder
    s. liver
    splanchnic venous s.
    s. syndrome
    s. ulceration
    venous s.
Statak suture
state
    asplenic s.
    central excitatory s.
    chronic hyperparathyroid s.
    dysphoric mood s.
    s. entropy
    exhaustion s.
    hypercoagulable s.
    inotropic s.
    International Classification of
      Diseases, Adapted for Use in the
      United S.'s (ICDA)
    local excitatory s.
    mood s.
    oxidation s.
    posthypercapnic s.
    presurgical s.
    thrombin-mediated consumptive s.
State-Trait
    S.-T. Anger Expression Inventory
      (STAXI)
    S.-T. Anxiety Inventory (STAI)
static
    s. closure pressure
    s. compliance
    s. compliance of the total
      respiratory system
    s. compression
    s. dilation technique
    s. evaluation
    s. fixation
    s. gangrene
    s. image
    s. method

S

static (*continued*)
    s. position
    s. relation
    s. storage allocation
station
    lymph nodal s.
    node s.
    perigastric node s.
    perihepatic lymph nodal s.
    s. pull-through (SPT)
    s. pull-through esophageal
      manometry technique
    s. pull-through technique
    s. test
stationary manometry
statoacoustic nerve
statoconia
statoconic membrane
status
    acid-base s.
    American Society of
      Anesthesiologists s.
    ASA physical s.
    cancer s.
    carrier s.
    s. cribrosus
    s. epilepticus
    s. evaluation
    hepatic intracellular energy s.
    hydration s.
    lymph node s.
    s. migrainosus
    mutation carrier s.
    nutritional s.
    performance s.
    premorbid performance s.
    respiratory s.
    semielective s.
    work s.
Stauffer
    S. modification
    S. syndrome
staurion
staving
    barrel s.
STAXI
    State-Trait Anger Expression Inventory
stay
    hospital s.
    length of s. (LOS)
    prolonged hospital s.
    s. suture technique
steady-state
    s.-s. infusion
    s.-s. ventilatory response
steal
    circulatory s.
    iliac s.
    s. phenomenon

    portal s.
    renal-splanchnic s.
    subclavian s.
steam autoclave sterilization
steamy appearance
steatocystoma
steatohepatitis
    chemotherapy-associated s.
    nonalcoholic s.
steatoma
steatosis
    hepatic s.
    liver s.
steatotic liver
steel
    S. correction
    S. maneuver
    s. mesh suture
    S. rule of thirds
    stainless s.
    s. suture
    S. triple innominate osteotomy
steep
    s. head-down tilt
    s. lateral decubitus position
    s. Trendelenburg position
steeple skull
steerable cystoscopy
Steffee
    S. spinal fusion instrumentation
      technique
    S. thumb arthroplasty
stegnosis
Steichen neurovascular free flap
Steinberg infiltration block
Steinbrocker arthritis functional
  classification
Steindler
    S. elbow flexion restoration
      procedure
    S. flexorplasty
    S. matrixectomy
Steinert disease
Steinmann pin fixation
stellate
    s. border breast lesion
    s. configuration
    s. ganglion
    s. ganglion block (SGB)
    s. ganglion blockade
    s. ganglion block anesthesia
    s. ganglion block anesthetic
      technique
    s. incision
    s. laceration
    s. ligament
    s. mass
    s. skull fracture
stellectomy

stem
- s. bronchus
- s. cell
- s. cell gene therapy
- s. cell mobilization
- s. removal

stem-loop structure
Stener-Gunterberg abdominal sacral rectal cancer resection
Stener lesion
stenion
stenobregmatic
stenocephalia (*var. of* stenocephaly)
stenocephalic (*var. of* stenocephalous)
stenocephalous, stenocephalic
stenocephaly, stenocephalia
stenocrotaphia (*var. of* stenocrotaphy)
stenocrotaphy, stenocrotaphia
Steno duct
stenopeic iridectomy
stenosal
stenosed
stenoses (*pl. of* stenosis)
stenosis, *pl.* **stenoses**
- acquired postintubation s.
- airway s.
- aortic s.
- arterial s.
- artery s.
- atherosclerotic renal artery s.
- calcific aortic s.
- carotid artery atherosclerotic s.
- cervical s.
- choledochoduodenal junctional s.
- chronic s.
- congenital cystic duct s.
- congenital pyloric s.
- discrete s.
- esophageal s.
- glottic s.
- granulation s.
- hypertrophic pyloric s.
- idiopathic hypertrophic subaortic s. (IHSS)
- ileostomy s.
- inflammatory-associated s.
- laryngotracheal s.
- mitral s.
- pulmonary valve s.
- pulmonic valve s.
- pyloric s
- renal artery s.
- short-segment tracheal s.
- spinal canal s. (SCS)
- stomal s.
- subglottic tracheal s.
- subvalvular aortic s.
- supravalvular aortic s.

- tracheal s.
- vessel s.

stenothorax
stenotic
- s. cricoid
- s. disease
- s. esophagogastric anastomosis
- s. lesion
- s. stoma

Stensen duct, Steno duct
stent
- s. apposition
- s. construction
- s. deployment
- s. dislodgment
- esophageal s.
- s. evaluation
- s. expansion
- s. graft
- s. implantation
- s. incrustation
- Palmaz s.
- s. patency
- s. placement
- s. retrieval
- self-expanding metallic s.

stented
- s. bovine pericardial xenograft
- s. porcine xenograft

stent-graft
- AAA s.-g.

stent-induced
- s.-i. intimal hyperplasia
- s.-i. pneumoperitoneum

stenting
- accessory duct s.
- antral s.
- biliary s.
- carotid s.
- carotid angioplasty with s.
- carotid artery s.
- endoluminal s.
- endoscopic ampullary s.
- endoscopic pancreatic s.
- endoscopic papillotomy and s.
- endoscopic retrograde biliary s.
- endovascular s.
- primary s.
- renal artery s.
- s. technique
- transhepatic s.
- tumor s.

stentless composite graft
stent-mounted
stent-through-wire mesh technique
Stenvers projection
step
- corneal graft s.
- diagnostic s.

S

step (*continued*)
    s. graft operation
    s. osteotomy
    s. preparation
    therapeutic s.
STEP
    serial transverse enteroplasty
    STEP procedure
2-step
    2-s. orchiopexy
    2-s. pancreatoduodenectomy
    2-s. procedure
    2-s. technique
step-by-step technique
step-cut
    s.-c. osteotomy
    s.-c. transection
stepdown
    s. osteotomy
    s. therapy
stephanial
stephanion
stepladder
    s. flap
    s. incision technique
step-sectioning
    nodal s.-s.
step-up in oxygen
  saturation
stercolith
stercoral
    s. abscess
    s. fecaloma
    s. fistula
    s. ulceration
stercoroma
stereoauscultation
stereochemistry
stereocolpogram
stereoencephalotomy
stereography
    3-dimensional s.
stereo-identical point
stereomagnification
stereoscopic interrogation
stereoscopy
stereoselective
stereoselectivity ratio
stereospecific action
stereotactic, stereotaxic
    s. aspiration
    s. aspiration biopsy
    s. automated technique
    s. brain biopsy
    s. catheter drainage
    s. cordotomy
    s. core biopsy method
    s. core biopsy technique
    s. core breast biopsy

    s. craniotomy
    s. guidance
    s. lesion
    s. localization
    s. needle core biopsy (SNCB)
    s. needle core biopsy
      procedure
    s. neurosurgery
    s. operation
    s. pallidotomy
    s. percutaneous needle biopsy
    s. puncture
    s. radiation therapy
    s. radiofrequency lesioning
    s. radiosurgery (SRS)
    s. surgery
    s. surgical ablation
    s. technique
    s. trigeminal tractotomy
    s. Vim thalamotomy
    s. VL thalamotomy
stereotactic-guided biopsy
stereotaxic (*var. of* stereotactic)
stereotaxis, stereotaxy
    frame-based s.
    frameless s.
    volumetric s.
stereotaxy (*var. of* stereotaxis)
sterile
    s. abscess
    s. field barrier
    s. granuloma
    s. matrix
    s. pericystectomy
    s. technique
    s. vaginal examination
sterility of solution
sterilization
    chemical vapor s.
    cold gas s.
    defined s.
    discontinuous s.
    dry heat oven s.
    ethylene oxide s.
    ETO s.
    flash s.
    fractional s.
    gas s.
    glutaraldehyde s.
    intermittent s.
    involuntary s.
    root canal s.
    steam autoclave s.
    tubal s.
    unsaturated chemical vapor s.
    voluntary s.
sterilized
    cold gas s.
Steri-Strip

steri-stripped incision
sternad
sternal
    s. angle
    s. artery
    s. branch
    s. cartilage
    s. click
    s. development
    s. fragment
    s. joint
    s. lifting
    s. line
    s. lymph node
    s. muscle
    s. notch
    s. override
    s. part of diaphragm
    s. plane
    s. position
    s. puncture
    s. rotation
    s. wire suture
sternal-occipital-mandibular
  immobilization (SOMI)
sternal-splitting incision
sternochondroscapularis
sternochondroscapular
  muscle
sternoclavicular
    s. angle
    s. disc
    s. joint
    s. joint dislocation
    s. joint reconstruction
    s. joint reduction
    s. junction
    s. ligament
    s. muscle
sternocleidal
sternocleidomastoid (SCM)
    s. artery
    s. hemorrhage
    s. muscle
    s. muscle origin
    s. region
    s. vein
sternocostal
    s. articulation
    s. head
    s. joint
    s. triangle
sternodynia
sternofascialis
sternoglossal
sternohyoideus
sternohyoid muscle
sternoid
sternomanubrial junction

sternomastoid
    s. artery
    s. muscle
sternopericardial ligament
sternoschisis
sternothyroid
    s. muscle
    s. muscle flap laryngoplasty
sternothyroideus
sternotomy
    complete s.
    concomitant median s.
    s. incision
    median s.
    s. scar
sternotracheal
sternotrypesis
sternovertebral
sternoxiphoid plane
sternum
    s. cartilage
    mobile s.
sternum-splitting approach
steroid
    s. concentration
    endogenous s.
    s. hormone
    s. injection
    lumbar epidural s.
steroid-dependent asthmatic
steroid-resistant proteinuria
stertorous respiration
stethalgia
stetharteritis
stethoscopy
Steward Recovery Score
Stewart
    S. collateral circulation test
    S. distal clavicular excision
    S. incision
    S. styloidectomy
Stewart-Hamilton cardiac output
  technique
Stewart-Treves syndrome
Stewart-Way bile duct injury
  classification
Stickler syndrome
stick-tie suture technique
Stieda
    S. fracture
    S. process
Stiegmann-Goff endoscopic esophageal
  varices ligation technique
stiff
    s. abdomen
    s. lung
stiffness
    fusion s.
stiff-person syndrome

S

stigma, *pl.* **stigmas,** *pl.* **stigmata**
    malpighian s.
    stigmata of recent hemorrhage
    (SRH)
stigmas (*pl. of* stigma)
stigmata (*pl. of* stigma)
stigmatization
stigmatoscopy
Stiles-Bunnell flexor digitorum
  superficialis transfer technique
Stilling
    canal of S.
Stillman
still radiography technique
stilus (*var. of* stylus)
Stimson
    S. anterior shoulder reduction
      technique
    gravity method of S.
    S. gravity shoulder dislocation
      reduction method
    S. posterior hip dislocation
      reduction maneuver
stimulated gracilis neosphincter technique
stimulating
    s. catheter
    s. effect
stimulation
    anal electrical s.
    anocutaneous s.
    antidromic s.
    biochemical s.
    brain s.
    calibrated electrical s.
    cervical carcinoma s.
    controlled disc s.
    cortical s.
    cutaneous s.
    deep brain s.
    direct brain s.
    direct electrical nerve s.
    direct neural s.
    dorsal column s. (DCS)
    dorsal cord s. (DCS)
    double-burst s.
    double simultaneous s.
    electric s.
    electrical nerve s.
    electrical surface s.
    electroacupoint s.
    electrogalvanic s.
    electronic bone s.
    electrophysiological s.
    external-coil electrical s.
    extradural cortical s.
    follicle maturation s.
    functional electrical s.
    functional neuromuscular s.
    galvanic s.

Ganzfeld s.
gastric electrical s.
gingival s.
high-voltage pulsed galvanic s.
hilum s.
implantable gastric s.
interferential current s.
intracranial s.
intraoperative cavernous nerve s.
intravaginal electrical s.
ischemic pain s.
juxtacrine s.
magnetic s.
magnetoelectric s.
mechanical s.
microamperage electrical nerve s.
microamperage neural s.
motor cortex s.
motor-evoked response to
  transcranial s. (tc-MER)
neurochemical s.
neuromuscular electrical s.
nociceptive s.
noninvasive programmed electrical s.
ovarian s.
ovulation s.
paired electrical s.
pelvic s.
percutaneous s.
percutaneous electrical nerve s.
  (PENS)
periaqueductal gray matter s.
periaqueductal-periventricular s.
peripheral nerve s.
photic s.
phrenic s.
precentral cortical s.
programmed electrical s.
punctate s.
repetitive magnetic s.
repetitive nerve s.
repetitive transcranial magnetic s.
s. scan
secretin s.
selective arterial s.
sensory s.
spinal cord s. (SCS)
subthreshold s.
supramaximal tetanic s.
tactile s.
s. test
tetanic s.
thermal s.
s. threshold
train-of-four s.
transcranial s. (TCS)
transcranial electrical s.
transcutaneous acupoint electrical s.
  (TAES)

transcutaneous cranial electrical s.
(TCES)
transcutaneous electric s. (TES)
transcutaneous electrical nerve s.
(TENS)
transesophageal atrial s.
transurethral electrical
bladder s.
ultrarapid subthreshold s.
vagal nerve s.
vaginal electrical s.
ventricular-programmed s.
vibroacoustic s.
visual s.
**stimulation-induced analgesia
(SIA)**
stimulator
cochlear s.
computerized thermal s.
implanted neural s.
interferential s.
neural s.
stimuli (*pl. of* stimulus)
stimulus, *pl.* **stimuli**
double extra s.
external s.
flicker-fusion s.
noxious s.
train-of-four s.
transcutaneous tetanic s.
stippled epiphysis
stippling
geographic s.
stitch
s. abscess
Alfieri s.
Allgöwer s.
angle s.
arthroscopic s.
baseball s.
bow-tie s.
box s.
Bunnell s.
Connell s.
continuous locked s.
corner s.
cuticular s.
deep s.
extramucosal s.
figure-of-8 s.
Fothergill s.
Frost s.
funnel s.
Heaney suture ligature s.
horizontal mattress s.
interrupted s.
interrupted corner s.
intracuticular s.
Lembert seromuscular s.

lock s.
locked s.
MaC s.
MaC s.
marker s.
mattress s.
McCall s.
modified Sturmdorf s.
O'Leary s.
roll s.
running s.
running locked s.
seromuscular s.
shoelace s.
simple interrupted s.
Sturmdorf s.
subcuticular s.
tagging s.
tilt s.
tracheal safety s.
triple-throw square knot s.
vertical mattress s.
STM
soft tissue mobilization
St. Mark polyposis registry
STO
surgical treatment objective
Stocker
S. line
S. operation
stocking anesthesia
stocking-glove
s.-g. anesthesia
s.-g. pain distribution
stocking-seam incision
Stock operation
**Stoffel spastic paralysis motor nerve
division**
stom
stomach
stoma, *pl.* **stomas, stomata**
abdominal s.
aberrant umbilical s.
anastomotic s.
Benchekroun s.
bowel s.
s. button
catheterizable s.
s. closure
colonoscopy per s.
concealed umbilical s.
diverting s.
double-barrel s.
dusky s.
end s.
endloop s.
gastroenterostomy s.
gastrointestinal s.
s. hernia

S

stoma (*continued*)
    ileostomy s.
    intestinal s.
    loop s.
    maturing the s.
    Mitrofanoff s.
    nippled s.
    permanent s.
    pleural s.
    prolapsed s.
    proximal diverting s.
    retracted s.
    rodless end-loop s.
    rosebud s.
    silastic collar-reinforced s.
    s. site
    stenotic s.
    s. therapist
    tracheostomy s.
    Turnbull loop s.
    ureteral s.
    ureteric s.
    Wang pleural s.
stomach
    s. acid
    s. adenocarcinoma
    bilocular s.
    s. cancer metastasis
    s. cardiomyotomy
    s. deformity
    Dieulafoy vascular malformation of s.
    drain-trap s.
    dumping s.
    hourglass s.
    insufflation of s.
    intrathoracic s.
    leather-bottle s.
    open eye-full s.
    posterior s.
    pyloric part of s.
    s. reefing
    s. resection
    sclerotic s.
    s. slippage
    thoracic s.
    totally intrathoracic s.
    trifid s.
    upside-down s.
    wallet s.
    watermelon s.
    water-trap s.
stomachal
stomachic
stomal
    s. colonoscopy
    s. complication
    s. intussusception
    s. invagination

    s. prolapse
    s. retraction
    s. stenosis
    s. ulceration
stomas (*pl. of* stoma)
stomata (*pl. of* stoma)
stomatal
stomatic
stomatodeum (*var. of* stomodeum)
stomatomy
stomatonoma
stomatoplastic
stomatoplasty
stomatoscopy
    diagnostic fiberoptic s.
    fiberoptic s.
stomatotomy
stomocephalus
stomodeum, stomatodeum
stone
    S. anoplasty procedure
    s. basket
    biliary tract s.
    bladder s.
    cholesterol s.
    common bile duct s.
    duct s.
    endoscopic extraction of pancreatic duct s.
    s. extraction
    extraction of bile duct s.
    extraction of pancreatic s.
    extrahepatic s.
    s. fragmentation
    s. granuloma formation
    kidney s.
    mounted point s.
    s. removal
    renal s.
    soft pigment s.
    s. surgery
    vein s.
stony-hard eye
Stookey-Scarff opening from third ventricular to prechiasmal and interpeduncular cistern
stool
    abdominal s.
    s. evacuation
    guaiac-negative s.
    guaiac-positive s.
    hard s.
    heme-negative s.
    heme-positive s.
    s. impaction
    soft s.
stopcock
    Medex Hi-Flo s.

Stoppa
S. bilateral inguinal hernia repair procedure
S. giant prosthetic reinforcement
S. giant prosthetic reinforcement of visceral sac
S. GPRVS
S. hernia repair
Stoppa-type laparoscopic repair
stopper
port s.
stop-valve airway obstruction
storage allocation
storm
thyroid s.
stove-in chest
strabismus
paralytic s.
s. surgery
strabotomy
straddle fracture
straight
s. canal
s. catheter test
s. graft
s. incision
s. leg raising test
s. seminiferous tubule
s. sinus
straightening maneuver
straight-in ventriculostomy
straight-leg raising (SLR)
strain
compression s.
lysogenic s.
s. pattern
strain/counterstrain technique
straining
excessive s.
Straith eyelid operation
Strampelli-Valvo operation
stranding
fascial s.
soft tissue s.
strangulated
s. hemorrhoid
s. hernia
s. incisional hernia
s. paraesophageal hernia
strangulation necrosis
stranguria (*var. of* strangury)
strangury, stranguria
strap muscle
strapping
Strasberg laparoscopic biliary tract injury classification

Strassman
S. bicornual uterus metroplasty technique
S. metroplasty
transverse fundal incision of S.
strata (*pl. of* stratum)
strategy
imaging s.
injury-prevention s.
management s.
pain-coping strategies
protective ventilatory s.
surgical s.
treatment s.
wound closure s.
stratification
stratified
s. clot
s. epithelium
stratiform fibrocartilage
stratum, *pl.* **strata**
Straub technique
Strauss method
strawberry angioma
straw-colored ascites
Strayer
S. gastrocnemius recession procedure
S. tendon technique
streak retinoscopy
stream
fecal s.
streamlined pharyngeal airway liner
Streatfield-Fox eyelid operation
Streatfield lid ptosis operation
Streatfield-Snellen operation
strength
bone-screw interface s.
cervical extension s.
extensor hallucis longus s.
extrinsic muscle s.
graft s.
isometric cervical extension s.
wound-breaking s.
strength-duration curve
strengthening exercise
Stren intraepiphysial osteotomy
streptococcal infection
***Streptococcus* infection**
stress
cold restraint s.
s. dorsiflexion projection
s. fracture
s. hormone response
s. lesion
s. loading
operative s.
s. reduction
s. relaxation
s. response

S

stress (*continued*)
    s. rupture
    surgical s.
    s. ulceration
    s. ulcer hemorrhage
    s. urethral pressure profile
    s. urinary incontinence
stress-induced
    s.-i. analgesia
    s.-i. gastric ulceration
    s.-i. hyperglycemia
    s.-i. hyperthermia (SIH)
stretch
    anal s.
    s. injury
stretch-and-spray technique
stretcher
stretch-induced neuropathy
stretching
    Brailey supraorbital nerve s.
    s. exercise
    soft tissue s.
Stretta
    S. GERD radiofrequency operation
    S. radiofrequency for GERD
    procedure
stria, *pl.* **striae**
    corneal s.
    cutaneous s.
    striae of Zahn
striae (*pl. of* stria)
striate
    s. artery
    s. body
striated
    s. duct
    s. muscle
    s. muscle innervation
    s. muscular sphincter
striation
    tabby-cat s.
    tigroid s.
Strickland
    S. flexor tendon repair
    technique
    S. modification
    S. tendon repair
stricture
    anastomotic s.
    benign s.
    bile duct s.
    biliary s.
    Bismuth type IV s.
    Caroli type I distal bile duct s.
    cicatricial s.
    clip-induced bile duct s.
    distal bile duct s.
    esophageal s.
    s. formation

    gastrointestinal s.
    high-grade s.
    iatrogenic biliary s.
    low-grade s.
    s. management
    peptic s.
    s. prophylaxis
    radiation-associated s.
    s. rate
    rectal s.
    reflux s.
    refractory s.
    short s.
stricturoplasty
    Finney s.
    Heineke-Mikulicz s.
    isoperistaltic s.
    stapled s.
    s. technique
    Thal s.
stricturotomy
    endoscopic s.
stridor
    biphasic s.
    nonorganic s.
    postextubation s.
stridulous respiration
string
    s. cell carcinoma
    s. test
string-of-beads appearance
strip
    autogenous s.
    s. biopsy
    s. biopsy resection technique
    circumferential s.
    s. craniectomy
    s. perforation
    s. procedure
    s. resection
    Suture Strip wound closure s.
stripe
    paratracheal tissue s.
    properitoneal flank s.
stripout
    screw s.
stripping
    Jackson-Babcock vein s.
    s. membrane
    s. program
    saphenous vein s.
stroboscope
stroboscopic evaluation
stroke
    acute ischemic s.
    s. ejection rate
    exploratory s.
    hemorrhagic s.
    ischemic s.

mitochondrial myopathy,
   encephalopathy, lactacidosis, s.
   (MELAS)
nonfatal s.
perioperative s.
s. volume
stroma, *pl.* **stromata**
stromal
   s. line
   s. neovascularization
stromata (*pl. of* stroma)
stromatolysis
stromatosis
Strombeck nipple transposition
Strong dorsal extension block splinting
strongyloma
strophocephaly
Stroud pectinated area
structural
   s. abnormality
   s. anomaly
   s. lesion
structure
   abdominal s.
   anatomic s.
   bony s.
   cord s.
   cystic s.
   echodense s.
   endosellar s.
   extraarticular s.
   graft s.
   helix-loop-helix s.
   implant s.
   infratentorial s.
   major vascular s.
   periesophageal s.
   retroclival s.
   retroperitoneal s.
   retrosellar s.
   ring s.
   sella s.
   sidewall s.
   soft tissue s.
   stem-loop s.
   underlying s.
   vascular s.
structured pain interview (SPI)
struma lymphomatosa
strumectomy
   median s.
strumiform
strut
   s. allograft
   s. fracture
   s. graft
   s. malposition
   s. plate fixation
   s. spinal fusion technique

struvite
   s. calculus
   s. crystal formation
STS
   soft tissue sarcoma
STSG
   split-thickness skin graft
STT
   spinothalamic tract
studding
   peritoneal s.
Studer
   S. neobladder
   S. pouch ileal neobladder procedure
   S. reservoir urinary diversion
study
   acoustic stimulation s.
   altitude simulation s.
   angiographic s.
   barium swallow s.
   bead chain s.
   bulb-tip retrograde s.
   contrast s.
   cytologic s.
   diagnostic s.
   Doppler s.
   electromyographic s.
   electrophysiology s.
   epidemiologic s.
   exercise s.
   histologic s.
   imaging s.
   injection s.
   localization s.
   manometric s.
   multicentric s.
   noninvasive localization s.
   noninvasive venous s.
   S. of the Efficacy of Nosocomial
      Infection Control (SENIC)
   postirradiation s.
   preoperative s.
   pressure s.
   pressure-flow electromyography s.
   prospective s.
   radiologic s.
   tissue s.
   T-tube s.
   venographic s.
   venous s.
   volumetric s.
Stulberg Legg-Calvé-Perthes disease
   classification
stump
   anastomotic s.
   cervical s.
   s. dehiscence
   distal s.
   duodenal s.

S

stump (*continued*)
    s. embolization syndrome
    Hartmann s.
    s. invagination
    jejunal s.
    s. leak
    s. ligation
    s. pain
    pancreatic s.
    pneumonectomy s.
    s. pressure
    rectal s.
    rectosigmoid s.
    Roux limb s.
    splenic vein s.
stunned myocardium
stunning
    myocardial s.
Sturge-Weber syndrome
Sturmdorf
    S. operation
    S. stitch
    S. suture technique
stuttering
    exteriorized s.
    urinary s.
stye
styliform
styloauricularis
styloauricular muscle
styloglossus muscle
stylohyal
stylohyoid
    s. branch
    s. ligament
    s. muscle
    s. process syndrome
styloid
    s. cornu
    s. prominence
    s. syndrome
styloidectomy
    Stewart s.
styloidei
    vagina processus s.
stylomandibular
    s. ligament
    s. membrane
stylomastoid
    s. artery
    s. foramen
    s. vein
stylomaxillary ligament
stylopharyngeal muscle
stylopharyngeus
stylostaphyline
stylosteophyte
stylus, stilus
styptic collodion

Suarez-Villafranca enucleation
Suave-Kapandji arthroplasty
subabdominal
subabdominoperitoneal
subacromial
    s. bursa
    s. space
subacute inflammation
subambient pressure
subanal
subanesthetic concentration
subanular mattress suture
subapical segment
subaponeurotic space
subarachnoid
    s. anesthesia
    s. block (SAB)
    s. cavity
    s. cistern
    s. hemorrhage
    s. injection
    s. migration
    s. space
subarcuata
subarcuate fossa
subareolar tenderness
subastragalar dislocation
subatmospheric epidural pressure
subaural
subauricular
subaxial
subaxillary
subcapital
    s. fracture
    s. osteotomy
subcapsular
    s. hemorrhage
    s. renal hematoma
    s. splenectomy
subcardiac cancer
subcartilaginous
subcatastrophic dose
subcaudate tractotomy
subcecal fossa
subchondral
subchorial
    s. hemorrhage
    s. space
subchorionic
    s. hematoma
    s. hemorrhage
subchoroidal approach
subciliary incision
subclassification
subclavia
    ansa s.
subclavian
    s. arteriovenous fistula
    s. artery

s. artery aneurysm
s. artery occlusion
s. central venous catheter insertion
s. duct
s. groove
s. injury
s. line
s. loop
s. lymphatic trunk
s. muscle
s. nerve
s. periarterial plexus
s. perivascular block
s. steal
s. steal syndrome (SSS)
s. sulcus
s. triangle
s. vein
s. vein catheterization
s. vein patch angioplasty
s. vessel exposure
subclavian-subclavian bypass
subclavicular approach
subclavius muscle
subclinical infection
subcoma therapy
subcomplete resection
subcondylar
s. deformity
s. oblique osteotomy
subconjunctival
s. hemorrhage
s. injection
subcoracoid
s. bursa
s. shoulder dislocation
s. space
subcorneal blister
subcortical hemorrhage
subcostal
s. artery
s. flank incision
s. groove
s. insufflation technique
s. line
s. muscle
s. nerve
s. plane
s. port
s. position
s. transperitoneal incision
s. vein
subcostosternal
subcranial
subcruralis
subcrureus
subcut
subcutaneous

subcutaneous (subcut)
s. acromial bursa
s. anastomosis
s. calcaneal bursa
s. catheter port system
s. cyst
s. dose
s. emphysema
s. fascia
s. fasciotomy
s. flap
s. fungal infection
s. hematoma
s. implantation
s. implanted injection port
s. infrapatellar bursa
s. infusion
s. injection
s. mastectomy
s. necrosis
s. necrotizing infection
s. olecranon bursa
s. operation
s. plane
s. portion
s. ring
s. route
s. scalp
s. suture
s. tibialis posterior tenotomy
s. tissue
s. transfusion
subcuticular
s. stitch
s. suture
s. suture technique
subcutis
subdeltoid
s. bursa
s. fat plane obliteration
subdiaphragmatic
s. abscess
s. event
s. space
subdigastric node
subdorsal
subduce, subduct
subduct (*var. of* subduce)
subdural
s. abscess
s. block
s. cavity
s. cleft
s. effusion
s. electrode array
s. grid implantation
s. hematoma
s. hematorrhachis
s. hemorrhage

S

subdural (*continued*)
- s. hygroma
- s. puncture
- s. space

subendocardial myocardial infarction

subependymal
- s. brain calcification
- s. brain nodule
- s. extension
- s. giant cell astrocytoma
- s. hemorrhage

subependymoma

subepithelial
- s. hemorrhage
- s. membrane

subepithelium

subfalcial herniation

subfascial
- s. endoscopic perforator surgery (SEPS)
- s. hematoma
- s. ligation
- s. perforator
- s. perforator surgery
- s. prepatellar bursa

subfrontal approach

subfrontal-transbasal approach

subgaleal
- s. abscess
- s. emphysema
- s. hematoma
- s. hemorrhage

subgingival space

subglenoid shoulder dislocation

subglottic
- s. cavity
- s. edema
- s. pressure
- s. tracheal stenosis

subgluteal hematoma

subgrundation

subhepatic
- s. abscess
- s. recess
- s. space

subhuman primate donor

subhyaloid hemorrhage

subhyoid bursa

subiliac

subilium

subimplant membrane

subinfection

subinguinal
- s. fossa
- s. incision
- s. microsurgical varicocelectomy
- s. salivary gland
- s. triangle

subintimal hemorrhage

subjacent tissue

subject
- human s.
- supine human s.

subjugal

sublabial
- s. incision
- s. midline rhinoseptal approach
- s. perforation

sublaminar
- s. fixation
- s. wiring

sublation

sublesional ulceration

sublethal x-ray damage repair

subligamentous dissection

sublimation

sublimis

sublingual
- s. artery
- s. bursa
- s. caruncula
- s. crescent
- s. cyst
- s. duct
- s. fold
- s. fossa
- s. ganglion
- s. gland
- s. hematoma
- s. papilla
- s. pit
- s. space
- s. space abscess
- s. vein

sublumbar

subluxation
- atlantoaxial s. (AAS)
- rotary s.
- s. stabilization

submammary incision

submandibular
- s. duct
- s. fossa
- s. ganglion
- s. gland
- s. node
- s. space
- s. space abscess
- s. triangle

submandibulectomy

submasseteric
- s. space
- s. space abscess

submassive PE

submaxillary
- s. duct
- s. fossa

s. ganglion
s. space
s. triangle
submembranous placental hematoma
submental
s. artery
s. fistula
s. hematoma
s. liposuction
s. node
s. space
s. space abscess
s. triangle
s. vein
s. vertex projection
submentovertical projection
submucosa
jejunal s.
small-intestine s. (SIS)
submucosal
s. collateral circulation
s. dissection
s. gastric hemorrhage
s. invasion
s. mass
s. plexus
s. space
s. urethral augmentation
s. vascular dilation
submucous, submucosal
s. membrane
s. resection (SMR)
submuscular implantation
subnarcotic
subnasal
subneural
suboccipital
s. decompression
s. muscle
s. nerve
s. region
s. triangle
s. venous plexus
suboccipital-subtemporal approach
suboccipital-transmeatal approach
suboptimal
s. examination
s. surgery
subparalyzing dose
subparietal
subpatellar
subpectoral
s. implantation
s. implantation technique
s. plane
s. pocket
subpelviperitoneal
subpericardial
subperichondrial excision

subperiosteal
s. abscess
s. dissection
s. exposure
s. fracture
s. hematoma
s. hemorrhage
s. implant abutment
s. implant 1-phase technique
s. infection
s. resection
subperiosteally
subperitoneal
s. fascia
s. space
subperitoneoabdominal
subperitoneopelvic
subpetrosal
subpharyngeal
subphrenic
s. abscess
s. fluid
s. recess
s. region
s. space
subpleural
subplexal
subpopliteal recess
subpopulation
subpreputial
subpubic
s. angle
s. hernia
subpubicus
subpulmonary
subpulmonic pleural space
subpylorici
subpyloric node
subretinal
s. damage
s. hemorrhage
s. neovascularization
s. neovascular membrane
s. space
s. surgery
subsarcolemma cisterna
subsartorial canal
subscale
catastrophizing s.
cognitive anxiety s.
fear s.
helplessness s.
subscapular
s. artery
s. branch
s. bursa
s. circumflex artery
s. fossa
s. muscle

S

subscapular (*continued*)
   s. nerve
   s. vein
subscapularis
   s. muscle
   s. tendon
subsector
subsegmental hepatectomy
subsegmentectomy
   hepatic s.
subselective embolization
subserosa
subserosal (*var. of* subserous)
subserous, subserosal
subspinous
substance
   s. abuse disorder
   cement s.
   compact s.
   s. concentration
   corneal s.
   cortical s.
   exogenous s.
   exophthalmos-producing s.
   extracellular ground s.
   glandular s.
   medullary s.
   müllerian inhibiting s. (MIS)
   muscular s.
   tumor polysaccharide s.
   vasoactive s.
substantia, *pl.* **substantiae**
substantiae (*pl. of* substantia)
substernal
   s. angle
   s. gland
substernomastoid
substitute
   blood s.
   bone graft s.
   hypooncotic plasma s.
   plasma s.
   red blood cell s.
   TransCyte temporary skin s.
substitutional cardiac surgery
substitution transfusion
substructure
subsuperior segment
subtalar
   s. articulation
   s. dislocation
subtemporal
   s. craniotomy
   s. decompression
   s. dissection
subtemporal-intradural approach
subtendinous
   s. iliac bursa
   s. prepatellar bursa

sub-Tenon block
subtentorial lesion
subthreshold stimulation
subtotal (ST)
   s. colectomy (SC, STC)
   s. distal pancreatectomy
   s. esophagectomy
   s. esophagoplasty
   s. gastrectomy
   s. gastric exclusion
   s. gastric resection
   s. glossectomy
   s. hepatectomy
   s. hysterectomy (STH)
   s. lateral meniscectomy
   s. maxillectomy
   s. pancreatoduodenectomy
   s. parathyroidectomy
   s. parenchymal resection
   s. proctectomy
   s. proctocolectomy
   s. somatectomy
   s. supraglottic laryngectomy
    (SSL)
   s. thyroidectomy (STT)
subtraction
   image s.
   s. technique
subtrochanteric
   s. femoral fracture
   s. incision
   s. osteotomy
subtrochlear
subtype
   comedo s.
   cribriform s.
   micropapillary s.
   papillary s.
   solid s.
   tumor s.
subumbilical
   s. incision
   s. infection
   s. space
subungual hematoma
suburethral rectus fascial sling procedure
subvaginal
subvalvular aortic stenosis
subvertebral
subvitrinal
subvolution
subvoxel accuracy
subxiphoid
   s. hernia
   s. limited pericardiotomy
   s. port
subzonal insemination
subzygomatic
succenturiate

success
    s. rate
    weaning s.
successive approximation
succinylcholine (SUX)
succinylcholine-related apnea
sucking chest wound
Sucquet
    S. anastomosis
    S. canal
Sucquet-Hoyer
    S.-H. anastomosis
    S.-H. canal
sucrose test
suction
    airway s.
    s. aspiration
    s. biopsy
    bulb s.
    s. coagulator
    continuous NG s.
    s. curettage
    diastolic s.
    s. dissection
    s. drainage
    Frazier s.
    Gomco s.
    s. injury
    lavage and s.
    low intermittent s. (LIS)
    s. method
    nasogastric s.
    nasopharyngeal s.
    nasotracheal s.
    NG s.
    orogastric s.
    perilimbal s.
    Rhoton s.
    s. suspension
suction-induced hemolysis
suctioning
    endotracheal s.
    nasotracheal s.
suction-irrigation technique
Suda papilla type I–III classification
sudation
sudden infant death syndrome (SIDS)
Sudeck critical point
sudomotor
    s. axon reflex testing
    s. evaluation
sudoriferous
    s. duct
    s. gland
sufentanil
sugammadex
Sugarbaker pseudomyxoma peritonei complete tumor removal
sugar-icing liver

suggillation
    postmortem s.
Sugioka transtrochanteric rotational osteotomy
Sugiura
    S. esophageal variceal transection
    S. esophageal varices operation
    S. esophageal varices repair procedure
suite
    endoscopy s.
sulcal artery
sulcate
sulci (*pl. of* sulcus)
sulciform
sulcomarginal tract
sulcus, *pl.* **sulci**
    ampullary s.
    atrioventricular s.
    calcaneal s.
    carotid s.
    cerebral s.
    chiasmatic s.
    cingulate s.
    coronary s.
    deltopectoral s.
    s. fixated position
    s. fixation
    implant gingival s.
    inferior petrosal s.
    internal spiral s.
    intertubercular s.
    mentolabial s.
    nymphocaruncular s.
    nymphohymenal s.
    paracolic s.
    preauricular s.
    pulmonary s.
    scleral s.
    sclerocorneal s.
    sigmoid s.
    subclavian s.
    superior petrosal s.
    supraacetabular s.
    talar s.
    terminalis s.
sulfacytine
sulfate
    protamine s.
sulfation
sulfonation
summation
    temporal s.
Summerskill operation
sump syndrome
sun
    s. and chemical combination damage
    s. exposure

S

SUNCT
short-lasting unilateral neuralgiaform headache with conjunctival injection and tearing
SUNCT syndrome
Sunderland nerve injury classification
Sunna circumcision
Supartz joint fluid therapy
superacromial
superanal
superciliary arch
superduct
superexcitation
superextended gastric cancer lymph node dissection (D3)
superfecundation
superfetation
superficial
s. angioma
s. anterior larynx
s. anterior wall
s. brachial artery
s. branch
s. burn
s. cardiac plexus
s. cervical artery
s. cervical plexus
s. circumflex iliac artery
s. desensitization technique
s. epigastric artery
s. excision
s. external pudendal artery
s. femoral artery (SFA)
s. forearm
s. head
s. implantation
s. inguinal fascia
s. keratectomy
s. lamellar keratoplasty
s. layer
s. lymphatic vessel
s. musculoaponeurotic system (SMAS)
s. neck
s. orbit
s. palmar arch
s. palmar artery
s. parotidectomy
s. perineal artery
s. perineal pouch
s. perineal space
s. peroneal branch block
s. radiation
s. renal cortical perfusion (SRCP)
s. subumbilical infection
s. suture technique
s. temporal artery (STA)
s. temporal artery to middle cerebral artery (STA-MCA)
s. temporal artery to middle cerebral artery bypass
s. temporal artery to middle cerebral artery revascularization
s. temporalis artery
s. temporal plexus
s. thrombophlebitis
s. type
s. volar artery
s. wound
superficialis
superficialization
supergenual
superimpregnation
superinfection
fungal s.
superior
s. aberrant ductule
s. alveolar artery
s. angle
s. arcuate bundle
s. articular process
s. boundary
s. carotid triangle
s. cerebellar artery
s. cervical cardiac branch
s. cervical ganglion
s. cervical ganglionectomy
s. costal facet
s. costal pit
s. dislocation
s. duodenal fold
s. duodenal fossa
s. duodenal recess
s. edge
s. epigastric artery
s. esophageal sphincter
s. face
s. fascia
s. flap
s. flexure
s. ganglion
s. gluteal artery
s. gluteal artery perforator
s. gluteal neurovascular bundle
s. hemorrhoidal artery
s. hemorrhoidal plexus
s. horn
s. hypogastric block
s. hypogastric plexus
s. hypophysial artery
s. ileocecal hernia
s. ileocecal recess
s. intercostal artery
s. internal parietal artery
s. joint space
s. labial artery
s. labial branch

s. labrum anterior and posterior (SLAP)
s. lacrimal duct
s. lacrimal papilla
s. lacrimal punctum
s. laryngeal cavity
s. laryngeal nerve external branch
s. laryngeal vein
s. larynx
s. lateral genicular artery
s. leaf
s. lingular segment
s. margin
s. meatus
s. medial genicular artery
s. mediastinum
s. mesenteric arterial system
s. mesenteric artery (SMA)
s. mesenteric ganglion
s. mesenteric lymph node
s. mesenteric plexus
s. mesenteric vein (SMV)
s. mesenterorenal bypass technique
s. oblique tendon
s. omental recess
s. orbit
s. orbital fissure
s. orbital fissure syndrome (SOFS)
s. pancreaticoduodenal artery
s. parathyroid
s. parietal lobe
s. pelvic aperture
s. peroneal retinaculum
s. petrosal sulcus
s. phrenic artery
s. pole
s. pubic ramotomy
s. pulmonary vein
s. rectal artery
s. rectal fold
s. rectal plexus
s. sector iridectomy
sinus petrosus s.
s. suprarenal artery
s. tarsus
s. thoracic aperture
s. thoracic artery
s. thyroid artery
s. thyroid notch
s. thyroid plexus
s. thyroid tubercle
s. thyroid vein
s. tibial articulation
s. ulnar collateral artery
s. vena cava (SVC)
s. vena cava syndrome
s. venal caval obstruction
s. vertebral notch
s. vesical artery

superior-intradural approach
superioris
    von Blaskovics resection and advancement of levator palpebrae s.
superlactation
supernate
supernumerary
    s. breast
    s. gland
    s. organ
    s. spleen
superobese
super-obese patient
superolateral
superovulation induction
superoxide scavenger
superpetrosal
superpigmentation
superselective
    s. microcoil embolization
    s. vagotomy
supersensitivity
superstructure
super-wet technique
supinate
supination
    s. deformity
    s. injury
    s. reflex
supination-adduction fracture
supination-eversion fracture
supination-external
    s.-e. rotation (SER)
    s.-e. rotation injury
    s.-e. rotation IV
    s.-e. rotation type I–IV fracture
supination-inversion rotation injury
supination-plantar flexion injury
supinator
    s. crest
    s. longus reflex
    s. muscle
supine
    s. human subject
    s. hypotensive syndrome
    s. position
    s. sciatic block
supine-oblique approach
supple bowel
supplementary
    s. analgesia
    s. canal
    s. oxygen
    s. respiration
    s. sling procedure

S

supplementation
    anabolic hormone s.
    calcitriol s.
    calcium carbonate s.
    leucine s.
    postoperative s.
    temporary postoperative s.
    vitamin D s.

supply
    arterial s.
    blood s.
    compensatory blood s.
    myocardial oxygen s.
    tumor blood s.

support
    advanced cardiac life s. (ACLS)
    advanced trauma life s. (ATLS)
    basic life s. (BLS)
    biologic liver s.
    blood pressure s.
    excessive lip s.
    external s.
    extracorporeal life s. (ECLS)
    inspiratory pressure s.
    mechanical ventilatory s.
    nonbiologic liver s.
    parenteral nutritional s.
    pediatric advanced life s. (PALS)
    pulmonary s.
    respiratory s.
    s. suture technique
    systemic pressure s.
    S. Team Assessment Schedule (STAS)
    vasopressor s.
    ventilator s.
    ventilatory s.
    volume-assured pressure s. (VAPS)

supporting tissue
suppository
suppressed respiration
suppression
    hypothalamic-pituitary-axis s.
    twitch s.

suppressor
    tumor s.

suppurant
suppurate
suppuration
    alveodental s.
    pulmonary s.

suppurativa
    hidradenitis s.

suppurative
    s. acute inflammation
    s. cholecystitis
    s. chronic inflammation
    s. exudate
    s. granulomatous inflammation
    s. infection

supraacetabular
    s. groove
    s. sulcus

supraacetabularis
supraacromial
supraanal
supraannular mitral valve replacement (SMVR)
supraaortic trunk
supraarytenoid cartilage
supraauricular point
supraaxillary
suprabuccal
suprabullar recess
supraceliac
    s. aorta
    s. aortic origin graft

supracerebellar approach
supracervical
    s. hysterectomy
    s. incision

suprachoroid
    s. lamina
    s. layer

suprachoroidal hemorrhage
suprachoroidea
supraciliary canal
supraclavicular (SC)
    s. approach
    s. brachial block
    s. brachial block anesthesia
    s. compression
    s. examination
    s. fracture
    s. lymph node biopsy
    s. muscle
    s. nerve
    s. node
    s. triangle

supraclinoid aneurysm
supracolic space
supracondylar (SC)
    s. amputation
    s. humeral fracture
    s. line
    s. process
    s. suspension
    s. varus osteotomy
    s. Y-shaped fracture

supracondyloid
supracostal
supracotyloid
supracrestal
    s. line
    s. plane

supracricoid partial laryngectomy
supracristal plane

supradiaphragmatic
    s. fundic wrap
    s. pouch
    s. pouch of esophagus
supraduodenal
    s. approach
    s. artery
supraepicondylar process
supraesophageal
    s. reflux changes
    s. reflux disease
supragenicular popliteal artery (SGPA)
supraglenoid tubercle
supraglottic
    s. airway (SGA)
    s. edema
    s. laryngectomy
supraglottoplasty
suprahepatic
    s. cuff
    s. inferior vena cava
    s. IVC
    s. space
    s. vena cava (SVC)
suprahyoid
    s. branch
    s. gland
    s. laryngeal release
    s. muscle
    s. neck dissection
    s. space
    s. triangle
suprainguinal vascular procedure
suprainterparietal bone
supraintestinal
supralevator
    s. anorectal space
    s. pelvic exenteration
    s. perirectal abscess
supralumbar
supramalleolar
    s. flap
    s. varus derotation osteotomy
supramammary
supramandibular
supramastoid fossa
supramaxillary
supramaximal tetanic stimulation
suprameatal
    s. pit
    s. triangle
supramental
supramentale
supramesocolic surgical procedure
Supramid
    S. Extra cable-type suture
    S. implant suture
    S. nylon monofilament suture
    S. suture

supranasal
Suprane
supraneural parotidectomy
supranormal
    s. cardiac index
    s. CI
    s. hemodynamic therapy
    s. resuscitation
    s. value
supranuclear lesion
supraomental
    s. region
    s. space
supraomohyoid neck dissection (SOHND)
supraoptic
    s. anastomosis
    s. canal
supraopticohypophysial tract
supraorbital
    s. arch
    s. artery
    s. canal
    s. foramen
    s. margin
    s. nerve
    s. notch
    s. pericranial flap
    s. point
    s. ridge
    s. vein
supraorbital-pterional approach
supraorbitomeatal
suprapapillary Roux-en-Y
  duodenojejunostomy
suprapatellar
    s. bursa
    s. pouch
suprapelvic
supraperiosteal flap
supraphysiologic, supraphysiological
    s. fluid
    s. fluid technique
    s. resuscitation
supraphysiological (*var. of*
  supraphysiologic)
suprapineal recess
suprapleural membrane
supraprostatectomy
suprapubic
    s. cystotomy
    s. extraction site
    s. hernia
    s. lithotomy
    s. midline recurrence
    s. needle aspiration
    s. Pfannenstiel incision
    s. port
    s. prostatectomy
    s. puncture

S

suprapubic (*continued*)
  s. region
  s. urethrovesical suspension
suprapyloric node
suprarenal
  s. body
  s. capsule
  s. cortex
  s. filter placement
  s. gland
  s. impression
  s. medulla
  s. plexus
  s. vein
suprarenalectomy
suprascapular
  s. artery
  s. ligament
  s. nerve
  s. nerve block (SSNB)
  s. nerve compression
  s. notch
  s. vein
suprasellar
  s. low-density lesion
  s. mass
  s. subarachnoid cistern
suprasphincteric fistula
supraspinale
  s. skinfold
  s. skinfold measurement
supraspinalis muscle
supraspinatus muscle
supraspinous
  s. fossa
  s. ligament
  s. muscle
suprasternal
  s. bone
  s. examination
  s. notch
  s. plane
  s. space
suprasymphysary
supratemporal
supratentorial
  s. approach
  s. arteriovenous malformation
  s. craniotomy
  s. lesion
  s. space
  s. tumor
suprathoracic
supratonsillar
  s. fossa
  s. recess
supratragic tubercle
supratrochlear
  s. artery

  s. nerve
  s. vein
supraumbilical incision
supravaginal
supravalvar, supravalvular
supravalvular (*var. of* supravalvar)
  s. aortic stenosis
supraventricular
  s. arrhythmia
  s. crest
  s. dysrhythmia
supraventricularis
supraversion
supravesical
  s. fossa
  s. hernia
supreme
  s. intercostal artery
  s. intercostal vein
sural
  s. artery
  s. nerve
  s. nerve biopsy
  s. nerve block
  s. region
surface
  acromial articular s.
  articular s.
  auricular s.
  s. biopsy
  buccal s.
  s. cooling technique
  costal s.
  cut s.
  denture foundation s.
  s. desensitization technique
  diaphragmatic s.
  s. disinfection
  dorsal s.
  s. electrode
  s. electromyogram
  endosteal s.
  s. epithelium
  extensor s.
  external s.
  foundation s.
  glenoid s.
  hepatic s.
  implant-bearing s.
  inferior s.
  internal s.
  s. irradiation
  s. landmark
  s. membrane
  orbital s.
  ovarian s.
  peritoneal s.
  posterior s.
  s. projection

raw hepatic s.
reconstruction occlusal s. (RecOS)
renal s.
s. replacement hip arthroplasty
temporal s.
s. tension theory of narcosis
tissue ingrowth s.
surface-projection rendering image
surfactant
s. dysfunction
hydrolysis of s.
surfer's ear
surgeon
American College of S.'s (ACS)
American Society for Colon and
Rectal S.'s (ASCRS)
American Society of Transplant S.'s
(ASTS)
board-certified s.
colorectal s.
endocrine s.
Fellow of American College of S.'s
(FACS)
general s.
S. General's Office (SGO)
gynecologic s.
oculoplastic s.
pancreatic s.
parathyroid s.
pediatric s.
plastic s.
primary s.
retinal s.
Society of American Gastrointestinal
Endoscopic S.'s (SAGES)
Society of Laparoendoscopic
Surgeons (SLS)
thoracic s.
thyroid s.
trauma s.
vascular s.
surgeon-dependent technique failure
surgeon's knot
surgery
ablative cardiac s.
adjustable suture strabismus s.
adult cardiovascular s.
adult scoliosis s.
AESOP-assisted laparoscopic s.
aesthetic s.
ambulatory s.
American Board of S. (ABS)
American Society for Aesthetic
Plastic S. (ASAPS)
American Society for Bariatric S.
(ASBS)
anorectal s.
anterior cervical spine s.
anterior cervicothoracic junction s.

anterior lower cervical spine s.
antiglaucoma s.
antireflux s.
aortic reconstructive s.
apically repositioned flap in
mucogingival s.
arterial reconstructive s.
arthroscopic laser s.
aseptic s.
asymmetric s.
bariatric s.
bat ear s.
beating-heart bypass s.
bench s.
breast-conserving s. (BCS)
bypass s.
cardiac s.
cardiothoracic s. (CTS)
cardiovascular s.
carotid s.
cataract s.
cervical decompression s.
cervical disc s.
cervicothoracic junction s.
ciliodestructive s.
clean-contaminated s.
closed s.
colon and rectal s.
colorectal s.
combination s.
s. complication
computer-assisted s. (CAS)
computer-assisted stereotactic s.
(CASS)
concomitant antireflux s.
conservation s.
conservative s.
conventional s.
corneal s.
cosmetic s.
craniofacial reconstructive s.
cranioorbital s.
curative-intent s.
cytoreductive s.
debulking s.
decompressive s.
definitive s.
dental s.
dentofacial s.
dialysis access s.
dirty s.
double jaw s.
ECA-PCA bypass s.
elective s.
elective cosmetic s. (ECS)
emergency s.
emergent s.
endocrine s.
endodontic s.

S

surgery *(continued)*
    endoscopic cardiac s.
    endoscopic sinus s. (ESS)
    endoscopic video-assisted s.
    endourologic laser s.
    endovascular s.
    epilepsy s.
    evidence-based s.
    excisional cardiac s.
    exploratory s.
    ex situ bench s.
    extracorporeal s.
    extracranial-intracranial bypass s.
    eyelid s.
    eye muscle s.
    failed s.
    fast track s.
    featural s.
    femorodistal reconstructive s.
    fetal s.
    filtration s.
    first ray s.
    fistulizing s.
    flexible endoscopic s.
    frameless stereotactic s.
    functional endoscopic sinus s.
      (FESS)
    gastric bypass s.
    gastric reduction s.
    gastrointestinal s.
    general thoracic s.
    glaucoma s.
    hand-assisted laparoscopic s. (HALS)
    hepatic resectional s.
    hepatobiliary s.
    hip replacement s.
    hypotensive s.
    hysteroscopic s.
    ileal pouch s.
    image-guided s. (IGS)
    inadequate s.
    intestinal s.
    intraabdominal s.
    intradural tumor s.
    intralacrimal s.
    intranasal sinus s.
    intraorbital s.
    iterative cytoreductive s.
    jejunoileal bypass s.
    keyhole s.
    knee replacement s.
    labyrinthine s.
    lacrimal s.
    laparoscopically assisted s.
    laparoscopic-assisted aortic
      reconstructive s.
    laparoscopic bariatric s.
    laparoscopic colorectal cancer s.
    laparoscopic Dorr antireflux s.

    laparoscopic Toupet antireflux s.
    laryngeal framework s.
    laser s.
    laser-filtering s.
    Lich-Gregoir kidney transplant s.
    limb-salvage s.
    limb-sparing s.
    local s.
    lower extremity s.
    lung volume reduction s.
    major abdominal s.
    major nonvascular abdominal s.
    mandibular s.
    maxillary s.
    maxillofacial s. (MFS)
    microscopically controlled s.
    minimal access general s.
    minimally invasive s. (MIS)
    minimally invasive robotic heart
      valve s.
    minor s.
    Mohs micrographic s.
    mucogingival s.
    nasal endoscopic s.
    navigated brain tumor s.
    navigational s.
    nephron-sparing s. (NSS)
    neurologic s.
    neurological s.
    neuroma relocation s.
    nonbench s.
    noncardiac s.
    nonvascular abdominal s.
    oculoplastic s.
    oncoplastic s.
    open antireflux s.
    open disc s.
    open heart s. (OHS)
    open neck s.
    oral and maxillofacial s. (OMS)
    orbital s.
    orthognathic s.
    osseous s.
    palliative s.
    pancreatic s.
    parathyroid s.
    parenchymal sparing s.
    pediatric cardiovascular s.
    pediatric ophthalmic s.
    pelvic colonic s.
    penile-preserving s.
    penile venous ligation s.
    periapical s.
    peripheral vascular s.
    plastic and reconstructive s.
    port-access technique for coronary
      bypass s.
    portal decompression s.
    portal-systemic shunt s.

posterior lower cervical spine s.
posterior lumbar spine and
  sacrum s.
posterior upper cervical spine s.
preprosthetic s.
primary perineal hypospadias s.
prophylactic s.
pure refractive s.
pylorus-preserving s.
radical curative s.
radioimmunoguided s. (RIGS)
reconstructive preprosthetic s.
rectal s.
rectovaginal s.
refractive s.
remedial s.
remedial parathyroid s.
renal-sparing s.
reoperative aesthetic s.
reoperative bariatric s.
reoperative carotid s.
reoperative pelvic s.
reparative cardiac s.
rescue s.
resective s.
retinal s.
retrograde intrarenal s. (RIRS)
reversal of jejunoileal bypass s.
right ventricle-pulmonary artery
  conduit s.
rigid endoscopic s.
robot-assisted s. (RAS)
robotic s.
robotic-assisted laparoscopic
  bariatric s.
salvage s.
sarcoma s.
scoliosis s.
secondary s.
second-look s.
segmental s.
sestamibi-directed parathyroid s.
sham s.
shunt s.
sinus s.
site-specific s.
sphincter-saving s.
spinal s.
STA-MCA bypass s.
stereotactic s.
stone s.
strabismus s.
subfascial endoscopic perforator s.
  (SEPS)
subfascial perforator s.
suboptimal s.
subretinal s.
substitutional cardiac s.
symmetric s.

targeted s.
telepresence s.
telerobotic-assisted laparoscopic s.
thoracic s.
thyroglossal cyst s.
total hip replacement s.
total knee replacement s.
tracheal s.
transperitoneal hand-assisted
  laparoscopic s.
transsexual s.
transsphenoidal s.
transsphincteric s.
trauma s. (TrS)
truly endocapsular microincision
  cataract s. (TECMIS)
tubal reconstruction s.
tumor s.
upper gastrointestinal tract s.
urologic s.
vaginal s.
valvular heart s.
vascular abdominal s.
video-assisted neck s.
video-assisted thoracoscopic s.
  (VATS)
videoscopic hernia s.
vitreoretinal s.
vitreous s.
volume reduction s.
  (VRS)
weight reduction s.
surgery-induced PGID
surgical
  s. abdomen
  s. access
  s. adjunct
  s. admitting unit
  s. airway
  s. anatomy
  s. anesthesia
  s. Apgar score (SAS)
  s. approach
  s. autoimmunization
  s. bone impression
  s. change
  s. cholecystectomy
  s. cholecystostomy
  s. chromic suture
  s. clinician
  s. closure
  s. correction
  s. crown lengthening
  s. cystogastrostomy
  s. débridement
  s. debulking
  s. defect
  s. diagnosis
  s. diathermy

surgical (*continued*)

s. drape combustion
s. dressing room
S. Education and Self-Assessment Program (SESAP)
s. emergency
s. emphysema
s. endarterectomy
s. endodontics
s. enucleation
s. enucleation method
s. enucleation procedure
s. enucleation technique
s. eruption
s. erysipelas
s. estrogen ablation
s. excision
s. excision biopsy
s. extirpation
s. failure
s. field
s. fire
s. flap
s. gastrostomy
s. gut suture
s. incision
s. indication
s. infection
S. Infection Society (SIS)
s. intervention
s. keratometry
s. ligation
s. linen suture
s. maggot
s. maggot therapy
s. management
s. maneuver
s. margin
s. marking solution
s. mesh
s. microscope navigation (SMN)
s. neck
s. neck fracture
s. neonate
s. neurangiographic technique
s. neurology
s. occlusion rim
s. oncologist
s. oncology
s. orthodontia
s. orthodontics
s. outcome
s. pancreatic disease
s. pathology
s. patient
s. perspective
s. placement
s. plication

s. portal decompression
s. portosystemic shunt
s. positioning
s. preparation
s. problem
s. pulp exposure
s. reduction
s. repair
s. resectability
s. resection
s. retention
s. risk
s. scar revision
s. sectioning
s. seeding
s. signature
s. silk suture
s. simulation
s. site infection (SSI)
s. specialty
s. staging
s. stapling
s. steel suture
s. strategy
s. stress
s. suture technique
s. thrombectomy
s. trauma
s. treatment
s. treatment objective (STO)
s. treatment option
s. tuberculosis
s. vagotomy
s. ventricular restoration (SVR)
s. weight loss
s. wound

surgically

s. corrected hypertension
s. implanted catheter
s. treated patient

surgical-pathologic staging
surgical-radiologic minicholecystostomy
SurgiChip
Surgidac suture
Surgilene suture
Surgilon braided nylon suture
Surgipro suture
surplus skin
surrenal
surveillance

endoscopic s.
s. endoscopy
Surveillance, Epidemiology, End Result (SEER)
graft s.
s. mechanism
s. program
s. technique

survey
>s. line
>s. program
>radiation s.

survival
>breast cancer-specific s.
>s. curve
>disease-free s. (DFS)
>distant recurrence-free s. (DRFS)
>graft s.
>locoregional recurrence-free s. (LRRFS)
>long-term s.
>postoperative s.
>s. probability
>recurrence-free s.
>specific s.
>trauma and injury severity scores probability of s.
>TRISS probability of s.

Surviving Sepsis Campaign
Susac syndrome
suspended
>s. animation
>s. inspiration

suspended-pedicle approach
suspension
>Aldridge-Studdefort urethral s.
>Alexander-Adams uterine s.
>Baldy-Webster uterine s.
>bladder neck s.
>Burch bladder s.
>Burch urethrovesical s.
>Coffey uterine s.
>corporeal sacrospinous s.
>corset s.
>cuff s.
>Donald-Fothergill uterine s.
>endoscopic bladder neck s. (EBNS)
>extraperitoneal laparoscopic bladder neck s.
>fingertrap s.
>flexible hinge s.
>Gilliam-Doleris uterine s.
>Gittes endoscopic bladder neck s.
>Gittes-Loughlin bladder neck s.
>s. laryngoscopy
>Manchester-Fothergill uterine s.
>minimal incision pubovaginal s.
>Olshausen uterine ligaments s.
>Pereyra bladder neck s.
>Pereyra needle s.
>Raz bladder neck s.
>Raz needle s.
>Raz 4-quadrant s.
>Raz urethral s.
>retropubic Lapides-Ball bladder neck s.
>sacrospinous ligament s.

>SC s.
>Stamey needle s.
>suction s.
>supracondylar s.
>suprapubic urethrovesical s.
>urethral s.
>uterine s.

suspension-type socket
suspensory
>s. ligament
>s. muscle
>s. sling operation

suspicion
>clinical s.

suspicious
>s. abnormality
>s. finding
>s. FNA
>s. lesion
>s. microcalcification

sustained
>s. pressure technique
>s. release (SR)

sustentacular tissue
sustentaculum tali
Sutherland-Greenfield osteotomy
Sutherland-Rowe incision
sutura, *pl.* **suturae**
>s. frontoethmoidalis
>s. frontolacrimalis
>s. frontomaxillaris
>s. frontonasalis

suturae (*pl. of* sutura)
sutural
>s. bone
>s. diastasis
>s. ligament

suture
>absorbable surgical s.
>Acier stainless steel s.
>Acufex bioabsorbable Suretac s.
>Acutrol s.
>Albert s.
>Albert-Lembert s.
>Alcon s.
>Allgöwer-Donati s.
>already-threaded s.
>American silk s.
>s. anastomosis
>Ancap braided silk s.
>s. anchor
>s. anchor technique
>angiocatheter with looped polypropylene s.
>antibody-coated s.
>antitorque s.
>apical s.
>Appolito s.
>Arroyo encircling s.

S

suture (*continued*)
    Arruga encircling s.
    arterial silk s.
    S. Assist
    Atraloc s.
    Aureomycin s.
    Auto S.
    Barraquer silk s.
    baseball s.
    basilar s.
    basting s.
    Bell s.
    bioabsorbable Dexon s.
    Bio-FASTak s.
    BioSorb s.
    Biosyn synthetic monofilament s.
    biparietal s.
    16-bite nylon s.
    black braided nylon s.
    black braided silk s.
    black silk bridle s.
    black silk sling s.
    blanket s.
    blue-black monofilament s.
    blue twisted cotton s.
    bolster s.
    Bondek absorbable s.
    bone wax s.
    braided s.
    braided Ethibond s.
    braided Mersilene s.
    braided Nurolon s.
    braided nylon s.
    braided polyamide s.
    braided polyester s.
    braided polyglactin s.
    braided silk s.
    braided Vicryl s.
    braided wire s.
    Bralon braided nylon s.
    bregmatomastoid s.
    s. bridge
    bridle s.
    Brown-Sharp gauge s.
    Bunnell wire pull-out s.
    s. button
    capitonnage s.
    caprolactam s.
    Caprosyn monofilament s.
    cardinal s.
    Cardioflon s.
    Cardionyl s.
    s. carrier
    catgut s.
    cervical s.
    Chinese fingertrap s.
    chromated catgut s.
    chromic s.
    chromic blue dyed s.

chromic catgut s.
chromic collagen s.
chromic gut s.
chromicized catgut s.
circular s.
circumcisional s.
s. clip forceps
s. closure
s. closure technique
coated polyester s.
coated Vicryl s.
coated Vicryl Rapide s.
collagen absorbable s.
compound s.
concha-mastoid s.
Connell s.
Cooley U s.
coronal s.
cotton nonabsorbable s.
cottony Dacron hollow s.
cranial s.
CT-1 needle s.
CT-2 needle s.
Cushing s.
Custodis s.
Cutalon nylon polyamide surgical s.
s. cutter
Czerny s.
Czerny-Lembert s.
Dacron s.
Dacron bolstered s.
Dacron traction s.
Dafilon s.
Dagrofil s.
Davis-Geck s.
Davis-Geck Softgut s.
Deklene II cardiovascular s.
Deklene polypropylene s.
Deknatel silk s.
dentate s.
DermaGlide oculoplastic s.
dermal s.
Dermalene polyethylene s.
Dermalon cuticular s.
Dexon s.
Dexon absorbable synthetic
  polyglycolic acid s.
Dexon II s.
Dexon Plus s.
DG s.
double-armed wire s.
double right-angle s.
double-running penetrating
  keratoplasty s.
Dulox s.
Endoknot s.
Endoloop s.
end-to-end s.
end-to-side s.

Ethibond s.
Ethibond polybutilate-coated
  polyester s.
Ethicon micropoint s.
Ethicon Sabreloc s.
Ethicon silk s.
Ethiflex retention s.
Ethilon nylon s.
ethmoidolacrimal s.
ethmoidomaxillary s.
everting mattress s.
extrachromic s.
eyelid crease s.
Faden s.
s. failure
false s.
s. fatigue
figure-of-8 s.
filament s.
fine chromic s.
fine silk s.
fingertrap s.
s. fixation
formaldehyde catgut s.
Foster s.
Fothergill s.
s. fracture
frontal s.
frontoethmoidal s.
frontomaxillary s.
frontonasal s.
frontoparietal s.
frontosphenoid s.
frontozygomatic s.
Frost s.
Gaillard-Arlt s.
Gambee s.
Gambee-type s.
gastrointestinal pop-off silk s.
gastrointestinal surgical gut s.
gastrointestinal surgical linen s.
gastrointestinal surgical silk s.
Gély s.
general closure s.
Gillies horizontal dermal s.
GI pop-off silk s.
glue-in s.
Gore-Tex s.
gossamer silk s.
Gould s.
green braided s.
green Mersilene s.
green monofilament polyglyconate s.
groove s.
guardian s.
s. guide
Gussenbauer s.
gut s.
Halsted mattress s.

harmonic s.
Heaney s.
heavy-gauge s.
heavy monofilament s.
heavy retention s.
heavy silk retention s.
heavy wire s.
helical s.
hemostatic s.
s. holder
Horsley s.
Hu-Friedy Perma Sharp s.
India rubber s.
infraorbital s.
interendognathic s.
intermaxillary s.
internasal s.
interparietal s.
interrupted pledgeted s.
intracorporeal s.
intraluminal s.
Investa s.
iodine catgut s.
Ivalon s.
s. joint
Kelly s.
Kessler s.
Kessler-Kleinert s.
Kirschner s.
Krackow s.
Küstner s.
L-25 absorbable
  surgical s.
lacrimoconchal s.
lacrimomaxillary s.
lambdoid s.
lancet s.
Lang s.
Lapra-Ty s.
large-caliber nonabsorbable s.
lateral trap s.
lead s.
Le Dentu s.
Lembert s.
s. ligated
s. ligation
Linatrix s.
Lindner corneoscleral s.
s. line
s. line cancer
s. line dehiscence
linen s.
lockout s.
Look Sharpoint Ophthalmic s.
Lukens catgut s.
malar periosteum-SMAS flap
  fixation s.
Mannis s.
Marlex s.

suture (*continued*)

mattress s.
Maxon s.
Maxon absorbable s.
Mayo linen s.
McCannel s.
McLean s.
Meigs s.
Mersilene braided nonabsorbable s.
Mersilk black silk s.
mesh s.
metal band s.
metallic s.
Micrins microsurgical s.
micropoint s.
Miralene s.
modified Frost s.
Monocryl s.
monofilament s.
monofilament absorbable s.
monofilament clear s.
monofilament green s.
monofilament nonabsorbable s.
monofilament nylon s.
monofilament polypropylene s.
monofilament skin s.
monofilament steel s.
monofilament wire s.
Monosoft s.
multifilament steel s.
multistrand s.
nasofrontal s.
nasomaxillary s.
natural s.
Needless Wound s.
nerve s.
neurocentral s.
neurosurgical s.
nonabsorbable surgical s.
Novafil s.
Nurolon s.
nylon 66 s.
nylon monofilament s.
nylon retention s.
occipital s.
occipitomastoid s.
occipitoparietal s.
occipitosphenoid s.
s. of lens
oiled silk s.
opaque wire s.
s. overlap
palatine s.
palatoethmoidal s.
palatomaxillary s.
Panacryl s.
Panalok absorbable s.
Pancoast s.
parietal s.

parietomastoid s.
s. passer
PDS II s.
Perlon s.
Permahand braided silk s.
Perma Sharp s.
petrobasilar s.
petrospheno-occipital s.
petrosquamous s.
petrotympanic s.
PGA synthetic absorbable s.
s. pickup hook
s. pickup spatula
pickup spatula s.
pin s.
pink twisted cotton s.
plain catgut s.
plain collagen s.
plain gut s.
plastic s.
pledget s.
pledgeted Ethibond s.
pledgeted mattress s.
s. plication
polyamide s.
polybutester s.
Polydek s.
polydioxanone s. (PDS)
polydioxanone surgical s.
polyester fiber s.
polyethylene s.
polyfilament s.
polygalactic acid s.
polyglactin 910 s.
polyglecaprone 25 s.
polyglycolate s.
polyglycolic acid s.
polyglyconate s.
polypropylene button s.
Polysorb s.
PolySyn Ophthalmic s.
polytetrafluoroethylene s.
pop-off s.
PremiCron nonabsorbable s.
Prolene s.
Pronova s.
Proxi-Strip s.
s. pulling
Pulvertaft weave s.
Quickert s.
Rapide s.
reabsorbable s.
s. repair
s. ring
rip-cord s.
rubber s.
Safil synthetic absorbable
  surgical s.
Serralnyl s.

Serralsilk s.
serrated s.
seton s.
Sharpoint ophthalmic
  microsurgical s.
Shirodkar s.
Shoch s.
shotted s.
SH pop-off s.
silicone-treated surgical silk s.
silk braided s.
silk nonabsorbable s.
silk pop-off s.
silk stay s.
silk traction s.
silkworm gut s.
silver s.
Sims s.
single-armed s.
s. slider system
slowly absorbable continuous s.
Snellen s.
Sofsilk coated braided silk s.
Sofsilk nonabsorbable silk s.
s. spacer
Spanish silk s.
sphenofrontal s.
sphenomaxillary s.
sphenooccipital s.
sphenoorbital s.
sphenoparietal s.
sphenosquamous s.
sphenovomerine s.
sphenozygomatic s.
squamomastoid s.
squamosal s.
squamous s.
SS s.
stainless steel s.
stainless steel wire s.
Statak s.
steel s.
steel mesh s.
sternal wire s.
S. Strip wound closure strip
subanular mattress s.
subcutaneous s.
subcuticular s.
Supramid s.
Supramid Extra cable-type s.
Supramid implant s.
Supramid nylon monofilament s.
surgical chromic s.
surgical gut s.
surgical linen s.
surgical silk s.
surgical steel s.
Surgidac s.
Surgilene s.

Surgilon braided nylon s.
Surgipro s.
swaged s.
swaged-on s.
Swiss silk s.
synthetic absorbable s.
Synthofil s.
s. tag forceps
tantalum wire tension s.
Tapercut s.
Teflon-coated s.
Teflon-pledgeted s.
temporal s.
tension-requiring s.
Tevdek s.
Tevdek pledgeted s.
Thiersch s.
through-and-through
  reabsorbable s.
through-the-wall mattress s.
tiger gut s.
TigerWire s.
S. Tram
transfixion s.
transosseous s.
transscleral s.
twisted virgin silk s.
s. tying platform forceps
tympanomastoid s.
tympanosquamosal s.
UltraFit PK s.
UltraGlide corneal transplant s.
umbilical tape s.
unabsorbable s.
undyed s.
Verhoeff s.
Vicryl pop-off s.
Vicryl Rapide s.
virgin silk s.
white braided silk s.
white nylon s.
white twisted s.
wing s.
s. wire
s. wire-cutting scissors
Worst artificial lens s.
ZF s.
Zimmer Statak s.
zygomaticofrontal s.
zygomaticomaxillary s.
zygomaticotemporal s.

suturectomy
sutured
  doubly s.
sutureless
  s. bowel anastomosis
  s. colostomy closure
  s. laparoscopic extraperitoneal
    inguinal herniorrhaphy

S

suturing
    Bard endoscopic s.
    conventional s.
    direct s.
    intracorporeal s.
    magnetic control s. (MCS)
    needleless s.
SUX
    succinylcholine
suxamethonium
SV
    sigmoid volvulus
SVB
    saphenous vein bypass
SVC
    superior vena cava
SVR
    systemic vascular resistance
swage
swaged-on suture
swaged suture
swallow
    barium s. (BaS, Ba swal, b.s., BS)
    s. method
swallowing dysfunction
swamp carcinoma
Swan-Ganz
    S.-G. catheter
    S.-G. tube
Swan incision
swan-neck
    s.-n. deformity reduction
    s.-n. finger
    s.-n. finger deformity
Swanson
    S. congenital limb anomalies
      classification
    S. convex condylar arthroplasty
    S. midfacial defect
      reconstruction
    S. radial head implant
      arthroplasty
    S. silicone wrist arthroplasty
    S. technique
sweat
    s. duct
    s. gland adenocarcinoma
    s. gland adenoma
sweating
    gustatory s.
Swedish
    S. approach
    S. massage
swelling
    external s.
    genital s.
    levator s.
    lysosomal s.
    scrotal s.

    soft tissue s.
    unilateral facial s.
Swenson
    S. colonic pullthrough procedure
    S. endorectal pull-through
    S. rectosigmoidectomy with coloanal
      anastomosis
Swiss silk suture
switch
    biliopancreatic diversion with
      duodenal s.
    compression s.
    duodenal s.
    s. operation
    s. procedure
switched B-gradient technique
swivel dislocation
SWL
    shock wave lithotripsy
SWMA
    segmental wall motion abnormality
sword-fighting
sycoma
sycosiform fungous infection
Sydney
    S. line
    S. system gastritis classification
sylvian
    s. approach
    s. aqueduct
    s. cistern
    s. dissection
    s. fissure
    s. fistula
    s. hematoma
    s. line
    s. point
    s. vein
Sylvius
    valve of S.
symblepharon ring
Syme
    S. ankle amputation procedure
    S. ankle disarticulation amputation
    S. external urethrotomy
    S. external urethrotomy procedure
Symington anococcygeal body
symmetric, symmetrical
    s. surgery
    s. thumb duplication
    s. vertebral fusion
symmetrical (*var. of* symmetric)
symmetry
    s. operation
    s. plane
sympathalgia
sympathectomy, sympathetectomy,
  sympathicectomy
    cervical perivascular s.

cervicothoracic s.
chemical s.
dorsal s.
endoscopic s.
high s.
Leriche s.
lumbar s.
periarterial s.
preganglionic s.
presacral s.
Smithwick s.
transdermal s.
upper dorsal s.
video-assisted lumbar s.
visceral s.
sympathetectomy (*var. of* sympathectomy)
sympathetic
s. blockade
s. blockade anesthetic technique
s. branch
s. cutaneous modulation
s. denervation
s. denitrogenation
s. efferent output channel
s. fiber
s. flow response
s. ganglion blockade
s. ganglion block anesthetic technique
s. hyperactivity
s. interruption
s. microneurography
s. nerve
s. nerve activity
s. nerve block
s. neurolysis
s. projection
s. sprouting
s. sweat response
s. trunk
sympathetically
s. independent pain (SIP)
s. maintained pain (SMP)
sympathetic-chain catheter
sympathetoblastoma
sympathic dystrophy
sympathicectomy (*var. of* sympathectomy)
sympathicoblastoma
sympathicogonioma
sympathicotripsy
sympathicus
sympathoadrenal response
sympathoblastoma
sympathoexcitation reflex
sympathoexcitatory response
sympathogonioma
sympatholysis
sympatholytic agent
sympathomimetic agent

symperitoneal
symphyseotomy (*var. of* symphysiotomy)
symphyses (*pl. of* symphysis)
symphysialis
symphysic
symphysion
symphysiotomy, symphyseotomy
symphysis, *pl.* **symphyses**
cardiac s.
intervertebral s.
mandibular s.
manubriosternal s.
mental s.
pleural s.
pubic s.
symptom
acute s.
autonomic s.
S. Checklist 90 (SCL90)
chronic reflux s.
S. Distress Scale (SDS)
s. experience stage
s. formation
insidious onset of s.'s
ipsilateral hemispheric s.
Knowles-Eccersley-Scott S. (KESS)
s. magnification syndrome
myelopathic s.
neurologic s.
nonspecific s.
postoperative s.
presenting s.
psychogenic s.
s. score
transient neurologic s. (TNS)
unremitting s.
symptomatic
s. abdominal aneurysm disease
s. embolization
s. gallstones
s. infection
s. patient
s. primary HPT
s. relief
s. spondylosis
s. traumatic dissection
symptomatology
symptothermal method
synadelphus
synanastomosis
synandrogenic
synapse
excitatory s.
synaptosome
synarthrodia
synarthrodial joint
synarthrosis

S

synbiotic
syncephalus
synchondrodial joint
synchondroseotomy
synchondrosis
    s. arycorniculata
    s. xiphosternalis
synchondrotomy
synchrocyclotron operation
synchronization
synchronized
    s. fibrillation
    s. intermittent mandatory ventilation
    (SIMV)
synchronous
    s. bladder reconstruction
    s. emergence
    s. hepatic metastasis
    s. intermittent mandatory ventilation
    s. lesion
    s. pathology
    s. resection
    s. scapuloclavicular rotation
    s. tumor
    s. urinary tract infection
syncope
syncytial knot
syndactylia, syndactylism, syndactyly
    Diamond-Gould reduction s.
    Kelikian-Clayton-Loseff surgical s.
    reduction s.
syndactylism (*var. of* syndactylia)
syndactylization
syndactylous
syndactyly (*var. of* syndactylia)
syndectomy
syndesmectomy
syndesmectopia
syndesmodial joint, syndesmotic joint
syndesmopexy
syndesmophyte
    bridging s.
syndesmoplasty
syndesmorrhaphy
syndesmotic joint
syndesmotomy
syndrome
    abdominal compartment s. (ACS)
    abdominal cutaneous nerve
     entrapment s.
    abdominal muscle deficiency s.
    acquired thoracic
     chondrodystrophy s.
    acrofacial s.
    acute coronary s. (ACS)
    acute disconnection s.
    acute tumor lysis s. (ATLS)
    adhesive s.
    adrenal feminization s.

afferent limb s.
afferent loop s. (ALS)
aglossia-adactylia s.
Alport s. (AS)
amniotic infection s. (AIS)
angio-osteohypertrophy s.
ankyloglossia superior s.
anomalous innominate artery
  compression s.
anterior cavernous sinus s.
anterior chest wall s.
anterior scalene compression s.
anterior spinal artery s.
antiphospholipid antibody s.
Apert s.
apical ballooning s.
apparent short leg s. (ASLS)
Arnold-Chiari s.
arterial compression s.
arterial steal s.
Ascher s.
Bannayan-Riley-Ruvalcaba s.
Beckwith-Wiedemann s.
Behçet s.
bent-nail s.
Bernard-Soulier s.
bile plug s.
biliary sump s.
billowing mitral valve s.
Birt-Hoss-Dube s.
black patch s.
blind loop s. (BLS)
blind pouch s.
Bloodgood s.
blue rubber bleb nevus s.
blue toe s.
body cast s.
Boerhaave s.
Bogorad s.
bowel bypass s.
brittle nail s.
bronchiolitis obliterans s. (BOS)
Brugada s.
Budd-Chiari s.
buried bumper s.
Burnett s.
burning feet s.
burning mouth s.
calcaneal spur s.
callosal disconnection s.
camptomelic s.
cancer susceptibility s.
capillary leak s.
capsular exfoliation s.
carcinoid s.
Caroli s.
carpal tunnel s. (CTS)
cauda equina s.
cavernous sinus s.

celiac artery compression s.
celiac axis compression s.
celiac band s.
central anticholinergic s.
central cord s.
central heel pad s.
cerebellomedullary malformation s.
cerebellopontine angle s.
cervical acceleration-deceleration s.
cervical compression s.
cervical facet s.
cervical fusion s.
Cheatle s.
Chiari II s.
chronic hyperventilation s.
chronic intestinal
  pseudoobstruction s.
classic multiple organ failure s.
clinical s.
clivus s.
cloverleaf skull s.
cluster tic s.
coarctation s.
Cogan s.
common peroneal nerve s.
compartment compression s.
compensatory antiinflammatory
  response s.
complex regional pain type I, II s.
  (CRPS)
compression s.
congenital central hypoventilation s.
congenital long QT s.
congenital pulmonary venolobar s.
congenital ring s.
Cooper s.
cord traction s.
coronary s.
Costen s.
costoclavicular compression s.
Cronkhite-Canada s.
Crouzon s.
crush s.
cubital tunnel s.
Cushing s.
cutaneomucouveal s.
Dandy-Walker s.
deafferentation pain s.
Dejerine-Roussy s.
delayed pulmonary toxicity s.
Denys-Drash s.
de Quervain s.
dialysis disequilibrium s.
dialysis encephalopathy s.
diffuse idiopathic skeletal
  hyperostosis s.
disconnection s.
DISH s.
dumping s.

Dunbar s.
dural shunt s.
Eagle s.
Eagle-Barrett s.
Eaton-Lambert s.
ectopic ACTH s.
efferent limb s.
Ehlers-Danlos s.
embryonic fixation s.
entrapment s.
euthyroid sick s.
excited skin s.
exertional anterior compartment s.
exertional deep posterior
  compartment s.
exfoliation s.
exploding head s.
extraarticular pain s.
extrapyramidal s.
facet joint s.
failed back surgery s. (FBSS)
familial aortic ectasia s.
familial atypical multiple mole
  melanoma s.
familial cardiac myxoma s.
familial cholestasis s.
familial polyposis s.
FAMM s.
FAM-M s.
fasciitis-panniculitis s.
Felty s.
female urethral s.
feminization s.
fetal aspiration s.
fibrocystic breast s.
fibrofascial compartment s.
first arch s.
flapping valve s.
floppy valve s.
Fraley s.
Franceschetti s.
Fraser s.
Frey s.
functional prepubertal castration s.
G s.
Gardner s.
gas-bloat s.
gastrojejunal loop obstruction s.
glomangiomatous osseous
  malformation s.
glucagonoma s.
Gorlin-Chaudhry-Moss s.
gray platelet s.
Hadju-Cheney acroosteolysis s.
Hallermann-Streiff s.
Hallermann-Streiff-François s.
Hanhart s.
head-bobbing doll s.
hemangioma-thrombocytopenia s.

S

syndrome (*continued*)

hemispheric disconnection s.
hemolytic uremic s. (HUS)
heparin-induced thrombocytopenia
  and thrombosis s. (HITTS)
hepatorenal s. (HRS)
hereditary cancer s.
hereditary flat adenoma s.
hereditary nonpolyposis colorectal
  cancer s.
Hermansky-Pudlak s.
Hinman s.
HNPCC s.
Horner s.
hungry bone s.
Hutchison s.
hyaline membrane s.
hymenal s.
hyoid s.
hypersensitive xiphoid s.
hyperventilation s.
hypoplastic left heart s.
hypothenar hammer s.
immotile cilia s. (ICS)
impaired regeneration s.
infantile choriocarcinoma s.
infant respiratory distress s. (IRDS)
inherited cancer s.
innominate artery compression s.
intersection s.
iridocorneal endothelial s.
iridocorneal epithelial s.
Jacod s.
Jeune s.
jugular foramen s.
Kasabach-Merritt s.
Klippel-Feil s.
Klippel-Trenaunay s.
Klippel-Trenaunay-Weber s.
lactic acidosis and strokelike s.
large vestibular aqueduct s.
Larsen s.
Leriche s.
levator ani s.
levator scapulae s.
lissencephaly s.
locked-in s.
loculation s.
loin pain hematuria s.
long QT s.
Louis-Bar s.
lower nephron s.
Luys body s.
Lynch s.
Maffucci s.
malignant carcinoid s.
malignant external otitis s.
Mallory-Weiss s.
mandibulofacial dysotosis s.

mangled extremity s.
Marfan s.
Marin Amat s.
MASS s.
massive bowel resection s.
maternal deprivation s.
May-Thurner s.
meconium aspiration s.
meconium plug s.
medial tibial stress s. (MTSS)
megacystis s.
megacystis-megaureter s.
megacystis-microcolon-intestinal
  hypoperistalsis s.
MEN s.
Mendelson s.
Ménière s.
mesenteric traction s.
minimal change nephrotic s.
minimal lesion nephrotic s.
Mirizzi s.
mitral valve prolapse s.
Mohr s.
monofixation s.
Morquio s.
mucocutaneous lymph node s.
mucocutaneous pigmentation of
  Peutz-Jeghers s.
mucosal neuroma s.
mucous plug s.
Muir-Torre s.
müllerian duct derivation s.
multiorgan dysfunction s. (MODS)
multiple hamartoma s.
multiple mucosal neuroma s.
multiple organ dysfunction s.
  (MODS)
multiple organ failure s.
multiple pterygium s.
myasthenic s. (MS)
myofascial pain s. (MPS)
myotonic s.
nail-patella s.
nail-patella-elbow s.
naviculocapitate fracture s.
nephritic s.
nephrotic s.
nerve compression-degeneration s.
neuroleptic malignant s. (NMS)
neurovascular compression s.
nevoid basal cell carcinoma s.
nonocclusive mesenteric
  ischemia s.
OAV s.
obesity hypoventilation s. (OHS)
occipital condyle s.
ocular-mucous membrane s.
oculoauriculovertebral s.
oculobuccogenital s.

oculomandibulofacial s.
oculovertebral s.
OFD s.
s. of inappropriate secretion of
  antidiuretic hormone (SIADH)
Ogilvie s.
optic tract s.
oral-facial-digital s.
orbital apex s.
organic short bowel s.
orofaciodigital s.
Ortner s.
osteogenesis imperfecta congenita s.
osteomyelofibrotic s.
osteopathia striata s.
osteoporosis pseudoglioma s.
Ostrum-Furst s.
otomandibular s.
ovarian hyperstimulation s.
ovarian overstimulation s.
ovarian vein s.
pacemaker s.
Paget-von Schrötter s.
pain s.
Papillon-Léage and Psaume s.
paraneoplastic s.
parasellar s.
paratrigeminal s.
Parsonage-Turner s.
patellofemoral pain s.
pectoralis minor s.
pelvic organ dysfunction s.
pericardiotomy s.
pericolic membrane s.
peritubal s.
peroneal compartment s.
persistent müllerian duct s.
Peutz-Jeghers s.
pharyngeal pouch s.
Phocas s.
piriformis s.
placental hemangioma s.
popliteal web s.
postadrenalectomy s.
postcardiotomy s.
postcholecystectomy s.
postcolonoscopy distention s.
postcommissurotomy s.
postembolization s.
posterior interosseous nerve
  compression s.
posterior reversible encephalopathy s.
posterior thalamic s.
postfundoplication s.
postgastrectomy s.
postirradiation s.
postlaminectomy s.
postpericardiotomy s.
postphlebitic s.

postpolypectomy coagulation s.
posttubal ligation s.
postural orthostatic tachycardia s.
  (POTS)
postvagotomy s.
preexcitation s.
prolapsed mitral valve s.
pronator teres s.
proximal loop s.
prune-belly s.
pseudo-blind loop s.
pseudoexfoliation s.
pseudolymphoma s.
pseudoobstruction s.
pseudoxanthoma elasticum s.
pterygopalatine fossa s.
pulmonary acid aspiration s.
pulmonary sulcus s.
quadrilateral space s.
radicular pain s.
Raeder s.
Ramsay Hunt s.
rapid tumor lysis s.
Rapunzel s.
Raynaud s.
Reclus I s.
recurrent abdominal pain s.
  (RAPS)
red ear s.
red-eyed shunt s.
red man s.
refeeding s.
Reifenstein s.
Reiter s.
renal crush s.
respiratory distress s. (RDS)
restless legs s. (RLS)
retained gastric antrum s.
retinoblastoma-mental retardation s.
retrolenticular s.
retrosphenoidal s.
rib tip s.
Rieger s.
Riley-Day s.
Riley-Smith s.
ring D chromosome s.
Roaf s.
Roberts s.
Roux stasis s.
Sakati-Nyhan s.
scalenus anticus s.
scapulocostal s.
scapuloperoneal s.
Scheie s.
scimitar s.
serotonin s.
Sertoli-cell-only s.
Sheehan s.
short bowel s.

S

syndrome (*continued*)
    short-lasting unilateral neuralgiaform headache with conjunctival injection and tearing s.
    sick building s.
    sick sinus s.
    Singleton-Merten s.
    sinus tarsi s.
    sleep apnea-hypoventilation s.
    slipped rib cartilage s.
    slipping rib s.
    slit ventricle s.
    small capillary s.
    Smith-Lemli-Opitz s.
    smooth-brain s.
    snapping hip s.
    solitary rectal ulcer s.
    somatostatinoma s.
    spectacular shrinking deficit s.
    spinal cord shock s.
    splenic sequestration s.
    SSRI discontinuation s.
    stagnant loop s.
    staphylococcal scalded skin s.
    stasis s.
    Stauffer s.
    Stewart-Treves s.
    Stickler s.
    stiff-person s.
    stump embolization s.
    Sturge-Weber s.
    stylohyoid process s.
    styloid s.
    subclavian steal s. (SSS)
    sudden infant death s. (SIDS)
    sump s.
    SUNCT s.
    superior orbital fissure s. (SOFS)
    superior vena cava s.
    supine hypotensive s.
    Susac s.
    symptom magnification s.
    systemic inflammatory response s. (SIRS)
    Takayasu s.
    talar compression s.
    tarsal tunnel s.
    terminal reservoir s.
    Terson s.
    testicular feminization s.
    tethered cord s.
    thalamic pain s.
    third and fourth pharyngeal pouch s.
    thoracic compression s.
    thoracic endometriosis s.
    thoracic outlet s. (TOS)
    Thorn s.
    Tietze s.

    Tillaux-Phocas s.
    Tolosa-Hunt s.
    tooth-and-nail s.
    Tourette s
    transient bone marrow edema s.
    transient compartment s.
    translocation Down s.
    transplant lung s.
    transurethral resection s. (TURS)
    Treacher Collins s.
    trisomy 8 s.
    trisomy C, D s.
    Trotter s.
    tumor lysis s. (TLS)
    Turcot s.
    Turner s. (TS)
    twin-twin transfusion s. (TTTS)
    ulnocarpal abutment s.
    Unverricht-Lundborg s.
    urethral s.
    Usher s.
    uterine hernia s.
    uveoencephalitic s.
    valgus extension overload s.
    vanished testis s.
    vanishing lung s. (VLS)
    vascular leak s. (VLS)
    vascular ring s.
    vasoplegic s.
    VATER association s.
    velocardiofacial s. (VCFS)
    venous leak s.
    Vernet s.
    vertebral subluxation s.
    vibration s.
    vibrator hand s.
    Villaret s.
    visual deprivation s.
    vitreoretinal traction s.
    Vogt-Koyanagi-Harada s.
    von Hippel-Lindau s.
    vulvar vestibulitis s.
    Wallenberg s.
    Wartenberg s.
    wasting s.
    Wernicke-Korsakoff s.
    Weyers-Thier s.
    white clot s.
    white dot s.
    Winchester s.
    yellow nail s.
    Yentl s.
    Zollinger-Ellison s. (ZES)
synechia, *pl.* **synechiae**
    s. formation
synechiae (*pl. of* synechia)
synechiotomy
    Paufique s.
synechotomy

synectenterotomy
synencephalocele
Synera topical anesthetic patch
synergism
synergistic
    s. drug interaction
    s. effect
    s. interaction
    s. muscle
synergy
    drug s.
syngeneic
    s. graft
    s. tissue
    s. transplant
syngenesioplastic transplant
syngenesioplasty
syngenesiotransplantation
syngnathia
syngraft
synonychia
synorchidism, synorchism
synorchism (*var. of* synorchidism)
synoscheos
synostectomy
synosteology
synosteosis (*var. of* synostosis)
synostosis, synosteosis
synotia
synovectomy
    Albright s.
    arthroscopic s.
    carpal s.
    dorsal s.
    Inglis-Ranawat-Straub elbow s.
    palmar s.
    6-portal s.
    Porter-Richardson-Vainio s.
    Smith-Petersen s.
    volar s.
    Wilkinson s.
synovial
    s. biopsy
    s. bursa
    s. cavity
    s. fistula
    s. fluid
    s. fluid examination
    s. fold
    s. frenula
    s. frenum
    s. fringe
    s. gland
    s. hernia
    s. herniation
    s. joint
    s. ligament
    s. membrane
    s. tendon sheath

    s. tissue
    s. villus
synovialis
synovioma
    benign giant cell s.
    malignant s.
synoviparous
synovitis
synovium
synpolydactyly
syntheses (*pl. of* synthesis)
synthesis, *pl.* **syntheses**
    collagen s.
    proinflammatory mediator s.
synthetic
    s. absorbable suture
    s. augmentation
    s. mesh
    s. method
    s. opioid receptor agonist
Synthofil suture
Synvisc
syphilid
syphilis
syphilitic fever
syphiloma of Fournier
syringadenoma
syringe
    s. infusion pump
    s. pump
    s. saddle
syringeal
syringectomy
syringes (*pl. of* syrinx)
syringoadenoma
syringocarcinoma
syringocele
syringocisternostomy
syringocystadenoma
syringocystoma
syringohydromyelic cavity
syringoma
syringomeningocele
syringomyelia
    cervical s.
syringomyelic
    s. dissociation
    s. hemorrhage
syringomyelocele
syringomyelus
syringotome
syringotomy
syrinx, *pl.* **syringes**
syssarcosic (*var. of* syssarcotic)
syssarcosis
syssarcotic, syssarcosic
system
    anesthetic s.
    arterial s.

S

system (*continued*)

Arthritis, Rheumatism, and Aging
 Medical Information S. (ARAMIS)
autologous melanoma s.
autonomic nervous s. (ANS)
behavioral inhibition s.
biliary s.
bioartificial liver support s.
Bismuth-Corlette staging s.
Blumgart T-staging s.
Breast Imaging Reporting and Data
 S. (BIRADS)
Bryan cervical disc s.
cartilaginous part of skeletal s.
Cavity Creation S.
celiac arterial s.
cell salvage s.
central nervous s. (CNS)
circle s.
circle breathing s.
Clinical Classification S. (CCS)
closed anesthesia s.
closed-loop s.
Cormack and Lehane laryngeal view
 scoring s.
coronary sinus perfusion s.
da Vinci robotic telemanipulation s.
digestive s.
duct s.
ductal s.
electromagnetic s.
emotional support s.
endogenous opioid s.
enteric nervous s.
externalized catheter s.
extracellular matrix s.
Facial Action Coding S. (FACS)
Fatal Accident Reporting S. (FARS)
force feedback s.
Fuhrman nuclear grading s.
hormone s.
implantable infusion s.
intracranial venous s.
intrathecal drug delivery s.
Ionsys fentanyl iontophoretic
 transdermal s.
J-Tip needleless injection s.
lacrimal s.
LENT-SOMA s.
LifeSite hemodialysis access s.
limbic s.
lymphatic s.
lymphoma s.
Mapleson-type ventilating s.
Maximally Discriminative Facial
 Coding S.
MELD severity assessment s.
mesenteric arterial s.
Moss Miami spinal s.

musculoskeletal s.
myocardial protection s.
National Nosocomial Infections
 Surveillance S.
navigation s.
needle-free s.
needleless intravenous administration
 s.
neoaortoiliac s. (NAIS)
Neonatal Facial Coding S. (NFCS)
nervous s.
neuroendocrine s.
neuronavigational s.
neurotransmitter s.
NNIS s.
noradrenergic s.
open anesthesia s.
opioid s.
optic s.
organ s.
Pain Relief Scoring S.
Pathway pain and sensory evaluation
 s.
patient-activated transdermal s.
 (PATS)
pediatric anesthesia s.
perfusion s.
peripheral access s. (PAS)
peripheral nervous s. (PNS)
pin-index safety s.
portal venous s.
preoperative scoring s.
renal collecting s.
reticular endothelial s.
reticuloendothelial s.
scavenging s.
scoring s.
serotonergic s.
static compliance of the total
 respiratory s.
subcutaneous catheter port s.
superficial musculoaponeurotic s.
 (SMAS)
superior mesenteric arterial s.
suture slider s.
Texas Scottish Rite Hospital
 hook-rod s.
therapeutic intervention scoring s.
 (TISS)
TNM staging s.
traditional circle breathing s.
trauma s.
trigeminocervical pain s.
United States Renal Data S.
 (USRDS)
Universal Spine S. (USS)
vascular s.
vein s.
venous s.

vertical vein s.
water-jet s.
wound surveillance s.
Zeus robotic s.

systema alimentarium

systematic
s. method
s. sextant biopsy

systematization

systemic
s. absorption
s. adjuvant therapy
s. antibiotic
s. anticoagulation
s. antifungal therapy
s. arteriovenous fistula
s. chemotherapy
s. condition
s. disease
s. dissection
s. drainage
s. endotoxemia
s. examination
s. fungal infection
s. hypoperfusion
s. hypotension
s. immunotherapy

s. inflammatory response syndrome (SIRS)
s. lesion
s. lupus
s. medication
s. oxygen extraction
s. perfusion
s. pressure support
s. radioimmunoglobulin therapy
s. sclerosis
s. sepsis
s. vascular disease
s. vascular resistance (SVR)
s. vascular resistance index
s. venodilation
s. venous circulation

systolic
s. arterial pressure (SAP)
s. blood pressure (SBP)
s. ejection murmur
s. ejection rate
s. left ventricular pressure
s. pressure time index
s. time

Szymanowski-Kuhnt ectropion repair with lid reconstruction

Szymanowski operation

S

T

    T cell
    T condylar fracture
    T fracture
    T incision
    T lesion
    T myelotomy
    T sign

T1

    first twitch height

T2

    T2 relaxation rate

T&A

    tonsillectomy and adenoidectomy

TAA

    total ankle arthroplasty

TAB

    temporal artery biopsy

tabby-cat striation
tabetic dissociation
tablature
table

    inner t.
    vitreous t.

tablet

    fentanyl buccal t.

tabulation
TAC

    total abdominal colectomy

TACC

    thoracic aortic cross-clamping

TACE

    transarterial chemoembolization

Tachdjian

    T. external fixation for cavus
      fixation procedure
    T. pediatric ankle fracture
      classification

tachistoscopy
tachycardia

    atrial ectopic t.
    atrioventricular reentry t.
    automatic ectopic t.
    bundle branch reentrant t.
    ectopic atrial t.
    endless-loop t.
    exercise-induced ventricular t.
    junctional ectopic t.
    pacemaker-mediated t.
    right ventricular outflow
      tract t.
    torsade de pointes ventricular t.
      (TdPVT)

tachyphylaxis
tack fixation

tacrolimus
tacrolimus-based immunosuppression
tactic

    thyroidectomy t.
    thyroid surgical t.

**Tactical Combat Casualty Care
(TCCC)**
tactile

    t. anesthesia
    t. stimulation

TAE

    total abdominal evisceration

taenia (*var. of* tenia)
taenial (*var. of* tenial)
TAES

    transcutaneous acupoint electrical
      stimulation

tag

    anal t.
    Crohn t.

tagging stitch
tagliacotian rhinoplasty operation
TAH

    total abdominal hysterectomy

TAHBSO

    total abdominal hysterectomy and
      bilateral salpingo-oophorectomy

tail

    artery of pancreatic t.
    axillary t.
    t. bone
    pancreatic t.
    t. tumor
    t. vertebra

tailbone
tailor bunionectomy
Tait vaginal flap
Tajima suture technique
Takayasu

    T. arteritis
    T. disease
    T. syndrome

takedown

    t. abdominal approach
    bilateral ureterostomy t.
    colostomy t.
    t. procedure

talar

    t. avulsion fracture
    t. canal
    t. compression syndrome
    t. dislocation
    t. neck fracture
    t. osteochondral fracture
    t. sulcus

talc
- t. insufflation
- t. operation
- t. peritonitis
- t. pleurodesis

talectomy
- Trumble t.

Talesnick scapholunate repair

tali (*pl. of* talus)

talipes
- t. cavus
- t. cavus deformity
- t. equinovarus

talocalcaneal, talocalcanean
- t. angle
- t. articulation
- t. fusion

talocalcanean (*var. of* talocalcaneal)

talocalcaneonavicular articulation

talocrural joint

talonavicular
- t. bone
- t. fusion

taloscaphoid

talotibial

talus, *pl.* **tali**
- sustentaculum tali

tamp
- bone t.

Tampa Scale of Kinesophobia (TSK)

tamponade, tamponage
- balloon tube t.
- delayed pericardial t.
- low-pressure t.
- t. needle tract
- pericardial t.
- tract t.

tamponage (*var. of* tamponade)

tamponing, tamponment

tamponment (*var. of* tamponing)

tamsulosin

Tanagho
- T. bladder flap urethroplasty
- T. bladder neck reconstruction

tandem
- t. clipping technique
- t. colonoscopy
- t. construction
- t. lesion

tangential
- t. biopsy
- t. colonic submucosal injection
- t. débridement
- t. excision
- t. incision
- t. projection
- t. section
- t. tract
- t. wound

tangent screen examination

Tanner stomach devascularization operation

Tansini osteomyocutaneous intercostal transposition flap operation

Tansley lid ptosis operation

tantalum
- t. cranioplasty
- t. wire tension suture

TAO
- thromboangiitis obliterans

tap
- abdominal t.
- peritoneal t.
- shunt t.

TAP
- transesophageal atrial pacing

tape mark

Tapercut suture

tapered tip

taper point

tapeta (*pl. of* tapetum)

tapetum, *pl.* **tapeta**

tapinocephalic

tapinocephaly

TAPP
- transabdominal preperitoneal

tapping
- glabellar t.

TAPVR
- total anomalous pulmonary venous return

TARA
- total articular resurfacing arthroplasty

tarda

target
- fixation t.
- t. gland
- t. lesion
- t. plasma
- t. plasma concentration (TPC)
- saccadic eccentric t.
- t. sign

target-controlled infusion (TCI)

targeted
- t. brain biopsy
- t. lobar deflation
- t. surgery

targeting
- tumor t.

Tarin space

tarsal
- t. amputation
- t. artery bypass
- t. bone fracture
- t. canal
- t. dislocation
- t. fold
- t. gland

t. joint infection
t. laceration
t. ligament
t. medullostomy
t. membrane
t. plate
t. strip procedure
t. tunnel syndrome
t. wedge osteotomy
tarsectomy
Beard t.
Blaskovics t.
Kuhnt t.
Tessier t.
tarsen
tarsi (*pl. of* tarsus)
tarsocheiloplasty
tarsoconjunctival flap
tarsometatarsal
t. amputation
t. articulation
t. dislocation
t. fracture-dislocation
t. truncated-wedge arthrodesis
tarsophalangeal
tarsoplasty
tarsorrhaphy
bilateral temporary t.
Leahey temporary t.
tarsotomy
transverse t.
tarsus, *pl.* **tarsi**
inferior t.
superior t.
tartrate
taste pathway
tattooing
colonic t.
Taussig-Bing anomaly
Taussig-Morton
T.-M. modified Blalock-Taussig
operation
T.-M. node dissection
Taussig operation
Tawara node
Taylor
T. combined spinal-epidural
anesthesia approach
T. suture technique
**Taylor-Daniel-Weiland free composite
iliac bone graft technique**
**Taylor-Townsend-Corlett iliac crest bone
graft**
TB
tuberculosis
TBI
traumatic brain injury
TBNA
transbronchial needle aspiration

TBSA
total body surface area
TCA
talocalcaneal angle
thymic carcinoma
total colonic aganglionosis
transluminal coronary angioplasty
99mTc
technetium-99m
TCCC
Tactical Combat Casualty Care
TCD
transcranial Doppler
TCD recanalization
T-cell-depleted bone marrow transplant
T-cell line
TCES
transcutaneous cranial electrical
stimulation
TCI
target-controlled infusion
TCM
thick cutaneous melanoma
tc-MER
motor-evoked response to transcranial
stimulation
T-configuration
TCRF
temperature-controlled radiofrequency
TCRFTA
temperature-controlled radiofrequency
tissue ablation
TCS
transcranial stimulation
TDCO
thermodilution cardiac output
TdPVT
torsade de pointes ventricular
tachycardia
TE
tracheoesophageal
TE fistula
TEA
thoracic epidural anesthesia
thromboendarterectomy
total elbow arthroplasty
teacup fracture
Teale-Knapp symblepharon operation
team
Burn Flight T.
trauma t.
2-team dissection
TEAP
transesophageal atrial pacing
TEAP threshold
tear
bucket-handle t.
capsular t.
esophageal t.

T

tear (*continued*)
  flap meniscal t.
  inadvertent serosal t.
  linear t.
  Mallory-Weiss t.
  mesenteric t.
  pulmonary circulation t.
  radial t.
  rotator cuff t.
  t. sac
  serosal t.
teardrop
  t. fracture
  t. line
tearing
  excessive t.
  short-lasting unilateral neuralgiaform
    headache with conjunctival
    injection and t. (SUNCT)
technetium-99m (^{99m}Tc)
technic
technical
  t. consideration
  t. factor
  t. failure
technician
  OR t.
technique, technic
  abdominal pressure t.
  abduction traction t.
  ablative t.
  Ace-Colles frame t.
  acid etch bonding t.
  adduction traction t.
  afterloading t.
  airbrasive t.
  air-gap t.
  airway occlusion t.
  Albert suture t.
  Alexander musculoskeletal
    relaxation t.
  Allison antireflux t.
  alternating suture t.
  American laryngectomy t.
  Amplatz coronary catheterization t.
  Amspacher-Messenbaugh cubitus
    varus correction t.
  Andrews strangulated hernia
    repair t.
  anesthetic t.
  angiographic road-mapping t.
  angle bisection t.
  angle suture t.
  antegrade double balloon-double
    wire t.
  antegrade/retrograde cardioplegia t.
  anterior quadriceps musculocutaneous
    flap t.
  anterior sandwich patch t.

anterograde transseptal t.
antireflux ureteral implantation t.
AO t.
APOLT t.
Appolito suture t.
apposition suture t.
approximation suture t.
arcuate suture t.
Argyll-Robertson suture t.
Arlt suture t.
Armistead distraction osteogenesis t.
Aronson-Prager supracondylar
  humerus fracture pinning t.
arrested-heart revascularization t.
arterial cannulation anesthetic t.
arthrographic capsular distention and
  rupture t.
ascending t.
aseptic t.
ASIF screw fixation t.
Asnis cannulated screw fixation t.
assisted reproductive t. (ART)
Atasoy V-Y t.
Atkinson cataract extraction t.
atraumatic suture t.
atrial-well t.
autosuture t.
Avila t.
avulsion t.
Axenfeld suture t.
axillary block anesthetic t.
axillary perivascular t.
Ayre spatula-Zelsmyr cytobrush
  cervical specimen collection t.
Babcock suture t.
back-and-forth suture t.
Badgley anterior cervical discectomy
  and fusion t.
bag-of-bones t.
Bailey-Badgley cervical spine
  interbody fusion t.
Bailey-Dubow internal fixation t.
Baker t.
Balacescu-Golden hallux valgus
  osteotomy t.
balanced anesthetic t.
balloon catheter t.
balloon-catheter and basket-
  retrieval t.
balloon tamponade t.
Banks-Laufman surgical exposure of
  extremities techniques
Barcat distal hypospadias repair t.
bare scleral t.
Barkan trabeculotomy t.
Barraquer suture t.
barrier t.
Barron hemorrhoidal banding t.
Barsky bilateral cleft lips repair t.

baseball suture t.
basic t.
basilar suture t.
basket extraction t.
basket fragmentation t.
basketing t.
Bassini herniorrhaphy t.
bastard suture t.
Batch-Spittler-McFaddin through-knee
   amputation t.
Bauer-Tondra-Trusler syndactyly skin
   release t.
Baumgard-Schwartz tennis elbow t.
Beckenbaugh biaxial wrist implant t.
Becker otoplasty t.
Béclard suture t.
Becton fracture fixation t.
Begg light wire differential force
   orthodontic t.
behavioral t.
Bell-Tawse open reduction t.
Belsey fundoplication t.
Belt radical prostatectomy t.
bench surgical t.
Bentall composite graft t.
Bentall inclusion t.
Bertrandi suture t.
Beverly-Douglas lip-tongue
   adhesion t.
bilateral inguinal hernia repair t.
Billroth I, II t.
bioprogressive t.
biopsy t.
biparietal suture t.
Bircher-Weber traditional
   orthopaedic t.
bisecting angle t.
bisecting-the-angle t.
bitewing t.
Black t.
Black-Broström staple t.
Blackburn t.
bladder neck preserving t.
Blair-Byars hypospadias t.
Blair hypospadias t.
blanket suture t.
Bleck midcalf lengthening by
   recession t.
blind nasal intubation anesthetic t.
blind nasotracheal intubation
   anesthetic t.
blind-spot projection t.
Bloom-Raney modification of
   Smith-Robinson anterior discectomy
   and interbody fusion t.
Blundell Jones t.
Bohlman triple-wire cervical
   fusion t.
bolster suture t.

bolus intravenous anesthetic t.
bone t.
Bonfiglio-Bardenstein bone grafting
   of femoral head and neck t.
Bonfiglio modification of Phemister
   bone graft of femoral neck t.
Bonola diaphyseal resection t.
boost t.
bootstrap 2-vessel t.
Bora t.
Borggreve-Hall tibial rotation
   plasty t.
bougienage t.
Bowers genital reassignment t.
Bowles breast conserving t.
Boyd-Anderson distal biceps tendon
   repair t.
Boyd-McLeod tennis elbow t.
Boyes brachioradialis transfer t.
Bozeman suture t.
Braasch bulb t.
brachial plexus block anesthetic t.
Brackett-Osgood-Putti-Abbott
   posterior knee t.
Brackin t.
Brady-Jewett proximal radial
   resection t.
Brain LMA-insertion t.
Brand tendon transfer t.
breast-conserving t.
breast reduction t.
bregmatomastoid suture t.
Brenner gastrojejunostomy t.
bridle suture t.
Brockenbrough transseptal left heart
   catheterization t.
Brockhurst scleral buckle t.
bronchoscopy anesthetic t.
Brooks atlantoaxial subluxation tape
   repair t.
Brooks-Jenkins atlantoaxial fusion t.
Brooks-Seddon tendon transfer t.
Brown-Beard oculoplastic t.
Brown endoscopic carpal tunnel
   release t.
Bruhat neosalpingostomy t.
Bruser lateral knee t.
Bryan-Morrey triceps-sparing
   humerus fracture repair t.
Buck-Gramcko dorsal rotational
   advancement flap t.
Bugg-Boyd Achilles tendon repair t.
bunching suture t.
Buncke microsurgical t.
Bunnell atraumatic t.
Bunnell suture t.
Bunnell tendon transfer t.
Burch bladder suspension t.
Burgess transtibial amputation t.

T

technique (*continued*)

buried mass far-and-near suture t.
Burkhalter modification of
  Stiles-Bunnell t.
Burkhalter transfer t.
Burrows triple fixation limb
  salvage t.
buttonhole suture t.
button suture t.
Buxton bolus suture t.
bypass t.
cable wire suture t.
Caldwell-Coleman flatfoot t.
Callahan posterior spinal fusion t.
Camitz palmaris longus tendon
  reconstruction t.
Campbell opening-wedge
  thoracostomy t.
Canale distal humerus fracture
  pinning t.
canal wall-up t.
Capello acetabular reconstruction t.
Cape Town injection sclerotherapy t.
capitonnage suture t.
capping t.
capsule flap t.
capsule forceps t.
cardiovascular imaging t.
Carnesale extremity amputation t.
carotid preservation t.
Carrell fibular substitution t.
Carrel suture t.
catheterization t.
catheter-securing t.
caudal epidural anesthetic t.
cavernosal alpha blockade t.
Cave-Rowe shoulder dislocation t.
celiac plexus block anesthetic t.
cement t.
cementless t.
central anesthetic t.
central slip-sparing t.
central venous cannulation
  anesthetic t.
cephalotrigonal t.
cervical plexus block anesthetic t.
cervical screw insertion t.
cervical spondylotic myelopathy
  fusion t.
chain suture t.
channel shoulder pin t.
Chaves-Rapp muscle transfer t.
Cherney suture t.
chevron t.
chew-in t.
Chiari pelvis osteotomy t.
Childress ankle fixation t.
chloramine T t.
cholangiographic t.

Cho tendon t.
Chow endoscopic carpal tunnel
  release t.
Chrisman-Snook ankle t.
Cierny-Mader single-stage
  osteomyelitis repair t.
Cincinnati pelvic osteotomy t.
circular suture t.
circulatory arrest anesthetic t.
circumcision suture t.
Clagett empyema t.
clamp-and-sew t.
clamp crushing t.
clamshell t.
Clancy ligament t.
Clark transfer t.
classic DSRS t.
clearance t.
Cleveland-Bosworth-Thompson t.
clip t.
closed circuit anesthetic t.
closed gloving t.
closed tubule fixation t.
Cloward anterior cervical discectomy
  and fusion t.
Coakley suture t.
coaptation suture t.
cobalt-60 moving strip t.
cobbler's suture t.
Cobb scoliosis measuring t.
Codivilla tendon lengthening t.
Coffey ureterosigmoid transplant t.
Coffey-Witzel jejunostomy t.
Cofield rotator cuff reconstruction t.
Cohen crosstrigonal t.
Colcher-Sussman x-ray pelvimetry t.
cold saline-induced paresthesia t.
Coleman flatfoot t.
Cole orthopaedic surgical t.
Collis broken femoral stem t.
Collis-Nissen fundoplication t.
Coltart fracture t.
combination of isotonics therapeutic
  exercise t.
combined spinal-epidural
  anesthetic t.
composite pelvic resection t.
compound suture t.
compression t.
computer-assisted continuous infusion
  anesthetic t.
computer-controlled drug
  administration anesthetic t.
computer-controlled infusion
  anesthetic t.
Connell suture t.
Connolly bone regeneration t.
continuous gum t.
continuous infusion anesthetic t.

continuous pullthrough t.
continuous spinal anesthetic t.
continuous suture t.
continuous wave t.
contoured anterior spinal plate t.
contract-relax t.
controlled release anesthetic t.
controlled water-added t.
conventional t.
Conyers t.
Coonse-Adams V-Y quadriceps turndown knee t.
Copeland arthroscopic rotator cuff repair t.
Cope transseptal left atrium catheterization t.
coracoclavicular t.
Corbin rhinoplasty t.
coronary button suture t.
coronary flow reserve t.
costotransversectomy t.
Counsellor-Flor modification of McIndoe vaginoplasty t.
Cozen-Brockway postaxial polydactyly t.
craniosacral t.
crash t.
Crawford graft inclusion t.
Crawford-Marxen-Osterfeld staged talipes equinovarus repair t.
Creech endoaneurysmorrhaphy t.
Crego tendon transfer t.
cricoid pressure anesthetic t.
cross-facial t.
Crown suture t.
cruciform suture t.
crushing t.
Crutchfield closed cervical spine fracture-dislocation t.
cryosurgical t.
CSEA t.
Cubbins shoulder dislocation t.
cup-patch ileocystoplasty t.
Curtis-Fisher knee t.
Curtis flexion contracture release t.
Cushing suture t.
cushioning suture t.
cut-and-sew t.
cutaneous suture t.
cutdown t.
cuticular suture t.
cystic duct marking t.
Czerny-Lembert suture t.
Czerny suture t.
Darrach-McLaughlin shoulder t.
Davey-Rorabeck-Fowler decompression t.
Davis drainage t.
decompression t.

decortication t.
Deisting prostatic dilation t.
delayed primary suture t.
deliberate hypotension anesthetic t.
demand-adapted administration anesthetic t.
Denis Browne urethroplasty t.
Dennis left atrium cannulation t.
de novo needle-knife t.
DePalma modified patellar t.
depth pulse t.
dermal suture t.
descending t.
Dewar-Barrington clavicular dislocation t.
Dewar-Harris shoulder t.
Dewar posterior cervical fusion t.
Deyerle femoral fracture t.
diagnostic t.
Dias-Giegerich fracture t.
Dickinson calcaneal bursitis t.
Dickson transplant t.
Dieffenbach-Duplay hypospadias t.
differential spinal block anesthetic t.
dilator-and-sheath t.
dilution-filtration t.
Dimon-Hughston intertrochanteric hip fracture reduction t.
Diprivan anesthetic t.
direct/indirect t.
direct insertion t.
distal splenorenal shunt t.
distraction t.
diversified chiropractic t.
Dolenc cavernous sinus exploration t.
Doll trochanteric reattachment t.
donor button t.
Doppler auto-correlation t.
Dor fundoplication t.
dot-blot t.
Dotter-Judkins superselective visceralangiography t.
Dotter percutaneous recanalization of arterial occlusion t.
double-armed suture t.
double-balloon t.
double-button suture t.
double-dummy t.
double-folded cup-patch ileocystoplasty t.
double-freeze t.
double-looped semitendinosus t.
double-needle t.
double-rod t.
double-sealant t.
double-staple t.
double-stapled ileoanal reservoir t.
double stapling t. (DST)

T

technique *(continued)*
    double-stick t.
    double-tube t.
    double-wire t.
    Douglas bag t.
    dowel t.
    doweling spondylolisthesis t.
    Drake tandem clipping t.
    DREZ modification of Eriksson
      ankle joint arthroscopy t.
    drilling t.
    Drummond interspinous wiring t.
    dry field t.
    DSRS t.
    dual impression t.
    duct-to-mucosa t.
    Dufourmentel pilonidal cyst and
      sinus closure t.
    dunking t.
    Dunn acromioclavicular joint t.
    Dunn-Brittain foot stabilization t.
    Duplay I, II hypospadias repair t.
    Dupuytren suture t.
    DuVries deltoid ligament
      reconstruction t.
    dye dilution cardiac output t.
    dynamic bolus tracking t.
    Eastwood anesthesia t.
    Eaton-Littler carpometacarpal thumb
      repair t.
    Eaton-Malerich fracture-dislocation t.
    Eberle contracture release t.
    Ecker-Lotke-Glazer tendon
      reconstruction t.
    edge-to-edge suture t.
    Eftekhar broken femoral stem t.
    Eggers tendon transfer t.
    Eisenberger t.
    elephant trunk aortic graft t.
    elliptical excision t.
    Ellis-Jones peroneal tendon t.
    Ellison iliotibial band transfer for
      ACL repair t.
    Ellis skin traction t.
    Emmet suture t.
    en bloc no-touch t.
    Ender femoral fracture t.
    endobronchial intubation anesthetic t.
    endodontic t.
    endofluoroscopic t.
    endorectal ileoanal pullthrough t.
    endoscope-assisted t.
    endoscopic-assisted microsurgical t.
    endoscopic mucosal resection t.
    endovascular stenting t.
    end-to-end reconstruction t.
    end-to-side vasoepididymostomy t.
    entangling t.
    enucleation t.

    epiaortic imaging t.
    epidural blood patch anesthetic t.
    epineural suture t.
    epithelialization t.
    Erickson-Leider-Brown 2-level spinal
      burst fracture repair t.
    Eriksson brachial block t.
    Eriksson ligament t.
    erysiphake t.
    esophageal banding t.
    Essex-Lopresti axial fixation t.
    Essex-Lopresti calcaneal
      fracture t.
    Evans ankle reconstruction t.
    eversion t.
    everting interrupted suture t.
    evoked potential t.
    exchange t.
    excisional biopsy t.
    excision-curettage t.
    ex situ-in situ t.
    extra-anatomical renal
      revascularization t.
    extraanatomic bypass t.
    extraarticular t.
    extracorporeal t.
    extraction balloon t.
    extradural anesthetic t.
    extravesical ureteral reimplantation t.
    extremity mobilization t.
    extubation anesthetic t.
    ex vivo t.
    facet excision t.
    Fahey t.
    Fahey-O'Brien unicameral bone cyst
      subtotal resection and grafting t.
    Fairbanks uvulopalatopharyngo-
      plasty t.
    Falk vesicovaginal fistula t.
    far-and-near suture t.
    Farmer t.
    fat-suppression t.
    feeder-frond ablative
      photocoagulation t.
    femoral 3-in-1 t.
    Ferkel torticollis t.
    fiberoptic bronchoscopy anesthetic t.
    fiberoptic endoscopy anesthetic t.
    fiberoptic tracheal intubation
      anesthetic t.
    Fick cardiac output t.
    Fielding modification of Gallie
      atlantoaxial instability spine
      fusion t.
    figure-of-8 suture t.
    filling first t.
    finger fracture t.
    Finochietto-Billroth I gastrectomy t.
    first line screening t.

first-pass t.
first rib resection via subclavicular approach t.
Fish cuneiform osteotomy t.
fixation t.
fixation suture t.
flap t.
Flatt hand surgery t.
Flick-Gould osteoarthritis dissecans of ankle repair t.
flip-flap t.
floppy Nissen fundoplication t.
flow detection t.
flow interruption t.
flow mapping t.
fluid loading anesthetic t.
fluoroscopic pushing t.
flush-and-bathe t.
flushing t.
Forbes modification of Phemister graft t.
fore-and-aft suture t.
forward triangle t.
Fowles dislocation t.
Frank permanent gastrotomy t.
Fraunfelder no-touch intraocular malignant melanoma t.
Freebody-Bendall-Taylor transperitoneal lumbar fusion t.
freehand suturing t.
free ligature suture t.
free-root insertion t.
French fracture t.
Fried-Hendel tendon t.
Froimson bicipital groove keyhole t.
frontalis sling t.
Frost suture t.
functional t.
furrier's suture t.
fusion t.
Gaenslen split-heel t.
Gallie atlantoaxial fusion wiring t.
Galveston spinopelvic reconstruction t.
Gambee suture t.
Ganley forefoot osseous reconstruction t.
Garceau tendon t.
gaseous laparoscopy t.
gasless laparoscopy t.
gastric valve tightening t.
gated t.
Gaur retroperitoneal balloon distention t.
Gély suture t.
general anesthetic t.
Giannestras modification of Lapidus hallux valgus t.
Gibson suture t.

gift wrap suture t.
Gilbert-Tamai-Weiland free fibular bone transfer t.
Gillies-Millard cocked-hat thumb reconstruction t.
Gill-Manning-White spondylolisthesis t.
Gill sliding graft t.
Gil-Vernet anti-vesicoureteral reflux t.
Gittes genitourinary t.
Glenn-Anderson perioscrotal transposition repair t.
gliding-hole-first t.
gloved-fist t.
Glover suture t.
Goebel-Frangenheim-Stoeckel urethrovesical t.
Goldberg clavicle fracture repair t.
Goldner-Clippinger multangular bone excision t.
gold plate t.
gold seed implantation t.
Goldstein spinal fusion t.
Gomco circumcision t.
Goodwin-Hohenfellner ureteric reimplantation t.
Goodwin orthotopic ileal neobladder t.
Goodwin-Scott plastic reconstruction of prepuce t.
Gordon-Broström t.
Gordon joint injection t.
Gordon-Taylor hip disarticulation t.
Gould suture t.
grabbing t.
gracilis flap t.
grasping t.
Graves t.
Greulich-Pyle skeletal age estimation t.
Grice-Green subtalar extraarticular arthrodesis t.
Gritti-Stokes knee amputation t.
groove suture t.
Grosse-Kempf tibial locked nailing t.
Groves-Goldner proximal median-radial palsy t.
Gruber suture t.
Grüntzig transaortic intraluminal angioplasty t.
Guhl ankle arthroscopy t.
guide wire and mini-snare t.
guide wire exchange t.
Gussenbauer suture t.
Guttmann t.
Guyon ankle amputation t.
guy suture t.

technique (*continued*)

Guyton-Friedenwald suture t.
Hackethal stacked nailing humeral shaft t.
Håkanson t.
half-mouth t.
half-Pringle t.
Hall preformed metal crown t.
Halsted suture t.
Hamas endoscopic facial rejuvenation t.
Hamou hysteroscopic endometrial ablation t.
Hardinge hip prosthesis measurement t.
harelip suture t.
Harmon transfer t.
Harris suture t.
Hartel trigeminal neuralgia alcohol injection t.
Hartmann reconstruction t.
Hassmann-Brunn-Neer elbow reconstruction t.
Hasson open trocar t.
Hauri penile revascularization t.
Hauser patellar realignment t.
Hawkins inside-out nephrostomy t.
Hawkins single-stick t.
head turn t.
Heaney vaginal hysterectomy t.
helical suture t.
hemostat t.
hemostatic suture t.
Hendler unitunnel ACL repair t.
Henning inside-to-outside meniscal repair t.
Henry acromioclavicular t.
hepatic vascular isolation t.
Hepp-Couinaud biliary reconstruction t.
Hermodsson internal rotation t.
Hey-Groves anterior cruciate ligament reconstruction t.
Hey-Groves fascia lata ACL repair t.
Heyman-Herndon-Strong correction of metatarsus varus t.
high-amplitude sucking t.
high-tension suturing t.
Hill-Nahai-Vasconez-Mathes tensor fasciae latae free flap t.
Hitchcock biceps tendon t.
Hodgson hypospadias repair t.
Hofmeister gastric resection t.
Hohl-Moore tibial plateau fracture repair t.
Hoke-Kite arthrodesis t.
hold-relax t.
hole-in-1 t.

Hoppenfeld-Deboer orthopaedic t.
Hori umbilicus reconstruction t.
horizontal mattress suture t.
hot biopsy t.
hot-dog ACL repair t.
Houghton-Akroyd fracture t.
House otosclerosis cochlear implant t.
Howard differential ureteral catheterization t.
Hughes modification of Burch colposuspension t.
Hughston-Jacobson tibial tunnel knee repair t.
Hunt-Early t.
Huntington tibial t.
hybridization-subtraction t.
hybridoma t.
hydroflow t.
hydrogen inhalation t.
hygroscopic t.
hypogastric plexus block anesthetic t.
hypothermia anesthetic t.
Ilizarov limb-lengthening t.
image-related screening t.
imaging t.
imbricate suture t.
immediate extension t.
immersion t.
implanted suture t.
impression t.
indirect t.
indocyanine green indicator dilution t.
induced hypotension anesthetic t.
induction anesthetic t.
infiltration anesthetic t.
Inglis-Cooper flexor slide t.
Inglis-Ranawat-Straub synovectomy and débridement of elbow t.
inhalation anesthetic t.
injection t.
inotrope resuscitation t.
Insall ligament reconstruction t.
insemination swim-up t.
insertion t.
inside-out t.
inside-to-outside t.
insufflation anesthetic t.
intercostal nerve block anesthetic t.
interference screw t.
interlocking suture t.
intermittent apnea t.
intermittent bolus t.
internal jugular vein cannulation anesthetic t.
internal jugular vein catheterization anesthetic t.

internal jugular vein puncture anesthetic t.
interpleural anesthetic t.
interpolation t.
interrupted suture t.
interscalene block anesthetic t.
interventional t.
intraarticular anesthetic t.
intracorporeal knotting t.
intradermal mattress suture t.
intradermal tattooing t.
intramuscular preanesthetic medication anesthetic t.
intraoperative computer-assisted spinal orientation t.
intraperitoneal t.
intraperitoneal onlay mesh t.
intrathecal cannulation anesthetic t.
intrathecal morphine anesthetic t.
intravenous cannulation anesthetic t.
intubation anesthetic t.
invaginating suture t.
invagination t.
invasive t.
inverting knot t.
ischemic-tourniquet t.
isolation t.
isometric t.
Jaboulay-Doyen-Winkleman hydrocele bottleneck t.
Jacobs locking-hook spinal rod t.
Jansey shoulder arthrodesis t.
Jeffery t.
jejunoileal bypass reversal t.
jet ventilation anesthetic t.
J-loop t.
Jobert suture t.
Johnson pelvic fracture t.
Johnson staple t.
Johnston pursestring suture t.
Jones and Jones wedge t.
Jorgensen anesthesia t.
Judd pyloroplasty t.
Judkins selective percutaneous transfemoral coronary arteriography t.
Judkins-Sones coronary arteriography t.
jugular t.
Kader-Senn gastrotomy t.
Kalt suture t.
kangaroo tendon suture t.
Kapandji distal radius fracture pinning t.
Kapel elbow dislocation t.
Kashiwagi elbow arthroplasty t.
Kates-Kessel-Kay forefoot arthroplasty t.
Kato thick smear t.

Kaufer tendon t.
Kaufmann subpial transection t.
Kehr biliary drainage t.
Kelikian-Clayton-Loseff surgical syndactylia of toes t.
Kelikian-Riashi-Gleason patellar tendon reconstruction t.
Kellogg-Speed fusion anterior interbody spinal fusion t.
Kelly suture t.
Kendrick-Sharma-Hassler-Herndon metatarsus adductus repair t.
Kennedy ligament t.
Kern lateral mass screw fixation t.
Kessler suture t.
Kety-Schmidt inert gas saturation t.
keyhole tenodesis t.
keystone anterior discectomy and fusion t.
Kidde cannula hysterosalpingogram t.
King contrast venography t.
King-Richards dislocation t.
King-Steelquist transiliac amputation t.
Kirk thigh amputation t.
Kirschner suture t.
kissing balloon t.
Krawkow-Cohn iliac crest bone harvest t.
Krawkow-Thomas-Jones locking suture t.
Krempen-Craig-Sotelo tibial nonunion t.
Krönig t.
Kugel hernia patch repair t.
Kumar-Cowell-Ramsey congenital vertical talus correction t.
Kumar spica cast t.
Küntscher intramedullary nailing t.
Kutler finger amputation t.
Labbé gastrotomy t.
labiolingual t.
lace suture t.
Lamb-Marks-Bayne upper limb repair t.
Lambrinudi triple arthrodesis for dropfoot t.
laparoscopic colposuspension t.
laparoscopic donor nephrectomy t.
laparoscopic lymph node dissection t.
laparoscopic Nissen fundoplication t.
laparoscopic no-trocar t.
laparoscopic paraaortic lymph node sampling t.
laparoscopic stripping t.
laparostomy t.
laparostomy with silo-bag t.

T

technique (*continued*)

Lapidus hammertoe t.
large-core t.
Larson posterolateral instability of knee repair t.
laryngeal mask insertion anesthetic t.
laryngoscopy anesthetic t.
laser welding t.
lateral bending t.
lateral window t.
layer t.
2-layer open t.
Lazarus-Nelson peritoneal lavage t.
LCVP-aided t.
LDN t.
Leach dual-imaging surgical planning t.
Leadbetter ureteroplasty modification t.
Le Dran suture t.
LeDuc ureteral tunneling t.
Lee laryngotracheal stenosis management t.
Lefèvre gastrectomy t.
Le Fort suture t.
Lehman endoscopic pancreatic sphincterotomy t.
Leibolt pantalar arthrodesis t.
Leksell stereotactic surgery t.
Lembert suture t.
lens suture t.
lesser sac t.
letterbox t.
Lewit stretch t.
Lich extravesical t.
Lich-Gregoir vesicoureteral reflux repair t.
Lichtman staging of Kienböck disease t.
lid-loading t.
Liebolt radioulnar t.
ligate-divide-staple t.
ligation suture t.
light-around-wire t.
Limberg pilonidal sinus flap repair t.
limb-saving t.
Lindholm Achilles tendon rupture repair t.
lingual split-bone t.
Lipscomb t.
Lister flexor tendon pulley reconstruction t.
Littler-Cooley opponensplasty t.
Littler swanneck deformity repair t.
Lloyd-Roberts fracture t.
localization t.
local standby anesthesia t.

locking suture t.
lock-stitch suture t.
Löffler suture t.
long cone t.
3-loop t.
loop gastric bypass t.
loop-on mucosa suture t.
Losee modification of MacIntosh ACL repair t.
Losee sling and reef ACL repair t.
loss-of-resistance t.
lost wax pattern t.
low-flow anesthetic t.
Lown cardioverter t.
Ludloff congenital hip dislocation repair t.
lumbar accessory movement t.
lumbar anesthetic t.
1-lung ventilation anesthetic t.
Luque instrumentation concave t.
Luque instrumentation convex t.
Luque sublaminar wiring t.
LUS scanning t.
Lyden real-time cerebral angiography t.
Lynn Achilles tendon rupture repair t.
MacIntosh laryngoscopy t.
macroelectrode recording t.
Madden modified radical mastectomy t.
Magerl translaminar facet screw fixation t.
Magilligan femoral anteversion measuring t.
Magnuson anterior dislocation of shoulder repair t.
Ma-Griffith Achilles tendon rupture repair t.
Maitland manual spinal therapy t.
Majestro-Ruda-Frost tendon t.
Malawer excision t.
mandibular swing t.
manometric t.
Manske radioulnar osteoclasis t.
manual push-pull t.
Marcus-Balourdas-Heiple ankle fusion t.
Marlex plug t.
Marshall ligament repair t.
Marshall-McIntosh ACL repair t.
marsupialization t.
Martin patellar wiring t.
Martin reduction t.
masking t.
masquerade t.
Mathieu hypospadias repair t.
Matti-Russe scaphoid nonunion bone graft t.

4-maximal breath preoxygenation t.
Mazet knee disarticulation t.
McCauley knee cartilage MRI t.
McConnell patellar taping t.
McElfresh-Dobyns-O'Brien extension
  block splinting t.
McElvenny orthopaedic t.
McFarland-Osborne hip joint lateral
  incision t.
McGoon double-switch TGA
  correction t.
McKeever-Buck elbow t.
McReynolds open reduction t.
McVay herniorrhaphy t.
Meares-Stamey chronic prostatitis t.
mechanical ventilation anesthetic t.
Meigs suture t.
membrane catheter t.
Menghini biopsy t.
Merendino incompetent mitral valve
  reconstruction t.
Messerklinger endoscopic sinus
  inflammation diagnostic t.
Meyerding orthopaedic t.
microelectrode recording t.
microinvasive t.
micromanipulation t.
microsurgery t.
microsurgical t.
microtransducer t.
microtubulotomy t.
microvascular t.
midface degloving t.
Milch cuff resection of ulna t.
Milch elbow t.
Milford mallet finger t.
Millen retropubic prostatectomy t.
mille pattes t.
Millesi modified nerve graft t.
minilaparotomy t.
minimal access t.
minimal leak t.
minimally invasive surgical t.
  (MIST)
Mital elbow release t.
miter t.
Mitrofanoff continent urinary
  diversion t.
Mizuno double-patch ventricular
  septal perforation repair t.
Mizuno-Hirohata-Kashiwagi pediatric
  distal humeral fracture-separation
  repair t.
modified Belsey fundoplication t.
modified brachial t.
modified Cantwell t.
modified Child t.
modified Hassan open t.
modified piggyback t.

modified Pomeroy t.
modified Sacks-Vine push-pull t.
modified Seldinger t.
modified Toupe t.
modified tumescent liposuction t.
modified V-Y advancement t.
Moe scoliosis t.
Mohs fresh tissue chemosurgery t.
Mohs microsurgery t.
molecular t.
monitored anesthesia care
  anesthetic t.
monitoring t.
Monticelli-Spinelli distraction
  epiphysiolysis limb lengthening t.
Moore t.
morcellation t.
Morgan-Casscells meniscus
  suturing t.
motor point block anesthetic t.
MPB t.
Mubarak-Hargens decompression t.
mucosal relaxing incision t.
multiple inert gas elimination t.
  (MIGET)
multiple-port incision t.
muscle energy t.
muscle-splitting t.
Nalebuff-Millender swan-neck
  deformity lateral band
  mobilization t.
nasotracheal intubation anesthetic t.
nasovesicular catheter t.
Nealon provisional dental
  restoration t.
near-and-far suture t.
2-needle t.
needle-knife t.
needle thoracentesis t.
needle-through-needle single
  interspace t.
negative pressure closure t.
nerve stimulator anesthetic t.
nerve suture t.
neural arch resection t.
neuroablative t.
neuroleptanalgesia anesthetic t.
neuromodulation t.
Neviaser acromioclavicular t.
Neviaser-Wilson-Gardner first dorsal
  interosseus replacement t.
Nicholas coracoclavicular congenital
  knee dislocation ligament t.
Nicholas 5-in-1 knee
  reconstruction t.
Niebauer-King congenital knee
  dislocation open reduction t.
Nikaidoh-Bex TGA with VSD
  repair t.

technique (*continued*)

 Nirschl lateral epicondylitis mini-open t.
 Nissen fundoplication t.
 Nissen-Rossetti fundoplication t.
 nitrous oxide-opioid-barbiturate anesthetic t.
 nitrous oxide-oxygen-opioid anesthetic t.
 no-leak t.
 noninvasive t.
 nonlaparoscopic t.
 nonoptimal t.
 nonprogressive dilational t.
 nonrib-spreading thoracotomy incision t.
 noose suture t.
 no-punch t.
 Norfolk phalloplasty t.
 no-touch t.
 Ober-Barr tendon transfer for footdrop t.
 Ober tendon transfer for footdrop t.
 O'Brien akinesia ocular anesthesia t.
 off-center isoperistaltic t.
 Okamura ACL repair t.
 Ollier transtrochanteric hip t.
 Omer-Capen proximal row carpectomy t.
 onlay t.
 onlay-tube-onlay urethroplasty t.
 open drop t.
 open flap t.
 open-gloving t.
 open Hasson t.
 open laparoscopic t.
 open palm t.
 open-sky t.
 operative t.
 O'Phelan t.
 opioid-based t.
 optimal t.
 oral anesthetic t.
 Orandi vascularized flap t.
 orbital exenteration gastroscopic access t.
 Orticochea scalping t.
 Osborne-Cotterill elbow t.
 Osgood modified t.
 Osmond-Clarke staged congenital vertical talus repair t.
 Ostrup bone graft harvesting t.
 out-in-out t.
 outside-to-outside arthroscopy t.
 over-and-over suture t.
 overlapping suture t.
 over-the-wire t.
 Oxford cleft palate repair t.
 oxygen washout t.

 Pacey anterior colporrhaphy t.
 Pagenstecher linen nonabsorbable suture t.
 palliative t.
 Palmer all-inside TFCC repair t.
 Palmer-Widen shoulder t.
 Palomo varicocele ligation t.
 Pancoast suture t.
 pants-over-vest t.
 Papineau open bone grafting t.
 Paquin ureterocystoneostomy t.
 paradoxical t.
 parallel t.
 paralleling t.
 paresthesia anesthetic t.
 Paré suture t.
 Parker-Kerr suture t.
 Parodi flow reversal t.
 Parrish-Mann hammertoe t.
 Parvin gravity t.
 passive gliding t.
 2-patch t.
 patch t.
 patient-controlled analgesia anesthetic t.
 Paulos ligament t.
 Pauwels osteotomy t.
 Peacock neurovascular island pedicle flap t.
 peg-and-socket t.
 pelviscopic clip ligation t.
 percutaneous insertion t.
 percutaneous interventional t.
 perfusion hypothermia t.
 perfusion measurement t.
 peribulbar anesthetic t.
 pericardial hood aortic flap t.
 pericostal suture t.
 peripheral nerve block anesthetic t.
 Perry-Nickel halo traction t.
 Perry-O'Brien-Hodgson orthopaedic t.
 Perry-Robinson cervical t.
 Petit suture t.
 1-phase subperiosteal implant t.
 Phemister-Bonfiglio femoral neck bone grafting t.
 Phemister onlay bone graft t.
 phrenic nerve block anesthetic t.
 Pichlmayer split liver transplantation t.
 Pierrot-Murphy tendon t.
 pinch-grasp injection t.
 pin suture t.
 plaque t.
 plastic matrix t.
 plastic suture t.
 plicating suture t.
 Pólya gastroduodenal anastomosis t.
 Ponsky pull PEG tube insertion t.

porcelain cervical ditching t.
Porstmann patent ductus
  arteriovenosus closure t.
4-port t.
2-portal t.
3-portal t.
Porter-Richardson-Vainio arthroscopic
  synovectomy t.
posterior flap t.
posterolateral costotransversectomy t.
postoperative analgesic t.
postresection filling t.
1-pour t.
2-pour t.
premuscular mesh t.
presaturation t.
preservation t.
pressure half-time t.
primary suture t.
Pringle vascular control t.
Proetz displacement sinus
  irrigation t.
prograde t.
progressive dilational t.
projection-reconstruction t.
projective t.
pseudobiopsy t.
Puddu tendon t.
pulley suture t.
pull-out wire suture t.
pull-through t.
pulmonary artery catheterization
  anesthetic t.
pulsed electromagnetic field t.
Pulvertaft weave tendon graft t.
puppet t.
pursestring suture t.
push-back t.
push plus refraction t.
push-pull T t.
quadrant sampling t.
Quartey pedicled penile flap
  urethroplasty t.
Quénu nail plate removal t.
quick angulation t.
Quickert 3-suture ectropion and
  entropin t.
quilt suture t.
radiographic t.
radioguided t.
radiologic t.
Ralston-Thompson pseudoarthrosis t.
Ranawat-DeFiore-Straub correction of
  Madelung deformity t.
rapid-flush t.
rapid pullthrough t.
rapid pullthrough esophageal
  manometry t.
rapid scan t.

rapid-sequence induction anesthetic t.
Rapoport renal function t.
Rashkind balloon t.
Ray-Clancy-Lemon semitendinosus
  tendon transfer t.
Rayhack ulnar shortening
  osteotomy t.
reattribution t.
rebreathing t.
Rebuck skin window t.
recanalization t.
reconstruction t.
reconstructive t.
rectal anesthetic t.
reduction t.
refractive operative t.
regional anesthetic t.
Reichel-Pólya gastric resection t.
Reichenheim elbow surgical
  stabilization t.
relaxation t.
reoperative laparoscopic t.
reoperative thoracotomy t.
rescue t.
resectional t.
restorative proctocolectomy t.
retained papilla t.
retention suture t.
retrobulbar anesthetic t.
retrograde tracheal intubation
  anesthetic t.
retromuscular prosthetic t.
reverse vein bypass t.
reverse wedge t.
rhythmic initiation t.
ribbon arch t.
Richardson suture t.
Richter suture t.
Ricketts-Abrams 2-catheter coronary
  arteriography t.
Rideau hip contracture release t.
right-angle t.
Riordan tendon transfer t.
Risser cast t.
Rives-Stoppa incisional hernia
  repair t.
Roberts fat grafting t.
Robinson-Southwick cervical spine
  fusion t.
Rockwood-Green orthopaedic
  casting t.
Rogers cervical fusion t.
rollerball t.
roll-tube t.
Rood neuromuscular facilitation t.
Ross mitral valve replacement t.
Royle-Thompson tendon transfer t.
RPT t.
running continuous suture t.

T

technique (*continued*)

running vascular t.

Russe scaphoid fracture t.

Russe scaphoid nonunion bone grafting t.

sacral bar t.

Saeed esophageal banding t.

Saenger suture t.

Saha trapezius muscle transfer t.

Sakellarides-DeWeese ulnar collateral ligament reconstuction t.

saline t.

Salter innominate osteotomy t.

Sammarco-DiRaimondo modification of Elmslie lateral ankle reconstruction t.

Sanders pediatric bronchoscopy t.

Sarmiento trochanteric fracture t.

Scaglietti closed reduction t.

scanning t.

Schaberg-Harper-Allen arthroscopic iliopsoas release t.

Schauwecker patellar wiring t.

Scheie cataract scleral flap t.

Schepens transvitreal probe testing t.

Schepsis-Leach hamstring reconstruction t.

Schlatter gastrectomy t.

Schnute wedge resection t.

Schober lumbar spine mobility measuring t.

Schonander imaging t.

Schoonmaker-King single-catheter t.

scleral search coil t.

Scott glenoplasty t.

screw insertion t.

scrubbing t.

Scudder energy-based healing t.

Scuderi ruptured quadriceps repair t.

sealed envelope t.

secondary suture t.

sectional t.

section freeze substitution t.

segmental blocking t.

segment-oriented t.

Seldinger percutaneous t.

Seldinger retrograde wire intubation t.

selective bronchial catheterization anesthetic t.

Sell-Frank-Johnson extensor shift t.

Semb nephrectomy t.

semitendinosus t.

Semm Z-stab laparoscope insertion t.

sensorineural acuity level t.

seromuscular suture t.

seroserous suture t.

Sewall-Boyden frontal sinus surgery t.

sewing machine t.

sextant t.

sharp dissection t.

Sharrard iliopsoas transfer t.

shave excision t.

Sherk-Probst pediatric humeral epiphysis fracture t.

Shirodkar suture t.

shish kebab t.

short-cone t.

short lever accessory movement t.

Shouldice hernia repair t.

Silber testicular autotransplantation t.

Silfverskiöld Achilles tendon lengthening t.

silver dollar t.

Simon suture t.

Simonton biofeedback t.

simple suture t.

Sims suture t.

Singer-Blom endoscopic tracheoesophageal puncture t.

single-armed suture t.

single-needle t.

single-port t.

single-pour dental material t.

single proximal portal t.

single space t.

skewer t.

skin expansion t.

skin surfacing t.

skin window t.

Skoog female genitalia construction t.

sleeve t.

2-sleeve t.

sling and blanket t.

sling and reef t.

sling suture t.

sling/wrapping t.

slit catheter t.

Slocum amputation t.

Slocum spinal fusion t.

slow pullthrough t.

smiley-face knotting t.

Smith Indian intracapsular cataract removal t.

Smith-Robinson anterior cervical discectomy and fusion t.

snare t.

Snellen suture t.

Sofield femoral deficiency leg-lengthening t.

soluble gas t.

Sones coronary arteriography t.

sonication t.

Speed-Boyd radial-ulnar fracture treatment t.

sperm microaspiration retrieval t. (SMART)

sphincter-saving t.

sphincter-sparing t.

Spiller-Frazier intracranial trigeminal neurotomy t.

spinal anesthetic t.

spinal fusion t.

spinal mobilization t.

spiral CT t.

spiral suture t.

Spivack gastrotomy t.

split-and-roll t.

split-bone t.

split-course t.

split-cuff nipple t.

spontaneous ventilation anesthetic t.

Sprague orthopaedic arthroscopic t.

SPT t.

stab avulsion microphlebotomy t.

staged pullthrough t.

2-stage tendon grafting t.

Staheli congenital hip dislocation containment t.

Stamm-Kader gastrotomy t.

standard t.

standard biopsy t.

Stanisavljevic knee reconstruction t.

stapled reconstruction t.

stapling t.

STAR t.

Stark-Moore-Ashworth-Boyes first metacarpotrapezial joint fusion t.

startle t.

Starzl intraluminal venous anastomosis t.

static dilation t.

station pull-through t.

station pull-through esophageal manometry t.

stay suture t.

Steffee spinal fusion instrumentation t.

stellate ganglion block anesthetic t.

stenting t.

stent-through-wire mesh t.

2-step t.

step-by-step t.

stepladder incision t.

stereotactic t.

stereotactic automated t.

stereotactic core biopsy t.

sterile t.

Stewart-Hamilton cardiac output t.

stick-tie suture t.

Stiegmann-Goff endoscopic esophageal varices ligation t.

Stiles-Bunnell flexor digitorum superficialis transfer t.

still radiography t.

Stimson anterior shoulder reduction t.

stimulated gracilis neosphincter t.

strain/counterstrain t.

Strassman bicornual uterus metroplasty t.

Straub t.

Strayer tendon t.

stretch-and-spray t.

Strickland flexor tendon repair t.

stricturoplasty t.

strip biopsy resection t.

strut spinal fusion t.

Sturmdorf suture t.

subcostal insufflation t.

subcuticular suture t.

subpectoral implantation t.

subperiosteal implant 1-phase t.

subtraction t.

suction-irrigation t.

superficial desensitization t.

superficial suture t.

superior mesenterorenal bypass t.

super-wet t.

support suture t.

supraphysiologic fluid t.

surface cooling t.

surface desensitization t.

surgical enucleation t.

surgical neurangiographic t.

surgical suture t.

surveillance t.

sustained pressure t.

suture anchor t.

suture closure t.

Swanson t.

switched B-gradient t.

sympathetic blockade anesthetic t.

sympathetic ganglion block anesthetic t.

Tajima suture t.

tandem clipping t.

Taylor-Daniel-Weiland free composite iliac bone graft t.

Taylor suture t.

telescoping suture t.

tendon suture t.

tension band wiring t.

tension suture t.

Terzis peripheral nerve microsurgery t.

test dose anesthetic t.

Teuffer Achilles tendon repair t.

Thal fundoplication t.

thermodilution t.

Thiersch suture t.

T

technique (*continued*)

thiopental-sufentanil-desflurane-nitrous oxide anesthetic t.
Thomas nipple reconstruction t.
Thomas-Thompson-Straub rotational transfer of vastus lateralis t.
Thompson-Loomer talar osteochondritis dissecans repair t.
thoracic epidural anesthetic t.
thoracolumbar spondylosis surgical t.
threaded-hole-first t.
through-and-through suture t.
thyroidectomy t.
thyroid surgical t.
tissue-sparing t.
titration t.
T-mesh closure t.
Todd-Evans stepladder tracheal dilatation t.
Tohen tendon t.
Tom Jones suture t.
tongue-and-groove suture t.
topical anesthetic t.
Torgerson-Leach modified tibial osteotomy t.
Torg tarsal navicular stress fracture repair t.
total etch t.
total fundoplication t.
total intravenous anesthetic t.
Toupe fundoplication t.
tracheal extubation anesthetic t.
tracheal intubation anesthetic t.
tracheal suction anesthetic t.
traction suture t.
transanal stapling t.
transarterial anesthetic t.
transcranial electrical stimulation anesthesia monitoring t.
transdermal anesthetic t.
transfixing suture t.
transiliac bar t.
translaryngeal guided intubation anesthetic t.
transmucosal drug administration anesthetic t.
transoral t.
transtracheal jet ventilation anesthetic t.
trapezius stimulation anesthetic t.
Traverso-Longmire pancreatoduodenectomy t.
Trethowan-Stamm-Simmonds-Menelaus-Haddad t.
triangulation t.
triple-wire t.
trocar t.
trocar-cannula t.
Trusler aortic valve t.

tubal ligation band t.
tube exchange t.
tube-shift t.
tube-within-tube t.
Tuffier morcellement t.
tumbling t.
tumescent liposuction t.
Turco clubfoot release t.
turn-and-suction biopsy t.
Turnbull temporary diverting ileostomy t.
Turner-Warwick and Ashken cecocystoplasty t.
twisted suture t.
twist-off t.
Uchida abdominal tubal sterilization t.
ultrasonographic t.
ultrasound anesthetic t.
uncut Collis-Nissen fundoplication t.
underlay fascia t.
unilateral inguinal hernia repair t.
uninterrupted suture t.
unitunnel t.
unlocking spiral t.
upgated t.
vacuum-pack laparostomy t.
van Lint modified t.
vascular isolation t.
Vastamäki wrist arthroscopy t.
Veleanu-Rosianu-Ionescu obturator neurectomy t.
velocity catheter t.
venous access t.
ventral bending t.
Verdan intrasynovial flexor tendon t.
Verhoeff suture t.
vertical-cut t.
vertical mattress suture t.
Vidal-Ardrey fracture t.
video-assisted t.
videofluoroscopic t.
video transurethral resection t.
Vim-Silverman needle biopsy t.
volumetric t.
Volz-Turner greater trochanter reattachment t.
von Haberer-Finney gastrectomy t.
Vulpius-Compere tendon t.
V-Y advancement t.
Wadsworth triceps tendon release t.
Wagner open reduction t.
Wagoner cervical spine t.
Waldhausen subclavian flap t.
Wallace ureteroileal anastomosis t.
Warner-Farber ankle fixation t.
wash t.
washed field t.
water-suppression MR imaging t.

Watkins intertransverse process lumbar spine fusion t.
Watson t.
Watson Cheyne wedge excision of toenail t.
wax matrix t.
wax pattern thermal expansion t.
Weaver-Dunn acromioclavicular t.
Weber-Brunner-Freuler-Boitzy pediatric orthopaedic t.
Weber-Vasey traction-absorption wiring of olecranon fracture t.
Weckesser tendon repair t.
Wertheim-Bohlman occipitocervical fusion t.
West and Soto-Hall patellar t.
whiplash t.
whipstitch suture t.
Whitesides-Kelly extraoral retropharyngeal cervical spine t.
whole blood lysis t.
Wick catheter t.
Williams-Haddad femoral nerve block for hip fracture t.
Willi glass crown t.
Wilson-Jacobs tibial fracture fixation t.
Wilson-McKeever shoulder t.
window t.
Windsor-Insall-Vince tissue grafting t.
Winograd lateral nail fold excision t.
Winter spondylolisthesis t.
wire removal t.
Wirth-Jager tendon t.
Wölfler suture t.
^{133}Xe intravenous injection t.
xenon washout t.
Young-Dees genitourinary system t.
Young urinary bladder repair t.
Y-suture t.
Z t.
Zancolli biceps tendon rerouting t.
Zarins-Rowe ACL reconstruction t.
Zavala pulmonary disease diagnostic t.
Zeier transfer t.
Zielke kyphotic deformity repair t.
Z-suture t.
Zuker and Manktelow facial muscle transplantation t.
technocausis
technologist
Certified Surgical T. (CST)
technology
assisted reproduction t.
endoluminal t.
endoscopic t.

endovascular t.
fluorescent optode t.
laparoscopic t.
minimal access spine t. (MAST)
signal extraction t. (SET)
TECMIS
truly endocapsular microincision cataract surgery
tectobulbar tract
tectocephalic
tectocephaly
tectology
tectonic
t. epikeratoplasty
t. keratoplasty
tectopontine tract
tectorial membrane
tectospinal
t. decussation
t. tract
TED
thromboembolic disease
TEE
transesophageal echocardiography
teeth (*pl. of* tooth)
TEF
tracheoesophageal fistula
Teflon-coated suture
Teflon granuloma
Teflon-pledgeted suture
teflurane
TEG
thromboelastogram
thromboelastograph
thromboelastography
Tegaderm
tegmentotomy
tela, *pl.* **telae**
telae (*pl. of* tela)
telangectasia
hereditary hemorhagic t.
telangiectasia
telangiectatic
t. angioma
t. vascular malformation
telangioma
telecobalt therapy
telelectrocardiogram
telemedicine
telementoring
telencephalic malformation
telencephalization
telepresence surgery
telerobotic-assisted
t.-a. laparoscopic colectomy
t.-a. laparoscopic surgery
t.-a. right hemicolectomy
telescope
laparoscopic t.

telescoping
- t. nail
- t. suture technique

telesurgery
televised radiofluoroscopy
television microscopy
TeLinde modified radical hysterectomy
telomerase
TEM
- transanal endoscopic microsurgery

temperature
- ambient t.
- axilla t.
- basal body t.
- bladder t.
- body t.
- brain t.
- core body t.
- esophagus t.
- t. exchange apparatus
- t. gradient
- heat production t.
- hyperthermic t.
- intraoperative core body t.
- normal body t.
- normothermic t.
- temperature, pulse, respiration (TPR)
- skin t.
- spiking t.
- t. threshold

temperature-compensated vaporizer
temperature-controlled
- t.-c. radiofrequency (TCR)
- t.-c. radiofrequency tissue ablation (TCRFTA)

templating
- digital t.

temporal
- t. aponeurosis
- t. apophysis
- t. arteritis
- t. artery
- t. artery biopsy (TAB)
- t. bone
- t. bone fracture
- t. bone tumor
- t. branch
- t. canal
- t. fascia
- t. flap
- t. fossa
- t. headache
- t. incision
- t. line
- t. lobectomy
- t. lobe radiation
- t. muscle
- t. nerve
- t. orientation
- t. plane
- t. process
- t. ridge
- t. space
- t. space infection
- t. squama
- t. summation
- t. summation pain
- t. surface
- t. suture
- t. vein
- t. wedge

temporal-cerebral arterial anastomosis
temporalis
- t. fascia flap
- t. fascial flap
- t. muscle flap
- t. tendon

temporary
- t. balloon occlusion
- t. cavity phenomenon
- t. diverting colostomy
- t. end colostomy
- t. fecal diversion
- t. loop ileostomy
- t. nerve blockade
- t. pacemaker placement
- t. palsy
- t. postoperative supplementation
- t. restoration

temporization
temporoauricular
temporofrontal tract
temporohyoid
temporomalar
temporomandibular
- t. articular disc
- t. disorder
- t. joint (TMJ)
- t. joint articulation
- t. joint dislocation
- t. ligament
- t. luxation
- t. muscle disorder (TMD)
- t. nerve
- t. pain

temporomandibularis
temporomaxillary vein
temporooccipital
temporoparietal
- t. fascial flap
- t. muscle

temporopontine tract
temporosphenoid
tempus
tenacious
- t. adhesion
- t. meconium

Tenckhoff peritoneal dialysis catheter

tendency
 thrombotic t.
tender
 t. line
 t. point (TeP)
 t. point examination
tenderness
 abdominal t.
 diffuse abdominal t.
 marked t.
 proximal bowel t.
 rebound t.
 subareolar t.
tendineae
 chordae t. (CT)
tendines (*pl. of* tendo)
tendinis (*gen. of* tendo)
tendinitis, tendonitis
tendinomyoplastic amputation
tendinoplasty, tenontoplasty, tenoplasty,
 tendoplasty
tendinosuture
tendinous
 t. arch
 t. cord
 t. inscription
 t. insertion
 t. opening
tendinum
tendo, *gen.* **tendinis** *pl.* **tendines**
 t. Achillis
 t. carcaneus communis
 vagina fibrosa tendinis
tendolysis (*var. of* tenolysis)
tendon
 abductor pollicis longus t.
 Achilles t.
 adductor magnus t.
 anterior tibialis t.
 attenuation of t.
 biceps t.
 calcaneal t.
 central t.
 t. centralization
 central perineum t.
 common annular t.
 common extensor t.
 conjoined t.
 conjoint t.
 cricoesophageal t.
 digital extensor t.
 elbow extensor t.
 erector spinae t.
 t. excursion
 extensor carpi radialis brevis t.
 extensor carpi radialis longus t.
 extensor carpi ulnaris t.
 extensor digiti minimi t.
 extensor digitorum t.

extensor digitorum brevis t.
extensor digitorum communis t.
extensor digitorum longus t.
extensor hallucis longus t.
extensor indicis proprius t.
extensor pollicis brevis t.
extensor pollicis longus t.
fibularis longus t.
fibularis tertius t.
t. flap
flexor carpi radialis t.
flexor digitorum longus t.
flexor digitorum profundus t.
flexor digitorum superficialis t.
flexor hallucis brevis t.
flexor hallucis longus t.
flexor pollicis longus t.
gracilis t.
t. graft
hamstring t.
heel t.
iliopsoas t.
intermediate digastric t.
intermediate omohyoid t.
t. interposition arthroplasty
lateral rectus t.
latissimus dorsi t.
t. lengthening
masseter t.
peroneal brevis t.
peroneal longus t.
plantaris t.
popliteus fossa muscle t.
posterior tibialis t.
pronator teres t.
psoas minor t.
quadriceps femoris t.
rectus femoris t.
t. repair
t. rupture
semimembranosus t.
semitendinosus t.
snapping iliopsoas t.
split anterior tibial t. (SPLATT)
stapedius t.
subscapularis t.
superior oblique t.
t. suture technique
temporalis t.
thumb extensor t.
toe extensor t.
t. transplant
trefoil t.
triceps t.
vastus medialis t.
wrist extensor t.
Zinn t.
tendonitis (*var. of* tendinitis)
tendoplasty (*var. of* tendinoplasty)

T

tendosynovitis (*var. of* tenosynovitis)
tendotomy (*var. of* tenotomy)
tendovaginal
tendovaginitis (*var. of* tenosynovitis)
tenectomy, tenonectomy
tenesmus
tenia, taenia, *pl.* **teniae**
    teniae coli
    free t.
    t. libera
    mesocolic t.
    omental t.
teniae (*pl. of* tenia)
tenial, taenial
teniamyotomy
tennis
    t. elbow
    t. racquet incision
Tennison-Randall lip repair
tenodesis
    calcaneal t.
    extensor t.
    MacIntosh extraarticular t.
    Watson-Jones t.
tenolysis, tendolysis
tenomyolasty (*var. of* tenontomyoplasty)
tenomyotomy
Tenon
    T. capsule
    T. membrane
    T. space
tenonectomy (*var. of* tenectomy)
tenontology
tenontomyoplasty, tenomyolasty
tenontomyotomy
tenontoplastic
tenontoplasty (*var. of* tendinoplasty)
tenophyte
tenoplastic reconstruction
tenoplasty (*var. of* tendinoplasty)
tenorrhaphy
tenosuture
tenosynovectomy
    dorsal t.
    flexor t.
tenosynovitis, tendosynovitis,
  tendovaginitis, tenovaginitis
    de Quervain t.
tenotomy, tendotomy
    adductor t.
    Arroyo t.
    Arruga t.
    Braun shoulder t.
    curb t.
    extensor t.
    free t.
    graduated t.
    intrasheath t.
    t. operation

    percutaneous t.
    semiopen sliding t.
    sliding t.
    subcutaneous tibialis posterior t.
    transverse t.
    Veleanu-Rosianu-Ionescu adductor t.
    Verhoeff multiple partial t.
    Z marginal t.
    Z-plasty t.
tenovaginitis (*var. of* tenosynovitis)
TENS
    transcutaneous electrical nerve
     stimulation
    high-frequency TENS
    low-frequency TENS
tensile
tension
    t. band fixation
    t. band wiring technique
    t. by applanation
    t. endothorax
    exhaled oxygen t.
    t. fracture
    t. headache
    isometric venous t.
    oxygen t.
    t. pneumopericardium
    t. pneumothorax
    running vascular technique
     without t.
    t. suture technique
    tissue oxygen t.
    twitch t.
tension-free
    t.-f. anastomosis
    t.-f. hernioplasty
    t.-f. hiatoplasty
    t.-f. mesh implantation
    t.-f. mesh repair
    t.-f. prosthetic mesh repair
tension-length relation
tension-requiring suture
tension-type headache
tensor
    t. fasciae latae
    t. fasciae latae muscle
    t. fascia lata muscle flap
    t. insertion
    t. tympani canal
tenth cranial nerve
tentoria (*pl. of* tentorium)
tentorial
    t. herniation
    t. laceration
    t. nerve
    t. notch
    t. pressure
    t. ring
    t. sinus

tentorium, *pl.* **tentoria**
Tenzel rotational cheek flap
TEP
    totally extraperitoneal
    tracheoesophageal puncture
        TEP repair
TeP
    tender point
tepa
TEPA
    totally extraperitoneal approach
teratoblastoma
teratocarcinoma
    pineal t.
teratogenic medication
teratogen-induced malformation
teratologic dislocation
teratoma
    epignathus t.
    mature t.
teratomatous
teratoneuroma
teratospermia
terebration
teres
    ligamentum t.
    t. major
    t. major (muscle)
    t. minor
    t. minor (muscle)
tergal
tergum
terlipressin
terminad
terminal
    t. bronchiole
    t. cisterna
    t. colostomy
    t. crest
    t. duct carcinoma
    t. head
    t. hinge position
    t. ileal limb
    t. ileal pouch
    t. ileal resection
    t. ileitis
    t. ileostomy
    t. ileum
    t. ileum intubation
    t. infection
    t. jaw relation record
    t. line
    t. neosalpingostomy
    nociceptor afferent peripheral t.
    t. plane
    t. reservoir syndrome
    t. sedation
    t. Syme toe-tip amputation
      procedure

    t. ventriculostomy
    t. web
terminalis sulcus
terminalization
termini (*pl. of* terminus)
terminolateral
Terminology
    Current Procedural T. (CPT)
terminoterminal anastomosis
terminus, *pl.* **termini**
    generales termini
territory
    hepatic t.
terror-induced multiple casualty injury
Terson
    T. ectropion operation
    T. syndrome
tertiary
    t. amputation
    t. care
    t. healing
    t. trauma center
    t. wound closure
Terzis peripheral nerve microsurgery
  technique
TES
    transcutaneous electric stimulation
Tesio catheter
Tessier
    T. craniofacial operation
    T. facial cleft classification
    T. osteotomy
    T. tarsectomy
test
    abduction external rotation t.
    acetowhite t.
    acoustic stimulation t.
    Adson t.
    air t.
    alcohol used disorders identification
      t.
    Allen blood supply to hand t.
    Ames mutagenic chemical t.
    anorectal function t.
    Apley compression t.
    articulation t.
    artificial erection t.
    Astrand 6-minute submaximal cycle
      ergometer t.
    axial compression t.
    balloon expulsion t.
    baroreceptor t.
    Behçet skin puncture t.
    Bernstein GERD t.
    Bielschowsky-Parks head-tilt 3-step t.
    Bielschowsky 3-step head-tilt t.
    bladder neck elevation t.
    Bonney urinary incontinence t.
    brachial plexus tension t. (BPTT)

test (*continued*)

breast stimulation contraction t. (BSCT)
breath excretion t.
Brodie-Trendelenburg tourniquet t.
bronchial inhalation challenge t.
bronchoprovocation t.
caffeine-halothane contracture t. (CHCT)
carpal compression t.
Casoni t.
cavity t.
4-chloro-m-cresol t.
circle system t.
closed patch t.
CO_2 inhalation t.
cold pressor t. (CPT)
compression t.
concentration performance t.
confrontation visual field t.
corneal staining t.
Cortrosyn stimulation t.
Crampton orthostatics t.
craniocervical flexion t.
deep articulation t.
diagnostic articulation t.
differential ureteral catheterization t.
Digit Symbol Substitution T.
direct immunofluorescence t.
disc space saline acceptance t.
t. dose anesthetic technique
double Maddox rod t.
Dupuy-Dutemps dacryocystorhinostomy dye t.
Durkan carpal compression t.
dye exclusion t.
dye reduction spot t.
ecarin-based t.
elevated arm stress t. (EAST)
epidural stimulation t.
ergonovine provocation t.
excitability t.
external rotation-abduction stress t.
external rotation-recurvatum t.
extrastimulus t.
extrinsic entrapment t.
fast-flush t.
Feagin shoulder dislocation t.
femoral nerve traction t.
fetal acoustic stimulation t.
Finger Oscillation T.
fistula t.
flexion-rotation-drawer knee instability t.
fluctuation t.
fluorescein instillation t.
fluorescein string t.
foramen compression t.
foraminal compression t.

forced duction t.
forced generation t.
forearm ischemic exercise t.
forearm supination t.
forward traction t.
Friberg microsurgical agglutination t.
gastric accommodation t.
germ tube t.
hair bulb incubation t.
halothane-caffeine contracture t.
head compression t.
head distraction t.
head-down tilt t.
head-dropping t.
head-tilt t.
head-up tilt t.
head-up tilt-table t.
hepaplastin t.
high-altitude simulation t. (HAST)
high-dose rate radiation t.
high-dose thrombin time t.
HiTT t.
Hollander insulin-induced hypoglycemia t.
1-hour office pad t.
Howard t.
Hughston external rotation recurvatum t.
human ovum fertilization t.
hyperventilation t.
iliac compression t.
immunodiffusion t.
immunofluorescence t.
implantation t.
indirect hemagglutination t.
indocyanine green retention t.
Ingram-Withers-Speltz motor t.
t. injection
invasive t.
in vitro contracture t. (IVCT)
Korotkoff collateral circulation t.
labyrinthine fistula t.
lacrimal irrigation t.
leak t.
1-legged stork t.
line t.
liver function t. (LFT)
localization t.
low-pressure circuit leak t.
lumbar extension t.
lumbar rotation t.
Luria-Delbruck fluctuation t.
Maddox rod t.
Maddox wing t.
Marshall bladder neck t.
Marshall-Marchetti urinary incontinence t.
matchstick t.
Maudsley Mentation T.

maximum stimulation t.
memory guidance saccade t.
Michigan Abuse Screening T. (MAST)
1-minute endoscopy room t.
mobilization t.
MUGA exercise stress t.
Multistage Maximal Effort exercise stress t.
nasal provocation t.
nerve excitability t.
neuropsychologic t.
neutralization t.
nipple stimulation t.
nonparametric t.
Noyes flexion rotation drawer t.
Object Classification T.
obturator t.
occlusive patch t.
open application t.
open patch t.
Pachon collateral circulation t.
parametric t.
Parks-Bielschowsky 3-step, head-tilt t.
Patrick sacroiliitis t.
penetration t.
percutaneous pressure ureteral perfusion t.
perimeter corneal reflex t.
perineal nerve terminal motor latency t.
peritoneal equilibration t.
Perthes deep femoral vein patency t.
2-point discrimination t.
postcoital t.
prick puncture t.
prism adaptation t.
promontory stimulation t.
prone extension t.
protection t.
protein truncation t.
provocation t.
provocative chelation t.
psychometric t.
Q-tip t.
Quantitative Sudomotor Axon Reflex T.
regurgitation t.
rotation drawer t.
rotation recurvatum t.
ryanodine t.
sag t.
scapular approximation t.
scarification t.
screening t.
serological t.
side-lying iliac compression t.

simple shoulder t.
skin puncture t.
SLR with external rotation t.
Spatial Orientation Memory T.
sperm immobilization t.
spinal flexibility t.
split renal function t.
station t.
Stewart collateral circulation t.
stimulation t.
straight catheter t.
straight leg raising t.
string t.
sucrose t.
thermoregulatory sweat t.
Thompson Achilles tendon rupture t.
thymol turbidity t.
tilt t.
tilt table t.
tissue compression t.
tourniquet t.
traction t.
transient hyperemic response t.
transillumination t.
Trieger hand-eye coordination t.
trunk incurvation t.
Tsui nerve stimulation catheter placement t.
tube dilution t.
tube precipitin t.
tumor skin t.
twitch height t.
University of Pennsylvania smell identification t. (UPSIT)
upper lip bite t.
vaginal cornification t.
vaginal mucification t.
Valpar whole body range of motion t.
vertical compression t.
vibration threshold t.
Visual-Motor Integration T.
von Frey touch t.
wake-up t.
walking ventilation t.
washout t.
Whitaker pressure-perfusion t.
wire-loop t.

testalgia
test-dose injection
testectomy
testes (*pl. of* testis)
testicle
solitary t.
testicular
t. adrenal-like tissue
t. appendage
t. artery
t. biopsy

testicular (*continued*)
    t. carcinoma
    t. cord
    t. duct
    t. ectopia
    t. feminization syndrome
    t. mass
    t. metastasis
    t. plexus
    t. rupture
    t. torsion
    t. tumor
    t. vein
testiculi (*pl. of* testiculus)
testiculus, *pl.* **testiculi**
testing
    antineural autoantibody t.
    compression t.
    confrontation t.
    Doppler ultrasound segmental blood
      pressure t.
    electrodiagnostic t.
    fecal occult blood t.
      (FOBT)
    genetic t.
    nucleic acid t.
    palpation t.
    patch t.
    penile injection t.
    Quantitative Sensory T. (QST)
    rotation t.
    sensory t.
    somatosensory t.
    sudomotor axon reflex t.
    tilt-table t.
    wake-up t.
testis, *pl.* **testes**
    t. cord
    cryptorchid t.
    t. fracture
    impalpable t.
    movable t.
    retractile t.
    torsion t.
    undescended t.
testitis (*var. of* orchitis)
testoid
TET
    tetralogy of Fallot
tetanic
    t. fade
    t. stimulation
    t. stimulation method
tetanization
tetanus
    cephalic t.
    extensor t.
    head t.
    traumatic t.

tetany
    duration t.
    hyperventilation t.
    postoperative t.
tethered
    t. cord syndrome
    t. spinal cord
tetracaine
    hyperbaric t.
    liposome-encapsulated t. (LET)
tetragonus
tetralogy of Fallot (TET, TOF)
Teuffer
    T. Achilles tendon repair technique
    T. tendo calcaneus repair
Teutleben ligament
TEVAP
    transurethral electrovaporization of
      prostate
Tevdek
    T. pledgeted suture
    T. suture
TEVP
    transesophageal ventricular pacing
Texas
    T. Scottish Rite Hospital (TSRH)
    T. Scottish Rite Hospital crosslink
      stabilization
    T. Scottish Rite Hospital hook-rod
      system
texture
    firm t.
    rubbery t.
textured fabric rub
T-fastener gastropexy
TFCC
    triangular fibrocartilage complex
TGA
    transposition of the great arteries
TGI
    tracheal gas insufflation
THA
    total hip arthroplasty
Thal
    T. esophageal stricture repair
    T. esophagogastroscopy
    T. esophagogastrostomy
    T. fundic patch
    T. fundic patch operation
    T. fundoplasty
    T. fundoplication
    T. fundoplication method
    T. fundoplication procedure
    T. fundoplication technique
    T. Quik tube
    T. stricturoplasty
thalamectomy
thalamencephalic
thalamencephalon

thalamic
- t. circulation
- t. lesion
- t. pain
- t. pain syndrome
- t. plane

thalamic-subthalamic hemorrhage
thalamocaudate arteriovenous malformation
thalamostriate vein
thalamotomy
- gamma t.
- staged bilateral stereotactic t.
- stereotactic Vim t.
- stereotactic VL t.
- Vim t.

thallium-technetium scanning
Thal-Nissen fundoplasty
Thal-Woodward antireflux procedure
thanatopsia (*var. of* thanatopsy)
thanatopsy, thanatopsia
Thane central sulcus of brain location method
THARIES
- total hip arthroplasty with internal eccentric shells

theater
- negative pressure operating t.
- operating t.
- twin operating t.

thebaine
thebesian
- t. circulation
- t. vein

thecal
- t. sac
- t. sac compression

theca lutein cyst
thecoma
- luteinized t.
- ovarian t.

Theden aneurysm and effusion treatment method
Theile muscle
Theirsch-Duplay hypospadias repair
thele
theleplasty
thenad
thenal
thenar
- t. eminence
- t. flap
- t. muscle
- t. prominence
- t. space

thenen
theory
- gate-control t.
- membrane expansion t.

neurogenic t.
piagetian t.
thoracic pump t.
vasogenic t.

therapeutic
- t. alternative
- t. anesthesia
- t. angiogenesis
- t. approach
- t. arsenal
- t. colonoscopy
- t. dissection
- t. effect
- t. efficacy
- t. endpoint
- t. hypothermia
- t. injection
- t. insemination
- t. intervention scoring system (TISS)
- t. iridectomy
- t. irradiation
- t. laparoscopy
- t. lymph node dissection (TLND)
- t. maneuver
- t. modality
- t. nerve block
- t. option
- t. phlebotomy
- t. step
- t. thyroidectomy
- t. trauma laparotomy
- t. upper endoscopy

therapia
therapist
- stoma t.

therapy
- ablation t.
- ablative laser t.
- active appliance t.
- active assistive motion t.
- adjunct t.
- adjunctive suppressive medical t.
- adjuvant t.
- adjuvant chemoradiation t.
- adjuvant drug t.
- aerosol t.
- albendazole t.
- alternate-day t.
- alternative t.
- anaclitic t.
- antiarrhythmic t.
- antibiotic t.
- anticoagulant t.
- anticoagulation t.
- antiemetic t.
- antifungal t.
- antihormonal t.
- antilymphoid t.

T

therapy (*continued*)

antimicrobial t.
antireflux t.
antispasmodic t.
antithrombotic t.
antiviral t.
apotreptic t.
aquatic t.
argon laser t.
around-the-clock oral maintenance
  bronchodilator t.
augmentation t.
balloon photodynamic t.
belly bath t.
biomagnetic t.
bite plane t.
Bragg peak proton-beam t.
breast conservation t. (BCT)
breast-conserving t. (BCT)
breast-preservation t.
brisement t.
bronchoscopic photodynamic t.
buprenorphine narcotic analgesic t.
cerebral protective t.
chest physical t.
chronic anticoagulation t.
chronic opioid analgesic t. (COAT)
Clinitron air-fluidized t.
coagulative laser t.
cobalt t.
cognitive-behavioral t. (CBT)
collateral meridian t.
combined chemoradiation t.
compartmental radioimmuno-globulin t.
complementary t.
concomitant t.
conditioning t.
conformal radiation t.
conservative t.
contact dissolution t.
continuous renal replacement t.
convulsive t.
3-cornered t.
corrective t.
craniosacral t.
Crozat orthodontic t.
deep chest t.
definitive local t.
device t.
diagnostic surgical t.
dialectical behavioral t.
diathermic t.
dilation t.
diuretic t.
dressing t.
dual t.
electrical stimulation t.
electric aversion t.
electric differential t.

electrotherapeutic sleep t.
empiric t.
endocavitary radiation t.
endoluminal t.
endoscopic hemostatic t.
endoscopic injection t.
endoscopic laser t.
endoscopic pancreatic t.
endoscopic photodynamic t.
endourological t.
endovascular t.
enterostomal t.
eradication t.
erythropoietin t.
esophageal photodynamic t.
ethanol injection t.
exercise t.
expansion and activator t.
external vacuum t.
external x-ray t.
ex vivo gene t.
factor replacement t.
fetal drug t.
focused radiation t.
fractionated radiation t.
frappage t.
frequency-difference interferential
  current t.
functional orthodontic t.
gene replacement t.
gene transfer t.
grenz ray t.
group t.
HBO t.
HDR intracavitary radiation t.
hemofiltration t.
hepatic arterial t.
herbal t.
high-dose radioiodine t.
high-dose rate radiation t.
high-voltage t.
horticulture t.
hydration t.
hyperbaric oxygen t.
hyperthermia t.
immunochemiluminescent t.
immunocompetent tissue t.
implosive t.
incremental t.
indirect pulpal t.
induction t.
infrared t.
inhalation t.
injection t.
innovative t.
instillation t.
insulin shock t.
integrated t.
interferential t.

interferon t.
interlesional t.
internal radiation t.
interstitial photodynamic t.
interstitial radiation t.
interventional t.
intraarterial t.
intracavernous injection t.
intracavitary radiation boost t.
intracorporeal injection t.
intradiscal electrothermal t. (IDET)
intralesional t.
intralesional steroid t.
intraoperative radiation t.
intraperitoneal radiation t.
intraspinal t.
intrathecal t.
intravascular fluid t.
intravascular volume t.
intravenous antibiotic t.
intravenous hydration t.
intravenous ozone t.
intraventricular t.
invasive t.
ischemia-guided medical t.
isolation perfusion t.
I.V. fluid t.
Kelsey unloading exercise t.
ketoprofen analgesic t.
laser t.
LDR intracavitary radiation t.
life-saving form of t.
Livingstone t.
local t.
locoregional t.
locoregional adjuvant t.
long-term opioid t.
long-term oxygen t.
low dose rate radiation t.
magnet t.
magnetic seizure t.
manipulative t.
manual t.
massage t.
medical t.
methyl-*tert*–butyl ether t.
microcurrent t.
microwave t.
microwave coagulation t.
migraine abortive t.
mind-body t.
morphine narcotic analgesic t.
MTBE t.
multimodal adjuvant t.
multimodality t.
multiple t.
myoablative t.
myofunctional t.
naprapathic t.

Nd:YAG laser t.
negative pressure t.
neoadjuvant t.
neutron beam t.
neutron capture t.
nonspecific t.
nonsurgical t.
occlusal t.
occlusion t.
occlusive t.
occupational t. (OT)
ocular radiation t. (ORT)
open surgical t.
operative t.
opioid t.
optimal t.
orthodontic t.
outpatient physical t.
oxygen t.
palliative t.
pancreatic intraluminal radiation t.
parenteral t.
particle beam radiation t.
pelvic floor physical t.
PEMF t.
penile injection t.
penile vein occlusion t.
percussion t.
percutaneous embolization t.
percutaneous ethanol injection t.
percutaneous local ablative t.
percutaneous microwave
  coagulation t.
percutaneous transcatheter t.
perfusion t.
periodontal t.
perioperative antibiotic t.
permanent anticoagulant t.
photodynamic t. (PDT)
photoradiation t.
physical t. (PT)
placebo t.
plasma exchange t.
pool t.
positional release t.
postnatal t.
postoperative anticoagulation t.
postradiation t.
posttransplant immunosuppression t.
postural t.
prenatal t.
preoperative t.
preventive intravesical t.
progestational t.
programmed t.
prophylactic t.
prophylactic antibiotic t.
protein shock t.
proton beam t.

T

therapy (*continued*)
    proton pump inhibition t.
    psychologic t.
    pulp canal t.
    pulsed electromagnetic field t.
    pulse dye laser t.
    pyretic t.
    quadrangular t.
    quadrantectomy, axillary dissection, radiation t. (QUART)
    quadruple t.
    radiation t.
    radical t.
    radioimmunoglobulin t.
    radioiodine ablation t.
    radiopharmaceutical t.
    red-filter t.
    reflex t.
    rehydration t.
    renal infusion t.
    renal replacement t.
    rescue t.
    respiratory kinetic t.
    rheologic t.
    root canal t.
    rotation t.
    saline injection t.
    salvage t.
    sandwich staghorn calculus t.
    sclerosing t.
    sedative t.
    skin lubrication t.
    soak t.
    social interaction t.
    sole laser t.
    somatic t.
    sparing t.
    stem cell gene t.
    stepdown t.
    stereotactic radiation t.
    subcoma t.
    Supartz joint fluid t.
    supranormal hemodynamic t.
    surgical maggot t.
    systemic adjuvant t.
    systemic antifungal t.
    systemic radioimmunoglobulin t.
    telecobalt t.
    thermal t.
    thrombolytic t.
    timed-sequential t.
    tocolytic t.
    tongue thrust t.
    total push t.
    transcatheter arterial embolization t.
    transfusion t.
    transgenic t.
    transurethral collagen injection t.
    transvenous t.

    triadic t.
    trial of conservative t.
    trimodality t.
    triple intrathecal t.
    tumor t.
    ultrasonic t.
    ultrasound t.
    ultrasound-guided shockwave t.
    unfractionated heparin t.
    vasodilatory t.
    vocal fold fixation t.
    voice t.
    volume t.
    whole-brain radiation t.
    wide-field radiation t.
    wide-range radiation t.
    xenogeneic cell t.
    x-ray t. (XRT)
therencephalous
thermal
    t. ablation
    t. allodynia
    t. anesthesia
    t. balance
    t. biofeedback
    t. coefficient expansion
    t. death point
    t. disinfection
    t. hypersensitivity
    t. injury
    t. injury-induced lung damage
    t. injury-induced vascular hypermobility
    t. keratoplasty
    t. necrosis
    t. pain threshold
    t. quenching
    t. rhizotomy
    t. sclerectomy
    t. stimulation
    t. therapy
thermal-assisted
    t.-a. capsular shift procedure
    t.-a. capsular shrinkage
thermal/perfusion balloon angioplasty
thermic anesthesia
thermoablation
    percutaneous radiofrequency t.
thermocauterectomy
thermocautery
thermochemotherapy
thermocoagulation
    intradiscal t.
    intradiscal radiofrequency t.
thermodilution
    bolus t. (BTD)
    t. cardiac output (TDCO)
    t. technique

thermodynamic theory of narcosis
thermogenesis
    nonshivering t.
thermogram
thermographic
    t. examination
    t. temperature measurement
thermography
thermokeratoplasty
thermolysis
thermometry
    tympanic t.
thermopenetration
thermoregulation
    perianesthetic t.
thermoregulatory
    t. defense
    t. sweat test
    t. vasoconstriction
thermorhizotomy
thermosclerectomy
thermosclerostomy
thermosclerotomy
thermotherapy
    microwave t.
    transurethral microwave t.
    (TUMT)
thick cutaneous melanoma (TCM)
thickened
    t. nail
    t. synovial membrane
thickening
    endocardial t.
    heel pad t.
    postlumpectomy skin t.
thickness
    Breslow t.
    endometrial t.
    end-systolic wall t. (ESWT)
    skinfold t.
    soft tissue t.
Thiersch
    T. anal incontinence operation
    T. anus procedure
    T. eyelid skin grafting method
    T. graft operation
    T. hand procedure
    T. medium split free graft
    T. skin graft procedure
    T. split-thickness skin graft
    T. suture
    T. suture technique
    T. thin split free graft
Thiersch-Duplay
    T.-D. proximal tube urethroplasty
    procedure
    T.-D. tube graft
    T.-D. urethral construction
    T.-D. urethroplasty

thigh
    t. bone
    t. graft arteriovenous fistula
    t. joint
    posterior t.
thimble valvotomy
thin
    t. basement membrane
    t. basement membrane disease
    t. glossy skin
    t. section
thin-needle biopsy
thinning
    corneal t.
thin-section
    t.-s. axial image
    t.-s. CT
thiol augmentation
thiopental-sufentanil-desflurane-nitrous
  oxide anesthetic technique
third
    t. and fourth pharyngeal pouch
     syndrome
    t. cranial nerve
    t. intention
    t. occipital nerve
    t. parallel pelvic plane
    t. space fluid accumulation
    t. space loss
    Steel rule of t.'s
    t. trochanter
    t. ventriculostomy
third-degree
    t.-d. burn
    t.-d. hemorrhoid
    t.-d. radiation injury
third-grade fusion
Thiry fistula
Thiry-Vella fistula
Thoma ampulla
Thomas
    T. body mass index and diastolic
     blood pressure classification
    T. extrapolated bar graft
    T. nipple reconstruction technique
    T. quadricepsplasty
    T. sign
Thomas-Thompson-Straub rotational
  transfer of vastus lateralis
  technique
Thomas-Warren incision
Thom flap laryngeal reconstruction
  method
Thompson
    T. Achilles tendon rupture test
    T. anterolateral hip approach
    T. anteromedial shoulder approach
    T. capsule flap pyeloplasty
    T. cleft lip repair procedure

T

Thompson (*continued*)
  T. correction of lymphedema
    procedure
  T. excision
  T. fascia
  T. ligament
  T. line
  T. posterior radial approach
  T. quadricepsplasty
  T. quadricepsplasty procedure
  T. resection
  T. telescoping V osteotomy
  T. thumb apposition with bone graft
    procedure
Thompson-Epstein femoral fracture
  classification
Thompson-Farley retractor
Thompson-Loomer talar osteochondritis
  dissecans repair technique
Thomson operation
thoracentesis
  needle t.
thoraces (*pl. of* thorax)
thoracic
  t. anesthesia
  t. aneurysm
  t. aorta
  t. aortic aneurysm repair
  t. aortic cross-clamping
    (TACC)
  t. aortic disease
  t. aortic dissection
  t. aortic ischemia reperfusion
  t. aortic plexus
  t. approach
  t. axis
  t. bioimpedance
  t. cage
  t. cardiac branch
  t. cardiac nerve
  t. cavity
  t. compression syndrome
  t. discectomy
  t. disc herniation
  t. duct
  t. duct fistula
  t. endometriosis syndrome
  t. epidural analgesia
  t. epidural anesthesia (TEA)
  t. epidural anesthetic technique
  t. epidural catheter
  t. epidural catheterization
  t. esophagogastrostomy
  t. esophagus
  t. facet fusion
  t. ganglion
  t. girdle
  t. great vessel
  t. index

  t. inlet
  t. inlet soft tissue
  t. inlet vascular injury
  t. interspinal muscle
  t. intertransverse muscle
  t. kidney
  t. lesion
  t. limb
  t. longissimus muscle
  t. motor paralysis
  t. outlet compression
  t. outlet decompression
  t. outlet syndrome (TOS)
  t. plane
  t. pump mechanism
  t. pump theory
  t. radiculopathy
  t. respiration
  t. rotator muscle
  t. short esophagomyotomy
  t. spinal fusion
  t. spinal nerve
  t. spine (T-spine)
  t. spine biopsy
  t. spine fracture
  t. spine kyphotic deformity
  t. spine landmark
  t. spine scoliotic deformity
  t. spine vertebral osteosynthesis
  t. stomach
  t. surgeon
  t. surgery
  t. trauma
  t. vein
  t. vertebra
  t. vertebral body
  t. wall
thoracicoabdominal
thoracicoacromial
thoracicohumeral
thoracoabdominal
  t. aneurysm
  t. aortic aneurysm
  t. aortic aneurysm repair
  t. artery
  t. esophagectomy
  t. esophagogastrectomy
  t. extrapleural approach
  t. gunshot wound
  t. incision
  t. injury
  t. intrapleural approach
  t. nerve
  t. region
  t. retroperitoneal lymphadenectomy
  t. trauma
thoracoacromial
  t. artery
  t. flap

t. trunk
t. vein
thoracoacromialis
thoracoceloschisis, thoracogastroschisis
thoracocentesis
thoracocyllosis
thoracocyrtosis
thoracodorsal
t. artery
t. nerve
thoracoepigastric
t. flap
t. vein
thoracofemoral bypass
thoracogastroschisis (*var. of*
thoracoceloschisis)
thoracograph
thoracolaparotomy
thoracolumbar
t. aponeurosis
t. burst fracture
t. fascia
t. junction surgical exposure
t. outflow
t. retroperitoneal approach
t. spine anterior exposure
t. spine fracture
t. spine fracture-dislocation
t. spine stabilization
t. spine vertebral osteosynthesis
t. spondylosis surgical technique
t. transdiaphragmatic approach
thoracolysis
thoracomelus
thoracopagus twin
thoracophrenolaparotomy
thoracoplasty
conventional t.
costoversion t.
Delorme t.
Schede t.
Wilms t.
thoracopneumoplasty
thoracoschisis
thoracoscopic
t. approach
t. discectomy
t. esophageal mobilization
t. esophagomyotomy
t. pericardiectomy
t. repair
t. splanchnicectomy
t. talc insufflation
thoracoscopic-assisted esophagectomy
thoracoscopy
single-trocar access t.
video t.
thoracostenosis
thoracosternotomy

thoracostomy
closed chest t.
tube t.
thoracotomy
anterior t.
anterolateral t.
t. approach
axillary t.
bilateral anterior t.
book t.
clamshell t.
emergency department t. (EDT)
emergency room t.
ER t.
esophagectomy with t.
t. incision
lateral t.
left-sided t.
Lewis t.
limited t.
limited anterior small t. (LAST)
median t.
muscle-sparing t.
open t.
resuscitative t.
right-sided t.
t. scar
standard t.
trapdoor t.
thorascopic
t. apical pleurectomy
t. drainage
Thoratec
thorax, *pl.* **thoraces**
left t.
Peyrot t.
right t.
Thorel bundle
thorn
T. fetal position maneuver
T. syndrome
Thornell microlaryngoscopy
THR
total hip replacement
threaded-hole-first technique
three-color
t.-c. concept
t.-c. concept of wound classification
three-field lymphadenectomy
threshold
apneic t.
atrial defibrillation t.
current perception t. (CPT)
defibrillation t.
detection t.
displacement t.
double-point t.
experimental t.
fibrillation t.

threshold (*continued*)
　　flicker-fusion t.
　　heat-pain t.
　　median detection t.
　　noise detection t.
　　pacemaker t.
　　pressure pain t. (PPT)
　　t. shift method
　　speech detection t.
　　stimulation t.
　　TEAP t.
　　temperature t.
　　thermal pain t.
　　ventilation t.
　　vibration detection t.
　　warm sensation t.
throat
　　t. anesthesia
　　t. pack retention
　　t. screen
thrombase
thrombasthenia
　　Glanzmann t.
Thrombate III blood product derivative
thrombectomy
　　chemical t.
　　early t.
　　mechanical t.
　　percutaneous t.
　　percutaneous mechanical t. (PMT)
　　percutaneous rotational t.
　　rheolytic catheter t.
　　rotational t.
　　surgical t.
　　venous t.
thrombelastography
thrombi (*pl. of* thrombus)
thrombin
　　t. formation
　　human t.
thrombin-mediated consumptive state
thromboangiitis obliterans (TAO)
thromboaspiration
　　transcatheter t.
thromboasthenia
thrombocythemia
thrombocytopenia
　　heparin-induced t. (HIT)
　　immune-mediated heparin-induced t.
　　unfractionated heparin-induced t.
thromboelastogram (TEG)
thromboelastograph (TEG)
thromboelastography (TEG)
thromboembolectomy
　　percutaneous aspiration t. (PAT)
　　rotating aspiration t.
thromboembolic
　　t. complication
　　t. disease (TED)

　　t. event
　　t. fistula
　　t. prophylaxis
　　t. risk factor
　　t. sequela
thromboembolism
　　recurrent t.
　　venous t.
thromboendarterectomy (TEA)
　　pulmonary t. (PTE)
　　renal t.
thrombogenesis
thrombogenic
　　t. disorder
　　t. foreign body
　　t. profile
thrombolysis
　　catheter-directed t.
　　coronary t.
　　T. in Myocardial Infarction (TIMI)
　　T. in Myocardial Infarction
　　　classification
　　selective intracoronary t. (SICT)
　　sonic t.
　　urokinase t.
thrombolytic
　　t. agent
　　t. therapy
thrombopathy
thrombophlebitis
　　recurrent t.
　　superficial t.
thromboplastin
　　tissue t.
thromboprophylaxis
thrombosed
　　t. graft
　　t. internal and external hemorrhoids
thromboses (*pl. of* thrombosis)
thrombosin
thrombosis, *pl.* **thromboses**
　　acute mesenteric venous t.
　　arterial t.
　　chronic t.
　　deep vein t. (DVT)
　　deep venous t. (DVT)
　　diffuse microvascular t.
　　early graft t.
　　effort t.
　　graft t.
　　graft limb t.
　　intimal t.
　　t. of IVC
　　portal t.
　　postoperative deep venous t.
　　　(PODVT)
　　recurrent t.
　　renal artery t.
　　vascular access t.

venous effort t.
widespread portal system t.
thrombostasis
thrombotic
t. complication
t. disease
t. episode
t. event
t. gangrene
t. process
t. tendency
t. thrombocytopenic purpura (TTP)
thrombus, *pl.* **thrombi**
deep venous t.
t. extension
peripheral t.
portal tumor t.
portal vein tumor t. (PVTT)
regression of t.
tumor t.
vein tumor t.
through-and-through
t.-a.-t. fracture
t.-a.-t. laceration
t.-a.-t. reabsorbable suture
t.-a.-t. suture technique
t.-a.-t. V-shaped horizontal osteotomy
through-knee amputation
through-the-scope (TTS)
t.-t.-s. balloon dilation
t.-t.-s. balloon removal
through-the-wall mattress suture
thrower's fracture
thrust manipulation
thumb
bifid t.
t. deformity
t. duplication
t. extensor tendon
t. metacarpophalangeal joint
approach
t. reconstruction
triphalangeal t.
t. web
thumb-in-palm
t.-i.-p. deformity
spastic t.-i.-p.
thumbprinting
thump
precordial t.
thymectomy
cervical t.
complete t.
neonatal t.
transcervical t.
video-assisted thoracoscopic t.
video-assisted thorascopic extended t.
(VATET)
thymi (*pl. of* thymus)

thymic
t. artery
t. branch
t. carcinoma
t. cyst
t. death
t. duct
t. mass
t. neoplasia
t. neoplasm
t. vein
thymica
mors t.
thymicolymphatic
Thymoglobulin
thymolipoma
thymol turbidity test
thymoma
spindle cell t.
thymus, *pl.* **thymi,** *pl.* **thymuses**
t. gland
t. gland excision
xenotransplantation t.
thymusectomy
thymuses (*pl. of* thymus)
thyroarytenoid muscle
thyrocele
thyrocervical
t. artery
t. trunk
thyrochondrotomy
thyroepiglottic
t. ligament
t. muscle
thyroepiglottidean
thyroglobulin
thyroglossal
t. cyst surgery
t. duct
t. duct carcinoma
t. duct cyst
t. fistula
thyrohyal
thyrohyoid
t. ligament
t. membrane
t. muscle
thyroid
t. adenoma
t. axis
t. body
t. cancer
t. carcinoma
t. cartilage
t. cyst
t. cystadenoma
t. disease
t. eminence
t. endocrine disorder

T

thyroid (*continued*)
    t. gland
    goitrous t.
    t. hormone serum
      concentration
    t. hyperplasia
    intratracheal ectopic t.
    t. isthmectomy
    t. isthmus
    t. lamina
    t. lobe
    t. lobectomy
    t. muscle
    t. needle biopsy
    t. neoplasia
    t. neoplasm
    t. nodule
    t. nodule ablation
    t. notch
    t. operation
    t. pathology
    t. plexus
    t. prominence
    pyramidal process of t.
    t. resection
    t. rest
    t. storm
    t. surgeon
    t. surgical tactic
    t. surgical technique
    t. tissue
    t. tumor
    t. ultrasound
    t. vein
thyroidal hernia
thyroidea
    levator glandulae t.
thyroidectomize
thyroidectomy
    breast approach t.
    complete t.
    completion t.
    gasless endoscopic t.
    Hartley-Dunhill subtotal t.
    near-total t.
    outpatient t.
    prophylactic t.
    provocative food t.
    scarless endoscopic t.
    subtotal t.
    t. tactic
    t. technique
    therapeutic t.
    total t.
    unilateral t.
    videoendoscopic t.
thyroiditis
    acute suppurative t.
    Riedel t.

thyrointoxication
thyrolaryngeal
thyrolingual duct
thyromental distance
thyropalatine
thyroparathyroidectomy
thyropharyngeal
thyroplasty
thyroptosis
thyrothymic
    t. ligament
    t. thyroid rest
thyrotomy
thyrotoxic coma
Ti
    titanium
TIA
    transient ischemic
    attack
tiagabine
tibia, *pl.* **tibiae**
tibiad
tibiae (*pl. of* tibia)
tibial
    t. acceleration
    t. angioplasty
    t. artery
    t. augmentation block
    t. bending fracture
    t. bone defect regeneration
    t. condyle fracture
    t. crest
    t. diaphysial fracture
    t. distractor
    t. epiphysis
    t. fracture fixation
    t. intertendinous bursa
    t. metaphysis
    t. muscle
    t. open fracture
    t. plafond fracture
    t. plateau fracture
    t. plateau fracture-dislocation
    t. recanalization
    t. shaft fracture
    t. triplane fracture
    t. tuberosity fracture
    t. tuberosity osteotomy
tibialis posterior dislocation
tibiocalcaneal
    t. arthrodesis
    t. medullary nailing
tibiofascialis
tibiofemoral articulation
tibiofibular
    t. articulation
    t. clear space
    t. diastasis
    t. fusion

t. joint dislocation
t. line
tibionavicular
tibioperoneal
t. trunk angioplasty
t. vessel angioplasty
tibioscaphoid
tibiotalar
t. fusion
posterior t.
tibiotalocalcaneal
t. arthrodesis
t. fusion
tic
t. douloureux
dystonic t.
tidal
t. drainage
t. volume
Tiedemann nerve
tier
remote t.
ties-over-stent
Tietze syndrome
tiger gut suture
TigerWire suture
tightening
gastric valve t.
tight Nissen repair
tight-to-shaft (TTS)
tigroid
t. appearance
t. striation
tigrolysis
Tikhoff-Linberg
T.-L. proximal humerus resection procedure
T.-L. shoulder girdle resection
tile
T. pelvic injury classification
t. plate facet replacement
Tillaux
T. apparatus
extraocular muscles of T.
T. fracture
T. sign
T. spiral
spiral of T.
Tillaux-Chaput fracture
Tillaux-Kleiger fracture
Tillaux-Phocas syndrome
Tillett blepharoptosis operation
tilt
base-ring t.
filter t.
head-down t.
head-up t.
steep head-down t.
t. stitch

t. table test
t. test
Trendelenburg t.
tilt-table testing
time
acceleration t.
activated clotting t. (ACT)
activated coagulation t. (ACT)
anesthesia t.
anesthetic t.
association t.
average extubation t.
bleeding t.
blood-brain equilibration t.
carotid ejection t.
celite-activated clotting t. (CACT)
cerebral circulation t.
circulation t.
cold ischemia t.
concentration times t.
context-sensitive decrement t.
correlation t.
deceleration t. (DCT)
decimal reduction t.
2D transit t.
Duke bleeding t.
duration t.
effect-site decrement t.
ejection t.
electrode response t.
evolution t.
execution t.
explosive doubling t.
followup t.
forced expiratory t. (FET)
helium equilibration t.
heparin neutralized thrombin t. (HnTT)
hepatic ischemic t.
high-dose thrombin t. (HiTT)
inspiration t.
inspiratory t.
interhemispheric propagation t.
isovolumetric relaxation t.
isovolumic relaxation t.
Ivy method of bleeding t.
kaolin-activated clotting t. (KACT)
lag t.
Lee-White clotting t.
mean circulation t.
Mielke bleeding t.
nucleation t.
t. of maximum concentration (Tmax)
operating t.
operative t.
plasma clotting t.
t. position scan
preoperative evolution t.

T

time (*continued*)
  preservation t.
  t. pressure
  procedure t.
  prolonged prothrombin t.
  prothrombin t. (protime, pro-time, PT)
  recalcification t.
  recovery t.
  recovery room t.
  relaxation t.
  saturation t.
  sensation t.
  systolic t.
  t. to recovery
  total respiratory t.
  total tourniquet t.
  tourniquet t.
  tumor doubling t.
  ventilator t.
  ventricular activation t.
  wait t.
  warm ischemic t.
time-concentration curve
time-cycled ventilation
timed
  t. forced expiratory volume
  t. intermittent rotation
timed-sequential therapy
time-of-flight (TOF)
  t.-o.-f. echoplanar imaging
TIMI
  Thrombolysis in Myocardial Infarction
  TIMI classification
Tim knot
timolol
Tinel sign
tip
  t. angle
  intraabdominal t.
  nasal t.
  overprojecting nasal t.
  papillary muscle t.
  TIPS procedure
  pyramidal t.
  rectal t.
  spleen t.
  tapered t.
TIPS
  transjugular intrahepatic portosystemic shunt
  TIPS procedure
Ti:sapphire
  titanium-sapphire
  Ti:sapphire laser
TISS
  therapeutic intervention scoring system
tissue
  abdominal adipose t.

aberrant t.
t. ablation
acellular pannus t.
acinar t.
acute wound granulation t.
t. adhesive
adipose connective t.
ampullary granulation t.
anechoic t.
aneurysm t.
aneurysmal t.
angiomatous neoplastic t.
anisotropic t.
aortic aneurysm t.
t. approximation
t. architecture
areolar connective t.
atrioventricular conduction t.
attenuating t.
t. bank
t. biopsy
t. blocking
border t.
breast biopsy t.
bronchial-associated lymphoid t. (BALT)
brown adipose t.
bursa-equivalent t.
bursal t.
cancellous t.
capsular support t.
cartilaginous t.
caseated t.
cementoid t.
cervical soft t.
chromaffin t.
cicatricial t.
t. coagulation
collagenous t.
t. compression
t. compression test
t. conductivity
t. confirmation
conjunctiva-associated lymphoid t. (CALT)
connective t.
corneal t.
coronal pulp t.
crushed t.
cutaneous t.
denuded connective t.
t. detritus
devitalized t.
diffuse lymphatic t.
t. dissection
donor t.
t. Doppler imaging
dorsal t.
earlobe adipose t.

echogenic t.
ectopic endometrial t.
elastic t.
enveloping scar t.
episcleral t.
t. expander
t. expansion
extraarticular t.
extracapsular t.
extraperitoneal t.
exuberant granulation t.
t. failure
fatty prostatic t.
fetal lymphoid t.
fibroadipose t.
fibroblastic t.
fibroelastic t.
fibrofatty breast t.
fibrotic t.
fibrous connective t.
fibrous scar t.
t. fluke
functional renal t.
t. fusion
Gamgee t.
ganglial t.
gastrointestinal-associated lymphoid t. (GALT)
gingival t.
glandular t.
granulation t.
granulomatous t.
gut-associated lymphoid t. (GALT)
hard and soft t.
healthy t.
hemangiomatous t.
hematopoietic t.
hilar structure scar t.
His-Purkinje t.
histiocytic t.
t. homogeneity
hyperplastic t.
hypertrophic granulation t.
hypocellular fibrous t.
t. hypoperfusion
t. hypoxia
t. imprint
t. ingrowth surface
interdental t.
interfascicular fibrous t.
t. interposition
interstitial t.
intervening connective t.
intralobular connective t.
intratracheal ectopic thyroid t.
isotropic t.
keratinized t.
ligamentous support t.
t. ligand

lipomalike t.
lipomatous t.
liver t.
t. loss
t. lymph
lymphatic t.
lymphoid t.
mammary t.
maternal t.
mesenchymal t.
mesothelial t.
mineralized t.
t. molding
mucosa-associated lymphoid t. (MALT, MALToma)
muscular t.
musculoskeletal t.
myeloid t.
myocardial t.
nasion soft t.
t. necrosis
necrotic/fibrotic t.
necrotic hyalinized t.
neoplastic t.
nephrogenetic t.
neural t.
nodal t.
nonviable t.
nonvital t.
normal t.
nuclear t.
t. nutrition
oral t.
orbital adipose t.
orbitonasal t.
osseous t.
t. oxygenation
t. oxygen delivery
t. oxygen tension
pancreatic t.
paracancerous t.
paraoral t.
parathyroid t.
paravaginal soft t.
parenchymatous t.
t. perfusion
periadventitial t.
periapical t.
periarticular t.
pericanalicular connective t.
periesophageal t.
periimplant t.
perilobular connective t.
perinephric t.
perineural t.
perinodal t.
periosteal t.
peripancreatic t.
peripancreatic necrotic t.

T

tissue (*continued*)
    peripheral lymphoid t.
    periprostatic t.
    petrotympanic t.
    pharyngeal t.
    t. pH monitoring
    placental t.
    polypoid t.
    preepiglottic soft t.
    t. preservation
    t. pressure
    t. pressure measurement
    pressure-sensitive t.
    pressure-tolerant t.
    prevertebral soft t.
    pulmonary t.
    redundant sac t.
    t. regeneration
    t. remodeling
    t. renewal
    t. repair
    residual ductal t.
    t. resistance
    t. respiration
    retained valvular t.
    retroperitoneal soft t.
    retropharyngeal soft t.
    revascularized t.
    rubber t.
    t. sampling
    scar t.
    skeletal t.
    t. slack
    slow exchange soft t.
    soft t.
    sonolucent t.
    t. space
    specialized intralobular connective t.
    splenic t.
    t. study
    subcutaneous t.
    subjacent t.
    supporting t.
    sustentacular t.
    syngeneic t.
    synovial t.
    testicular adrenal-like t.
    t. texture abnormality (TTA)
    thoracic inlet soft t.
    t. thromboplastin
    thyroid t.
    t. tolerance
    t. tolerance dose
    t. transfer
    t. transplant
    t. transplant
    t. trauma
    t. trimming
    trophoblastic t.

    tuberculosis granulation t.
    t. typing
    vascular t.
    viable t.
    viscoelastic t.
    vital t.
    t. water content
    t. welding
    xenogeneic t.
tissue-base relationship
tissue-bearing area
tissue-borne
tissue-equivalent
tissue-sparing technique
tissue-supported base
tissue-tissue-supported base
titanium (Ti)
    t. clip
    t. flexible humeral nail
    t. vocal fold medialization implant
titanium-sapphire (Ti:sapphire)
titratable
titration
    Dean and Webb t.
    potentiometric t.
    Rinkel serial endpoint t.
    t. technique
titubation
    head t.
TIVA
    total intravenous anesthesia
    total intravenous anesthetic
TKA
    total knee arthroplasty
    total knee arthroscopy
TLND
    therapeutic lymph node dissection
TLS
    tumor lysis syndrome
T-lymphocyte
    cytotoxic T-l. (CTL)
TM
    tympanic membrane
Tmax
    time of maximum concentration
TMD
    temporomandibular muscle disorder
TME
    total mesenteric excision
    total mesorectal excision
T-mesh closure technique
TMJ
    temporomandibular joint
TMLR
    transmyocardial laser revascularization
TMR
    transmyocardial laser revascularization
TMT
    tarsometatarsal

TNM

tumor, node, metastasis
TNM classification
TNM staging system
TNM system for tumor staging

TNS

transient neurologic symptom

to-and-fro anesthesia

tocolysis

tocolytic therapy

Todd-Evans stepladder tracheal dilatation technique

toddler's fracture

toe

Butler procedure to correct overlapping t.'s
catheter t.
t. extensor
t. extensor muscle
t. extensor tendon
great t.
mallet t.

toe-block anesthesia

toenail

embedded t.
ingrowing t.

toe-phalanx transplant

TOF

tetralogy of Fallot
time-of-flight
train-of-four
TOF ratio

TOF-Watch SX accelerometer

Tohen tendon technique

toilet

cavity t.
peritoneal t.
pulmonary t.

tolazoline

Toldt

T. fascia
line of T.
T. membrane
white fascial line of T.

tolerance

acute opioid t.
anesthetic t.
Fletcher rule of irradiation t.
histologic t.
poor exercise t.
pressure t.
tissue t.

Tolosa-Hunt syndrome

tomentum, tomentum cerebri

Tom Jones suture technique

tomography

chest computed t.
computed t. (CT)
contrast-enhanced computed t.
expiratory computed t.
multidetector computed t. (MDCT)
positron emission t. (PET)
ultrafast CT electron beam t.
ultrafast spiral computed t.

tone

airway t.

tongue

t. base reduction
t. bone
t. fasciculation
t. flap
t. fracture
mandibular t.
t. plication
t. pressure
t. thrust classification
t. thrust therapy

tongue-and-groove suture technique

tongue-in-groove operation

tongue-jaw-neck dissection

tongue-splitting transmandibular approach

tonic spasm

tonometer

Goldmann applanation t. (GAT)
indentation t.

tonometry

applanation t.
gastric t.
indentation t.
intraluminal t.
nasogastric t.
Schiotz t.

tonsil

Gerlach t.
palatine t.
quinsy t.

tonsilla pharyngealis

tonsillar, tonsillary

t. branch
t. crypt
t. fold
t. fossa
t. hernia
t. herniation

tonsillary (*var. of* tonsillar)

tonsillectomy

t. and adenoidectomy (T&A)
contact diode laser t.
intracapsular partial t.
Sluder guillotine t.

tonsilloadenoidectomy

tool

Malnutrition Universal Screening T. (MUST)

tooth, *pl.* **teeth**

anatomic t.
canine teeth

tooth (*continued*)
    central incisor teeth
    t. extraction
    extruded teeth
    t. fracture
    t. hemisection
    t. immobilization
    teeth ligation
    t. mass
    t. migration
    molar teeth
    t. perforation
    t. plane
    t. position
    premolar teeth
    t. sac
    t. transplant
tooth-and-nail syndrome
tooth-to-tooth position
TOPA
    topical oropharyngeal anesthesia
topectomy
Topel knot
tophi (*pl. of* tophus)
tophus, *pl.* **tophi**
topical
    t. anesthetic
    t. anesthetic technique
    t. antibacterial agent
    t. antibiotic
    t. cooling
    t. hemostatic agent
    t. iodine application
    t. oropharyngeal anesthesia
    (TOPA)
Topinard facial angle
topistic
topographic
    t. anatomy
    t. projection
top-up
    epidural t.-u.
Torek
    T. cryptorchidism orchidopexy
    T. esophagus operation
    T. orchiopexy
    T. thoracic esophagus cancer
    resection
Torg
    T. knee reconstruction
    T. metatarsal fracture classification
    T. tarsal navicular stress fracture
    repair technique
Torgerson-Leach modified tibial osteotomy technique
tori (*pl. of* torus)
toric ablation
Torkildsen ventriculocisternostomy
Tornwaldt cyst

Torode-Zieg pediatric pelvic fracture classification
Toronto pelvic fracture classification
Torpin cul-de-sac resection
torque
    t. control endobronchial blocker
    light-wire t.
    translation of t.
    t. tube catheter
    unwanted screw t.
torr
torrential hemorrhage
torsade de pointes ventricular tachycardia (TdPVT)
torsion
    angle of femoral t.
    bilateral t.
    biliary tract t.
    extravaginal testicular t.
    intravaginal t.
    lobar t.
    neonatal testicular t.
    perinatal t.
    postnatal t.
    prenatal t.
    testicular t.
    t. testis
    unilateral testicular t.
torsional fracture
torso
    t. crease
    t. injury
torsoclusion
tortipelvis
tortuous
    t. intercostal artery
    t. megaesophagus
toruloma
Torulopsis **infection**
torus, *pl.* **tori**
    t. fracture
TOS
    thoracic outlet syndrome
total
    t. abdominal colectomy (TAC)
    t. abdominal evisceration (TAE)
    t. abdominal hysterectomy (TAH)
    t. abdominal hysterectomy and bilateral salpingo-oophorectomy (TAHBSO)
    t. abdominal vagotomy
    t. ankle arthroplasty (TAA)
    t. anomalous pulmonary venous return (TAPVR)
    t. articular replacement arthroplasty (TARA)
    t. articular resurfacing arthroplasty (TARA)
    t. axial node irradiation

t. bilateral vagotomies
t. bilirubin level
t. biopsy
t. body fat
t. body fluid loss
t. body hypothermia
t. body irradiation
t. body scanning
t. body solute
t. body surface area (TBSA)
t. body water
t. body weight
t. breech extraction
t. closed cystopericystectomy
t. colectomy
t. colonic aganglionosis
t. colonoscopy
t. continence
t. cystectomy
t. dehiscence
t. ear obliteration
t. elbow arthroplasty (TEA)
t. endoscopic coronary artery bypass
t. endoscopic esophagectomy
t. erythrocyte volume
t. etch technique
t. ethmoidectomy
t. exchangeable potassium measurement
t. excisional operation
t. fundoplication
t. fundoplication method
t. fundoplication procedure
t. fundoplication technique
t. gastrectomy
t. gastric pull-up
t. gastric wrap
t. glossectomy
t. graft area
t. graft area rejection
t. hepatic venous exclusion
t. hip arthroplasty (THA)
t. hip arthroplasty with internal eccentric shells (THARIES)
t. hip replacement (THR)
t. hip replacement surgery
t. hypophysectomy
t. hysterectomy
t. internal reflection
t. intravenous anesthesia (TIVA)
t. intravenous anesthetic (TIVA)
t. intravenous anesthetic technique
t. joint replacement
t. keratoplasty
t. knee arthroplasty (TKA)
t. knee arthroscopy (TKA)
t. knee replacement
t. knee replacement surgery
t. laparoscopic esophagectomy

t. laryngectomy
t. laryngopharyngectomy
t. L-chain concentration
t. left hepatectomy
t. lobectomy
t. lymphoid irradiation
t. mastectomy
t. maxillectomy
t. meniscectomy
t. mesenteric excision (TME)
t. mesorectal excision (TME)
t. nodal irradiation
t. open cystopericystectomy
T. Pain Rating Score
t. pancreatectomy
t. parathyroidectomy
t. parenteral alimentation (TPA)
t. parenteral nutrition (TPN)
t. parotidectomy
t. patellectomy
t. patellofemoral joint arthroplasty
t. pelvic exenteration (TPE)
t. pericystectomy
t. perineal prostatectomy
t. perineal rupture
t. petrosectomy
t. proctectomy
t. proctocolectomy
t. prostatoseminal vesiculectomy
t. protein concentration
t. pulpotomy
t. push therapy
t. respiratory time
t. retrocolic end-to-side gastrojejunostomy
t. scrotectomy
t. shoulder arthroplasty (TSA)
t. space analysis
t. spinal anesthesia
t. surgical removal
T. Tenderness Score
t. thoracic esophagectomy
t. thyroidectomy
t. time to intubation (TTI)
t. tourniquet time
t. transfusion
t. vascular exclusion
t. vascular isolation (TVI)
t. wrist arthroplasty (TWA)
t. wrist fusion

totally

t. extraperitoneal (TEP)
t. extraperitoneal approach
t. extraperitoneal inguinal herniorrhaphy
t. extraperitoneal prosthetic
t. extraperitoneal repair
t. intrathoracic stomach
t. stapled restorative proctocolectomy

T

Toti
- T. dacryocystorhinostomy procedure
- T. operation

Toti-Mosher operation

touch
- 3-point t.

touch-up procedure

Toupe
- T. fundoplication procedure
- T. fundoplication technique
- T. pharyngocolonic anastomosis method

Toupet
- T. antireflux procedure
- T. fundoplasty
- T. hemifundoplication
- T. hemifundoplication fundoplication
- T. wrap

Tourette syndrome

tourniquet
- chemical t.
- t. control
- t. ischemia
- t. ischemic pain
- t. occlusion
- t. pain
- t. paralysis
- t. pressure
- t. test
- t. time

tourniquet-induced pain

tourniquet-related nerve damage

Tourtual
- T. canal
- T. membrane

Towako transvaginal-transmyometrial embryo transfer method

tower skull

Towne projection

Townley-Paton corneal transplant

toxemia, toxicemia

toxic
- t. adenoma
- t. epidermal necrolysis
- t. granulation
- t. megacolon
- t. multinodular goiter

toxicemia (*var. of* toxemia)

toxicity
- acute t.
- aluminum t.
- aminoglycoside t.
- citrate t.
- endocrine t.
- extramedullary t.
- glutamate t.
- neostigmine t.

oxygen t.
radiation-induced pulmonary t.
transient t.

toxic-traumatized patient

toxin
- botulinum t. (BTX)
- botulinum t. A (BTA)
- t. exposure
- extracellular t.
- omega-conopeptide t.

Toynbee muscle

TPA
- total parenteral alimentation

TPC
- target plasma concentration

TPE
- total pelvic exenteration

T-penia
- thrombocytopenia

TPI
- trigger point injection

TPN
- total parenteral nutrition

T-pouch ileal neobladder

TPR
- temperature, pulse, respiration

trabecula, *pl.* **trabeculae**

trabeculae (*pl. of* trabecula)

trabecular
- t. arachnoid component
- t. bone fracture
- t. membrane
- t. network

trabeculated
- t. bladder
- t. bone lesion

trabeculation

trabeculectomy
- Cairns t.
- t. operation
- Redmond Smith ab externo t.
- Smith t.

trabeculopexy
- argon laser t. (ALT)

trabeculoplasty
- argon laser t. (ALT, ALTP)
- laser t.

trabeculotomy
- Harms-Dannheim t.

trabeculotomy-trabeculectomy
- Silva Costa combined t.-t.

trace anesthetic

tracer dilution

trach
- tracheostomy
- tracheotomy

trachea, *pl.* **tracheae**
- saber-sheath t.

tracheae (*pl. of* trachea)

tracheal
- t. adenoma
- t. agenesis
- t. aspiration
- t. bifurcation angle
- t. block
- t. blood flow
- t. branch
- t. cartilage
- t. compression
- t. extubation
- t. extubation anesthetic technique
- t. fenestration
- t. fracture
- t. gas insufflation (TGI)
- t. gland
- t. injury
- t. intubation
- t. intubation anesthetic technique
- t. ligation
- t. node
- t. reconstruction
- t. repair
- t. resection
- t. ring
- t. safety stitch
- t. secretion
- t. stenosis
- t. suction anesthetic technique
- t. surgery
- t. topical analgesia
- t. triangle
- t. tug
- t. tumor
- t. ulceration
- t. web

tracheal-bronchial tree
trachealis muscle
tracheitis, trachitis
trachelectomy
trachelematoma
trachelian
trachelocele (*var. of* tracheocele)
tracheloclavicularis
tracheloclavicular muscle
trachelomastoid
trachelomastoideus
trachelopexy
tracheloplasty
trachelorrhaphy
trachelos
tracheloschisis
trachelotomy
tracheoaerocele
tracheobiliary fistula
tracheobronchial
- t. anomaly
- t. foreign body
- t. node
- t. tree

tracheobronchitis
tracheobronchoesophageal fistula
tracheobronchomalacia
tracheobronchoscopy
tracheocele, trachelocele
tracheocutaneous fistula
tracheoesophageal (TE)
- t. fistula (TEF)
- t. groove
- t. puncture (TEP)
- t. puncture repair

tracheolaryngeal
tracheomalacia
tracheo-oesophageal,
tracheopharyngeal
tracheoplasty
- slide t.

tracheostomy
- definitive t.
- elective dilatational t.
- emergency t.
- flap t.
- Great Ormond Street t.
- Montgomery t.
- percutaneous dilational t. (PDT)
- t. stoma
- tube-free t.

tracheotomy
- awake t.
- pediatric t.
- percutaneous t.

trachitis (*var. of* tracheitis)
trachoma gland
track
- bleeding t.
- pin t.
- radial suture t.

tracking
- electromagnetic t.
- optic t.

Tracrium
tract
- abnormal fetal urogenital t.
- aerodigestive t.
- alimentary t.
- Arnold t.
- association t.
- atriodextrofascicular t.
- atriofascicular t.
- atrionodal bypass t.
- auditory t.
- bile t.
- biliary t.
- bronchial t.
- Burdach t.
- bypass t.
- central tegmental t.

T

tract (*continued*)
    cerebellorubral t.
    cerebellothalamic t.
    cholinergic t.
    Collier t.
    concealed bypass t.
    corticobulbar t.
    corticopontine t.
    corticospinal t.
    crossed pyramidal t.
    cuneocerebellar t.
    dead t.
    deep liver t.
    deiterospinal t.
    dental sinus t.
    dentatothalamic t.
    dermal sinus t.
    digestive t.
    t. dilation
    direct pyramidal t.
    dopaminergic t.
    dorsolateral t.
    extrapyramidal t.
    fastigiobulbar t.
    fetal urogenital t.
    fistulous t.
    Flechsig t.
    frontopontine t.
    frontotemporal t.
    gastrointestinal t.
    geniculocalcarine t.
    geniculotemporal t.
    genital t.
    genitourinary t.
    GI t.
    Gowers t.
    habenulointerpeduncular t.
    hepatic outflow t.
    high blind t.
    Hoche t.
    hypothalamohypophysial t.
    ileal inflow t.
    ileal outflow t.
    iliopubic t.
    iliotibial t.
    infected t.
    inflammatory sinus t.
    inflow t.
    intestinal t.
    intramural fistulous t.
    lateral corticospinal t.
    left ventricular outflow t. (LVOT)
    Lissauer t.
    liver t.
    Loewenthal t.
    mamillothalamic t.
    Marchi t.
    mesolimbic-mesocortical t.
    Monakow t.

    nasal t.
    needle t.
    neotrigeminothalamic t.
    nerve t.
    nigrostriatal t.
    nodoventricular t.
    occipitocollicular t.
    occipitopontine t.
    occipitotectal t.
    t. of Münzer and Wiener
    t. of Schütz
    olfactory t.
    olivocerebellar t.
    olivospinal t.
    optic t.
    ororespiratory t.
    outflow t.
    paleotrigeminothalamic t.
    pancreaticobiliary t.
    parietopontine t.
    perineal sinus t.
    portal t.
    posterior spinocerebellar t.
    prepyramidal t.
    pulmonary outflow t.
    pyramidal t.
    reproductive t.
    respiratory t.
    reticulospinal t.
    retrochiasmal optic t.
    right ventricular outflow t. (RVOT)
    rubrobulbar t.
    rubroreticular t.
    rubrospinal t.
    seminal t.
    sensory t.
    septomarginal t.
    serotonergic t.
    sinus t.
    solitary t.
    sphincteroid t.
    spinal dermal sinus t.
    spinocerebellar t.
    spinoolivary t.
    spinotectal t.
    spinothalamic t. (STT)
    spiral foraminous t.
    Spitzka marginal t.
    sulcomarginal t.
    supraopticohypophysial t.
    t. tamponade
    tamponade needle t.
    tangential t.
    tectobulbar t.
    tectopontine t.
    tectospinal t.
    temporofrontal t.
    temporopontine t.

tree-barking urinary t.
T-tube t.
tuberoinfundibular t.
Türck t.
UGI t.
upper aerodigestive t.
upper gastrointestinal t.
upper respiratory t.
urinary t.
urogenital t.
uveal t.
ventral spinocerebellar t.
ventral spinothalamic t.
ventricular outflow t.
vestibulospinal t.
vocal t.
Waldeyer t.
wound t.

traction
t. alopecia
t. aneurysm
t. application
t. atrophy
t. detachment
t. diverticulum
t. epiphysis
t. fracture
gentle t.
t. headache
t. suture technique
t. test

tractotomy
anterolateral t.
bulbar cephalic pain t.
dorsal column t.
intramedullary t.
medullary spinothalamic t.
mesencephalic t.
pontine spinothalamic t.
pyramidal t.
Schwartz t.
Sjöqvist intramedullary t.
spinal t.
spinothalamic t.
stereotactic trigeminal t.
subcaudate t.
trigeminal t.
Walker t.

traditional
t. Chinese medicine
t. circle breathing system
t. method

trafficking
membrane t.

tragi (*pl. of* tragus)
tragicus muscle
tragus, *pl.* **tragi**
trainer
conventional video t.

virtual endoscopic surgery t.
(VEST)
virtual reality t.

training
autogenic t.
joint protection t.
prophylactic inspiratory muscle t.
stabilization t.

train-of-four (TOF)
t.-o.-f. ratio
t.-o.-f. stimulation
t.-o.-f. stimulus
t.-o.-f. transmission

Trainor operation
trajector
trajectory
bullet t.
missile t.

TRALI
transfusion-related acute lung
injury

tram line
TRAM
transverse rectus abdominis muscle
TRAM flap
TRAM flap procedure

tramadol
trampoline fracture
trance coma
tranquilization
tranquilizer
transabdominal
t. approach
t. laparoscopic herniorrhaphy
t. mucosectomy
t. onlay mesh
t. preperitoneal (TAPP)
t. preperitoneal hernioplasty
t. preperitoneal repair
t. proctopexy
t. ultrasonography

transacromial approach
transactivation
transaminase
glutamic-oxaloacetic t.
glutamic pyruvic t.

transampullary
t. drainage
t. septectomy

transanal
t. approach
t. endoscopic microsurgery (TEM)
t. endoscopic microsurgical
resection
t. excision
t. mucosectomy
t. mucosectomy with handsewn
anastomosis
t. pouch advancement

transanal (*continued*)
    t. stapling technique
    t. ultrasonography
transanimation
transantral
    t. approach
    t. ethmoidal approach
    t. ethmoidectomy
transaortic
    t. endarterectomy
    t. mesenteric endarterectomy
    t. valve gradient
transarterial
    t. anesthetic technique
    t. axillary block
    t. chemoembolization (TACE)
transarticular wire fixation
transaxial scan plane
transaxillary
    t. apical bullectomy
    t. approach
transbrachioradialis approach
transbronchial
    t. lung biopsy
    t. needle aspiration (TBNA)
transcallosal transventricular approach
transcanine approach
transcaphoid fracture
transcapillary hydrostatic pressure gradient
transcapitate
    t. fracture
    t. fracture-dislocation
transcapitellar wire fixation
transcardiac membranotomy
transcarpal amputation
transcatheter
    t. ablation
    t. arterial embolization therapy
    t. closure
    t. device closure
    t. thromboaspiration
transcavernous transpetrous apex approach
transcerebellar hemispheric approach
transcervical
    t. approach
    t. balloon tuboplasty
    t. femoral fracture
    t. intrafallopian tube transfer
    t. resection
    t. thymectomy
    t. tubal access
transchondral fracture
transclavicular approach
transcoccygeal approach
transcochlear
    t. approach

    t. cochleovestibular neurectomy
    t. vestibular neurectomy
transcondylar fracture
transcortical transventricular approach
transcranial
    t. Doppler (TCD)
    t. Doppler recanalization
    t. electrical stimulation
    t. electrical stimulation anesthesia monitoring technique
    t. frontal-temporal-orbital approach
    t. stimulation (TCS)
transcranial-supraorbital approach
transcubital approach
transcutaneous
    t. access
    t. acupoint electrical stimulation (TAES)
    t. biopsy
    t. cranial electrical stimulation (TCES)
    t. electrical nerve stimulation (TENS)
    t. electric stimulation (TES)
    t. oxygen monitoring
    t. oxygen pressure measurement
    t. partial pressure of oxygen
    t. tetanic stimulus
    t. tissue oxygen level
transcylindrical cholecystectomy
transcystic
    t. approach
    t. choledochoscopy
    t. drain
    t. drainage
TransCyte temporary skin substitute
transdermal
    t. administration
    t. analgesic
    t. anesthesia
    t. anesthetic technique
    t. scopolamine
    t. sympathectomy
Transderm Scop antiemetic patch
transdiaphragmatic approach
transducer
    differential variable reluctance t.
transduction
    complex signal t.
transduodenal
    t. approach
    t. endoscopic decompression
    t. pancreatectomy
    t. sphincteroplasty
    t. sphincterotomy
transect
transected
    t. ductule
    t. vertical gastric bypass

transection, transsection
  aortic t.
  atlantooccipital t.
  esophageal t.
  hepatic parenchymal t.
  t. incision
  intracorporeal rectal t.
  parenchymal t.
  t. plane
  step-cut t.
  Sugiura esophageal variceal t.
  traumatic aortic t.
transendoscopic
  t. electrocoagulation
  t. laser photocoagulation
  t. procedure
  t. sphincterotomy
transepiphysial fracture
transesophageal
  atrial pacing t.
  t. atrial pacing (TEAP)
  t. atrial stimulation
  t. color Doppler echocardiography
  t. echocardiograph-guided left
    ventricular oximetry
  t. echocardiograph-guided right
    ventricular oximetry
  t. echocardiography (TEE)
  t. echocardiography scan
  t. echocardiography with pacing
  t. endoscopy
  t. ligation of varix
  t. varix ligation
  t. ventricular pacing (TEVP)
transethmoidal
transfemoral
  t. liver biopsy
  t. venous catheterization
transfer
  adenoviral t.
  barber pole stripe t.
  composite free tissue t.
  dermal fat free tissue t.
  free flap t.
  free tissue t.
  gamete intrafallopian tube t. (GIFT)
  in vitro fertilization-embryo t.
  island nail t.
  maternal-placental-fetal drug t.
  microvascular free flap t.
  Ober-Barr procedure for
    brachioradialis t.
  placental t.
  pronuclear stage t. (PROST)
  saturation t.
  single-stage tissue t.
  SPLATT t.
  split anterior tibial tendon t.
    (SPLATTT)

tissue t.
transcervical intrafallopian tube t.
wraparound neurovascular composite
  free tissue t.
zygote intrafallopian t. (ZIFT)
transferrin
  melanoma t.
transfibular approach
transfixation
  Fuchs iris bombé t.
transfixing suture technique
transfixion suture
transforaminal passage
transform
transformary mass
transformation
  hemorrhagic t.
  malignant t.
  neoplastic t.
  t. zone
transfrontal approach
transfuse
transfusion
  acute blood t.
  acute normovolemic hemodilution t.
  allogenic blood t.
  arterial t.
  blood product t.
  coagulation factor t.
  direct t.
  double-volume exchange t.
  drip t.
  exchange t.
  exsanguination t.
  homologous blood t.
  immediate t.
  indirect t.
  intraperitoneal blood t.
  intraperitoneal fetal t.
  intrauterine intraperitoneal fetal t.
  mediate t.
  perioperative t.
  peritoneal t.
  t. reaction
  simple t.
  subcutaneous t.
  substitution t.
  t. therapy
  total t.
transfusion-related
  t.-r. acute lung injury (TRALI)
  t.-r. air embolism
  t.-r. lung injury (TRLI)
transgastric
  t. fine-needle aspiration biopsy
  t. laparoscopic resection
  t. ligation
  t. plication
transgastrostomic enteroscopy

T

transgenic therapy
transglomerular hydrostatic filtration
 pressure
transgluteal approach
transhamate
    t. fracture
    t. fracture-dislocation
transhepatic
    t. antegrade biliary drainage
     procedure
    t. approach
    t. catheterization
    t. stenting
transhiatal
    t. blunt esophagectomy
    t. esophagectomy
    t. esophagectomy approach
    t. esophagojejunostomy
    t. pyloroplasty
transhyoid pharyngotomy
transient
    t. ataxia
    t. azotemia
    t. bone marrow edema syndrome
    t. cavitation
    t. compartment syndrome
    t. edema
    t. hiatal hernia
    t. hyperemic response
    t. hyperemic response test
    t. hypocalcemia
    t. ischemic attack (TIA)
    t. lesion
    t. motor blockade
    t. neurologic deficit
    t. neurologic symptom (TNS)
    t. osteoporosis of hip
    t. paralysis
    t. profound neurologic deficit
    t. toxicity
    t. visual obscuration
transiliac
    t. amputation
    t. bar technique
    t. fracture
    t. rod fixation
transilluminated power phlebectomy
transillumination test
transischiac
transit
    hepatopulmonary t.
transition
    cervicothoracic t.
    t. zone
transitional
    t. cell carcinoma
    t. epithelium
    t. respiration
    t. zone biopsy

transjugular
    t. hepatic biopsy
    t. insertion
    t. intrahepatic portosystemic shunt
    (TIPS)
    t. intrahepatic portosystemic shunt
    procedure
    t. liver access
    t. liver biopsy
translabyrinthine and suboccipital
 approach
translaryngeal
    t. guided intubation anesthetic
    technique
    t. tracheal intubation
translation
    anterior t.
    anteroposterior t.
    caudal t.
    cephalad t.
    coronal plane deformity sagittal t.
    dorsal t.
    force t.
    t. injury
    t. mobility
    t. motion
    t. of torque
    posterior t.
    pure t.
    ulnar t.
    vertical t.
translational
    t. fracture
    t. movement
    t. position
translocation
    bacterial t.
    t. Down syndrome
transluminal
    t. coronary angioplasty
    t. extraction atherectomy
    t. valve
transmandibular-glossopharyngeal
 approach
transmandibular projection
transmastoid approach
transmeatal
    t. approach
    t. tympanoplasty incision
transmembrane hydraulic pressure
transmesenteric
    t. hernia
    t. plication
transmetatarsal amputation
transmission
    double-burst t.
    t. electron microscopy
    excitatory synaptic t.
    glutamatergic t.

iatrogenic t.
t. image
neuromuscular t.
pressure t.
train-of-four t.

transmucosal
t. administration
t. delivery
t. drug administration anesthetic technique

transmural
t. approach
t. closure
t. hydrostatic pressure gradient
t. inflammation
t. pressure

transmutation
transmyocardial
t. carbon dioxide laser revascularization
t. laser revascularization (TMLR, TMR)
t. perfusion pressure

transnasal
t. administration
t. bile duct catheterization
t. biopsy
t. endoscopy

transocular
transodontoid screw fixation
transolecranon approach
transomental hernia
transoral
t. approach
t. endoscopy
t. odontoid excision
t. odontoid resection
t. technique

transorbital
t. leukotomy
t. lobotomy
t. projection

transosseous suture
transpalatal
t. approach
t. exposure

transpapillary
t. approach
t. biopsy
t. cannulation
t. catheterization
t. drainage
t. endoscopic cholecystotomy

transparent adhesive dressing
transparietal
transpedicular
t. approach
t. percutaneous vertebroplasty
t. screw-rod fixation

transpelvic
t. amputation
t. gunshot wound

transperineal palladium-103 (^{103}Pd)
transperineurial passage
transperitoneal
t. approach
t. cesarean section
t. exposure
t. hand-assisted laparoscopic surgery
t. laparoscopic adrenalectomy
t. laparoscopic nephrectomy
t. laparoscopic nephroureterectomy

transplacental hemorrhage
transplant, transplantation
acute rejection of liver t.
adrenal medulla t.
adult-to-adult living related donor living t.
allogenic t.
allograft t.
anhepatic stage of liver t.
Arlt-Jaesche eyelash t.
autogenous tooth t.
autologous blood stem cell t.
autologous bone marrow t. (ABMT)
autologous lymph node t.
autologous osteochondral allograft t.
autologous ovarian t.
auxiliary t.
auxiliary partial orthotopic liver t. (APOLT)
Barnard heart t.
bilateral sequential lung t.
bladder-drained pancreas t.
Bosworth femoroischial t.
bowel t.
brain t.
bridge organ t.
cadaveric hand t.
cadaveric whole organ t.
cardiac t.
clinical intestinal t.
composite tissue t.
corneal t.
Cowen-Loftus toe-phalanx t.
cryopreserved extrapelvic ovarian t.
Del Toro hematopoietic stem cell t.
domino t.
double-lung t.
femoroischial t.
fetal cell t.
fetal liver t.
fetal thymus t.
fetal tissue t.
fresh extrapelvic ovarian t.
Gallie t.
heart t.
heart and lung t.

T

transplant (*continued*)
    hepatic t.
    hepatocyte t.
    heterotopic t.
    homogenous tooth t.
    homotopic t.
    intestinal t.
    kidney t.
    lamellar corneal t.
    liver t.
    living donor lobar lung t.
    living donor renal t.
    living-related donor t.
    living-related liver t. (LRLT)
    living-related small-bowel t.
    lung t.
    t. lung syndrome
    multivisceral t.
    muscle-tendon t.
    neonatal pulmonary t.
    t. nephrectomy
    Nizetic corneal t.
    organ t.
    orthoptic t.
    orthotopic heart t. (OHT)
    orthotopic liver t. (OLT)
    osteoarticular allograft t.
    PAK t.
    pancreas t. (PTX)
    pancreas-kidney t.
    pancreatic t.
    penetrating corneal t.
    piggyback liver t.
    pigment cell t.
    pituitary gland t.
    placental tissue t.
    post-living donor liver t.
    primarily vascularized organ t.
    pulmonary t.
    t. recipient
    reduced liver t. (RLT)
    reduced-size t.
    t. rejection
    rejection cardiomyopathy t.
    simultaneous kidney-pancreas t. (SKPT)
    simultaneous pancreas-kidney t.
    single-lung t. (SLT)
    SPK t.
    split-liver t. (SLT)
    syngeneic t.
    syngenesioplastic t.
    T-cell-depleted bone marrow t.
    tendon t.
    tissue t.
    tissue t.
    toe-phalanx t.
    tooth t.
    Townley-Paton corneal t.
    vein valve t.
    whole organ pancreas t.
    WOP t.
    xenograft t.

transplantation
    adult-to-adult live donor liver t.
    bone marrow t. (BMT)
    pancreaticoduodenal t.
    renal t.

transplantectomy

transplanted stamp graft

transpleural approach

transpleurodiaphragmatic

transport
    air critical care t.
    alveolar fluid t.
    bronchial mucus t.
    mitochondrial electron t.
    splanchnic oxygen t.

transportation

transposition
    carotid t.
    t. flap
    Jensen abducens palsy muscle t.
    t. of the great arteries (TGA)
    omentum-to-brain t.
    penoscrotal t.
    Strombeck nipple t.
    vein segment t.
    Z-plasty t.

transpubic incision

transpupillary cyclophotocoagulation

transpyloric plane

transradial approach

transrectal
    t. approach
    t. surgical treatment
    t. ultrasound-guided sextant biopsy (TRUS)

transrectus incision

transsacral
    t. fracture
    t. proctectomy

transsacrococcygeal ganglion impar block

transscaphoid
    t. dislocation fracture
    t. perilunate dislocation

transscleral suture

transscrotal

transsection (*var. of* transection)

transseptal
    t. approach
    t. left heart catheterization
    t. orchiopexy
    t. puncture

transsexualism

transsexual surgery

transsinus approach

transsphenoidal

t. approach
t. evacuation
t. hypophysectomy
t. microsurgical resection
t. operation
t. pituitary resection
t. removal
t. surgery
transsphincteric
t. anal fistula
t. approach
t. surgery
transstenotic pressure gradient measurement
transsternal approach
transsylvian approach
transtentorial
t. approach
t. herniation
transthermia
transthoracic
t. antireflux procedure
t. approach
t. discectomy
t. dissection
t. echocardiography
t. esophageal leak
t. esophagectomy
t. mediastinoscopy
t. needle aspiration (TTNA)
t. needle aspiration biopsy
t. Nissen fundoplication
t. percutaneous fine-needle aspiration biopsy
t. repair
t. route
t. ultrasonography
t. vertebral body resection
transthoracotomy
transtorcular approach
transtracheal
t. aspirate
t. aspiration (TTA)
t. jet
t. jet ventilation (TTJV)
t. jet ventilation anesthetic technique
transtriquetral
t. fracture
t. fracture-dislocation
transtrochanteric
t. approach
t. rotational osteotomy
transtubercular plane
transtympanic neurectomy
transubstantiation
transudation
transudative
t. ascites
t. inflammation

transumbilical breast augmentation (TUBA)
transureteroureteral anastomosis
transureteroureterostomy (TUU)
transurethral
t. ablative prostatectomy
t. balloon dilation
t. collagen injection therapy
t. electrical bladder stimulation
t. electrovaporization of prostate (TEVAP, TUEP, TUEVP, TUVP, TVP)
t. laser incision
t. marsupialization
t. microwave thermotherapy (TUMT)
t. needle ablation (TUNA)
t. resection
t. resection of bladder tumor (TURBT)
t. resection of prostate (TURP)
t. resection syndrome (TURS)
t. sphincterotomy
t. ultrasound-guided laser-induced prostatectomy (TULIP)
t. ureterorenoscopy
t. vaporization of prostate (TUVP)
transvaginal
t. approach
t. Burch procedure
t. fallopian tube catheterization
t. oocyte retrieval (TVOR)
t. tubal catheterization
t. ultrasonically guided oocyte retrieval
t. ultrasonographic examination
t. urethrolysis
transvalvular
t. gradient
t. pressure gradient
transvector
transvenous
t. approach
t. liver biopsy
t. therapy
transventricular
t. approach
t. mitral valve commissurotomy
transversalis fascia
transverse
t. abdominal muscle
t. anthelicine groove
apical t.
t. aponeurotic arch
t. approach
t. arytenoid muscle
t. cervical artery
t. cervical nerve
4-chamber t. (4C-T)
5-chamber t. (5C-T)

transverse (*continued*)
t. colectomy
t. colon
t. colostomy
t. comminuted fracture
t. costal facet
deep gastric t. (DG-T)
t. duodenotomy
t. facial
t. facial artery
t. facial fracture
t. fascia
t. fixation
t. fixator application
t. foramen
t. fundal incision
t. fundal incision of Strassman
t. head
t. incision
t. ligament rupture
t. loop rod colostomy
lower uterine segment t. (LUST)
t. magnetization phase
t. mastectomy
t. mastectomy incision
t. maxillary fracture
t. mesocolon
t. oval pelvis
t. palatine fold
t. pancreatic artery
t. pericardial sinus
t. plane
t. plane motion insufficiency
t. process
t. process fracture
t. projection
t. rectal fold
t. rectus abdominis muscle (TRAM)
t. rectus abdominis muscle flap
t. rectus abdominis muscle flap procedure
t. relaxation
t. relaxation rate
t. resection
t. scan
t. scanning
t. scapular artery
t. section
t. section imaging
t. section of heart
t. septum
t. skin incision
t. suture of Krause
t. tarsotomy
t. tenotomy
t. venous sinus
t. vesical fold
transversectomy

transversely oriented endplate compression fracture
transversocostal
transversospinal muscle
transversostomy
transversovertical index
transversus
t. abdominis aponeurosis
t. abdominis muscle
t. abdominis plane block
transxiphoid approach
Trantas operation
trapdoor
t. approach
t. fragment
t. incision
t. thoracotomy
trapezial
trapeziform
trapeziometacarpal
t. fusion
t. silicone arthroplasty
trapezium fracture
trapezius
t. flap
t. (muscle)
t. stimulation anesthetic technique
trapezoid
t. body
t. line
t. method
t. ridge
trapezoidal
t. incision
t. keratotomy
t. osteotomy
trapezoideum
trap incision
trapped lung
trapping
gas t.
Traube-Hering curve
Traube semilunar space
trauma
American Association for the Surgery of T. (AAST)
t. and injury severity scores probability of survival
avulsion t.
blunt abdominal t.
blunt hepatic t.
t. care
t. center
corneal t.
external t.
focused abdominal sonography for t. (FAST)
focused assessment with sonography for t. (FAST)

foreign body t.
genital tract t.
head t.
t. hemorrhage
hepatic t.
inadvertent t.
intraoral t.
pancreatic t.
t. patient
penetrating t.
penile t.
perineal impact t.
t. recidivism
renal t.
t. room
T. Score and Injury Severity Score (TRISS)
t. service
spinal t.
t. surgeon
t. surgery
surgical t.
t. system
t. team
thoracic t.
thoracoabdominal t.
tissue t.
truncal t.
t. victim
trauma-related death
traumasthenia
traumatic
t. amputation
t. anesthesia
t. aortic rupture
t. aortic transection
t. atlantooccipital dislocation
t. brain injury (TBI)
t. cardiac arrest
t. cervical disc herniation
t. choroidal rupture
T. Coma Data Bank
t. corneal abrasion
t. diaphragmatic hernia
t. false aneurysm
t. fistula
t. fracture
t. gangrene
t. hernia
t. inflammation
t. internal carotid artery dissection
t. intracranial hematoma
t. lesion
t. optic neuropathy
t. perforation
t. progressive encephalopathy
t. pseudomeningocele
t. renal mass

t. shear force
t. tetanus
traumatism
traumatize
traumatologist
orthopedic t.
traumatology
traumatonesis
traumatopathy
traumatopnea
traumatosepsis
traumatotherapy
Trautmann triangular space
Traverso-Longmire pancreatoduodenectomy technique
Treacher Collins syndrome
treadmill
t. exercise (TE)
t. exercise capacity
treatment
acidification t.
acorn t.
allocation of t.
alternative t.
anoplasty t.
antifungal t.
behavioral t.
bioelectric t.
chemotherapeutic t.
cholecystectomy t.
chronic anoplasty t.
coadjuvant t.
complementary t.
compression rod t.
computer-assisted t.
conservative surgical t.
continuous medical t.
definitive t.
diabetic retinal t.
dialysis t.
distraction/compression scoliosis t.
dual compression scoliosis t.
early active t.
endoscopic t.
endovascular graft t.
esophageal dilation t.
extracorporeal shock wave t. (ESWT)
ex utero intrapartum t. (EXIT)
ex vivo marrow t.
ferromagnetic microembolization t.
Gelfoam particles transarterial embolization t.
graft t.
hemodialysis t.
hepatic intraarterial yttrium-90 microspheres t.
insulin coma t.
intracavernosal injection t.

treatment (*continued*)
    intravesical chemotherapeutic t.
    iodine t.
    laparoscopic t.
    lipiodol transarterial embolization t.
    local t.
    locoregional t.
    medical t.
    mitomycin transarterial
      embolization t.
    t. modality
    multidisciplinary pain t. (MPT)
    neoadjuvant t.
    nonsurgical t.
    open surgical t.
    operative t.
    t. option
    palliative t.
    paraffin-film t.
    percutaneous endovascular t.
    photocoagulation t.
    placebo t.
    prophylactic antifungal t.
    radiation t.
    radioiodine t.
    rectovaginal surgical t.
    t. regimen
    retinal t.
    root canal t.
    t. sequencing
    sham t.
    t. strategy
    surgical t.
    transrectal surgical t.
    ureteral surgical t.
treatment-resistant rejection
tree
    biliary t.
    bronchial t.
    cannulation of biliary t.
    endobronchial t.
    extrahepatic biliary t.
    iliac arterial t.
    intrahepatic biliary t.
    tracheal-bronchial t.
    tracheobronchial t.
tree-barking urinary tract
trefoil
    t. deformity
    t. tendon
Treitz
    T. arch
    T. fascia
    T. fossa
    T. hernia
    T. ligament
    T. muscle
trellis formation
trema

trematode infection
tremor
    essential t.
    parkinsonian t.
    pill-rolling t.
Trendelenburg
    T. II great saphenous vein ligation
      operation
    T. I pulmonary embolism operation
    T. position
    T. tilt
trepanation (*var. of* trephination)
trepanning
    Argyll-Robertson glaucomatous
      eye t.
    Turner t.
trephination, trepanation
    corneal t.
    dental t.
    Elliot sclerocornea t.
    open-sky t.
trephine needle biopsy
***Treponema pallidum* immobilization**
  (TPI)
Trethowan metatarsal osteotomy
Trethowan-Stamm-Simmonds-Menelaus-
  Haddad technique
Treves
    T. appendicitis operation
    T. fold
    T. lumbar and last dorsal vertebrae
      operation
    T. psoas abscess operation
triad
    acute compression t.
    Beck t.
    Charcot t.
    hepatic t.
    t. knee repair
    portal t.
    Virchow t.
    wall-echo shadow t.
    Whipple t.
triadic therapy
triage
triaging
trial
    t. cementation
    European Carotid Surgery T.
      (ECST)
    Initiative on Methods, Measurement,
      and Pain Assessment in Clinical
      T.'s (IMMPACT)
    neuraxial medication t.
    neurostimulation t.
    t. of conservative therapy
    t. point
    random controlled t.
    t. reduction

triangle
anal t.
Assézat t.
auricular t.
axillary t.
Béclard t.
Burow t.
Calot t.
carotid t.
cephalic t.
cervical t.
Charcot t.
digastric t.
Elaut t.
facial t.
Farabeuf t.
femoral t.
fire t.
frontal t.
gastrinoma t.
Grynfeltt t.
Henke t.
Hesselbach t.
inferior carotid t.
inferior occipital t.
infraclavicular t.
inguinal t.
interscalene t.
Koch t.
Labbé t.
Langenbeck t.
Lesser t.
Lesshaft t.
Lieutaud t.
lumbar t.
lumbocostoabdominal t.
Macewen t.
Malgaigne t.
Marcille t.
muscular t.
occipital t.
omoclavicular t.
omotracheal t.
Petit lumbar t.
Pirogoff t.
posterior t.
pubourethral t.
retromolar t.
sacral t.
scalene t.
Scarpa t.
sternocostal t.
subclavian t.
subinguinal t.
submandibular t.
submaxillary t.
submental t.
suboccipital t.
superior carotid t.

supraclavicular t.
suprahyoid t.
suprameatal t.
tracheal t.
umbilicomammillary t.
urogenital t.
vesical t.
Weber t.
triangular
t. advancement flap
t. aponeurosis
t. bone
t. capsulotomy
t. cartilage
t. fascia
t. fibrocartilage complex (TFCC)
t. fold
t. fossa
t. ligament
t. ligament of liver
t. muscle
t. space
triangular-shaped skin
triangulation
indirect t.
t. stapling method
t. technique
triarticular complex
triaxial total elbow arthroplasty
tributary
venous t.
triceps
t. bursa
t. flap
t. tendon
trichangion
trichiasis repair
trichilemmoma, tricholemomma
desmoplastic t.
trichion
trichobezoar
trichodiscoma
tricholemmoma
tricholemomma (*var. of* trichilemmoma)
trichoma
Trichomonas **infection**
trichoscopy
trichrome-stained specimen
tricipital
trick
cough t.
triclofos
tricorn
tricornute
tricorrectional bunionectomy
tricuspid, tricuspidal, tricuspidate
t. insufficiency
t. position
t. regurgitation

tricuspid (*continued*)
    t. valve anuloplasty
    t. valve anulus
    t. valve area
    t. valve disease
    t. valve flow
    t. valve repair
    t. valvoplasty
tricuspidal (*var. of* tricuspid)
tricuspidate (*var. of* tricuspid)
tridermoma
Trieger hand-eye coordination test
triethiodide
    gallamine t.
trifacial nerve
trifid stomach
trifurcation
    t. injury
    t. involvement
    popliteal artery t.
trigastric
trigeminal
    t. cave
    t. cavity
    t. decompression
    t. dermatome
    t. ganglion
    t. impression
    t. nerve
    t. nerve block
    t. nerve root
    t. neuralgia
    t. nucleus caudalis
    t. rhizotomy
    t. tractotomy
trigeminocervical pain system
trigeminus
trigger
    t. point
    t. point deactivation
    t. point injection (TPI)
    t. point massage
triggered ventilation
triggering agent
trigger-point inactivation
trigona (*pl. of* trigonum)
trigonal ring
trigone
    habenular t.
    inguinal t.
    Lieutaud t.
    retromolar t.
    right fibrous t.
    vertebrocostal t.
trigonectomy
trigonitis
trigonocephaly
trigonum, *pl.* **trigona**
Trillat shoulder bone block procedure

trilobate, trilobed
trilobed (*var. of* trilobate)
trimalleolar ankle fracture
trimming
    tissue t.
trimodality therapy
triophthalmos
triotus
triphalangeal
    t. thumb
    t. thumb deformity
triphosphate
Tripier
    T. foot amputation
    T. operation throw square knot
triplane
    t. osteotomy
    t. tibial fracture
triple
    t. anastomosis
    t. arthrodesis
    t. heater meridian
    t. hemisection
    t. innominate osteotomy
    t. intrathecal therapy
    t. ligamentous repair
    t. lobe hepatectomy
    t. loop pouch
    t. point
triple-balloon valvoplasty
triple-lumen
    t.-l. catheter
    t.-l. infusion
triple-throw square knot stitch
triple-wire
    t.-w. procedure
    t.-w. technique
triplication
tripod
    t. fracture
    Haller t.
tripodia
tripoint
triquetral
    t. bone
    t. fracture
triquetrolunate dislocation
triquetropisiform articulation
triquetrous cartilage
triquetrum
triradial, triradiate
triradiate (*var. of* triradial)
    t. acetabular extensile approach
    t. line
    t. transtrochanteric approach
triradius
triscaphe fusion
trisection
    pulse t.

trisectionectomy
trisectorectomy
trisegmentectomy
trismus spasm
trisomy
    t. C, D syndrome
    t. 8 syndrome
trisplanchnic
TRISS
    Trauma Score and Injury Severity Score
    TRISS probability of survival
tristichia
triticeal cartilage
triticeum
trituration
trivalve
TRLI
    transfusion-related lung injury
trocar
    t. cystostomy
    t. drainage method
    t. gas leak
    t. injury
    t. placement
    t. site hernia
    t. technique
    t. wound
    t. wound bleeding
    t. wound site complication
trocar-cannula technique
2-trocar laparoscopic cholecystectomy
trocar-related injury
3-trocar technique cholecystectomy
trochanter
    greater t.
    lesser t.
    t. major
    t. minor
    small t.
    third t.
trochanterian (*var. of* trochanteric)
trochanteric, trochanterian
    t. bursa
    t. crest
    t. migration
    t. osteotomy
trochanterica
    bursa t.
trochanterplasty
trochantin
trochantinian
trochlea
trochlear
    t. fossa
    t. fovea
    t. nerve
    t. process
    t. synovial bursa

trochleariform
trochleariformis
trochlearis
trochleiform
trochoid
    t. articulation
    t. joint
Trolard vein
tromethamine
    ketorolac t.
Tronzo intertrochanteric fracture classification
trophectoderm biopsy
trophic
    t. fracture
    t. lesion
trophoblastic tissue
tropic hormone
tropisetron
tropism
    facet t.
    negative t.
    positive t.
Trotter syndrome
trough line
Trousseau
    T. point
    T. sign
Troutman radial keratotomy
Truc
    T. flap
    T. operation
Tru-Cut needle biopsy
true
    t. aneurysm
    t. diverticulum
    t. exfoliation
    t. hernia
    t. knot
    t. lymphedema
    t. muscle
    t. mutation
    t. negative
    t. pelvis
    t. positive
    t. rib
    t. size
    t. vertebra
    t. vocal cord
true-negative result
true-positive result
truly endocapsular microincision cataract surgery
Trumble talectomy
trumpet
    nasal t.
truncal
    t. lesion
    t. melanoma

truncal (*continued*)
  t. trauma
  t. vagotomy
  t. vagotomy and gastroenterostomy
  t. vagotomy and pyloroplasty
truncated
  t. exponential voltage
  t. tarsometatarsal wedge arthrodesis
truncated-wedge arthrodesis
truncation
  t. phenomenon
  protein t.
  uterine positioning via ligament
    investment fixation and t.
    (UPLIFT)
trunci (*pl. of* truncus)
truncus, *pl.* **trunci**
  t. (lymphaticus) bronchiomediastinalis
  t. medius
trunk
  accessory nerve t.
  anterior vaginal t.
  brachiocephalic t.
  bronchomediastinal t.
  celiac t.
  costocervical t.
  t. duplication
  hepatic venous t.
  hepatosplenomesenteric t.
  t. incurvation test
  intestinal t.
  jugular lymphatic t.
  linguofacial t.
  lumbar t.
  lumbosacral t.
  nerve t.
  posterior vaginal t.
  pulmonary t.
  subclavian lymphatic t.
  supraaortic t.
  sympathetic t.
  thoracoacromial t.
  thyrocervical t.
  upper t.
  vagal t.
  venous t.
TRUS
  transrectal ultrasound-guided sextant
    biopsy
Trusler
  T. aortic valve technique
  T. technique of aortic valvoplasty
trypsin
  crystallized t.
trypsinization
TSA
  total shoulder arthroplasty
Tsai-Stillwell distal radioulnar joint
  repair procedure

Tscherne-Gotzen tibial fracture and soft
  tissue damage classification
Tscherne soft tissue injury in closed
  fracture classification
T-shaped
  T-s. capsulotomy
  T-s. constriction ring
  T-s. incision
TSK
  Tampa Scale of Kinesophobia
T-spine
  thoracic spine
TSRH
  Texas Scottish Rite Hospital
  TSRH crosslink stabilization
  TSRH double-rod construct
  TSRH rod fixation
Tsui nerve stimulation catheter
  placement test
Tsuji laminoplasty
TTA
  tissue texture abnormality
  transtracheal aspiration
T-tack gastropexy
TTI
  total time to intubation
TTJV
  transtracheal jet ventilation
TTNA
  transthoracic needle aspiration
TTS
  through-the-scope
  TTS balloon dilation
TTTS
  twin-twin transfusion syndrome
T-tube
  T-t. drainage
  T-t. placement
  T-t. study
  T-t. tract
  T-t. tract choledochofiberoscopy
  T-t. tract choledochoscopy
tuba, *pl.* **tubae**
TUBA
  transumbilical breast augmentation
tubae (*pl. of* tuba)
tubage
tubal
  t. branch
  t. cannulation
  t. insufflation
  t. ligation
  t. ligation band technique
  t. permeability
  t. reconstruction surgery
  t. rupture
  t. sterilization
tubaria, *pl.* **tubariae**
  glandulae tubariae

tubariae (*pl. of* tubaria)
tubatorsion
tube
    auditory t.
    Baker t.
    Cantor t.
    t. cecostomy
    cholecystostomy t.
    t. decompression
    diagnostic t.
    digestive t.
    t. dilution test
    direct percutaneous endoscopic
      jejunostomy t.
    dislodged t.
    double-lumen endotracheal t.
    DPEJ t.
    embryonic neural t.
    end t.
    endothelial t.
    eustachian t.
    Ewald t.
    t. exchange technique
    t. extrusion
    fallopian t.
    t. feeding
    t. flap graft
    G t.
    gastric t.
    gastrojejunostomy t.
    t. gastrostomy
    gastrostomy t. (G tube)
    germ t.
    GJ t.
    Gowen decompression t.
    intestinal decompression t.
    King laryngeal t.
    knuckle of t.
    t. leakage
    Levin t.
    Magill-tip endotracheal t.
    t. malposition
    medullary t.
    t. migration
    Miller-Abbott t.
    molar t.
    Murphy eye of endotracheal t.
    Murphy-tip endotracheal t.
    nasoenteric feeding t.
    nasogastric t. (NGT)
    nasojejunal t.
    nasotracheal tube fixation using
      infant feeding t.
    neural t.
    obstructed t.
    PEG-J t.
    percutaneous endoscopic
      gastrojejunostomy t.
    t. placement

    t. precipitin test
    t. removal
    t. replacement
    retrograde percutaneous gastrostomy
      t.
    Robinson nephrostomy t.
    RPG t.
    S-B t.
    Sengstaken-Blakemore t.
    SG t.
    Swan-Ganz t.
    Thal Quik t.
    t. thoracostomy
    Univent t.
tube-carina distance
tubectomy
tubed
    t. free skin graft
    t. groin flap
    t. pedicle flap
    t. urethroplasty
tube-fed patient
tube-free tracheostomy
tube-over-needle airway insertion
tube-patient distance
tuber
    calcaneal t.
    cortical t.
    frontal t.
    omental t.
    parietal t.
tubercle
    accessory t.
    anatomic t.
    anterior t.
    auricular t.
    calcaneal t.
    carotid t.
    Chassaignac t.
    conoid t.
    corniculate t.
    cuneiform t.
    dental t.
    dissection t.
    dorsal radius t.
    genial t.
    genital t.
    Gerdy t.
    hard t.
    iliac t.
    inferior thyroid t.
    infraglenoid t.
    jugular t.
    labial t.
    Lisfranc t.
    Lister t.
    mamillary t.
    marginal t.
    maxillary t.

tubercle (*continued*)
    mental t.
    Morgagni t.
    obturator t.
    t. osteotomy
    pharyngeal t.
    Princeteau t.
    prosector t.
    pterygoid t.
    pubic t.
    quadrate femoral t.
    scalene t.
    soft t.
    superior thyroid t.
    supraglenoid t.
    supratragic t.
    wedge-shaped t.
    Whitnall orbital t.
    Wrisberg t.
    Zuckerkandl t.
tubercula (*pl. of* tuberculum)
tuberculation
tuberculization
tuberculocele
tuberculoma
tuberculosis (TB, TBC)
    central nervous
      system t.
    endobronchial t.
    endometrial t.
    extraarticular t.
    extrapulmonary t.
    extrathoracic t.
    exudative t.
    t. granulation tissue
    inhalation t.
    peritoneal t.
    reactivation t.
    reinfection t.
    splenic t.
    surgical t.
tuberculous
    t. abscess
    t. arthritis
    t. caseation
    t. empyema
    t. infiltration
    t. lesion
tuberculum, *pl.* **tubercula**
    first-degree t.
    t. impar
    Zuckerkandl t.
tuberoinfundibular tract
tuberositas
tuberosity
    costal t.
    t. fragment
    masseteric t.
    pterygoid t.

    reduction t.
    t. reduction
tuberous
    t. sclerosis
    t. sclerosis-associated renal cell
      carcinoma
    t. sclerosis-associated tumor
    t. sclerosis complex
tube-shift technique
tube-to-film distance
tube-within-tube technique
tubi (*pl. of* tubus)
tuboabdominal
tuboligamentous
tuboovarian abscess
tuboperitoneal
tuboplasty
    balloon t.
    transcervical balloon t.
    ultrasound transcervical t.
tubotorsion, tubatorsion
tubouterine implantation
tubovaginal
tubular
    t. aneurysm
    t. basement membrane
    t. carcinoma
    t. colonic duplication
    t. excretory mass
    t. reconstruction
    t. regeneration
    t. respiration
    t. vertical gastroplasty
tubularized
    t. bladder neck
      reconstruction
    t. cecal flap
tubulation
tubule
    Albarran y Dominguez t.
    convoluted seminiferous t.
    Henle t.
    mesonephric t.
    paragenital t.
    straight seminiferous t.
    uriniferous t.
tubuli (*pl. of* tubulus)
tubulization
    gastric t.
tubulovillous
    t. adenoma
    t. lesion
tubulus, *pl.* **tubuli**
tubus, *pl.* **tubi**
Tu cardiac surgery risk
  score
tuck
    t. position
    t. procedure

Tudor-Thomas
    T.-T. corneal graft
    T.-T. operation
TUEP
    transurethral electrovaporization of
    prostate
TUEVP
    transurethral electrovaporization of
    prostate
Tuffier morcellement technique
tufted angioma
tuft fracture
tug
    tracheal t.
tularemia
TULIP
    transurethral ultrasound-guided
    laser-induced prostatectomy
tumbler
    t. flap
    t. graft
tumbling
    t. procedure
    t. technique
    t. technique operation
tumescent
    t. liposuction technique
    t. technique breast reduction
tummy tuck flap
tumor
    abdominal t.
    t. ablation
    Abrikosov t.
    adenoid t.
    adrenal gland t.
    alveolar t.
    ampullary t.
    t. angiogenesis
    t. antigen
    antral t.
    aortic body t.
    t. ascites
    t. bed
    benign bone t.
    benign germ cell t.
    biliary tract t.
    Bismuth classification I-IV of
      Klatskin t.
    bleeding t.
    blood t.
    t. blood supply
    blood vessel t.
    t. blush
    body t.
    bone t.
    brain t.
    brown-fat t.
    t. bulk
    t. burden

Buschke-Löwenstein t.
t. capsule
carcinoid t.
cardiac t.
carotid body t.
celiac t.
t. cell
t. cell-host bone relationship
t. cell purging
cervical t.
colon t.
colorectal primary t.
debulking of t.
deep t.
t. defect
diffuse t.
discrete t.
distal t.
t. dormancy mode
t. doubling time
dumbbell t.
dumbbelling of t.
duodenal t.
t. embolism
embryonal t.
t. encapsulation
endocrine t.
t. erosion
esophageal t.
exogenous t.
extrahepatic t.
eye t.
eyelid t.
t. feature
focal t.
focus of t.
t. formation
fungating t.
gastric stromal t.
gastrointestinal stromal t.
  (GIST)
genital tract t.
glial t.
glomus t.
t. grade
t. grading
gritty t.
t. growth
gynecologic t.
hepatic t.
hyperplastic t.
hypervascular t.
t. hypoxia
t. imaging
t. infiltration
infratentorial t.
t. initiation
t. in situ
intracranial t.

T

tumor (*continued*)

intraductal papillary mucinous t. (IPMT)
intraluminal t.
intramedullary t.
intramyocardial t.
t. invasion
invasive t.
islet cell t.
isolated metastatic t.
t. kinetic model
Klatskin t.
lacrimal gland t.
liver t.
t. location
lumbar t.
lung t.
t. lysis syndrome
malignant t.
margins free of t.
margins with t.
t. marker
t. mass
mediastinal t.
metastatic t.
midbody t.
mixed t.
mucoepidermoid t.
multifocal t.
musculoskeletal t.
t. necrosis
t. neovasculature
neuroendocrine t.
tumor, node, metastasis (TNM)
tumor, node, metastasis classification
tumor, node, metastasis staging
nonfamilial malignant endocrine t.
nonfunctional malignant t.
nonfunctioning islet cell t.
nonpolypoid t.
nonseminomatous testicular t.
ocular t.
optic nerve t.
oral cavity t.
orbital t.
t. origin
ovarian t.
t. oxygenation
Pancoast t.
pancreatic endocrine t.
pancreatic neuroendocrine t.
parathyroid t.
periampullary t.
phyllodes t.
pituitary t.
t. ploidy
t. plop
polypoid t.
t. polysaccharide substance

potato t.
primary parathyroid hyperplastic t.
t. progression
t. promoter
proximal t.
pulmonary t.
t. receptor protein negative
t. recurrence
recurrent t.
t. registry
t. regression
t. removal
renal t.
t. resectability
resectable t.
t. resection
resection margin free of t. (R0)
retroperitoneal t.
retrorectal t.
sacral bone t.
sacrococcygeal t.
salivary gland t.
t. seeding
sellar t.
t. shrinkage
Siewert type I–III t.
sinonasal t.
t. site
t. size
t. skin test
skull base t.
solid t.
space-occupying t.
t. specific
t. spillage
spinal cord t.
sporadic islet cell t.
t. stage
t. stage grouping
t. staging
t. stenting
t. subtype
t. suppressor
t. suppressor oncogene
supratentorial t.
t. surgery
synchronous t.
tail t.
t. targeting
temporal bone t.
testicular t.
t. therapy
t. thrombus
thyroid t.
t. to cerebellum ratio
tracheal t.
transurethral resection of bladder t. (TURBT)

tuberous sclerosis-associated t.
t. ulceration
unresectable t.
vascular t.
t. vascularity
vasoactive intestinal polypeptide t.
   (VIPoma)
t. vessel
t. volume
von Hippel-Lindau t.
Wilms t.
Wilms renal t.
tumor-bearing kidney
tumor-cell product
tumorectomy
tumor-free margin
tumorigenesis
   foreign body t.
tumorlike bone condition
tumor-related death
tumor-targeting ability
TUMT
   transurethral microwave
      thermotherapy
TUNA
   transurethral needle ablation
tunable dye laser lithotripsy
tunic, tunica
   mucosal t.
   muscular t.
tunica (*var. of* tunic)
   t. muscularis
tunicae
tunicary hernia
tunnel
   t. and sling fixation
   axillofemoral t.
   catheter t.
   t. creation
   t. graft
   t. infection
   t. of Wertheim
   Witzel t.
tunneled
   t. epidural catheter
   t. ventriculostomy
tunneling
Tupper arthroplasty
turbid peritoneal fluid
turbinal
turbinate, turbinated
turbinated (*var. of* turbinate)
   t. bone
turbinectomy
turbinoplasty
turbo spin-echo sequence
TURBT
   transurethral resection of bladder
      tumor

Türck
   T. bundle
   T. tract
Turco
   T. clubfoot release technique
   T. release of joint capsule in
      clubfoot procedure
Turco-Spinella tendo calcaneus repair
Turcot syndrome
Turkish saddle
Türk line
turn-and-suction biopsy technique
Turnbull
   T. blowhole operation
   T. colostomy
   T. end-loop ileostomy
   T. loop stoma
   T. ostomy operation
   T. temporary diverting ileostomy
      technique
turned-down tendon flap
turned-up pulp deformity
Turner
   T. syndrome
   T. trepanning
Turner-Warwick and Ashken
   cecocystoplasty technique
turnover flap
TURP
   transurethral resection of prostate
TURS
   transurethral resection syndrome
turunda, *pl.* **turundae**
turundae (*pl. of* turunda)
tuss
   cough
tutamen, *pl.* **tutamina**
tutamina (*pl. of* tutamen)
TUU
   transureteroureterostomy
TUVP
   transurethral electrovaporization of
      prostate
   transurethral vaporization of
      prostate
TVI
   total vascular isolation
TVOR
   transvaginal oocyte retrieval
TVP
   transurethral electrovaporization of
      prostate
TWA
   total wrist arthroplasty
Tweed dentofacial analysis method
T1-weighted spin-echo image
T2-weighted spin-echo image
twelfth cranial nerve
twilight sleep

T

twin
- t. bracket tooth rotation
- t. formation
- t. method
- t. operating theater
- thoracopagus t.

Twining line
twin-twin transfusion syndrome (TTTS)
twirling scalp acupuncture method
twisted
- t. fundoplication
- t. suture technique
- t. virgin silk suture

twist-off technique
twitch
- t. depression
- evoked t.
- t. height
- t. height test
- t. response
- t. suppression
- t. tension

two-compartment pharmacokinetic model
Tycos pressure infusion line
tylectomy
tylion
tyloma
tympana (*pl. of* tympanum)
tympani
- chorda t.

tympanic
- t. bone
- t. canal
- t. canaliculus
- t. cavity
- t. membrane (TM)
- t. membrane measurement
- t. neurectomy
- t. notch
- t. plexus
- t. ring
- t. sinus
- t. thermometry

tympanitic abdomen
tympanohyal bone
tympanomastoid
- t. fissure
- t. suture

tympanomastoidectomy
tympanomeatal flap
tympanoplasty
- t. mastoidectomy
- t. ossiculoplasty
- staged t.
- type I–V t.

tympanosquamosal suture
tympanosquamous fissure
tympanotemporal
tympanum, *pl.* **tympana,** *pl.*
tympanums
tympanums (*pl. of* tympanum)
tyndallization
type
- t. B-1, -2 lesion
- depressed t.
- histologic t.
- 5-hydroxytryptamine t. 3
- t. II endoleak
- t. I, II, III, IIIA, IIIB, IIIC open fracture
- t. I–IV canal
- t. I–V tympanoplasty
- macroscopic t.
- superficial t.
- ulcerated t.

typhlectasis
typhlectomy
typhlodicliditis
typhloempyema
typhlolithiasis
typhlon
typhlopexia (*var. of* typhlopexy)
typhlopexy, typhlopexia
typhlorrhaphy
typhlostomy
typhlotomy
typhloureterostomy
typhoidal cholecystitis
typical skin lesion
typing
- tissue t.

tyroma
Tyrrell fascia
Tyson gland

U

U pouch
U pouch construction

UA

umbilical arterial
umbilical artery
uterine artery
UA blood

UAL

ultrasonic-assisted liposuction

UAO

upper airway obstruction

UC

ulcerative colitis

Uchida abdominal tubal sterilization technique

UE

upper extremity

UESR

upper esophageal sphincter relaxation

UGCR

ultrasound-guided compression repair

UGI

upper gastrointestinal
UGI endoscopy
UGI tract

Uhl

U. anomaly
U. malformation

UICC

Union Internationale Contre le Cancer
UICC tumor classification

UID

unilateral interfacetal dislocation

ulcer

aphthous u.
arterial insufficiency u.
u. bed
bleeding duodenal u.
cervical u.
collar-buttonlike u.
Cruveilhier u.
diabetic neuropathic u.
duodenal u.
gastric u.
genital u.
ischemic u.
neuropathic u.
oral aphthous u.
penetrating u.
peptic u.
perforated peptic u.
postsclerotherapy u.
pressure u.
ring u.

scrotal skin u.
skin u.
solitary rectal u.
venous stasis u.

ulcerated

u. mucosa
u. type

ulceration

acetylsalicylic acid-induced gastric u.
acute hemorrhagic u.
anal u.
anastomotic u.
aphthous u.
ASA-induced gastric u.
catarrhal marginal u.
CMV-associated u.
CMV-induced esophageal u.
collar-button u.
corneal u.
diffuse u.
duodenal u.
esophageal u.
gastric u.
gastrointestinal u.
genital u.
herpes epithelial tropic u.
intertrigo with u.
intestinal u.
ischemic infected u.
labial u.
linear u.
marginal u.
mucosal u.
mucous membrane u.
nasal mucosal u.
necrotic u.
oral u.
patchy colonic u.
plaque u.
postbulbar u.
radiation-induced u.
rectal u.
rheumatoid-related u.
serpiginous u.
stasis u.
stercoral u.
stomal u.
stress u.
stress-induced gastric u.
sublesional u.
tracheal u.
tumor u.

ulcerative

u. colitis (UC)
u. inflammation

U

ulcerogenic fistula
ulcerogranuloma
ulectomy
ulegyria
uletomy
Ullmann line
ulna, *pl.* **ulnae**
ulnae (*pl. of* ulna)
ulnar
    u. artery
    u. branch
    u. bursa
    u. collateral ligament rupture
    u. deviation deformity
    u. drift deformity
    u. fracture
    u. head
    u. head excision
    u. hemiresection interposition
      arthroplasty
    u. motor neurectomy
    u. translation
ulnari
ulnaris
    extensor carpi u. (ECU)
ulnocarpal abutment syndrome
ulocarcinoma
uloid
U-loop nephrostomy
ulotomy
Ultane
Ultiva
ultrabrachycephalic
ultrafast
    u. CT electron beam tomography
    u. magnetic resonance imaging
      (UMRI)
    u. spiral computed tomography
ultrafiltration
    continuous arteriovenous u. (CAVU)
    dialytic u.
    extracorporeal u. (ECU)
    glomerular u.
    modified u.
    spontaneous dialytic u.
UltraFit PK suture
UltraGlide corneal transplant suture
ultrahigh-frequency ventilation
ultrahigh-magnification endoscopy
ultraligation
ultralow
    u. anterior resection
    u. anterior resection parastomal
      infection
ultramicroscopy
ultrarapid subthreshold stimulation
ultrasonic
    u. aspiration
    u. attenuation

    u. cutting
    u. dissection
    u. endovaginal finding
    u. fragmentation
    u. lithotresis
    u. lithotripsy
    u. nebulizer
    u. therapy
ultrasonic-assisted liposuction (UAL)
ultrasonication
ultrasonographic
    u. data
    u. examination
    u. technique
ultrasonographically guided injection
ultrasonography
    carotid duplex u.
    color duplex u.
    contrast-enhanced u.
    Doppler duplex u.
    duplex u.
    endoanal u.
    endoscopic u. (EUS)
    high-resolution u.
    intraoperative u. (IOUS)
    laparoscopic u. (LUS)
    laparoscopic intracorporeal u. (LICU)
    laparoscopic intraoperative u.
      (LIOUS)
    open intraoperative u.
    transabdominal u.
    transanal u.
    transthoracic u.
    venous duplex u.
ultrasonography-guided fine-needle
aspiration biopsy
ultrasonosurgery
ultrasound
    u. anesthetic technique
    cervical u.
    Doppler u.
    endoscopic u. (EUS)
    endoscopic esophageal u. (EUS)
    u. examination
    u. guidance
    u. image
    intraoperative u. (IOUS)
    in vivo duplex u.
    laparoscopic u. (LUS)
    preoperative u.
    u. therapy
    thyroid u.
    u. transcervical tuboplasty
ultrasound-assisted percutaneous
endoscopic gastrostomy
ultrasound-guided
    u.-g. anterior subcostal liver biopsy
    u.-g. automated large-core breast
    biopsy

u.-g. bronchoscopy
u.-g. caudal epidural needle placement
u.-g. compression
u.-g. compression repair (UGCR)
u.-g. core breast biopsy
u.-g. core needle biopsy (US-CNB)
u.-g. echo biopsy
u.-g. fine-needle aspiration
u.-g. fine-needle aspiration biopsy (US-FNAB)
u.-g. lumbar facet nerve block
u.-g. needle biopsy
u.-g. nephrostomy puncture
u.-g. regional anesthesia
u.-g. shockwave therapy
u.-g. stereotactic biopsy
ultraterminal excementosis
ultrathin
ultraviolet (UV)
u. blood irradiation
ultropaque rapid tissue analysis method
umbilectomy
umbilical
aberrant u.
u. arterial (UA)
u. artery (UA)
u. artery blood
u. artery catheterization
u. circulation
u. cord
u. cord anomaly
u. cord blood stem cells
u. cord hematoma
u. fissure
u. fistula
u. flap
u. fossa
u. hernia
u. hernia rupture
u. herniorrhaphy
u. mass
u. notch
u. plane
u. plate
u. port
u. prevesical fascia
u. region
u. ring
u. skin-knife incision
u. tape suture
u. vein (UV)
u. vein blood
u. vein catheterization
u. vein recanalization
u. vein to maternal vein
u. vein to maternal vein ratio (UV:MV)
u. venous

umbilicate, umbilicated
umbilicated (*var. of* umbilicate)
umbilication
umbilici (*pl. of* umbilicus)
umbilicomammillary triangle
umbilicovesical fascia
umbilicus, *pl.* **umbilici**
umbo
umbrascopy
umbrella closure
UMRI
ultrafast magnetic resonance imaging
UMSS
University of Michigan Sedation Scale
unabsorbable suture
unanticipated hepatic disease
unattended laboratory operation
unavoidable hemorrhage
unbanded gastroplasty
uncal herniation
unci (*pl. of* uncus)
unciform bone
uncinate
u. bundle of Russell
u. groove
u. pancreas
u. process
u. process fracture
u. process mass
uncinectomy
uncipressure
uncomminuted fracture
uncommitted metaphysial lesion
uncomplicated
u. acute cholecystitis
u. angiomyolipoma
unconstrained shoulder arthroplasty
uncontained
u. hemorrhage
u. leak
uncontrollable glaucoma
uncontrolled hemorrhage
uncoupling
cardiac u.
uncovertebral joint
uncus, *pl.* **unci**
uncut
u. Collis-Nissen fundoplication
u. Collis-Nissen fundoplication method
u. Collis-Nissen fundoplication procedure
u. Collis-Nissen fundoplication technique
underangulation
undercorrection
undercut
soft tissue u.

U

underlay fascia technique
underlying
  u. cardiomyopathy
  u. cause
  u. structure
underresuscitated
underresuscitation
undersensing
  pacemaker u.
underventilation
underwater seal for pneumothorax
undescended testis
undifferentiated
  u. adenocarcinoma
  u. connective tissue disease
  u. embryonal sarcoma
  u. lesion
  u. squamous cell carcinoma
undifferentiation
undisplaced fracture
undiversion
Undritz anomaly
undulating, undulatory
  u. membrane
undulatory (*var. of* undulating)
undyed suture
unfiltered
  u. preparation
  u. radioisotope
unfractionated
  u. heparin antibody
  u. heparin-induced thrombocytopenia
  u. heparin reversal
  u. heparin therapy
ungual
  u. fibroma
  u. labia
  u. labia fold
ungues (*pl. of* unguis)
unguis, *pl.* **ungues**
uniaxial joint
unicaliceal kidney
unicanalicular sphincter
unicompartmental knee arthroplasty
  (UKA)
unicondylar fracture
unidirectional valve
unification
unifocal optic nerve lesion
unilateral
  u. adrenalectomy
  u. aldosteronoma
  u. amputee
  u. anesthesia
  u. cyst
  u. diaphragmatic elevation
  u. facial swelling
  u. hemidysplasia cornification
  disorder

  u. hemilaminectomy
  u. hernia
  u. hypophysectomy
  u. inguinal hernia repair
  u. inguinal hernia repair method
  u. inguinal hernia repair procedure
  u. inguinal hernia repair technique
  u. interfacetal dislocation (UID)
  u. laryngeal paralysis
  u. lavage
  u. lobectomy
  u. neck exploration
  u. nephrectomy
  u. pallidotomy
  u. parathyroidectomy
  u. pedicle cannulation
  u. pneumoretroperitoneum
  u. resection
  u. sacroiliac approach
  u. salpingo-oophorectomy
  u. subcostal incision
  u. supraglottic edema
  u. testicular torsion
  u. thyroidectomy
  u. vocal cord paralysis
unilobar disease
unilocular
  u. cyst
  u. cystic lesion
  u. joint
unimalleolar fracture
uninhibited neurogenic bladder
uninterrupted suture technique
union
  delayed fracture u.
  fibrous u.
  U. Internationale Contre le Cancer
  (UICC)
  osteonal bone u.
  primary u.
  secondary u.
  vicious u.
unipedicled flap
unipedicle transverse rectus abdominus
  flap
unipennate muscle
unipolar
  u. cauterization
  u. disorder
uniportal arthroscopic microdiscectomy
unique
  u. NCRLM
  u. noncolorectal liver metastasis
unit
  autologous blood u.
  autologous RBC u.
  cardiac surgical recovery u.
  Confusion Assessment Method for
  Intensive Care U. (CAM-ICU)

day care surgical u. (DCSU)
electrosurgery u. (ESU)
inpatient dialysis u.
intensive care u. (ICU)
low-grade suction u.
u. membrane
neurosurgical intensive care u. (NSICU)
u. of mass
postanesthesia care u. (PACU)
surgical admitting u.

united
U. Kingdom Heart Valve Registry
U. Network for Organ Sharing (UNOS)
U. States Renal Data System (USRDS)

uniting
u. canal
u. cartilage
u. duct

unitunnel technique
Univent tube
Universal Spine System (USS)
University
U. of Michigan Sedation Scale (UMSS)
U. of Pennsylvania smell identification test (UPSIT)

unlocking spiral technique
unmonitored local anesthesia
Unna boot
UNOS
United Network for Organ Sharing
unplanned valgus osteotomy
unreamed nailing
unreduced dislocation
unremitting symptom
unrepositioned flap
unresectability
unresectable
u. extrahepatic disease
u. hepatoblastoma
u. lesion
u. metastasis
u. periampullary cancer
u. tumor

unresuscitated
unroofing
unsaturated chemical vapor sterilization
unsex
unshuntable portal hypertension
unstable
u. angina
u. bladder
u. fracture
u. fracture-dislocation

unstrained jaw relation
unstriated muscle, unstriped muscle

unstriped muscle
untethering procedure
untreated
u. HPT
u. hyperparathyroidism
u. tetralogy of Fallot

ununited fracture
unusual opportunistic infection
Unverricht-Lundborg syndrome
unwanted screw torque
up-and-down staircases procedure
UPF
uvulopalatal flap
upgated technique
UPJ
ureteropelvic junction
UPLIFT
uterine positioning via ligament investment fixation and truncation
UPLIFT procedure
UPP
uvulopalatoplasty
upper
u. abdominal evisceration
u. adenoma
u. aerodigestive tract
u. airway obstruction (UAO)
u. alimentary endoscopy
u. arm straight graft
u. cervical spine anterior exposure
u. cervical spine fusion
u. cervical spine procedure
u. dorsal sympathectomy
u. end
u. endoscopy and colonoscopy
u. esophageal sphincter relaxation (UESR)
u. extremity (UE)
u. extremity lymphedema
u. extremity nerve block
u. eyelid
u. gastrointestinal (UGI)
u. gastrointestinal bleeding
u. gastrointestinal endoscopy
u. gastrointestinal hemorrhage
u. gastrointestinal panendoscopy
u. gastrointestinal tract
u. gastrointestinal tract foreign body
u. gastrointestinal tract surgery
u. genital tract infection
u. incisor angulation
u. intestinal endoscopy
u. jaw
u. jaw bone
u. jejunal motility
u. jejunal motor pattern
u. jejunum
u. lateral quadrant
u. lid

upper (*continued*)
    u. lip
    u. lip bite test
    u. medial quadrant
    u. mediastinum
    u. midline incision
    u. respiratory infection
    u. respiratory tract
    u. respiratory tract infection
    u. respiratory tract mucosa
    u. small-bowel motor disturbance
    u. sternal split
    u. subscapular nerve
    u. thoracic wall
    u. thorax aperture
    u. tract disease
    u. trapezius flap
    u. trunk

UPPP
    uvulopalatopharyngoplasty

upright
    u. position
    u. reflux

upright-Y incision

upside-down stomach

upsiloid

UPSIT
    University of Pennsylvania smell
    identification test

uptake
    local lymphatic u.
    lymphatic u.
    placental u.
    radioactive iodine u.
    (RAIU, RIU)
    radioisotope u.

upward

urachal
    u. carcinoma
    u. fistula
    u. fold
    u. ligament

urachi
    plica u.

uraniscoplasty

uraniscorrhaphy

uranoplasty
    Wardill-Kilner 4-flap u.

uranorrhaphy

uranostaphyloplasty,
  Uranostaphylorrhaphy

uranostaphylorrhaphy, uranostaphyloplasty

uraroma

urate

urate-associated inflammation

uratoma

urban
    U. operation
    u. trauma center

Urbaniak
    U. neurovascular free
    flap
    U. scapular flap

urea hydrolysis

urea-impermeable membrane

urecchysis

uredema, uroedema

urelcosis

uremia, urinemia

uremia-related coagulopathy

uremic
    u. coma
    u. gastrointestinal lesion
    u. inflammation

ureter
    curlicue u.
    ectopic u.
    extravesical infrasphincteric
    ectopic u.
    u. implantation
    postcaval u.
    retrocaval u.
    retroiliac u.

ureteral, ureteric
    u. bladder augmentation
    u. branch
    u. carcinoma
    u. catheterization
    u. colic
    u. duplication
    u. ectopia
    u. fistula
    u. infarction
    u. injury
    u. leak
    u. meatotomy
    u. meatus
    u. obstruction
    u. patch procedure
    u. perforation
    u. plexus
    u. pressure
    u. reimplantation
    u. spatulation
    u. stent placement
    u. stoma
    u. stoma removal
    u. surgical treatment

ureteralgia

ureterectasia

ureterectomy
    distal u.

ureteric
    u. branch
    u. colic
    u. fold
    u. pelvis
    u. stoma

ureteris
    orificium u.
ureteritis
ureterocalicostomy
ureterocele
    ectopic u.
    orthotopic u.
    pyoureter ectopic u.
ureterocelorraphy
ureterocolic fistula
ureterocolonic anastomosis
ureterocolostomy, ureterosigmoidostomy
    ileocecal u.
    Maydl u.
ureterocutaneous fistula
ureterocystoneostomy
    Gil-Vernet u.
ureterocystoplasty
ureterocystostomy
ureteroendoscopy
ureteroenteric
ureteroenterostomy
ureterohydronephrosis
ureteroileal anastomosis
ureteroileocecoproctostomy
ureteroileoneocystostomy
ureteroileostomy
    Bricker u.
ureterointestinal urinary diversion
ureterolithiasis
ureterolithotomy
    laparoscopic u.
ureterolysis
    combined u.
    extravesical u.
    intravesical u.
    Lich-Gregoir u.
    Pacquin u.
    Politano-Leadbetter u.
ureteroneocystostomy
    Glenn-Anderson u.
    u. herniation
    Hutch u.
    Politano-Leadbetter u.
    reoperative u.
ureteroneopyelostomy,
  ureteropyeloneostomy
ureteronephrectomy
ureteropelvic
    u. junction (UPJ)
    u. obstruction
ureteropelvioneostomy
ureteropelvioplasty (*var. of*
  ureteropyeloplasty)
ureteroperitoneal fistula
ureteroplasty
    ileal patch u.
ureteroproctostomy, ureterorectostomy
ureteropyelitis

ureteropyeloneostomy (*var. of*
  ureteroneopyelostomy)
ureteropyelonephrostomy
ureteropyeloplasty, ureteropelvioplasty
ureteropyeloscopy
    flexible u.
ureteropyelostomy
ureteropyosis
ureterorectostomy (*var. of*
  ureteroproctostomy)
ureterorenoscopy
    transurethral u.
ureterorrhagia
ureterorrhaphy
ureteroscopy
    rigid u.
ureterosigmoid anastomosis
ureterosigmoidostomy
ureterostegnosis (*var. of* ureterostenosis)
ureterostenoma
ureterostenosis, ureterostegnosis,
  ureterostenoma
ureterostoma
ureterostomy
    cutaneous loop u.
    Davis intubated u.
    high-loop cutaneous u.
    low-loop cutaneous u.
    retroperitoneal cutaneous u.
ureterotomy
    Davis intubated u.
    intubated u.
ureterotrigonoenterostomy
ureterotubal anastomosis
ureteroureteral anastomosis
ureteroureterostomy
ureterouterine fistula
ureterovaginal fistula
ureterovesical obstruction
ureterovesicoplasty
    Leadbetter-Politano u.
ureterovesicostomy
urethane
urethra
    anterior u.
    female u.
    fixed drain pipe u.
    male u.
    membranous u.
    penile u.
    posterior u.
    prostatic u.
    spongy u.
urethral
    u. artery
    u. atresia
    u. calculus
    u. carcinoma
    u. caruncle

U

urethral (*continued*)
    u. closure mechanism
    u. closure pressure profile
    u. coaptation
    u. crest
    u. dilation
    u. diverticulectomy
    u. gland
    u. groove
    u. lacuna
    u. opening
    u. papilla
    u. pressure
    u. pressure measurement
    u. sphincter
    u. sphincterotomy
    u. suspension
    u. syndrome
    u. vesicle suspension procedure
urethralgia
urethralis
urethrectomy
urethremorrhagia (*var. of* urethrorrhagia)
urethrism, urethrismus, urethrospasm
urethrismus (*var. of* urethrism)
urethritis
urethrobalanoplasty
urethrobulbar
urethrocavernous fistula
urethrocele
urethrocystometry
urethrocystopexy, urethropexy
    Gittes u.
    Lapides u.
    Marshall-Marchetti-Krantz u.
    retropubic u.
    Stamey u.
urethrocystoscopy
urethrodynia
urethrography
urethrohymenal fusion
urethrolysis
    retropubic u.
    transvaginal u.
urethropenile
urethroperineal fistula
urethroperineoscrotal
urethropexy (*var. of* urethrocystopexy)
urethroplasty
    Badenoch u.
    Cantwell-Ransley u.
    Cecil u.
    modified Young u.
    onlay island flap u.
    pedicle flap u.
    prostatic u.
    retrograde transurethral prostatic u.
    Tanagho bladder flap u.

    Thiersch-Duplay u.
    tubed u.
urethroprostatic
urethrorectal fistula
urethrorrhagia, urethremorrhagia
urethrorrhaphy
urethrorrhea
urethroscopic
urethroscopy
    retropubic u.
urethrospasm
urethrostaxis
urethrostenosis
urethrostomy
    perineal u.
    Poncet perineal u.
urethrotomy
    direct-vision internal u.
    endoscopic optical u.
    external u.
    internal u.
    perineal u.
    Syme external u.
    Wheelhouse perineal u.
urethrovaginal fistula
urethrovesical (UV)
    u. anastomosis
urethrovesicopexy
urge incontinence
urgency incontinence
URI
    upper respiratory infection
    upper respiratory tract infection
uricosuria
urinariae
    cervix vesicae u.
urinarius
    meatus u.
urinary
    u. apparatus
    u. bladder
    u. bladder rupture
    u. calcium excretion
    u. calculus
    u. catheterization
    u. conduit
    u. diversion
    u. EGF
    u. exertional incontinence
    u. extravasation
    u. extraversion
    u. fistula
    u. incontinence
    u. organ
    u. retention
    u. sand

u. stuttering
u. tract
u. tract abnormality
u. tract anomaly
u. tract disease
u. tract disorder
u. tract infection (UTI)
u. tract injury
u. tract obstruction
u. tract reconstruction
urinary-rectal fistula
urinary-umbilical fistula
urinary-vaginal fistula
urination
delayed u.
urine
extravasated u.
u. specimen collection
urinemia (*var. of* uremia)
uriniferous tubule
urinogenital
urinogenous, urogenous
urinoma
urinoscopy
urinosexual
urocele
urocheras (*var. of* uropsammus)
urochesia
urocyst
urocystic
urocystis
urodynamics
urodynia
uroedema (*var. of* uredema)
urogenital
u. anomaly
u. apparatus
u. canal
u. cleft
u. diaphragm
u. fistula
u. membrane
u. region
u. ridge
u. septum
u. sinus
u. tract
u. triangle
urogenous
urogram
excretory u.
urokinase thrombolysis
urolith
urolithiasis
urolithic
urolithology
urologic, urological
u. anesthesia
u. complication

u. evaluation
u. laparoscopic surgical procedure
u. oncology
u. operation
u. surgery
u. system cancer
urological (*var. of* urologic)
urologist
pediatric u.
urology
pediatric u.
uroncus
uronephrosis
uronoscopy (*var. of* uroscopy)
uropathy
obstructive u.
uropoiesis
uropoietic
uropsammus, urocheras
urorectal
u. membrane
u. septum
uroschesis
uroscopy, uronoscopy
urosepsin
urosepsis
urostomy
urothelial
u. basement membrane
u. carcinoma
urothelium
urothorax
urticaria
blue u.
urtication
USAISR
U.S. Army Institute of Surgical
Research
**U.S. Army Institute of Surgical
Research (USAISR)**
US-CNB
ultrasound-guided core needle biopsy
U-SCOPE
ureteroscopy
use
off-label u.
US-FNAB
ultrasound-guided fine-needle aspiration
biopsy
U-shaped
U-s. incision
U-s. jejunal pouch
U-s. scalp flap
Usher syndrome
USRDS
United States Renal Data System
USS
Universal Spine System
uterectomy

U

uteri (*pl. of* uterus)
uterina
>placenta u.

uterinae
>plicae tubariae tubae u.

uterine
>u. adenocarcinoma
>u. anomaly
>u. artery (UA)
>u. aspiration
>u. cavity
>u. compression
>u. dehiscence
>u. evaluation
>u. fibromyoma
>u. gland
>u. hernia
>u. hernia syndrome
>u. incision
>u. infection
>u. lysosome level
>u. mass
>u. myoma
>u. papillary serous carcinoma
>u. perforation
>u. positioning via ligament investment fixation and truncation (UPLIFT)
>u. positioning via ligament investment fixation and truncation procedure
>u. prolapse
>u. relaxation
>u. rupture
>u. sarcoma metastasis
>u. suspension
>u. vein
>u. venous plexus
>u. window

uteroabdominal
uterocervical
uterocystostomy
uterofixation
uterolysis
>laparoscopic u.

uteroovarian
uteroparietal
uteropelvic
uteroperitoneal fistula
uteropexy
uteroplacental circulation
uteroplasty
uterosacral
>u. block
>u. fold
>u. ligament

uteroscopy
uterotomy
uterotubal

uterovaginal
>u. canal
>u. plexus

uteroventral
uterovesical
>u. fold
>u. ligament
>u. pouch

uterus, *pl.* uteri
>masculine u.

UTI
>urinary tract infection

utilization
>impaired oxygen u.
>oxygen u.

utricle
>prostatic u.

utricular spot
utriculitis
utriculosaccular duct
U-turn maneuver
UV
>ultraviolet
>umbilical vein
>urethrovesical
>UV blood
>UV irradiation
>UV to MV ratio (UV:MV)

UVCP
>unilateral vocal cord paralysis

uveal
>u. metastasis
>u. tract

uveitides (*pl. of* uveitis)
uveitis, *pl.* uveitides
>anterior u.
>endogenous u.
>posterior u.

uveoencephalitic syndrome
uveoplasty
uviofast
uvioresistant
uviosensitive
UV:MV
>umbilical vein to maternal vein ratio
>UV to MV ratio

uvula, *pl.* uvuli
>Lieutaud u.

uvular muscle
uvulectomy
uvuli (*pl. of* uvula)
uvulopalatal flap (UPF)
uvulopalatopharyngoplasty (UPPP)
uvulopalatoplasty (UPP)
>laser u. (LUPP)
>laser-assisted u. (LAUP)

uvulotomy
Uyemura operation

v.
vein
vena
VA
alveolar ventilation
volume of alveolar gas
VAC
vacuum-assisted closure
vaccinia
v. infection
v. melanoma oncolysate
(VMO)
vaccinization
VACTERL
vertebral, anal, cardiac, tracheal,
esophageal, renal, limb
VACTERL anomaly
vacuolation, vacuolization
basket-weave v.
isometric tubular v.
vacuole
vacuolization (*var. of* vacuolation)
vacuum
v. aspiration
constant v.
v. extraction
v. extractor delivery
vacuum-assisted
v.-a. closure (VAC)
v.-a. core biopsy
v.-a. wound closure
(VAWC)
vacuum-pack laparostomy
technique
VAD
ventricular assist device
Abiomed BVS 500 VAD
DeBakey VAD
VAE
venous air embolism
vagal
afferent v.
v. arrest
v. body
v. nerve stimulation (VNS)
v. trunk
vagectomy
vagi (*pl. of* vagus)
vagina, *pl.* **vaginae**
azygos artery of v.
v. fibrosa tendinis
v. masculina
posterior fornix of v.
v. processus styloidei
vaginae (*pl. of* vagina)

vaginal
v. adenocarcinoma
v. anomaly
v. artery
v. birth after cesarean (VBAC)
v. carcinoma
v. celiotomy
v. column
v. condyloma
v. cone biopsy
v. construction
v. cornification test
v. cuff
v. cuff cellulitis
v. cystourethropexy
v. ectopic anus
v. electrical stimulation
v. examination
v. fistula
v. fixation
v. foreign body
v. fornix
v. gland
v. hernia
v. hysterectomy
v. hysterotomy
v. infection
v. inflammation
v. laceration
v. lithotomy
v. mass
v. mucification test
v. myomectomy
v. needle suspension procedure
v. nerve
v. opening
v. orifice
v. perineorrhaphy
v. process
v. rhabdomyosarcoma
v. surgery
v. vault prolapse
v. venous plexus
v. vesicostomy
v. wall approach
v. wall repair
v. wall sling procedure
vaginal-psoas suspension repair
vaginapexy
vaginate
vaginectomy
vaginitides (*pl. of* vaginitis)
vaginitis, *pl.* **vaginitides**
vaginoabdominal
vaginocele

V

vaginofixation
>Dührssen v.

vaginogram
vaginohysterectomy
vaginolabial hernia
vaginoperineal
vaginoperineoplasty
vaginoperineorrhaphy
vaginoperineotomy
vaginoperitoneal
vaginopexy
>Norman Miller v.

vaginoplasty
>cutback-type v.
>Fenton v.
>posterior flap v.

vaginoscopy
>pediatric v.

vaginotomy
vaginourethroplasty
vaginovesical
vaginovulvar
vagoaccessorius
vagoglossopharyngeal neuralgia
vagolysis
vagotomy
>v. and antrectomy with
>   gastroduodenostomy
>v. and pyloroplasty (V&P)
>bilateral vagotomies
>gastric v.
>highly selective v. (HSV)
>laparoscopic v.
>laparoscopic highly selective v.
>laser laparoscopic v.
>medical v.
>parietal cell v.
>posterior truncal v.
>proximal gastric v.
>Roux-en-Y procedure with v.
>selective proximal v. (SPV)
>superselective v.
>surgical v.
>total abdominal v.
>total bilateral v.'s
>truncal v.

vagovagal reflex
vagus, *pl.* **vagi**
>v. nerve
>v. nerve root

**Vaino metacarpophalangeal joint
  arthroplasty**
valdecoxib
Valentine position
valgum
>genu v.

valgus
>v. angulation
>cubitus v.

>v. deformity
>v. extension overload syndrome
>hallux v.
>v. wedge osteotomy
>v. Y-shaped osteotomy

valgus-external rotation injury
validation
>histopathologic v.

vallate papilla
vallecula, *pl.* **valleculae**
valleculae (*pl. of* vallecula)
Valleix point
**Valls-Ottolenghi-Schajowicz bone
  neoplasm needle biopsy**
Valpar whole body range of motion test
Valsalva
>V. maneuver
>V. muscle

value
>acid-base v.
>diagnostic v.
>high predictive v.
>intracranial pressure v.
>negative predictive v. (NPV)
>positive predictive v. (PPV)
>postprandial v.
>predictive v.
>pressure v.
>prognostic v.
>standardized uptake v.
>supranormal v.

value-based anesthesia practice
valva, *pl.* **valvae**
valvae (*pl. of* valva)
valve
>v. ablation
>Amussat v.
>APL v.
>v. bladder
>Bochdalek v.
>Cabot trumpet v.
>Carpentier-Edwards stented bovine
>   pericardial v.
>Carpentier-Edwards stented porcine
>   xenograft v.
>v. cinefluoroscopy
>v. cusp
>v. cutter
>v. debris
>expiratory v.
>fail-safe v.
>Gerlach v.
>Heimlich v.
>ileocecal v.
>v. leaflet
>left coronary v.
>mitral v. (MV)
>v. of Bauhin
>v. of Guérin

v. of Hasner
v. of Heister
v. of Houston
v. of Rosenmüller
v. of Sylvius
v. of Vieussens
v. orifice area
parachute mitral v.
v. patency
pop-off v.
pressure relief v.
v. replacement
right coronary v.
right septal v.
v. rupture
slit v.
transluminal v.
unidirectional v.
v. wrapping

valvectomy, valvulectomy
valved conduit anastomosis
valve-sparing aortic root
  replacement
valve-transverse
mitral v.-t.
Valvo full-thickness lid operation
valvoplasty, valvuloplasty
aortic v.
bailout v.
balloon aortic v.
balloon dilation v.
balloon mitral v.
balloon pulmonary v.
Carpentier tricuspid v.
catheter balloon v.
double-balloon v.
intracoronary thrombolysis balloon v.
mitral v.
multiple-balloon v.
percutaneous balloon aortic v.
  (PBAV)
percutaneous balloon mitral v.
percutaneous balloon pulmonic v.
percutaneous transluminal balloon v.
pulmonary v.
single-balloon v.
sliding v.
tricuspid v.
triple-balloon v.
Trusler technique of aortic v.
valvotomy, valvulotomy
aortic v.
balloon aortic v.
balloon mitral v.
balloon pulmonary v.
balloon tricuspid v.
Brock closed transventricular v.
double-balloon v.
Inoue balloon mitral v.

Longmire v.
mitral balloon v.
mitral valve v.
percutaneous mitral balloon v.
v. procedure
rectal v.
repeat balloon mitral v.
single-balloon v.
thimble v.

valvula (*var. of* valvule), *pl.* **valvulae**
Amussat v.
Gerlach v.
valvulae (*pl. of* valvula)
valvular
v. aortic disease
v. competence
v. heart disease
v. heart surgery
v. septum
valvule, valvula
lymphatic v.
valvulectomy (*var. of* valvectomy)
valvuloplasty (*var. of* valvoplasty)
valvulotome
Mills v.
retrograde v.
valvulotomy (*var. of* valvotomy)
VAMP
venous/arterial management protection
Baxter VAMP
van
v. Andel catheter
v. Buren artificial anus operation
v. Buren disease
v. Herick modification
v. Hoorn delivery maneuver
v. Horne canal
v. Lint anesthesia
v. Lint flap
v. Lint injection
v. Lint lid block
v. Lint modified technique
v. Ness lower limb amputation with
  foot reversal procedure
v. Ness rotationplasty
Vancouver fracture
vanilloid
v. agonist
v. receptor
vanished testis syndrome
vanishing lung syndrome (VLS)
Vannas capsulotomy
VAP
ventilator-associated pneumonia
vapor
anesthetic v.
v. density
partial pressure of water v.
v. pressure

V

vaporization
    contact laser v.
    laser v.
vaporize
vaporizer
    draw-over v.
    flow-over v.
    temperature-compensated v.
VAPS
    visual analog pain score
    volume-assured pressure support
variability
    heart rate v. (HRV)
    index of v.
    interpretation v.
variable
    v. positive airway pressure
      (VPAP)
    v. screw placement (VSP)
variable-dose patient-controlled anesthesia (VDPCA)
variable-release compression
variation
    biliary anatomic v.
varication
variceal
    v. band ligation
    v. bleeding
    v. column
    v. decompression
    v. eradication
    v. hemorrhage
    v. pressure
    v. sclerotherapy
    v. wall
varicella infection
varicella-zoster virus infection
varicelliform lesion
varices (*pl. of* varix)
varicocele
varicocelectomy
    laparoscopic v.
    microsurgical inguinal v.
    Palomo v.
    subinguinal microsurgical v.
varicose
    v. aneurysm
    v. vein stripping and
      ligation
varicotomy
variety
    diffuse v.
    multifocal v.
variolation, variolization
variolization (*var. of* variolation)
varix, *pl.* **varices**
    actively bleeding v.
    aneurysmal v.
    coil-shaped v.

    ectopic v.
    esophageal v.
    v. ligation
    Okuda transhepatic obliteration of v.
    percutaneous transhepatic obliteration
      of esophageal v.
    peristomal v.
    transesophageal ligation of v.
Varolius sphincter
varum
    genu v.
varus
    v. hindfoot
    v. hindfoot deformity
    v. rotation shortening osteotomy
varus-valgus plane
vas, *pl.* **vasa**
    v. deferens
    v. efferens
VAS
    visual analog scale
vasa (*pl. of* vas)
vascular
    v. abdominal surgery
    v. abnormality
    v. access
    v. access patient
    v. access thrombosis
    v. accident
    v. air embolism
    v. anastomosis
    v. anatomy
    v. anomaly
    v. bed
    v. bundle
    v. cannulation
    v. circle
    v. closure device
    v. complication
    v. compression
    v. control
    v. decompensation
    v. disease
    v. disease death
    v. dysfunction
    v. ectasia
    v. endothelium
    v. exclusion
    v. fold
    v. injury
    v. invasion
    v. isolation technique
    v. laceration
    v. laceration repair
    v. lamina
    v. leak syndrome (VLS)
    v. loop
    v. malformation
    v. manifestation

v. medicine
v. metastasis
v. neoplasia
v. nerve
v. net
v. occlusion
v. pedicle
v. perforation
v. plexus
v. pressure
v. procedure
v. radiologist
v. reconstruction
v. rejection
v. renal mass
v. ring
v. ring division
v. ring syndrome
v. shear
v. sheath
v. space
v. spider
v. structure
v. surgeon
V. Surgery Board
v. system
v. tissue
v. tumor
v. watershed
v. zone

vascular-endothelial growth factor (VEGF)
vascularity
parathyroid v.
tumor v.
vascularization
vascularize
vascularized
v. bone graft
v. free flap
v. omentum
v. pericranial flap
vasculature
extracranial cerebral v.
vasculitic lesion
vasculitis
diffuse v.
leukocytoclastic v.
widespread v.
vasculo-Behçet disease
vasculobiliary pedicle
vasculocardiac
vasculogenesis
vasculogenic impotence
vasculomyelinopathy
vasculopathy
allograft v.
cardiac-allograft v.
graft v.

vasectomy
no-scalpel v.
v. reversal
vasoactive
v. instability and flushing
v. intestinal peptide (VIP)
v. intestinal polypeptide tumor (VIPoma)
v. medication
v. substance
vasoconstriction
hypoxic pulmonary v. (HPV)
isoflurane-induced v.
peripheral v.
thermoregulatory v.
vasocutaneous fistula
vasodilatation (*var. of* vasodilation)
vasodilation, vasodilatation
afferent v.
efferent v.
vasodilator
v. administration
v. agent
arterial-selective intravenous v.
v. infusion
mesenteric v.
vasodilatory
v. property
v. therapy
vasoepididymostomy
vasoganglion
vasogenic theory
vasoinvasive growth
vasoligation
vasomotor nerve
vasoneuropathy
vasoneurosis
vasoplegic syndrome
vasopressin
intravenous v.
vasopressor support
vasoproliferation
vasopuncture
vasoreflex
vasorelaxation
vasorum
vasosection
vasostimulant
vasostomy
vasotomy, vasosection
vasovagal
vasovasostomy
vasovesiculectomy
VASPI
visual analog scale of pain intensity score
VASPI score
Vastamäki wrist arthroscopy technique
vastus medialis tendon

V

Vater
>   ampulla of V.
>   V. association
>   V. association syndrome
>   V. fold
>   V. papilla

VATER
>   vertebral, anus, tracheoesophageal,
>   radial, renal

VATET
>   video-assisted thorascopic extended
>   thymectomy

VATS
>   video-assisted thoracoscopic
>   surgery
>   VATS approach
>   VATS lobectomy
>   VATS procedure
>   VATS wedge resection

vault
>   cranial v.
>   rectal v.

vaulting gait

VAWC
>   vacuum-assisted wound closure

V-banded gastroplasty

VBG
>   vascularized bone graft
>   venous blood gas
>   vertical banded gastroplasty
>   VBG pouch

VCFS
>   velocardiofacial syndrome

VCP
>   vocal cord paralysis

VCV
>   volume-controlled ventilation

VDPCA
>   variable-dose patient-controlled
>   anesthesia

Veau congenital malformation of lip and palate classification

Veau-Wardill-Kilner

Vecchietti
>   V. neovagina construction
>   method
>   V. neovagina operation

VECO$_2$
>   pulmonary carbon dioxide
>   elimination

vection

vector
>   v. phase
>   v. product
>   v. profile
>   v. quantity

vecuronium
>   v. neuromuscular blocking

vegetative lesion

VEGF
>   vascular-endothelial growth factor

veil
>   aqueduct v.

vein (v.)
>   aberrant obturator v.
>   accessory cephalic v.
>   adrenal v.
>   anastomotic v.
>   angular v.
>   appendicular v.
>   aqueous v.
>   arcuate v.
>   arterial v.
>   ascending lumbar v.
>   auricular v.
>   autogenous v.
>   autologous internal jugular v.
>   axillary v.
>   azygos v.
>   basal v.
>   basilic v.
>   basivertebral v.
>   brachiocephalic v.
>   bronchial v.
>   Browning v.
>   buccal v.
>   Burow v.
>   canaliculus v.
>   capillary v.
>   cardiac v.
>   central v.
>   cephalic v.
>   cerebellar v.
>   cerebral v.
>   cervical v.
>   choroid v.
>   ciliary v.
>   circumflex v.
>   colic v.
>   collateral v.
>   comitans v.
>   common basal v.
>   common facial v.
>   condylar emissary v.
>   v. confluence
>   coronary v.
>   costoaxillary v.
>   cremasteric v.
>   v. cuff
>   v. decompression
>   deep cervical v.
>   descending genicular v.
>   digital v.
>   diploic v.
>   dorsispinal v.
>   dumbbelling of v.'s
>   emissary v.
>   epigastric v.

esophageal v.
ethmoidal v.
facial v.
femoral v.
femoropopliteal v.
fetal intrahepatic v.
frontal v.
gastric v.
gastrocolic v.
gastroepiploic v.
gonadal v.
v. graft
great saphenous v.
hemiazygos v.
hemorrhoidal v.
hepatic portal v.
human umbilical v. (HUV)
hypogastric v.
hypophyseoportal v.
ileal v.
ileocolic v.
iliac v.
inferior alveolar v.
inferior interosseous v.
inferior lateral genicular v.
inferior medial genicular v.
inferior mesenteric v. (IMV)
inferior pancreatic v.
infraorbital v.
innominate cardiac v.
intercapitular v.
intercostal v.
internal auditory v.
internal jugular v.
internal maxillary v.
internal pudendal v.
internal thoracic v.
intervertebral v.
intestinal v.
intraportal v.
jugular v.
juxtahepatic v.
Labbé v.
labial v.
labyrinthine v.
lacrimal v.
laryngeal v.
left brachiocephalic v.
left subclavian v. (LSCV)
lesser saphenous v.
lingual v.
long thoracic v.
lumbar v.
Marshall oblique v.
mediastinal v.
meningeal v.
mesenteric v.
musculophrenic v.
nasofrontal v.

native portal v.
v. obstruction
occipital cerebral v.
occipital emissary v.
v. occlusion
v. of Galen malformation
ophthalmic v.
orbital v.
v. orifice
ovarian v.
palatal v.
pancreatic v.
pancreaticoduodenal v.
paratonsillar v.
paraumbilical v.
parietal emissary v.
parotid v.
v. patch
v. patch angioplasty
patent portal v.
perforator v.
pericardiacophrenic v.
pericardial v.
peripheral v.
peritoneal v.
peroneal v.
petrosal v.
pharyngeal v.
phrenic v.
popliteal v.
portal v.
portal-systemic collateral v.
posterior anterior jugular v.
posterior auricular v.
posterior facial v.
posterior intercostal v.
posterior interosseous v.
posterior labial v.
posterior parotid v.
posterior scrotal v.
prepyloric v.
proximal v.
proximal saphenous v.
pudendal v.
pulmonary v.
pyloric v.
rectosigmoid v.
renal v.
reticular v.
retrohepatic v.
retromandibular v.
Retzius v.
right gastric v.
right gastroepiploic v.
right gastroomental v.
right hepatic v.
rolandic v.
Rolando v.
Rosenthal v.

V

vein (*continued*)
 Santorini v.
 saphenous v.
 scrotal v.
 v. segment transposition
 short gastric v.
 short hepatic v.
 short saphenous v.
 spermatic v.
 sphenoid emissary v.
 spider v.'s
 spigelian v.
 spinal v.
 splenic v.
 sternocleidomastoid v.
 v. stone
 stylomastoid v.
 subclavian v.
 subcostal v.
 sublingual v.
 submental v.
 subscapular v.
 superior laryngeal v.
 superior mesenteric v. (SMV)
 superior pulmonary v.
 superior thyroid v.
 supraorbital v.
 suprarenal v.
 suprascapular v.
 supratrochlear v.
 supreme intercostal v.
 sylvian v.
 v. system
 temporal v.
 temporomaxillary v.
 testicular v.
 thalamostriate v.
 thebesian v.
 thoracic v.
 thoracoacromial v.
 thoracoepigastric v.
 thymic v.
 thyroid v.
 Trolard v.
 v. tumor thrombus
 umbilical v. (UV)
 umbilical vein to maternal v.
 uterine v.
 v. valve transplant
 v. valve wrapping
 vertebral v.
 vertebral plexus of v.'s
 vertical v.
 Vesalius v.
 vesical v.
 vestibular v.
 vidian v.
 Vieussens v.
 vitelline v.
 vorticose v.
 v. wall
vein-sparing dissection
VeinViewer vein locator
Veirs canaliculus repair
vela (*pl. of* velum)
velamen
velamentous insertion
velamentum
velar
Veleanu-Rosianu-Ionescu
 V.-R.-I. adductor tenotomy
 V.-R.-I. obturator neurectomy
  technique
veliform
Vella fistula
vellication
vellus olivae inferioris
velocardiofacial syndrome (VCFS)
velocity
 v. catheter technique
 cerebrospinal fluid v.
 migration v.
velopharyngeal
 v. closure
 v. port
 v. sphincter
veloplasty
 functional v.
 intravelar v.
Velpeau
 V. canal
 V. deformity
 V. fossa
 V. hernia
velum, *pl.* **vela**
 corneal v.
ven
vena (v.), vein, *pl.* **venae**
 v. comitans
 venae pancreaticae
 venae pericardiacae
 venae peroneae
venacavaplasty
 face to face v.
venae (vv.) (*pl. of* vena)
venectomy
venereal
 v. condyloma
 v. disease
 v. sore
venereology
venesection
venipuncture
Venn-Watson polydactyly
 classification
venoablation
 percutaneous v.
venobiliary fistula

venoconstriction
    mesenteric v.
    reflex v.
venodilation
    nitrate-induced v.
    systemic v.
venogram
venographic study
venography
    contrast v.
    wedge hepatic v.
venolysis
    circumferential v.
venom extract
venoperitoneostomy
venostasis
venostomy
venosum
    ligamentum v.
venosus
    sinus v. (SV)
venotomy
venous (V)
    v. access
    v. access technique
    v. admixture
    v. air embolism (VAE)
    v. anastomosis
    v. angioma
    v. angle
    v. blood gas
    v. bypass procedure
    v. cannulation
    v. cannulation pain
    v. channel
    v. circulation
    circulus v.
    v. collateral
    v. compression
    v. confluence
    v. cutdown
    v. dialysis pressure
    v. drainage
    v. duplex ultrasonography
    v. effort thrombosis
    v. embolization
    v. foramen
    v. gangrene
    v. groove
    v. hemorrhage
    v. hypercapnia
    v. injury
    v. insufficiency
    v. interposition graft
    v. intravasation
    v. invasion
    v. leak syndrome
    v. ligament
    v. line

    v. loop
    v. malformation
    maternal v.
    v. occlusion
    v. outflow
    v. outflow recording
    v. pathology
    v. plexus
    v. pressure
    v. puncture
    v. reflux
    v. return
    v. sampling
    v. saturation
    v. segment
    v. sheath patch
    v. sinus
    v. stasis
    v. stasis disease
    v. stasis ulcer
    v. study
    v. system
    v. thrombectomy
    v. thromboembolism
    v. thromboembolism prophylaxis
    v. tributary
    v. trunk
    umbilical v.
    v. web
    v. web disease
venous/arterial management protection (VAMP)
venous-filling index
venous-occlusion volume plethysmography
venous-related complication
venous-to-venous anastomosis (VVA)
venovenostomy
venovenous
    v. bypass (VVB)
    v. extracorporeal bypass
vent
venter
ventilation
    v. agent
    airway pressure release v. (APRV)
    alveolar v. (Va)
    apneustic v.
    artificial v.
    assist-control mode v.
    assisted v.
    bag-and-mask v.
    bagged mask v.
    Biot v.
    v. circuit
    v. collateralization
    continuous flow v.
    continuous mandatory v. (CMV)
    continuous positive pressure v. (CPPV)

V

ventilation (*continued*)
    controlled v.
    controlled mechanical v. (CMV)
    control-mode v.
    control of v.
    cuirass v.
    decreased alveolar v.
    v. defect
    difficult v.
    emergency v.
    v. equivalent
    extended mandatory minute v.
      (EMMV)
    forced mandatory intermittent v.
      (FMIV)
    hand v.
    heart synchronized v.
    high-frequency v. (HFV)
    high-frequency jet v. (HFJV)
    high-frequency oscillation v. (HFOV)
    high-frequency oscillatory v. (HFOV)
    high-frequency percussive v.
    high-frequency positive-pressure v.
      (HFPPV)
    hyperoxic v.
    inadequate postoperative v.
    v. index (VI)
    inspired v. (VI)
    intermittent demand v.
    intermittent mandatory v. (IMV)
    intermittent positive-pressure v.
      (IPPV)
    intratracheal pulmonary v.
    inverse-ratio v.
    jet v.
    local exhaust v.
    low-frequency jet v.
    1-lung v. (OLV)
    2-lung v.
    v. lung scan
    manual v.
    mask v.
    maximal voluntary v. (MVV)
    maximum voluntary v. (MVV)
    mechanical v.
    monopulmonary v.
    mouth-to-mouth v.
    negative pressure v. (NPV)
    neonate v.
    noninvasive positive-pressure v.
      (NPPV)
    oscillatory v.
    partial liquid v.
    v. peak pressure
    percutaneous transtracheal v.
    percutaneous transtracheal jet v.
      (PTJV)
    positive-pressure v. (PPV)
    postoperative v.

    pressure-control v. (PCV)
    pressure control inverse ratio v.
      (PCIRV)
    pressure controlled v. (PCV)
    pressure controlled inverse ratio v.
      (PCIRV)
    pressure-limited v.
    pressure-regulated volume
      control v.
    pressure-support v. (PSV)
    prolonged postoperative v.
    proportional assist v. (PAV)
    pulmonary v.
    regional v.
    single lung v.
    split-lung v.
    spontaneous v.
    spontaneous intermittent mandatory
      v. (SIMV)
    synchronized intermittent mandatory
      v. (SIMV)
    synchronous intermittent
      mandatory v.
    v. threshold
    time-cycled v.
    transtracheal jet v. (TTJV)
    triggered v.
    ultrahigh-frequency v.
    volume-controlled v. (VCV)
    volume-cycled decelerating-flow v.
    volume-limited v.

ventilation/perfusion
    v. abnormality
    v. defect
    v. distribution
    v. imaging
    v. inequality
    v. lung scan
    v. mismatch
    v. quotient
    v. ratio
    v. relation
    v. relationship

ventilator (*var. of* respirator)
    v. breathing
    v. dependency
    high-frequency jet v.
    high-frequency positive-pressure v.
    v. management
    proportional assist v. (PAV)
    v. support
    v. time
    v. weaning

ventilator-assisted respiration
ventilator-associated pneumonia (VAP)
ventilator-induced
    v.-i. lung injury (VILI)
    v.-i. pneumopericardium
    v.-i. pneumothorax

ventilatory
    v. depression
    v. flow rate
    v. response
    v. support
venting percutaneous gastrostomy (VPG)
ventral
    v. abdominal hernia
    v. bending technique
    v. decubitus position
    v. hernia
    v. herniorrhaphy
    v. incisional hernia
    v. root
    v. sacrococcygeal ligament
    v. sacrococcygeus muscle
    v. spinocerebellar tract
    v. spinothalamic tract
    v. tegmental decussation
Ventralex patch
ventricle
    laryngeal v.
    lateral v.
    left v.
    Morgagni v.
    right v.
ventricular
    v. aberration
    v. access
    v. activation time
    v. assist device (VAD)
    v. canal
    v. depolarization abnormality
    v. diastolic pressure
    v. dilation
    v. dysrhythmia
    v. endoaneurysmorrhaphy
    v. endomyocardial biopsy
    v. end-systolic pressure-volume
      relation
    v. fibrillation/pulseless ventricular
      tachycardia resuscitation algorithm
    v. filling pressure
    v. fold
    v. inflow anomaly
    v. inflow tract obstruction
    v. ligament
    v. outflow tract
    v. outflow tract obstruction
    v. perforation
    v. peritoneal
    v. peritoneal shunt
    v. preexcitation
    v. puncture
    v. relaxation
    v. restoration
    v. septal defect (VSD)
    v. septal defect closure
    v. septal rupture
    v. septal wound defect
    v. septum
    v. tachycardia/ventricular fibrillation
ventricularization
ventricular-programmed stimulation
ventriculectomy
    partial left v.
ventriculi (*pl. of* ventriculus)
ventriculoarterial concordance
ventriculocisternostomy
    Torkildsen v.
ventriculocordectomy
ventriculography
    bubble v.
ventriculomastoidostomy
ventriculomegaly
ventriculoperitoneal (VP)
    v. shunt
    v. shunting procedure
    v. shunt placement
ventriculoplasty
    reduction v.
ventriculopuncture
ventriculoscopy
ventriculostomy
    Dandy third v.
    straight-in v.
    terminal v.
    third v.
    tunneled v.
ventriculotomy
    encircling endocardial v. (EEV)
    partial encircling endocardial v.
ventriculus, *pl.* **ventriculi**
ventrocystorrhaphy
ventroinguinal
ventrolateral (VL)
    v. hernia
ventroposterolateral (VPL)
ventroptosia (*var. of* ventroptosis)
ventroptosis, ventroptosia
ventroscopy
ventrotomy
ventrum penis flap
Venturi principle
venula, *pl.* **venulae**
venulae (*pl. of* venula)
venular lesion
venule
    high endothelial v.
vera
    polycythemia v.
verapamil
veratridine
verbal
    v. descriptor scale
    v. pain score
    v. stress score
verbal-rank scale

V

Verdan
  V. intrasynovial flexor tendon
    technique
  V. osteoplastic thumb reconstruction
Veress needle
Verga
  accessory venous sinus of V.
verge
  anal v.
Verhoeff
  V. multiple partial tenotomy
  V. suture
  V. suture technique
Verhoeff-Chandler
  V.-C. capsulotomy
  V.-C. operation
verification
  intraoperative v.
Vermale operation
vermian fossa
vermicular colic
vermiculation
vermiform
  v. appendage
  v. appendix
  v. body
  v. process
vermiformis
  appendix v.
  processus v.
vermilion border
vermilionectomy
Vermont spinal fixator articulation
Vernet syndrome
Verneuil
  V. canal
  V. operation
vernix membrane
verrucous lesion
vertebra, *pl.* **vertebrae**
  basilar v.
  caudal v.
  cervical v.
  coccygeal v.
  dorsal v.
  false v.
  lumbar v.
  picture frame v.
  v. plana fracture
  sacral v.
  tail v.
  thoracic v.
  true v.
  wedge-shaped v.
vertebrae (*pl. of* vertebra)
vertebral
  vertebral, anal, cardiac, tracheal,
    esophageal, renal, limb
    (VACTERL)

vertebral, anus, tracheoesophageal,
    radial, renal (VATER)
  v. arch
  v. artery
  v. artery disease
  v. artery reconstruction
  v. aspiration
  v. body
  v. body anterior cortex
  v. body corpectomy
  v. body decompression
  v. body fracture
  v. bone mass
  v. canal
  v. column
  v. compression
  v. compression fracture
  v. dissection
  v. epidural space
  v. exposure
  v. foramen
  v. fusion
  v. ganglion
  v. groove
  v. hemangioma
  v. interbody fusion
  v. mobilization
  v. notch
  v. osteosynthesis
  v. osteosynthesis fusion
    rate
  v. plexus of veins
  v. region
  v. resection
  v. rib
  v. ring apophysis
  v. rotation
  v. spine infectious process
  v. stable burst fracture
  v. subluxation complex
  v. subluxation syndrome
  v. vein
  v. venous plexus
  v. wedge compression fracture
vertebrated
vertebrectomy
  Bohlman anterior cervical v.
  cervical spondylotic myelopathy v.
vertebroarterial foramen
vertebrochondral rib
vertebrocostal trigone
vertebrofemoral
vertebroiliac
vertebropelvic ligament
vertebroplasty
  percutaneous v.
  transpedicular percutaneous v.
vertebrosacral
vertebrosternal rib

vertex, *pl.* **vertices**
    v. position
vertical
    v. adjustable banded gastroplasty
    v. angulation
    v. banded gastroplasty (VBG)
    v. banded gastroplasty pouch
    v. canal
    v. compression
    v. compression test
    v. condensation root canal filling
    method
    v. divergence position
    v. flap
    v. gastric bypass
    v. illumination
    v. incision
    v. index
    v. lip biopsy
    v. mastopexy
    v. mattress stitch
    v. mattress suture technique
    v. maxillary excess
    v. midline incision
    v. osteotomy
    v. partial laryngectomy
    v. pedicle technique breast
    reduction
    v. plane
    v. reduction rectoplasty
    v. relation
    v. ring gastroplasty (VRG)
    v. section
    v. shear fracture
    v. silastic ring gastroplasty
    v. suspension reflex
    v. tooth fracture
    v. translation
    v. uterine incision
    v. vein
    v. vein system
    v. versus horizontal preparation
vertical-cut
    v.-c. method
    v.-c. technique
vertically acquired infection
vertices (*pl. of* vertex)
verticomental
vertiginous migraine
vertigo
    benign paroxysmal positional v.
    cyclic v.
    positional v.
verumontanum
Verwey eyelid operation
very
    v. large scale integration
    v. late activation
    v. long-limb Roux gastric bypass

Vesalius
    V. bone
    canal of V.
    V. foramen
    V. vein
vesica, *pl.* **vesicae**
vesicae (*pl. of* vesica)
vesical
    v. calculus
    v. diverticulectomy
    v. fistula
    v. flap
    v. gland
    v. lithotomy
    v. nerve
    v. plexus
    v. triangle
    v. vein
vesication
vesicle
    air v.
    brush-border
      membrane v.
    v. hernia
    optic v.
    otic v.
    seminal v.
vesicoabdominal
vesicoacetabular fistula
vesicobullous lesion
vesicocele
vesicocervical space
vesicoclysis
vesicocolic fistula
vesicocutaneous fistula
vesicoenteric fistula
vesicofixation
vesicoinguinal hernia
vesicointestinal fistula
vesicolithiasis
vesicomyectomy
vesicomyotomy
vesicoovarian fistula
vesicoprostatic
vesicopubic
vesicorectal fistula
vesicorectostomy
vesicosalpingovaginal
    fistula
vesicosigmoid
vesicosigmoidostomy
vesicospinal
vesicostomy
    cutaneous v.
    preputial continent v.
    vaginal v.
vesicotomy
vesicoumbilical ligament
vesicoureteral reflux

V

vesicourethral
- v. anastomosis
- v. canal

vesicouterine
- v. fistula
- v. ligament
- v. pouch

vesicouterovaginal

vesicovaginal
- v. fistula
- v. repair

vesicovaginorectal fistula

vesicovaginostomy

vesicovisceral

vesicula, *pl.* **vesiculae**

vesiculae (*pl. of* vesicula)

vesicular
- v. acute inflammation
- v. appendage
- v. granulomatous inflammation
- v. venous plexus
- v. viral infection

vesiculation

vesiculectomy
- prostatoseminal v.
- total prostatoseminal v.

vesiculitis

vesiculocavernous respiration

vesiculoprostatectomy
- retropubic v.

vesiculoprostatitis

vesiculotomy

Vesling line

vessel
- aberrant v.
- abnormally feeding blood v.
- absorbent v.
- afferent lymphatic v.
- anterior great v.
- atheromatous v.
- bleeding v.
- blood v.
- celiac v.
- chyle v.
- collateral v.
- deep lymphatic v.
- v. disruption
- v. distention
- ectatic v.
- endosteal v.
- v. exposure
- gastric v.
- gastroepiploic v.
- inflow v.
- infrapopliteal v.
- innominate v.
- intercostal v.
- lacteal v.
- v. ligation

- lumbar v.
- lymph v.
- lymphatic v.
- mesenteric v.
- nutrient v.
- pancreaticoduodenal arcade v.
- parent v.
- periesophageal blood v.
- portal v.
- posterior great v.
- renal v.
- right subclavian v.
- segmental v.
- short gastric v.
- splanchnic v.
- v. stenosis
- superficial lymphatic v.
- thoracic great v.
- tumor v.
- v. wall

vessel-containing plate

VEST
- virtual endoscopic surgery trainer

vestibular
- v. blind sac
- v. canal
- v. canaliculus
- v. crest
- v. fissure
- v. fold
- v. ganglion
- v. gland
- v. labyrinth
- v. ligament
- v. membrane
- v. nerve
- v. nerve section
- v. neurectomy
- v. vein
- v. window

vestibule
- esophagogastric v.
- gastroesophageal v.
- labial v.
- nasal v.

vestibuli
- rima v.

vestibulitis

vestibulocochlear nerve

vestibuloplasty

vestibulospinal tract

vestibulourethral

vestibulum

vestige

vestigial muscle

vest-over-pants
- v.-o.-p. hernia repair
- v.-o.-p. herniorrhaphy

V-flap meatoplasty

VI
    inspired ventilation
    ventilation index
viability
    flap v.
viable tissue
vial
    multidose v.
    scintillation v.
vibrating line
vibration
    v. condensation
    v. detection threshold
    v. disease
    v. neuritis
    v. syndrome
    v. threshold test
vibrational angioplasty
vibrator hand syndrome
vibrissa, *pl.* **vibrissae**
vibrissae (*pl. of* vibrissa)
vibroacoustic stimulation
vibrotactile display
vicarious respiration
vicious union
Vicq d'Azyr bundle
Vicryl
    V. mesh
    V. pop-off suture
    V. Rapide suture
victim
    trauma v.
Victor Gomel microsurgical reconstruction method
Vidal-Ardrey fracture technique
video
    v. image
    v. mediastinoscopy
    v. small-bowel enteroscopy
    v. thoracoscopic drainage
    v. thoracoscopy
    v. transurethral resection technique
video-assisted
    v.-a. excisional biopsy
    v.-a. gastrectomy
    v.-a. lobectomy
    v.-a. lumbar sympathectomy
    v.-a. neck surgery
    v.-a. technique
    v.-a. thoracic surgical procedure
    v.-a. thoracoscopic surgery (VATS)
    v.-a. thoracoscopic thymectomy
    v.-a. thoracoscopic wedge resection
    v.-a. thorascopic extended thymectomy
    v.-a. transsternal radical esophagectomy

videoendoscopic-assisted microsurgery
videoendoscopic thyroidectomy
videoendoscopy
videoesophagogoscopy
videoesophagram
videofluoroscopic technique
videofluoroscopy
videolaparoscopic
    v. cardiomyotomy
    v. guidance
videolaparoscopy
videolaseroscopy
video-Macintosh laryngoscope
videomicroscopy
videoscopic
    v. evaluation
    v. fundoplication
    v. hernia surgery
    v. repair
videoscopy
    3-dimensional v.
videostroboscopy
videothoracoscopy
videourodynamic evaluation
vidian
    v. canal
    v. nerve
    v. neuralgia
    v. vein
Viers punctoplasty
Vieussens
    V. ansa
    V. ganglion
    V. limbus
    V. ring
    valve of V.
    V. vein
view
    abdominal v.
    anterior v.
    apical lordotic v.
    Boehler calcaneal v.
    Boehler lumbosacral v.
    Breuerton v.
    cine v.
    coned-down v.
    decubitus v.
    frontal x-ray v.
    laparoscopic transhiatal v.
    lateral x-ray v.
    1-plane v.
vigil
    coma v.
vigilance monitoring
vigorous hydration
VILI
    ventilator-induced lung injury
Villaret syndrome
villi (*pl. of* villus)

villose (*var. of* villous)
villous, villose
    v. atrophy
    v. epithelium
villus, *pl.* **villi**
    arachnoid v.
    intestinal v.
    peritoneal v.
    pleural v.
    synovial v.
villusectomy
Vim-Silverman
    V.-S. needle biopsy technique
    V.-S. technique for liver biopsy
Vim thalamotomy
Vincent infection
vinculum
Vineberg internal mammary artery implantation procedure
violaceous lesion
violation
    peritoneal v.
    pleural v.
VIP
    vasoactive intestinal peptide
VIPoma
    vasoactive intestinal polypeptide tumor
Virag operation
viral
    v. cirrhosis
    v. marker
    v. replication
    v. respiratory infection
Virchow
    V. metastasis
    V. triad
Virchow-Robin
    V.-R. space
    V.-R. space dilation
virgin
    v. neck
    v. silk suture
virginal membrane
Virginia Mason pancreatic cancer approach
virginity
virilia
virilization
virtual
    v. colonoscopy
    v. cystoscopy
    v. endoscopic surgery trainer (VEST)
    v. endoscopy
    v. implantation
    v. point
    v. reality
    v. reality trainer

virus
    adenoidal-pharyngeal-conjunctival v.
    coxsackievirus A, B v.
    Epstein-Barr v. (EBV)
    hepatitis C v. (HCV)
    human immunodeficiency v. (HIV)
    human T-lymphotrophic v.
viscera (*pl. of* viscus)
viscerad
visceral
    v. anesthesia
    v. angiomyolipoma
    v. artery
    v. biplanar arteriography
    v. edema
    v. hamartoma
    v. herniation
    v. hyperalgesia
    v. hypersensitivity
    v. injury
    v. layer
    v. lesion
    v. muscle
    v. nerve
    v. node
    v. pain
    v. pelvic fascia
    v. perforation
    v. perfusion
    v. pericardiectomy
    v. pericardium
    v. peritoneum
    v. pleura
    v. postsurgical disturbance
    v. pouch
    v. rotation
    v. space
    v. sympathectomy
    v. traction reflex
    v. vessel endarterectomy
visceralgia
viscerobronchial cardiovascular anomaly
viscerocranium
visceroinhibitory
visceroparietal
visceroperitoneal
visceropleural
visceroptosia (*var. of* visceroptosis)
visceroptosis, visceroptosia
viscerosensory
visceroskeletal
visceroskeleton
viscerosomatic
viscerotomy
viscerum
    situs inversus v.
viscoelastic tissue
viscosity

viscosupplementation
viscus, *pl.* **viscera**
    abdominal v.
    abdominal viscera
    abdominopelvic v.
    herniated v.
    hollow v.
    v. injury
    intraperitoneal v.
    viscera retention
    retroperitoneal v.
Visick dysphagia classification
vision
    central v.
    direct laparoscopic v.
    laparoscopic v.
    presbyopic v.
visiting nurse
visor flap
visual
    v. analog pain score (VAPS)
    v. analog scale (VAS)
    v. analog scale of pain intensity
      score (VASPI)
    v. analysis
    v. association area
    v. closure
    v. compromise
    v. deprivation syndrome
    v. direction
    v. extinction
    v. function evaluation
    v. laser ablation
    v. laser ablation of prostate (VLAP)
    v. laser-assisted prostatectomy
      (VLAP)
    v. line
    v. method
    v. orientation
    v. pathway
    v. plane
    v. point
    v. preservation
    v. projection
    v. stimulation
visualization
    contrast v.
    3D v.
    4D v.
    direct fluoroscopic v.
    double-contrast v.
    endoscopic v.
    fluoroscopic v.
    4-gland parathyroid v.
    inadequate v.
visually triggered headache
Visual-Motor Integration Test
vital
    v. capacity

    v. knot
    v. tissue
vitamin D supplementation
vitelline
    v. duct anomaly
    v. fistula
    v. membrane
    v. sac
    v. vein
vitellointestinal cyst
vitiation
vitreal
    v. hemorrhage
    v. membrane
vitrectomy
    anterior v.
    closed system pars
      plana v.
    core v.
    open-sky v.
    port v.
    posterior v.
    Weck-Cel v.
vitreolysis
vitreoretinal
    v. surgery
    v. traction syndrome
vitreoretinopathy
    exudative v.
    familial exudative v.
vitreous
    v. aspiration
    v. breakthrough hemorrhage
    v. cavity
    v. foreign body
    v. hernia
    v. herniation
    v. humor
    v. membrane
    v. neovascularization
    v. surgery
    v. table
vitreum
vitrification
vividialysis
vividiffusion
vivification
vivo
    ex v.
    in v.
VL
    ventrolateral
VLAP
    visual laser ablation of prostate
    visual laser-assisted prostatectomy
V line
VLS
    vanishing lung syndrome
    vascular leak syndrome

V

VMO
vaccinia melanoma oncolysate
polyvalent VMO
VO$_2$
oxygen consumption
peak exercise oxygen consumption
vocal
v. cord
v. cord atrophy
v. cord damage
v. cord injection
v. cord movement
v. cord palsy
v. cord paralysis (VCP)
v. dysfunction
v. fold
v. fold approximation
v. fold fixation therapy
v. ligament
v. muscle
v. process
v. process granuloma
v. shelf
v. tract
vocalis muscle
vocational
v. counseling
v. rehabilitation
Vogt cyclodiathermy operation
Vogt-Koyanagi-Harada syndrome
voice
v. disorder
v. restoration
v. therapy
voiding
v. flow rate
v. urethral pressure measurement
Voigt line
vola
volar
v. angulation
v. angulation deformity
v. aspect
v. epineurolysis
v. finger approach
v. interosseous artery
v. midline approach
v. midline oblique incision
v. plate
v. plate arthroplasty
v. plate arthroplasty technique
fracture-dislocation
v. plate repair
v. radial approach
v. semilunar wrist dislocation
v. synovectomy
v. ulnar approach
v. V-Y flap
v. zig-zag finger incision

volaris
volarward approach
volatile
v. anesthesia
v. anesthetic
v. anesthetic agent
volatilization
volitional saccade
Volkmann
V. canal
V. clawhand
V. clawhand deformity
V. fracture
V. ischemic contracture
Volpicelli functional ambulation scale
volsella
voltage
truncated exponential v.
voltage-gated ion channel
volume
abdominal v.
biopsy v.
blood transfusion v.
circulation v.
compartmental v.
drain v.
end-expiratory lung v. (EELV)
end-inspiratory v.
estimated blood v.
v. expansion
expiratory reserve v.
expiratory residual v.
extracellular v.
extracellular fluid v. (ECFV)
fiber bundle v.
forced expiratory v. (FEV)
gland v.
gross tumor v. (GTV)
injection v.
intracellular v.
intraperitoneal v.
intravascular v.
intravascular blood v.
left ventricular v.
liver v.
lung v.
maximal expiratory flow v.
median biopsy v.
minute v.
v. of alveolar gas (V$_A$)
pelvic hemorrhage v.
peritoneal exchange v.
v. plethysmography
presystolic pressure and v.
v. reduction surgery (VRS)
remnant liver v.
respiratory minute v.
resuscitated by v.
rib-cage v.

v. segmentation
specimen v.
stroke v.
v. therapy
tidal v.
timed forced expiratory v.
total erythrocyte v.
tumor v.
weight-based peritoneal exchange v.
volume-assured pressure support (VAPS)
volume-controlled ventilation (VCV)
volume-cycled decelerating-flow ventilation (VCDF)
volume-limited ventilation
volumetric
v. analysis
v. capnometry
v. method
v. solution
v. stereotaxis
v. study
v. technique
volumetry
CT v.
voluntary
v. area
v. guarding
v. sterilization
volutrauma
Voluven
volvulus
cecal v.
colonic v.
gastric v.
mesenteroaxial v.
midgut v.
organoaxial v.
v. reduction
sigmoid v. (SV)
Volz arthroplasty
Volz-Turner greater trochanter reattachment technique
vomer cartilagineus
vomerine canal
vomerobasilar canal
vomeronasal
v. cartilage
v. nerve
vomerorostral canal
vomerovaginal
v. canal
v. groove
vomit
bilious v.
vomiting, vomition
bilious v.
intractable v.
postdischarge nausea and v.
postoperative nausea and v. (PONV)

vomition (*var. of* vomiting)
vomiturition (*var. of* retching)
vomitus
coffee-grounds v.
von
v. Ammon cheek flap blepharoplasty
v. Ammon epichanthus operation
v. Bergman hernia
v. Blaskovics-Doyen vesicouterine fistula operation
v. Blaskovics resection and advancement of levator palpebrae superioris
v. Ebner gland
v. Ebner line
v. Economo disease
v. Frey monofilament
v. Frey touch test
v. Giordano suburethral sling operation
v. Graefe operation
v. Haberer-Finney anastomosis
v. Haberer-Finney gastrectomy technique
v. Haberer gastroenterostomy
v. Hippel keratoplasty
v. Hippel-Lindau disease
v. Hippel-Lindau syndrome
v. Hippel-Lindau tumor
v. Langenbeck bipedicle mucoperiosteal flap
v. Langenbeck palatal closure
v. Langenbeck pedicle flap
v. Noorden incision
v. Willebrand factor (vWF)
vortices (*pl. of* vortex)
vortex, *pl.* **vortices**
vorticose vein
Vostal radial fracture classification
V-osteotomy
Japas V-o.
off-set V-o.
V&P
vagotomy and pyloroplasty
VP
ventricular peritoneal
ventriculoperitoneal
VPAP
variable positive airway pressure
VPG
venting percutaneous gastrostomy
VPL
ventroposterolateral
VPL pallidotomy
V/Q
ventilation/perfusion
VRG
vertical ring gastroplasty

V

VRS
    volume reduction surgery
VSD
    ventricular septal defect
V-shaped
    V-s. configuration
    V-s. incision
    V-s. osteotomy
V-sign of Naclerio
V-slope method
VSP
    variable screw placement
V-to-Y closure
Vulpius
    V. and Strofel inverted V slide lengthening of distal gastrocnemius/soleus aponeurosis
    V. lengthening of gastrocnemius muscle procedure
Vulpius-Compere tendon technique
Vulpius-Stoffel gastrocnemius intramuscular aponeurotic recession procedure
vulsella, vulsellum
vulsellum (*var. of* vulsella)
vulva, *pl.* **vulvae**
vulvae (*pl. of* vulva)
vulval (*var. of* vulvar)
vulvar, vulval
    v. adenoid cystic adenocarcinoma
    v. biopsy
    v. carcinoma
    v. infection
    v. pigmented lesion
    v. slit
    v. vestibulitis syndrome

vulvectomy
    Basset radical v.
    Parry-Jones v.
    radical v.
    simple v.
    skinning v.
vulvitis
vulvocrural
vulvodynia
vulvoplasty
vulvouterine
vulvovaginal
    v. carcinoma
    v. cystectomy
    v. gland
    v. lesion
    v. premenarchal infection
vulvovaginoplasty
    Williams v.
vv.
    venae
VVA
    venous-to-venous anastomosis
VVB
    venovenous bypass
vWF
    von Willebrand factor
V-Y
    V-Y advancement
    V-Y advancement flap
    V-Y advancement technique
    V-Y gastroplasty
    V-Y Kutler flap
    V-Y plasty
    V-Y procedure
    V-Y quadricepsplasty
Vypro mesh

W

W hernia
W pelvic pouch
W position
W pouch
W procedure
W sitting

Wachendorf membrane
Wackenheim clivus canal line
WAD

whiplash-associated disorder

Waddell nonorganic sign
Wadsworth

W. elbow approach
W. posterolateral approach
W. triceps tendon release technique

Wagner

W. closed pinning
W. diabetic foot disease
classification
W. modification of Syme
amputation
W. open reduction technique
W. skin incision
W. 2-stage Syme amputation

Wagoner

W. cervical spine technique
W. posterior spinal approach

wagon-wheel fracture
Wagstaffe fracture
wait

w. list
w. time

wake-up

w.-u. evaluation
w.-u. test
w.-u. testing

Walcher position
Waldeyer

W. fossa
W. gland
W. ring
W. sheath
W. space
W. throat ring lesion
W. tract

Waldhauer entropion operation
Waldhausen

W. subclavian flap angioplasty
procedure
W. subclavian flap technique

Walker tractotomy
walking

w. epidural
w. epidural anesthetic

w. program
w. ventilation test

wall

anterior abdominal w.
anterior aortic w. (AAW)
anterior rectus sheath w.
anterior thoracic w.
aortic w.
bile duct w.
bowel w.
cavity w.
chest w.
cyst w.
deep anterior w.
duct w.
edematous bowel w.
fibrotic w.
gastric w.
gingival cavity w.
intermediate anterior w.
w. invasion
lateral w.
nail w.
nasal w.
nontumoral gastric w.
w. of body
orbital w.
oropharyngeal w.
parietal w.
peripheral cavity w.
posterior oropharyngeal w.
posterior rectus sheath w.
pulpal w.
w. push maneuver
rectus sheath w.
soft w.
splanchnic w.
superficial anterior w.
thoracic w.
upper thoracic w.
variceal w.
vein w.
vessel w.

wallaby pouch
Wallace ureteroileal anastomosis
technique
wall-echo shadow triad
Wallenberg syndrome
wallet stomach
Wallstent
Walsh radical retropubic prostatectomy
Walter

W. Reed HIV infection
classification
W. Reed operation

W

Walther
  W. canal
  W. duct
  W. fracture
  W. ganglion
  W. plexus
waltzed flap
wandering
  w. abscess
  w. kidney
  w. liver
  w. organ
  w. spleen
Wangensteen drainage
Wang pleural stoma
ward
  observation w.
Wardill
  W. 4-flap method
  W. pharyngoplasty
Wardill-Kilner
  W.-K. advancement flap
    method
  W.-K. 4-flap uranoplasty
  W.-K. palatoplasty procedure
Ward-Mayo vaginal hysterectomy
Wardrop aneurysm ligation
  method
warm
  w. autoimmune hemolytic anemia
  w. condensation
  w. ischemia
  w. ischemic time
  w. sensation threshold
warmer
  Belmont buddy fluid w.
  fluid w.
  high-capacity fluid w.
  inspiratory w.
warming
  forced air w.
  in-line intravenous fluid w.
  w. needle
  preanesthetic skin-surface w.
  preoperative skin-surface w.
Warner-Farber ankle fixation technique
warning
  black box w.
  w. headache
Warren
  W. incision
  W. splenorenal shunt operation
  W. vaginal anal incontinence flap
Warren-Marshall gastritis classification
Warren-Zeppa shunt
Wartenberg syndrome
wartlike excrescence
washed
  w. clot

  w. field technique
  w. intrauterine insemination
washing
  cytologic w.
  endometrial jet w.
  peritoneal w.
washout
  peritoneal w.
  seminal tract w.
  w. test
wash technique
Wasmann gland
Wassel
  W. thumb duplication
  W. thumb duplication classification
wasting
  muscle w.
  w. syndrome
Watanabe
  W. classification of discoid meniscus
  W. discoid meniscus classification
watchband incision
water
  degasified distilled w.
  w. density line
  w. displacement
  w. dissection
  distilled w. (aq. dist, DW)
  extracellular w. (ECW)
  W.'rs extraperitoneal cesarean section
  extravascular lung w. (EVLW)
  hydration layer w.
  lung w.
  W.'s projection
  total body w. (TBW, TBWA)
  w. vapor monitoring
Waterhouse transpubic urethroplasty
  procedure
water-jet system
Waterman osteotomy
watermelon stomach
watershed
  vascular w.
water-soluble
  w.-s. contrast enema
  w.-s. contrast esophagram
Waterston
  W. aorto-to-right pulmonary artery
    closure method
  W. extrapericardial anastomosis
  W. operation
Waterston-Cooley aorto-to-right
  pulmonary artery anastomosis
  procedure
water-suppression MR imaging technique
watertight closure
water-trap stomach
Watkins intertransverse process lumbar
  spine fusion technique

Watson
W. capsule biopsy
W. Cheyne-Burghard segmental matrix toenail excision procedure
W. Cheyne wedge excision of toenail technique
W. operation
W. scapholunate treatment method
W. scaphotrapeziotrapezoidal fusion
W. technique

Watson-Jones
W.-J. ankle reconstruction
W.-J. anterolateral total hip approach
W.-J. fracture repair
W.-J. incision
W.-J. shoulder procedure
W.-J. tenodesis
W.-J. tibial tubercle avulsion fracture classification

Watzke scleral buckling

Waugh abdominoanal pullthrough operation

Waugh-Clagett pancreatoduodenostomy

wave
abdominal fluid w.
contraction w.
phasic pressure w.
pressure w.

waveform
aortic root velocity w.
electrical stimulator w.
epidural pressure w. (EPWF)
photoplethysmographic w.
pressure w.

wavelength frequency

wavy respiration

wax
w. expansion
w. matrix technique
w. pattern thermal expansion technique

waxy
w. exudate
w. kidney
w. liver

Wayne County General Hospital reduction

weakened bowel

weakness
contralateral w.
muscle w.

weaning
on-off w.
w. success
ventilator w.

weapon
stand-off w.

wear
3-body w.

Weaver-Dunn
W.-D. acromioclavicular joint stabilization procedure
W.-D. acromioclavicular technique
W.-D. distal clavicle resection

weaving
head w.

web
antral w.
arterial w.
cell w.
w. corn
duodenal w.
esophageal w.
w. eye
finger w.
w. formation
hepatic w.
intestinal w.
laryngeal w.
mucosal w.
postcricoid w.
pulmonary arterial w.
w. space
w. space flap
w. space incision
w. space infection
terminal w.
thumb w.
tracheal w.
venous w.

webbed penis

Weber
W. humeral osteotomy
W. organ
W. physical injury classification
W. point
W. subcapital osteotomy
W. triangle

Weber-Brunner-Freuler-Boitzy pediatric orthopaedic technique

Weber-Brunner-Freuler open reduction

Weber-Danis ankle injury classification

Weber-Fergusson
W.-F. incision
W.-F. maxillofacial skeleton exposure procedure

Weber-Vasey traction-absorption wiring of olecranon fracture technique

Webril immobilization

Webster
W. 3D-degree flap
W. operation

Weck-Cel vitrectomy

Wecker iridectomy

Weckesser tendon repair technique

weddellite calculus

W

Wedensky facilitation
wedge
    arterial w.
    ball w.
    w. bone
    bone w.
    closing base w.
    compensatory w.
    w. compression fracture
    dental w.
    disconnect w.
    w. excision
    w. graft
    w. hepatectomy
    w. hepatic biopsy
    w. hepatic venography
    w. incision
    light-reflecting w.
    w. liver biopsy
    Livingston peribulbar w.
    mediastinal w.
    open w.
    w. osteotomy
    w. pressure
    pulmonary artery w. (PAW)
    w. resection
    temporal w.
wedge-and-groove joint
wedged
    w. hepatic vein pressure (WHVP)
    w. hepatic venous pressure
      (WHVP)
wedge-shaped
    w.-s. erosion
    w.-s. fasciculus
    w.-s. osteotomy
    w.-s. tubercle
    w.-s. uncomminuted tibial plateau
      fracture
    w.-s. vertebra
Weekers peripheral iridectomy
weeping lesion
Wegner line
Wei composite maxillary defect
  reconstruction flap
weight
    body w.
    w. estimation and assessment
    graft w.
    gut mucosal w.
    ideal body w.
    lean body w.
    w. loading
    mucosal w.
    percentage of ideal body w.
    w. reduction
    w. reduction surgery
    total body w.
weight-based peritoneal exchange volume

Weiland
    W. iliac crest bone graft
    W. osteomyelitis classification
Weinberg
    W. modification
    W. modification of pyloroplasty
Weinstock desyndactylization
Weir
    W. appendectomy
    W. appendicostomy procedure
    W. correction of nostrils procedure
    W. incision
Weiss epidural needle
Weissman intraoperative therapeutic
  intensity score classification
Weitbrecht
    W. cartilage
    W. cord
weld
    laser tissue w.
welding
    fusion w.
    laser tissue w.
    pressure w.
    tissue w.
well-circumscribed lesion
well-defined mass
well-localized adenoma
Wells posterior rectopexy
Wendell Hughes cataract operation
Wepfer gland
Werb operation
Wernekinck decussation
Wernicke-Korsakoff syndrome
Wernicke radiation
Wertheim
    W. operation
    tunnel of W.
Wertheim-Bohlman occipitocervical fusion
  technique
Wertheim-Schauta operation
West
    W. and Soto-Hall patellar technique
    W. and Soto-Hall patellectomy
    W. operation
Westberg space
Westhaven-Yale Multidimensional Pain
  Inventory (WHYMPI)
Westin-Hall incision
wet
    w. colostomy
    w. field cautery
    w. gangrene
    w. lung
    w. technique with liposuction breast
      reduction
wetting solution
Weve operation
Weyers-Thier syndrome

Wharton
> W. duct
> W. Jones operation

Wheeler
> W. cicatricial ectropion correction method
> W. entropion repair procedure
> W. halving repair
> W. operation

Wheelhouse perineal urethrotomy
wheel rotation
wheezing
> expiratory w.

whewellite calculus
whip
> catheter w.

whiplash
> w. injury
> w. technique

whiplash-associated disorder (WAD)
whipping condensation
Whipple
> W. incision
> W. operation
> W. pancreaticoduodenostomy
> W. pancreatic resection
> W. pancreatoduodenectomy
> W. pancreatoduodenostomy
> W. radical pancreatoduodenectomy procedure
> W. triad

whipstitch suture technique
whipworm infection
whispered pectoriloquy, whispering pectoriloquy
whispering pectoriloquy
whistle-tip catheter
whistling deformity
Whitacre spinal needle
Whitaker pressure-perfusion test
white
> w. braided silk suture
> w. cell
> w. clot syndrome
> W. diabetes mellitus in pregnancy classification
> w. dot syndrome
> w. epidermoidoma
> w. fascial line of Toldt
> w. fixation
> w. gangrene
> w. graft
> w. lesion
> w. line
> w. line response
> w. matter
> w. muscle
> w. nylon suture

> w. patch
> w. point
> W. posterior ankle fusion
> w. pulp
> w. ring
> W. slide lengthening of tendo Achillis
> W. slide lengthening of tendo Achillis procedure
> w. twisted suture
> w. without pressure

white-centered hemorrhage
Whitecloud-LaRocca fibular strut graft
whitegraft reaction
Whitehead
> W. deformity
> W. gastritis classification
> W. operation

Whitesides-Kelly extraoral retropharyngeal cervical spine technique
white-spot lesion
whitlow
> melanotic w.

Whitman
> W. femoral neck reconstruction
> W. osteotomy
> W. talectomy procedure

Whitmore-Jewett (W-J)
> W.-J. classification for prostate cancer
> W.-J. classification prostate cancer staging
> W.-J. prostate cancer classification

Whitnall
> W. ligament
> W. orbital tubercle
> W. sling operation

WHO
> World Health Organization
> WHO analgesic ladder
> WHO gastric carcinoma classification

whole
> w. abdomen irradiation
> w. abdominal radiation
> w. abdominopelvic irradiation
> w. blood lysis technique
> w. body irradiation
> w. lobar graft
> w. organ pancreas (WOP)
> w. organ pancreas transplant
> w. pelvis irradiation

whole-arm fusion
whole-body
> w.-b. cooling
> w.-b. extract
> w.-b. hyperthermia
> w.-b. radiation

W

whole-body (*continued*)
    w.-b. scanning
    w.-b. titration curve
whole-brain radiation therapy
whole-cell patch clamp recording
whole-gut
    w.-g. irrigation
    w.-g. lavage activating solution
whorl
    coccygeal w.
whorled appearance
WHVP
    wedged hepatic vein pressure
    wedged hepatic venous pressure
WHYMPI
    Westhaven-Yale Multidimensional Pain
    Inventory
Wiberg patellar classification
Wicherkiewicz eyelid operation
Wick catheter technique
wide
    w. elliptical anastomosis
    w. internal inguinal ring
    w. local excision
    w. mucosa-to-mucosa Roux-en-Y
      hepaticojejunostomy
    w. plane
wide-field
    w.-f. radiation therapy
    w.-f. total laryngectomy
wide-mouthed cystic duct
wide-mouth sac
widened retrogastric space
wide-open anastomosis
wide-range radiation therapy
widespread
    w. portal system thrombosis
    w. vasculitis
Widman gingival flap
width
    line w.
    pulse w.
Wiener
    tract of Münzer and W.
Wies
    W. lower lid entropion operation
    W. transconjunctival lower eyelid
      involutional entropion repair
      procedure
Wigand fetal position maneuver
Wilde incision
Wilkie artery
Wilkinson synovectomy
Wilkins radial fracture classification
will
    living w.
William
Williams
    W. copulating pouch operation

    W. discectomy
    W. microlumbar disc excision
    W. vaginal construction procedure
    W. vulvovaginoplasty
Williams-Haddad femoral nerve block
 for hip fracture technique
Willi glass crown technique
Willis
    W. antrum
    artery of W.
    W. cord
    W. pancreas
    W. pouch
willow fracture
Willy Meyer mastectomy incision
Wilmer lens extraction
Wilms
    W. amputation
    W. renal tumor
    W. thoracoplasty
    W. tumor
Wilson
    W. angulation osteotomy for hallux
      valgus procedure
    W. ankle fusion
    W. bone graft
    W. bunionectomy
    W. fracture
    W. muscle
    W. oblique displacement osteotomy
Wilson-Jacobs
    W.-J. patellar graft
    W.-J. tibial fracture fixation
      technique
Wilson-McKeever
    W.-M. arthroplasty
    W.-M. shoulder technique
Wiltberger
    W. anterior cervical approach
    W. posterior interbody fusion
Wiltse
    W. ankle osteotomy
    W. bilateral lateral fusion
    W. system double-rod construct
    W. system H construct
    W. system single-rod construct
    W. varus supramalleolar osteotomy
Wiltse-Spencer paraspinal approach
Winberger line
Winchester syndrome
windblown deformity
window
    aortic-pulmonic w.
    aortopulmonary w. (APW)
    dilating w.
    oval w.
    pericardial w.
    peritoneal w.
    soft tissue w.

w. technique
uterine w.
vestibular w.
windpipe
windsock deformity
Windsor-Insall-Vince
W.-I.-V. bone graft
W.-I.-V. tissue grafting technique
windswept deformity
wind-up (*var. of* windup)
windup, wind-up
neuronal w.
second pain w.
winged
w. scapula deformity
w. V double flap
wing suture
Winiwarter-Buerger disease
Winiwarter operation
Winkelmann rotationplasty
Winkler body
Winkler-Waldeyer
closing ring of W.-W.
Winograd
W. ingrown nail procedure
W. lateral nail fold excision
technique
W. nail plate removal
W. partial matrixectomy
**Winquist femoral shaft fracture
classification**
**Winquist-Hansen femoral fracture
classification**
Winslow
epiploic foramen of W.
W. pancreas
Winter
W. convex fusion
W. priapism repair procedure
W. spastic hemiplegic cerebral palsy
classification
W. spondylolisthesis technique
Wintrobe
wire
w. arch
w. contour preparation
w. extrusion
w. insertion
w. knot
w. localization
w. osteosynthesis
w. passage
w. removal technique
w. stabilization
suture w.
wire-guided
w.-g. balloon-assisted endoscopic
biliary stent exchange
w.-g. biopsy sample

w.-g. breast biopsy
w.-g. cricothyrotomy
w.-g. dilation
w.-g. endobronchial blocker
w.-g. placement
wireless biomedical sensor
wire-loop
w.-l. fixation
w.-l. lesion
w.-l. test
wire-reinforced airway barrel
4-wire trochanter reattachment
wiring
compression w.
continuous loop w.
craniofacial suspension w.
facet fracture stabilization w.
facet subluxation stabilization w.
interspinous w.
Ivy loop w.
sublaminar w.
Wirsung
W. canal
W. dilation
W. duct
Wirsung-choledochus junction
Wirth-Jager tendon technique
Wise
W. mastopexy
W. operation
W. pattern mammaplasty
within-list recognition (WLR)
Witzel
W. decompression of Roux-en-Y
loop maneuver
W. duodenostomy
W. enterostomy
W. gastrostomy
W. jejunostomy
W. operation
W. tunnel
W-J
Whitmore-Jewett
W-J classification for staging of
prostate cancer
WLE
wide local excision
WLR
within-list recognition
WOB
work of breathing
Wolfe
W. full-thickness fat-free skin graft
method
W. mammogram classification
W. ptosis operation
Wolfe-Kawamoto bone graft
**Wolfe-Krause full-thickness fat-free skin
graft**

W

wolffian
- w. body
- w. cyst
- w. duct
- w. duct carcinoma

Wölfler
- W. gastroenterostomy
- W. gland
- W. suture technique

Womack portal systemic shunting procedure

womb

wood
- W. light examination
- W.'s screw fetal position maneuver
- w. wool

Woodward
- W. esophagogastroscopy
- W. esophagogastrostomy
- W. operation
- W. release of high-riding scapula procedure

Woofry-Chandler classification of Osgood-Schlatter lesion

Wookey laryngopharyngeal reconstruction

wool
- wood w.

Wooler-type anuloplasty

WOP
- whole organ pancreas
- WOP transplant

work
- w. hardening program
- w. of breathing (WOB)
- preload recruitable stroke w.
- w. status

working
- w. bite relation
- w. memory
- w. port

workup
- diagnostic w.
- hematologic w.

world
- W. Health Organization (WHO)
- W. Health Organization classification

wormian bone

Worst
- W. artificial lens suture
- W. operation

Worth ptosis operation

wound
- abdominal gunshot w.
- abraded w.
- w. abscess
- acute w.
- anterior w.
- w. approximation
- avulsed w.
- back gunshot w.
- w. biopsy
- bullet w.
- w. cavity
- central hepatic gunshot w.
- w. closure
- w. closure strategy
- w. complication
- w. contaminant
- crease w.
- w. dehiscence
- w. disruption
- w. drainage
- w. dressing
- exit w.
- w. failure
- w. fibroblast
- flank gunshot w.
- w. fluid
- fresh w.
- full-thickness w.
- glancing w.
- gunshot w. (GSW)
- gutter w.
- w. healing
- w. hematoma
- hepatic gunshot w.
- w. hernia
- incised w.
- w. infection
- w. irrigation
- laparoscopic trocar w.
- lateral w.
- mature w.
- nonpenetrating w.
- open w.
- penetrating w.
- perforating w.
- precordial w.
- primarily healing w.
- w. problem
- puncture w.
- w. recurrence
- remodeling of w.
- w. retraction
- w. sealing
- seton w.
- shotgun w.
- w. site
- skin deficit w.
- stab w.
- sucking chest w.
- superficial w.
- surgical w.
- w. surveillance system
- tangential w.
- thoracoabdominal gunshot w.
- w. tract

transpelvic gunshot w.
trocar w.
wound-breaking strength
W-plasty
W-pouch
    ileal W-p.
wrap
    cardiac muscle w.
    fundic w.
    gastric w.
    gastric fundus w.
    w. hematoma
    Nissen fundoplication w.
    rectus fascial w.
    smooth w.
    supradiaphragmatic fundic w.
    total gastric w.
    Toupet w.
wraparound
    w. neurovascular composite free
      tissue transfer
    w. neurovascular free flap
    w. periapical lesion
wrapping
    fascial w.
    omental pedicle w.

pedicle w.
valve w.
vein valve w.
Wright
    W. caries of spine operation
    W. maneuver
wrinkler muscle
wrinkling membrane
Wrisberg
    W. cartilage
    W. lesion
    W. nerve
    W. tubercle
wrist
    w. block
    w. deformity
    w. disarticulation
    w. dislocation
    w. extensor
    w. extensor tendon
wry neck (*var. of* wryneck)
wryneck, wry neck
W-shaped
    W-s. ileal pouch-anal anastomosis
    W-s. incision
W-sitting position

W

X

X body

Xa

chiasma

xanthoastrocytoma
xanthogranuloma
xanthogranulomatous

x. cholecystitis
x. panniculitis
x. pyelonephritis (XGP)

xanthomatosis

cerebrotendinous x.

xanthosarcoma
Xe

xenon
^{133}Xe intravenous injection technique

xenogeneic, xenogenous, xenogenic

x. cell therapy
x. graft
x. infection
x. tissue

xenogenic (*var. of* xenogeneic)
xenogenous (*var. of* xenogeneic)
xenograft

x. graft
stented bovine pericardial x.
stented porcine x.
x. transplant

xenografting
xenon (Xe)

x. arc photocoagulation
x. gas
x. lung ventilation imaging
x. washout technique

xenon-enhanced cerebral blood flow
xenotransplantation

cellular x.
x. thymus

xenozoonosis
xerocytosis
xerogram (*var. of* xeroradiogram)
xerography

soft tissue x.

xeroma
xeronosus

xeroradiogram, xerogram
xerosis
xerostomia
XFS

exfoliation syndrome

XGP

xanthogranulomatous pyelonephritis

xiphicostal (*var. of* xiphocostal)

x. angle

xiphisternal

x. joint
x. junction
x. junction chondritis

xiphisternum
xiphocostal, xiphicostal
xiphodynia
xiphoid

x. cartilage
x. process

xiphoidalgia
xiphoid-to-pubis midline abdominal incision
xiphoid-to-umbilicus incision
xiphopubic laparotomy
xiphosternalis

synchondrosis x.

X-leg

crossleg

X-line atlantooccipital dislocation diagnostic method
X-pattern exotropia
XR

extended release

x-radiation
x-ray

abdominal x-r. (AXR)
anteroposterior chest x-r.
barium contrast x-r.
chest x-r. (CXR)
x-r. control
frontal x-r.
lateral chest x-r.
x-r. therapy (XRT)

XRT

x-ray therapy

Xta

chiasmata

Y

- Y angle
- Y body
- Y cartilage
- Y configuration
- Y fracture (Y-Fx)
- Y graft
- Y incision
- Y mesh hernia repair
- Y piece

⁹⁰Y

yttrium-90

Yacoub and Radley-Smith congenital heart disease classification

YAG

yttrium-aluminum-garnet
YAG laser

Yale Optimal Observation Score

Yancey osteotomy

y-angle

Yasargil craniotomy

year

quality adjusted life y. (QALY)

yeast infection

Yee posterior shoulder approach

yellow

- y. atrophy
- y. body
- y. hepatization
- y. lesion
- y. ligament
- y. nail
- y. nail syndrome

yellow-ochre hemorrhage

Yentl syndrome

yield

nodal y.

yoke

- alveolar y.
- y. block
- y. bone
- cricoid y.
- y. hanger
- y. transposition procedure

yolk

- y. membrane
- y. sac

y. sac carcinoma
y. space

York-Mason

- Y.-M. incision
- Y.-M. rectourinary fistula approach
- Y.-M. rectourinary fistula repair
- Y.-M. repair of postoperative rectoprostatic-urethral fistula procedure

Y-osteotomy

Pauwels Y-o.

young

- y. cyst
- Y. epispadias repair procedure
- Y. pelvic fracture classification
- Y. perineal prostatectomy
- Y. type epispadias repair
- Y. urinary bladder repair technique

Young-Dees

- Y.-D. bladder neck reconstruction
- Y.-D. bladder neck repair
- Y.-D. bladder neck repair procedure
- Y.-D. genitourinary system technique

Young-Dees-Leadbetter bladder neck reconstruction

young-onset cancer

Yount

- Y. fasciotomy
- Y. gluteal-iliotibial fasciotomy procedure

Y-plasty

ypsiliform

Y-shaped incision

Y-suture technique

Y-T fracture

yttrium-90 (⁹⁰Y)

yttrium-aluminum-garnet (YAG)

holmium: y.-a.-g. (Ho:YAG)

Yu

- Y. osteotomy
- Y. pyloroplasty

Y-V

- Y-V anoplasty
- Y-V plasty
- Y-V plasty incision
- Y-V rotational flap

Z

Z band
Z direction
Z fashion
Z incision
Z line
Z marginal tenotomy
Z myotomy
Z point
Z procedure
Z technique

Zadik total matrixectomy
Zaglas ligament
Zahn

anomaly of Z.
Z. line
striae of Z.

Zaias nail biopsy
Zancolli

Z. biceps tendon rerouting technique
Z. biceps tendon transfer procedure
Z. capsuloplasty
Z. clawhand deformity repair
Z. procedure for clawhand
    deformity
Z. upper limb reconstruction

Zang space
Zarins-Rowe

Z.-R. ACL reconstruction technique
Z.-R. semitendinosus and iliotibial
    band knee repair procedure

**Zavala pulmonary disease diagnostic
technique**
**Zazapen-Gamidov anteromedial lesser
trochanter approach**
Z-dimension
ZEEP

zero end-expiratory pressure

Zeier transfer technique
Zeis gland
Zemuron
Zenapax
Zenker

Z. diverticulum
Z. pouch

zero

z. end-expiratory pressure (ZEEP)
z. end-inspiratory pressure
z. line

ZES

Zollinger-Ellison syndrome

zeta
zeugmatography

rotating frame z.
rotating-frame z.

Zeus robotic system
ZF

zygomaticofrontal
ZF suture

Z-flap incision
Zickel

Z. fracture classification
Z. nail
Z. subtrochanteric fracture operation

Ziegler

Z. operation
Z. puncture

**Zielke kyphotic deformity repair
technique**
ZIFT

zygote intrafallopian transfer

zig-zag

z.-z. approach
z.-z. compensatory deformity
z.-z. finger incision

Zimany bilobed flap
Zimmerman colpocleisis
Zimmer Statak suture
Zinn

Z. ligament
Z. membrane
Z. tendon
Z. zonule

zipped canal
zipper

fascial z.
z. sphincterotomy

**Zlotsky-Ballard acromioclavicular injury
classification**
Zm

zygomaxillare

**Zoellner-Clancy sliding fibular graft
repair of peroneal tendon procedure**
Zofran
Zollinger-Ellison syndrome (ZES)
Zollinger hernia classification
Zöllner line
zona, *pl.* **zonae**

z. pectinata
z. pellucida

zonae (*pl. of* zona)
zonal anatomy
zone

abdominal z.
adherent z.
anal high pressure z.
anal transition z. (ATZ)
arcuate z.
barrier z.
basement membrane z.

Z

893

zone (*continued*)
    calcification z.
    cervical transformation z.
    chemoreceptor trigger z.
    ciliary z.
    dorsal root entry z. (DREZ)
    echo z.
    entry z.
    exudative z.
    gingival z.
    Head z.
    hemorrhoidal z.
    high pressure z. (HPZ)
    normal transformation z.
    orbicular z.
    pectinate z.
    proliferation z.
    pupillary z.
    transformation z.
    transition z.
    vascular z.
zonoskeleton
zonula, *pl.* **zonulae**
    fibrae zonulares
zonulae (*pl. of* zonula)
zonular
    z. band
    z. fiber
    z. space
zonule
    ciliary z.
    Zinn z.
zonulolysis, zonulysis, zonulysis
    Barraquer z.
    Barraquer enzymatic z.
    enzymatic z.
zonulotomy
zonulysis (*var. of* zonulolysis)
zoodermic
zoograft
zoografting
zoonotic infection
zooplastic graft
zooplasty
zoospermia
Z-osteotomy
    scarf Z-o.
Z-osteotomy-bunionectomy
    scarf Z-o.-b.
Z-plasty
    Z-p. approach
    Broadbent-Woolf 4-limb Z-p.
    Cozen-Brockway Z-p.
    4-flap Z-p.
    Gudas scarf Z-p.
    Z-p. incision
    4-limb Z-p.
    Z-p. local flap graft
    Peet Z-p.

    Z-p. procedure
    scarf Z-p.
    Spencer-Watson Z-p.
    Z-p. tenotomy
    Z-p. transposition
Z-point pressure
Z-shaped
    Z-s. anastomosis
    Z-s. incision
    Z-s. suture line
Z-suture technique
Z-type deformity
Zuckerkandl
    Z. diverticulum
    Z. fascia
    organ of Z.
    Z. perforating canal
    Z. tubercle
    Z. tuberculum
Zuker and Manktelow facial muscle transplantation technique
Zung Depression Scale
Zusanli acupoint
Zy
    zygion
zygapophyseal (*var. of* zygapophysial)
zygapophysial, zygapophyseal
    z. joint
    z. joint pain
zygapophysis
zygion (Zy)
zygoma
zygomatic
    z. arch
    z. arch fracture
    z. bone
    z. branch
    z. fossa
    z. injury
    z. nerve
    z. region
zygomatic-maxillary complex fracture
zygomaticoauricular index
zygomaticofacial
    z. artery
    z. branch
    z. canal
    z. foramen
zygomaticofrontal (ZF)
    z. suture
zygomaticomaxillary
    z. fracture
    z. suture
zygomaticoorbital
    z. artery
    z. foramen
zygomatico-orbitalis
    arteria z.-o.

zygomaticosphenoid
zygomaticotemporal
    z. branch
    z. canal
    z. foramen
    z. space
    z. suture
zygomaticus

    z. major muscle
    z. minor muscle
zygomaxillare (Zm)
zygomaxillary point
zygopodium
zygote intrafallopian transfer
 (ZIFT)
Zylik operation

Z

Contents: The Appendices

Anatomical Illustrations

Direction of Fracture Lines

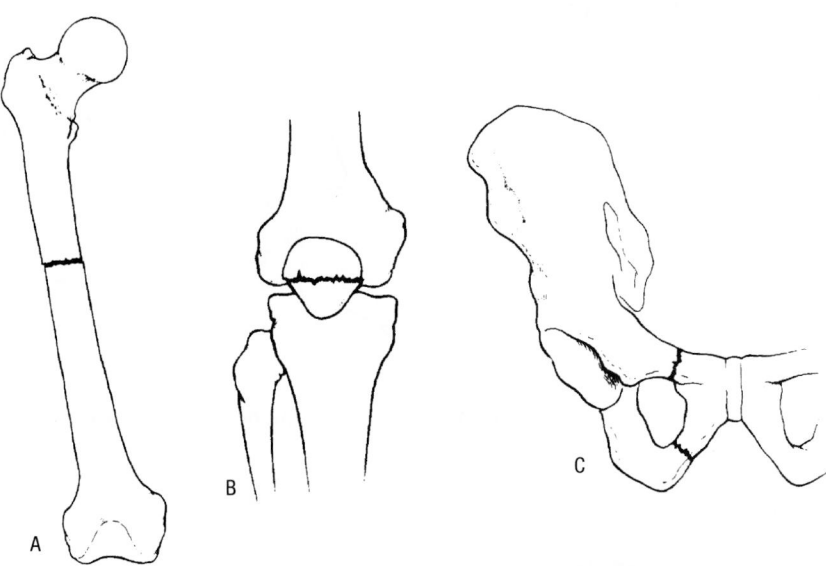

transverse fractures: (A) transverse fracture of the middle third of the femur; (B) transverse fracture of the midpatella; (C) transverse fracture of the superior and inferior pubic rami

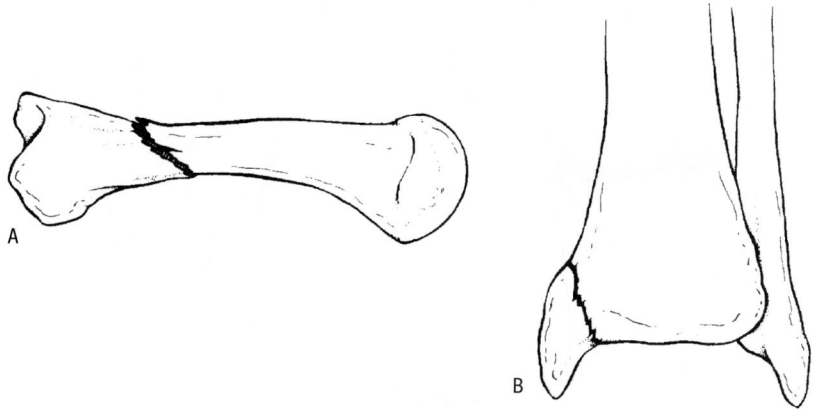

oblique fractures: (A) oblique fracture of the proximal third of metacarpal; (B) oblique fracture of the medial malleolus

Appendix 1

spinal fractures

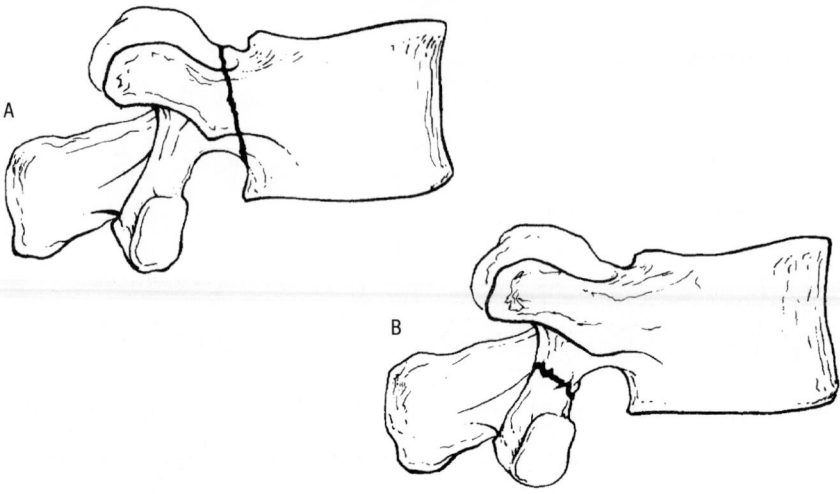

(A) fracture through the pedicle; (B) fracture through the pars interartricularis

shoulder fractures

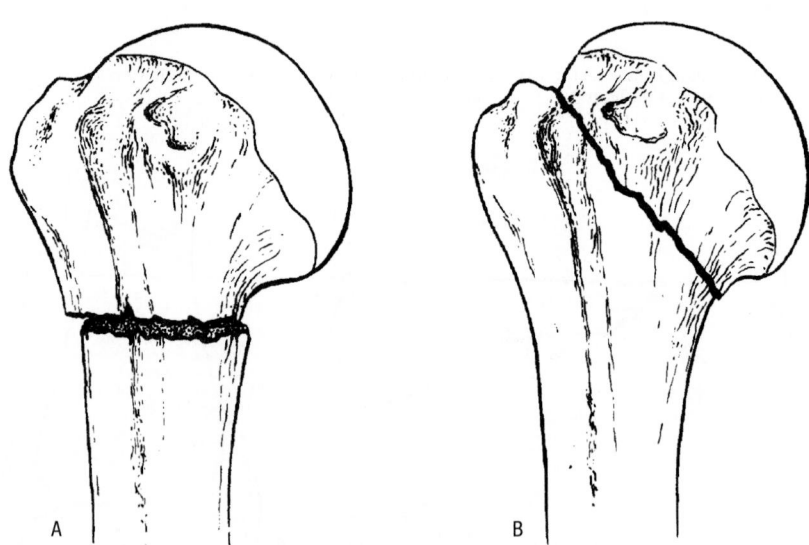

(A) transverse fracture of the surgical neck of the humerus; (B) fracture of the anatomic neck of the humerus

elbow fractures

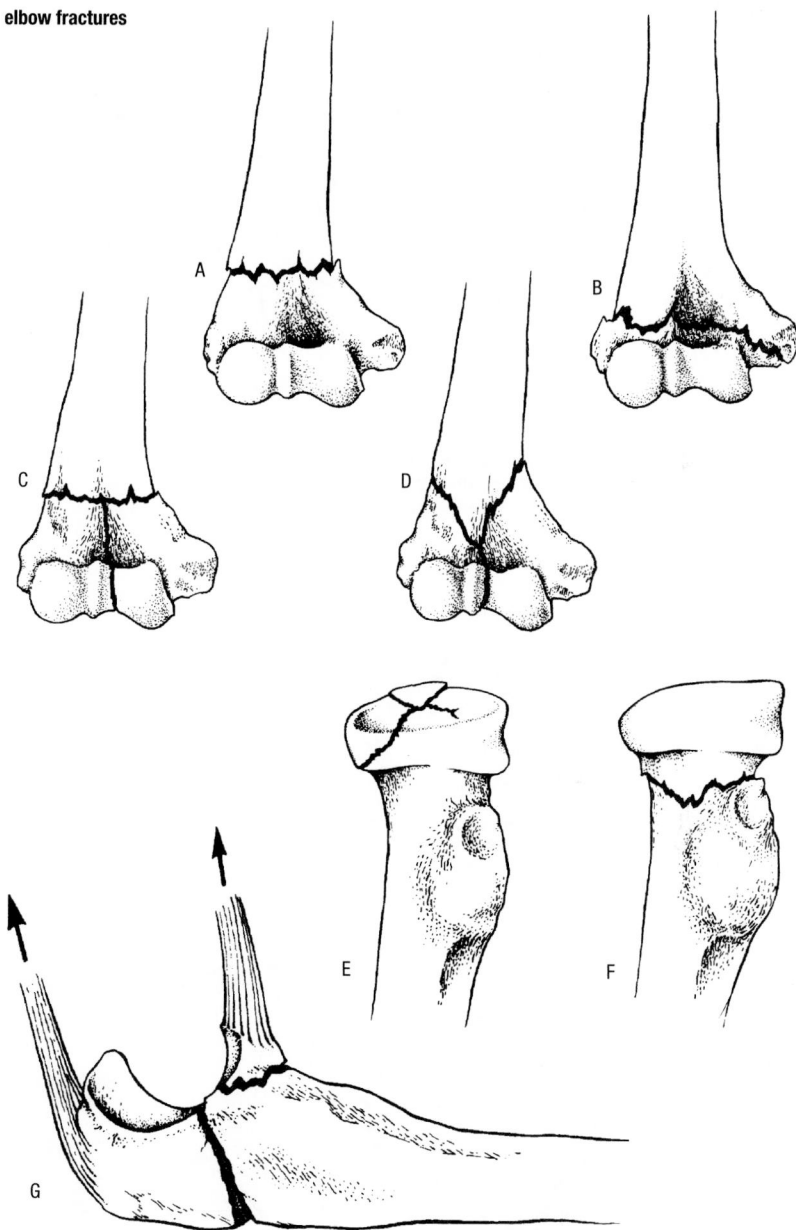

(A) supracondylar fractures are fractures that occur above the level of the condyles; (B) transcondylar fracture; note that the fracture extends through both condyles. **comminuted intraarticular fractures of the distal humerus; (C) T-shaped fracture; (D) Y-shaped fracture; (E) comminuted fracture of the head of the radius; (F) transverse nondisplaced fracture of the neck of the radius; (G) fracture of the olecranon and coronoid process;** muscle contraction can cause distraction of fracture fragments.

pelvic fractures

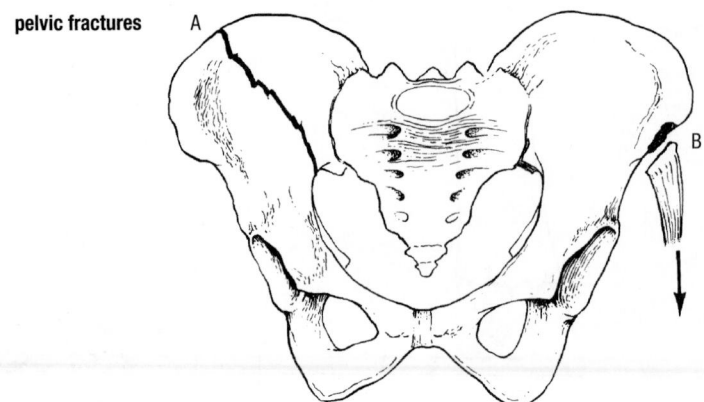

fractures of the ilium: (A) oblique fracture through the wind of the ilium; (B) avulsion fracture of the anteroinferior iliac spine

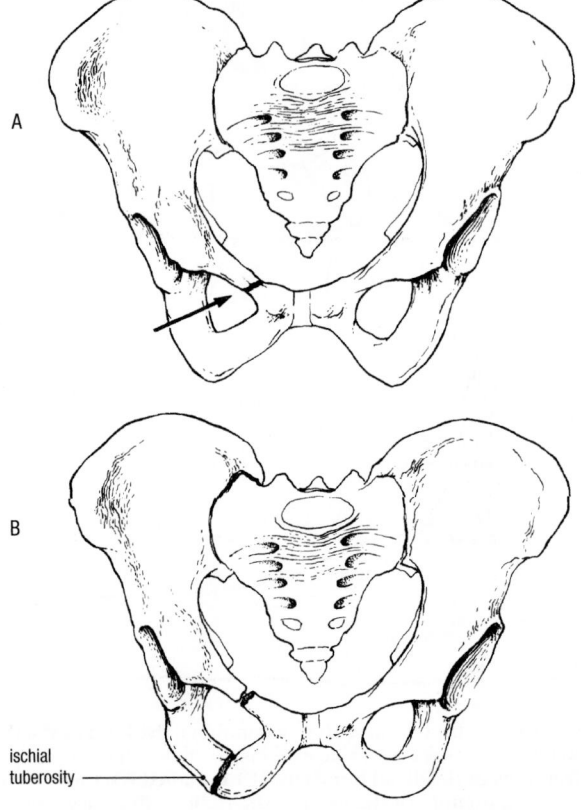

ischial tuberosity

(A) oblique fracture of the superior pubic ramus; (B) transverse fractures of the inferior ischial ramus and superior pubic ramus

hip fractures

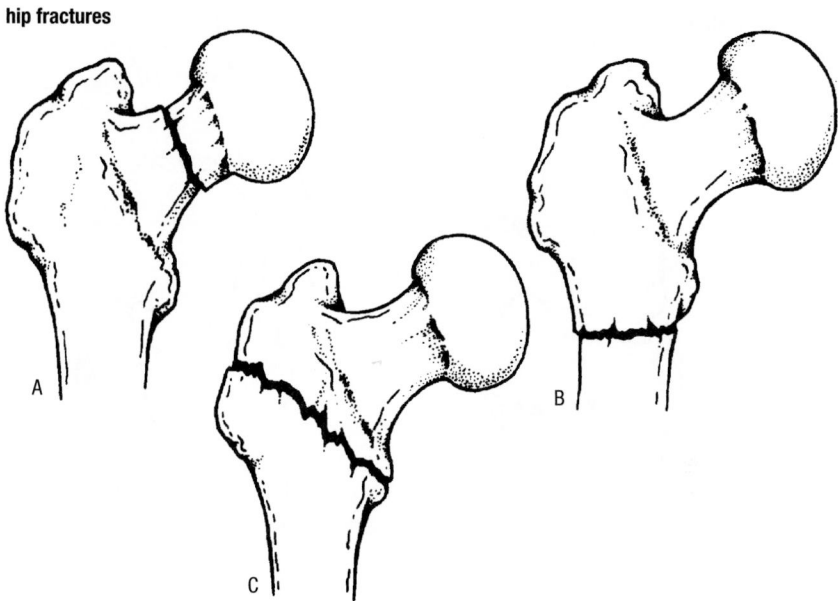

fractures of the hip described by the location in which they occur: (A) transverse intracapsular fracture; (B) oblique intertrochanteric fracture; (C) transverse subtrochanteric fracture

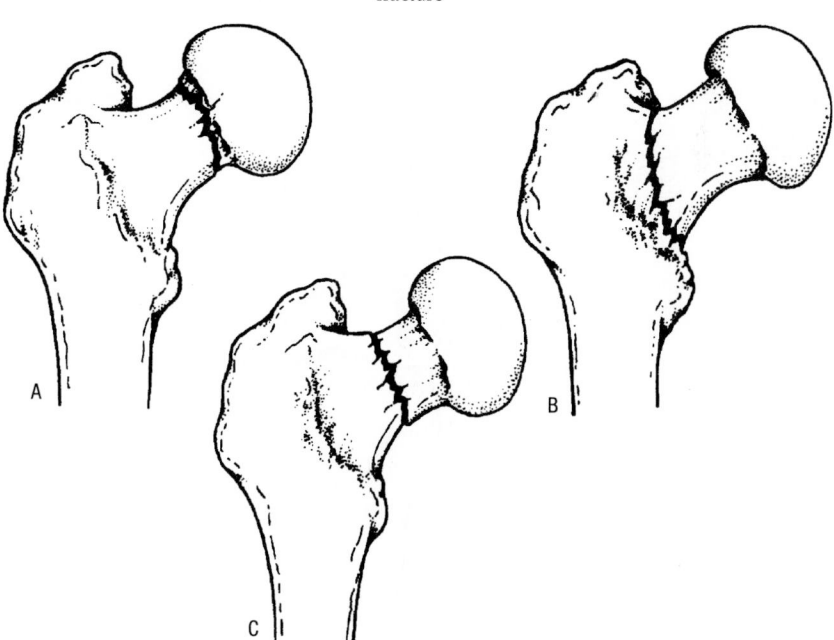

subclassification of intracapsular fractures: (A) subcapital fracture; (B) transcervical fracture; (C) base of neck fracture

knee fractures

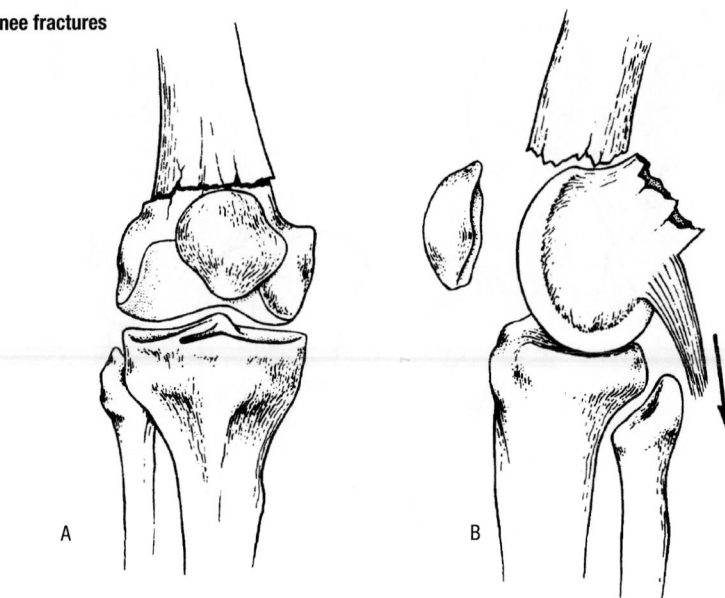

A   B

supracondylar fracture: transverse supracondylar fracture of the femur; note the pull of the gastrocnemius muscle, causing the distal fragment to be rotated posteriorly

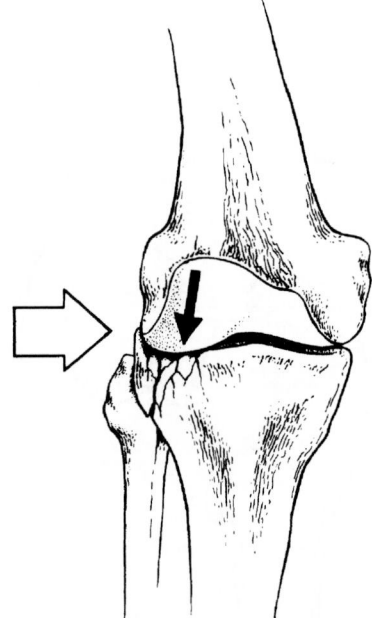

a valgus force applied to the knee causes the hard femoral condyle to be driven into the softer tibial plateau, resulting in depression of the tibial plateau

ankle fractures

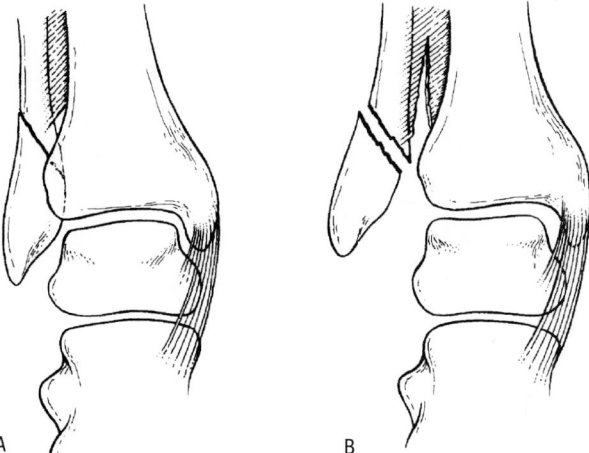

(A) fracture of the lateral malleolus occurring above its articular surface; thus, the ankle mortise is not involved; (B) similar fracture as in (A), above the articular surface with disturbance of the mortise is due to separation of the syndesmosis

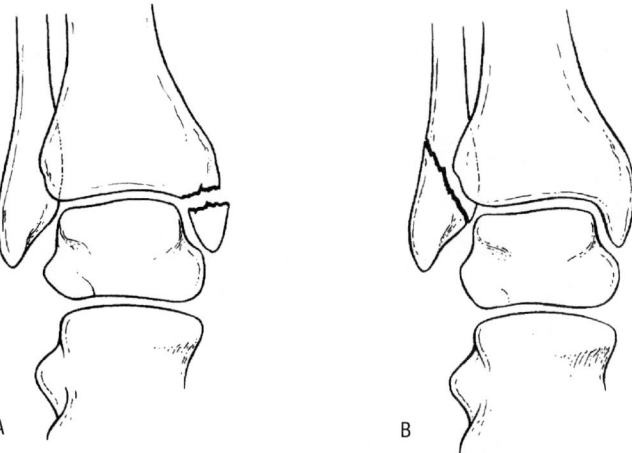

fractures of the malleoli: (A) transverse fracture of the medial malleolus; (B) oblique fracture of the lateral malleolus

Appendix 1

ankle fractures

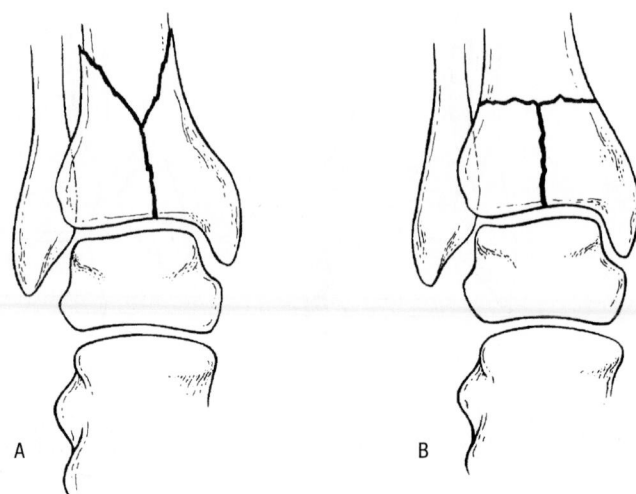

(A) Y-shaped comminuted intraarticular fracture of the distal tibia; (B) T-shaped comminuted intraarticular fracture of the distal tibia

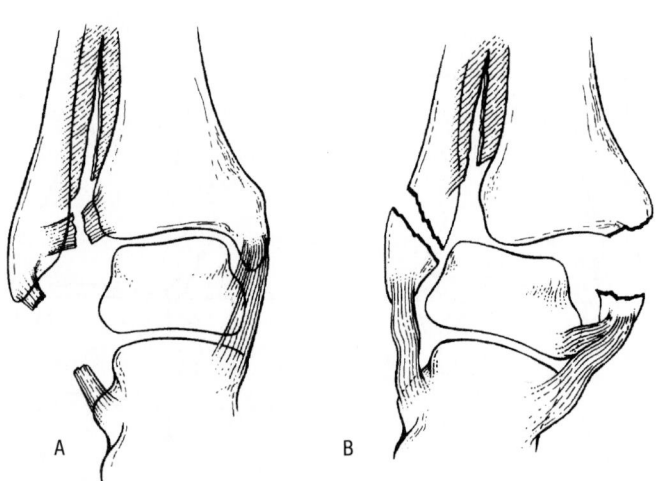

separation of the distal tibiofibular syndesmosis: (A) separation of the tibiofibular syndesmosis without an accompanying fracture; (B) separation of the syndesmosis associated with fracture of the medial and lateral malleoli

leg fractures

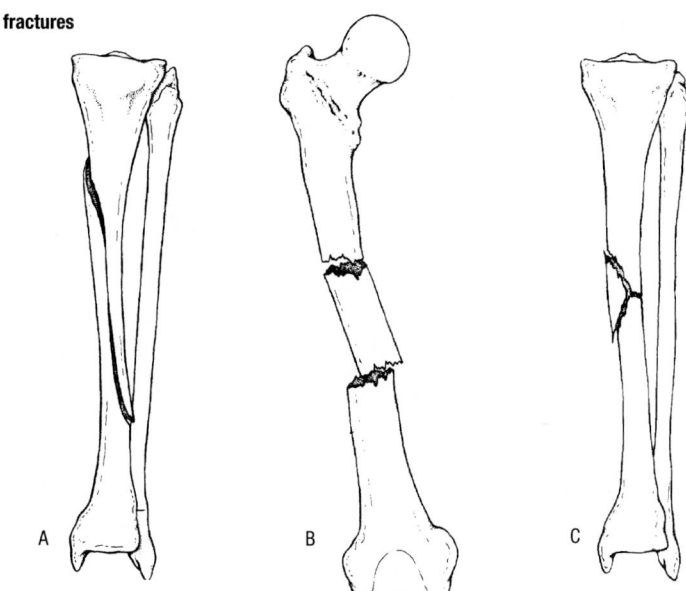

(A) spiral fractures of the middle third of the tibia; (B) segmental fracture of the femur; (C) butterfly fragment

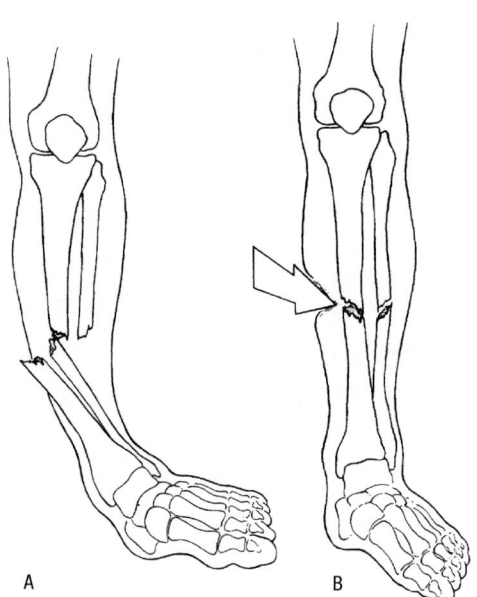

(A) compound fracture caused by an inside-out injury; the skin defect is caused, following the fracture, by the bone perforating the skin from within; **(B) outside-in compound fracture;** in this injury, the skin defect is produced by the fracturing agent entering from without

ankle fractures

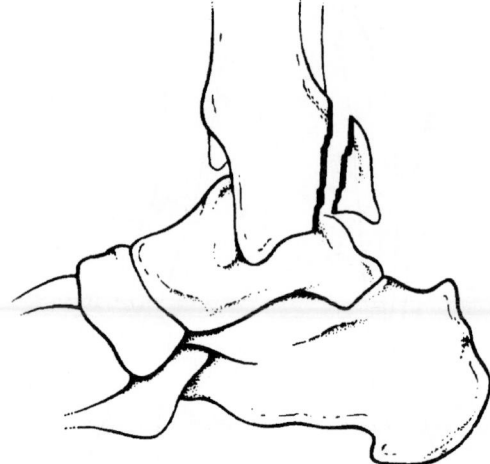

fracture of the posterior malleolus

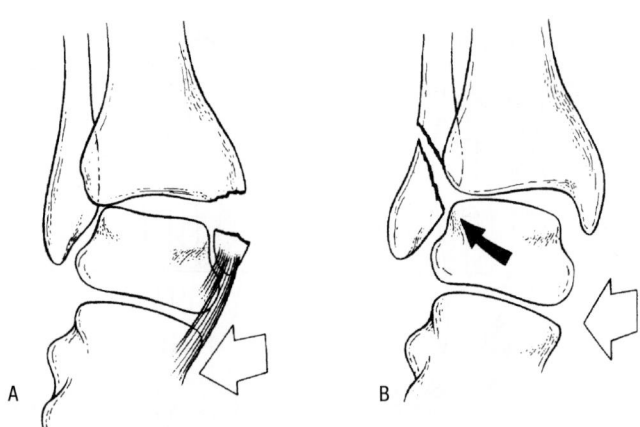

(A) avulsion fracture of the medial malleolus; (B) oblique fracture of the lateral malleolus

foot fractures

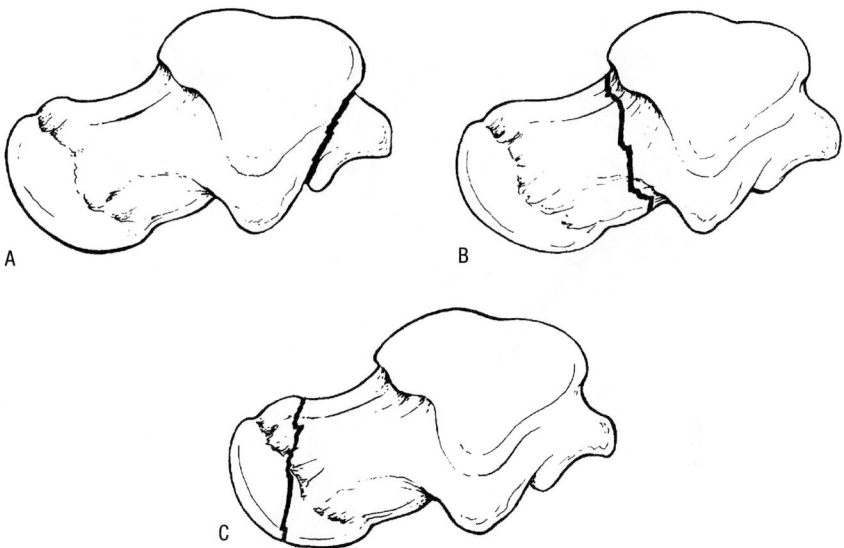

fractures of the talus can be described by the anatomic area involved; (A) fracture of the posterior process; (B) fracture of the body; (C) fracture of the head

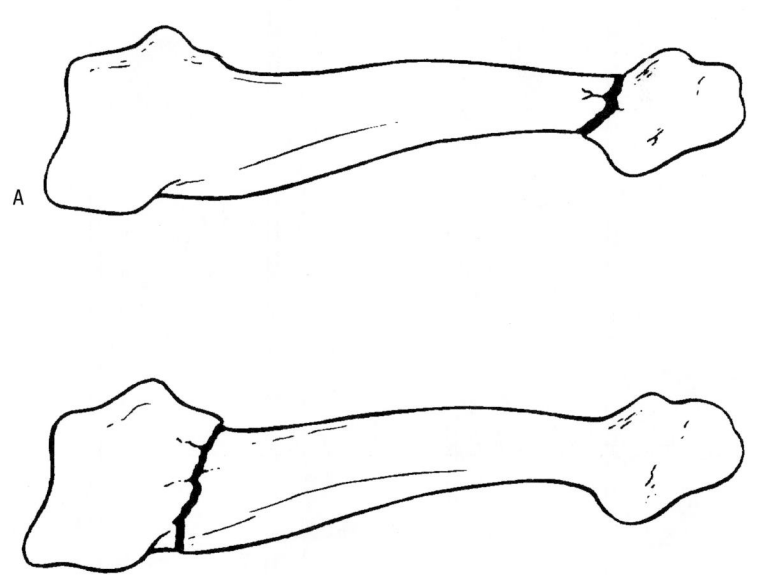

(A) fracture of the head of a metatarsal; (B) fracture of the base of a metatarsal bone

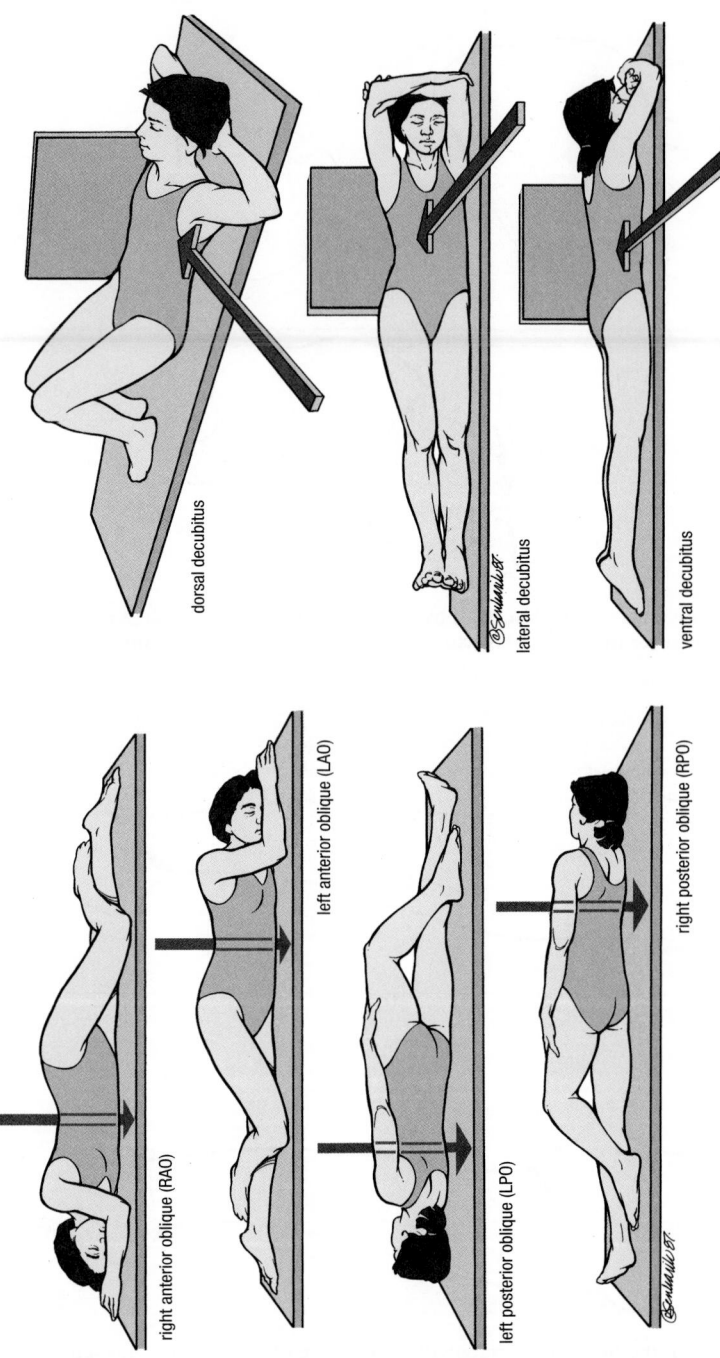

right anterior oblique (RAO)

left anterior oblique (LAO)

left posterior oblique (LPO)

right posterior oblique (RPO)

dorsal decubitus

lateral decubitus

ventral decubitus

patient positions

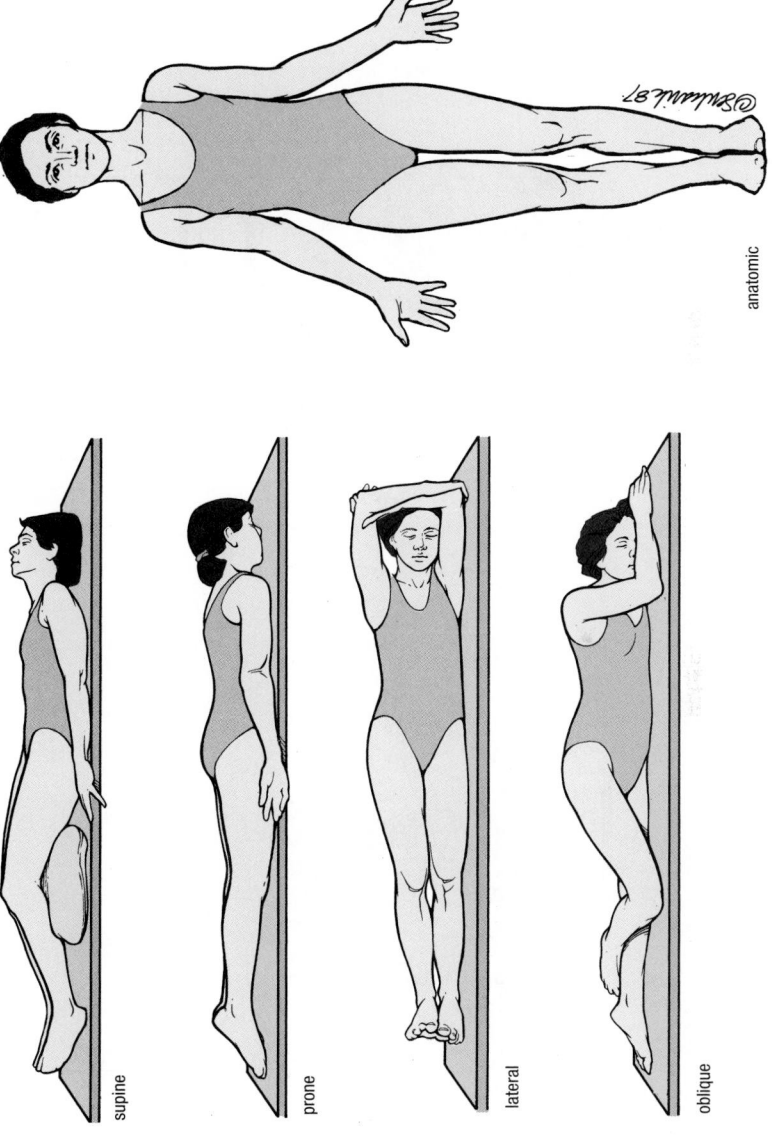

anatomic

supine

prone

lateral

oblique

patient positions

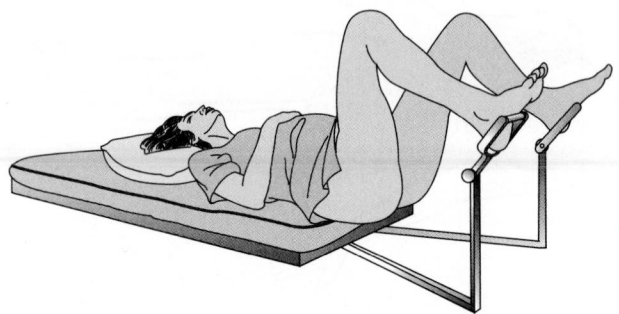

lithomy position, inferolateral view

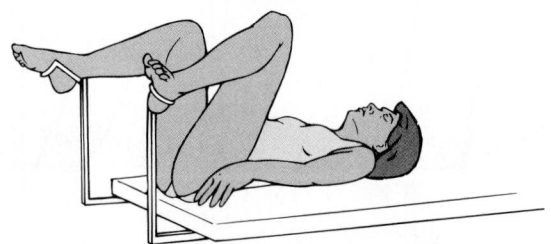

dorsal lithomy position

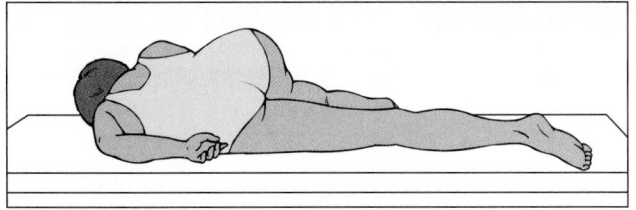

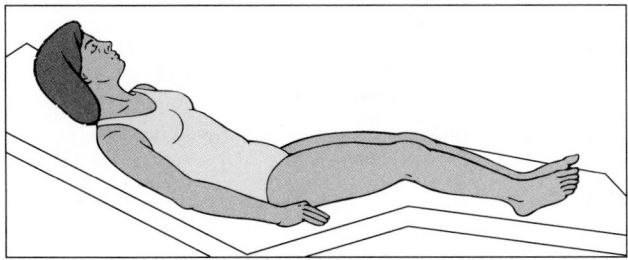

Fowler position

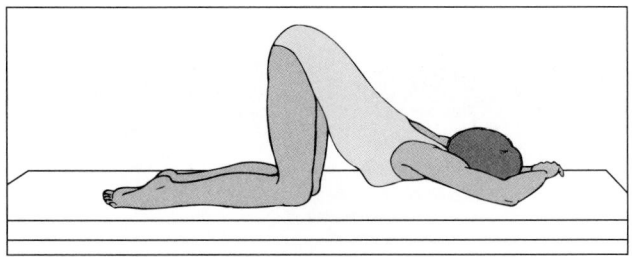

knee-chest position

Assessment of chest pain				
Ailment	**Character, location, and radiation**	**Duration**	**Precipitating conditions**	**Relieving measures**
angina pectoris	Substernal or retrosternal pain spreading across chest May radiate to inside of arm, neck, or jaws	5–15 min	Usually related to exertion, emotion, eating, cold	Rest, nitroglycerin, oxygen
myocardial infarction	Substernal pain or pain over precordium May spread widely throughout chest Painful disability of shoulders and hands may be present	>15 min	Occurs spontaneously but may be sequela to unstable angina	Morphine sulfate, successful reperfusion of blocked coronary artery
pericarditis	Sharp, severe substernal pain or pain to the left of sternum May be felt in epigastrium and may be referred to neck, arms, and back	Intermittent	Sudden onset Pain increases with inspiration, swallowing, coughing, and rotation of trunk	Sitting upright, analgesia, antiinflammatory medications
pulmonary pain	Pain arises from inferior portion of pleura May be referred to costal margins or upper abdomen Patient may be able to localize the pain	30+ min	Often occurs spontaneously Pain occurs or increases with inspiration	Rest, time Treatment of underlying cause, bronchodilation
esophageal pain (Hiatus hernia, reflux esophagitis, or spasm)	Substernal pain May be projected around chest to shoulders	5–60 min	Recumbency, cold liquids, exercise May occur spontaneously	Food, antacid Nitroglycerin relieves spasm
anxiety	Pain over left chest May be variable Does not radiate Patient may complain of numbness and tingling of hands and mouth	2–3 min	Stress, emotional tachypnea	Removal of stimulus, relaxation

assessment of chest pain

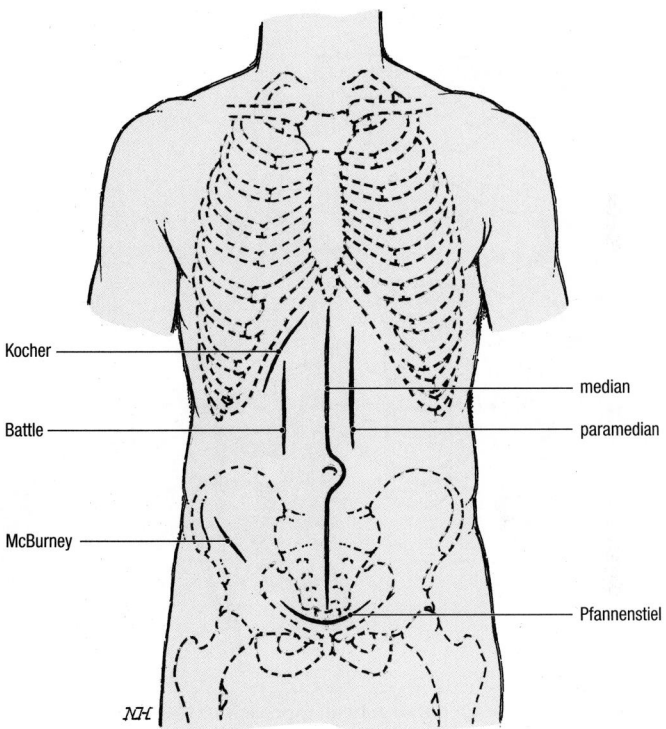

Kocher

Battle

McBurney

median

paramedian

Pfannenstiel

NH

surgical incisions

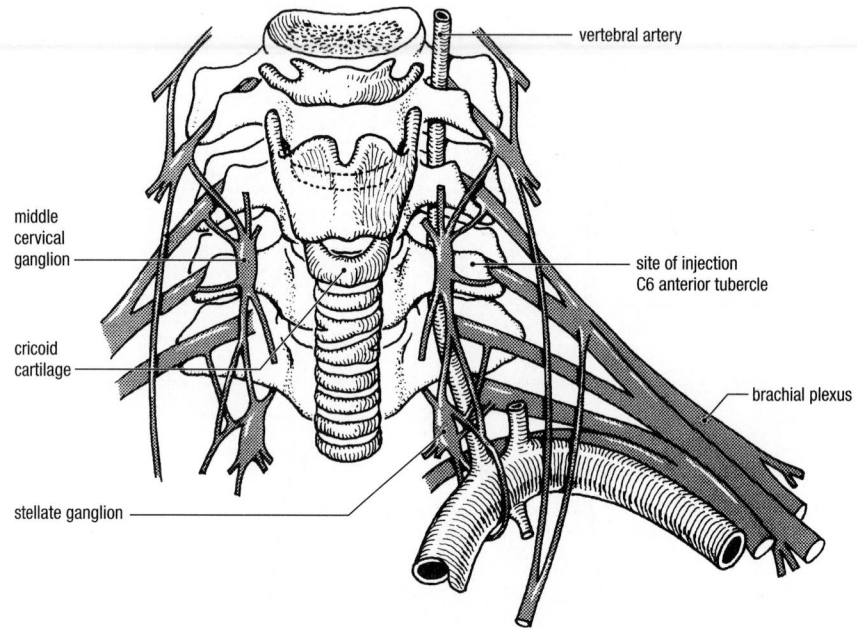

middle
cervical
ganglion

cricoid
cartilage

stellate ganglion

vertebral artery

site of injection
C6 anterior tubercle

brachial plexus

site of injection for the C6 paratracheal approach to the stellate ganglion block

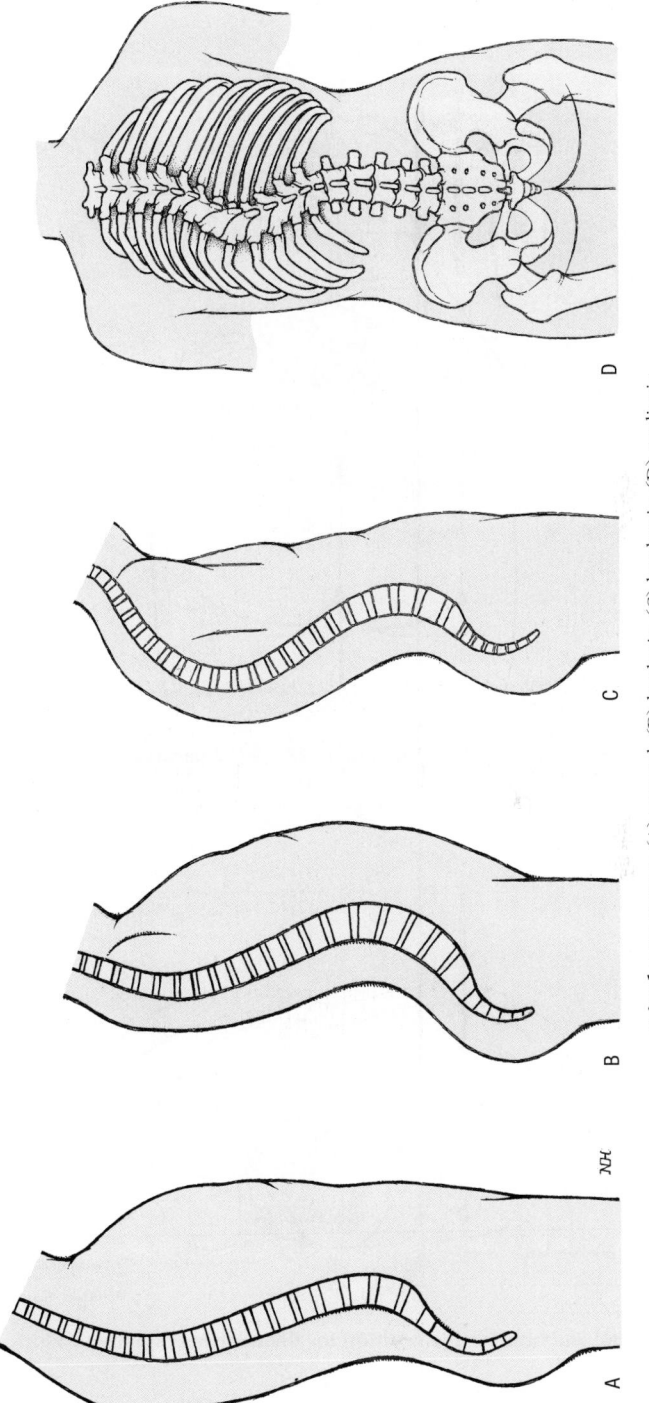

spinal curvatures: (A) normal; (B) lordosis; (C) kyphosis; (D) scoliosis

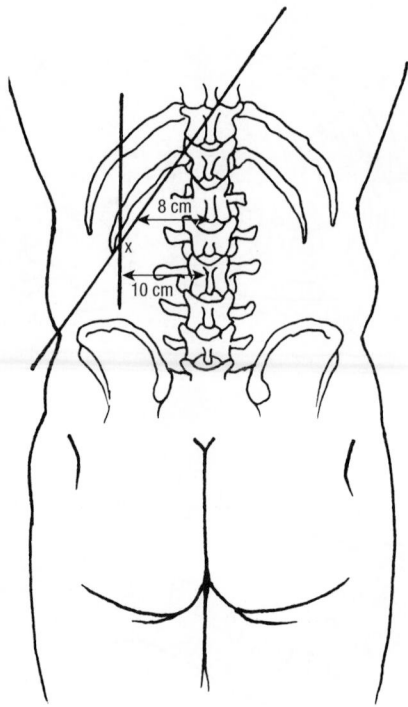

landmarks for the lumbar sympathetic block (L2 paravertebral approach)

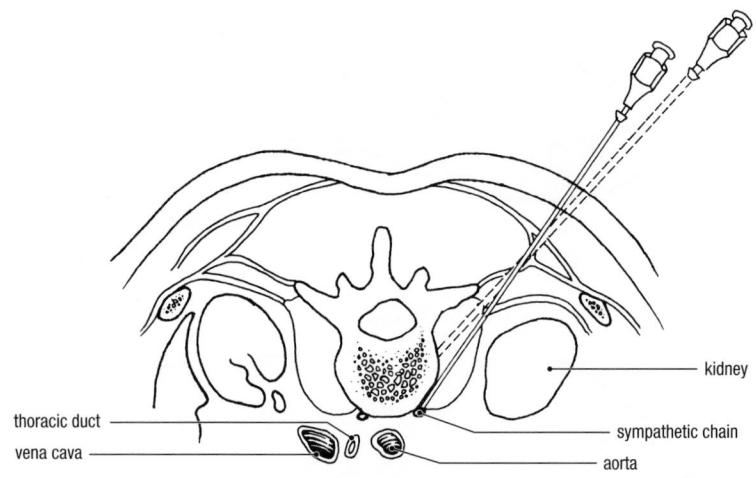

initial and final needle position for the lumbar sympathetic block

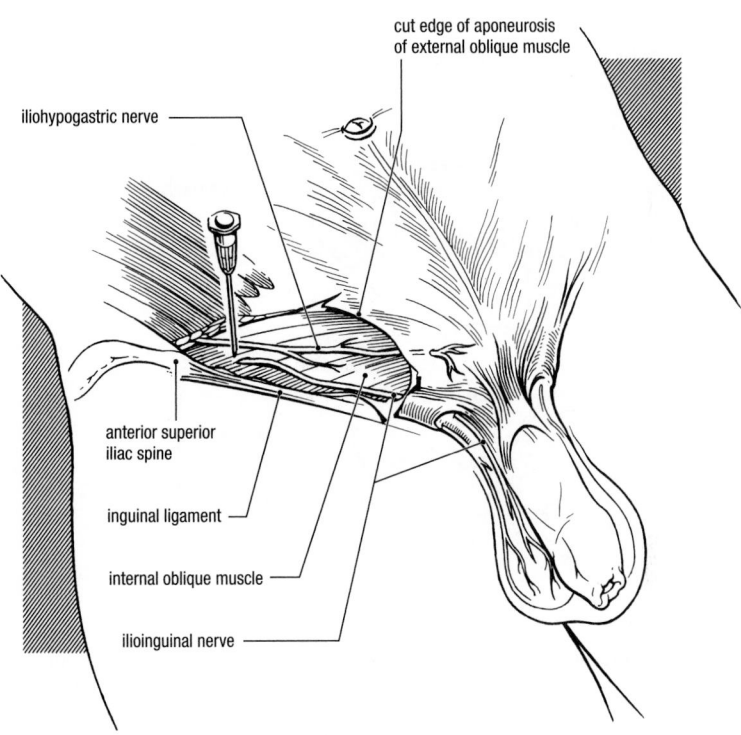

ilioinguinal and iliohypogastric nerve block

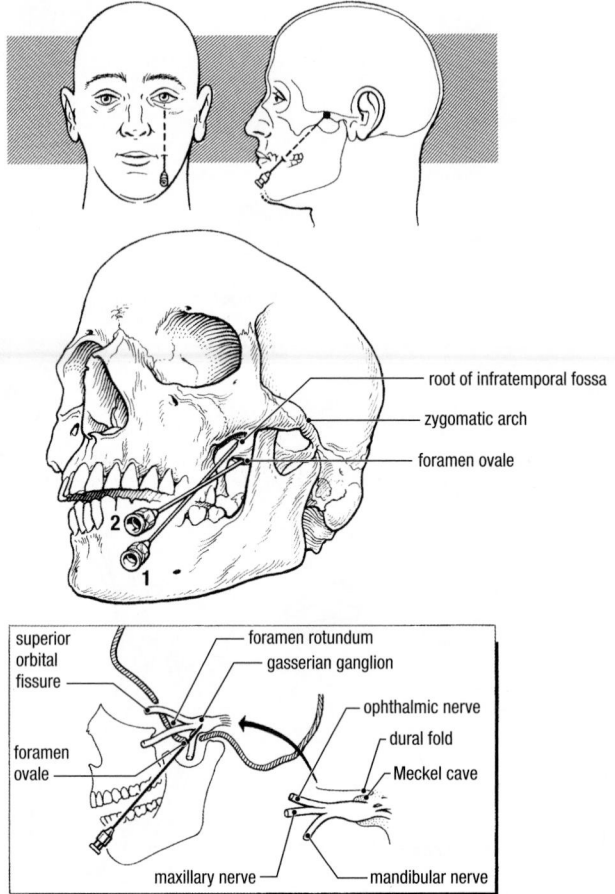

gasserian ganglion block: top panel: needle is inserted in the cheek about 1 cm posterior to the angle of the mouth as shown and directed toward the pupil in the anterior view and the midpoint of the zygoma in the lateral view. In patients with teeth, needle insertion in the cheek is superficial to the teeth of the upper jaw. In edentulous patients, this may lie a variable distance between the angle of the mouth and the line midway between upper lip and nose. A palpating finger in the mouth helps to prevent needle penetration into the mouth. Middle panel: (1) as the needle is advanced into the infratemporal fossa, it will usually strike the roof of the infratemporal fossa initially; this is the correct depth to seek the foramen ovale; (2) the needle is then directed slightly posteriorly to obtain a mandibular nerve (V3) paresthesia. Lower panel: the needle can then be advanced through the foramen ovale into the middle cranial fossa, where it will be adjacent to the gasserian ganglion, as shown. Note the relationships of the dural fold and Meckel cave, containing cerebrospinal fluid. A needle advanced too far through the foramen ovale can enter the Meckel cave, and subsequent injections could enter the cranial CSF and produce total spine anesthesia.

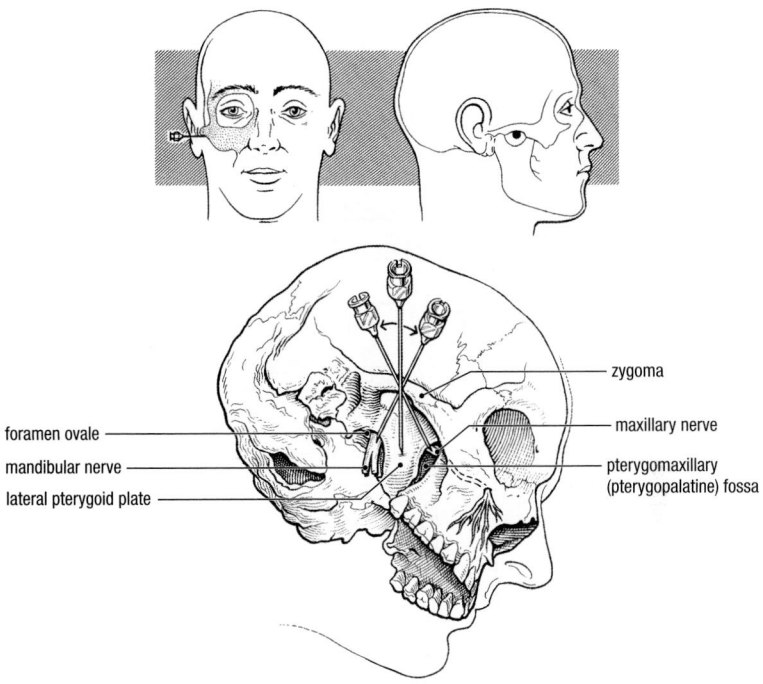

gasserian ganglion block

zygoma

foramen ovale

maxillary nerve

mandibular nerve

pterygomaxillary
(pterygopalatine) fossa

lateral pterygoid plate

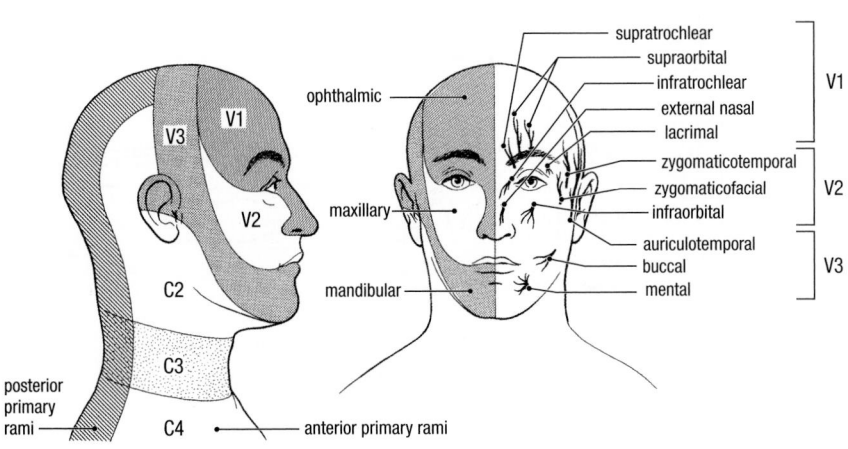

dermatomes and cutaneous nerves of head, neck, and face

supratrochlear

supraorbital

infratrochlear

external nasal

lacrimal

V1

zygomaticotemporal

zygomaticofacial

infraorbital

V2

auriculotemporal

buccal

mental

V3

ophthalmic

maxillary

mandibular

V3

V1

V2

C2

C3

C4

posterior primary rami

anterior primary rami

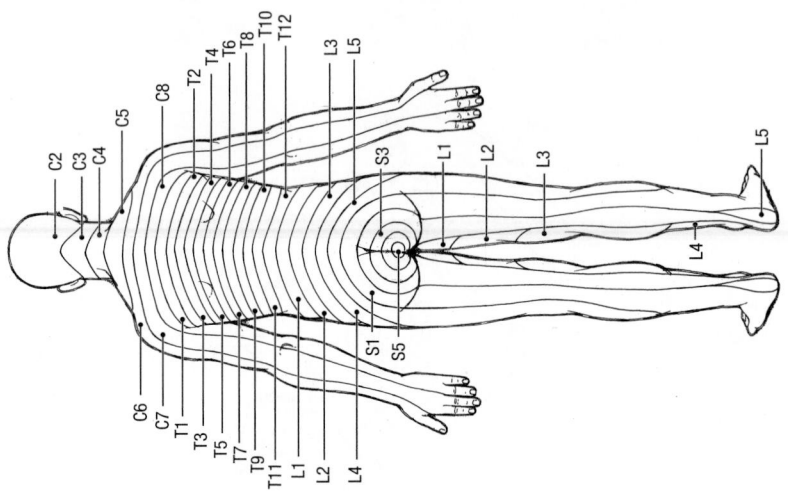

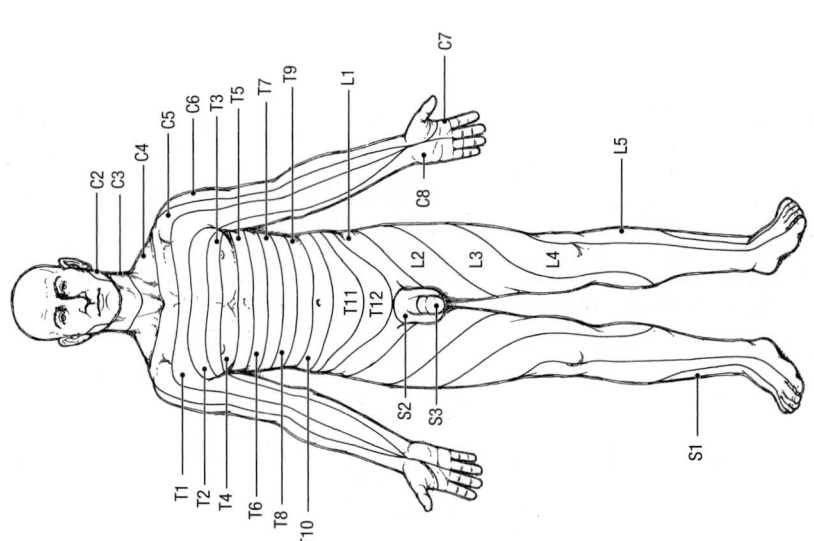

dermatomes

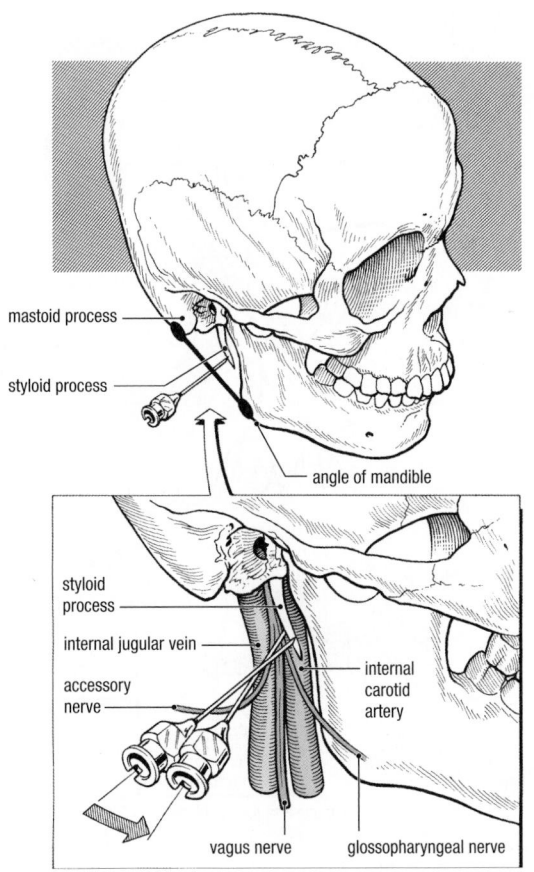

mastoid process

styloid process

angle of mandible

styloid process

internal jugular vein

accessory nerve

internal carotid artery

vagus nerve

glossopharyngeal nerve

glossopharyngeal nerve block

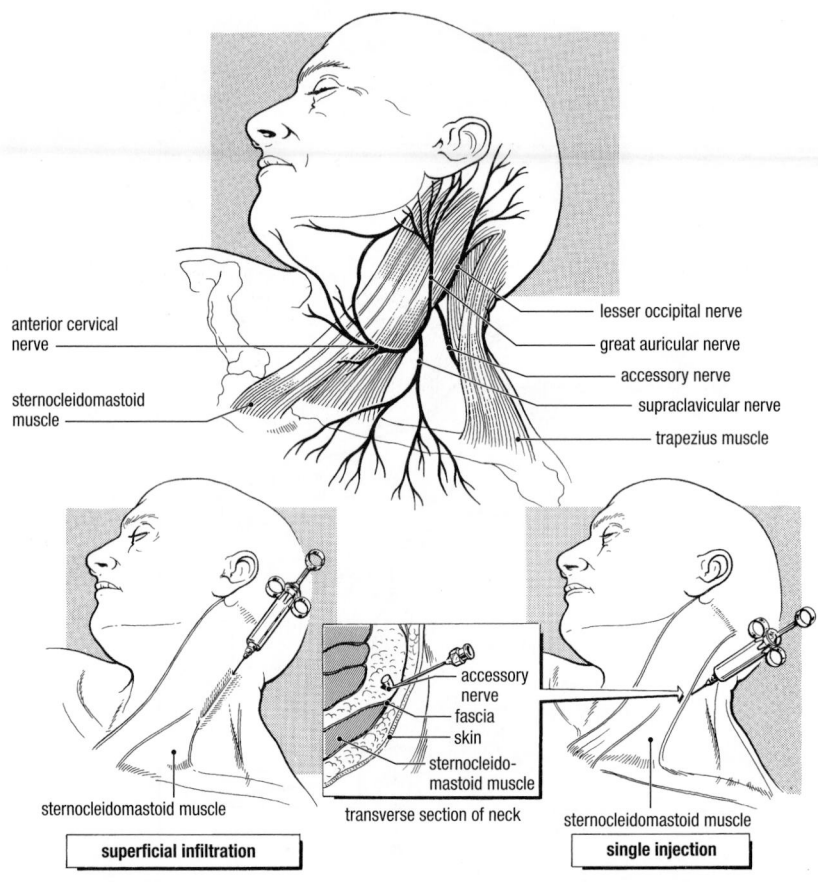

anterior cervical nerve

sternocleidomastoid muscle

lesser occipital nerve

great auricular nerve

accessory nerve

supraclavicular nerve

trapezius muscle

sternocleidomastoid muscle

superficial infiltration

accessory nerve

fascia

skin

sternocleido-mastoid muscle

transverse section of neck

sternocleidomastoid muscle

single injection

the superficial cervical plexus, which is blocked in the posterior triangle of the neck as it emerges adjacent to the midpoint of the posterior border of the sternocleidomastoid muscle

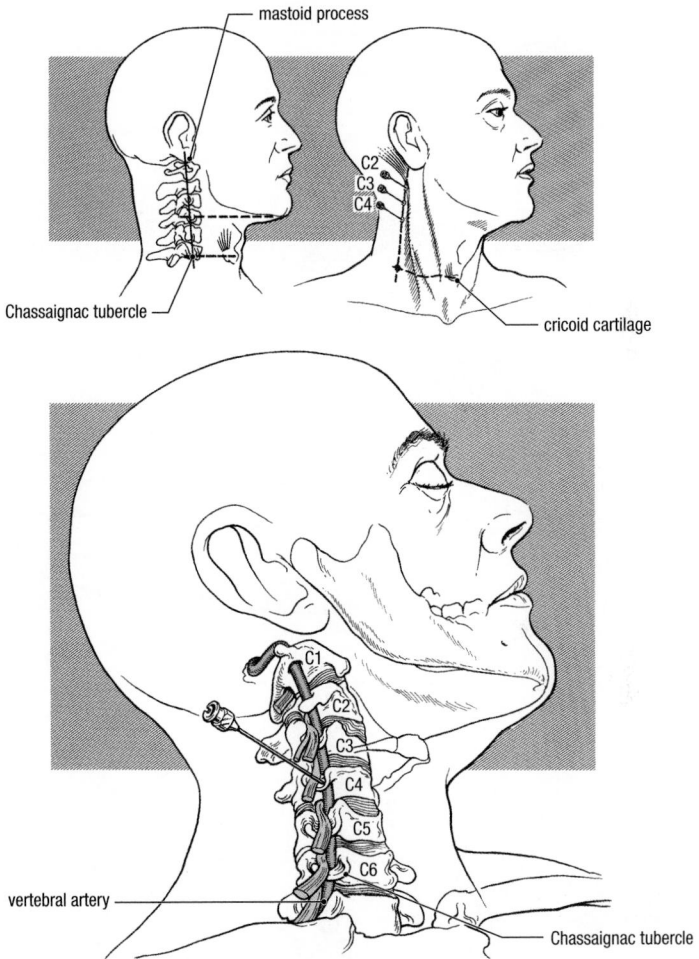

deep cervical plexus block

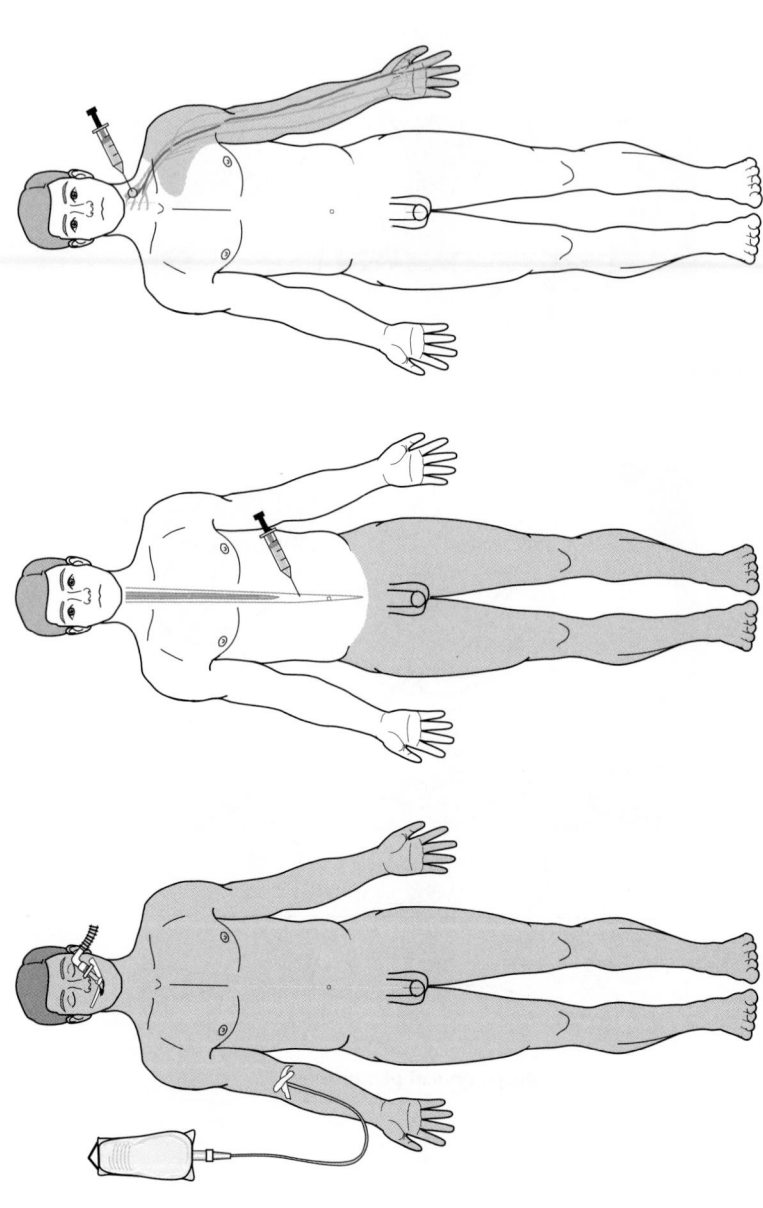

3-part illustration showing the regions affected by 3 types of anesthesia: (left) general, (middle) regional, and (right) peripheral

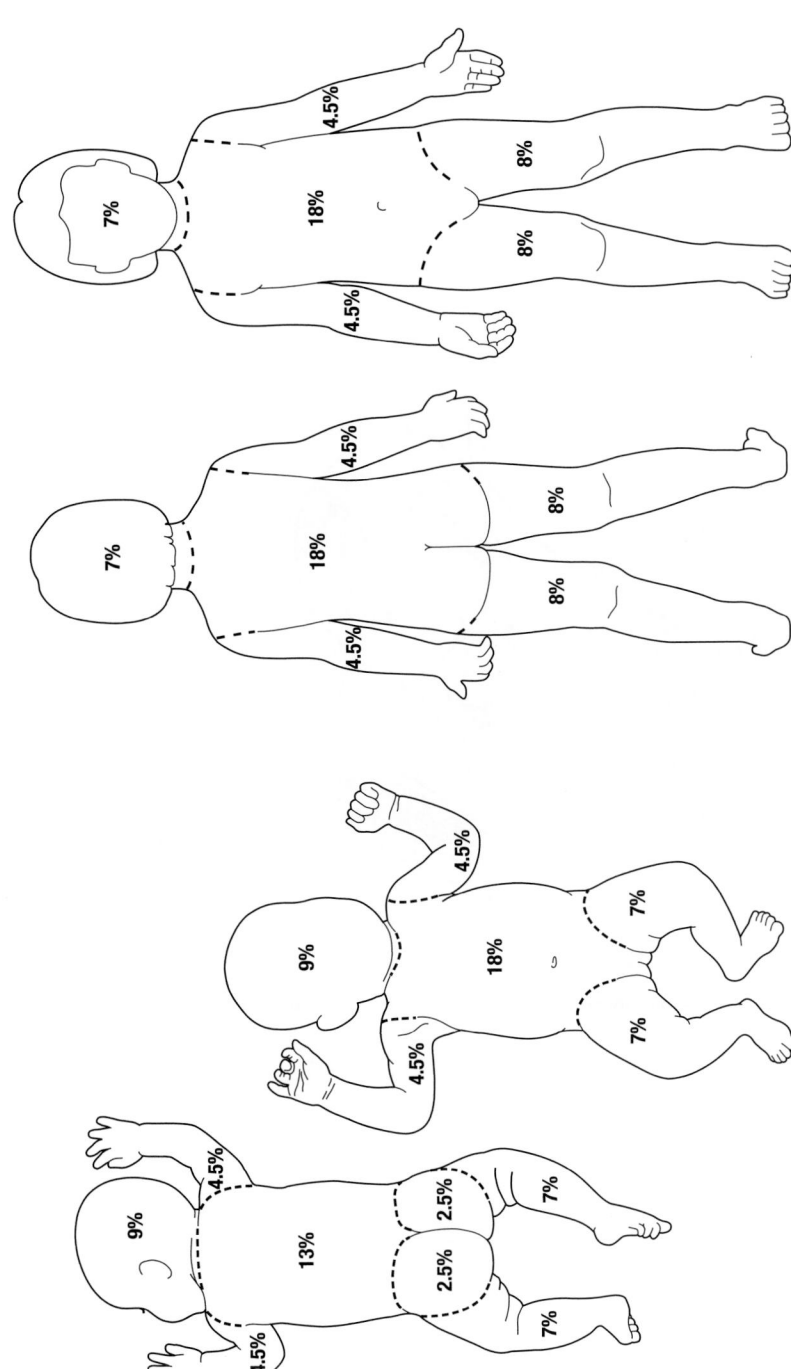

rule of nines (child, 5–9 years): outline of child's body with areas and percentages indicated to calculate total burn surface area

rule of nines (infant): outline of infant's body with areas and percentages indicated to calculate total burn surface area

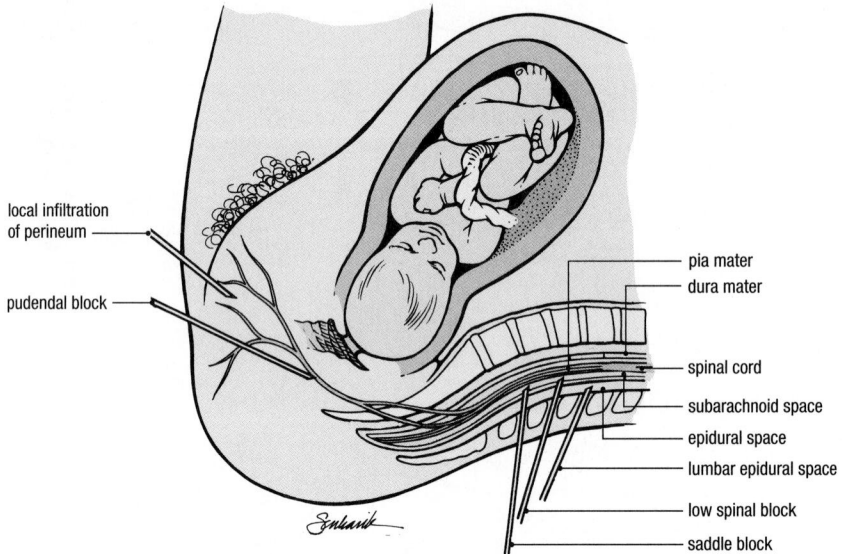

local infiltration
of perineum

pudendal block

pia mater
dura mater

spinal cord
subarachnoid space
epidural space
lumbar epidural space
low spinal block
saddle block

regional anesthesia for child birth, sites of injection

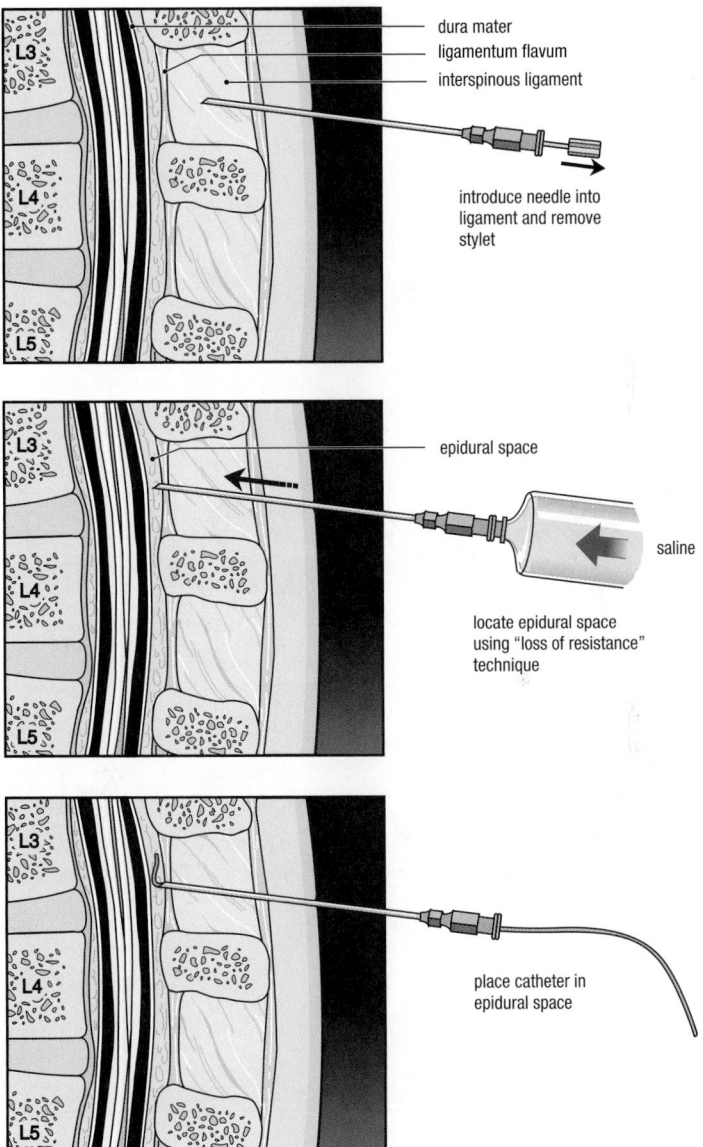

3-step illustration showing the procedure used in giving an epidural

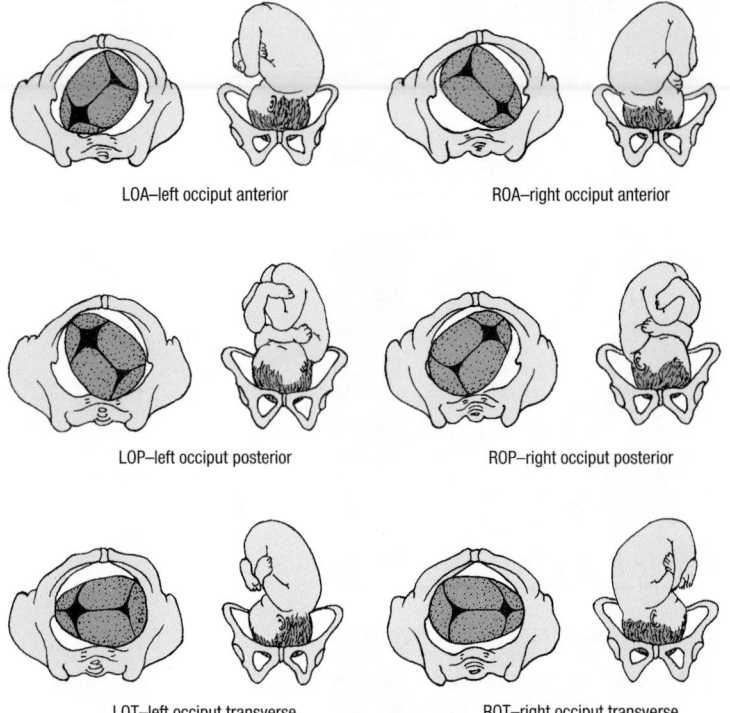

LOA–left occiput anterior

ROA–right occiput anterior

LOP–left occiput posterior

ROP–right occiput posterior

LOT–left occiput transverse

ROT–right occiput transverse

vertex presentation: fetal head position within the pelvic girdle in a vertex presentation

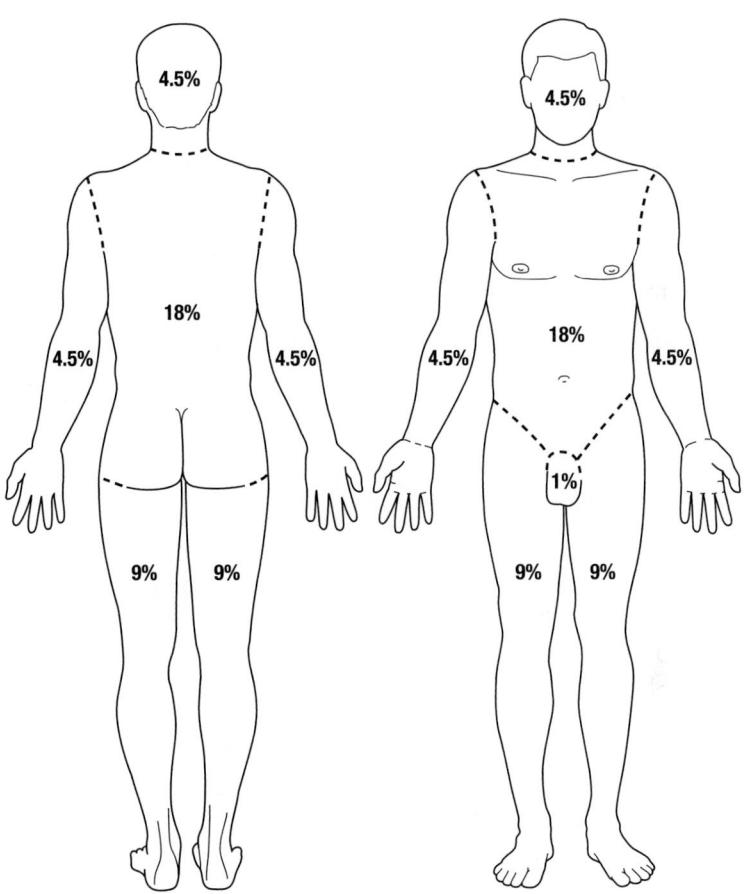

rule of nines (adult): outline of adult's body with areas and percentages indicated to calculate total burn surface area

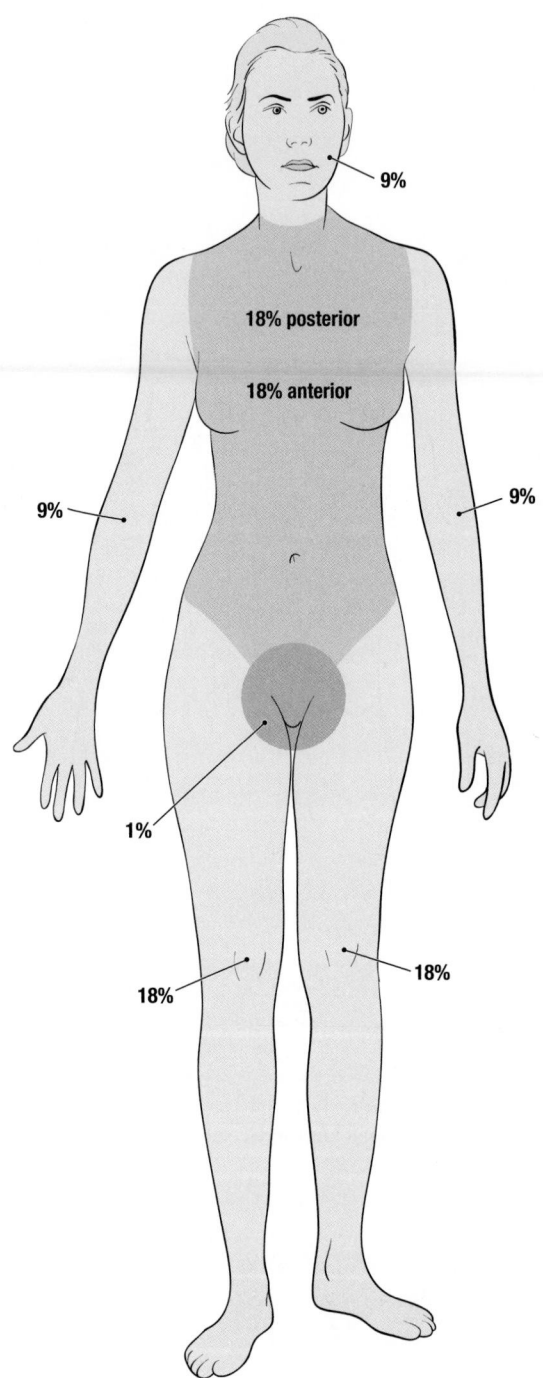

adult female illustrating the rule of nines used when assessing burn damage to various body parts

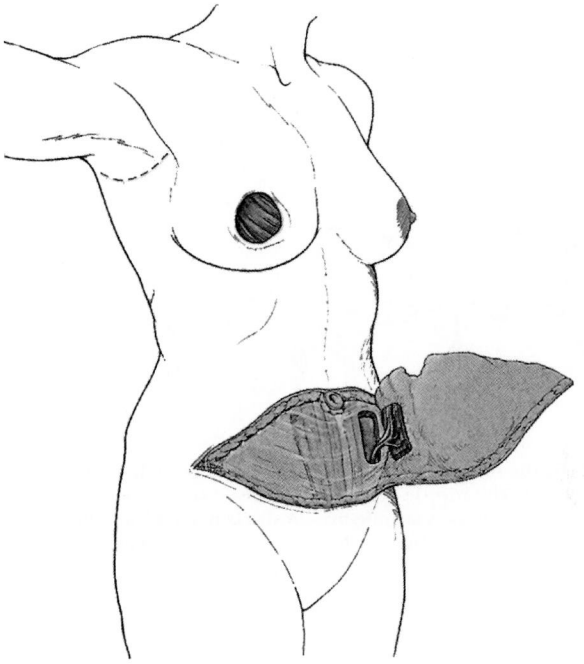

concept of the skin-sparing mastectomy by using the periareolar approach: in this case, the depicted free TRAM flap is based on the deep inferior epigastric artery and vein

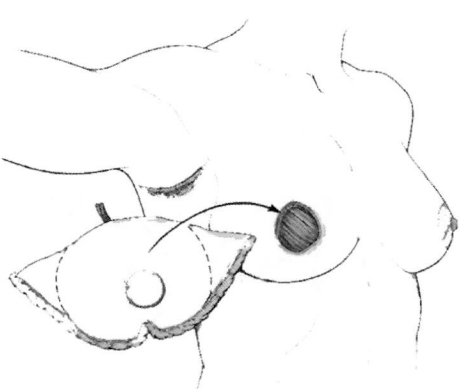

the flap is then passed through the periareolar incision, with the microvascular anastomoses performed through small separate axillary incision

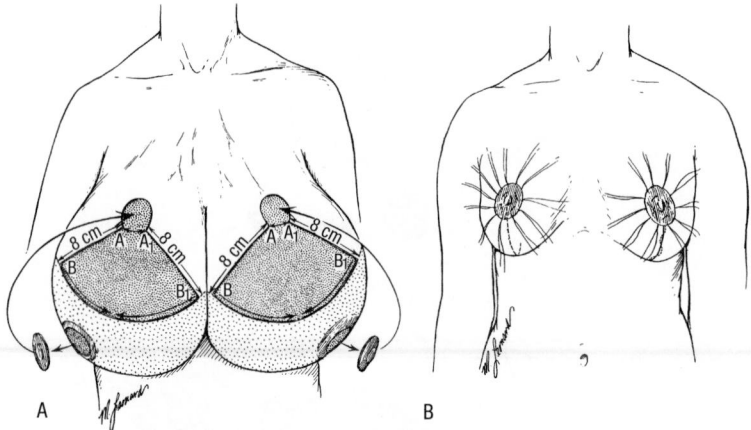

(A) the width of the breast amputation and dermal pedicle may vary depending on the size of each breast. The nipple-areolas are excised from the breast tissue specimen; (B) the position of the new nipple-areola site is determined with the patient in a semi-upright position and the nipple-areola specimen placed on the dermal base as a free graft

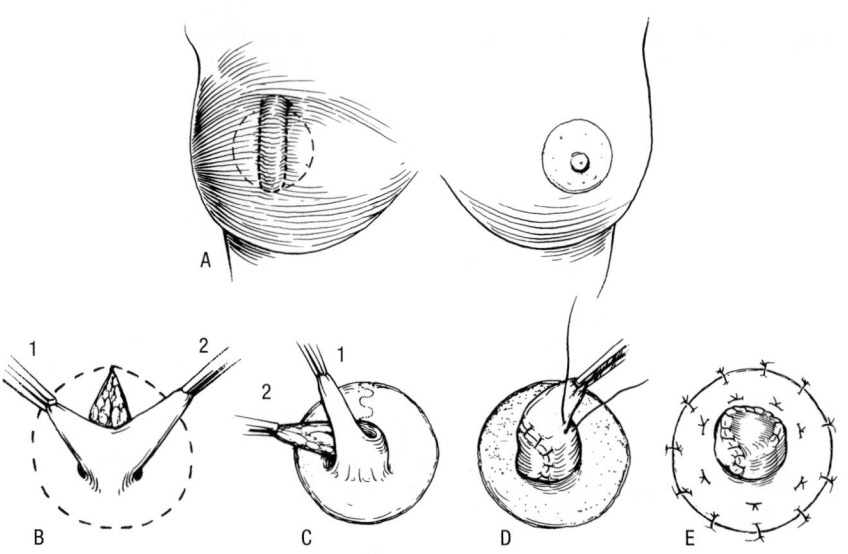

(A) the redundant area of a TRAM flap is marked for the position of a new areola; (B) flaps 1 and 2 are elevated utilizing the redundant TRAM flap tissue; (C) flaps 1 and 2 are now interpolated; (D) the position of new flaps 1 and 2. the surrounding area is deepithelialized; (E) the newly reconstructed nipple and full-thickness skin graft

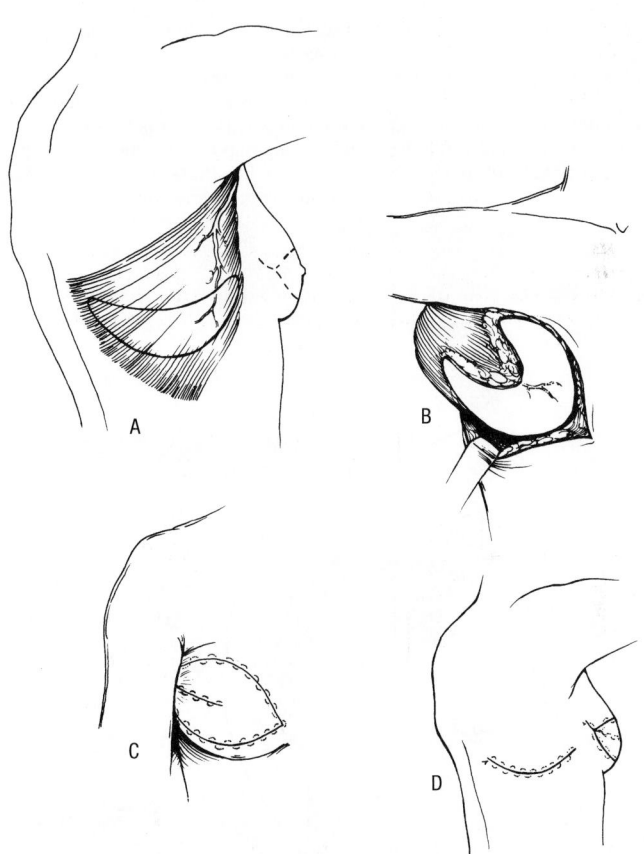

(A) the latissimus myocutaneous flap outline; (B) myocutaneous flap being transferred beneath a lateral axillary skin bridge; (C) transferred flap in its new position; (D) location of the final incisions

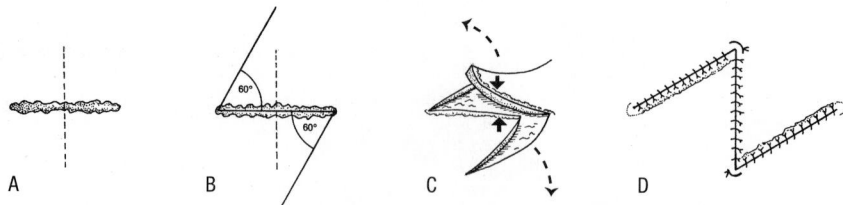

the classic Z-plasty: (A) a thick, contracted scar crosses a skin fold. Design is begun by drawing a perpendicular line at the midpoint of the scar; this line helps establish flap incisions, but it is not itself incised; (B) completing the design, the limbs of flaps are equal to each other and to the length of the scar; angles of the flaps are 60°; (C) flaps are elevated, preserving the subdermal plexus undermining is accomplished around flap bases. The scar is excised unless it is too wide; here a portion of the scar is left for clarity in showing flap transposition; (D) flaps are transposed and sutured; a 3-corner suture (half-buried horizontal mattress) is used to anchor narrow tips, avoiding necrosis that could result from simple sutures near tips

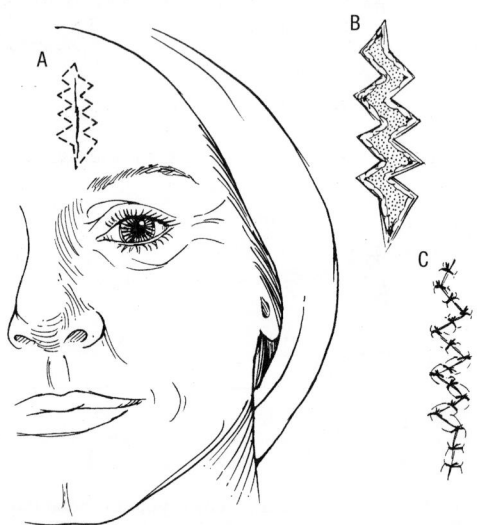

the W-plasty: (A) dotted lines show the design for the excision of the scar; (B) flaps have now been developed and are ready for interdigitation; (C) the W-flaps are in position

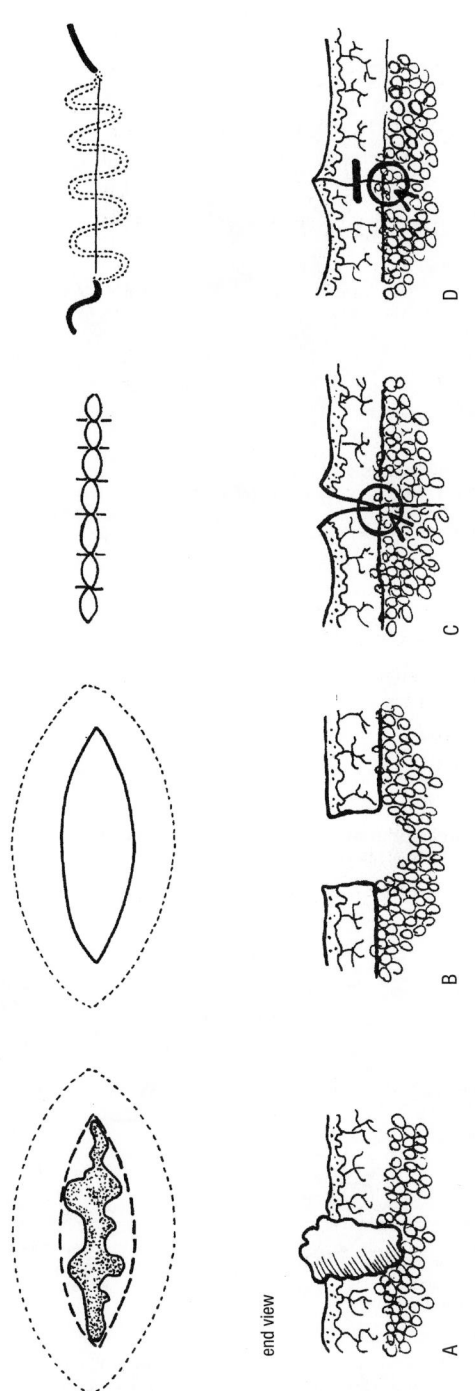

linear scar revision: (A) outline for planned repair; (B) excision and undermining; (C) deep layer closure, the end view shows that the wound should be almost fully closed; (D) final closure, buried running subcuticular Prolene. The top view shows suture weaving back and forth across wound in dermis, piercing the epidermis only at each end; the thickness of the suture is exaggerated for clarity

end view

A   B   C   D

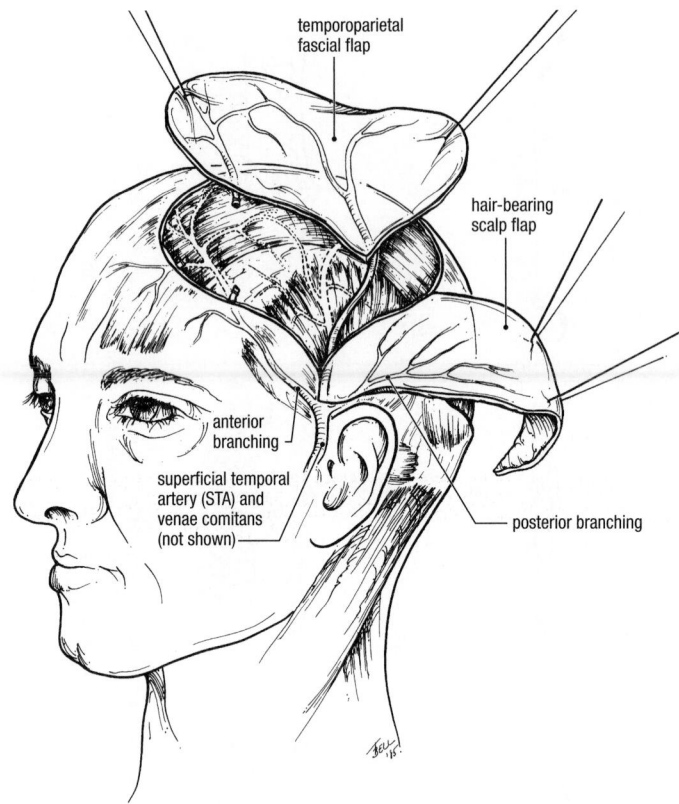

surgical anatomy of scalp and facial flap

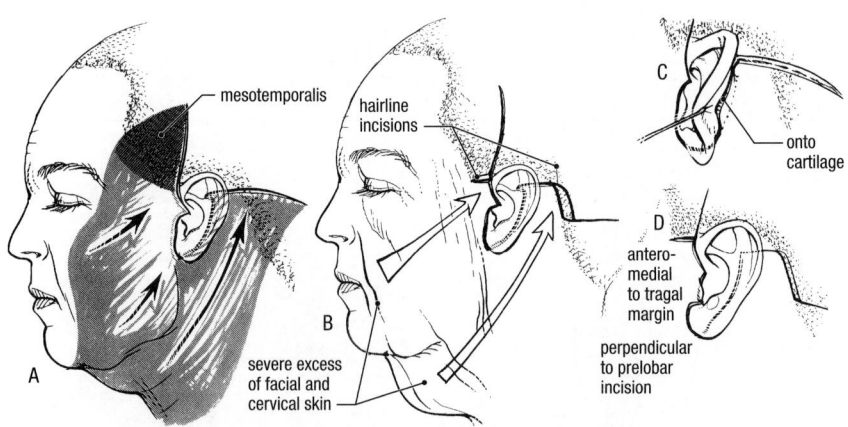

classic facelift incisions: (A) areas of incision; (B) hairline incisions; (C) postauricular incision for redrape; (D) retrotragal approach for redrape

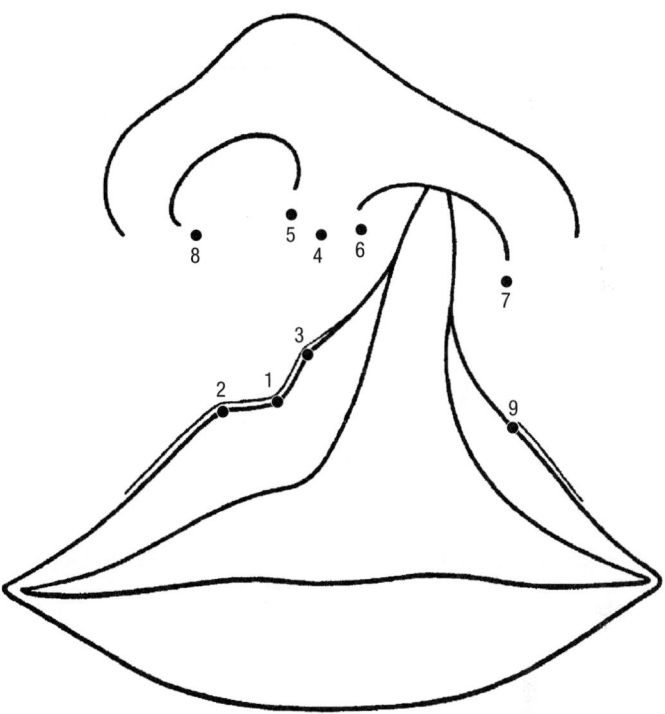

anatomy of the normal and unrepaired unilateral cleft lip indicating key points used for planning repair: (1) lowest point in arch of Cupid's bow, midline of the lip; (2) peak of Cupid's bow on the noncleft side; (3) proposed peak of Cupid's bow; (4) midpoint of the columella; (5, 6) base of columella laterally; (7, 8) inset of alar base into nostril sill; (9) a point on the well-developed vermilion cutaneous roll of the lateral lip and the same horizontal plane as the peak of Cupid's bow on the noncleft side

Appendix 1

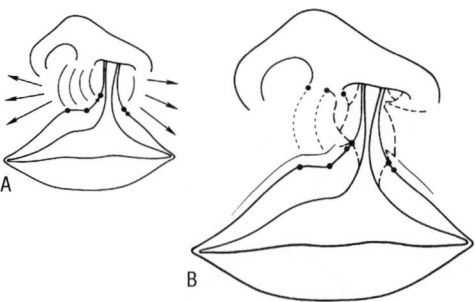

cleft lip repair: (A) unrepaired cleft lip stresses; (B) incorportating stresses into repair

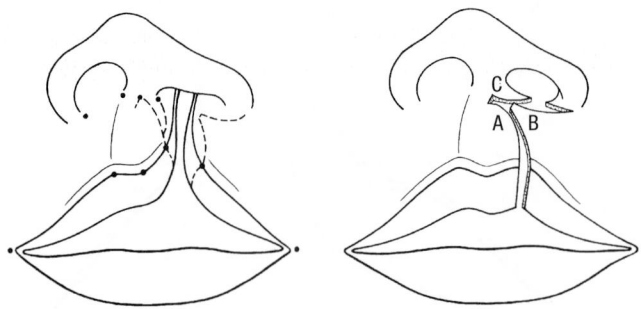

rotation advancement flap technique: (A) medial lip element; (B) lateral lip element; (C) small medial flap

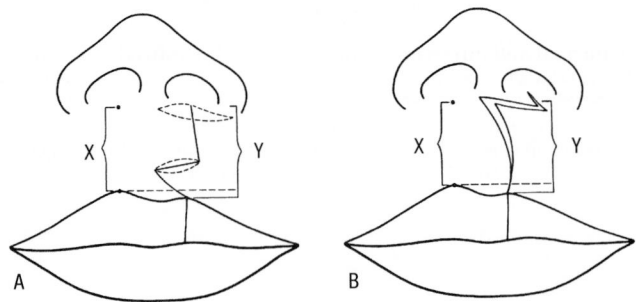

cleft lip redo surgery: (A) previous triangular or quadrangular repair flap; (B) rotation advancement flap redo technique

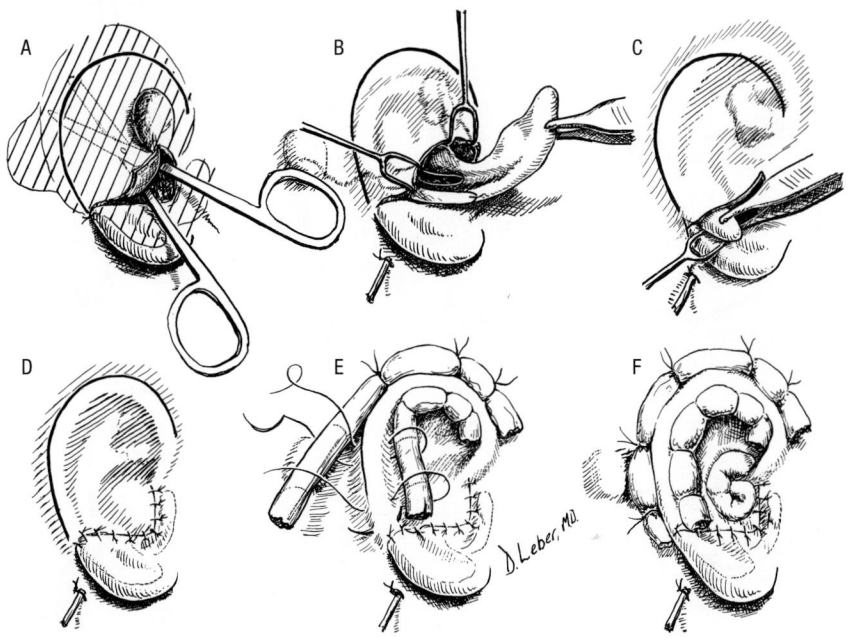

otoplasty techniques: (A) preparing subcutaneous pocket; (B) placing cartilage graft material; (C) incorportating helix; (D) separate placement of tragal material; external sutures; (E) stent placement for external shaping; (F) conchal floor pressure dressing

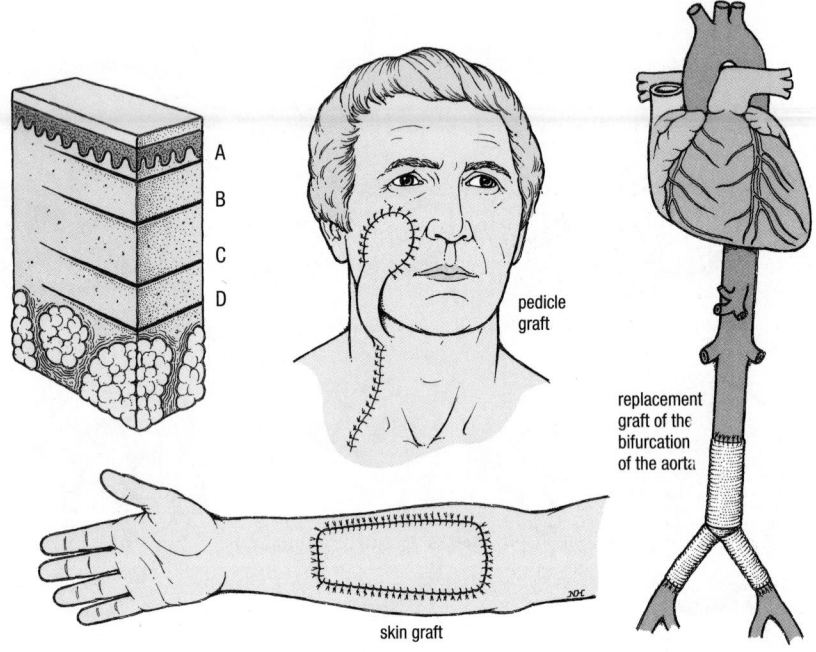

pedicle
graft

replacement
graft of the
bifurcation
of the aorta

skin graft

graft types: (A,B,C) split-thickness graft; (D) full-thickness graft

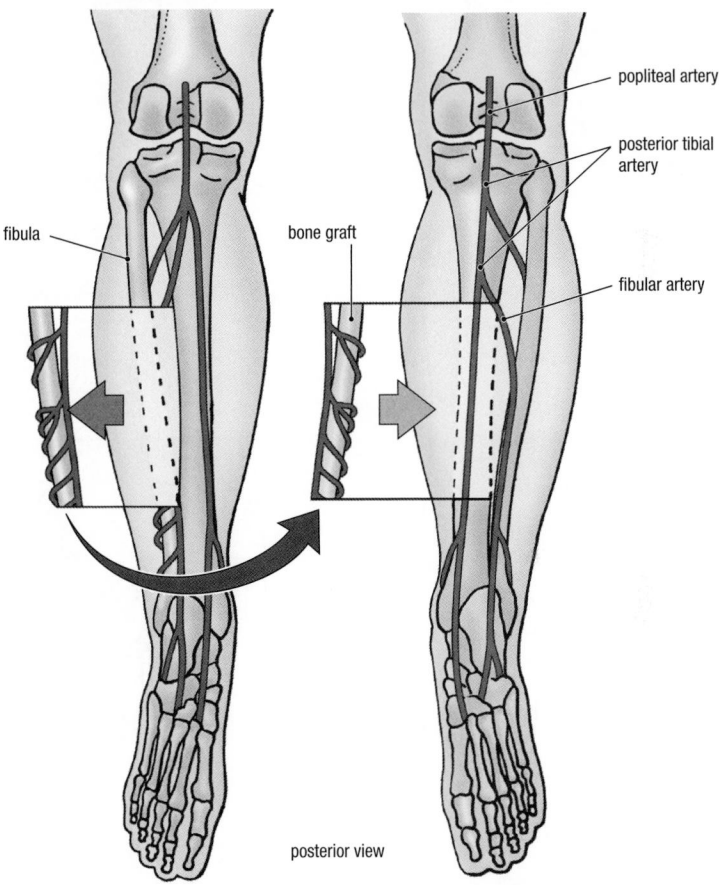

fibula

bone graft

popliteal artery

posterior tibial artery

fibular artery

posterior view

bone grafts: the fibula is a common source of bone for grafting

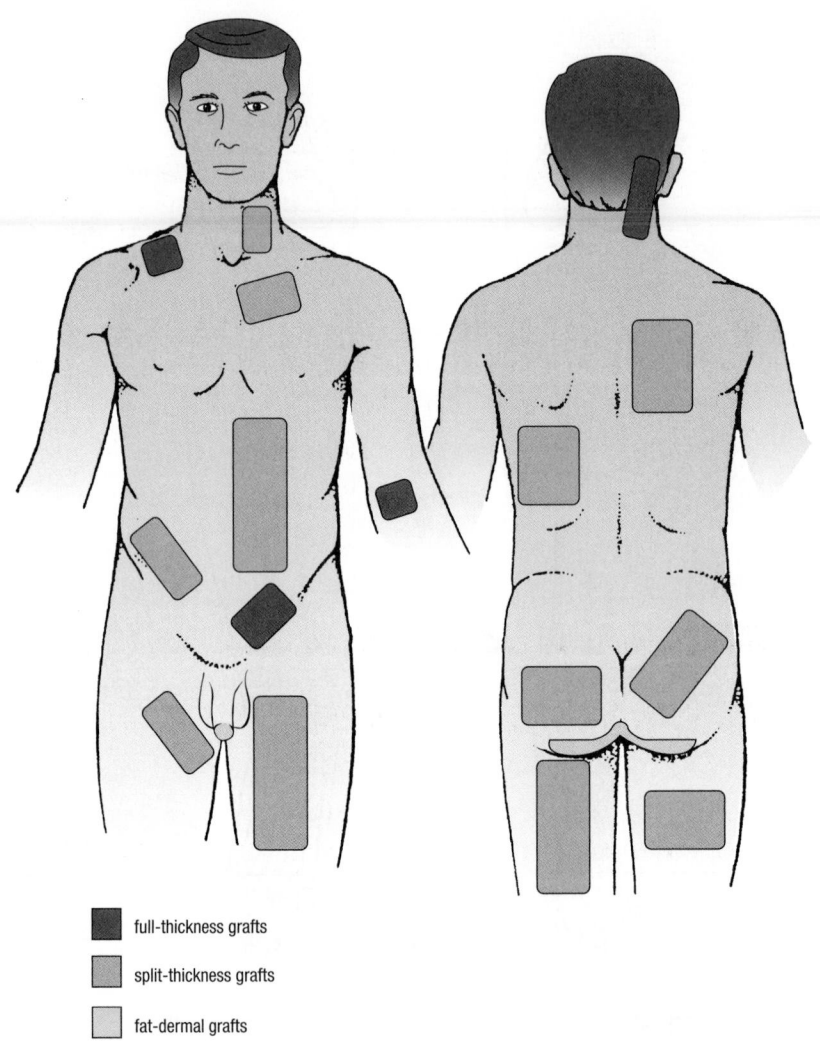

full-thickness grafts

split-thickness grafts

fat-dermal grafts

common donor skin graft sites: dark gray skin areas are appropriate for full-thickness grafts; medium gray areas are used for split-thickness grafts, and light gray sites are used for fat-dermal grafts

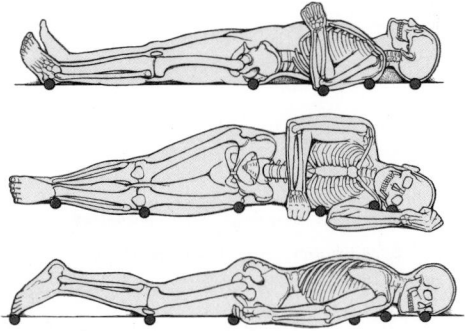

decubitus ulcer: dots indicate most common sites due to proximity of bone to skin

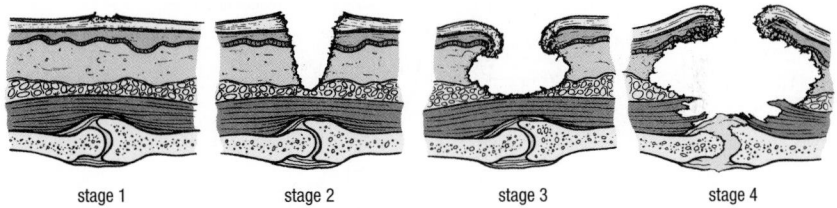

stage 1   stage 2   stage 3   stage 4

cross-section of skin showing 4 stages of pressure sore and ulcer classification: stage 1: inflammation, redness of epidermis; stage 2: loss of epidermis, damage to dermis; stage 3: involvement of subcutaneous tissue; stage 4: damage to tendon, muscle and bone

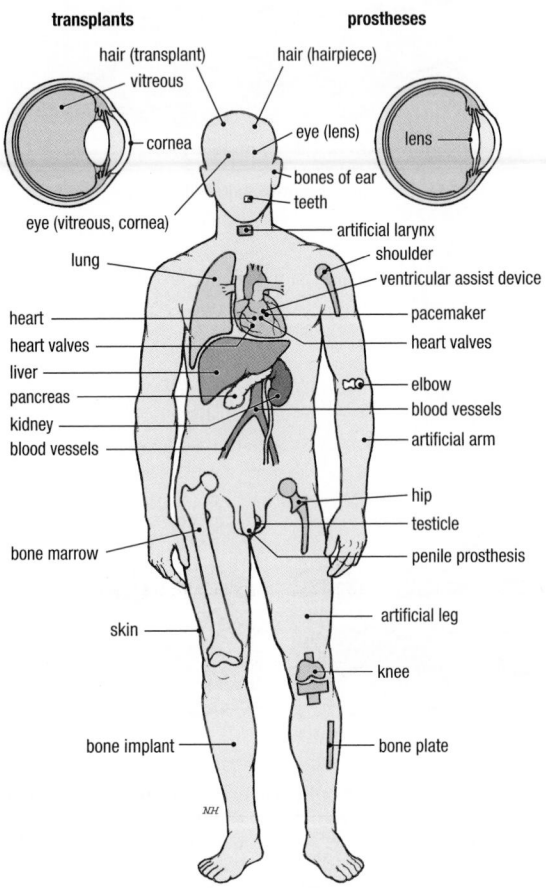

transplants and prostheses

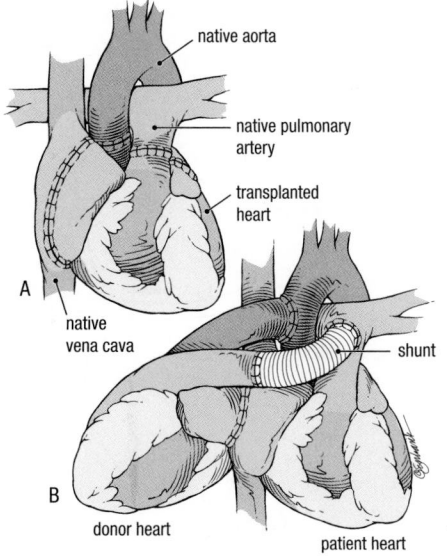

heart transplantation: (A) orthotopic method; (B) heterotopic method

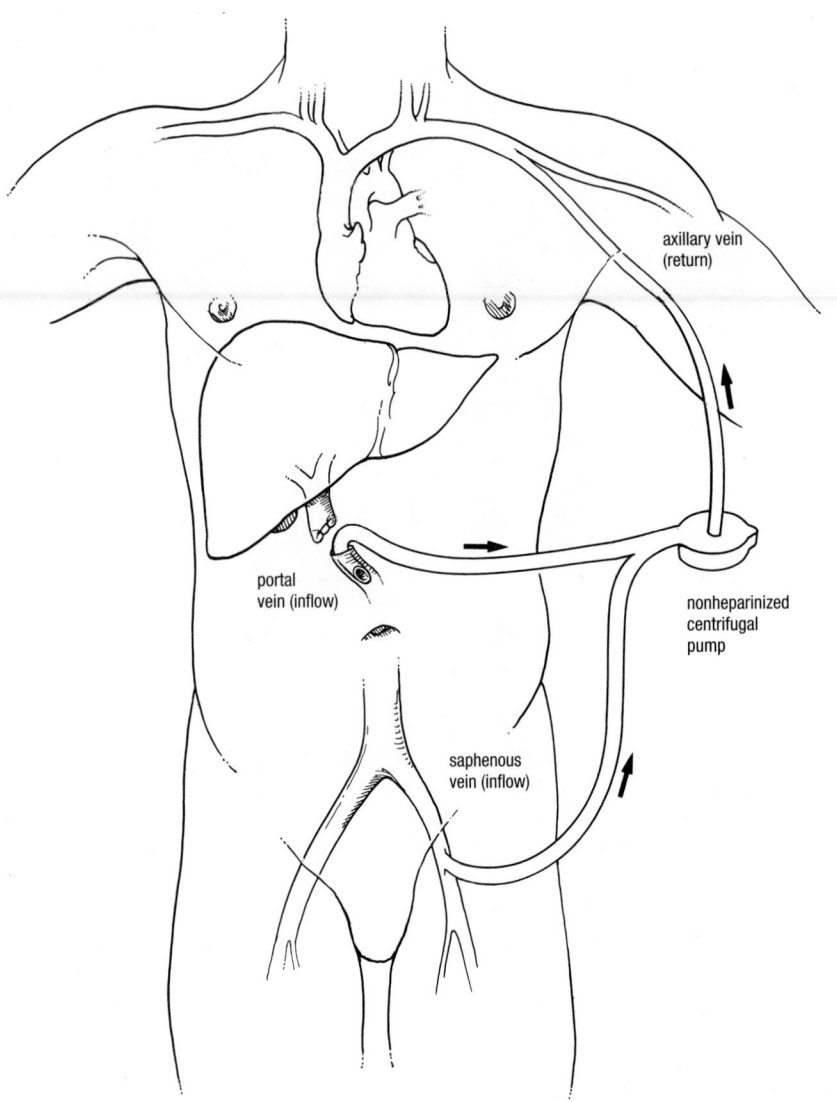

axillary vein
(return)

portal
vein (inflow)

nonheparinized
centrifugal
pump

saphenous
vein (inflow)

venous bypass: the portal vein is divided and cannulated, and a second cannula is placed into the inferior vena cava. the blood is pumped in a nonheparinized system and returned to the patient via cannula in the axillary vein.

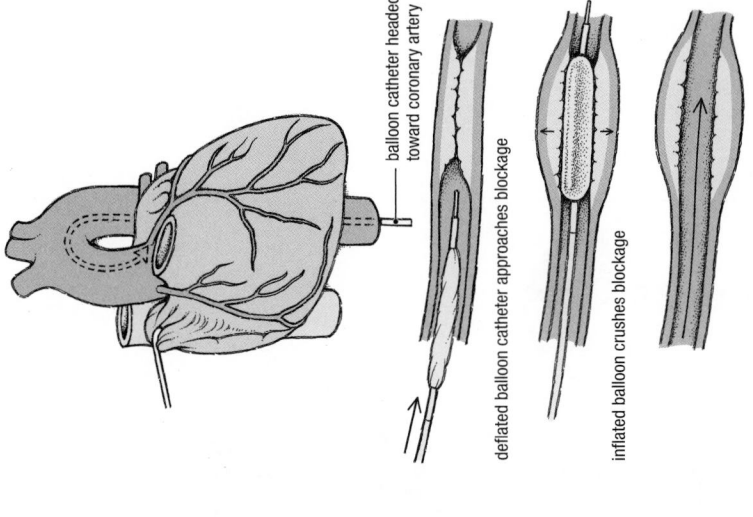

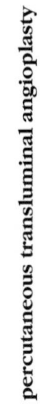

balloon catheter headed toward coronary artery

deflated balloon catheter approaches blockage

inflated balloon crushes blockage

catheter removed and circulation reestablished

percutaneous transluminal angioplasty

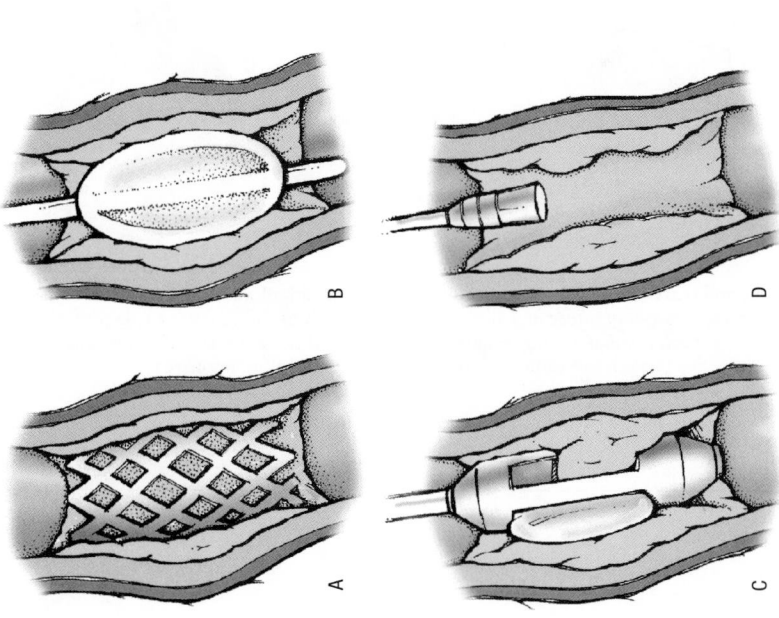

close-up views of coronary arteries showing a variety of procedures to improve blood supply to the heart: (A) stent; (B) balloon angioplasty; (C) atherectomy; (D) laser ablation

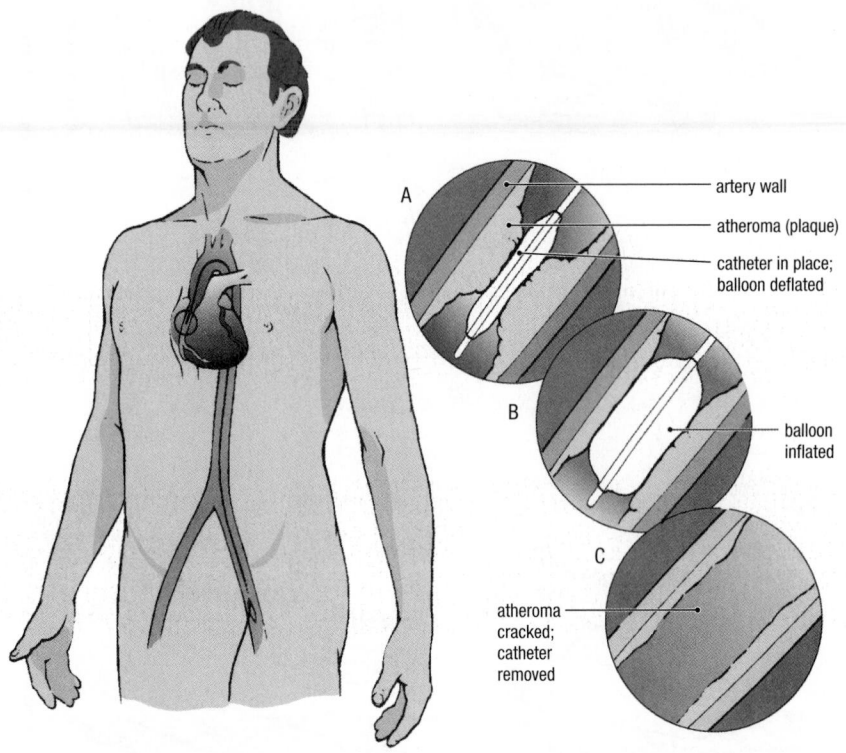

percutaneous transluminal coronary angioplasty: (A) a balloon-tipped catheter is passed into the affected coronary artery and placed within the area of the atheroma (plaque); (B) the balloon is then rapidly inflated and deflated with controlled pressure; (C) after the atheroma is cracked, the catheter is removed, and blood flow improves

Appendix 2
Pain Glossary and Types of Pain

afterpain	painful cramplike contractions of the uterus occurring after childbirth
algesthesia	hypersensitivity to pain
allodynia	condition in which ordinarily nonpainful stimuli evoke pain
analgesia	neurologic or pharmacologic state in which painful stimuli are so moderated that, though still perceived, they are no longer painful
anesthesia dolorosa	severe spontaneous pain occurring in an anesthetic area
arthralgia	pain in a joint, especially one not inflammatory in character
arthrodynia	arthralgia
bearing-down pain	a uterine contraction accompanied by straining and tenesmus; usually appearing in the second stage of labor
causalgia	persistent severe burning pain, usually following injury of a peripheral nerve (especially median and tibial) or the brachial plexus, accompanied by trophic changes
central pain syndrome	neurological condition caused by damage to or dysfunction of the central nervous system, which includes the brain, brainstem, and spinal cord
dysesthesia	impairment of sensation short of anesthesia; a condition in which a disagreeable sensation is produced by ordinary stimuli, caused by lesions of the sensory pathways, peripheral or central; abnormal sensations experienced in the absence of stimulation
expulsive pain	effective labor pains, associated with contraction of the uterine muscle
false pain	ineffective uterine contractions, preceding and sometimes resembling true labor, but distinguishable from it by the lack of progressive effacement and dilation of the cervix

(continued)

girdle pain	a painful sensation encircling the body like a belt, occurring in tabes dorsalis or other spinal cord disease
growing pains	aching pains, frequently felt at night, in the limbs of children; cause is unclear, but the condition is benign
hunger pain	cramp in the epigastrium associated with hunger
hypalgesia	decreased sensibility to pain
hyperalgesia	extreme sensitivity to painful stimuli
hyperesthesia	abnormal acuteness of sensitivity to touch, pain, or other sensory stimuli
hyperpathia	exaggerated subjective response to painful stimuli, with a continuing sensation of pain after the stimulation has ceased
hypesthesia	diminished sensitivity to stimulation
intractable pain	pain resistant or refractory to ordinary analgesic agents
neuralgia	pain of a severe, throbbing, or stabbing character in the course or distribution of a nerve
neuritis	inflammation of a nerve
neuropathy	a disease involving the cranial nerves or the peripheral or autonomic nervous system
nociceptor	a peripheral nerve organ or mechanism for the reception and transmission of painful or injurious stimuli
noxious stimulus	stimulus that is potentially or actually damaging to body tissue
night pain	nyctalgia
nyctalgia	pain that characteristically occurs at night (e.g., nocturnal bone pain experienced by patients with syphilis)
organic pain	pain caused by an organic lesion
pain	unpleasant sensation associated with actual or potential tissue damage and mediated by specific nerve fibers to the brain where its conscious appreciation may be modified by various factors

pain reaction	dilation of the pupil or any other involuntary act occurring in response to a stimulus causing sharp pain anywhere
pain threshold	the smallest intensity of a painful stimulus at which the subject perceives pain
pain tolerance	the greatest intensity of painful stimulation that an individual is able to tolerate
paralgesia	painful paresthesia; any disorder or abnormality of the sense of pain
paralgia	abnormal or unusual pain
paresthesia	an abnormal sensation, such as of burning, pricking, tickling, or tingling
phantom limb pain	the sensation that an amputated limb is still present, often associated with painful paresthesia
post ɔrandial pain	pain occurring after eating, typical of malignancy in esophagus or stomach
pseudesthesia	phantom limb pain
psychalgia	psychogenic pain
psychogenic pain	pain that is associated or correlated with a psychologic, emotional, or behavioral stimulus
referred pain	pain from deep structures perceived as arising from a surface area remote from its actual origin; the area where the pain is appreciated is innervated by the same spinal segment(s) as the deep structure
respirophasic pain	pain, often mistakenly termed pleuritic, that occurs or worsens synchronously with the respiratory cycle
rest pain	pain occurring, usually in the extremities, during rest in the sitting or lying position
somatoform pain	psychogenic pain
telalgia	referred pain

Pain Glossary

Appendix 3
Pain Management Techniques

PHARMACOLOGIC THERAPY
adjuvant analgesics
  alpha-adrenergic agonist
  anticonvulsants
  antispasmodics
  corticosteroids
  local anesthetics
  topical agents
  nonsteroidal antiinflammatory drugs
    (NSAIDs)
opioids
psychopharmacology
  antidepressants
  antipsychotics
  anxiolytics
  mood stabilizers
  psychostimulants

NONPHARMACOLOGIC THERAPY
blocks
  central nerve blocks
  epidural steroid injections
  facet joint blocks
  intravenous regional sympathetic
    blocks
  peripheral nerve blocks
  sacroiliac joint blocks
  sympathetic nerve blocks
  trigger point injections
  visceral nerve blocks
    (Bier blocks)
intravenous lidocaine injections
intravenous phentolamine infusions

INTERVENTIONAL THERAPY
angiogenesis inhibitor therapy
bone marrow transplantation
cryosurgery
discography
gene therapy
hyperthermia
intradiscal electrothermal therapy
intrathecal therapy
laser therapy
photodynamic therapy
spinal cord stimulation
targeted cancer therapy
vertebroplasty

NEUROSURGICAL THERAPY
ablative procedures
augmentation procedures

PHYSICAL THERAPY
electrical stimulation
endurance exercises
joint mobilization
local cooling
local heat
soft tissue mobilization
strengthening exercises
stretching exercises
ultrasound

ACUPUNCTURE
auricular acupuncture
electrical stimulation
electroacupuncture (EA)
laser stimulation
moxibustion
transcutaneous nerve stimulation (TNS)

RADIOTHERAPY AND RADIOPHARMACEUTICALS FOR CANCER PAIN
chemotherapy for reduction of tumor
  size
hemibody irradiation
palliative treatment
radiation therapy for bone metastases
systemic radioisotopes

Sample Reports

BREAST BIOPSY – RIGHT BREAST EXCISIONAL BIOPSY WITH WIRE-GUIDED LOCALIZATION

PREOPERATIVE DIAGNOSIS: Microcalcifications, right breast.

POSTOPERATIVE DIAGNOSIS: Microcalcifications, right breast.

PROCEDURE PERFORMED: Excisional biopsy, right breast, with wire-guided localization.

INDICATIONS: This is a 70-year-old female who presented with right breast microcalcifications which had increased on her recent mammogram. A core biopsy was performed and suggested the diagnosis was benign. Due to the increased number of microcalcifications, the decision was made to perform an excisional biopsy with wire localization.

FINDINGS: There were no complications encountered during the procedure. The specimen was sent to radiology for imaging, and it appeared the area of microcalcifications was within the specimen.

PROCEDURE: The patient was taken to the operating room and placed in the supine position. She was placed under general anesthesia after endotracheal intubation. The patient was then prepped and draped appropriately in sterile fashion.

A small elliptical incision was made in the right breast around the wire that had been placed by radiology. Cautery was used to divide through the dermis, and skin hooks were used for retraction in order to undermine the skin superiorly and inferiorly. Cautery was used to dissect a segment of breast tissue circumferentially around the wire extending relatively deep, however, not all the way down to the pectoralis muscle. The specimen was excised, and there appeared to be a firm area within the specimen likely representative of microcalcifications. The tip of the wire was never seen during the surgery.

The specimen was sent to radiology, and imaging was performed. It appeared the area of concern was within the specimen.

Hemostasis was maintained with electrocautery, and deep dermal approximation was done with interrupted 3-0 Vicryl sutures. The skin incision was closed with running subcuticular 4-0 Monocryl sutures. Steri-Strips were applied to the wound.

Needle, sponge and instrument counts were correct by the nursing staff on 2 occasions, and this was confirmed by visual and manual inspection. The estimated blood loss through the procedure was minimal, and the patient was taken to recovery in stable condition.

Breast Biopsy – Left Breast Needle-Localized Excisional Biopsy

Preoperative Diagnosis: Left breast mass.

Postoperative Diagnosis: Left breast mass.

Procedure Performed: Left breast needle-localized excisional biopsy.

Anesthesia: Local with IV sedation.

Specimens: Left breast mass short suture superior, long suture lateral.

Operative Findings: Recent mammogram showed a mass. The mass is palpable.

Indications: This is a 51-year-old female who had an enlarging left breast mass. A core biopsy showed fibroadenoma; however, the recommendation was for excision because the mass was enlarging. Indication for surgery and possible complications were explained to the patient who consented. The mass was vaguely palpable on physical exam, so it was localized with a wire.

Procedure: The patient went to mammography where she had a wire placed to localize the mass. She then came to the operating room and was prepped and draped. She was placed on the operating table in the supine position. Under IV sedation, the left breast was prepped and draped in the sterile fashion.

Lidocaine 1% was injected subcutaneously, and an incision was made in the upper inner quadrant of the left breast. Skin flaps were raised, and the breast tissue surrounding the wire was excised with Bovie cautery. The mass was palpable. The specimen was oriented with a short suture superior and a long suture lateral and sent to mammography where specimen mammogram showed the mammographic mass. The specimen was sent to pathology.

The wound was irrigated. Hemostasis was obtained with Bovie cautery. The wound was closed with simple interrupted 3-0 Vicryl suture and a running 4-0 Monocryl suture. There were no complications.

Cholecystectomy, Laparoscopic

Preoperative Diagnosis: Gallstone pancreatitis.

Postoperative Diagnosis: Gallstone pancreatitis.

Surgical Procedure: Laparoscopic cholecystectomy.

INDICATIONS: The patient is a 24-year-old female who presented to the emergency room with gallstone pancreatitis, which resolved with conservative management. She did not wish to stay in the hospital at that time for a laparoscopic cholecystectomy, because she has an infant at home. She presents today for an elective laparoscopic cholecystectomy. Her liver enzymes are now normal.

FINDINGS: The patient had a minimally-inflamed gallbladder which was removed without any complications. There were gallstones within the gallbladder.

PROCEDURE: The patient was taken to operating room, placed in the supine position and given general anesthesia after endotracheal intubation. The patient was then prepped and draped in the usual sterile fashion.

Using a scalpel, a small, transverse supraumbilical incision was made, and 2 Kocher clamps were used to grasp the fascia. A scalpel was used to make an incision in the fascia. Two #0 Vicryl sutures were placed on either end of the cut fascia, and a Hasson introducer was placed into the abdominal cavity which was insufflated with carbon dioxide gas. An 11-mm subxiphoid port and two 5-mm right lateral ports were then inserted under direct vision. The gallbladder was grasped and retracted to the right upper quadrant. A few adhesions were taken down with L-hook cautery as well as with the Maryland grasper. L-hook cautery was used to divide the peritoneum off the gallbladder posteriorly as well as anteriorly. The Maryland was used to dissect within the hepatocystic triangle and clearly identified the cystic duct and cystic artery. There was some bleeding from the cystic artery during dissection, and this was controlled with 3 clips on the cystic artery proximally and 1 distally, and scissors were used to divide it. The cystic duct was clipped by applying 3 clips distally and 1 proximally, and the laparoscopic Metzenbaum scissors were used to divide the duct. The remainder of the gallbladder was divided off the hepatic bed using the L-hook cautery. The gallbladder was removed through the supraumbilical incision with mother-in-law graspers and sent to pathology.

The right upper quadrant was suctioned to remove the small amount of blood from the bleeding that had been encountered with the cystic artery. There was no need for any irrigation. The ports were then removed, and the supraumbilical fascia was closed using a running #0 Vicryl suture. The skin incisions were then closed using a running subcuticular 4-0 Monocryl suture, as well as interrupted subcuticular 4-0 Monocryl sutures followed by the application of Steri-Strips. A total of 20 mL of Marcaine 0.25% with epinephrine was used for local wound injection. Tegaderm dressings were then applied to the wounds.

Needle, sponge and instrument counts were correct by the nursing staff on 2 occasions, and this was confirmed by visual and manual inspection. The estimated blood loss for the procedure was minimal. The patient was transferred to recovery in stable condition.

CONTROL OF GASTROINTESTINAL HEMORRHAGE

PREOPERATIVE DIAGNOSIS: Acute gastrointestinal bleed.

POSTOPERATIVE DIAGNOSIS: Visible artery, Dieulafoy at the gastroesophageal junction.

PROCEDURE PERFORMED: Control of gastrointestinal hemorrhage.

DETAILS: Premedication consisting of multiple doses of Versed and fentanyl was administered by the ICU nurse. The Olympus therapeutic scope was passed without difficulty; however, on reaching the gastroesophageal junction, it was clear there was a huge blood clot and fresh blood present in the mid esophagus. The scope was ultimately passed into the stomach and then down to the third part of the duodenum. The duodenum was sequentially washed from the distal duodenum back to the bulb, and no lesions were noted apart from 2 or 3 small superficial erosions, which were oozing, but were not actively spurting and were not thought to be the source of the GI blood loss.

The antrum and body of the stomach were cleansed, and there were 2 superficial ulcers in the gastric antrum on the anterior wall, each about 1 cm in size, with some debris and some mucus and eschar on the surface; there was no visible vessel, no stigmata of recent hemorrhage. There was a large blood clot in the fundus and the midbody. After repeated attempts to clear the clot, which were unsuccessful, the scope was removed. An Edlich tube was inserted, and the stomach was lavaged with about 6 L of sterile water. The stomach was reasonably clean, but there was still a moderate amount of residual clot present in the fundus. Therefore 2 separate washes with 10 mL of 3% peroxide were administered in order to dissolve the clot. It was then washed with sterile saline, and eventually the fundus was reasonably visualized. The patient was on her left side, and then placed on her back and finally on her right side in order for us to see well. There was a bulge in the cardia on the lateral wall, and as the scope was being withdrawn an ulcerated area just above this area was noted. The scope was then withdrawn, and at the gastroesophageal junction, after adequate cleansing, there was a visible vessel about 5 mm in size which was noted with some submucosal tissue protruding around it.

A surgery consultant was then called, and we discussed possibilities including a Dieulafoy lesion versus a possible varix. After visualizing the area for several minutes, we felt the lesion was pulsating, and it was likely to be an artery. An injection with a total of 7 mL of 1:10,000 epinephrine was undertaken, and application of 3 clips to the visible vessel was performed. We then observed for a further 2–3 minutes, and there was no bleeding from the site. This was washed, and the scope was then withdrawn.

The remaining esophageal mucosa was normal. The site of bleeding was likely this visible vessel at the gastroesophageal junction. The bleeding appears to be successfully stopped.

The patient should not have any nasogastric tube passed for at least 48 hours. She may begin her J-feeds. If bleeding recurs, and we are unable to undertake any further procedures to stop the bleeding, the alternative measure could include insertion of a Linton tube.

Needle, sponge and instrument counts were correct. The patient tolerated the procedure well and was in stable condition when taken to recovery.

CYSTIC MASS EXCISION, RIGHT AXILLA

PREOPERATIVE DIAGNOSIS: Complex cystic mass of the right axilla.

POSTOPERATIVE DIAGNOSIS: Complex cystic mass of the right axilla, pending pathology report.

OPERATION PERFORMED: Excision cystic mass, right axilla, with cystic tract.

FINDINGS: The patient had a cystic mass in the right axilla confirmed on sonogram and read as cystic with a solid component inside. Intraoperative revealed the cystic mass was below the vessels, both the vein and the axillary artery, and the cystic component measured about 2.5 cm in greatest diameter and had 1-cm intracystic solid lesions. This was attached to the tract, which extended all the way out to the axillary apex.

OPERATIVE PROCEDURE: Under effective general anesthesia, the patient was prepped and draped in the usual fashion.

An incision was made in the right axilla, and the incision was carried down to the subcutaneous tissue. The axillary vessels were then identified. The cystic mass was palpated just inferior to the axillary vein. This was separated from the surrounding tissue by means of blunt dissection. After the cyst was separated, mucoid content was found within, along with a solid component, and this was removed. However, this was attached to a tract that was followed all the way up to the apex of the axilla. It seemed to be a questionable ganglion because of the distance of this tract. The tract was cut very proximal to the axillary apex and left open. There was no bleeding.

The specimen was sent for frozen section, which came back benign, however, pending permanent section.

Interrupted sutures of 2-0 chromic catgut were then used to approximate the subcutaneous tissues, and the skin edges were approximated with subcuticular sutures of 4-0 Monocryl. A dry sterile dressing was applied to the wound, and the operation was terminated. All counts were correct.

The patient tolerated the procedure well and was sent to the recovery room.

SPECIMEN: Cystic mass and tract sent to pathology.

GASTROSCOPY

PREOPERATIVE DIAGNOSIS: Ascites, hematemesis, coffee-ground emesis and melena.

POSTOPERATIVE DIAGNOSIS: Antral gastric ulcer.

PROCEDURE PERFORMED: Gastroscopy.

ANESTHESIA: General.

INDICATIONS: This is a 35-year-old gentleman with known alcohol abuse, progressive jaundice and ascites who presented with hematemesis, coffee-ground emesis and melena. His hemoglobin fell from 11.9 to 8.9. His INR was prolonged at 1.5. He had also been having recurrent nosebleeds. He drinks up to 3 bottles of sherry per day. The patient also has a past history of frostbite.

Physical exam reveals gross ascites, pitting edema with anasarca, grade 4. He has hypoalbuminemia, massive splenomegaly, bilateral distal foot amputations from frostbite, and left hemiparesis.

PROCEDURE: The Olympus endoscope was passed without difficulty through the esophagus, stomach and into the third part of the duodenum.

The duodenum and bulb were normal apart from some anterior wall gastric metaplasia. The antrum and body of the stomach had well-defined portal hypertensive gastropathy. On the anterior wall of the antrum, about 3-4 cm from the pylorus, there was a deep 2-cm chronic-looking ulcer with central clot. There was possibly a small white-appearing visible vessel adjacent to the small clot, although this could not be determined exactly. We washed the clot several times and were unable to remove it. The ulcer was very deep and chronic looking; however, there was no bleeding. Four injections each of 2 mL 1:10,000 epinephrine were undertaken in 4 quadrants around the ulcer base. The area blanched well, and there was a tiny amount of oozing from 1 of the injection sites, which stopped within 1 minute. The remaining stomach was normal. There may have been some fundal varices, which were small and well supported. There appeared to be grade 1-2 varices at the gastroesophageal junction; there were 2 or 3 columns which extended proximally to about 35 cm from the incisors. There were no stigmata of bleeding from these.

IMPRESSION: The patient likely bled from his anterior wall antral gastric ulcer. Should he bleed again, we should perform another gastroscopy. He may require either addition of a clip, if he has an obvious visible vessel at that time, or coagulation with electrocautery with the gold probe. He should be scoped again in 2-3 days' time to ensure there is no continuing bleeding. He should continue IV proton pump inhibitor for 72 hours.

Hernia Repair – Incisional Hernia Repair With Mesh

Preoperative Diagnosis: Incisional hernia.

Postoperative Diagnosis: Incisional hernia.

Procedure Performed: Incisional hernia repair with mesh.

Indications: This 49-year-old obese female had a previous hysterectomy and developed an incisional hernia just to the right of the umbilicus, medial to the rectus muscle. She had a CT scan of the abdomen performed in the emergency department. The hernia was approximately 3 cm in diameter and contained preperitoneal fat and omentum; otherwise there was no strangulated bowel. She presents today for elective repair.

Findings: The patient had a 3-cm fascial defect just to the right of the umbilicus and medial to the rectus muscle. Once the hernia sac was reduced, which simply contained preperitoneal fat and omentum, a primary repair was performed. Mesh was sutured over the top of the repair. There were no complications encountered during the procedure.

Procedure: The patient was taken to the operating room, placed in the supine position and general anesthesia was administered after endotracheal intubation. The patient was then prepped and draped appropriately in sterile fashion.

Using a scalpel, a midline vertical incision was made in the area of the patient's previous scar, and this was extended slightly above and below the umbilicus. Cautery was used to dissect through the subcutaneous fat down to the fascia. Initially it was difficult to locate the hernia itself due to the patient's size; however, upon further dissection and clearing of the adipose tissue off the fascia, a hernia defect was noted just medial to the rectus muscle on the right side and just to the right of the umbilicus on the superior aspect. The defect was approximately 3 cm in diameter. The hernia sac was separated off the fascia circumferentially with cautery, and the hernia sac was then reduced. There was no entry into the abdominal cavity during this dissection. The hernia sac had been opened up slightly, and a portion of the hernia sac had been removed; however, the contents simply consisted of preperitoneal fat and omentum.

The fascial defect was then closed using a running #1 PDS suture. Following this, a piece of 3 × 6 Prolene mesh was cut to appropriate size, placed over the top of the repair and sutured to the fascia circumferentially using several interrupted 0 Prolene sutures. The subcutaneous fat was then reapproximated using a running 2-0 Vicryl suture. The wound was irrigated with saline, and following this the incision was closed with staples.

Needle, sponge and instrument counts were correct by the nursing staff on 2 occasions, and this was confirmed by visual and manual inspection of the wound.

The estimated blood loss during the procedure was minimal, and the patient was taken to the recovery room in stable condition.

LAPAROTOMY FOR ABDOMINAL TRAUMA

PREOPERATIVE DIAGNOSIS: Gunshot wound to the abdomen.

POSTOPERATIVE DIAGNOSIS: Gunshot wound to the abdomen.

SURGICAL PROCEDURE PERFORMED: Laparotomy for abdominal trauma.

INDICATIONS FOR PROCEDURE: This man suffered a gunshot wound just above the pubis earlier today.

PROCEDURE: The patient was taken to the operating room, and under general anesthesia the abdomen was prepared and draped and opened through a lower midline incision. I cut right down to the pubis through the entrance wound, which had some powder burns in it and was just above the midline at the symphysis.

On entering the abdomen, there was no blood or feculent material. I ran the small bowel for its entire length, and it was completely normal. I had a good look at the cecum, lower ascending colon and the appendix, and these were normal. The sigmoid colon at its apex had a little bleeding spot where an appendix of fat had been injured. I am not sure if this occurred during the opening of the abdomen or was caused by the gunshot wound. In any event, it was bleeding slightly, and I placed a stitch in it. The bowel itself was not injured. I looked down in the pelvis quite carefully, and there were no signs of injury to the rectum down to the peritoneal reflection. The back and dome of the bladder looked okay, but on the anterior aspect of the dome there was a small rent in the superficial musculature which was likely made by the bullet and not by us opening. I tried to follow a track where the bullet might have gone, but I could not identify such a track. X-rays had been taken in any case, and there was no sign of the bullet, which I suspect may have gone obliquely and inferiorly into one of the thighs.

Having satisfied myself there was no significant intraabdominal or urological trauma, I then closed the abdomen with heavy Vicryl for the fascia and clips for the skin. I packed the lower 2 cm of the incision in the region of the gunshot wound.

All counts were correct and verified. The patient was stable throughout and was taken to ICU in good condition.

OPEN CAPSULECTOMY, LEFT BREAST

PREOPERATIVE DIAGNOSIS: Left breast implant displacement.

POSTOPERATIVE DIAGNOSIS: Left breast implant displacement.

PROCEDURE: Left breast open capsulectomy.

INDICATIONS FOR OPERATION: This woman had cohesive gel implants inserted several years ago and has had a significant scar contracture with medial displacement of the left implant. She is brought to the OR for open capsulectomy.

OPERATIVE PROCEDURE: In the operating room under general endotracheal anesthesia with the patient supine, the chest was prepped and draped in the usual fashion. Preoperative markings had been made for lateral extension of the pocket with medial plication.

The skin was incised along the previous scar, and the inferior portion of the periprosthetic capsule was identified and incised. The capsule was then separated from the implant, which was removed intact. Following this, capsulectomy was carried out as marked laterally from the superior to the inferior pole of the breast. Hemostasis was secured with electrocautery. The pocket was then instilled with Kefzol solution, agitated and thoroughly suctioned. The implant was then replaced in anatomic position, nicely filling the area of capsulectomy laterally.

The incision was closed in 3 layers with 2 subcutaneous layers of 3-0 Vicryl, and the skin was closed with running subcuticular 4-0 Prolene. The operative area was cleaned and dried and Steri-Strips applied. A sterile Bactigras dressing was applied, followed by 4×8 gauze over the incision. Two large wraps were placed over the sternum to maintain position of the implant. Additional 4×4 gauze was then applied followed by Elastoplast bandage.

The patient tolerated the entire procedure well. She received 1 g of Kefzol intravenously during the procedure. She tolerated the procedure well and left the operating room in good condition. All counts were correct.

PELVIC MASS RESECTION, LYSIS OF ADHESIONS AND APPENDECTOMY

PREOPERATIVE DIAGNOSIS: Pelvic mass.

POSTOPERATIVE DIAGNOSIS: Pelvic mass.

OPERATION PERFORMED: Exploratory laparotomy, lysis of adhesions, resection of pelvic mass and appendectomy.

FINDINGS: The patient had previous colon cancer, and a CT scan revealed a new pelvic mass. Exploration revealed a pelvic mass at the level of the right ovarian area, suspicious for metastatic cancer from her previous colon cancer. A resection of the mass was performed, and an appendectomy was performed after lysis of multiple adhesions (the patient had multiple previous surgeries).

PROCEDURE: Under satisfactory general anesthesia, the patient was prepped and draped in the usual manner.

A midline incision was performed and carried down subcutaneously. Massive adhesions were encountered. They were lysed off progressively to enable entrance into the abdominal cavity. One small bowel opening was identified and was sutured with running chromic and Prolene sutures. After mobilization of the small bowel completely, the right adnexa was identified. There appeared to be a mass at that level, and it was progressively dissected.

An appendectomy was also performed by removal of the appendix, inverting the stump and removing the appendix by clamping the mesoappendix.

Following this, hemostasis was achieved. The wounds were closed in layers with sutures and staples for the skin.

The patient's operative course was satisfactory.

DRAINS: None.

DISPOSITION: To recovery.

ESTIMATED BLOOD LOSS: Minimal.

SPECIMEN: Appendix and pelvic mass were sent to pathology.

REDUCTION MAMMOPLASTY, BILATERAL

PREOPERATIVE DIAGNOSIS: Bilateral macromastia.

POSTOPERATIVE DIAGNOSIS: Bilateral macromastia.

SURGICAL PROCEDURE: Bilateral reduction mammoplasty.

INDICATIONS FOR OPERATION: This woman was admitted for elective reduction mammoplasty.

OPERATIVE PROCEDURE: In the operating room, under general endotracheal anesthesia with the patient supine, the chest was prepped and draped in the usual fashion. Preoperative markings were made, and these were revised and reinforced with a Codman surgical marker. An inferiorly based nipple-carrying pedicle was designed.

Beginning on the right side, skin was incised as marked. The nipple-carrying pedicle was deepithelialized. Using cutting and coagulation cautery, glandular resection was carried out medially, laterally and superiorly. A total of 930 g of breast tissue was removed. Hemostasis was secured throughout and a tacking subcutaneous closure completed using interrupted 3-0 Vicryl. Skin closure was accomplished with running subcuticular 3-0 white Vicryl.

Attention was then turned to the opposite side where essentially an identical procedure was carried out removing 1190 g of breast tissue to correct for preoperative asymmetry. Closure was identical.

The operative area was then cleaned and dried, and Steri-Strips were applied to the incisions. This was followed by dressings of Bactigras, 4 × 8 gauze, large lap pads and Elastoplast bandage.

The patient tolerated the procedure well. Blood loss was not excessive. No problems were encountered, and she left the OR in good condition. Instrument, needle and sponge counts were correct.

RETROGRADE PYELOGRAM WITH REMOVAL OF DOUBLE-J STENT, LEFT

PREOPERATIVE DIAGNOSIS: Left ureteral ileal obstruction.

POSTOPERATIVE DIAGNOSIS: Left ureteral ileal obstruction.

OPERATION: Left retrograde pyelogram and removal of left double-J stent.

FINDINGS: The patient is a 68-year-old male status post cystoprostatectomy. For the last year he has had an indwelling double-J stent, because he developed a left ureteral ileal stricture. The patient has been dilated multiple times.

PROCEDURE: On this occasion, we filled up his stent and noted a normal-looking collecting system. We watched the pulsations of the dye go down the ureter, and we felt there were sufficient pulsations and no gross signs of hydronephrosis.

After observing for 10 minutes, I removed the ureteral stent. The patient will be followed in our office with IVP and ultrasounds.

FINAL DIAGNOSIS: Patent left ureteral stent.

Common Terms by Procedure

BREAST BIOPSY – RIGHT BREAST EXCISIONAL BIOPSY WITH WIRE-GUIDED LOCALIZATION

benign
breast tissue
cautery
core biopsy
deep dermal approximation
dermis
electrocautery
elliptical incision
endotracheal intubation
excisional biopsy
hemostasis
interrupted 3-0 Vicryl suture
mammogram
microcalcification
pectoralis muscle
retraction
running subcuticular 4-0 Monocryl
  suture
skin hook
specimen
Steri-Strips
wire-guided localization

BREAST BIOPSY – LEFT BREAST NEEDLE-LOCALIZED EXCISIONAL BIOPSY

Bovie cautery
breast mass
breast tissue
core biopsy
fibroadenoma
hemostasis
interrupted 3-0 Vicryl suture

IV sedation
Lidocaine
mammogram
mammographic mass
mammography
needle-localized excisional biopsy
pathology
running 4-0 Monocryl suture
skin flap

CHOLECYSTECTOMY, LAPAROSCOPIC

#0 Vicryl suture
abdominal cavity
adhesion
carbon dioxide gas
cystic artery
cystic duct
dissection
endotracheal intubation
epinephrine
fascia
gallbladder
gallstone pancreatitis
gallstones
Hasson introducer
hepatic bed
hepatocystic triangle
interrupted subcuticular 4-0 Monocryl
  suture
Kocher clamp
laparoscopic cholecystectomy
laparoscopic Metzenbaum scissors
lateral port
L-hook cautery
liver enzymes
Marcaine
Maryland grasper
mother-in-law grasper
pathology

peritoneum
running #0 Vicryl suture
running subcuticular 4-0 Monocryl
    suture
scalpel
Steri-Strips
subxiphoid port
supraumbilical fascia
supraumbilical incision
Tegaderm dressing
transverse supraumbilical incision

CONTROL OF GASTROINTESTINAL HEMORRHAGE

3% peroxide
antrum
blood clot
body of the stomach
bulb
cardia
debris
Dieulafoy lesion
duodenum
Edlich tube
epinephrine
eschar
esophageal mucosa
fentanyl
fundus
gastric antrum
gastroesophageal junction
gastrointestinal bleed
gastrointestinal hemorrhage
J-feeds
lesion
Linton tube
mucus
nasogastric tube
Olympus therapeutic scope
sterile saline
sterile water
stigma
stomach

submucosal tissue
superficial erosion
superficial ulcer
varix
Versed
visible vessel

CYSTIC MASS EXCISION, RIGHT AXILLA

2-0 chromic catgut
4-0 Monocryl
axilla
axillary apex
axillary artery
axillary vein
benign
blunt dissection
cystic mass
cystic tract
frozen section
ganglion
interrupted suture
intracystic solid lesion
mucoid content
permanent section
sonogram
subcutaneous tissue
subcuticular suture

GASTROSCOPY

antrum
ascites
bulb
clip
clot
coagulation
coffee-ground emesis
duodenum
electrocautery
epinephrine
esophagus
fundal varix
gastric metaplasia
gastric ulcer

gastroesophageal junction
gastroscopy
gold probe
hematemesis
hemoglobin
incisor
melena
Olympus endoscope
portal hypertensive gastropathy
proton pump inhibitor
pylorus
stigma
stomach
ulcer
visible vessel

HERNIA REPAIR – INCISIONAL HERNIA REPAIR WITH MESH

abdominal cavity
adipose tissue
cautery
dissection
fascia
fascial defect
hernia defect
hernia sac
incisional hernia
interrupted 0 Prolene suture
mesh
omentum
preperitoneal fat
Prolene mesh
rectus muscle
running #1 PDS suture
running 2-0 Vicryl suture
scalpel
strangulated bowel
umbilicus

LAPAROTOMY FOR ABDOMINAL TRAUMA

abdomen
apex

appendix
ascending colon
bladder
cecum
dome of the bladder
intraabdominal trauma
laparotomy
lower midline incision
pelvis
peritoneal reflection
rectum
rent
sigmoid colon
small bowel
superficial musculature
symphysis
urological trauma
Vicryl

OPEN CAPSULECTOMY, LEFT BREAST

3-0 Vicryl
Bactigras dressing
breast implant
cohesive gel implant
Elastoplast bandage
electrocautery
hemostasis
Kefzol
open capsulectomy
periprosthetic capsule
pocket
running subcuticular 4-0 Prolene
scar contracture
Steri-Strips
sternum

PELVIC MASS RESECTION, LYSIS OF ADHESIONS AND APPENDECTOMY

abdominal cavity
adnexa
appendectomy
chromic suture

laparotomy
lysis of adhesions
mesoappendix
pelvic mass
Prolene suture
small bowel
stump

REDUCTION MAMMOPLASTY, BILATERAL

Bactigras
coagulation cautery
Codman surgical marker
Elastoplast bandage
glandular resection
hemostasis
macromastia
mammoplasty
nipple-carrying pedicle

preoperative asymmetry
Steri-Strips
tacking subcutaneous closure
interrupted 3-0 Vicryl
running subcuticular 3-0 white Vicryl

RETROGRADE PYELOGRAM WITH REMOVAL OF DOUBLE-J STENT, LEFT

collecting system
double-J stent
dye
hydronephrosis
pulsation
retrograde pyelogram
stent
ureter
ureteral ileal obstruction
ureteral stent

Appendix 6

Dermatomal Explanation

Dermatome	Area Innervated and Reflex Elicited	Nerve Affected
C2	occiput, top part of neck	greater occipital and anterior cutaneous of neck
C3	lower part of neck to clavicle	supraclavicular
C4	area just below the clavicle, deltoids	supraclavicular
C5	lateral arm, at and above the elbow, brachioradialis, infraspinatus, supraspinatus, deltoid, biceps	axillary
C6	forearm, radial side of hand wrist extensors	radial and median
C7	pronator teres, flexor carpi ulnaris, latissimus dorsi, triceps, long finger, elbow extensors	median
C8	lateral aspect of hand, wrist extensors and flexors, finger flexors	ulnar
T1	medial forearm, little finger adductors	medial brachial cutaneous
T2	sternal notch	intercostal and medial cutaneous
T3-T12	chest and back to hip girdle	
T4	nipples	intercostal
T6	xiphoid process	intercostal
T10	umbilicus	intercostal
L1	inguinal ligament	ilioinguinal, iliohypogastric
L2	iliopsoas, hip flexors	anterior femoral, lateral femoral
L3	adductor longus, hip adductors, quadriceps, patellar reflex, knee extensors	obturator

Dermatome	Area Innervated and Reflex Elicited	Nerve Affected
L4	vastus lateralis, knee extensors, vastus medialis, ankle dorsiflexors, anterior tibialis, patellar reflex	saphenous
L5	hip abductors, ankle dorsiflexion, eversion and inversion, long toe extensors, hallucis longus	lateral cutaneous
S1	hip extensors, ankle plantar flexors, gastrocnemius, heel, middle of back of leg, Achilles reflex	sural
S2	back of thigh	posterior cutaneous
S3	medial side of buttocks	posterior cutaneous
S4/5	perineal region, anal sphincter	pudendal
S5	skin at and adjacent to anus	pudendal

Dermatomal Explanation

American Academy of Pain Management (AAPM) Accredited Pain Programs

This list includes facilities that have passed the American Academy of Pain Management's rigorous pain program accreditation testing and on-site inspection and participate in additional AAPM services and status. For additional information, please visit www.aapainmanage.org.

COLORADO
Craniofacial Diagnostic Center
1660 S. Albion, Ste. 1008
Denver, CO 80222

FLORIDA
Lee Memorial Health System
Pain Management Center Cape Coral
708 Del Prado Blvd, Suite 7
Cape Coral, FL 33990

Lee Memorial Health System
Pain Management Center HealthPark
16281 Bass Rd. Suite 300
Ft. Myers, FL 33908

Wuesthoff Pain Management Center
2400 N. Courtenay Pkwy.
Merritt Island, FL 32953

GEORGIA
Pain Control and Rehabilitation Institute
  of Georgia
2784 N. Decatur Rd., Ste. 120
Decatur, GA 30033

ILLINOIS
Advanced Pain Management Institute
7309 N. Knoxville Ave.
Peoria, IL 61614

Central Illinois Pain Center
OSF Center for Health
8600 N. State Route 91, Ste. 250
Peoria, IL 61615

Kishwaukee Community Hospital Pain
  Management Program
626 Bethany Rd.
DeKalb, IL 60115

INDIANA
Oliver Headache and Pain Clinic
2828 Mt. Vernon Ave.
Evansville, IN 47712

KENTUCKY
Ephraim McDowell Regional Medical
  Center
Pain Management Center
217 S. Third St.
Danville, KY 40422

Murphy Pain Center
3020 Eastpoint Pkwy.
Louisville, KY 40223

Spine & Brain Neurosurgical Center
5001 Houston Rd.
Florence, KY 41042

Spine & Brain Neurosurgical Center
524 East Main St.
Hazard, KY 41701

Spine & Brain Neurosurgical Center
1721 Nicholasville Rd.
Lexington, KY 40503

Spine & Brain Neurosurgical Center
189 West Hwy 192 Bypass
London, KY 40741

Spine & Brain Neurosurgical Center
7160 North Mayo Trail
Pikeville, KY 41501

MASSACHUSETTS

Catholic Memorial Home Pain
  Management Program
2446 Highland Ave.
Fall River, MA 02720

Madonna Manor Pain Program
85 N. Washington St.
North Attleboro, MA 02760

Marian Manor Pain Management
  Program
33 Summer St.
Taunton, MA 02780-3491

Our Lady's Haven Pain Management
  Program
71 Center St.
Fairhaven, MA 02719

Sacred Heart Home Pain Management
  Program
359 Summer St.
New Bedford, MA 02740

MINNESOTA

United Pain Center
280 N. Smith Ave., Ste. 600
St. Paul, MN 55102

MISSISSIPPI

Pain Treatment Center
Rush Foundation Hospital
1314 19th Ave.
Meridian, MS 39301

MISSOURI

Headache Care Center
3805 S. Kansas Expressway
Springfield, MO 65807

St. Francis Medical Center Pain
  Management Program
211 St. Francis Dr.
Cape Girardeau, MO 63703

MONTANA

Frances Mahon Deaconess Hospital
621 Third St. S.
Glasgow, MT 59230

NEW HAMPSHIRE

Cottage Hospital Pain Clinic
PO Box 2001
90 Swiftwater Rd.
Woodsville, NH 03785

NEW YORK

Healthworks of Staten Island
1428 Victory Blvd.
Staten Island, NY 10301

The Kingston Hospital-Pain
  Management Service
358 Broadway
Kingston, NY 12401

NORTH CAROLINA

Pitt County Memorial Hospital
Pain Management Center
2010 W. Arlington Blvd.
Greenville, NC 27835

OHIO

Doctors Pain Clinic
1011 Boardman-Canfield Road
Youngstown, OH 44512

Grandview Hospital & Medical
  Center
Pain Management Center
405 Grand Ave.
Dayton, OH 45405-4796

The St. Joseph Pain Management
  Center
662 Eastland Ave.
Eastland Medical II Building, #201
Warren, OH 44484

PENNSYLVANIA

Gettysburg Rehabilitation Services
124 Carlisle St.
Gettysburg, PA 17325

AAPM

Jefferson Pain & Rehabilitation Center
4735 Clairton Blvd.
Pittsburgh, PA 15236

Dr. Joseph L. Kaczor, INC. P.C.
2606 Broad Ave.
Altoona, PA 16601

Latrobe Area Hospital-Pain Control
 Center
121 W. Second Ave.
Latrobe, PA 15650

Michael S. Melnick, D.M.D., M.A.G.D.
The Park Plaza, Ste. 207
128 N. Craig St.
Pittsburgh, PA 15213

Montgomery Surgical Center
One Abington Plaza, Ste. 100
Jenkintown, PA 19046

Oral & Maxillofacial Surgery and Pain
 Mgmt.
2606 Broad Ave
Altoona, PA 16601

Pinnacle Health Rehab Options
2501 N. 3rd Street

Landis 3
Harrisburg, PA 17110

Sarah and Benjamin Lincow Pain
 Foundation
7622 Ogontz Ave.
Philadelphia, PA 19150

TEXAS

Acute & Chronic Pain Management
 Center
24 Care Circle
Amarillo, TX 79124

American College of Acupuncture &
 Oriental Medicine
9100 Park West Dr.
Houston, TX 77063

Pain Man Serv of Central Imaging of
 Arlington
3100 Matlock Rd. Suite 105
Arlington, TX 76105

Tri-County Pain Management
 Centre
PO Box 758
200 N. Arch St.
Royse City, TX 75189

Drugs by Indication

ABORTION
Antiprogestin
Mifeprex(R) [US]
mifepristone
Oxytocic Agent
oxytocin
Pitocin(R) [US/Can]
Syntocinon(R) [Can]
Prostaglandin
carboprost tromethamine
Cervidil(R) [US/Can]
dinoprostone
Hemabate(R) [US/Can]
Prepidil(R) [US/Can]
Prostin E2(R) [US/Can]

ANESTHESIA (GENERAL)
Anesthetic, Gas
nitrous oxide
Barbiturate
Brevital(R) [Can]
Brevital(R) Sodium [US]
methohexital
General Anesthetic
Amidate(R) [US/Can]
Compound 347(TM) [US]
desflurane
Diprivan(R) [US/Can]
enflurane
Ethrane(R) [US]
etomidate
Forane(R) [US]
halothane
isoflurane
Ketalar(R) [US/Can]
ketamine
Ketamine Hydrochloride Injection,
USP [Can]
propofol
sevoflurane
Sevorane(TM) [Can]
Suprane(R) [US/Can]
Terrell(TM) [US]
Ultane(R) [US]

ANESTHESIA (LOCAL)
Local Anesthetic
Alcaine(R) [US/Can]
Americaine(R) [US-OTC]
Americaine(R) Hemorrhoidal
[US-OTC]
Ametop(TM) [Can]
Anestacon(R) [US]
articaine and epinephrine
Astracaine(R) [Can]
Astracaine(R) Forte [Can]
Band-Aid(R) Hurt-Free(TM)
Antiseptic Wash [US-OTC]
benzocaine
benzocaine, butyl aminobenzoate,
tetracaine, and benzalkonium
chloride
Benzodent(R) [US-OTC]
Betacaine(R) [Can]
bupivacaine
bupivacaine and epinephrine
Burnamycin [US-OTC]
Burn Jel [US-OTC]
Burn-O-Jel [US-OTC]
Carbocaine(R) [US/Can]
Carbocaine(R) 2% with
Neo-Cobefrin(R) [US]
Cetacaine(R) [US]
cetylpyridinium
chloroprocaine
Citanest(R) Plain
[US/Can]
cocaine
Curasore [US-OTC]
Cylex(R) [US-OTC]
Cēpacol(R) Dual Action Maximum
Strength [US-OTC]

Dermoplast(R) Antibacterial [US-OTC]
Dermoplast(R) Pain Relieving [US-OTC]
Detane(R) [US-OTC]
dibucaine
Diocaine(R) [Can]
Duocaine(TM) [US]
dyclonine
ethyl chloride
ethyl chloride and dichlorotetrafluoroethane
Flucaine(R) [US]
Fluoracaine(R) [US]
Fluro-Ethyl(R) [US]
Foille(R) [US-OTC]
Gebauer's Ethyl Chloride(R) [US]
hexylresorcinol
Hurricaine(R) [US-OTC]
L-M-X(TM) 4 [US-OTC]
L-M-X(TM) 5 [US-OTC]
Lanacane(R) [US-OTC]
Lanacane(R) Maximum Strength [US-OTC]
LidaMantle(R) [US]
lidocaine
lidocaine and bupivacaine
lidocaine and epinephrine
Lidodan(TM) [Can]
Lidoderm(R) [US/Can]
LidoSite(TM) [US]
LTA(R) 360 [US]
Marcaine(R) [US/Can]
Marcaine(R) Spinal [US]
Marcaine(R) with Epinephrine [US]
mepivacaine
mepivacaine and levonordefrin
Mycinettes(R) [US-OTC]
Naropin(R) [US/Can]
Nesacaine(R) [US]
Nesacaine(R)-CE [Can]
Nesacaine(R)-MPF [US]
Novocain(R) [US]
Nupercainal(R) [US-OTC]

Ophthetic(R) [US]
Oticaine [US]
Otocaine(TM) [US]
Outgro(R) [US-OTC]
Polocaine(R) [US/Can]
Polocaine(R) 2% and Levonordefrin 1:20,000 [Can]
Polocaine(R) Dental [US]
Polocaine(R) MPF [US]
Pontocaine(R) [US/Can]
Pontocaine(R) Niphanoid(R) [US]
Pontocaine(R) With Dextrose [US]
pramoxine
Prax(R) [US-OTC]
Premjact(R) [US-OTC]
prilocaine
procaine
ProctoFoam(R) NS [US-OTC]
proparacaine
proparacaine and fluorescein
ropivacaine
Sarna(R) Sensitive [US]
Sensorcaine(R) [US/Can]
Sensorcaine(R)-MPF [US]
Sensorcaine(R)-MPF with Epinephrine [US]
Sensorcaine(R) with Epinephrine [US/Can]
Septanest(R) N [Can]
Septanest(R) SP [Can]
Septocaine(R) [US]
S.T. 37(R) [US-OTC]
Tanac(R) [US-OTC]
tetracaine
tetracaine and dextrose
Topicaine(R) [US-OTC]
Trocaine(R) [US-OTC]
Tronolane(R) [US-OTC]
Ultracaine(R) D-S [Can]
Ultracaine(R) D-S Forte [Can]
Xylocaine(R) [US/Can]
Xylocaine(R) MPF [US]
Xylocaine(R) MPF With Epinephrine [US]
Xylocaine(R) Viscous [US]

Xylocaine(R) With Epinephrine
[US/Can]
Xylocard(R) [Can]
Zilactin(R) [Can]
Zilactin-L(R) [US-OTC]
Zilactin(R)-B [US-OTC/Can]
Zilactin Baby(R) [Can]
Zorcaine(TM) [US]

ANESTHESIA (OPHTHALMIC)
Local Anesthetic
Flucaine(R) [US]
Fluoracaine(R) [US]
proparacaine and fluorescein

ANGIOGRAPHY (OPHTHALMIC)
Diagnostic Agent
AK-Fluor [US]
Angiscein(R) [US]
Fluor-I-Strip(R) [US]
Fluor-I-Strip-AT(R) [US]
fluorescein sodium
Fluorescite(R) [US/Can]
Fluorets(R) [US]
Ful-Glo(R) [US]

ANXIETY
Antianxiety Agent
Apo-Buspirone(R) [Can]
BuSpar(R) [US/Can]
Buspirex [Can]
buspirone
Gen-Buspirone [Can]
Lin-Buspirone [Can]
Novo-Buspirone [Can]
Nu-Buspirone [Can]
PMS-Buspirone [Can]
Antianxiety Agent, Miscellaneous
meprobamate
Novo-Mepro [Can]
Benzodiazepine
alprazolam
Alprazolam Intensol(R) [US]
Alti-Alprazolam [Can]

Apo-Alpraz(R) [Can]
Apo-Bromazepam(R) [Can]
Apo-Chlordiazepoxide(R) [Can]
Apo-Clorazepate(R) [Can]
Apo-Diazepam(R) [Can]
Apo-Lorazepam(R) [Can]
Apo-Oxazepam(R) [Can]
Apo-Temazepam(R) [Can]
Ativan(R) [US/Can]
bromazepam (Canada only)
chlordiazepoxide
clorazepate
CO Temazepam [Can]
Diastat(R) [US/Can]
Diastat(R) AcuDial(TM) [US]
Diastat(R) Rectal Delivery System
[Can]
Diazemuls(R) [Can]
diazepam
Diazepam Intensol(R) [US]
Gen-Alprazolam [Can]
Gen-Bromazepam [Can]
Gen-Temazepam [Can]
Lectopam(R) [Can]
Librium(R) [US]
lorazepam
Lorazepam Injection, USP [Can]
Lorazepam Intensol(R) [US]
Niravam(TM) [US]
Novo-Alprazol [Can]
Novo-Bromazepam [Can]
Novo-Clopate [Can]
Novo-Dipam [Can]
Novo-Lorazepam [Can]
Novo-Temazepam [Can]
Novoxapram(R) [Can]
Nu-Alprax [Can]
Nu-Bromazepam [Can]
Nu-Loraz [Can]
Nu-Temazepam [Can]
oxazepam
Oxpam(R) [Can]
Oxpram(R) [Can]
PMS-Lorazepam [Can]
PMS-Oxazepam [Can]

PMS-Temazepam [Can]
ratio-Temazepam [Can]
Restoril(R) [US/Can]
Riva-Lorazepam [Can]
Riva-Oxazepam [Can]
Serax(R) [US]
temazepam
Tranxene(R) SD(TM) [US]
Tranxene(R) SD(TM)-Half Strength
[US]
Tranxene(R) T-Tab(R) [US]
Valium(R) [US/Can]
Xanax(R) [US/Can]
Xanax TS(TM) [Can]
Xanax XR(R) [US]

BLADDER IRRIGATION
Antibacterial, Topical
acetic acid

BOWEL CLEANSING
Electrolyte Supplement, Oral
Fleet(R) Accu-Prep(R) [US-OTC]
Fleet Enema(R) [Can]
Fleet(R) Phospho-Soda(R) [US-OTC]
Fleet(R) Phospho-Soda(R) Oral
Laxative [Can]
OsmoPrep(TM) [US]
sodium phosphates
Visicol(R) [US]
Laxative
castor oil
Citro-Mag(R) [Can]
Colyte(R) [US/Can]
Fleet(R) Accu-Prep(R) [US-OTC]
Fleet Enema(R) [Can]
Fleet(R) Phospho-Soda(R) [US-OTC]
Fleet(R) Phospho-Soda(R) Oral
Laxative [Can]
GoLYTELY(R) [US]
Klean-Prep(R) [Can]
magnesium citrate
NuLYTELY(R) [US]
OsmoPrep(TM) [US]
PegLyte(R) [Can]

polyethylene glycol-electrolyte
solution
Purge(R) [US-OTC]
sodium phosphates
TriLyte(TM) [US]
Visicol(R) [US]
Laxative, Bowel Evacuant
HalfLytely(R) and Bisacodyl
[US]
polyethylene glycol-electrolyte
solution and bisacodyl
Laxative, Stimulant
HalfLytely(R) and Bisacodyl [US]
polyethylene glycol-electrolyte
solution and bisacodyl

BOWEL STERILIZATION
Aminoglycoside (Antibiotic)
Neo-Fradin(TM) [US]
neomycin
Neo-Rx [US]

CARDIAC DECOMPENSATION
Adrenergic Agonist Agent
dobutamine
Dobutamine Injection, USP [Can]
Dobutrex(R) [Can]

CARDIOGENIC SHOCK
Adrenergic Agonist Agent
dobutamine
Dobutamine Injection, USP [Can]
Dobutrex(R) [Can]
dopamine
Antiarrhythmic Agent, Miscellaneous
Digitek(R) [US]
digoxin
Digoxin CSD [Can]
Lanoxicaps(R) [US/Can]
Lanoxin(R) [US/Can]
Novo-Digoxin [Can]
Pediatric Digoxin CSD [Can]
Cardiac Glycoside
Digitek(R) [US]

digoxin
Digoxin CSD [Can]
Lanoxicaps(R) [US/Can]
Lanoxin(R) [US/Can]
Novo-Digoxin [Can]
Pediatric Digoxin CSD [Can]

CATARACT
Adrenergic Agonist Agent
AK-Dilate(R) [US]
Altafrin [US]
Anu-Med [US-OTC]
Dionephrine(R) [Can]
Formulation R(TM) [US-OTC]
Medicone(R) [US-OTC]
Mydfrin(R) [US/Can]
Neo-Synephrine(R) [Can]
Neo-Synephrine(R) Extra Strength
  [US-OTC]
Neo-Synephrine(R) Mild [US-OTC]
Neo-Synephrine(R) Regular Strength
  [US-OTC]
Nāsop(TM) [US]
phenylephrine
Rectacaine [US-OTC]
Relief(R) [US-OTC]
Rhinall [US-OTC]
Tronolane(R) Suppository
  [US-OTC]
Nonsteroidal Anti-inflammatory Drug
  (NSAID), Ophthalmic
nepafenac
Nevanac(TM) [US]

COLONIC EVACUATION
Laxative
Alophen(R) [US-OTC]
Apo-Bisacodyl(R) [Can]
Bisac-Evac(TM) [US-OTC]
bisacodyl
Bisacodyl Uniserts(R) [US-OTC]
Carter's Little Pills(R) [Can]
Correctol(R) Tablets [US-OTC]
Doxidan(R) (reformulation)
  [US-OTC]

Dulcolax(R) [US-OTC/Can]
Femilax(TM) [US-OTC]
Fleet(R) Bisacodyl Enema [US-OTC]
Fleet(R) Stimulant Laxative
  [US-OTC]
Gentlax(R) [Can]
Modane Tablets(R) [US-OTC]
Veracolate [US-OTC]

CONGESTION (NASAL)
Adrenergic Agonist Agent
Afrin(R) Sinus [US-OTC]
AK-Con(TM) [US]
AK-Dilate(R) [US]
Albalon(R) [US]
Allersol(R) [US]
Altafrin [US]
Anu-Med [US-OTC]
Balminil Decongestant [Can]
Benylin(R) D for Infants [Can]
Benzedrex(R) [US-OTC]
Biofed [US-OTC]
Claritin(R) Allergic Decongestant
  [Can]
Contac(R) Cold 12 Hour Relief Non
  Drowsy [Can]
Contact(R) Cold [US-OTC]
Dimetapp(R) 12-Hour Non-Drowsy
  Extentabs(R) [US-OTC]
Dimetapp(R) Decongestant Infant
  [US-OTC]
Dionephrine(R) [Can]
Dristan(R) Long Lasting Nasal [Can]
Drixoral(R) Nasal [Can]
Drixoral(R) ND [Can]
Duramist(R) Plus [US-OTC]
Duration(R) [US-OTC]
ElixSure(TM) Congestion [US-OTC]
Eltor(R) [Can]
ephedrine
Formulation R(TM) [US-OTC]
Genaphed(R) [US-OTC]
Genasal [US-OTC]
Kidkare Decongestant [US-OTC]

Kodet SE [US-OTC]
Medicone(R) [US-OTC]
Murine(R) Tears Plus [US-OTC]
Mydfrin(R) [US/Can]
naphazoline
Naphcon(R) [US-OTC]
Naphcon Forte(R) [Can]
NRS(R) [US-OTC]
Nāsop(TM) [US]
Nōstrilla(R) [US-OTC]
Oranyl [US-OTC]
oxymetazoline
PediaCare(R) Decongestant Infants
    [US-OTC]
phenylephrine
PMS-Pseudoephedrine [Can]
Pretz-D(R) [US-OTC]
Privine(R) [US-OTC]
propylhexedrine
pseudoephedrine
Pseudofrin [Can]
Rectacaine [US-OTC]
Relief(R) [US-OTC]
Rhinall [US-OTC]
Robidrine(R) [Can]
Silfedrine Children's [US-OTC]
Simply Stuffy(TM) [US-OTC]
Sudafed(R) [US-OTC]
Sudafed(R) 12 Hour [US-OTC]
Sudafed(R) 24 Hour [US-OTC]
Sudafed(R) Children's [US-OTC]
Sudafed(R) Decongestant [Can]
Sudafed PE(TM) [US-OTC]
Sudodrin [US-OTC]
SudoGest [US-OTC]
Sudo-Tab(R) [US-OTC]
tetrahydrozoline
Tronolane(R) Suppository [US-OTC]
Tyzine(R) [US]
Tyzine(R) Pediatric [US]
Vasocon(R) [Can]
Vicks Sinex(R) 12 Hour [US-OTC]
Vicks Sinex(R) 12 Hour Ultrafine
    Mist [US-OTC]
Vicks(R) Sinex(R) Nasal Spray
    [US-OTC]
Vicks(R) Sinex(R) UltraFine Mist
    [US-OTC]
4-Way(R) 12 Hour [US-OTC]

CYCLOPLEGIA
Anticholinergic Agent
  AtroPen(R) [US]
  atropine
  Atropine-Care(R) [US]
  Buscopan(R) [Can]
  Cyclogyl(R) [US/Can]
  cyclopentolate
  Cylate(R) [US]
  Diopentolate(R) [Can]
  Dioptic's Atropine Solution
      [Can]
  Diotrope(R) [Can]
  homatropine
  Isopto(R) Atropine [US/Can]
  Isopto(R) Homatropine [US]
  Isopto(R) Hyoscine [US]
  Mydral(TM) [US]
  Mydriacyl(R) [US/Can]
  Sal-Tropine(TM) [US]
  Scopace(TM) [US]
  scopolamine derivatives
  Transderm-V(R) [Can]
  Transderm Scōp(R) [US]
  Tropicacyl(R) [US]
  tropicamide

DEBRIDEMENT OF
CALLOUS TISSUE
Keratolytic Agent
  Tri-Chlor(R) [US]
  Trichlor Fresh Pac(TM) [US]
  trichloroacetic acid

DEBRIDEMENT OF
ESCHAR
Protectant, Topical
  Granulex(R) [US]
  Optase(TM) [US]

trypsin, balsam peru, and castor oil
Xenaderm(TM) [US]

DECUBITUS ULCERS

Enzyme
collagenase
Santyl(R) [US]
Enzyme, Topical Debridement
Accuzyme(R) [US]
Allanzyme [US]
Allanzyme 650 [US]
Ethezyme(TM) [US]
Ethezyme(TM) 830 [US]
Gladase(R) [US]
Kovia(R) [US]
papain and urea
Protectant, Topical
Granulex(R) [US]
Optase(TM) [US]
trypsin, balsam peru, and castor oil
Xenaderm(TM) [US]
Topical Skin Product
Accuzyme(R) [US]
Allanzyme [US]
Allanzyme 650 [US]
Ethezyme(TM) [US]
Ethezyme(TM) 830 [US]
Gladase(R) [US]
Kovia(R) [US]
papain and urea

DEPRESSION (RESPIRATORY)

Respiratory Stimulant
Dopram(R) [US]
doxapram

EROSIVE ESOPHAGITIS

Proton Pump Inhibitor
esomeprazole
Nexium(R) [US/Can]

ESOPHAGEAL VARICES

Hormone, Posterior Pituitary
Pitressin(R) [US]
Pressyn(R) [Can]

Pressyn(R) AR [Can]
vasopressin
Sclerosing Agent
Ethamolin(R) [US]
ethanolamine oleate
sodium tetradecyl
Sotradecol(R) [US]
Trombovar(R) [Can]
Variceal Bleeding (Acute) Agent
somatostatin (Canada only)
Stilamin(R) [Can]

ESOPHAGITIS

Gastric Acid Secretion Inhibitor
Apo-Omeprazole(R) [Can]
lansoprazole
Losec(R) [Can]
Losec MUPS(R) [Can]
omeprazole
Prevacid(R) [US/Can]
Prevacid(R) SoluTab(TM) [US]
Prilosec(R) [US]
Prilosec OTC(TM) [US-OTC]

GAG REFLEX SUPPRESSION

Local Anesthetic
Americaine(R) [US-OTC]
Ametop(TM) [Can]
Anbesol(R) [US-OTC]
Anestacon(R) [US]
Band-Aid(R) Hurt-Free(TM)
Antiseptic Wash [US-OTC]
benzocaine
benzocaine, butyl aminobenzoate,
tetracaine, and benzalkonium
chloride
Benzodent(R) [US-OTC]
Betacaine(R) [Can]
Burnamycin [US-OTC]
Cetacaine(R) [US]
Cylex(R) [US-OTC]
Cēpacol(R) Dual Action Maximum
Strength [US-OTC]

Dermoplast(R) Antibacterial
[US-OTC]
Dermoplast(R) Pain Relieving
[US-OTC]
Detane(R) [US-OTC]
dyclonine
Foille(R) [US-OTC]
Hurricaine(R) [US-OTC]
L-M-X(TM) 4 [US-OTC]
L-M-X(TM) 5 [US-OTC]
Lanacane(R) [US-OTC]
Lanacane(R) Maximum Strength
[US-OTC]
LidaMantle(R) [US]
lidocaine
Lidodan(TM) [Can]
Lidoderm(R) [US/Can]
LTA(R) 360 [US]
Mycinettes(R) [US-OTC]
Pontocaine(R) [US/Can]
Pontocaine(R) Niphanoid(R) [US]
Premjact(R) [US-OTC]
tetracaine
Topicaine(R) [US-OTC]
Trocaine(R) [US-OTC]
Xylocaine(R) [US/Can]
Xylocaine(R) MPF [US]
Xylocaine(R) Viscous [US]
Xylocard(R) [Can]
Zilactin(R) [Can]
Zilactin-L(R) [US-OTC]
Zilactin(R)-B [US-OTC/Can]

GALL BLADDER DISEASE (DIAGNOSTIC)
Diagnostic Agent
Kinevac(R) [US]
sincalide

GASTRITIS
Antacid
Alamag [US-OTC]
aluminum hydroxide and magnesium
hydroxide

Diovol(R) [Can]
Diovol(R) Ex [Can]
Gelusil(R) Extra Strength [Can]
Mylanta(TM) [Can]
Rulox [US-OTC]
Histamine H2 Antagonist
Alti-Ranitidine [Can]
Apo-Cimetidine(R) [Can]
Apo-Ranitidine(R) [Can]
BCI-Ranitidine [Can]
cimetidine
CO Ranitidine [Can]
Gen-Cimetidine [Can]
Gen-Ranidine [Can]
Novo-Cimetidine [Can]
Novo-Ranidine [Can]
Nu-Cimet [Can]
Nu-Ranit [Can]
PMS-Cimetidine [Can]
PMS-Ranitidine [Can]
ranitidine
Ranitidine Injection, USP [Can]
Rhoxal-ranitidine [Can]
Sandoz-Ranitidine [Can]
Tagamet(R) [US]
Tagamet(R) HB [Can]
Tagamet(R) HB 200 [US-OTC]
Zantac(R) [US/Can]
Zantac 75(R) [US-OTC/Can]
Zantac 150(TM) [US-OTC]
Zantac(R) EFFERdose(R) [US]

GASTROESOPHAGEAL REFLUX DISEASE (GERD)
Cholinergic Agent
bethanechol
Duvoid(R) [Can]
Myotonachol(R) [Can]
PMS-Bethanechol [Can]
Urecholine(R) [US]
Gastric Acid Secretion Inhibitor
AcipHex(R) [US/Can]
Apo-Omeprazole(R) [Can]
lansoprazole

Losec(R) [Can]
Losec MUPS(R) [Can]
omeprazole
Pariet(R) [Can]
Prevacid(R) [US/Can]
Prevacid(R) SoluTab(TM) [US]
Prilosec(R) [US]
Prilosec OTC(TM) [US-OTC]
rabeprazole
Gastrointestinal Agent, Prokinetic
Apo-Metoclop(R) [Can]
cisapride
metoclopramide
Metoclopramide Hydrochloride
    Injection [Can]
Nu-Metoclopramide [Can]
Propulsid(R) [US]
Reglan(R) [US]
Histamine H2 Antagonist
Alti-Ranitidine [Can]
Apo-Cimetidine(R) [Can]
Apo-Famotidine(R) [Can]
Apo-Famotidine(R) Injectable [Can]
Apo-Nizatidine(R) [Can]
Apo-Ranitidine(R) [Can]
Axid(R) [US/Can]
Axid(R) AR [US-OTC]
BCI-Ranitidine [Can]
cimetidine
CO Ranitidine [Can]
famotidine
Famotidine Omega [Can]
Gen-Cimetidine [Can]
Gen-Famotidine [Can]
Gen-Nizatidine [Can]
Gen-Ranidine [Can]
nizatidine
Novo-Cimetidine [Can]
Novo-Famotidine [Can]
Novo-Nizatidine [Can]
Novo-Ranidine [Can]
Nu-Cimet [Can]
Nu-Famotidine [Can]
Nu-Nizatidine [Can]

Nu-Ranit [Can]
Pepcid(R) [US/Can]
Pepcid(R) AC [US-OTC/Can]
Pepcid(R) I.V. [Can]
PMS-Cimetidine [Can]
PMS-Nizatidine [Can]
PMS-Ranitidine [Can]
ranitidine
Ranitidine Injection, USP [Can]
Rhoxal-ranitidine [Can]
Riva-Famotidine [Can]
Sandoz-Ranitidine [Can]
Tagamet(R) [US]
Tagamet(R) HB [Can]
Tagamet(R) HB 200 [US-OTC]
Ulcidine [Can]
Zantac(R) [US/Can]
Zantac 75(R) [US-OTC/Can]
Zantac 150(TM) [US-OTC]
Zantac(R) EFFERdose(R) [US]
Proton Pump Inhibitor
Panto(TM) IV [Can]
Pantoloc(R) [Can]
pantoprazole
Protonix(R) [US/Can]

HEMORRHAGE

Adrenergic Agonist Agent
Adrenalin(R) [US/Can]
epinephrine
EpiPen(R) [US/Can]
EpiPen(R) Jr [US/Can]
Primatene(R) Mist [US-OTC]
Raphon [US-OTC]
S2(R) [US-OTC]
Twinject(TM) [US]
Antihemophilic Agent
Bebulin(R) VH [US]
factor IX complex (human)
Profilnine(R) SD [US]
Proplex(R) T [US]
Ergot Alkaloid and Derivative
ergonovine
Ergotrate(R) [US]

Hemostatic Agent
  Amicar(R) [US]
  aminocaproic acid
  aprotinin
  Avitene(R) [US]
  Avitene(R) Flour [US]
  Avitene(R) Ultrafoam [US]
  Avitene(R) UltraWrap(TM)
    [US]
  cellulose, oxidized regenerated
  collagen hemostat
  EndoAvitene(R) [US]
  gelatin (absorbable)
  Gelfilm(R) [US]
  Gelfoam(R) [US]
  Helistat(R) [US]
  Helitene(R) [US]
  Instat(TM) [US]
  Instat(TM) MCH [US]
  Surgicel(R) [US]
  Surgicel(R) Fibrillar [US]
  Surgicel(R) NuKnit [US]
  SyringeAvitene(TM) [US]
  Thrombin-JMI(R) [US]
  thrombin (topical)
  Trasylol(R) [US/Can]
Progestin
  Alti-MPA [Can]
  Apo-Medroxy(R) [Can]
  Aygestin(R) [US]
  Camila(TM) [US]
  Crinone(R) [US/Can]
  Depo-Prevera(R) [Can]
  Depo-Provera(R) [US/Can]
  Depo-Provera(R) Contraceptive [US]
  depo-subQ provera 104(TM) [US]
  Errin(TM) [US]
  Gen-Medroxy [Can]
  Jolivette(TM) [US]
  medroxyprogesterone
  Micronor(R) [US/Can]
  Nora-BE(TM) [US]
  norethindrone
  Norlutate(R) [Can]

Nor-QD(R) [US]
Novo-Medrone [Can]
Prochieve(TM) [US]
progesterone
Prometrium(R) [US/Can]
Provera(R) [US/Can]
Provera-Pak [Can]
Sclerosing Agent
  sodium tetradecyl
  Sotradecol(R) [US]
  Trombovar(R) [Can]
Vitamin, Fat Soluble
  AquaMEPHYTON(R) [Can]
  Konakion [Can]
  Mephyton(R) [US/Can]
  phytonadione

HEMORRHAGE (POSTPARTUM)

Ergot Alkaloid and Derivative
  ergonovine
  Ergotrate(R) [US]
  Methergine(R) [US/Can]
  methylergonovine
Oxytocic Agent
  oxytocin
  Pitocin(R) [US/Can]
  Syntocinon(R) [Can]
Prostaglandin
  carboprost tromethamine
  Hemabate(R) [US/Can]

HEMORRHAGE (PREVENTION)

Antihemophilic Agent
  Cyklokapron(R) [US/Can]
  tranexamic acid
  Tranexamic Acid Injection BP [Can]

HEMORRHAGE (SUBARACHNOID)

Calcium Channel Blocker
  nimodipine
  Nimotop(R) [US/Can]

HEMOSTASIS
Hemostatic Agent
  Crosseal(TM) [US]
  fibrin sealant kit
  Tisseel(R) VH [US/Can]

HYPERTENSION
Adrenergic Agonist Agent
  inamrinone
Alpha-Adrenergic Agonist
  Apo-Clonidine(R) [Can]
  Carapres(R) [Can]
  Catapres(R) [US]
  Catapres-TTS(R) [US]
  clonidine
  Dixarit(R) [Can]
  Duraclon(TM) [US]
  guanabenz
  guanfacine
  Novo-Clonidine [Can]
  Nu-Clonidine [Can]
  Tenex(R) [US/Can]
  Wytensin(R) [Can]
Alpha-Adrenergic Blocking Agent
  Alti-Doxazosin [Can]
  Alti-Terazosin [Can]
  Apo-Doxazosin(R) [Can]
  Apo-Methyldopa(R) [Can]
  Apo-Prazo(R) [Can]
  Apo-Terazosin(R) [Can]
  Cardura(R) [US]
  Cardura-1(TM) [Can]
  Cardura-2(TM) [Can]
  Cardura-4(TM) [Can]
  Cardura(R) XL [US]
  Dibenzyline(R) [US/Can]
  doxazosin
  Gen-Doxazosin [Can]
  Hytrin(R) [US/Can]
  methyldopa
  Minipress(R) [US/Can]
  Novo-Doxazosin [Can]
  Novo-Prazin [Can]
  Novo-Terazosin [Can]

Nu-Medopa [Can]
Nu-Prazo [Can]
Nu-Terazosin [Can]
phenoxybenzamine
phentolamine
PMS-Terazosin [Can]
prazosin
Regitine(R) [Can]
Rogitine(R) [Can]
terazosin
Alpha-/Beta-Adrenergic Blocker
  Apo-Labetalol(R) [Can]
  labetalol
  Labetalol Hydrochloride Injection,
    USP [Can]
  Normodyne(R) [Can]
  Trandate(R) [US/Can]
Angiotensin II Antagonist Combination
  eprosartan and hydrochlorothiazide
  Teveten(R) HCT [US/Can]
  Teveten(R) Plus [Can]
Angiotensin II Receptor Antagonist
  Atacand(R) [US/Can]
  Avapro(R) [US/Can]
  Benicar(R) [US]
  Benicar HCT(R) [US]
  candesartan
  Cozaar(R) [US/Can]
  Diovan(R) [US/Can]
  eprosartan
  irbesartan
  losartan
  Micardis(R) [US/Can]
  olmesartan
  olmesartan and hydrochlorothiazide
  telmisartan
  Teveten(R) [US/Can]
  valsartan
Angiotensin-Converting Enzyme (ACE)
  Inhibitor
  Accupril(R) [US/Can]
  Altace(R) [US/Can]
  Alti-Captopril [Can]
  Apo-Benazepril(R) [Can]

Apo-Capto(R) [Can]
Apo-Fosinopril(R) [Can]
Apo-Lisinopril(R) [Can]
benazepril
Capoten(R) [US/Can]
captopril
cilazapril (Canada only)
enalapril
fosinopril
fosinopril and hydrochlorothiazide
Gen-Captopril [Can]
Inhibace(R) [Can]
lisinopril
Lotensin(R) [US/Can]
Mavik(R) [US/Can]
moexipril
moexipril and hydrochlorothiazide
Monopril(R) [US/Can]
Monopril-HCT(R) [US/Can]
Novo-Captopril [Can]
Novo-Cilazapril [Can]
Novo-Fosinopril [Can]
Nu-Capto [Can]
PMS-Captopril [Can]
Prinivil(R) [US/Can]
quinapril
ramipril
ratio-Fosinopril [Can]
Riva-Rosinopril [Can]
trandolapril
Uniretic(R) [US/Can]
Univasc(R) [US]
Vasotec(R) [US/Can]
Zestril(R) [US/Can]
Antihypertensive Agent
  diazoxide
  eplerenone
  Hyperstat(R) [US]
  Inspra(TM) [US]
  Proglycem(R) [US/Can]
Antihypertensive Agent, Combination
  Accuretic(R) [US/Can]
  Aldactazide(R) [US]
  Aldactazide 25(R) [Can]

Aldactazide 50(R) [Can]
Aldoril(R) [US]
amlodipine and benazepril
Apo-Methazide(R) [Can]
Apo-Triazide(R) [Can]
Atacand HCT(TM) [US]
Atacand(R) Plus [Can]
atenolol and chlorthalidone
Avalide(R) [US/Can]
benazepril and hydrochlorothiazide
bisoprolol and hydrochlorothiazide
candesartan and hydrochlorothiazide
Capozide(R) [US/Can]
captopril and hydrochlorothiazide
clonidine and chlorthalidone
Clorpres(R) [US]
Diovan HCT(R) [US/Can]
Dyazide(R) [US]
enalapril and felodipine
enalapril and hydrochlorothiazide
eprosartan and hydrochlorothiazide
hydralazine and hydrochlorothiazide
hydrochlorothiazide and
  spironolactone
hydrochlorothiazide and triamterene
Hyzaar(R) [US/Can]
Hyzaar(R) DS [Can]
Inderide(R) [US]
irbesartan and hydrochlorothiazide
Lexxel(R) [US/Can]
lisinopril and hydrochlorothiazide
losartan and hydrochlorothiazide
Lotensin(R) HCT [US]
Lotrel(R) [US]
Maxzide(R) [US]
Maxzide(R)-25 [US]
methyldopa and hydrochlorothiazide
Micardis(R) HCT [US]
Micardis(R) Plus [Can]
Minizide(R) [US]
Novo-Spirozine [Can]
Novo-Triamzide [Can]
Nu-Triazide [Can]
Penta-Triamterene HCTZ [Can]

prazosin and polythiazide
Prinzide(R) [US/Can]
propranolol and hydrochlorothiazide
quinapril and hydrochlorothiazide
Quinaretic [US]
Riva-Zide [Can]
Tarka(R) [US/Can]
telmisartan and hydrochlorothiazide
Tenoretic(R) [US/Can]
Teveten(R) HCT [US/Can]
Teveten(R) Plus [Can]
trandolapril and verapamil
valsartan and hydrochlorothiazide
Vaseretic(R) [US/Can]
Zestoretic(R) [US/Can]
Ziac(R) [US/Can]
Beta-Adrenergic Blocker
acebutolol
Alti-Nadolol [Can]
Alti-Timolol [Can]
Apo-Acebutolol(R) [Can]
Apo-Atenol(R) [Can]
Apo-Bisoprolol(R) [Can]
Apo-Carvedilol(R) [Can]
Apo-Metoprolol(R) [Can]
Apo-Nadol(R) [Can]
Apo-Pindol(R) [Can]
Apo-Propranolol(R) [Can]
Apo-Timol(R) [Can]
Apo-Timop(R) [Can]
atenolol
Betaloc(R) [Can]
Betaloc(R) Durules(R) [Can]
betaxolol
Betimol(R) [US]
Betoptic(R) S [US/Can]
bisoprolol
Blocadren(R) [US]
Brevibloc(R) [US/Can]
carteolol
Cartrol(R) [US/Can]
carvedilol
Coreg(R) [US/Can]
Corgard(R) [US/Can]

esmolol
Gen-Acebutolol [Can]
Gen-Atenolol [Can]
Gen-Pindolol [Can]
Gen-Timolol [Can]
Inderal(R) [US/Can]
Inderal(R) LA [US/Can]
InnoPran XL(TM) [US]
Istalol(TM) [US]
Kerlone(R) [US]
Lopressor(R) [US/Can]
metoprolol
Metoprolol Tartrate Injection, USP
  [Can]
Monitan(R) [Can]
Monocor(R) [Can]
nadolol
Novo-Acebutolol [Can]
Novo-Atenol [Can]
Novo-Bisoprolol [Can]
Novo-Carvedilol [Can]
Novo-Metoprolol [Can]
Novo-Nadolol [Can]
Novo-Pindol [Can]
Novo-Pranol [Can]
Nu-Acebutolol [Can]
Nu-Atenol [Can]
Nu-Metop [Can]
Nu-Pindol [Can]
Nu-Propranolol [Can]
Nu-Timolol [Can]
Ocupress(R) Ophthalmic
  [Can]
oxprenolol (Canada only)
Phoxal-timolol [Can]
pindolol
PMS-Atenolol [Can]
PMS-Carvedilol [Can]
PMS-Metoprolol [Can]
PMS-Pindolol [Can]
PMS-Timolol [Can]
propranolol
Propranolol Hydrochloride Injection,
  USP [Can]

RAN(TM)-Carvedilol [Can]
ratio-Carvedilol [Can]
Rhotral [Can]
Rhoxal-acebutolol [Can]
Rhoxal-atenolol [Can]
Riva-Atenolol [Can]
Sandoz-Acebutolol [Can]
Sandoz-Atenolol [Can]
Sandoz-Betaxolol [Can]
Sandoz-Bisoprolol [Can]
Sandoz-Metoprolol [Can]
Sandoz-Timolol [Can]
Sectral(R) [US/Can]
Slow-Trasicor(R) [Can]
Tenolin [Can]
Tenormin(R) [US/Can]
Tim-AK [Can]
timolol
Timoptic(R) [US/Can]
Timoptic(R) in OcuDose(R)
  [US]
Timoptic-XE(R) [US/Can]
Toprol-XL(R) [US/Can]
Trasicor(R) [Can]
Visken(R) [Can]
Zebeta(R) [US/Can]
Beta Blocker, Beta1 Selective
  Lopressor HCT(R) [US]
  metoprolol and hydrochlorothiazide
Calcium Channel Blocker
  Adalat(R) XL(R) [Can]
  Adalat(R) CC [US]
  Afeditab(TM) CR [US]
  Alti-Verapamil [Can]
  amlodipine
  amlodipine and atorvastatin
  Apo-Nifed(R) [Can]
  Apo-Nifed PA(R) [Can]
  Apo-Verap(R) [Can]
  Apo-Verap(R) SR [Can]
  Caduet(R) [US/Can]
  Calan(R) [US/Can]
  Calan(R) SR [US]

Cardene(R) [US]
Cardene(R) I.V. [US]
Cardene(R) SR [US]
Chronovera(R) [Can]
Covera(R) [Can]
Covera-HS(R) [US/Can]
DynaCirc(R) [Can]
DynaCirc(R) CR [US]
felodipine
Gen-Verapamil [Can]
Gen-Verapamil SR [Can]
Isoptin(R) SR [US/Can]
isradipine
nicardipine
Nifediac(TM) CC [US]
Nifedical(TM) XL [US]
nifedipine
nisoldipine
Norvasc(R) [US/Can]
Novo-Nifedin [Can]
Novo-Veramil SR [Can]
Nu-Nifed [Can]
Nu-Verap [Can]
Plendil(R) [US/Can]
Procardia(R) [US/Can]
Procardia XL(R) [US]
Renedil(R) [Can]
Riva-Verapamil SR [Can]
Sular(R) [US]
verapamil
Verapamil Hydrochloride Injection,
  USP [Can]
Verelan(R) [US]
Verelan(R) PM [US]
Diagnostic Agent
  phentolamine
  Regitine(R) [Can]
  Rogitine(R) [Can]
Diuretic, Combination
  amiloride and hydrochlorothiazide
  Apo-Amilzide(R) [Can]
  Gen-Amilazide [Can]
  Moduret [Can]

Novamilor [Can]
Nu-Amilzide [Can]
Diuretic, Loop
  Apo-Furosemide(R) [Can]
  bumetanide
  Bumex(R) [US/Can]
  Burinex(R) [Can]
  Demadex(R) [US]
  Edecrin(R) [US/Can]
  ethacrynic acid
  furosemide
  Furosemide Injection, USP
    [Can]
  Furosemide Special [Can]
  Lasix(R) [US/Can]
  Lasix(R) Special [Can]
  Novo-Semide [Can]
  torsemide
Diuretic, Miscellaneous
  Apo-Chlorthalidone(R) [Can]
  Apo-Indapamide(R) [Can]
  chlorthalidone
  Gen-Indapamide [Can]
  indapamide
  Lozide(R) [Can]
  Lozol(R) [US/Can]
  metolazone
  Mykrox(R) [Can]
  Novo-Indapamide [Can]
  Nu-Indapamide [Can]
  PMS-Indapamide [Can]
  Thalitone(R) [US]
  Zaroxolyn(R) [US/Can]
Diuretic, Potassium Sparing
  Aldactone(R) [US/Can]
  Dyrenium(R) [US]
  Novo-Spiroton [Can]
  spironolactone
  triamterene
Diuretic, Thiazide
  Apo-Hydro(R) [Can]
  Aquatensen(R) [Can]
  Benicar HCT(R) [US]

chlorothiazide
Diuril(R) [US/Can]
Enduron(R) [Can]
eprosartan and hydrochlorothiazide
hydrochlorothiazide
Lopressor HCT(R) [US]
methyclothiazide
metoprolol and hydrochlorothiazide
Microzide(TM) [US]
moexipril and hydrochlorothiazide
Novo-Hydrazide [Can]
olmesartan and hydrochlorothiazide
PMS-Hydrochlorothiazide [Can]
Teveten(R) HCT [US/Can]
Teveten(R) Plus [Can]
Uniretic(R) [US/Can]
Ganglionic Blocking Agent
  Inversine(R) [US/Can]
  mecamylamine
Miscellaneous Product
  Aceon(R) [US]
  Coversyl(R) [Can]
  Coversyl(R) Plus [Can]
  perindopril and indapamide (Canada
    only)
  perindopril erbumine
  Preterax(R) [Can]
Rauwolfia Alkaloid
  reserpine
Selective Aldosterone Blocker
  eplerenone
  Inspra(TM) [US]
Vasodilator
  Apo-Gain(R) [Can]
  Apo-Hydralazine(R) [Can]
  Apresoline(R) [Can]
  hydralazine
  Loniten(R) [US]
  Minox [Can]
  minoxidil
  Nitropress(R) [US]
  nitroprusside
  Novo-Hylazin [Can]

Nu-Hydral [Can]
Rogaine(R) [Can]
Rogaine(R) Extra Strength for Men
  [US-OTC]
Rogaine(R) for Men [US-OTC]
Rogaine(R) for Women [US-OTC]

HYPERTENSION (ARTERIAL)

Beta-Adrenergic Blocker
  Levatol(R) [US/Can]
  penbutolol

HYPERTENSION (CEREBRAL)

Barbiturate
  Pentothal(R) [US/Can]
  thiopental
Diuretic, Osmotic
  Amino-Cerv(TM) [US]
  Aquacare(R) [US-OTC]
  Aquaphilic(R) With Carbamide
    [US-OTC]
  Carmol(R) 10 [US-OTC]
  Carmol(R) 20 [US-OTC]
  Carmol(R) 40 [US]
  Carmol(R) Deep Cleaning [US]
  Cerovel(TM) [US]
  DPM(TM) [US-OTC]
  Gormel(R) [US-OTC]
  Keralac(TM) [US]
  Keralac(TM) Nailstik [US]
  Lanaphilic(R) [US-OTC]
  mannitol
  Nutraplus(R) [US-OTC]
  Osmitrol(R) [US/Can]
  Rea-Lo(R) [US-OTC]
  Resectisol(R) [US]
  Ultra Mide(R) [US-OTC]
  UltraMide 25(TM) [Can]
  Umecta(R) [US]
  urea
  Ureacin(R) [US-OTC]
  Uremol(R) [Can]

Urisec(R) [Can]
Vanamide(TM) [US]

HYPERTENSION (CORONARY)

Vasodilator
  Gen-Nitro [Can]
  Minitran(TM) [US/Can]
  Nitrek(R) [US]
  Nitro-Bid(R) [US]
  Nitro-Dur(R) [US/Can]
  nitroglycerin
  Nitrol(R) [Can]
  Nitrolingual(R) [US]
  NitroQuick(R) [US]
  Nitrostat(R) [US/Can]
  NitroTime(R) [US]
  Rho-Nitro [Can]
  Transderm-Nitro(R) [Can]
  Trinipatch(R) 0.2 [Can]
  Trinipatch(R) 0.4 [Can]
  Trinipatch(R) 0.6 [Can]

HYPERTENSION (EMERGENCY)

Antihypertensive Agent
  Corlopam(R) [US/Can]
  fenoldopam

HYPERTENSION (OCULAR)

Alpha2-Adrenergic Agonist Agent,
  Ophthalmic
  Alphagan(R) [Can]
  Alphagan(R) P [US]
  brimonidine
  PMS-Brimonidine Tartrate [Can]
  ratio-Brimonidine [Can]
Beta-Adrenergic Blocker
  Apo-Levobunolol(R) [Can]
  Betagan(R) [US/Can]
  levobunolol
  Novo-Levobunolol [Can]
  Optho-Bunolol(R) [Can]
  PMS-Levobunolol [Can]
  Sandoz-Levobunolol [Can]

HYPOTENSION
Adrenergic Agonist Agent
  Adrenalin(R) [US/Can]
  dopamine
  ephedrine
  epinephrine
  isoproterenol
  Isuprel(R) [US]
  Levophed(R) [US/Can]
  norepinephrine
  Primatene(R) Mist [US-OTC]

INTRACRANIAL PRESSURE
Barbiturate
  Pentothal(R) [US/Can]
  thiopental
Diuretic, Osmotic
  mannitol
  Osmitrol(R) [US/Can]
  Resectisol(R) [US]

INTRAOCULAR PRESSURE
Ophthalmic Agent, Miscellaneous
  Bausch & Lomb(R) Computer Eye
    Drops [US-OTC]
  Colace(R) Adult/Children
    Suppositories [US-OTC]
  Colace(R) Infant/Children
    Suppositories [US-OTC]
  Fleet(R) Babylax(R) [US-OTC]
  Fleet(R) Glycerin Suppositories
    [US-OTC]
  Fleet(R) Glycerin Suppositories
    Maximum Strength
    [US-OTC]
  Fleet(R) Liquid Glycerin
    Suppositories [US-OTC]
  glycerin
  Sani-Supp(R) [US-OTC]

LABOR INDUCTION
Oxytocic Agent
  oxytocin
  Pitocin(R) [US/Can]
  Syntocinon(R) [Can]

Prostaglandin
  carboprost tromethamine
  Cervidil(R) [US/Can]
  dinoprostone
  Hemabate(R) [US/Can]
  Prepidil(R) [US/Can]
  Prostin E2(R) [US/Can]

LABOR (PREMATURE)
Adrenergic Agonist Agent
  Brethine(R) [US]
  Bricanyl(R) [Can]
  terbutaline

MUSCLE SPASM
Analgesic, Nonnarcotic
  Norgesic(TM) [Can]
  Norgesic(TM) Forte [Can]
  orphenadrine, aspirin, and caffeine
Skeletal Muscle Relaxant
  Apo-Cyclobenzaprine(R) [Can]
  carisoprodol
  carisoprodol and aspirin
  carisoprodol, aspirin, and codeine
  chlorzoxazone
  cyclobenzaprine
  Flexeril(R) [US]
  Flexitec [Can]
  Gen-Cyclobenzaprine [Can]
  metaxalone
  methocarbamol
  Mivacron(R) [Can]
  mivacurium
  Norflex(TM) [US/Can]
  Norgesic(TM) [Can]
  Norgesic(TM) Forte [Can]
  Novo-Cycloprine [Can]
  Nu-Cyclobenzaprine [Can]
  Orphenace(R) [Can]
  orphenadrine
  orphenadrine, aspirin, and caffeine
  Parafon Forte(R) [Can]
  Rhoxal-orphendrine [Can]
  Robaxin(R) [US/Can]
  Skelaxin(R) [US/Can]

Soma(R) [US/Can]
Soma(R) Compound [US]
Soma(R) Compound w/Codeine [US]
Strifon Forte(R) [Can]

MYDRIASIS
Adrenergic Agonist Agent
  AK-Dilate(R) [US]
  Mydfrin(R) [US/Can]
  Neo-Synephrine(R) [Can]
  phenylephrine
Anticholinergic/Adrenergic Agonist
  Cyclomydril(R) [US]
  cyclopentolate and phenylephrine
  Murocoll-2(R) [US]
  phenylephrine and scopolamine
Anticholinergic Agent
  AtroPen(R) [US]
  atropine
  Atropine-Care(R) [US]
  Cyclogyl(R) [US/Can]
  cyclopentolate
  Cylate(R) [US]
  Diopentolate(R) [Can]
  Dioptic's Atropine Solution [Can]
  Diotrope(R) [Can]
  homatropine
  Isopto(R) Atropine [US/Can]
  Isopto(R) Homatropine [US]
  Mydral(TM) [US]
  Mydriacyl(R) [US/Can]
  Tropicacyl(R) [US]
  tropicamide

NAUSEA
Anticholinergic Agent
  Buscopan(R) [Can]
  Isopto(R) Hyoscine [US]
  Scopace(TM) [US]
  scopolamine derivatives
  Tebamide(TM) [US]
  Tigan(R) [US/Can]
  Transderm-V(R) [Can]
  Transderm Scōp(R) [US]
  trimethobenzamide

Antiemetic
  Aloxi(R) [US]
  aprepitant
  dronabinol
  droperidol
  Emend(R) [US]
  Emetrol(R) [US-OTC]
  Especol(R) [US-OTC]
  Formula EM [US-OTC]
  fructose, dextrose, and phosphoric
    acid
  Inapsine(R) [US]
  Kalmz [US-OTC]
  Marinol(R) [US/Can]
  Nausea Relief [US-OTC]
  palonosetron
  Phenadoz(TM) [US]
  Phenergan(R) [US/Can]
  promethazine
  Promethegan(TM) [US]
  Tebamide(TM) [US]
  Tigan(R) [US/Can]
  trimethobenzamide
Antihistamine
  Apo-Dimenhydrinate(R) [Can]
  Children's Motion Sickness Liquid
    [Can]
  Diclectin(R) [Can]
  dimenhydrinate
  Dinate(R) [Can]
  doxylamine and pyridoxine (Canada
    only)
  Dramamine(R) [US-OTC]
  Gravol(R) [Can]
  Jamp(R) Travel Tablet [Can]
  Nauseatol [Can]
  Novo-Dimenate [Can]
  SAB-Dimenhydrinate [Can]
Antipsychotic Agent, Butyrophenone
  droperidol
  Inapsine(R) [US]
Gastrointestinal Agent, Prokinetic
  Apo-Metoclop(R) [Can]
  metoclopramide

Metoclopramide Hydrochloride
Injection [Can]
Nu-Metoclopramide [Can]
Reglan(R) [US]
Phenothiazine Derivative
Apo-Perphenazine(R) [Can]
Apo-Prochlorperazine(R) [Can]
chlorpromazine
Compazine(R) [Can]
Compro(TM) [US]
Largactil(R) [Can]
Novo-Chlorpromazine [Can]
Nu-Prochlor [Can]
perphenazine
Phenadoz(TM) [US]
Phenergan(R) [US/Can]
prochlorperazine
promethazine
Promethegan(TM) [US]
Stemetil(R) [Can]
Selective 5-HT3 Receptor Antagonist
Aloxi(R) [US]
granisetron
Kytril(R) [US/Can]
ondansetron
palonosetron
Zofran(R) [US/Can]
Zofran(R) ODT [US/Can]
Vitamin
Diclectin(R) [Can]
doxylamine and pyridoxine (Canada
only)

NERVE BLOCK

Local Anesthetic
Ametop(TM) [Can]
Anestacon(R) [US]
Band-Aid(R) Hurt-Free(TM)
Antiseptic Wash [US-OTC]
Betacaine(R) [Can]
bupivacaine
Burnamycin [US-OTC]
Burn Jel [US-OTC]
Burn-O-Jel [US-OTC]

Carbocaine(R) [US/Can]
chloroprocaine
Citanest(R) Plain [US/Can]
L-M-X(TM) 4 [US-OTC]
L-M-X(TM) 5 [US-OTC]
LidaMantle(R) [US]
lidocaine
lidocaine and epinephrine
Lidodan(TM) [Can]
Lidoderm(R) [US/Can]
LidoSite(TM) [US]
LTA(R) 360 [US]
Marcaine(R) [US/Can]
Marcaine(R) Spinal [US]
mepivacaine
Nesacaine(R) [US]
Nesacaine(R)-CE [Can]
Nesacaine(R)-MPF [US]
Novocain(R) [US]
Polocaine(R) [US/Can]
Polocaine(R) Dental [US]
Polocaine(R) MPF [US]
Pontocaine(R) [US/Can]
Pontocaine(R) Niphanoid(R)
[US]
Pontocaine(R) With Dextrose
[US]
Premjact(R) [US-OTC]
prilocaine
procaine
Sensorcaine(R) [US/Can]
Sensorcaine(R)-MPF [US]
Solarcaine(R) Aloe Extra Burn Relief
[US-OTC]
tetracaine
tetracaine and dextrose
Topicaine(R) [US-OTC]
Xylocaine(R) [US/Can]
Xylocaine(R) MPF [US]
Xylocaine(R) MPF With Epinephrine
[US]
Xylocaine(R) Viscous [US]
Xylocaine(R) With Epinephrine
[US/Can]

Xylocard(R) [Can]
Zilactin(R) [Can]
Zilactin-L(R) [US-OTC]

NEURALGIA

Analgesic, Nonnarcotic
Asaphen [Can]
Asaphen E.C. [Can]
Ascriptin(R) [US-OTC]
Ascriptin(R) Extra Strength
[US-OTC]
Aspercin [US-OTC]
Aspercin Extra [US-OTC]
aspirin
Bayer(R) Aspirin [US-OTC]
Bayer(R) Aspirin Extra Strength
[US-OTC]
Bayer(R) Aspirin Regimen Adult
Low Strength [US-OTC]
Bayer(R) Aspirin Regimen Children's
[US-OTC]
Bayer(R) Aspirin Regimen Regular
Strength [US-OTC]
Bayer(R) Plus Extra Strength
[US-OTC]
Bayer(R) Women's Aspirin Plus
Calcium [US-OTC]
Bufferin(R) [US-OTC]
Bufferin(R) Extra Strength
[US-OTC]
Buffinol [US-OTC]
Buffinol Extra [US-OTC]
Easprin(R) [US]
Ecotrin(R) [US-OTC]
Ecotrin(R) Low Strength
[US-OTC]
Ecotrin(R) Maximum Strength
[US-OTC]
Entrophen(R) [Can]
Halfprin(R) [US-OTC]
Novasen [Can]
St. Joseph(R) Adult Aspirin
[US-OTC]
Sureprin 81(TM) [US-OTC]

ZORprin(R) [US]
Analgesic, Opioid
acetaminophen, codeine, and
doxylamine (Canada Only)
Mersyndol(R) With Codeine
[Can]
Analgesic, Topical
Antiphlogistine Rub A-535 No Odour
[Can]
ArthriCare(R) for Women Extra
Moisturizing [US-OTC]
ArthriCare(R) for Women
Multi-Action [US-OTC]
ArthriCare(R) for Women Silky Dry
[US-OTC]
Aspercreme(R) [US-OTC]
Capsagel(R) [US-OTC]
capsaicin
Capzasin-HP(R) [US-OTC]
Capzasin-P(R) [US-OTC]
Flex-Power [US-OTC]
Mobisyl(R) [US-OTC]
Myoflex(R) [US-OTC/Can]
Sportscreme(R) [US-OTC]
trolamine
Zostrix(R) [US-OTC/Can]
Zostrix(R)-HP [US-OTC/Can]

OPHTHALMIC SURGERY

Nonsteroidal Antiinflammatory Drug
(NSAID)
Apo-Diclo(R) [Can]
Apo-Diclo Rapide(R) [Can]
Apo-Diclo SR(R) [Can]
Cataflam(R) [US/Can]
diclofenac
Novo-Difenac [Can]
Novo-Difenac K [Can]
Novo-Difenac-SR [Can]
Nu-Diclo [Can]
Nu-Diclo-SR [Can]
Pennsaid(R) [Can]
PMS-Diclofenac [Can]
PMS-Diclofenac SR [Can]

Riva-Diclofenac [Can]
Riva-Diclofenac-K [Can]
Solaraze(R) [US]
Voltaren(R) [US/Can]
Voltaren Ophtha(R) [Can]
Voltaren Ophthalmic(R) [US]
Voltaren Rapide(R) [Can]
Voltaren(R)-XR [US]

OPHTHALMIC SURGICAL AID

Ophthalmic Agent, Miscellaneous
Cellugel(R) [US]
GenTeal(R) [US-OTC/Can]
GenTeal(R) Mild [US-OTC]
Gonak(TM) [US-OTC]
Goniosoft(TM) [US]
hydroxypropyl methylcellulose
Isopto(R) Tears [US-OTC/Can]
Tearisol(R) [US-OTC]
Tears Again(R) MC [US-OTC]

OVULATION INDUCTION

Gonadotropin
chorionic gonadotropin (human)
chorionic gonadotropin (recombinant)
Humegon(R) [Can]
Menopur(R) [US]
menotropins
Novarel(R) [US]
Ovidrel(R) [US/Can]
Pregnyl(R) [US]
Profasi(R) HP [Can]
Repronex(R) [US/Can]
Ovulation Stimulator
chorionic gonadotropin (recombinant)
Clomid(R) [US/Can]
clomiphene
Milophene(R) [Can]
Ovidrel(R) [US/Can]
Serophene(R) [US/Can]

PAIN

Analgesic Combination (Narcotic)
propoxyphene, aspirin, and caffeine

Analgesic Combination (Opioid)
acetaminophen, caffeine, and dihydrocodeine
Panlor(R) DC [US]
Panlor(R) SS [US]
pentazocine and acetaminophen
Talacen(R) [US]
ZerLor(TM) [US]
Analgesic, Miscellaneous
acetaminophen and tramadol
Tramacet [Can]
Ultracet(TM) [US]
Analgesic, Narcotic
acetaminophen and codeine
Actiq(R) [US/Can]
Alfenta(R) [US/Can]
alfentanil
Alfentanil Injection, USP [Can]
Anexsia(R) [US]
Apo-Butorphanol(R) [Can]
Astramorph/PF(TM) [US]
Avinza(TM) [US]
Balacet 325(TM) [US]
Bancap HC(R) [US]
belladonna and opium
B&O Supprettes(R) [US]
Buprenex(R) [US/Can]
buprenorphine
butalbital, aspirin, caffeine, and codeine
butorphanol
Capital(R) and Codeine [US]
Ceta-Plus(R) [US]
codeine
Codeine Contin(R) [Can]
Co-Gesic(R) [US]
Damason-P(R) [US]
Darvocet A500(TM) [US]
Darvocet-N(R) 50 [US/Can]
Darvocet-N(R) 100 [US/Can]
Darvon(R) [US]
Darvon-N(R) [US/Can]
Demerol(R) [US/Can]
DepoDur(TM) [US]

dihydrocodeine, aspirin, and caffeine
Dilaudid(R) [US/Can]
Dilaudid-HP(R) [US/Can]
Dilaudid-HP-Plus(R) [Can]
Dilaudid(R) Sterile Powder [Can]
Dilaudid-XP(R) [Can]
Dolophine(R) [US/Can]
Duragesic(R) [US/Can]
Duramorph(R) [US]
Endocet(R) [US/Can]
Endodan(R) [US/Can]
ETH-Oxydose(TM) [Can]
fentanyl
Fentanyl Citrate Injection, USP [Can]
Fiorinal(R)-C 1/2 [Can]
Fiorinal(R)-C 1/4 [Can]
Fiorinal(R) With Codeine [US]
hycet(TM) [US]
hydrocodone and acetaminophen
hydrocodone and aspirin
hydrocodone and ibuprofen
Hydromorph Contin(R) [Can]
Hydromorph-IR(R) [Can]
hydromorphone
Hydromorphone HP [Can]
Hydromorphone HP(R) 10 [Can]
Hydromorphone HP(R) 20 [Can]
Hydromorphone HP(R) 50 [Can]
Hydromorphone HP(R) Forte [Can]
Hydromorphone Hydrochloride
    Injection, USP [Can]
Infumorph(R) [US]
Ionsys(TM) [US]
Kadian(R) [US/Can]
Levo-Dromoran(R) [US]
levorphanol
Lorcet(R) 10/650 [US]
Lorcet(R) Plus [US]
Lortab(R) [US]
Margesic(R) H [US]
Maxidone(TM) [US]
meperidine
meperidine and promethazine
Meperitab(R) [US]

M-Eslon(R) [Can]
Metadol(TM) [Can]
methadone
Methadone Diskets(R) [US]
Methadone Intensol(TM) [US]
Methadose(R) [US/Can]
Morphine HP(R) [Can]
Morphine LP(R) Epidural [Can]
morphine sulfate
M.O.S.(R) 10 [Can]
M.O.S.(R) 20 [Can]
M.O.S.(R) 30 [Can]
M.O.S.-S.R.(R) [Can]
M.O.S.-Sulfate(R) [Can]
MS Contin(R) [US/Can]
MS-IR(R) [Can]
nalbuphine
Norco(R) [US]
Nubain(R) [US]
Numorphan(R) [US]
opium tincture
Oramorph SR(R) [US]
Oxycocet(R) [Can]
Oxycodan(R) [Can]
oxycodone
oxycodone and acetaminophen
oxycodone and aspirin
OxyContin(R) [US/Can]
OxyFast(R) [US]
Oxy.IR(R) [Can]
oxymorphone
paregoric
pentazocine
Percocet(R) [US/Can]
Percocet(R)-Demi [Can]
Percodan(R) [US/Can]
Phrenilin(R) With Caffeine and
    Codeine [US]
PMS-Butorphanol [Can]
PMS-Hydromorphone [Can]
PMS-Morphine Sulfate SR [Can]
PMS-Oxycodone-Acetaminophen
    [Can]
Pronap-100(R) [US]

propoxyphene
propoxyphene and acetaminophen
ratio-Emtec [Can]
ratio-Lenoltec [Can]
ratio-Morphine SR [Can]
remifentanil
Reprexain(TM) [US]
RMS(R) [US]
Roxanol(TM) [US]
Roxanol 100(TM) [US]
Roxicet(TM) [US]
Roxicet(TM) 5/500 [US]
Roxicodone(R) [US]
Stadol(R) [US]
Stagesic(R) [US]
Statex(R) [Can]
Sublimaze(R) [US]
Subutex(R) [US/Can]
Sufenta(R) [US/Can]
sufentanil
Supeudol(R) [Can]
Synalgos(R)-DC [US]
642(R) Tablet [Can]
Talwin(R) [US/Can]
Talwin(R) NX [US]
Tecnal C 1/2 [Can]
Tecnal C 1/4 [Can]
Triatec-8 [Can]
Triatec-8 Strong [Can]
Triatec-30 [Can]
Tylenol(R) Elixir with Codeine [Can]
Tylenol(R) No. 1 [Can]
Tylenol No. 1 Forte [Can]
Tylenol(R) No. 2 with Codeine [Can]
Tylenol(R) No. 3 with Codeine [Can]
Tylenol(R) No. 4 with Codeine [Can]
Tylenol(R) With Codeine [US]
Tylox(R) [US]
Ultiva(R) [US/Can]
Vicodin(R) [US]
Vicodin(R) ES [US]
Vicodin(R) HP [US]
Vicoprofen(R) [US/Can]
Zomorph(R) [Can]

Zydone(R) [US]

Analgesic, Nonnarcotic
Abenol(R) [Can]
Acephen(TM) [US-OTC]
Aceta-Gesic [US-OTC]
acetaminophen
acetaminophen and diphenhydramine
acetaminophen and phenyltoloxamine
acetaminophen and tramadol
acetaminophen, aspirin, and caffeine
Acular(R) [US/Can]
Acular LS(TM) [US/Can]
Acular(R) PF [US]
Advil(R) [US-OTC/Can]
Advil(R) Children's [US-OTC]
Advil(R) Infants' [US-OTC]
Advil(R) Junior [US-OTC]
Aleve(R) [US-OTC]
Alti-Flurbiprofen [Can]
Amigesic(R) [US/Can]
Anaprox(R) [US/Can]
Anaprox(R) DS [US/Can]
Ansaid(R) [Can]
Apo-Acetaminophen(R) [Can]
Apo-Diclo(R) [Can]
Apo-Diclo Rapide(R) [Can]
Apo-Diclo SR(R) [Can]
Apo-Diflunisal(R) [Can]
Apo-Etodolac(R) [Can]
Apo-Flurbiprofen(R) [Can]
Apo-Ibuprofen(R) [Can]
Apo-Indomethacin(R) [Can]
Apo-Keto(R) [Can]
Apo-Keto-E(R) [Can]
Apo-Ketorolac(R) [Can]
Apo-Ketorolac Injectable(R) [Can]
Apo-Keto SR(R) [Can]
Apo-Mefenamic(R) [Can]
Apo-Nabumetone(R) [Can]
Apo-Napro-Na(R) [Can]
Apo-Napro-Na DS(R) [Can]
Apo-Naproxen(R) [Can]
Apo-Naproxen EC(R) [Can]
Apo-Naproxen SR(R) [Can]

Apo-Oxaprozin(R) [Can]
Apo-Piroxicam(R) [Can]
Apo-Sulin(R) [Can]
Apra Children's [US-OTC]
Asaphen [Can]
Asaphen E.C. [Can]
Ascriptin(R) [US-OTC]
Ascriptin(R) Extra Strength
  [US-OTC]
Aspercin [US-OTC]
Aspercin Extra [US-OTC]
Aspergum(R) [US-OTC]
aspirin
Aspirin Free Anacin(R) Maximum
  Strength [US-OTC]
Atasol(R) [Can]
Bayer(R) Aspirin [US-OTC]
Bayer(R) Aspirin Extra Strength
  [US-OTC]
Bayer(R) Aspirin Regimen Adult
  Low Strength [US-OTC]
Bayer(R) Aspirin Regimen Children's
  [US-OTC]
Bayer(R) Aspirin Regimen Regular
  Strength [US-OTC]
Bayer(R) Plus Extra Strength
  [US-OTC]
Bayer(R) Women's Aspirin Plus
  Calcium [US-OTC]
Bufferin(R) [US-OTC]
Bufferin(R) Extra Strength [US-OTC]
Buffinol [US-OTC]
Buffinol Extra [US-OTC]
Cataflam(R) [US/Can]
Cetafen(R) [US-OTC]
Cetafen Extra(R) [US-OTC]
choline magnesium trisalicylate
Clinoril(R) [US]
Comtrex(R) Sore Throat Maximum
  Strength [US-OTC]
Daypro(R) [US/Can]
diclofenac
diflunisal
Dologesic(R) [US]

Dom-Mefenamic Acid [Can]
Easprin(R) [US]
EC-Naprosyn(R) [US]
Ecotrin(R) [US-OTC]
Ecotrin(R) Low Strength
  [US-OTC]
Ecotrin(R) Maximum Strength
  [US-OTC]
ElixSure(TM) IB [US-OTC]
Entrophen(R) [Can]
etodolac
Excedrin(R) Extra Strength
  [US-OTC]
Excedrin(R) P.M. [US-OTC]
Feldene(R) [US]
Fem-Prin(R) [US-OTC]
fenoprofen
FeverAll(R) [US-OTC]
Flextra 650 [US]
Flextra-DS [US]
flurbiprofen
Froben(R) [Can]
Froben-SR(R) [Can]
Genaced(TM) [US-OTC]
Genapap(TM) [US-OTC]
Genapap(TM) Children [US-OTC]
Genapap(TM) Extra Strength
  [US-OTC]
Genapap(TM) Infant [US-OTC]
Genebs [US-OTC]
Genebs Extra Strength [US-OTC]
Genesec(TM) [US-OTC]
Gen-Nabumetone [Can]
Gen-Naproxen EC [Can]
Gen-Piroxicam [Can]
Genpril(R) [US-OTC]
Goody's(R) Extra Strength Headache
  Powder [US-OTC]
Goody's(R) Extra Strength Pain
  Relief [US-OTC]
Goody's PM(R) [US-OTC]
Halfprin(R) [US-OTC]
Hyflex-DS(R) [US]
Ibu-200 [US-OTC]

ibuprofen
Indocid(R) P.D.A. [Can]
Indocin(R) [US/Can]
Indocin(R) SR [US]
Indo-Lemmon [Can]
indomethacin
Indotec [Can]
Infantaire [US-OTC]
I-Prin [US-OTC]
ketoprofen
ketorolac
Ketorolac Tromethamine Injection,
    USP [Can]
Legatrin PM(R) [US-OTC]
Lodine(R) [Can]
Mapap [US-OTC]
Mapap Children's [US-OTC]
Mapap Extra Strength [US-OTC]
Mapap Infants [US-OTC]
meclofenamate
Meclomen(R) [Can]
Mefenamic-250 [Can]
mefenamic acid
Midol(R) Cramp and Body Aches
    [US-OTC]
Midol(R) Extended Relief [US]
Motrin(R) [US]
Motrin(R) Children's [US-OTC/Can]
Motrin(R) IB [US-OTC/Can]
Motrin(R) Infants' [US-OTC]
Motrin(R) Junior Strength [US-OTC]
nabumetone
Nalfon(R) [US]
Naprelan(R) [US]
Naprosyn(R) [US/Can]
naproxen
Naxen(R) [Can]
Naxen(R) EC [Can]
NeoProfen(R)
Norgesic(TM) [Can]
Norgesic(TM) Forte [Can]
Nortemp Children's [US-OTC]
Novasen [Can]
Novo-Difenac [Can]

Novo-Difenac K [Can]
Novo-Difenac-SR [Can]
Novo-Diflunisal [Can]
Novo-Flurprofen [Can]
Novo-Gesic [Can]
Novo-Keto [Can]
Novo-Keto-EC [Can]
Novo-Ketorolac [Can]
Novo-Methacin [Can]
Novo-Nabumetone [Can]
Novo-Naproc EC [Can]
Novo-Naprox [Can]
Novo-Naprox Sodium [Can]
Novo-Naprox Sodium DS [Can]
Novo-Naprox SR [Can]
Novo-Pirocam [Can]
Novo-Profen [Can]
Novo-Sundac [Can]
Nu-Diclo [Can]
Nu-Diclo-SR [Can]
Nu-Diflunisal [Can]
Nu-Flurprofen [Can]
Nu-Ibuprofen [Can]
Nu-Indo [Can]
Nu-Ketoprofen [Can]
Nu-Ketoprofen-E [Can]
Nu-Mefenamic [Can]
Nu-Naprox [Can]
Nu-Pirox [Can]
Nu-Sundac [Can]
Ocufen(R) [US/Can]
orphenadrine, aspirin, and caffeine
Oruvail(R) [Can]
oxaprozin
Pain-Eze [US-OTC]
Pain-Off [US-OTC]
Pamprin(R) Maximum Strength All
    Day Relief [US-OTC]
Pediatrix [Can]
Pennsaid(R) [Can]
Percogesic(R) [US-OTC]
Percogesic(R) Extra Strength
    [US-OTC]
Pexicam(R) [Can]

Phenagesic [US-OTC]
Phenylgesic [US-OTC]
piroxicam
PMS-Diclofenac [Can]
PMS-Diclofenac SR [Can]
PMS-Mefenamic Acid [Can]
Ponstan(R) [Can]
Ponstel(R) [US]
Prialt(R) [US]
Proprinal [US-OTC]
ratio-Ketorolac [Can]
Relafen(R) [Can]
RhinoFlex(TM) [US]
RhinoFlex 650 [US]
Rhodacine(R) [Can]
Rhodis(TM) [Can]
Rhodis-EC(TM) [Can]
Rhodis SR(TM) [Can]
Rhoxal-nabumetone [Can]
Riva-Diclofenac [Can]
Riva-Diclofenac-K [Can]
Riva-Naproxen [Can]
Salflex(R) [Can]
salsalate
Sandoz-Nabumetone [Can]
Silapap(R) Children's
    [US-OTC]
Silapap(R) Infants [US-OTC]
Solaraze(R) [US]
Staflex [US]
St. Joseph(R) Adult Aspirin
    [US-OTC]
sulindac
Sureprin 81(TM) [US-OTC]
Tempra(R) [Can]
Tolectin(R) [US]
tolmetin
Toradol(R) [US/Can]
Toradol(R) IM [Can]
Tramacet [Can]
tramadol
Tycolene [US-OTC]
Tycolene Maximum Strength
    [US-OTC]

Tylenol(R) [US-OTC/Can]
Tylenol(R) 8 Hour [US-OTC]
Tylenol(R) Children's [US-OTC]
Tylenol(R) Children's with Flavor
    Creator [US-OTC]
Tylenol(R) Extra Strength [US-OTC]
Tylenol(R) Infants [US-OTC]
Tylenol(R) Junior [US-OTC]
Tylenol(R) PM [US-OTC]
Tylenol(R) Severe Allergy [US-OTC]
Ultracet(TM) [US]
Ultram(R) [US/Can]
Ultram(R) ER [US]
Ultraprin [US-OTC]
Utradol(TM) [Can]
Valorin [US-OTC]
Valorin Extra [US-OTC]
Vanquish(R) Extra Strength Pain
    Reliever [US-OTC]
Voltaren(R) [US/Can]
Voltaren Ophtha(R) [Can]
Voltaren Ophthalmic(R) [US]
Voltaren Rapide(R) [Can]
Voltaren(R)-XR [US]
ziconotide
ZORprin(R) [US]
Analgesic, Opioid
    acetaminophen, codeine, and
        doxylamine (Canada Only)
    Mersyndol(R) With Codeine [Can]
Decongestant/Analgesic
    Advil(R) Cold, Children's [US-OTC]
    Advil(R) Cold & Sinus
        [US-OTC/Can]
    Children's Advil(R) Cold [Can]
    Dristan(R) Sinus [US-OTC]
    Motrin(R) Cold and Sinus
        [US-OTC]
    Motrin(R) Cold, Children's
        [US-OTC]
    Proprinal(R) Cold and Sinus
        [US-OTC]
    pseudoephedrine and ibuprofen
    Sudafed(R) Sinus Advance [Can]

PAIN (ANOGENITAL)
Anesthetic/Corticosteroid
  Analpram-HC(R) [US]
  Enzone(R) [US]
  Epifoam(R) [US]
  Pramosone(R) [US]
  Pramox(R) HC [Can]
  pramoxine and hydrocortisone
  ProctoFoam(R)-HC [US/Can]
  Zone-A(R) [US]
  Zone-A Forte(R) [US]
Local Anesthetic
  Americaine(R) [US-OTC]
  Ametop(TM) [Can]
  Anbesol(R) [US-OTC]
  Anbesol(R) Baby [US-OTC/Can]
  Anbesol(R) Jr. [US-OTC]
  Anbesol(R) Maximum Strength
    [US-OTC]
  Anusol(R) Ointment [US-OTC]
  benzocaine
  Benzodent(R) [US-OTC]
  Cylex(R) [US-OTC]
  Cēpacol(R) Dual Action Maximum
    Strength [US-OTC]
  Dentapaine [US-OTC]
  Dermoplast(R) Antibacterial
    [US-OTC]
  Dermoplast(R) Pain Relieving
    [US-OTC]
  Detane(R) [US-OTC]
  dibucaine
  dyclonine
  Foille(R) [US-OTC]
  Lanacane(R) [US-OTC]
  Lanacane(R) Maximum Strength
    [US-OTC]
  Mycinettes(R) [US-OTC]
  Nupercainal(R) [US-OTC]
  Orabase(R) with Benzocaine
    [US-OTC]
  Orajel PM(R) [US-OTC]
  Pontocaine(R) [US/Can]
  Pontocaine(R) Niphanoid(R) [US]
  pramoxine
  Prax(R) [US-OTC]
  ProctoFoam(R) NS [US-OTC]
  Sucrets(R) [US-OTC]
  Tanac(R) [US-OTC]
  tetracaine
  Trocaine(R) [US-OTC]
  Tronolane(R) [US-OTC]

PAIN (BONE)
Radiopharmaceutical
  Metastron(R) [US/Can]
  strontium-89

PAIN (DIABETIC NEUROPATHY NEURALGIA)
Analgesic, Topical
  ArthriCare(R) for Women Extra
    Moisturizing [US-OTC]
  ArthriCare(R) for Women
    Multi-Action [US-OTC]
  ArthriCare(R) for Women Silky Dry
    [US-OTC]
  Capsagel(R) [US-OTC]
  capsaicin
  Capzasin-HP(R) [US-OTC]
  Capzasin-P(R) [US-OTC]
  Zostrix(R) [US-OTC/Can]
  Zostrix(R)-HP [US-OTC/Can]

PAIN (LUMBAR PUNCTURE)
Analgesic, Topical
  EMLA(R) [US/Can]
  lidocaine and prilocaine
  Oraquix(R)

PAIN (MUSCLE)
Analgesic, Topical
  dichlorodifluoromethane and
    trichloromonofluoromethane

PAIN (SKIN GRAFT HARVESTING)
Analgesic, Topical
  EMLA(R) [US/Can]

lidocaine and prilocaine
Oraquix(R)

PAIN (VENIPUNCTURE)

Analgesic, Topical
EMLA(R) [US/Can]
lidocaine and prilocaine
Oraquix(R)

PEPTIC ULCER

Antibiotic, Miscellaneous
Apo-Metronidazole(R) [Can]
Flagyl(R) [US/Can]
Flagyl ER(R) [US]
Flagyl(R) I.V. RTU(TM)
[US]
Florazole(R) ER [Can]
MetroCream(R) [US/Can]
MetroGel(R) [US/Can]
MetroGel-Vaginal(R) [US]
MetroLotion(R) [US]
metronidazole
Nidagel(TM) [Can]
Noritate(R) [US/Can]
Trikacide [Can]
Vandazole(TM) [US]
Anticholinergic Agent
Anaspaz(R) [US]
Apo-Chlorax(R) [Can]
AtroPen(R) [US]
atropine
Atropine-Care(R) [US]
Cantil(R) [Can]
clidinium and chlordiazepoxide
Cystospaz(R) [US/Can]
Dioptic's Atropine Solution [Can]
Donnatal(R) [US]
Donnatal Extentabs(R) [US]
glycopyrrolate
hyoscyamine
hyoscyamine, atropine, scopolamine,
and phenobarbital
Hyosine [US]
Isopto(R) Atropine [US/Can]
Levbid(R) [US]

Levsin(R) [US/Can]
Levsinex(R) [US]
Levsin/SL(R) [US]
Librax(R) [US/Can]
mepenzolate
methscopolamine
NuLev(TM) [US]
Pamine(R) [US/Can]
Pamine(R) Forte [US]
propantheline
Robinul(R) [US]
Robinul(R) Forte [US]
Sal-Tropine(TM) [US]
Symax SL [US]
Symax SR [US]
Gastric Acid Secretion Inhibitor
Apo-Omeprazole(R) [Can]
lansoprazole
lansoprazole and naproxen
Losec(R) [Can]
Losec MUPS(R) [Can]
omeprazole
Prevacid(R) [US/Can]
Prevacid(R) NapraPAC(TM) [US]
Prevacid(R) SoluTab(TM) [US]
Prilosec(R) [US]
Prilosec OTC(TM) [US-OTC]
Gastrointestinal Agent, Gastric or
Duodenal Ulcer Treatment
Carafate(R) [US]
Novo-Sucralate [Can]
Nu-Sucralate [Can]
PMS-Sucralate [Can]
sucralfate
Sulcrate(R) [Can]
Sulcrate(R) Suspension Plus
[Can]
Gastrointestinal Agent, Miscellaneous
bismuth subsalicylate
Children's Kaopectate(R)
(reformulation) [US-OTC]
Colo-Fresh(TM) [US-OTC]
Diotame(R) [US-OTC]
Kaopectate(R) [US-OTC]

Kaopectate(R) Extra Strength
[US-OTC]
Pepto-Bismol(R) [US-OTC]
Pepto-Bismol(R) Maximum Strength
[US-OTC]
Histamine H2 Antagonist
Alti-Ranitidine [Can]
Apo-Cimetidine(R) [Can]
Apo-Famotidine(R) [Can]
Apo-Famotidine(R) Injectable [Can]
Apo-Nizatidine(R) [Can]
Apo-Ranitidine(R) [Can]
Axid(R) [US/Can]
Axid(R) AR [US-OTC]
BCI-Ranitidine [Can]
cimetidine
CO Ranitidine [Can]
famotidine
Famotidine Omega [Can]
Gen-Cimetidine [Can]
Gen-Famotidine [Can]
Gen-Nizatidine [Can]
Gen-Ranidine [Can]
nizatidine
Novo-Cimetidine [Can]
Novo-Famotidine [Can]
Novo-Nizatidine [Can]
Novo-Ranidine [Can]
Nu-Cimet [Can]
Nu-Famotidine [Can]
Nu-Nizatidine [Can]
Nu-Ranit [Can]
Pepcid(R) [US/Can]
Pepcid(R) AC [US-OTC/Can]
Pepcid(R) I.V. [Can]
PMS-Cimetidine [Can]
PMS-Nizatidine [Can]
PMS-Ranitidine [Can]
ranitidine
Ranitidine Injection, USP [Can]
Rhoxal-ranitidine [Can]
Riva-Famotidine [Can]
Sandoz-Ranitidine [Can]
Tagamet(R) [US]

Tagamet(R) HB [Can]
Tagamet(R) HB 200 [US-OTC]
Ulcidine [Can]
Zantac(R) [US/Can]
Zantac 75(R) [US-OTC/Can]
Zantac 150(TM) [US-OTC]
Zantac(R) EFFERdose(R) [US]
Macrolide (Antibiotic)
Biaxin(R) [US/Can]
Biaxin(R) XL [US/Can]
clarithromycin
ratio-Clarithromycin [Can]
Penicillin
amoxicillin
Amoxil(R) [US]
Apo-Amoxi(R) [Can]
Gen-Amoxicillin [Can]
Lin-Amox [Can]
Novamoxin(R) [Can]
Nu-Amoxi [Can]
PHL-Amoxicillin [Can]
PMS-Amoxicillin [Can]

PERCUTANEOUS TRANSLUMINAL CORONARY ANGIOPLASTY (PTCA)
Anticoagulant (Other)
Angiomax(R) [US/Can]
bivalirudin

POSTPARTUM HEMORRHAGE
Uteronic Agent
carbetocin (Canada only)
Duratocin(TM) [Can]

PREECLAMPSIA
Anticonvulsant
magnesium sulfate
Electrolyte Supplement, Oral
magnesium sulfate
Laxative
magnesium sulfate

PREOPERATIVE SEDATION

Analgesic, Narcotic
Actiq(R) [US/Can]
Demerol(R) [US/Can]
Duragesic(R) [US/Can]
fentanyl
Fentanyl Citrate Injection, USP [Can]
Ionsys(TM) [US]
Levo-Dromoran(R) [US]
levorphanol
meperidine
Meperitab(R) [US]
Sublimaze(R) [US]
Anticonvulsant
Luminal(R) Sodium [US]
phenobarbital
PMS-Phenobarbital [Can]
Antiemetic
Apo-Hydroxyzine(R) [Can]
Atarax(R) [Can]
hydroxyzine
Hydroxyzine Hydrochloride
Injection, USP [Can]
Novo-Hydroxyzin [Can]
PMS-Hydroxyzine [Can]
Vistaril(R) [US/Can]
Antihistamine
Apo-Hydroxyzine(R) [Can]
Atarax(R) [Can]
hydroxyzine
Hydroxyzine Hydrochloride
Injection, USP [Can]
Novo-Hydroxyzin [Can]
PMS-Hydroxyzine [Can]
Vistaril(R) [US/Can]
Barbiturate
Luminal(R) Sodium [US]
Nembutal(R) [US]
pentobarbital
phenobarbital
PMS-Phenobarbital [Can]
Benzodiazepine
Apo-Midazolam(R) [Can]
midazolam

SHOCK

Adrenal Corticosteroid
Apo-Dexamethasone(R)
[Can]
Apo-Prednisone(R) [Can]
Aristocort(R) [US/Can]
Aristospan(R) [US/Can]
Betaject(TM) [Can]
betamethasone (systemic)
Bubbli-Pred(TM) [US]
Celestone(R) [US]
Celestone(R) Soluspan(R)
[US/Can]
Cortef(R) [US/Can]
corticotropin
cortisone acetate
Decadron(R) [US]
Depo-Medrol(R) [US/Can]
Dexamethasone Intensol(R)
[US]
dexamethasone (systemic)
Dexasone(R) [Can]
DexPak(R) TaperPak(R) [US]
Diodex(R) [Can]
Diopred(R) [Can]
H.P. Acthar(R) Gel [US]
Hydeltra T.B.A.(R) [Can]
hydrocortisone (systemic)
Kenalog(R) [US/Can]
Kenalog-10(R) [US]
Kenalog-40(R) [US]
Medrol(R) [US/Can]
methylprednisolone
Novo-Prednisolone [Can]
Novo-Prednisone [Can]
Oracort [Can]
Orapred(R) [US]
Pediapred(R) [US/Can]
PMS-Dexamethasone [Can]
prednisolone (systemic)
prednisone
Prednisone Intensol(TM) [US]
Prelone(R) [US]
Sab-Prenase [Can]

Solu-Cortef(R) [US/Can]
Solu-Medrol(R) [US/Can]
Sterapred(R) [US]
Sterapred(R) DS [US]
triamcinolone (systemic)
Winpred(TM) [Can]
Adrenergic Agonist Agent
dopamine
isoproterenol
Isuprel(R) [US]
Levophed(R) [US/Can]
norepinephrine
Blood Product Derivative
Albumarc(R) [US]
albumin
Albuminar(R) [US]
Albutein(R) [US]
Buminate(R) [US]
Flexbumin [US]
Plasbumin(R) [US]
Plasbumin(R)-5 [Can]
Plasbumin(R)-25 [Can]
Plasmanate(R) [US]
plasma protein fraction
Plasma Volume Expander
dextran
Gentran(R) [US/Can]
Hespan(R) [US]
hetastarch
Hextend(R) [US/Can]
LMD(R) [US]
Voluven(R) [Can]

SKELETAL MUSCLE RELAXANT (SURGICAL)

Skeletal Muscle Relaxant
atracurium
cisatracurium
doxacurium
Nimbex(R) [US/Can]
Nuromax(R) [US]
pancuronium
Quelicin(R) [US/Can]
rocuronium

succinylcholine
Tracrium(R) [US]
vecuronium
Zemuron(R) [US/Can]

SURGICAL AID (OPHTHALMIC)

Ophthalmic Agent, Viscoelastic
chondroitin sulfate and sodium
hyaluronate
Viscoat(R) [US]

TOPICAL ANESTHESIA

Analgesic, Topical
Anestacon(R) [US]
Band-Aid(R) Hurt-Free(TM)
Antiseptic Wash [US-OTC]
Betacaine(R) [Can]
Burnamycin [US-OTC]
Burn Jel [US-OTC]
Burn-O-Jel [US-OTC]
L-M-X(TM) 4 [US-OTC]
L-M-X(TM) 5 [US-OTC]
LidaMantle(R) [US]
lidocaine
Lidodan(TM) [Can]
Lidoderm(R) [US/Can]
LTA(R) 360 [US]
Premjact(R) [US-OTC]
Solarcaine(R) Aloe Extra Burn Relief
[US-OTC]
Topicaine(R) [US-OTC]
Xylocaine(R) [US/Can]
Xylocaine(R) MPF [US]
Xylocaine(R) Viscous [US]
Xylocard(R) [Can]
Zilactin(R) [Can]
Zilactin-L(R) [US-OTC]

TRANSURETHRAL SURGERY

Genitourinary Irrigant
sorbitol
Laxative
sorbitol

ULCER (DUODENAL)
Proton Pump Inhibitor
    Panto(TM) IV [Can]
    Pantoloc(R) [Can]
    pantoprazole
    Protonix(R) [US/Can]

ULCER (GASTRIC)
Proton Pump Inhibitor
    Panto(TM) IV [Can]
    Pantoloc(R) [Can]
    pantoprazole
    Protonix(R) [US/Can]

Appendix 9
Anesthesia Methods

Anesthesia is defined as the loss of sensation resulting from pharmacologic depression of nerve function or from neurologic dysfunction. Anesthetics are used to block pain, induce sleep, relax muscles, inhibit memory and for sedation. Their use enables a patient to be comfortable during surgery or a procedure, and they are also used for other reasons, including for preoperative, postoperative and chronic pain. There are various types of anesthesia, including medications given intravenously (IV), applied topically or injected directly into the surgical site, and gases given through a face mask or a nasal tube. The method of anesthesia and the type of anesthetic used is based on the situation and the desired result.

acupuncture anesthesia – percutaneous insertion of, and stimulation by, needles placed in critical areas of the body to produce loss of sensation in another area.

balanced anesthesia – a technique of general anesthesia based on the concept that administration of a mixture of small amounts of several neuronal depressants summates the advantages, but not the disadvantages of, the individual components of the mixture.

basal anesthesia – parenteral administration of one or more sedatives to produce a state of depressed consciousness short of a general anesthesia.

block anesthesia (see conduction anesthesia)

brachial anesthesia – anesthetization of an upper extremity by injection of local anesthetic solution about the brachial plexus.

caudal anesthesia – regional anesthesia by injection of local anesthetic solution into the epidural space via the sacral hiatus.

cervical anesthesia – regional anesthesia of the neck by injection of a local anesthetic solution about the cervical nerves or into the cervical epidural space.

circle absorption anesthesia – inhalation anesthesia in which a circuit with carbon dioxide absorbent is used for complete (closed) or partial (semiclosed) rebreathing of exhaled gases.

closed anesthesia – inhalation anesthesia in which there is total rebreathing of all exhaled gases, except carbon dioxide which is absorbed; gas flow into the anesthetic circuit consists only of oxygen, in amounts equal to the patient's metabolic consumption, plus small amounts of other gases (e.g., nitrous oxide) that undergo continued uptake by and distribution in the patient.

conduction anesthesia – regional anesthesia in which local anesthetic solution is injected about nerves to inhibit nerve transmission; includes spinal, epidural, nerve block, and field block anesthesia, but not local or topical anesthesia; Syn. block anesthesia

continuous epidural anesthesia – insertion of a catheter into the lumbar or caudal epidural space for the repeated injection of local anesthetic solutions as a means of prolonging duration of anesthesia; Syn. fractional epidural anesthesia

continuous spinal anesthesia – insertion of a catheter into the spinal subarachnoid space and leaving it in situ to permit serial intermittent injection of local anesthetic solution for prolonged spinal anesthesia; Syn. fractional spinal anesthesia

crossed anesthesia – anesthesia of one side of the head and the other side of the body due to a brainstem lesion.

cryoanesthesia – localized application of cold as a means of producing regional anesthesia; Syn. refrigeration anesthesia

dental anesthesia – general, conduction, local, or topical anesthesia for operations upon the teeth, gingivae, or associated structures.

diagnostic anesthesia – anesthesia induced for evaluation of the mechanism responsible for a painful condition.

differential spinal anesthesia – a form of diagnostic spinal anesthesia producing blockade of different types of nerves in the subarachnoid space, based upon their differences in sensitivity to local anesthetics; also observed during surgical spinal anesthesia.

dissociative anesthesia – a form of general anesthesia, but not necessarily complete unconsciousness, characterized by catalepsy, catatonia, and amnesia, especially that produced by phenylcyclohexylamine compounds, including ketamine.

electric anesthesia – anesthesia, usually general anesthesia, produced by application of an electrical current.

endotracheal anesthesia – inhalation anesthesia technique in which anesthetic and respiratory gases pass through a tube placed in the trachea via the mouth or nose; Syn. intratracheal anesthesia

epidural anesthesia – regional anesthesia produced by injection of local anesthetic solution into the peridural space; Syn. peridural anesthesia

extradural anesthesia – anesthetization, by local anesthetics, of nerves near the spinal canal external to the dura mater; often refers to epidural anesthesia, but may include paravertebral anesthesia.

field block anesthesia – conduction anesthesia in which small nerves are not anesthetized individually, as in nerve block anesthesia, but instead are blocked en masse by local anesthetic solution injected to form a barrier proximal to the operative site.

fractional epidural anesthesia (see continuous epidural anesthesia)

fractional spinal anesthesia (see continuous spinal anesthesia)

general anesthesia – loss of ability to perceive pain associated with loss of consciousness produced by intravenous or inhalation anesthetic agents.

girdle anesthesia – anesthesia distributed as a band encircling the trunk.

hemianesthesia – anesthesia on one side of the body. Syn: unilateral anesthesia

high spinal anesthesia – spinal anesthesia in which the level of sensory denervation extends to the second or third thoracic dermatome.

hyperbaric anesthesia – inhalation of depressant gases or vapors at pressures greater than 1 atmosphere, especially as a means of producing general anesthesia with agents too weak to produce anesthesia at 1 atmosphere.

hyperbaric spinal anesthesia – spinal anesthesia in which spread of local anesthetic solution in the subarachnoid space is controlled by adjusting the position of the patient when the density of local anesthetic is made greater than the density of cerebrospinal fluid (i.e., hyperbaric) by the addition of glucose.

hypobaric spinal anesthesia – spinal anesthesia in which spread of local anesthetic solution in the subarachnoid space is controlled by adjusting the position of the patient when the density of the local anesthetic solution is made less than the density of cerebrospinal fluid (i.e., hypobaric) by the addition of distilled water.

hypotensive anesthesia – anesthesia in which arterial hypotension is deliberately induced as a means of decreasing operative blood loss.

hypothermic anesthesia – general anesthesia administered in conjunction with artificial lowering of body temperature.

infiltration anesthesia – anesthesia produced by injection of local anesthetic solution directly into an area that is painful or about to be operated upon.

inhalation anesthesia – general anesthesia resulting from breathing of anesthetic gases or vapors.

insufflation anesthesia – maintenance of inhalation anesthesia by delivery of anesthetic gases or vapors directly to the airway of a spontaneously breathing patient.

intercostal anesthesia – regional anesthesia produced by injection of local anesthetic solution about intercostal nerves.

intramedullary anesthesia – rarely used method of general anesthesia by injection of intravenous anesthetic agent(s) into the medullary canal of long bones; Syn. intraosseous anesthesia

intranasal anesthesia – insufflation anesthesia in which an inhalation anesthetic is added to inhaled air passing through the nose or nasopharynx; anesthesia of nasal passages by infiltration and topical application of local anesthetic solution to nasal mucosa.

intraoral anesthesia – insufflation anesthesia in which an inhalation anesthetic is added to inhaled air passing through the mouth; regional anesthesia of the mouth and associated structures when local anesthetic solutions are used by topical application to oral mucosa, by local infiltration, or as nerve blocks.

intraosseous anesthesia (see intramedullary anesthesia)

intraspinal anesthesia – inaccurate synonym for spinal anesthesia; local anesthetic solutions are not injected into the spinal cord.

intratracheal anesthesia (see endotracheal anesthesia)

intravenous anesthesia – general anesthesia produced by injection of central nervous system depressants into the venous circulation.

intravenous regional anesthesia – regional anesthesia by intravenous injection of local anesthetic solution distal to an occlusive tourniquet in an extremity previously exsanguinated by pressure or gravity. Syn: Bier method

isobaric spinal anesthesia – spinal anesthesia of same density as cerebrospinal fluid so that the level of anesthesia is not influenced by a change in the position of the patient.

local anesthesia – a general term referring to topical, infiltration, field block, or nerve block anesthesia but usually not to spinal or epidural anesthesia.

low spinal anesthesia – spinal anesthesia in which the level of sensory denervation extends to the 10th or 11th thoracic dermatome.

nerve block anesthesia – conduction anesthesia in which local anesthetic solution is injected about nerves, nerve trunks, or nerve plexuses.

nonrebreathing anesthesia – a technique for inhalation anesthesia in which valves exhaust all exhaled air from the circuit.

open drop anesthesia – inhalation anesthesia by vaporization of a liquid anesthetic placed drop by drop on a gauze mask covering the mouth and nose. outpatient anesthesia (see patient-controlled anesthesia)

paracervical block anesthesia – regional anesthesia of the cervix uteri by injection of local anesthetic solution into tissues adjacent to the cervix.

paravertebral anesthesia – anesthesia by injection of local anesthetic solution about nerves as they exit from the vertebral canal; combined presynaptic, postsynaptic, and ganglionic sympathetic block by injection of local anesthetic solution about paravertebral sympathetic chains.

patient-controlled anesthesia – a method for control of pain based upon a pump for the constant intravenous or, less frequently, epidural infusion of a dilute narcotic solution that includes a mechanism for the self-administration at predetermined intervals of a predetermined amount of the narcotic solution should the infusion fail to relieve pain.

peridural anesthesia (see epidural anesthesia)

periodontal anesthesia – anesthesia of the periodontal ligament, produced by injection of a local anesthetic drug.

presacral anesthesia – injection of local anesthetic solution anterior to the sacrum, to block nerves as they exit from the sacral foramina.

pudendal anesthesia – local anesthesia produced by blocking the pudendal nerves near the spinal processes of the ischium; used in obstetrics.

rebreathing anesthesia – a technique for inhalation anesthesia in which a portion or all of the gases that are exhaled are subsequently inhaled after carbon dioxide has been absorbed.

rectal anesthesia – general anesthesia produced by instillation into the rectum of a solution containing a central nervous system depressant.

refrigeration anesthesia (see cryoanesthesia)

regional anesthesia – use of local anesthetic solution(s) to produce circumscribed areas of loss of sensation; a generic term including conduction, nerve block, spinal, epidural, field block, infiltration, and topical anesthesia.

retrobulbar anesthesia – injection of a local anesthetic behind the eye to produce sensory denervation of the eye.

sacral anesthesia – regional anesthesia limited to those areas innervated by sacral sensory nerves.

saddle block anesthesia – a form of spinal anesthesia limited in area to the buttocks, perineum, and inner surfaces of the thighs.

spinal anesthesia – loss of sensation produced by injection of local anesthetic solution(s) into the spinal subarachnoid space; Syn: subarachnoid anesthesia

subarachnoid anesthesia (see spinal anesthesia)

surgical anesthesia – any anesthesia administered for the purpose of permitting performance of an operative procedure, as differentiated from obstetrical, diagnostic, and therapeutic anesthesia; loss of sensation with muscle relaxation adequate for an operative procedure.

therapeutic anesthesia – administration of an anesthetic as a means of treatment.

to-and-fro anesthesia – anesthesia using of a valveless closed anesthesia circuit in which respired gases pass back and forth through a carbon dioxide absorbent interposed between patient and respiratory reservoir bag.

topical anesthesia – superficial loss of sensation in conjunctiva, mucous membranes or skin, produced by direct application of local anesthetic solutions, ointments, or jellies.

total spinal anesthesia – spinal anesthesia extensive enough to produce loss of sensation in all extracranial sensory roots.

unilateral anesthesia (see hemianesthesia)

Anesthesia Methods

Common Suture Techniques & Materials

SUTURE TECHNIQUES & TYPES

absorbable surgical suture – a surgical suture material prepared from a substance that can be dissolved by body tissues and is therefore not permanent; it is available in various diameters and tensile strengths; the rate of disappearance of strength depends on the characteristics of the suture material.

Albert suture – a modified Czerny suture, the 1st row of stitches passing through the entire thickness of the wall of the gut.

apposition suture – a suture of the skin only; Syn. coaptation suture.

approximation suture – a suture that pulls together the deep tissues.

atraumatic suture – a suture swaged onto the end of an eyeless needle.

blanket suture – a continuous lock–stitch used to approximate the skin of a wound.

bridle suture – a suture passed beneath the superior rectus muscle to rotate the globe downward in eye surgery.

Bunnell suture – a method of tenorrhaphy using a pull–out wire affixed to buttons.

buried suture – any suture placed entirely below the surface of the skin.

button suture – a suture in which the threads are passed through the holes of a button and then tied; used to reduce the danger of the threads cutting through the flesh.

coaptation suture (see apposition suture)

cobbler's suture (see doubly armed suture)

Connell suture – a continuous suture used for inverting the gastric or intestinal walls in performing an anastomosis.

continuous suture – an uninterrupted series of stitches using one suture; the stitching is fastened at each end by a knot; Syn. spiral suture, uninterrupted suture.

control release suture – eyeless suture with thread attached to a needle such that the 2 separate when tension is applied to the thread.

Cushing suture – a running horizontal mattress suture used to approximate 2 adjacent surfaces.

Czerny suture – the 1st row of the Czerny–Lembert intestinal suture; the needle enters the serosa and passes out through the submucosa or muscularis, and then enters the submucosa or muscularis of the opposite side and emerges from the serosa.

Czerny-Lembert suture – an intestinal suture in 2 rows combining the Czerny suture (1st) and the Lembert suture (2nd).

delayed suture – a suturing of a wound after an interval of days.

doubly armed suture – a suture with a needle attached at both ends; Syn. cobbler's suture

Dupuytren suture – a continuous Lembert suture.

end-on mattress suture – a vertical mattress suture used for exact skin approximation.

Faden suture – a suture placed between an ocular rectus muscle and the posterior sclera to limit excessive action of the eyeball.

far-and-near suture – an interrupted suture using alternate near and far stitches, used to approximate fascial edges.

figure-of-8 suture – a suture using criss–cross stitches to approximate fascial edges or the musculofascial and outer layers of an abdominal wound.

Frost suture – intermarginal suture between the eyelids to protect the cornea.

Gély suture – a cobbler's suture used in closing intestinal wounds.

glover suture – a continuous suture in which each stitch is passed through the loop of the preceding one.

Gould suture – an intestinal mattress suture in which each loop is invaginated in such a way that the tissue at the loop is bulged out, becoming convex instead of concave.

Gussenbauer suture – a figure–of–8 suture for the intestine, resembling the Czerny–Lembert suture but not including the mucous membrane.

Halsted suture – a suture placed through the subcuticular fascia; used for exact skin approximation; Syn. subcuticular suture

implanted suture – passage of a pin through each lip of the wound parallel to the line of incision, the pins then being looped together with sutures.

interrupted suture – a series of single stitches, the ends of each suture tied together.

Jobert de Lamballe suture – an interrupted intestinal suture, used for invaginating the margins of the intestines in circular enterorrhaphy.

Lembert suture – the 2nd row of the Czerny–Lembert intestinal suture; an inverting suture for intestinal surgery, used either as a continuous suture or interrupted suture, producing serosal apposition and including the collagenous submucosal layer but not entering the lumen of the intestine.

locking suture – a running suture in which the suture material is made to pass through the loop made from the previous stitch; Syn. lock stitch.

mattress suture – a suture utilizing a double stitch that forms a loop about the tissue on both sides of a wound, producing eversion of the edges when tied; Syn. quilted suture.

nonabsorbable surgical suture – surgical suture material that is relatively unaffected by the biologic activities of the body tissues and is therefore permanent unless removed; e.g., stainless steel, silk, cotton, nylon, and other synthetic materials.

Paré suture – the approximation of the edges of a wound by pasting strips of cloth to the surface and stitching them instead of the skin.

Parker-Kerr suture – a continuous inverting suture used to close an open end of intestine.

pledgetted suture – a suture supported by a small piece of fabric or tissue so that the suture will not tear through the tissue.

purse-string suture – a continuous suture placed in a circular manner either for inversion (as for an appendiceal stump) or closure (as for a hernia).

quilted suture (see mattress suture)

Common Suture Techniques

relaxation suture – a suture so arranged that it may be loosened if the tension of the wound becomes excessive.

retention suture – a heavy reinforcing suture placed deep within the muscles and fasciae of the abdominal wall to relieve tension on the primary suture line; Syn. tension suture.

secondary suture – delayed closure of a wound.

shotted suture – a suture in which the ends are fastened by passing through a split shot (a partially divided lead pellet) which is then compressed.

spiral suture (see continuous suture)

subcuticular suture (see Halsted suture)

tension suture (see retention suture)

transfixion suture – a criss–cross stitch so placed as to control bleeding from a tissue surface or small vessel when tied; a suture used to fix the columella to the nasal septum.

uninterrupted suture (see continuous suture)

SUTURE MATERIALS

absorbable
Biosyn
catgut
chromic catgut
cotton
Dexon
Maxon
Monocryl
PDS (polydioxanone)
Vicryl

nonabsorbable
cotton
Dacron
Ethibond polyester
Ethilon nylon
Prolene
stainless steel
surgical silk

COMMON SUTURE SIZES & USES – Suture material size is measured by width and diameter. The smaller the number, the larger and heavier the suture material.

1–0 and 2–0: large and strong; good retention; used for deep fascia repairs and very large wounds.

3–0: strong with medium retention; used for smaller wounds, such as torso, hands, feet and scalp.

4–0: minimal retention and medium strength; used for superficial wounds.

5–0: very minimal retention and minimal strength; commonly used for the ears, eyelids, eyebrows, nose and face.

6–0: little or no retention and minimal strength; used in cosmetic procedures and repairs.

Appendix 11

Common Intubation Techniques

Intubation is defined as insertion of a tubular device into a canal, hollow organ, or cavity; specifically, passage of an orotracheal or nasotracheal tube for anesthesia or for control of pulmonary ventilation.

Anesthesia or Ventilator Intubation

awake fiberoptic intubation	intratracheal
blind	lighted stylet-guided oral
blind nasotracheal	nasal
bronchoscope-guided	nasal endotracheal
catheter-guided endoscopic	nasogastric
direct laryngoscopy	nasotracheal
double-lumen	oral
endobronchial	oral endotracheal
endotracheal	oral lighted-stylet
esophageal	orotracheal
esophagogastric	rapid sequence
fiberoptic	rapid sequence induction orotracheal
flexible fiberoptic	retrograde
flexible lightwand-guided	tracheal
intraluminal	translaryngeal tracheal

Therapeutic Intubation

altercursive intubation: rarely used term for diversion of secretion intermittently to the exterior from its normal destination, e.g., of the bile from the intestine.

aqueductal intubation: insertion of a tube in the sylvian aqueduct to relieve atresia or narrowing of the aqueduct.

awake aqueductal intubation: a technique of aqueductal intubation.

endobronchial: a single- or double-lumen tube with an inflatable cuff at the distal end that, after being passed through the larynx and trachea, is positioned so that ventilation is restricted to one lung; a single-lumen tube is placed in the mainstem bronchus of the lung; a double-lumen tube is positioned at the tracheal carina to permit ventilation of either or both lungs.

esophagogastric: passage of tube or stent into esophagus to reduce stricture.

Appendix 12
Common Surgical Fluids

antihemophilic human plasma
calcium
chloride
citrated plasma
colloid
crystalloid
dextran
dextrose
electrolytes (sodium, potassium, chloride)
fresh frozen plasma
human serum albumin
hydroxyethyl starch
insulin
lactated Ringer

magnesium
normal human plasma
normal saline
oxalate plasma
packed red blood cells
plasma
plasma protein solution
plasma volume expander
pooled plasma
potassium
salt plasma
sodium
true plasma
whole blood